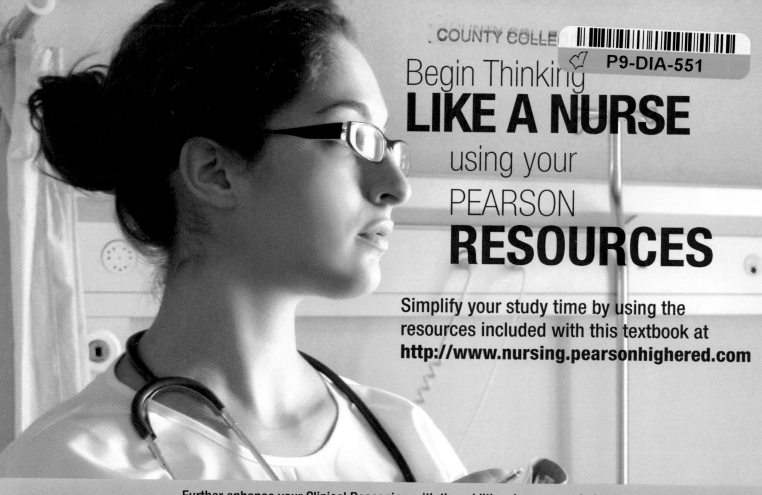
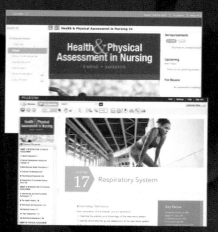
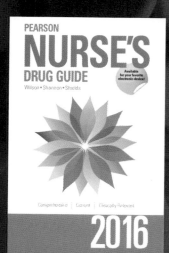
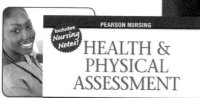

MyNursingLab®

www.mynursinglab.com
Learn more about and purchase
access to MyNursingLab.

myPEARSONstore

www.mypearsonstore.com
Find your textbook and everything
that goes with it.

Health&Physical Assessment in Nursing

D'AMICO • BARBARITO

3rd EDITION

Health&Physical Assessment in Nursing

D'AMICO • BARBARITO

3rd EDITION

Donita D'Amico, MEd, RN

Associate Professor

William Paterson University

Wayne, New Jersey

Colleen Barbarito, EdD, RN

Associate Professor

William Paterson University

Wayne, New Jersey

PEARSON

Boston   Columbus   Indianapolis   New York   San Francisco   Hoboken
Amsterdam   Cape Town   Dubai   London   Madrid   Milan   Munich   Paris   Montreal   Toronto
Delhi   Mexico City   São Paulo   Sydney   Hong Kong   Seoul   Singapore   Taipei   Tokyo

Publisher: Julie Levin Alexander
Publisher's Assistant: Sarah Henrich
Executive Editor: Pamela Fuller
Development Editor: Jill Rembetski, iD8-TripleSSS Media Development, LLC
Editorial Assistant: Erin Sullivan
Project Manager: Cathy O'Connell
Program Manager: Erin Rafferty
Director, Product Management Services: Etain O'Dea
Team Lead, Program Management: Melissa Bashe
Team Lead, Project Management: Cynthia Zonneveld
Full-Service Project Manager: Roxanne Klaas, S4Carlisle Publishing Services
Manufacturing Buyer: Maura Zaldivar-Garcia

Art Director: Maria Guglielmo
Interior and Cover Design: Wanda Espana
Vice President of Sales & Marketing: David Gesell
Vice President, Director of Marketing: Margaret Waples
Senior Product Marketing Manager: Phoenix Harvey
Field Marketing Manager: Debi Doyle
Marketing Specialist: Michael Sirinides
Marketing Assistant: Amy Pfund
Media Product Manager: Travis Moses-Westphal
Media Project Manager: Lisa Rinaldi
Composition: S4Carlisle Publishing Services
Printer/Binder: LSC Communications
Cover Printer: LSC Communications
Cover Image: Pete Saloutos/Corbis

Credits and acknowledgments borrowed from other sources and reproduced, with permission, in this textbook appear on appropriate page within text or on page PC-1.

Many of the designations by manufacturers and sellers to distinguish their products are claimed as trademarks. Where those designations appear in this book, and the publisher was aware of a trademark claim, the designations have been printed in initial caps or all caps.

Notice: Care has been taken to confirm the accuracy of information presented in this book. The authors, editors, and the publisher, however, cannot accept any responsibility for errors or omissions or for consequences from application of the information in this book and make no warranty, express or implied, with respect to its contents.

The authors and publisher have exerted every effort to ensure that drug selections and dosages set forth in this text are in accord with current recommendations and practice at time of publication. However, in view of ongoing research, changes in government regulations, and the constant flow of information relating to drug therapy and drug reactions, the reader is urged to check the package inserts of all drugs for any change in indications of dosage and for added warnings and precautions. This is particularly important when the recommended agent is a new and/or infrequently employed drug.

Library of Congress Cataloging-in-Publication Data
D'Amico, Donita, author.
 [Health & physical assessment in nursing]
Health and physical assessment in nursing / Donita D'Amico, Colleen Barbarito.—Third edition.
 p. cm.
Includes bibliographical references and index.
ISBN 978-0-13-387640-6—ISBN 0-13-387640-3
I. Barbarito, Colleen, author. II. Title.
 [DNLM: 1. Nursing Assessment—methods—Case Reports. 2. Physical Examination--nursing—Case Reports. 3. Holistic Nursing—methods—Case Reports. WY 100.4]
RT48
616.07'5—dc23
2014043375

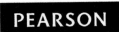

ISBN-10: 0-13-387640-3
ISBN-13: 978-0-13-387640-6

About the Authors

Donita D'Amico, MEd, RN

Donita D'Amico, a diploma nursing school graduate, earned her baccalaureate degree in Nursing from William Paterson College. She earned a master's degree in Nursing Education at Teachers College, Columbia University, with a specialization in Adult Health. Ms. D'Amico has been a faculty member at William Paterson University for more than 30 years. Her teaching responsibilities include physical assessment, medical-surgical nursing, nursing theory, and fundamentals in the classroom, skills laboratory, and clinical settings.

Ms. D'Amico coauthored several textbooks, including *Health Assessment in Nursing* and its companion clinical handbook by Sims, D'Amico, Stiesmeyer, and Webster, as well as *Comprehensive Health Assessment: A Student Workbook* and *Modules for Medication Administration* with Dr. Colleen Barbarito.

Ms. D'Amico is active in the community. Within the university, she is a charter member of the Iota Alpha Chapter of Sigma Theta Tau International. She also serves as a consultant and contributor to local organizations.

Colleen Barbarito, EdD, RN

Colleen Barbarito received a nursing diploma from Orange Memorial Hospital School of Nursing, graduated with a baccalaureate degree from William Paterson College, and earned a master's degree from Seton Hall University, all in New Jersey. She received her Doctor of Education from Teachers College, Columbia University. Prior to a position in education, Dr. Barbarito's clinical experiences included medical-surgical, critical care, and emergency nursing. Dr. Barbarito has been a faculty member at William Paterson University since 1984, where she has taught Physical Assessment and a variety of clinical laboratory courses for undergraduate nursing students and curriculum development at the graduate level.

Dr. Barbarito coauthored two books with Donita D'Amico—*Modules for Medication Administration* and *Comprehensive Health Assessment: A Student Workbook*. She published articles on anaphylaxis in *American Journal of Nursing* and *Coping with Allergies and Asthma*. Her research includes physical assessment and collaboration on revising a physical assessment project with results published as a brief in *Nurse Educator*. As a faculty member, Dr. Barbarito participated in committees to explore curricular change and to develop multimedia learning modules for critical thinking.

Dr. Barbarito is a member of Sigma Theta Tau International Honor Society of Nursing and the National League for Nursing.

Thank You

Contributors

We extend a sincere thanks to our contributors, who gave their time, effort, and expertise so tirelessly to the development and writing of chapters and resources that helped foster our goal of preparing student nurses for evidence-based practice.

Third Edition Contributors

Michelle Aebersold, PhD, RN
Clinical Assistant Professor/
Director—Clinical Learning Center
University of Michigan
Ann Arbor, Michigan
Case Studies

L. S. Blevins, MS, MFA, ELS, RN
WilliamsTown Communications
Zionsville, Indiana

Dorothy J. Dunn, PhD, RN, FNP-BC, AHN-BC
Assistant Professor, School of Nursing
President Lambda Omicron Chapter of Sigma Theta Tau
Northern Arizona University
Flagstaff, Arizona
Chapter 6, Assessment of Vulnerable Populations

Karen Kassel, PhD, ELS
WilliamsTown Communications
Zionsville, Indiana

Sheila Tucker, MA, RD, CSSD, LDN
Executive Dietitian, Auxiliary Services
Nutritionist, Office of Health Promotion
Performance Nutritionist, Athletics
Part-time Faculty, Connell School of Nursing
Part-time Faculty, Woods College of Advancing Studies
Boston College
Boston, Massachusetts
Chapter 12, Nutritional Assessment

Linda D. Ward, PhD, ARNP
Assistant Professor
Washington State University College of Nursing
Spokane, Washington
Genetics and Genomics in Chapter 8, The Health History

Previous Edition Contributors

Vicki Lynn Coyle, RN, MS
Assistant Professor
William Paterson University
Wayne, New Jersey
Chapter 27, The Pregnant Female

Dawn Lee Garzon, PhD, APRN, BC, CPNP
Clinical Associate Professor
University of Missouri–St. Louis
Ladue, Missouri
Pediatrics content in assessment chapters

Advisory Board

We could not have created this revision without the guidance of the talented faculty on our advisory board. They helped us to develop this third edition by providing valuable feedback and responding to myriad questions throughout the development process, and we are endlessly grateful for their assistance.

Patricia J. Bishop, PhD, MSN, RN
Faculty Chair
Chamberlain College of Nursing
Phoenix, Arizona

Cindy Fenske, DNP, RN, CNE
Clinical Assistant Professor
University of Michigan
Ann Arbor, Michigan

Anne F. Meyer, MS, FNP-BC
Instructor
Fitchburg State University
Fitchburg, Massachusetts

Kate Watkins, MSN, RN, CPNP, CNE
Associate Clinical Professor
Northern Arizona University
Flagstaff, Arizona

Reviewers

Our heartfelt thanks go out to our colleagues from schools of nursing across the country who have given their time generously to help create this exciting new edition of our health and physical assessment textbook. These individuals helped us plan and shape our book and resources by reviewing art, design, and more. *Health & Physical Assessment in Nursing*, Third Edition, has reaped the benefit of your collective knowledge and experience as nurses and teachers, and we have improved the materials due to your efforts, suggestions, objections, endorsements, and inspiration. Among those who gave their time generously to help us are the following:

Michelle Aebersold, PhD, RN
Clinical Assistant Professor/
Director—Clinical Learning Center
University of Michigan
Ann Arbor, Michigan

Joanne Affinito, MSN, APRN-BC
Adjunct Professor
William Paterson University
Wayne, New Jersey

Maria M. Baptiste, MSN, APRN-BC, NP-C, CCRN-CMC
Nurse Practitioner, Division of Cardiothoracic Surgery
University Hospital
Newark, New Jersey

Linda Cook, PhD, RN, CCRN, CCNS, ACNP, APRN-BC
Professor
Prince George's Community College
Largo, Maryland

Lori A. Cook, MS, RN, CNE
Faculty
Regis University
Denver, Colorado

Colleen A. D'Angiolillo, MSN, RN, CNOR
Adjunct Professor
William Paterson University
Wayne, New Jersey

Eileen A. Dehouske, MSN, RN-BC
WilliamsTown Communications
Zionsville, Indiana

Jennifer L. DeJong, PhD, FNP-BC, CNE, IBCLC
Associate Professor
Concordia College
Moorhead, Minnesota

David J. Derrico, RN, MSN
Clinical Assistant Professor
University of Florida
Gainesville, Florida

Hobie Etta Feagai, EdD, MSN, FNP-BC, APRN-Rx
Professor and Coordinator
Hawai'i Pacific University
Kaneohe, Hawaii

Cathy Franklin-Griffin, PhD, MA, MSN, RN, CHPN
Interim Director, RN-BSN Option
Winston-Salem State University
Winston-Salem, North Carolina

Catherine D. Hall, MSN, RN, OCN, CNE
Assistant Professor
Albany State University
Albany, Georgia

Becky Hauserman, RN-BC, MSN, CLNC, EMT-I, CHEP
Teaching Assistant, RN-BSN Program
Ohio University
Athens, Ohio

Karen L. Hessler, PhD, FNP-C
Associate Professor
University of Northern Colorado
Greeley, Colorado

Mary Alice Hodge, PhD, RN
Associate Professor
University of South Carolina Upstate
Spartanburg, South Carolina

Sandra Kuebler, MS, RN, PhD(c)
Continuing Lecturer
Purdue University
West Lafayette, Indiana

Susan L. Lindner, RNC-OB, MSN
Clinical Assistant Professor
Virginia Commonwealth University
Richmond, Virginia

Marie P. Loisy, RN, MSN, FNP-BC
Associate Professor
Chattanooga State Community College
Chattanooga, Tennessee

Rosemary Macy, PhD, RN, CNE
Associate Professor
Boise State University
Boise, Idaho

Andrea Mann, MSN, RN, CNE
Interim Dean, Level Chair
ARIA Health
Trevose, Pennsylvania

Lizy Mathew, EdD, RN
Associate Professor
William Paterson University
Wayne, New Jersey

Peggy McGannon, RN, MSN, MBA
Faculty (Online Division)
University of Phoenix
Tempe, Arizona

Debby Nolan, MSN, RN, CNE
Assistant Clinical Professor and Course Manager of Assessment
Texas Woman's University
Dallas, Texas

Jean Pastorello, RN, MSN, FNP-C, DNP-C
Lecturer and Lab Instructor
University of Massachusetts
Boston, Massachusetts

Kim C. Phillips, RN, BSN, MSN, PhD
Adjunct Faculty, RN-BSN Program
Winston-Salem State University
Winston-Salem, North Carolina

Colleen M. Quinn, EdD, MSN, RN
Professor
Broward College
Pembroke Pines, Florida

Margaret Quinn, DNP, RN-BC, CPNP, CNE, NCSN
Clinical Associate Professor
Rutgers University
Newark, New Jersey

Jacqueline Robinson, PhD(c), MBA, MSN, CCRN, ACNS-BC
Faculty/Manager of Nursing Resource Laboratory
Cleveland State University
Cleveland, Ohio

Ruth E. Schumacher, DNP, RN, CPN
Assistant Professor
Elmhurst College
Elmhurst, Illinois

Christy Seckman, DNP, RN
Associate Professor
Goldfarb School of Nursing at Barnes-Jewish College
St. Louis, Missouri

Joyce A. Shanty, PhD, RN
Associate Professor and Coordinator of the Allied Health Professions
Indiana University of Pennsylvania
Indiana, Pennsylvania

Caroline "Cari" Spettel, RN, MSN, NP-C
Section Faculty, Adult Health FNP Program
Ohio University College of Nursing
Athens, Ohio

Ann St. Germain, MSN, ANP-BC, WHNP-BC
Associate Clinical Professor
Texas Woman's University
Houston, Texas

Twila Sterling-Guillory, RN, CFNP-BC, PhD
Associate Professor
McNeese State University
Lake Charles, Louisiana

Linda Stone, MS, RN, CPNP
Adjunct Clinical Instructor
Roxbury Community College
Boston, Massachusetts

Tina M. Turner, DHA, MSN, RN
Assistant Professor
Miami Dade College
Homestead, Florida

Lynn M. Underwood, RN, MSN, PhD(c)
Assistant Professor
University of North Alabama
Florence, Alabama

Marjorie A. Vogt, PhD, DNP, CNP, CNE, FAANP
Professor
Otterbein University
Westerville, Ohio

Amber Young-Brice, MSN, RN
Clinical Instructor
Marquette University
Milwaukee, Wisconsin

Preface

We wrote *Health & Physical Assessment in Nursing* and developed its rich media package to help instructors mentor students in the art and skills of health and physical assessment, as well as to help students develop and refine the assessment skills they need to care for a diverse population of patients in a variety of settings. The focus of this book is patient assessment, recognizing that patients present a variety of physical, cultural, and spiritual experiences to nurses today. We approach assessment holistically, advocating the principles of health promotion and patient education. We introduce concepts related to health, wellness, communication, culture, and education. As long-time teachers of assessment, we developed a system that extends the textbook—a way to help students learn the material effectively through true integration of the textbook and the media.

Organization of This Textbook

Health & Physical Assessment in Nursing is comprised of four units. Unit I, Introduction to Health Assessment, introduces health assessment concepts. The chapters within this unit establish a focus for comprehensive health assessment to promote health and well-being across the life span. Nursing assessment includes all of the factors that impact the patient and health. Chapter 1 describes the knowledge, skills, and processes that professional nurses use in holistic health assessment and health promotion. Among these processes is evidence-based practice (EBP). This is introduced in unit I, and references to evidence-based guidelines, recommendations, and practices are addressed throughout the textbook. The professional nurse functions within the healthcare delivery system and has a responsibility to partner with other professionals and patients to maximize health. We introduce information about the goals of *Healthy People 2020* to eliminate preventable diseases, disability, injury, and premature death; achieve health equity; and create environments that promote good health across the life span. In later chapters, we present *Healthy People 2020* objectives along with recommended interventions aimed at health promotion. Chapter 2 discusses the importance of growth, development, and aging as factors that impact physical and psychosocial well-being. Chapter 3 explains the concepts of health and wellness, applying examples of several health promotion models. The patient's heritage and spirituality have significant influences on the individual's health-related activities. Chapter 4 provides an overview of cultural concepts and describes methods to incorporate and address the patient's culture, values, and beliefs in the assessment process. Chapter 5 describes psychological and social phenomena that the nurse must consider during a comprehensive assessment. Chapter 6 discusses the assessment of vulnerable patient groups, including factors that place certain populations at risk for health disparities.

Unit II, Introduction to Physical Assessment, introduces physical assessment concepts. The nurse's ability to communicate effectively is essential to the interview process. Subjective data refers to the patient's own perceptions and recollections about health, illness, values, beliefs, and practices. In chapter 7 we discuss the communication process and provide examples of effective communication techniques. Chapter 8 builds on this knowledge by reviewing the parts of the health history. We describe techniques and equipment required for physical assessment in chapter 9. Chapter 10 provides an in-depth explanation of the initial steps of physical assessment—the general survey and measurement of vital signs. Chapters 11 and 12 discuss two important aspects of health assessment—pain and nutrition. Each chapter describes concepts related to these areas and includes measurements, methods, and tools to guide data gathering and interpretation of findings for patients across the life span.

Unit III, Physical Assessment, introduces the methods and techniques that nurses use to obtain objective data. Objective data refer to measurable and observable behaviors. The chapters in unit III are organized by body system, and each chapter begins with a review of anatomy and physiology. This is followed by a Special Considerations section discussion of the issues the nurse must consider when collecting data, including health promotion, age, developmental level, race, ethnicity, work history, living conditions, socioeconomic status, and emotional wellness. This section includes specific *Healthy People 2020* objectives related to a particular body system. Recommended interventions based on these objectives are then discussed later in the Gathering the Data section.

These highly structured chapters use a consistent format to walk students through the steps of assessment and build their skills step by step:

Gathering the Data

▶ Gathering the Data

Health assessment of the ears, nose, mouth, and throat includes gathering subjective and objective data. Recall that subjective data collection occurs during the patient interview, before the actual physical assessment. During the interview the nurse uses a variety of communication techniques to elicit general and specific information about the state of health or illness of the patient's ears, nose, mouth, and throat. Health records, the results of laboratory tests, and x-rays are important secondary sources to be reviewed and included in the data-gathering process. The techniques of inspection, palpation, and percussion will be used in the physical assessment of the ears, nose, mouth, and throat. Before proceeding, it may be helpful to review the information about each of the data-gathering processes and practice the techniques of health assessment. Some special equipment and assessments are included—for example, the use of the otoscope. See Table 16.2 for information on potential secondary sources of patient data.

In Gathering the Data, students learn how to gather subjective data while conducting a patient interview. We provide Focused Interview Questions that ask the patient about general health, illness, symptoms, behaviors, pain, and life span–related issues. We also provide follow-up questions to help the student gather more data from the interview as well as Rationales and supporting Evidence so the student understands why the nurse needs to ask these questions. We provide reminders about specific communication techniques to increase student confidence and competence while performing the health assessment.

Patient Education

ENVIRONMENTAL CONSIDERATIONS	
Risk Factors	**Patient Education**
• Diabetes increases the risk for vascular diseases including hypertension, arterial or venous insufficiency, and coronary artery disease (CAD).	► Advise those with a family history of diabetes about screening. Early diagnosis can reduce risks for complications.
• The use of oral contraceptives increases the risk for development of thrombosis, especially in females who smoke.	► Explain the risks of oral contraceptives to female patients, provide information about the signs of thrombosis, and advise them to seek health care if symptoms arise.
• Peripheral vascular disease (PVD) can result in slow-healing ulcers. Risks for PVD include obesity, family history, diabetes, CAD, aging, and high cholesterol.	► Educate patients with diabetes or PVD about skin assessment and care, particularly of the feet.
• Medications for hypertension may have side effects including nausea, headache, dizziness, decreased sex drive, and impotence in males. Noncompliance with treatment increases the risks for complications of hypertension.	► Educate patients about the importance of following recommended treatment for hypertension. Advise patients to discuss side effects with their healthcare provider so that effective treatment can be provided.

BEHAVIORAL CONSIDERATIONS	
Risk Factors	**Patient Education**
• Hypertension increases the risk for cardiac disease and stroke. Risk factors for hypertension include obesity, lack of exercise, alcohol consumption, smoking, and stress.	► Advise all patients to have blood pressure screening. African Americans and those in the prehypertensive category must receive information about blood pressure monitoring and activities to reduce risks including healthy dietary practices, weight reduction, and exercise.
• Prolonged immobility is a risk factor for development of deep vein thrombosis (DVT), which can occur in those who are severely ill, postsurgery, involved in prolonged sitting at work, or in travel.	► Provide general education about immobility as a risk for DVT, especially to older patients and those who are involved in air or other travel. Include advice to get up and walk and to increase intake of water when traveling.
• Smoking is associated with increased risk for PVD and hypertension.	► Educate patients about the risks of smoking and encourage them to join a cessation program.

The Patient Education section describes risk factors for physiologic, behavioral, cultural, and life span considerations that affect the health of a specific body system. The left column presents bulleted risk factors, many of which relate to the *Healthy People 2020* objectives, while the right column offers teaching points for patients on ways they can reduce their risks.

Physical Assessment

Techniques and Normal Findings	Abnormal Findings Special Considerations
2. **Auscultate the patient's chest with the bell of the stethoscope.**	► Low-pitched sounds are best auscultated with light application of the bell. Sounds such as S3, S4, murmurs (originating from stenotic valves), and gallops are best heard with the bell.
• Place the bell of the stethoscope lightly on each of the five key landmark positions shown with step 1.	
• Listen for softer sounds over the five key landmarks. Start with the bell and listen for the S3 and S4 sounds. Then listen for murmurs.	
3. **Auscultate the carotid arteries.**	► A **bruit**, a loud blowing sound, is an abnormal finding. It is most often associated with a narrowing or stricture of the carotid artery usually associated with atherosclerotic plaque.
• Listen with the diaphragm and bell of the stethoscope. Have the patient hold the breath briefly. You may hear heart tones. This finding is normal.	
4. **Compare the apical pulse to a carotid pulse.**	
• Auscultate the apical pulse.	
• Simultaneously palpate a carotid pulse.	
• Compare the findings. The two pulses should be synchronous. The carotid artery is used because it is closest to the heart and most accessible (see Figure 19.22 ■).	► An apical pulse greater than the carotid rate indicates a pulse deficit. The rate, rhythm, and regularity must be evaluated.

In Physical Assessment, we show the student how to collect objective data and conduct a physical assessment—from the preparation of the room and gathering of equipment, to greeting the patient and the examination, to sharing findings with the patient. The left column demonstrates step-by-step instruction for patient preparation,

position, details for each technique in assessment, and the expected findings. The right column includes corresponding abnormal findings and special considerations, such as an alternate method, technique, or finding in relation to age, development, culture, or specific patient condition such as obesity. This format helps the student differentiate normal from abnormal findings while interpreting and analyzing data to plan nursing care. Hundreds of photos and illustrations help the student envision how to perform the techniques precisely and thoroughly. Documentation samples for each Physical Assessment section can be found in the *Applications Manual for Health & Physical Assessment in Nursing*. This allows the student to review and practice charting for each body system.

Abnormal Findings

► Abnormal Findings

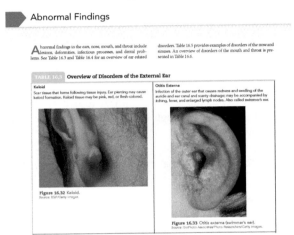

Abnormal findings in the ears, nose, mouth, and throat include lesions, deformities, infectious processes, and dental problems. See Table 16.3 and Table 16.4 for an overview of ear-related disorders. Table 16.5 provides examples of disorders of the nose and sinuses. An overview of disorders of the mouth and throat is presented in Table 16.6.

TABLE 16.3 Overview of Disorders of the External Ear	
Keloid	**Otitis Externa**
Scar tissue that forms following tissue injury. Ear piercing may cause keloid formation. Keloid tissue may be pink, red, or flesh-colored.	Infection of the outer ear that causes redness and swelling of the auricle and ear canal and scanty drainage; may be accompanied by itching, fever, and enlarged lymph nodes. Also called swimmer's ear.

Figure 16.32 Keloid.
Source: BSIP/Getty Images.

Figure 16.33 Otitis externa (swimmer's ear).
Source: BioPhoto Associates/Photo Researchers/Getty Images.

In Abnormal Findings, we provide a vivid atlas of illustrations and photographs that feature examples of abnormal findings, diseases, and conditions. This section helps the student recognize these conditions and distinguish them from normal findings before they see them in the clinical setting.

Application Through Critical Thinking

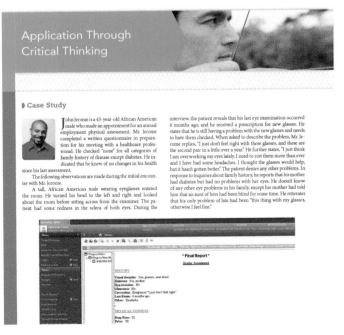

Application Through Critical Thinking

► Case Study

John Jerome is a 45-year-old African American male who made an appointment for an annual employment physical assessment. Mr. Jerome completed a written questionnaire in preparation for his meeting with a healthcare professional. He checked "none" for all categories of family history of disease except diabetes. He indicated that he knew of no changes in his health since his last assessment.

The following observations are made during the initial encounter with Mr. Jerome.

A tall, African American male wearing eyeglasses entered the room. He turned his head to the left and right and looked about the room before sitting across from the examiner. The patient had some redness in the sclera of both eyes. During the interview, the patient reveals that his last eye examination occurred 6 months ago, and he received a prescription for new glasses. He states that he is still having a problem with the new glasses and needs to have them checked. When asked to describe the problem, Mr. Jerome replies, "I just don't feel right with these glasses, and these are the second pair in a little over a year." He further states, "I just think I am overworking my eyes lately. I need to rest them more than ever and I have had some headaches. I thought the glasses would help, but it hasn't gotten better." The patient denies any other problems. In response to inquiries about family history, he reports that his mother had diabetes but had no problems with her eyes. He doesn't know of any other eye problems in his family, except his mother had told him that an aunt of hers had been blind for some time. He reiterates that his only problem of late had been "this thing with my glasses, otherwise I feel fine."

In Application Through Critical Thinking, we challenge students to apply critical thinking and diagnostic reasoning by working through a Case Study. After a detailed patient scenario, students will answer critical thinking questions, prepare documentation, and create a sample teaching plan.

Unit IV, Focused Assessment, contains two chapters that provide information about physical assessment of specialized patient groups. These chapters describe how to conduct comprehensive head-to-toe assessments of pregnant females and hospitalized patients. Chapter 29 provides a comprehensive overview of the content to foster assessment of all systems.

New to This Edition

- New Chapter: Chapter 6, "Assessment of Vulnerable Populations," walks the student through the recommended assessment procedure for vulnerable populations, which are groups that are not well integrated into the healthcare system because of ethnic, cultural, economic, geographic, or health characteristics.

- New Chapter: Chapter 7, "Interviewing and Communication Techniques," helps students to understand and develop their interviewing and communication skills in order to develop healthy nurse–patient relationships and collect data appropriately.

- Content related to assessment of pediatric and older-adult populations has been integrated throughout the body systems chapters to provide students with a more comprehensive view into assessing common populations.

- Health promotion is now integrated into the chapters more seamlessly through inclusion of related concepts and *Healthy People 2020* information in the Special Considerations and newly expanded Patient Education sections.

- The end-of-chapter case studies throughout the text have been updated to provide new practice exercises for students.

- Updated documentation examples throughout the text are now shown in a realistic electronic health record format.

- More advanced skills are clearly labeled as such to indicate to students that, while less common, they may still be performed in certain situations.

- Additional evidence has been provided to support the rationales for Focused Interview questions, and references have been moved to the end of each chapter to provide easier access to further resources.

More Features

We have shown you how to use the major sections and features of the textbook and media to be successful in this course. In addition, we offer the following features to further enhance the learning process and help you use this book successfully:

Key Terms

Key Terms at the beginning of the chapter identify the terminology that the student encounters in conducting assessment and the pages where the student can find the definitions. We bold key terms and define them in the text.

Patient-Centered Interaction

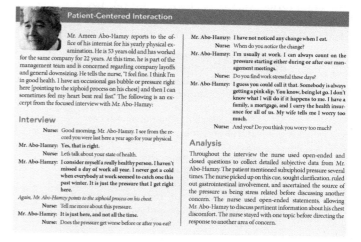

This feature teaches effective communication skills. It presents a brief clinical scenario and interaction between the patient and nurse. The Patient Interaction includes assessment cues to help the student develop strong communication skills by addressing body language, cultural sensitivity and values, language barriers, and noncompliant patients. These are common issues that present challenges to nurses, and the Analysis at the end of the interaction offers the student goals that the nurse needs to obtain with this specific patient.

"Alert!" boxes remind students of specific nursing care tips or signs to be aware of when performing a physical assessment and identify critical findings that the nurse should report immediately.

> **ALERT!**
>
> *The patient may tire during these procedures. If this happens, stop the assessment and continue at a later time. Be sure to test corresponding body parts. Take a distal-to-proximal approach along the extremities. When the patient describes sensations accurately at a distal point, it is usually not necessary to proceed to a more proximal point. If a deficit is detected at a distal point, then it becomes imperative to proceed to proximal points while attempting to map the specific area of the deficit. Repeat testing to determine accuracy in areas of deficits.*

Equipment

Equipment boxes help you prepare for the assessment by identifying the equipment you will need to conduct the assessment.

> **EQUIPMENT**
>
> - visual acuity charts (Snellen or E for distant vision, Rosenbaum for near vision). For patients who cannot read, including children, charts with pictures or numbers are used (MedlinePlus, 2013).
> - opaque card or eye cover
> - penlight
> - cotton-tipped applicator
> - ophthalmoscope

At the beginning of the Physical Assessment section, the Helpful Hints provide suggestions and reminders about conducting the physical assessment. We offer clinical guidance to prepare the student for the assessment and promote patient comfort.

HELPFUL HINTS

- The patient should don an examination gown, but undergarments may remain in place.
- The patient should remove watches and jewelry that may interfere with assessment.
- Socks and stockings should be removed.
- The patient will sit, stand, and lie in a supine position during various aspects of the assessment. The nurse should provide assistance and support when required and ensure that the patient's respiratory effort will not be affected by moving about or when lying flat.
- Use Standard Precautions.

A table titled "Potential Secondary Sources for Patient Data" is included in each of the assessment chapters in unit III. The table includes laboratory tests with the normal values and other possible diagnostic tests relevant to the particular system.

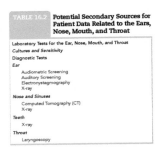

Resources for Student Success

- **Online Resources** are available for download at www.pearsonhighered.com/nursingresources, including:
  - NCLEX-RN®-Style Review questions
  - Sample Teaching Plans
  - Answers to Critical Thinking questions, and more!
- **Clinical Pocket Guide**—This portable, quick-reference to health assessment offers tools to use in class or in clinical settings to help develop students' health assessment skills.
- **Applications Manual**—This popular study tool incorporates strategies for students to focus their study and increase comprehension of concepts of nursing assessment.

Resources for Faculty Success

Pearson is pleased to offer a complete suite of resources to support teaching and learning, including:

- **TestGen Test Bank**
- **Lecture Note PowerPoints**
- **Instructor's Resource Manual**
- **New! Annotated Instructor's eText**—This version of the eText is designed to help instructors maximize their time and resources in preparing for class. The annotated eText contains suggestions for classroom and clinical activities and key concepts to integrate into the classroom in any way imaginable. Additionally, each chapter has recommendations for integrating other digital Pearson Nursing resources, including The Neighborhood 2.0, Real Nursing Skills 2.0, and MyNursingLab.

Acknowledgements

The third edition of this book would not have been possible without the support and dedication of many individuals. We especially want to thank Julie Alexander, our publisher, who is a true visionary in the field of educational publishing. Thanks also goes to executive editor Pamela Fuller for her commitment to excellence in nursing education and dedication to shaping this book into the greatest possible resource for students. Cathy O'Connell, project manager, and Erin Rafferty, program manager, moved parts in all directions, problem-solved, and monitored quality. Special thanks goes to editorial assistant Erin Sullivan for coordinating many pieces of this project. Designer Maria Guglielmo Walsh created the stunning layout for this edition, again proving her unparalleled creative skills.

Our gratitude goes out to Jill Rembetski for her impressive development work, attention to detail, and tireless efforts throughout this project. The staff at S4Carlisle Publishing Services, especially Roxanne Klaas, kept us on schedule during this process. Last but not least, thanks to Michal Heron and her staff for the wonderful photography that you will find in the pages of this book.

We dedicate this book to our students.
You have provided us with the inspiration to write a book that
makes sense and can truly guide you in developing skills that you
will use throughout your professional lives.

Contents

UNIT IV
Focused Assessment

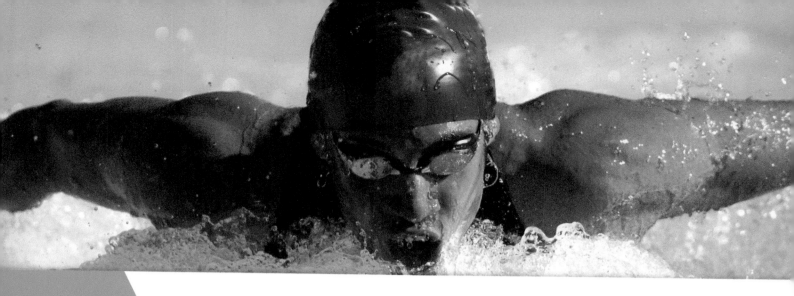

Health Assessment

Learning Outcomes

Upon completion of the chapter, you will be able to:

1. Distinguish various definitions of health.

2. Relate the goals and objectives of *Healthy People 2020* to health assessment in nursing.

3. Explain the steps of the nursing process.

4. Identify the key components of health assessment in nursing.

5. Explain the role of the professional nurse in health assessment.

6. Apply the critical thinking process to health assessment in nursing.

7. Outline the key elements of an effective teaching plan.

Key Terms

assessment, 12
communication, 10
confidentiality, 5
critical thinking, 14
focused interview, 4
formal teaching, 18
health, 3
health assessment, 4
health history, 4
holism, 10
informal teaching, 18
interpretation of findings, 8
interview, 4
nursing diagnosis, 12
nursing process, 11
objective data, 5
patient record, 5
physical assessment, 5
subjective data, 4
uniform language, 5
wellness, 3

largely due to changes in the United States healthcare system, the nurse's role is expanding. Historically, health care has focused on treating patients' illnesses and symptoms. In contrast, today's healthcare model emphasizes wellness promotion and disease prevention. Increased knowledge, rising healthcare costs, and shifts in practice areas have all caused changes. These changes have been the impetus for the nurse to develop an expanded knowledge base, greater flexibility, and the ability to work in a variety of settings. The patient is no longer the passive recipient of care. Patients today take a more active role in the planning, decision making, and treatment modalities used in their care. Factors that influence changes in the healthcare delivery system are described in the following sections.

Legislation, professional organizations, nurses, and consumers nationally and internationally have influenced reform of the healthcare delivery system. In 1978 the World Health Organization (WHO) prepared a primary healthcare report that emphasized health or well-being as a fundamental right and a social goal worldwide. Within the report is a stipulation that public institutions, governments, and consumers be involved in planning and delivering health care.

The American Nurses Association (ANA) outlined the profession's recommendations for reform of the healthcare system in 2005. The recommendations included restructuring the system to enhance access to primary care in community settings, fostering consumer responsibility in self-care and decision making about health, and facilitating the use of cost-effective providers. Further recommendations included the development of standardized services to be provided to all U.S. residents (to be financed through private and public sources), planned change to reflect changes in demographics, reduction in healthcare costs, insurance reform, provision of long-term care, and the institution of essential services.

Consumers are encouraging reform of the healthcare system to include wellness and quality of life, rather than simply treatment of disease. In addition, consumers value community health, health promotion, and disease prevention. These many changes in the delivery of health care impact the role of the nurse providing care. As a result, these aspects of nursing care are explained in this chapter and incorporated throughout this text. Nurses are taking on more responsibilities. Health assessment has become an integral part of the expanded role of the nurse. Health assessment was always performed in a limited manner in the acute care setting. Today, however, nurses perform assessment in all settings and with patients of all ages and diversity. A description of the assessment process is included in a later section of this chapter. The subsequent chapters address specific areas of concern in the assessment of the whole individual. The chapters in unit III provide step-by-step guides for learning how to perform physical assessment of each of the systems. ∞ Nurses use the nursing process and critical thinking skills as the bases for the implementation of safe, competent patient care.

The United States Department of Health and Human Services (USDHHS) joined the healthcare reform movement by developing the *Healthy People* initiatives. These initiatives are based on the premise that individual health is closely related to the health of the community. Accordingly, the interactions of governments, professionals, communities, and individuals are required to improve access to health care and change the nation's health. Promotion of individual and community health is an important focus of nursing practice. As such, nurses are an integral part of initiatives that address the health status of individuals and groups in the communities in which they live and work. One important initiative is *Healthy People*. Since 1979, the USDHHS has developed a 10-year plan for each decade, striving to improve and increase the quality of life and years of health while decreasing health disparities across the nation. This plan incorporates public input, scientific knowledge, and outcome evaluation from previous years. *Healthy People 2020* addresses the risk factors and determinants of health and the diseases and disorders affecting our communities.

Healthy People 2020

Healthy People 2020 (*About Healthy People 2020*, USDHHS, 2012) presents a 10-year strategy intended to eliminate preventable disease, disability, injury, and premature death; achieve health equity; create environments that promote good health; and promote healthy development and behaviors at every stage of life. *About Healthy People 2020* proposes science-based national objectives to improve health. The objectives are organized into topic areas that reflect public health concerns in the United States. These topics include but are not limited to:

- Physical Activity
- Nutrition
- Tobacco Use
- Alcohol and Substance Abuse
- Sexual and Reproductive Health
- Mental Health
- Injury and Violence Prevention
- Occupational Safety and Health
- Environmental Health
- Oral Health
- Emerging Issues
- Preventive Services

Each topic area is linked to objectives related to health improvement. The objectives serve as a foundation for the development of plans to improve health for both individuals and communities. Many of the plans to improve health incorporate the promotion of screening for health problems as well as implementation of preventive measures including immunization, increased physical activity, and education regarding all aspects of health. In relation to health problems and plans to improve health, *Healthy People 2020* addresses the changing demographics in the United States as well as cultural, ethnic, geographic, linguistic, and socioeconomic differences that impact health. The *Healthy People 2020* initiative is so significant that it is incorporated throughout this text.

Units I and II of this text introduce the essential elements of health assessment in nursing, while unit III discusses the fundamentals of assessment for each body system. Unit IV describes assessment considerations related to special populations, including pregnant patients and hospitalized patients. ∞ Recommended interventions aimed at health promotion are linked with the related topics or objectives of *Healthy People 2020*. For example, the objectives related to tobacco use and respiratory diseases are linked with chapter 17, "Respiratory System." ∞

Evidence-Based Practice

Evidence-based nursing practice integrates the best available evidence, nursing expertise, and the preferences and values of the individuals, families, and communities who are receiving care (Sigma Theta Tau International, 2005). Through application of evidence-based practice (EBP), the nurse delivers quality health care to specific patient populations by implementing critically appraised interventions that are supported by scientific evidence (Majid et al., 2011).

The evidence-based movement is intended to influence outcomes in health care through the development of best practice policies and guidelines. The Agency for Healthcare Research and Quality (AHRQ), through Evidence-based Practice Centers (EPCs) in the United States and Canada, reviews scientific literature on clinical, behavioral, organization, and financing topics to produce evidence reports and technology assessments. The resulting evidence reports and technology assessments are used by federal and state agencies, private sector professional societies, health delivery systems, providers, payers, and others committed to evidence-based health care (AHRQ, n.d.).

The work of the AHRQ is intended to improve health care through the support of research on the quality of services and patient outcomes. Further, the AHRQ translates research into practice through the provision of information needed to make critical decisions about health care (AHRQ, n.d.).

To promote the use of EBP and to facilitate achievement of the best possible patient outcomes, numerous clinical practice guidelines and recommendations have been developed. Among the sources of information about specific practice guidelines and recommendations are the National Guideline Clearinghouse (NGC), Evidence-based Resources for Nurses through the AHRQ, and Evidence-based Practice Guidelines for Nurses through the University of Iowa, College of Nursing. Use of best evidence enables nurses to provide care and assist patients, families, and communities to achieve optimum health outcomes.

This chapter provides an overview of the aspects of nursing practice and nursing skills required for the expanding role of the nurse. These include comprehensive assessment, nursing process, critical thinking, communication, documentation, and teaching. The skills and approaches required to meet the needs of diverse patients seeking advice and care in the changing healthcare system are illustrated throughout this text. Case studies provide opportunities to apply developing critical thinking skills. Simulated patient interactions with analyses illustrate communication techniques. Teaching plans, derived from case studies, provide examples of one of the most important interventions in health promotion and illness prevention. The process of health assessment is carefully explained in regard to the interview and hands-on physical assessment of the patient in general and for each system of the body. Samples of documentation for each aspect of assessment provide guidelines and exemplify the requirements for documentation explained in this initial chapter.

The succeeding chapters provide information about the developmental, cultural, psychosocial, and environmental factors that impact health and influence approaches to assessment. Additionally, each chapter provides rationales to support the evidence-based practice that serves as a foundation for assessment and nursing care

of patients. The illustrations, photographs, tables, and figures in each chapter enhance learning about assessment and all related factors.

Health

Traditionally, **health** has been thought of as the absence of disease. The terms *health* and *wellness* have been used interchangeably to describe the state when one is not sick. However, the concept of health extends beyond freedom from physical illness; considered from a holistic approach, health encompasses psychosocial and spiritual components, as well. **Wellness** describes a state of life that is balanced, personally satisfying, and characterized by the ability to adapt and to participate in activities that enhance quality of life. Wellness, which incorporates personal responsibility and choices regarding lifestyle and environmental factors, is discussed in depth in chapter 3 , "Wellness and Health Promotion." ∞

Definitions of Health

In 1947, the World Health Organization (WHO) presented a definition of health that remains active and relevant today. Health is defined as a state of complete physical, mental, and social well-being (WHO, 1947). Further, WHO describes health from a holistic approach in which the individual is viewed as a total person interacting with others. The individual functions within his or her physical, psychologic, and social fields. These fields interact with each other and the external environment. The individual has the capability of maximizing the potential and fostering the most positive aspects of health. Models and principles related to wellness and health promotion are described in chapter 3 of this text. ∞ Today, many definitions and models of health and wellness have been designed using these concepts. It is evident that health is far more than the absence of illness, disease, and symptoms.

The following definitions of health reflect the work of nursing theorists:

- A process and a state of being and becoming whole and integrated in a way that reflects person and environment mutuality (Roy & Andrews, 1999).

- The state of a person as characterized by soundness or wholeness of developed human structures and mental and bodily functioning that requires therapeutic self-care (Orem, 1971).

- A culturally defined, valued, and practiced state of well-being reflective of the ability to perform role activities (Leininger, 2007).

- A state of well-being and use of every power the person possesses to the fullest extent (Nightingale, 1860/1969).

Models of Health

The following are examples of models that explain the concept of health:

- The ecologic model developed by Leavell and Clark (1965) examines the interaction of agent, host, and environment. Health is present when these three variables are in harmony. When this harmony is disrupted, health is not maintained at its highest level and illness and disease occur.

- In the clinical model, health is defined as the absence of disease or injury. The aim of the care by the health professional is to relieve signs and symptoms of disease, relieve pain, and eliminate malfunction of physiologic symptoms.

- The eudaemonistic model views health as the actualization of a person's potential. Actualization refers to fulfillment and complete development. Illness would prevent self-actualization.

- According to Pender, Murdaugh, and Parsons (2011), the health promotion model defines health as the actualization of inherent and acquired human potential through goal-directed behavior, competent self-care, and satisfying relationships with others, while adjustments are made to maintain structural integrity and harmony with relevant environments.

Health is highly individualized and the definition one develops for self will be influenced by many factors. These factors will include but not be limited to age, gender, race, family, culture, religion, socioeconomic conditions, environment, previous experiences, and self-expectations.

Nurses must recognize that each patient will have a personal definition for health, illness, and wellness. Likewise, health-related behaviors will be unique for each patient. Nurses must be aware of their own personal definition of health while also accepting and respecting the patient's definition of health. When health is defined in terms of physical change, the practice focus is on improvement of physical function. When health is considered to be reflective of physical, cultural, environmental, psychologic, and social factors, the focus of nursing practice is more holistic and wide ranging. Any of the previously mentioned health models could be used by the professional nurse and other members of the health team as a paradigm for the design and delivery of health care.

Health Assessment

Health assessment may be defined as a systematic method of collecting data about a patient for the purpose of determining the patient's current and ongoing health status, predicting risks to health, and identifying health-promoting activities. The data include physical, social, cultural, environmental, and emotional factors that impact the overall well-being of the patient. The health status will include wellness behaviors, illness signs and symptoms, patient strengths and weaknesses, and risk factors. The scope of focus must be more than problems presented by the patient. The nurse will use a variety of sources to gather the objective and subjective data. Knowledge of the natural and social sciences is a strong foundation for the nurse. Effective communication techniques and use of critical thinking skills are essential in helping the nurse to gather detailed, complete, relevant, objective, subjective, and measurable data needed to formulate a plan of care to meet the needs of the patient. Health assessment includes the interview, physical assessment, documentation, and interpretation of findings. Each of these components is described in detail in units II and III of this text. ∞ All planning for care is directed by interpretation of findings from the objective and subjective data collected throughout the assessment process. This chapter offers an overview of basic considerations related to health assessment of the ambulatory patient. Hospitalized and critically ill patients may require considerably more in-depth assessment processes. Assessment of the hospitalized patient is discussed in detail in chapter 28. ∞

The Interview

The **interview,** in which subjective data are gathered, includes the health history and focused interview. The data collected will come from primary and secondary sources. The primary source from which data are collected is the patient, and the patient is considered to be the direct source. An indirect or secondary source would include a significant other, family members, caregivers, other members of the health team, and medical records.

Subjective data are information that the patient experiences and communicates to the nurse. Perceptions of pain, nausea, dizziness, itching sensations, or feeling nervous are examples of subjective data. Only the patient can describe these feelings. Subjective data are usually referred to as covert (hidden) data or as a symptom when they are perceived by the patient and cannot be observed by others. Family members or caregivers could report subjective data based on perceptions the patient has shared with them. This information is most helpful when the patient is very ill or unable to communicate, and it is required when the patient is an infant or a child. However, to ensure accuracy the nurse must validate subjective data obtained from other sources. The accuracy of subjective data depends on the nurse's ability to clarify the information gathered with follow-up questions and to obtain supporting data from other pertinent sources.

The Health History

The purpose of the **health history** is to obtain information about the patient's health in his or her own words and based on the patient's own perceptions. Biographic data, perceptions about health, past and present history of illness and injury, family history, a review of systems, and health patterns and practices are the types of information included in the health history. The health history provides cues regarding the patient's health and guides further data collection. The health history is a most important aspect of the assessment process. Detailed information regarding the health history is presented in chapter 8 of this text. ∞

The Focused Interview

The **focused interview** enables the nurse to clarify points, to obtain missing information, and to follow up on verbal and nonverbal cues identified in the health history. The nurse does not use a prepared set of questions for the focused interview. The nurse applies knowledge and critical thinking when asking specific and detailed questions or requesting descriptions of symptoms, feelings, or events. Therefore, the focused interview provides the means and opportunity to expand the subjective database regarding specific strengths, weaknesses, problems, or concerns expressed by the patient or required by the nurse to begin to make reliable judgments about information and observations as part of planning care. In-depth information about the focused interview in health assessment is included in each chapter in unit III of this text. ∞

Physical Assessment

Physical assessment is hands-on examination of the patient. Components of the physical assessment are the survey and examination of systems. Objective data gathered during the physical assessment, when combined with all other reliable sources of information, provide a sound database from which care planning may proceed. **Objective data** are observed or measured by the professional nurse. Because they are detected by the nurse, they are also known as overt data or signs. These data can be seen, felt, heard, or measured by the professional nurse. For example, skin color can be seen, a pulse can be felt, a cough can be heard, and a blood pressure can be measured. These objective data are needed to validate the subjective data and to complete the database. The accuracy of the objective data depends on the nurse's ability to avoid reaching conclusions without substantive evidence. The accuracy of the objective data is also increased by attention to detail and verification. Unit II of this text provides information about the general survey and techniques for physical assessment. ∞ Unit III includes detailed descriptions of the physical assessment process for each body system. ∞

In addition, data from all secondary sources including charts, reports from diagnostic and laboratory testing, family, and all healthcare professionals involved in patient care are part of the database from which decisions about care are derived. Both subjective and objective data may further be categorized as constant or variable. *Constant data* are information that does not change over time such as race, sex, or blood type. *Variable data* may change within minutes, hours, or days. Blood pressure, pulse rate, blood counts, and age are examples of variable data.

Documentation

Documentation of data from the health assessment creates a patient record or becomes an addition to an existing health record. The **patient record** is a legal document used to plan care, to communicate information between and among healthcare providers, and to monitor quality of care. Further, the patient record provides information used for reimbursement of services, is often a source of data for research, and is reviewed by accrediting agencies to determine adherence to standards.

Documentation is used to communicate information between and among the health professionals involved in the care of the patient. In order for that communication to be effective, the nurse must adhere to the following guidelines for documentation: Documentation must be accurate, confidential, appropriate, complete, and detailed. When documenting, the nurse must use standard and accepted abbreviations, symbols, and terminology and must reflect professional and organizational standards (Box 1.1). To help ensure the safety of patient care, The Joint Commission (TJC) has published a "Do Not Use" list, which specifically outlines abbreviations that are not acceptable for use in healthcare documentation.

Accuracy means that documentation is limited to facts or factual accounts of observations rather than opinions or interpretations of observations. When recording subjective data, it is important to use quotation marks and to quote a patient exactly rather than interpret the statement. In health assessment, accuracy also requires the use of accurate measurement and location of symptoms and

Box 1.1	Standard Abbreviations
abd	Abdomen
ADL	Activities of daily living
BP	Blood pressure
CBC	Complete blood count
CNS	Central nervous system
CVA	Costovertebral angle, cerebrovascular accident
Dx	Diagnosis
Ht	Height
Hx	History
LMP	Last menstrual period
P	Pulse
RR	Respiratory rate
T	Temperature
VS	Vital signs
WBC	White blood cell
Wt	Weight

physical findings. For example, rather than writing that the patient had severe pain and swelling in the left lower extremity, the nurse would document that a patient had pain rated 8 on a scale of 0 to 10, and edema and redness on the dorsal surface of the foot over the first through third phalanges. Accuracy in documentation requires the use of accepted terminology, symbols, and abbreviations. Accepted terminology for documentation of findings includes the use of anatomic planes. These are imaginary lines separating the body into parts. The planes are as follows: the frontal plane, indicating the anterior and posterior sections of the body; the median plane, separating the body into right and left halves; the horizontal plane, dividing the superior and inferior parts of the body; and the sagittal plane, referring to any plane parallel to the median. Additional terms for documentation of findings relative to the anatomic planes are included in Table 1.1. In health care, **uniform language** refers to the consistent use of accepted terminology by all individuals involved in documenting any aspect of the patient's care, including patient data that pertains to assessment and treatment. The use of uniform language in documentation provides for consistent interpretation of data as it is reviewed and used by healthcare professionals to monitor and oversee healthcare planning and delivery.

Confidentiality means that information sharing is limited to those directly involved in patient care. Information is considered appropriate for inclusion in a health record only if it has direct bearing on the patient's health. Complete documentation means that all information required to develop a plan of care for the patient has been included. In comprehensive health assessment, data from the health history, focused interview, and physical assessment are required for a complete record.

Protection of an individual's health information is regulated federally through the Health Insurance Portability and Accountability Act (HIPAA). Regulations under this law became effective in April 2003. The aim of the law was to create a national standard for privacy and to provide individuals with greater control over personal health information. Title II of the law, also known as Administrative Simplification, stipulates the requirements for maintaining the security and privacy of medical information. Healthcare

TABLE 1.1	Terminology in Relation to Anatomic Planes

TERM	DEFINITION
Anterior (ventral)	toward the front
Cephalad	toward the head
Distal	farthest from the center, or a medial line
Deep	below the surface
External	outside of
Medial	closer to the midline
Superior	upper
Supine	face up
Posterior (dorsal)	toward the back
Caudad	toward the feet
Proximal	closest to the center or a medial line
Superficial	on or above the surface
Internal	inside of
Lateral	farther from the midline; toward or on the side
Inferior	lower
Prone	face down

providers, hospitals, and health insurance providers are required to follow policies to protect the privacy of health information. The HIPAA regulations protect medical records and other individually identifiable health information whether communicated in writing, orally, or electronically. Identifiable health information includes demographic information and any information that could identify an individual. For further information about HIPAA regulations, contact the USDHHS. The types and amounts of documentation are determined by the purpose of the healthcare service and often by the setting. In emergency situations, data collection and documentation focus on the immediate problem and factors that may influence or impact care decisions related to the emergency. For example, for an unconscious patient, one would want to know if the altered level of consciousness was a result of a head injury in an otherwise healthy individual or associated with a previously diagnosed problem. In nonemergency situations in which a comprehensive health assessment will be conducted, documentation will include all subjective and objective data.

Data recorded during visits to healthcare providers or clinics for continued management of an existing condition are generally limited to findings indicating change, progress, or problems associated with the existing condition. Documentation for health screening and health promotion is often limited to the results of the screening process and referral information.

Documentation of health assessment data should be completed as promptly as possible. Recollection of details becomes difficult as time elapses. The nurse should record some details and notes during the data collection process, particularly direct patient quotes and precise information, such as the location of a lesion, a wound, or an abnormal finding. Immediacy of recording increases the accuracy of the information. The nurse should inform the patient that documentation will be used to record pertinent information. Most facilities use some type of computerized documentation system to maintain an electronic health record (EHR). Specific methods of documentation include narrative notes, problem-oriented charting, scales, flow sheets or check sheets, charting by exception, and focus documentation. Each of these documentation methods is described in the following paragraphs, and additional documentation exercises are provided throughout this text. Examples of each type of documentation appear in Figures 1.1 through 1.5 and are based on the following case study. Documentation may involve using paper or electronic (computerized) records, as well as a combination of the two formats.

Janet Lewis, a 20-year-old female, came to the university health center. Ms. Lewis told the nurse, "I feel bloated and achy in my left side and it has increased over the past 3 or 4 days." In response to questions about appetite, Ms. Lewis responded, "I really don't feel like eating and I'm worried because I'm supposed to eat carefully. I recently had anemia and have been taking pills for it for a month." When asked about bowel elimination, she said, "My last BM was 4 days ago; it was hard pellets and dark colored." She responded to questions about gastrointestinal symptoms with the following: "I'm not nauseous and I haven't vomited." She further reported, "I had my last period 10 days ago." She told the nurse that her voiding was normal in amount and number of voids. Ms. Lewis brought the medication with her. The label read "ferrous gluconate 300 mg by mouth three times daily." Her physician instructed her to take the medication and have a follow-up visit in 1 month.

The physical assessment revealed the presence of bowel sounds in all quadrants, dullness to percussion in the left upper and lower quadrants, firm distention, and tenderness in the left lower quadrant. There was no tenderness at the costovertebral angle (CVA). Hard, dry stool high in the rectum was identified on the rectal examination and a sample applied to a slide for occult blood testing. Blood was drawn for a complete blood count (CBC).

A rectal suppository was administered with a result, within 15 minutes, of a moderate amount of hard, dark stool. Ms. Lewis stated, "I feel a little better, but still achy." She was discharged to her dormitory with 30 mL of milk of magnesia (MOM) to take at bedtime. Ms. Lewis was advised to increase her fluid intake and continue to take the ferrous gluconate as ordered. She was instructed to call the health center in the morning as a follow-up measure and to call her physician to schedule a visit and to discuss her laboratory results.

The nurse provided education as follows:

- Constipation and change in stool color are side effects of ferrous gluconate.
- Ferrous gluconate should be taken 2 hours after meals, with a full glass of water or juice.
- Increasing roughage by adding fresh fruits to the diet will help to reduce the constipation.

Narrative Notes

When implementing narrative notes, the nurse utilizes words, phrases, sentences, and paragraphs to record information. The

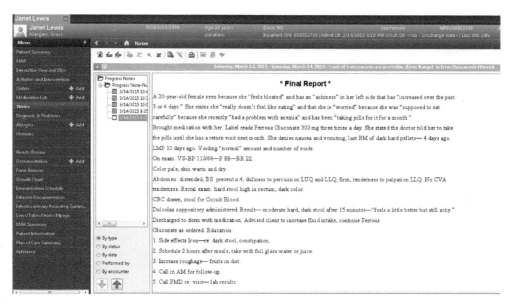

Figure 1.1 Narrative notes.
Source: From Cerner Electronic Health Record. Copyright © by Cerner Corporation. Used by permission of Cerner Corporation.

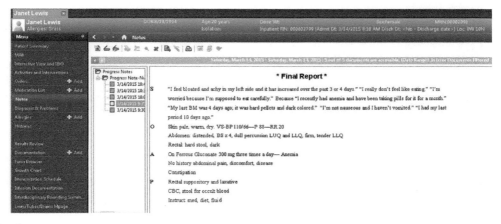

Figure 1.2 SOAP notes.
Source: From Cerner Electronic Health Record. Copyright © by Cerner Corporation. Used by permission of Cerner Corporation.

information may be recorded in chronologic order from initial contact through conclusion of the assessment, or in categories according to the type of data collected. The narrative record includes words, sentences, phrases, or lists to indicate judgments made about the data, plans to address concerns, and actions taken to meet the health needs of the patient (see Figure 1.1 ■).

Problem-Oriented Charting

Problem-oriented records include the SOAP and APIE methods. The letters SOAP refer to recording **S**ubjective data, **O**bjective data, **A**ssessment, and **P**lanning. Subjective data are those reported by the patient or a reliable informant. Objective data are derived from the physical assessment, patient records, and reports. Assessment refers to conclusions drawn from the data. Planning indicates the actions to be taken to resolve problems or address patient needs (see Figure 1.2 ■). The letters APIE refer to **A**ssessment, **P**roblem, **I**ntervention, and **E**valuation. When using this method, documentation of assessment includes combining the subjective and objective data. The nurse will draw conclusions from the data, identify and record the problem or problems, and

plan to address these problems. Interventions are documented as they are carried out. Evaluation refers to documentation of the response to the plan (see Figure 1.3 ■).

Flow Sheets

Documentation of health assessment data can be accomplished through the use of scales, check sheets, or flowcharts. Whether in paper or electronic form, these methods of documentation are usually formatted for a specific purpose or need. They may use columns or categories for recording data and may include lists of expected findings with associated qualifiers for ranges of normal or abnormal findings. Charts and check sheets often provide space for narrative descriptions or comments (see Figure 1.4 ■).

Focus Documentation

Focus documentation is a method that does not limit documentation to problems and can include patient strengths. This type of documentation is intended to address a specific purpose or focus, that is, a symptom, strength, or need. A comprehensive health assessment may result in one or more foci for documentation.

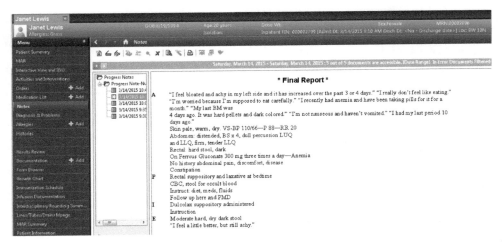

Figure 1.3 APIE notes.
Source: From Cerner Electronic Health Record. Copyright © by Cerner Corporation. Used by permission of Cerner Corporation.

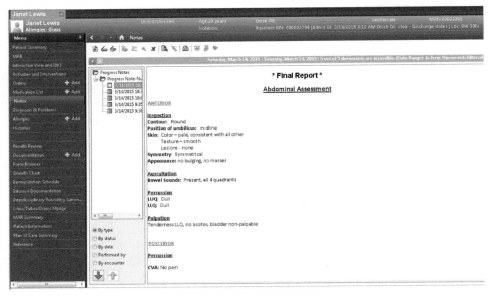

Figure 1.4 Check sheet.
Source: From Cerner Electronic Health Record. Copyright © by Cerner Corporation. Used by permission of Cerner Corporation.

The format for focus documentation is a column to address subjective and objective data, nursing action, and patient response (see Figure 1.5 ■).

Charting by Exception

Charting by exception is a system in which documentation is limited to exceptions from pre-established norms or significant findings. Flow sheets with appropriate information and parameters are completed. This type of documentation eliminates much of the repetition involved in narrative and other forms of documentation.

Electronic Health Records (EHRs)

Electronic health records (EHRs) may include all of the previously mentioned methods for recording data. The amount and types of information to be documented vary according to the EHR format and institutional policies and standards. Most EHRs benefit healthcare providers in numerous ways, including decreasing the time spent determining correct terms, spelling, and descriptors.

Development of confidence and competence in documentation is an important part of nursing education. This text provides samples of recording for the patient interview. Documentation of subjective and objective data collection for body systems is provided to guide and assist in the development of these skills.

Interpretation of Findings

Interpretation of findings can be defined as making determinations about all of the data collected in the health assessment process. One must determine if the findings fall within normal and expected ranges in relation to the patient's age, gender, and race and then the significance of the findings in relation to the patient's health status and immediate and long-range, health-related needs. Interpretation of findings is influenced by a number of factors. These factors include the ability to obtain, recall, and apply knowledge; to communicate effectively; and to use a holistic approach. Each of these factors is discussed in the following sections.

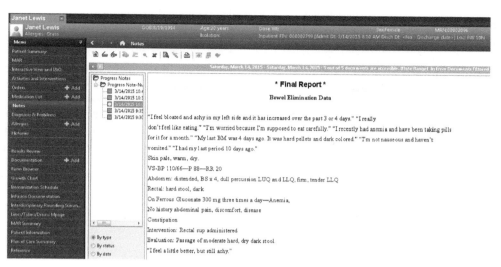

Figure 1.5 Focus notes.
Source: From Cerner Electronic Health Record. Copyright © by Cerner Corporation. Used by permission of Cerner Corporation.

Knowledge

Nurses obtain, recall, and apply knowledge from physical and social sciences, nursing theory, and all areas of research that impact current nursing practice. For example, knowledge would include human anatomy and physiology and the differences that are associated with growth and development across the life span as well as characteristics specific to gender and race. Further, knowledge includes health-related and healthcare trends in groups and populations, such as the increased incidence of risk factors or actual illnesses in certain groups or populations. In the United States, for example, trends include increased longevity and increased incidence of obesity in children and particularly in adults. The nurse must be able to access and use reliable resources in interpretation of findings. Resources include research; scientific literature; and charts, scales, and graphs to indicate ranges of norms and expectations about physical and psychologic development. Examples include Denver Developmental Screening Test scores, mental status examinations, weight and body composition charts, and growth charts prepared by centers for health statistics. Examples of charts and scales or links to information about measures are provided in each of the chapters in this text. Additionally, the nurse must be able to communicate effectively, to think critically, to recognize and act on patient cues, to incorporate a holistic perspective, and to determine the significance of data in meeting immediate and long-term patient needs.

Expectations about interpretation of findings change as one gains experience in nursing practice and with advanced practice preparation. The nurse must be able to recognize situations that require immediate attention and initiate care or seek appropriate assistance. For example, if a patient presented to an urgent care clinic complaining of dyspnea, the nurse would focus on alleviating the patient's acute symptoms through implementing interventions such as positioning the patient to promote optimal ventilatory exchange and loosening constrictive clothing. Many facilities have protocols in place to allow for implementation of emergent or urgent interventions, such as oxygen administration. While attending to the patient's acute needs, the nurse would also notify the primary care provider of the patient's need for immediate attention. A nursing student is expected to recall and apply knowledge to discriminate between

normal and abnormal findings and to use resources to understand the findings in relation to wellness or illness for a particular patient. Consider the findings from an assessment of 12-year-old Julie Connor: asymmetric shoulders and elevated right scapula on inspection of the posterior thorax, and right lateral curvature of the thoracic spine on palpation of the vertebrae. The student would recall that the scapulae should be symmetric and the vertebrae should be aligned. The findings are interpreted as a deviation from the normal. The student would refer to available resources and learn that the findings are associated with scoliosis. A primary care provider would determine Julie's medical diagnosis, formulate a medical plan of care, and evaluate the impact on Julie's current and future health. The nursing plan of care would incorporate dependent nursing interventions, including those ordered by the primary care provider and implemented by the nurse, as well as independent nursing interventions, such as wellness promotion strategies and patient teaching.

Continued learning and actual experiences promote the ability to discriminate between normal and abnormal findings. In addition, one can recognize patterns that predispose individuals to illness or are indicative of specific illnesses, and implement and evaluate appropriate nursing care. Consider the following findings from an assessment of James Long, a 46-year-old African American male: height 5'9", weight 220 lb, BP 156/94, mother died at age 62 from cerebral vascular accident (CVA, stroke, brain attack), father died at age 42 from myocardial infarction (MI, heart attack). Using knowledge of normal ranges of findings for vital signs, height, and weight, the BP and weight would be interpreted as abnormal findings. The findings indicate that this patient has high blood pressure and is obese. The nurse applies knowledge of patterns associated with health problems to interpret the significance of the findings for this patient. The nurse knows that hypertension occurs more frequently in African American males than in Caucasians and that a family history of coronary artery disease, hypertension, and obesity increases the risk of acquiring both hypertension and its associated complications. Recommendations and plans for Mr. Long's care will be developed in collaboration with other healthcare professionals to address the immediate and long-term healthcare needs of reducing blood pressure and weight.

Communication

Effective communication is essential to the data-gathering process. **Communication** refers to the exchange of information, feelings, thoughts, and ideas. Communication occurs through nonverbal means such as facial expression, gestures, and body language. Verbal methods include spoken or written communication. A variety of verbal techniques, such as open-ended and closed questions, statements, clarification, and rephrasing, are used to gather information. The communication techniques must incorporate regard for the individual in relation to the purposes of the data gathering, the patient's age, and the level of anxiety. In addition, the nurse must use techniques that accommodate language differences or difficulties, cultural influences, cognitive ability, affect, demeanor, and special needs. Interviewing and communication techniques in health assessment are discussed in chapter 7 of this text. ∞ Sample patient-nurse interactions appear in each chapter of unit III. ∞

Holistic Approach

A holistic approach is an essential characteristic of nursing practice. **Holism** can best be defined as considering more than the physiologic health status of a patient. Holism includes all factors that impact the patient's physical and emotional well-being. In a holistic approach, the nurse recognizes that developmental, psychologic, emotional, family, cultural, and environmental factors will affect immediate and long-term actual and potential health goals, problems, and plans.

Developmental Factors

The patient's developmental level significantly impacts health assessment. The primary source of patient data may vary depending on the patient's age and developmental level. For patients with developmental alterations, findings related to intellectual ability must be interpreted according to the assessed developmental level, not the patient's age. Parents or guardians are the primary sources for information about children. The patient's developmental level also influences the approach to assessment, including the words and terminology that are used. For example, the assessment of a pregnant adolescent would be different from that of a 38-year-old woman who is pregnant with her third child.

Psychologic and Emotional Factors

Psychologic and emotional factors impact physiologic health and must be considered as predisposing or contributing factors when interpreting health assessment findings. One needs only to recall that anxiety triggers an autonomic response resulting in increased pulse and blood pressure to understand that relationship. Conversely, physical problems can impact emotional health. For example, childhood obesity can lead to problems with self-esteem and impact socialization and development. Psychologic problems such as anxiety and depression may interfere with the ability to fully participate in a health assessment. Grieving may limit one's ability to carry out required health practices or to recognize health problems.

Family Factors

A family history of illness or health problems must be considered in the health assessment and interpretation of findings. Individuals with a family history of some illnesses are considered at high risk for contracting that disease. For example, a female with a first-degree relative (mother, sister, daughter) with breast cancer has a risk almost three times higher than others of developing breast cancer. The nurse must recognize that family dynamics may influence one's approach to health care. In some families, health-related decisions are not made independently but rather by the family leader or by group consensus. Family dynamics can impact both physical and emotional health and must be considered as part of the health assessment. For example, children of alcoholics are at risk for developing alcoholism, as well as for experiencing emotional issues not encountered by other children. Unexpected physical or emotional behaviors should be interpreted in the context of the patient's family dynamics and psychosocial influences.

Cultural Factors

Culture impacts language, expression, emotional and physical well-being, and health practices. Findings regarding physical and emotional health must be interpreted in relation to the cultural norms for the patient. For example, in many Asian cultures, direct eye contact is considered to be disrespectful (Dayer-Berenson, 2011). As such, for a patient who is of Asian descent, avoidance of eye contact would not be indicative of an inability to interact or depression; rather, this would be a normal finding. The nurse should provide clear explanations of abnormal findings, illnesses, and treatments because views of illness, causality, and treatment may have cultural influences. Refer to chapter 4 of this text for further discussion of culture and cultural competence in nursing care. ∞

Environmental Factors

Internal and external environmental factors impact the health assessment and interpretation of findings. The data must always be considered in relation to norms and expectation for age, race, and gender and in relation to factors impacting the individual patient. It is essential then to gather and use data from the health history, focused interview, and physical assessment when interpreting data.

INTERNAL ENVIRONMENTAL FACTORS comprise a variety of patient-specific variables. Health assessment data provide cues about the patient's internal environment, including emotional state, response to medication and treatment, and physiologic or anatomic alterations that influence findings and interpretation. For example, consider Mrs. Bernice Hall, 49, whose assessment included the patient's report of passing dark, almost black, formed stools. Typically, this would be considered an abnormal finding. However, Mrs. Hall stated during her health history that she has taken iron pills and eaten a lot of spinach and greens for years, and her stools have been that way ever since. Therefore, considering the internal environment of medication and diet, both of which darken the stool, the nurse interprets this as a normal finding for Mrs. Hall.

EXTERNAL ENVIRONMENTAL FACTORS can also impact health, health assessment, and interpretation of findings. External factors include but are not limited to inhaled toxins such as smoke, chemicals, and fumes; irritants that can be inhaled, ingested, or contacted through the skin; noise, light, and motion; and any objects or substances one may encounter in the home, in schools, in workplaces, while shopping, or while traveling and carrying out normal activities. Consider the assessment of Martha Whitman, a 22-year-old with back pain whose physical assessment findings are all within normal limits. Ms. Whitman stated that the pain started 2 weeks ago and has been getting worse. Aspirin provides temporary pain relief. While recognizing that Ms. Whitman's primary care provider may order diagnostic studies, during the patient interview the nurse explored external environmental factors that may contribute to Ms. Whitman's back pain. The nurse asked about any activities or events associated with the onset of the pain. Ms. Whitman revealed that she had taken up quilting about 2 weeks ago and has been sitting and working with an embroidery hoop almost every day for an hour or so. The additional information assists the nurse in the interpretation of the back pain. The nurse recommends ways to sit and perform the quilting without straining the muscles of the back and will follow up to see if this relieves the pain. Consider the assessment of a toddler with nausea and vomiting. The nurse must consider gathering information about the circumstances surrounding the onset of the problem. For example, was the child in a new environment in which he could have ingested medications, cleaning fluids, or other toxic substances?

Health assessment includes the interview, physical assessment, documentation, and interpretation of findings. The preceding discussion with the accompanying examples illustrates the importance of knowledge, communication, and a holistic approach in health assessment. Collection of information and interpretation of findings are important components of nursing practice. Nursing practice is concerned with health promotion, wellness, illness prevention, health restoration, and care for the dying. The nursing process in which the nurse uses comprehensive assessment to identify a patient's health status and actual or potential needs guides the practice of nursing. The nursing process then guides the nurse in identifying desired patient outcomes and implementing nursing interventions to promote achievement of those outcomes.

Nursing Process

The **nursing process** is a systematic, rational, dynamic, and cyclic process used by the nurse for assessing, planning, and implementing care for the patient. When first developed, the nursing process had four steps or phases: assessment, planning, implementation, and evaluation. Many nursing theorists have taken the original steps and expanded and clarified the meaning and action of each step. Most experts today recognize a five-step process (see Figure 1.6 ■). These steps are assessment, diagnosis, planning, implementation, and evaluation. The nursing process can be used in any setting, with patients of all ages, and in all levels of health and illness.

Since the nursing process is patient centered, the approach to nursing care is patient specific. The patient can be an individual, family, community, or population. The nursing process combines critical thinking, therapeutic communication skills, and knowledge of many arts and sciences. Each step of the process is defined here; however, greatest emphasis is placed on assessment.

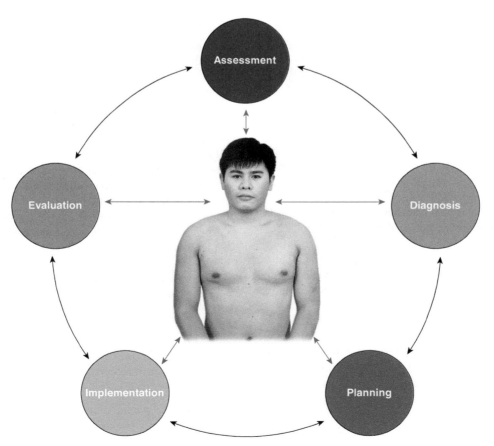

Figure 1.6 The nursing process.

In the following sections, the steps of the nursing process are identified as discrete actions. However, in practice they are interrelated and overlap to some degree. The application and effective use of the nursing process is influenced by the ability of the nurse to obtain comprehensive, accurate data.

Assessment

Assessment, step 1 of the nursing process, is the collection, organization, and validation of subjective and objective data. The data collected form the database used by the nurse. As the data change, the nurse must update the database. The database will describe the physical, emotional, and spiritual health status of the patient. Strengths and weaknesses are identified, as are responses to any treatment modalities.

Assessment begins when the nurse meets the patient and starts to gather information. Each piece of information collected about a patient is a cue, because it hints at the total health status of the patient. The baseline data act as a marker during future assessments. These data become a guide for the nurse as to what questions to ask and what additional information is needed.

For example, consider Mrs. Martha Jacobs, a 70-year-old female patient. Mrs. Jacobs tripped at home 1 week ago and sustained a right ankle sprain. Her initial treatment included an Ace bandage wrap, ice, and ibuprofen (a nonsteroidal anti-inflammatory drug, or NSAID) for reduction of pain and swelling. She was instructed to elevate the extremity for 3 days and to gradually increase weight-bearing activity. She is being seen in a follow-up visit at her physician's office and reports that her ankle is feeling much better, but she has abdominal discomfort.

When questioned about her gastrointestinal complaint, Mrs. Jacobs stated, "My stomach has been cramping and it really started to get worse a couple of days ago." She denied nausea or vomiting. She also denied having a current or past problem with bowel elimination and stated, "I usually go once a day and it's soft." According to the patient, her stools are normal in color and consistency, and she has not noticed any visible blood in her stools. When asked about her food intake, she reported a decreased appetite and stated, "I haven't been eating much, because I'm sitting around a lot and I don't feel like fixing meals." She also reported that she had been taking her ibuprofen every 6 hours, regardless of whether or not she had eaten. According to the patient, her fluid intake and urinary elimination patterns were normal. She verbalized understanding of the relationship between decreased fluid intake and risk for dehydration. She also verbalized a desire to learn more about what she could do to help her ankle heal as effectively as possible.

A physical assessment revealed the following findings: bowel sounds were present in all quadrants and percussion revealed no unusual sounds. The abdomen was soft, nondistended, and nontender to palpation.

Assessment refers to the collection of subjective and objective data in order to plan and provide patient care. Recall that subjective data are information that the patient experiences and reports to the nurse. Subjective data for Mrs. Jacobs include the following: stomach cramps for several days, normal stool elimination, decreased appetite, decreased food intake, and taking ibuprofen on an empty stomach.

Objective data are observed or measured by the nurse. The objective data for Mrs. Jacobs include the following: bowel sounds in all four abdominal quadrants, no unusual findings with abdominal percussion, and no abdominal tenderness or distention.

Diagnosis

Step 2 of the nursing process is nursing diagnosis. The nurse uses critical thinking and applies knowledge from the sciences and other disciplines to analyze and synthesize the data. Data are compared to normative values and standards. Normative values and standards include but are not limited to charts for growth and development; laboratory values (hemoglobin, hematocrit, total cholesterol, blood glucose, etc.); the rate and quality of pulses; blood pressure; heart sounds; skin texture; core body temperature; language development; role performance; and interdependent functions.

Similar data are clustered or grouped together. After analyzing and synthesizing the collected data, the nurse identifies an applicable **nursing diagnosis,** which is the basis for planning and implementing nursing care.

The following is an analysis of the data from the previously cited assessment of Mrs. Jacobs. The analysis describes the comparison to normative values and standards for the subjective and objective data, respectively. Stomach cramping represents a deviation from normal, because the abdomen is pain-free under normal conditions. She denies any abnormalities related to bowel elimination. However, her decreased appetite is a deviation from normal. She also reports taking ibuprofen regularly, regardless of food intake. Ibuprofen and many other NSAIDs can cause stomach pain and cramping, breakdown of the stomach's mucosal lining, and gastrointestinal bleeding (Wilson, Shannon, & Shields, 2013). To help reduce the risk of developing these side effects, patients usually are advised to take NSAIDs with food. She denies any visible blood in her stools. Bloody stools may be reflective of numerous gastrointestinal alterations, including ulceration of the mucosal lining of the stomach. A reduction in food intake can lead to alterations in nutrition, impaired healing, and alterations in elimination. In addition, decreased mobility increases the risk for physical problems including alterations in elimination, weakness, and joint discomfort. Psychologically, the older adult may lose independence or become socially isolated. The patient understands the relationship between the amount of intake and the frequency and amount of urination. She also verbalizes a desire to learn more about promoting physical healing of her injury.

The findings from the physical assessment include the presence of bowel sounds in all four abdominal quadrants. This is a normal finding. Bowel sounds are indicative of peristaltic activity. Abdominal percussion reveals no abnormal findings. The abdomen is nontender to palpation and nondistended, both of which are normal findings. If abdominal distention were present, this finding may be indicative of stool and flatus accumulation in the bowel. The patient reports passage of moist stools that are normal in appearance. Moisture of the feces is related to fluid intake. The patient denies any alterations in fluid intake or urinary elimination.

The analysis of assessment data includes clustering of information. The clusters consist of related pieces of information. The following clusters can be developed from the analysis of the objective and subjective data for Mrs. Jacobs:

- Stomach cramping with nondistended abdomen and normal passage of nonbloody stool
- Self-administration of ibuprofen with and without food

- Decreased appetite and food intake
- Verbalization of desire to learn more about promoting physical healing of injury

After clustering and analyzing the data, nursing diagnoses are formulated. Nursing diagnoses may be reflective of actual problems or potential problems. Additionally, nursing diagnoses may represent a state of wellness that the patient wants to enhance or optimize.

A taxonomy, a conceptual framework for the formulation of nursing diagnoses, has been developed by the North American Nursing Diagnosis Association International (NANDA-I).

Each NANDA-I diagnosis is composed of four components: a diagnostic label, a definition, defining characteristics, and risks or related factors. *Anxiety* is an example of a diagnostic label. Anxiety is defined as a state of mental uneasiness, apprehension, or dread in response to a perceived threat to oneself. Defining characteristics for anxiety include a verbal statement of anxiety ("I feel anxious") or observed evidence including trembling, pallor, or a change in vital signs. Risks or related factors include physical or other factors that promote anxiety. For example, uncertainty about the outcome of a physical assessment, uncertainty about the cause of a physical symptom such as a severe and prolonged headache, a job interview, or public speaking may promote anxiety.

NANDA-I diagnoses that represent actual problems are formulated using a three-part PES statement. The problem (P) is the diagnostic label, the etiology (E) includes the cause and contributing factors, and the signs and symptoms (S) are the defining characteristics. An example of an actual nursing diagnosis from the case study for Mrs. Jacobs would contain the following three components: Impaired Comfort (P) related to stomach cramping (E) as evidenced by patient reports of abdominal pain (S).

Nursing diagnoses that represent potential problems—or risks—are written as two-part statements. Risk nursing diagnoses identify problems that the patient is at risk for developing based on the patient's current physical or psychosocial status. Because these problems are potential and have not yet occurred, risk nursing diagnoses are written as two-part statements that include the potential problem ("Risk for") followed by the related potential cause and contributing risk factors. It is important to note that a risk nursing diagnosis may take priority over an actual nursing diagnosis. For example, a risk nursing diagnosis from the case study for Mrs. Jacobs would contain the following two components: Risk for Bleeding (P) related to side effects of NSAID medication (ibuprofen) (E). Because this risk nursing diagnosis poses a threat to Mrs. Jacobs' physiologic health, it takes priority over the actual nursing diagnosis related to Impaired Comfort.

Finally, wellness-related nursing diagnoses are written as one-part statements. Wellness-related nursing diagnoses begin with "Readiness for Enhanced," followed by an aspect of health that the patient wishes to optimize. In many cases, wellness diagnoses are reflective of areas in which the patient is seeking to learn more about some aspect of self-care.

In summary, the following are selected examples of nursing diagnoses that may be appropriate for inclusion in Mrs. Jacobs' nursing care plan:

1. Risk for bleeding related to side effects of NSAID medication (ibuprofen)

2. Impaired comfort related to stomach cramping as evidenced by patient reports of abdominal pain

3. Deficit knowledge related to self-administration of NSAID medication as evidenced by patient reports of taking ibuprofen without food

4. Risk for imbalanced nutrition: less than body requirements related to decreased appetite and decreased food intake

5. Readiness for enhanced health management.

Source: Nursing Diagnoses—Definitions and Classification 2015–2017 International. Copyright © 2014, 1994–2014 by NANDA International. Used by arrangement with John Wiley & Sons Limited.

Each chapter in unit III of this text includes a case study. ∞ The reader will be expected to analyze the data from the case studies in relation to critical thinking and the nursing process.

Planning

Planning, which is step 3 of the nursing process, involves setting priorities, identifying measurable patient goals or outcomes, and selecting evidence-based nursing interventions that promote achievement of the measurable patient goals or outcomes. When possible, these activities need to include input from the patient. Consultation or additional input may be needed from other healthcare professionals and family members.

In continuing with the case study featuring Mrs. Jacobs, one priority of care involves reducing her risk for gastrointestinal bleeding related to her medication. Related evidence-based nursing interventions should address the factors that contribute to the problem. The nurse uses the diagnostic statements to develop measurable patient goals and interventions. The goal is stated in terms of the expected patient outcome, includes a time frame, and is derived from the first part of the diagnosis. The interventions are developed by determining strategies to address the causes of the problem and are derived from the second part of the diagnostic statement.

As an example, consider the nursing diagnosis Deficit knowledge related to self-administration of NSAIDs as evidenced by patient reports of taking ibuprofen without food. This nursing diagnosis will generate the following measurable patient goal: The patient will correctly explain the risks associated with taking NSAIDs on an empty stomach prior to discharge from the physician's office.

Nursing interventions are focused on achievement of the patient goal. For example, nursing interventions for Mrs. Jacobs' nursing diagnosis related to a knowledge deficit will include teaching her about the side effects of NSAID medications.

Implementation

Implementation is step 4 of the nursing process. During implementation, the nurse carries out the nursing interventions. Implementation of evidence-based nursing interventions promotes the patient's achievement of the goals or outcomes.

The intervention prescribed for Mrs. Jacobs, as previously stated, involves teaching. In this case, the nurse will teach Mrs. Jacobs about the side effects of NSAID medications, including their potential for damaging the stomach lining and causing gastrointestinal bleeding. Ensuring that Mrs. Jacobs understands the importance of taking these medications with food would be included in the intervention.

Evaluation

Step 5, the final step of the nursing process, is evaluation. During this phase of the nursing process, the nurse evaluates the degree to which the patient has accomplished the identified goals or outcomes. Based on the evaluation, the nurse will need to revise certain elements of the nursing care plan. For example, revisions may include adding or discontinuing nursing diagnoses or nursing interventions.

Recall that the goal for Mrs. Jacobs was to correctly explain, prior to discharge from the physician's office, the risks associated with taking NSAIDs on an empty stomach. The nurse must evaluate Mrs. Jacobs's ability to explain the information; for example, by asking Mrs. Jacobs to perform a "teachback" during which she uses her own words to explain her understanding of the teaching. If Mrs. Jacobs cannot successfully explain the risks associated with taking NSAIDs on an empty stomach, the goal is not met. In that case, the nursing care plan must be modified and further action is required.

It is important to point out that a single nursing diagnosis may generate more than one patient goal. Likewise, achievement of a single patient goal may require multiple nursing interventions.

Critical Thinking

Critical thinking is a cognitive skill that is central to all nursing activities. The nurse's use of critical thinking skills enhances the application of the nursing process. Alfaro-LeFevre (2013) defined and explained the critical thinking process. This work provided the foundation for the following discussion. **Critical thinking** is a process of purposeful and creative thinking about resolutions of problems or the development of ways to manage situations. Critical thinking is more than problem solving; it is a way to apply logic and cognitive skills to the complexities of patient care. It demands that nurses avoid bias and prejudice in their approach while using all of the knowledge and resources at their disposal to assist patients in achieving health goals or maintaining well-being.

When critically thinking about the patient's health status, problems, or situations, one applies essential elements and skills. The five essential elements of critical thinking are collection of information, analysis of the situation, generation of alternatives, selection of alternatives, and evaluation. Figure 1.7 ■ depicts the elements of critical thinking.

Each element has working skills to help the nurse be complete, thorough, and competent with the cognitive processes of critical thinking. Critical thinking skills are linked with each of the essential elements. The following discussion provides information and examples of the linkage of the elements and skills of critical thinking as they are applied in health assessment. Additionally, each chapter of unit III includes a case study and questions to provide opportunities to apply critical thinking skills. ∞

Collection of Information

Collection of information, the first of the elements in critical thinking, involves the five skills of identifying assumptions, organizing data collection, determining the reliability of the data, identifying relevant versus irrelevant data, and identifying inconsistencies in the data (see Figure 1.8 ■). In use of this first skill, the nurse must be able to identify assumptions that can misguide or misdirect the

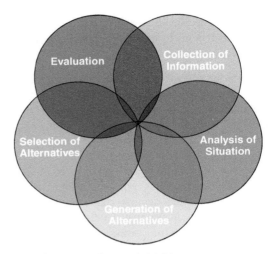

Figure 1.7 Elements of critical thinking.

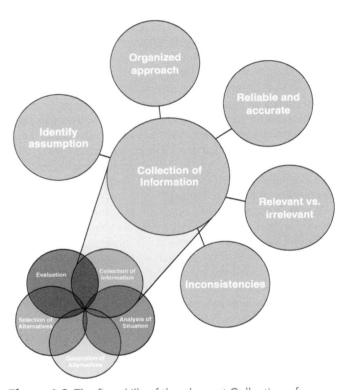

Figure 1.8 The five skills of the element Collection of Information.

assessment and intervention processes. For example, when interviewing a patient, one must not assume that lack of eye contact indicates lack of attention, dishonesty, or apathy when it occurs in Asian, Native American, and other individuals (Dayer-Berenson, 2011).

The second skill of collection of information is organizing data collection. Collection of subjective and objective data must be carried out in an organized manner. In health assessment the nurse first determines the patient's current health status, level of distress, and ability to participate in the assessment process. The aim of data gathering in a patient in acute distress is rapid identification of the problem and significant predisposing and contributory factors in order to select and initiate interventions to alleviate the distress.

In nonacute situations, assessment follows an accepted and organized framework of survey, interview, and physical assessment.

The third skill of collection of information is determining the reliability of the data. One must recall that patient information is valuable if it is reliable and accurate. The patient is generally the best source of information, especially historic. However, physical and psychologic factors may interfere with that capability. Information is then sought from a family member or caregiver who can provide reliable information. Other reliable sources of information include charts, medical records, and notes from other health professionals. One must also be certain that the objective data are accurate. Measuring devices must be standardized, calibrated, and applied correctly.

A wealth of information is obtained when carrying out a comprehensive health assessment. One then applies the fourth critical thinking skill, which is to determine the relevance of the information in relation to the patient's current, evolving, or potential condition or situation. Consider the relevance of nonimmunization or contraction of German measles in a male patient seeking care for a fracture versus a 26-year-old sexually active female having an annual examination.

Identifying inconsistencies is the last of the skills associated with the element of collection of information. The nurse must be able to recognize discrepancies in the information. Further, one must determine if the inconsistency is a result of an oversight, misunderstanding, linguistic factor, or cultural factor. Indication of confusion, memory impairment, and subtle or overt communication indicating discomfort with a topic or area of questioning must also be considered. The following is an example of an inconsistency indicating misunderstanding: During the interview a patient failed to identify a surgical repair of a fracture when asked about surgical procedures, but reported it when asked about treatment for accidents or injuries. The inconsistency may not become apparent until the physical assessment takes place. A patient may say that he or she has never used street drugs, but during the assessment the nurse may see track marks on the arms. The nurse must use care in communication while dealing with the inconsistency.

Analysis of the Situation

The second element of critical thinking is analysis of the situation. The following five skills are linked to this element: distinguishing data as normal or abnormal, clustering related data, identifying patterns in the data, identifying missing information, and drawing valid conclusions (see Figure 1.9 ■).

The first of the skills is distinguishing normal from abnormal data. The nurse uses knowledge of human behavior as well as anatomy and physiology to compare findings with established norms in these areas. The nurse will use standards for laboratory results, diagnostic testing, charts, scales, and measures related to development and aging. The data must be analyzed in relation to expected ranges for the age, gender, genetic background, and culture of the patient. Consider the following situation: In a regularly scheduled checkup, John Morgan, age 31, undergoes a complete health assessment. He is found to have alopecia (hair loss) at the anterior hairline and thinning of the hair that has increased since his last visit. The nurse knows that alopecia occurs more frequently in men than in women, that in male pattern baldness the alopecia begins at the

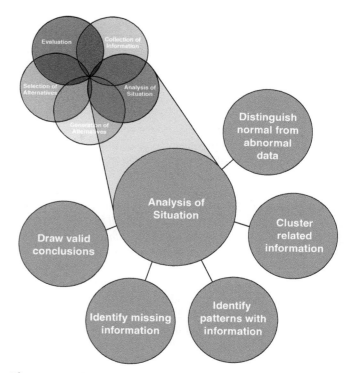

Figure 1.9 The five skills of the element Analysis of Situation.

anterior hairline, and that alopecia is genetic and begins in early adulthood. When all other findings are within the normal limits for a 31-year-old male, the nurse considers the alopecia a normal finding in this patient.

If the previously mentioned finding had occurred during an assessment of Margaret Lane, a 31-year-old female, the nurse would apply the same knowledge and consider alopecia an abnormal finding. Further, other findings would be carefully examined. In this situation, Ms. Lane stated in the health history, "I'm tired all the time. I must be anemic because I'm cold all the time and on top of all that I'm constipated." Additionally, she said, "I think I'm becoming irregular because I'm too tired to exercise and don't eat right and I guess that has messed up my periods, too; it lasts much longer than it ever did." Findings during the physical assessment included pallor, weight gain, dry skin, and brittle nails. The nurse must now begin to apply the other skills associated with analysis of the situation.

When using the second analysis skill, the nurse will cluster related information by sorting and categorizing information into groupings that may include but are not limited to cues, symptoms, body systems, or health practices. The following are clusters derived from the data about Ms. Lane:

- Skin dry, nails brittle, hair thinning and loss
- Constipation, irregularity, weight gain, "not eating right"
- Lack of exercise, tired, cold, pallor, "I must be anemic"
- Prolonged menstruation

Once the clustering has been completed, the nurse must apply the third skill of identifying patterns in the information. Use of this skill enables the nurse to get an idea about what is happening with the patient and to determine if more information is required. The nurse must rely on knowledge and resources in identifying patterns.

One might consider a pattern suggesting a nutritional or abdominal problem since information includes changes in eating, changes in bowel elimination, fatigue, and changes in the skin and hair. The data also suggest a metabolic or hormonal problem. However, the information is incomplete.

At this point the nurse would identify missing information, the fourth skill. Missing information would include but is not limited to onset of symptoms, medication history, family history of similar problems, and measures the patient has taken to alleviate the problems. Additional information would include laboratory studies of hematologic, metabolic, or hormonal function.

The following is subjective data from the interview of Ms. Lane: *The symptoms had been going on for over a year, gradually getting worse. She didn't take any medications except Advil for a headache now and then. She knows of no one in her family with a problem like hers and she hasn't done anything except take laxatives sometimes, use hand cream, and try all kinds of hair care products that friends recommend.* The nurse explained the need for diagnostic studies. Ms. Lane obtained the requested laboratory and diagnostic testing and returned for a follow-up visit. The reports of several laboratory studies were as follows: Hgb 10 g/dL (grams per deciliter), Hct 30%, RBC 3.6 cells/ mcL (million cells per microliter), free T_3 64 ng/dL (nanograms per deciliter), T_4 0.7 microgram/dL, TSH 6.0 microunits/mL, glucose 126 mg/dL (milligrams per deciliter).

The nurse has acquired the information necessary to apply the last skill of drawing valid conclusions. This skill requires using all of one's knowledge and reasoning skills to draw logical conclusions about a problem or situation. The nurse concludes, based on history, objective findings in physical assessment, and diagnostic testing, that Ms. Lane has hypothyroidism. The critical thinking process continues as the nurse works with the patient to develop a treatment plan for her problem.

Assessment is the focus of this chapter, and students will be applying the previously mentioned steps in the critical thinking process. To identify the importance of critical thinking to future practice, a discussion of the remaining elements and skills is included. These skills are essential to delivery of competent nursing care. The nurse gathers data, determines the meaning of the data, and decides what to do once information gathering is completed. The nursing actions depend on the level of practice. For example, autonomous decisions such as diagnosis and treatment of disease by prescription of medication are within the role of the advanced practice nurse. For the generalist, data are shared with physicians who prescribe medical treatment. The generalist develops interventions such as education, support, and some modes for symptom relief as part of professional practice. Furthermore, the nurse brings a holistic approach to the patient situation. Therefore, the nurse will collaborate with all healthcare professionals to be sure that plans are developed to meet individual physical and psychosocial needs.

Generation of Alternatives

Articulating options and establishing priorities are the two skills associated with the critical thinking element of generation of alternatives (see Figure 1.10 ■). Articulation of options is simply stating possible paths to follow or actions to take to resolve a problem. There are several options for treatment of the patient, Ms. Lane, cited previously: (1) Begin treatment with thyroid medication immediately as prescribed by the nurse practitioner, (2) delay the treatment with thyroid medication while continuing with diagnostic testing to

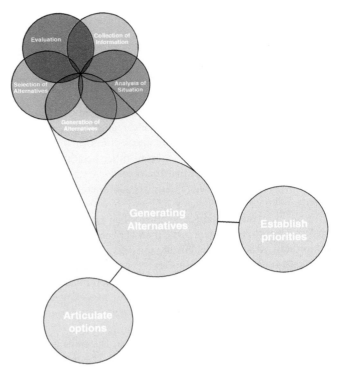

Figure 1.10 The two skills of the element Generation of Alternatives.

establish the cause of the problem, (3) delay treatment with thyroid medication and seek a referral with an endocrinologist, or (4) initiate treatments to relieve symptoms.

Once the options have been enumerated, the nurse and patient work together to establish priorities. This process must reflect the acuity of the problem and the patient's ability to interpret the information required to weigh the advantages and disadvantages of each of the options in relation to health, lifestyle, cultural, and socioeconomic factors. The nurse knows that the aim of therapy in hypothyroidism is to achieve and maintain normal thyroid functioning by administering thyroid replacement for the life of the patient. Symptoms associated with hypothyroidism subside with thyroid replacement therapy. Immediate relief of discomfort can be achieved through dietary and activity modifications. The nurse shares this knowledge with Ms. Lane and priorities are established.

Selection of Alternatives

Selection of alternatives is the next element of critical thinking, and linked with it are the skills of developing outcomes and developing plans (see Figure 1.11 ■). Outcomes are statements of what the patient will do or be able to do in a specific time. The plan includes all of the actions required by the patient independently or in coordination with healthcare professionals and others to achieve the stated outcomes. An overall outcome for Ms. Lane could be stated as follows: Ms. Lane will have and maintain normal thyroid levels within 5 weeks of initial dose of thyroid replacement. The plan for the outcome includes taking the prescribed medication as directed, having drug levels monitored, and reporting problems with the medication. The nurse must be sure that Ms. Lane has the knowledge and skills required to follow the plan. Therefore, the nurse may have to provide education, follow-up, and support for the patient.

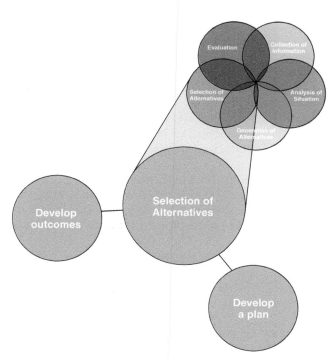

Figure 1.11 The two skills of the element Selection of Alternatives.

Some outcomes for Ms. Lane could include weight loss, return of normal bowel function, and improved nutritional status. A time frame would be determined for achievement of each outcome and a plan developed to guide the patient toward meeting expectations in the stated outcomes.

Evaluation

The last element in critical thinking is evaluation (see Figure 1.12 ■). This element includes the skills of determining if the expected outcomes have been achieved and review of application of each of the critical thinking skills to be sure that omissions and misinterpretations did not occur. In addition, the nurse must evaluate thinking and judgment in the situation. One must be sure that decisions and actions were based on knowledge and the use of reliable resources and information. Furthermore, one must be sure that acts are based on moral and ethical principles and that the effects of values and biases have been considered. The nurse would follow up with Ms. Lane to determine if each of the expected outcomes has been achieved in a timely manner.

Role of the Professional Nurse

The professional nurse provides care to the patients needing and seeking help. Nursing care is based on a strong knowledge base and the application of critical thinking. The knowledge base of the professional nurse is developed over time using information from the humanities and the biologic, natural, and social sciences. Using research data, standards of care, and the nursing process, the professional nurse provides competent care. The patient will be the individual, family, or community. The individual could be any age and at any developmental level. The actions of the professional nurse will be directed to promote health and wellness, treat and care for the ill, and care for the dying individual while being supportive to family

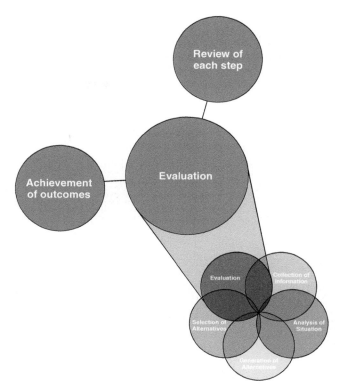

Figure 1.12 The two skills of the element Evaluation.

members. To perform these actions, the nurse works in a variety of settings including hospitals, clinics, nursing homes, patients' homes, schools, and workplaces.

Regardless of the setting, the role of the professional nurse is multifaceted. Each situation requires the professional nurse to use critical thinking and the nursing process. To provide care and utilize the nursing process, the professional nurse must develop strong assessment skills. The gathering of complete, accurate, and relevant data is required. While gathering the subjective and objective data from the patient, the nurse must be attuned to the signs, symptoms, behaviors, and cues offered by the patient. As the status of the patient changes, the collected data will vary. The professional nurse functions as a teacher, caregiver, patient advocate, and manager of patient care.

Teacher

As a teacher, the nurse helps the patient to acquire knowledge required for health maintenance or improvement, to prevent illness or injury, to manage therapies, and to make decisions about health and treatment. Teaching occurs in all settings and for a variety of reasons and may be informal or formal. Teaching is an important intervention to promote wellness and prevent illness. This intervention is enacted when collection and analysis of patient data reveal a knowledge deficit, a need for education about an identified risk, or readiness to learn to enhance health. These three conditions represent the three types of diagnoses in the NANDA-I taxonomy: actual, risk, and wellness. Teaching is such an important intervention that each chapter of unit III of this text includes a section called Health Promotion Considerations in which common risk factors and intervention strategies are identified. ∞ Further, each assessment chapter includes a teaching plan. The teaching plans included in this text are derived from case study information and are intended to illustrate this important nursing intervention.

Informal Teaching

Informal teaching generally occurs as a natural part of a patient encounter. This type of teaching may be to provide instructions, to explain a question or procedure, or to reduce anxiety. For example, while asking about medications and the use of natural, herbal, or home remedies during the health history interview, the nurse may offer an explanation as follows: "This information is important because medications may interact with each other or with herbs and natural substances. The interaction can sometimes be harmful or change the effectiveness of one of your prescribed medications." The same information may be offered in response to a patient statement or question such as, "What is so important that I have to go over my medications every time I come here?"

Explanations are offered to inform the patient and often reduce anxiety. When performing a physical assessment, the nurse provides explanations. For example, "I would like you to take a deep breath in and out through your mouth each time I place the stethoscope on your chest. This will help me to clearly hear the air as it moves in and out of your lungs." The nurse may explain a technique during assessment of the musculoskeletal system as follows: "You will notice that I've asked you to push with both arms against my hands; that is so I can compare the strength of the left and right arms."

The following are additional examples of informal teaching. In response to parents' concerns about their infant's height and weight, the nurse explains how charts are used to assess growth and development and assists them to compare their child's data with that on the chart. A child with food allergies may approach the school nurse and ask, "I forgot my lunch today. Can I eat this packaged tuna thing from the machine?" The nurse will explain that the ingredients must be checked and may state, "I'll help you look at the container and we can determine if it is okay to eat."

Formal Teaching

Formal teaching occurs in response to an identified learning need of an individual, group, or community. Teaching plans are developed for formal teaching sessions. There are six components in teaching plans: the identified learning need, goal, objectives, content, teaching strategies and rationales, and evaluation, as noted in Box 1.2. The following sections address each of the components of the teaching plan.

LEARNING NEEDS are identified as discrete knowledge deficits for an individual or as common needs of individuals and groups. Individual learning needs can be identified through the interview or in communication with a patient throughout the assessment process. Consider the following situation. James Dempsey, a 20-year-old male, states during the health history, "I do not perform self testicular examinations; I don't know how to do it." Testicular self-examination is an important part of health promotion and disease prevention. Therefore, James Dempsey has a need to learn about self-examination of the testicles.

Box 1.2 Elements of a Teaching Plan

- Learning Need
- Goal
- Objectives
- Content
- Teaching Strategy/Rationale
- Evaluation

The need for learning in individuals, families, and groups arises in response to lack of knowledge about common changes or risks that occur with aging, role change and development, illness, health promotion, and disease prevention. The following provides an example of a learning need for a group. The wellness center at a university provides health promotion classes for students. The sessions are planned in collaboration with healthcare providers in the community. One session was developed to address the need for information about testicular cancer because of the increased incidence of testicular cancer in young males.

GOALS are based on identified learning needs. The goal is written as a broad statement of the expected outcome of the learning. When considering the need for James Dempsey, the goal would be broadly stated as follows: The patient will accurately perform testicular self-examination every month.

A goal for a group is developed as well in response to identification of a learning need. The goal for the male students in the at-risk age group would be: The participants will follow recommended guidelines for testicular cancer screening.

OBJECTIVES identify specific, measurable behaviors or activities expected of the patient or group. Action verbs are used to denote the behavior or activity. Table 1.2 provides examples of action verbs. The objectives may include criteria or conditions under which the behavior must occur. Objectives should also be measurable. A measurable objective for James Dempsey is written as follows: The patient will correctly demonstrate testicular self-examination at the conclusion of the patient teaching session. An example of a measurable objective for a group that is learning about testicular health would be written as follows: At the completion of the learning session, the participants will identify three measures to detect testicular cancer.

The type of learning or behavior that is expected of the patient also determines objectives. Objectives, therefore, are in the cognitive, psychomotor, or affective domains. Cognitive objectives include those concerning the acquisition of knowledge. Psychomotor objectives include the acquisition of skills. The affective domain refers to attitudes, feelings, values, and opinions. The expectation for James Dempsey is that he will be able to perform a skill. The objective for performance of testicular self-examination is in the psychomotor domain. The example of an objective for the group learning about testicular health is in the cognitive domain because it calls for the participants to identify three measures for testicular cancer detection.

CONTENT within a teaching plan refers to what will actually be taught. The objective for James Dempsey states: The patient will correctly demonstrate testicular self-examination at the conclusion of the patient teaching session. Therefore, the content must include the steps and actions required for self-examination of the testicles. Examples of content that addresses the objective of identifying three measures for testicular cancer detection would include information about self-examination, annual examination by a healthcare provider, blood tests, ultrasonic examination, and biopsy.

TEACHING METHODS or strategies are the channels or avenues used to present the content. They must be suited to the needs of the learner and the type of learning that is expected. Psychomotor learning requires, for example, in the case of James Dempsey, demonstration as one teaching methodology. One-on-one discussion is a common strategy for individual patient teaching. Group teaching

TABLE 1.2	**Action Verbs for Development of Objectives**	
DOMAIN	**ACTION VERBS**	
Cognitive	Appraises	Explains
	Changes	Generates
	Composes	Matches
	Concludes	Modifies
	Converts	Names
	Creates	Reorganizes
	Criticizes	Separates
	Defines	Solves
	Designs	States
	Diagrams	Subdivides
	Discriminates	Summarizes
Affective	Acts	Greets
	Adheres	Justifies
	Describes	Modifies
	Discusses	Presents
	Displays	Proposes
	Explains	
Psychomotor	Assembles	Fixes
	Calibrates	Makes
	Changes	Manipulates
	Demonstrates	Operates
	Dismantles	

strategies may include lecture, discussion, or role-play. Table 1.3 includes information about teaching methods.

RATIONALES explain and support the selection of specific teaching strategies. Teaching plans are developed to meet the distinct needs of individual patients or the common needs of individuals, groups, or communities. When developing or using previously developed teaching plans, the nurse must consider the age, gender, developmental level, culture, linguistic ability, dexterity, physical ability or limitations, and resources of the patient or group. The selection of the content and methods for teaching and evaluation of learning should be influenced by the previously mentioned factors. For example, use of printed materials would be inappropriate for a patient with impaired vision or with limited literacy. The nurse would not include referral to Internet sites for patients without computer access. It would be best to suggest walking in a park or using a public facility for exercise rather than a health club for those with limited income.

EVALUATION of learning is incorporated into the teaching plan. In evaluation, one determines if the learning objectives have been achieved. The learning domain of the objective determines the methods for evaluation. Cognitive learning may be evaluated verbally through questions or in discussion with the patient or by use of written measurements. Written evaluations include short answer, true-false, fill-in, multiple-choice, and other types of tests.

Members of the group learning about testicular cancer detection, as described earlier, could be evaluated by a short answer quiz at the end of the session. Psychomotor learning is best evaluated by a demonstration of the skill expected in the objective. James Dempsey would be evaluated through a return demonstration of testicular self-examination. When evaluation reveals that learning has not occurred, the nurse should repeat all or part of the teaching.

Caregiver

The caregiver role has always been the traditional role of the nurse. Historically, physical care was the primary focus. Today, the nurse uses a holistic approach to nursing care. Using critical thinking and the nursing process, the professional nurse provides direct and indirect care to the patient. Indirect care is accomplished with the delegation of activities to other members of the team. As patient advocate the nurse acts as a protector. Patients are kept informed of their rights, given information to make informed decisions, and encouraged to speak for themselves. As a case manager, the professional nurse helps to coordinate care, manages the multidisciplinary team, and plans patient outcomes within a specific time frame. Providing care, containing costs, and identifying the effectiveness of the plan are all responsibilities of the case manager.

Advanced Practice Roles

The advanced formal education and expanded roles of the nurse permit the professional nurse to function in advanced roles. These advanced roles include but are not limited to nurse researcher, practitioner, anesthetist, clinical specialist, administrator, and educator.

Nurse Researcher

The nurse researcher identifies problems regarding patient care, designs plans of study, and develops tools. Findings are analyzed and knowledge is disseminated. The nurse performing the research adds to the body of knowledge of the profession, gives direction for future research, and improves patient care.

Nurse Practitioner

The nurse practitioner, with advanced degrees and certified by the American Nurses Credentialing Center or by the American Academy of Nurse Practitioners, practices independently in a variety of situations. At an agency or community-based setting, one could find a family nurse practitioner (FNP), gerontological nurse practitioner (GNP), or psychiatric-mental health nurse practitioner (PMHNP) meeting the healthcare needs of patients seeking assistance.

Nurse Anesthetist

In addition to undergraduate nursing education, the certified registered nurse anesthetist (CRNA) has completed an accredited nurse anesthesia education program and passed a national certification examination. In collaboration with other healthcare providers, including anesthesiologists and surgeons, CRNAs provide a full range of anesthesia services. CRNAs are the sole providers of anesthesia care in most rural hospitals (American Association of Nurse Anesthetists [AANA], n.d.). CRNAs must maintain registered nurse licensure, as well as credentialing by the National Board of Certification and Recertification for Nurse Anesthetists (NBCRNA).

TABLE 1.3	Teaching Methods		
TEACHING METHOD	**DOMAIN**	**ADVANTAGES**	**DISADVANTAGES**
Explanation	Cognitive	May be used for individual or group.	Passive learning.
One-on-One Discussion	Cognitive Affective	Learner participation. Clarification can be provided. Questions can be answered.	Requires time for discussion and to allow for questions.
Lecture	Cognitive	Useful for large groups. Facts presented in logical manner.	Passive learning.
Group Discussion	Cognitive Affective	Learners are more comfortable in groups. Allows participation of all members.	Can easily lose focus in a group discussion.
Case Study	Cognitive	Develops problem-solving skills. Allows learners to explore complex concepts.	Difficult to develop. Learners may have difficulty applying information to their own situation.
Role-Play	Cognitive Affective	Allows learners to appreciate different points of view. Learners actively participate.	Learners may be too anxious to participate. Effective in small groups only.
Demonstration	Psychomotor	Can be used with individuals and groups.	Passive learning.
Practice	Psychomotor	Learners actively involved. Hands-on experience.	Time consuming. Effective with small groups only to provide feedback.
Printed Material	Cognitive	Efficiently presents important information. Can supplement other teaching methods.	May not meet needs of low-literacy learners or those with language differences. Passive learning.
Media Audiovisual Presentation	Cognitive Affective Psychomotor	Can be used in all types of learning. Can supplement other teaching methods. Provides aural and visual stimulation.	Time consuming. Passive learning. Requires proficiency with digital technology. Requires careful selection of authoritative content.
Computer-Assisted Instruction (CAI)	Cognitive Affective Psychomotor	Can be used with individuals and groups. Learning is active. Provides immediate feedback. Provides an opportunity to apply knowledge to patient-care scenarios without the need for a patient simulator.	Requires equipment. Time consuming. Favors knowledge retention as opposed to hands-on practice (Feng et al., 2013).

Clinical Nurse Specialist

Clinical nurse specialists have advanced education and degrees in a specific aspect of practice. They provide direct patient care, direct and teach other team members providing care, and conduct nursing research within their area of specialization.

Nurse Administrator

Today, the role of the nurse administrator varies. Professional titles include vice president of nursing services, supervisor, or nurse manager of a specific unit. The responsibilities vary and could include staffing, budgets, patient care, staff performance evaluations, consulting, and ensuring that the goals of the agency are being accomplished. Advanced degrees are usually required for these positions. It is common to find nurse administrators with advanced degrees in several disciplines such as nursing and business administration.

Nurse Educator

The nurse educator, a nurse with advanced degrees, is employed to teach in a nursing program. This could be at a university, community college, or department of staff development in an agency providing nursing care. The educator is responsible for didactic and clinical teaching, curriculum development, clinical placement, and practice for students. The educator provides the student with the opportunity to practice assessment skills in a variety of settings with a diverse patient population.

This chapter has presented an overview of concepts and processes important to health assessment. Aspects of nursing practice, knowledge, and skills required for the changing role of the nurse in today's healthcare arena have been introduced. These include health, comprehensive assessment, nursing process, critical thinking, communication, documentation, and teaching. An in-depth discussion of these important concepts is presented in succeeding chapters of this book. Development of knowledge, skills, and techniques is enhanced through the use of clinical examples and case studies. *Healthy People 2020,* the initiative to promote the health of individuals and communities, is incorporated as a feature in this text to facilitate awareness of population-based goals related to health and wellness.

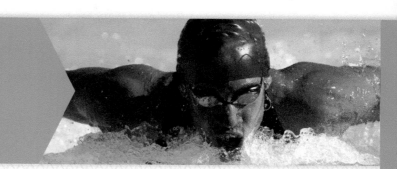

Application Through Critical Thinking

▶ Case Study

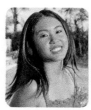

Mary Wong is a 19-year-old college freshman living in the dormitory. She has come to the University Health Center with the following complaints: nausea, vomiting, abdominal pain increasing in severity, diarrhea, a fever, and dry mouth. She tells you, the nurse, "I have had abdominal pain for about 12 hours with nausea, vomiting, and diarrhea." These symptoms, she tells you, "all started after supper in the student cafeteria on campus."

You conduct an interview and follow it with a physical assessment, which reveals the following: symmetric abdomen, bowel sounds in all quadrants, tender to palpation in the lower quadrants, guarding. Mary's skin is warm and moist, her lips and mucous membranes are dry.

▶ Critical Thinking Questions

1. Identify the findings as objective or subjective data.
2. Prepare a narrative nursing note from the data.
3. What factors must be considered in conducting the comprehensive health assessment of Mary Wong? Provide rationale.
4. How would you cluster the data you obtained from your history and physical examination of Mary?
5. Prior to developing a nursing diagnosis, what must you do?

▶ References

Agency for Healthcare Research and Quality. (n.d.). *Evidence-based practice centers (EPC) program overview.* Retrieved from http://www.ahrq.gov/research/findings/evidence-based-reports/overview/index.html

Alfaro-LeFevre, R. (2013). *Critical thinking, clinical reasoning, and clinical judgment: A practical approach* (5th ed.). St. Louis, MO: Elsevier.

American Association of Nurse Anesthetists (AANA). (n.d.). *Become a CRNA.* Retrieved from http://www.aana.com/ceandeducation/becomeacrna/pages/default.aspx

Berman, A., & Snyder, S. (2012). *Kozier and Erb's fundamentals of nursing: Concepts, process and practice* (9th ed.). Upper Saddle River, NJ: Prentice Hall.

Dayer-Berenson, L. (2011). *Cultural competencies for nurses: Impact on health and illness.* Sudbury, MA: Jones & Bartlett.

Feng, J. Y., Chang, Y. T., Chang, H. Y., Erdley, W. S., Lin, C. H., & Chang, Y. J. (2013). Systematic review of effectiveness of situated e-learning on medical and nursing education. *Worldviews on Evidence-Based Nursing, 10*(3), 174–183.

Herdman, T. H. (Ed.). (2014). *NANDA International nursing diagnoses: Definitions and classification, 2015–2017* (10th ed.). Oxford: Wiley-Blackwell.

Leavell, H. R., & Clark, E. G. (1965). *Preventive medicine for the doctor in the community.* New York: McGraw-Hill.

Leininger, M. M. (Ed.). (2007). *Culture care diversity and universality: A theory of nursing* (2nd ed.). New York: National League for Nursing Press.

LeMone, P., Burke, K., & Bauldoff, G. (2011). *Medical-surgical nursing: Critical thinking in patient care.* (5th ed.). Upper Saddle River, NJ: Pearson.

Majid, S., Foo, S., Luyt, B., Zhang, X., Theng, Y. L., Chang, Y. K., & Mokhtar, I. A. (2011). Adopting evidence-based practice in clinical decision making: nurses' perceptions, knowledge, and barriers. *Journal of the Medical Library Association, 99*(3), 229.

Nightingale, F. (1969). *Notes on nursing: What it is and what it is not.* New York: Dover Books. (Original work published 1860)

Orem, D. E. (1971). *Nursing: Concepts of practice.* Hightstown, NJ: McGraw-Hill.

Osborn K. S., Wraa, C. E., Watson, A., & Holleran, R. S. (2013). *Medical-surgical nursing: Preparation for practice.* (2nd ed.). Upper Saddle River, NJ: Pearson.

Pender, N. J., Murdaugh, C. L., & Parsons, M. J. (2011). *Health promotion in nursing practice* (6th ed.). Upper Saddle River, NJ: Pearson.

Roy, C., & Andrews, H. (1999). *The Roy adaptation model* (2nd ed.). Stamford, CT: Appleton & Lange.

Sigma Theta Tau International. (2005). *Evidence-based nursing position statement.* Retrieved from http://www.nursingsociety.org/aboutus/PositionPapers/Pages/EBN_positionpaper.aspx

U.S. Department of Health and Human Services (USDHHS). (2012). *About healthy people.* Retrieved from http://healthypeople.gov/2020/about/default.aspx

Wilson, B. A., Shannon, M. T., & Shields, K. M. (2013). *Pearson nurse's drug guide.* Upper Saddle River, NJ: Pearson.

World Health Organization (WHO). (1947). *Constitution of the World Health Organization.* Geneva: Author.

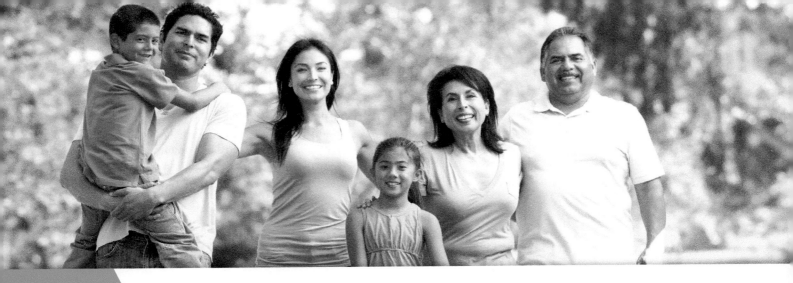

Human Development Across the Life Span

▶ Learning Outcomes

Upon completion of the chapter, you will be able to:

1. Relate the principles of growth and development to the nursing process.

2. Examine theories of development.

3. Appraise stages of development.

4. Differentiate between various tools used for measurement of growth and development across the age span.

5. Examine growth and development in relation to health assessment.

6. Appraise factors that influence growth and development.

Knowledge of growth and development provides a framework for nursing assessment and planning effective nursing interventions. The focus of assessment is not a specific aspect of an individual's health. Rather, nursing assessment requires the ability to interpret how the complex interactions of heredity; environment; and physiologic, cognitive, and psychologic development affect an individual at a particular time. By developing an image of what is usual or expected of children and adults of various ages, the nurse has a basis for a comparison with the norm. This knowledge and an understanding of individual variations provide a foundation for assessment and appropriate nursing interventions that help individuals attain their maximum level of wellness.

The selected nursing interventions will support wellness and, at the same time, reflect the objectives and goals of *Healthy People 2020.* The goals of *Healthy People 2020* are to eliminate preventable diseases, disability, injury, and premature death; achieve health equity; create environments that promote good health; and promote healthy development and behaviors across the life span. Objectives, derived from the goals, have been formulated to assist the nurse to implement primary and secondary prevention strategies. Each of the assessment chapters in unit III of this text provides information about specific focus areas and actions to promote health as outlined in *Healthy People 2020.* ∞

Growth and development are dynamic processes that describe how people change over time. The two processes are interdependent and interrelated. **Growth** involves measurable physical change and increase in size. Indicators of growth include height, weight, bone size, and dentition. Growth is rapid during the prenatal, neonatal, infancy, and adolescent stages of life; slows during childhood; and is minimal during adulthood. **Development** is an orderly, progressive increase in the complexity of the total person. It involves the continuous, irreversible, complex evolution of intelligence, personality, creativity, sociability, and morality. Development is continuous throughout the life cycle as the individual progresses through stages in physiologic maturation, cognitive development, and personality development.

The pattern of growth and development is consistent in all individuals; however, the rate of growth and development varies as a result of heredity and environmental factors. Heredity is a determinant of physical characteristics such as stature, gender, and race. It may also play an important role in personality development as the determinant of temperament. Environmental factors affecting growth and development include nutrition, family, religion, climate, culture, school, community, and socioeconomic status.

Principles of Growth and Development

Four commonly accepted principles define the orderly, sequential progression of growth and development in all individuals:

1. Growth and development proceed in a **cephalocaudal**, or head to toe, direction (see Figure 2.1 ■). An infant's head grows and becomes functional before the trunk or limbs. A baby's hands are able to grasp before the legs and feet are used purposefully.

2. Growth and development occur in a proximal to distal direction, or from the center of the body outward. A child gains the

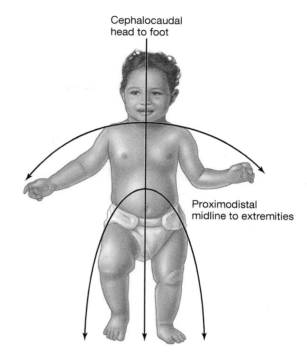

Figure 2.1 Cephalocaudal growth proceeds in a head to toe direction.

ability to use the hand as a whole prior to being able to control individual fingers.

3. Development proceeds from simple to complex or from the general to specific. To accomplish an integrated act such as putting something in the mouth, the infant must first learn to reach out to the object, grasp it, move it to the open mouth, and insert it.

4. Differentiated development begins with a generalized response and progresses to a skilled specific response. An infant responds to stimuli with the entire body. An older child responds to specific stimuli with happiness, anger, or fear.

Although the classic theories of human development provide the foundation for nursing assessment, researchers are continuously evolving developmental theories that further define and explain human behavior. Additionally, interpretation of the classic theories broadens as societal changes and advances in technology redefine individuals' relationships, expectations, and goals. Behavior that is widely accepted or even the norm today was often considered unusual or abnormal a generation ago. For instance, the family unit is no longer assumed to be two parents with children but may now consist of a single parent, stepsiblings, half siblings, a surrogate mother, same-sex parents, or other configurations. What are the implications for development? Researchers also study innovations in technology. Children are educated and entertained by various forms of stimuli, and they interact extensively with mobile devices, tablets, and computers. How do these affect the development of interpersonal skills? Advances in healthcare knowledge and technology have increased life expectancy, thus prolonging the span of productive years. This profoundly affects development, which continues until the individual dies.

Theories of Development

Three of the most influential classic theories of development are discussed here to provide a basic framework for nursing assessment. Although no one theory encompasses all aspects of human development, each is valuable as a framework for understanding, predicting, or guiding behavior.

Cognitive Theory

Cognitive theory explores how people learn to think, reason, and use language. Jean Piaget theorized that cognitive development is an orderly, sequential process that occurs in four stages in the growing child. Each stage demonstrates a new way of thinking and behaving. Piaget believed that a child's thinking develops progressively from simple reflex behavior into complex, logical, and abstract thought. All children move through the same stages, in the same order, with each stage providing the foundation for the next. At each stage, the child views the world in increasingly complex terms. Piaget's stages of cognitive development are summarized below and discussed in more detail with each specific developmental stage later in this chapter.

Stage 1: Sensorimotor (Birth to 2 Years) The infant progresses from responding primarily through reflexes to purposeful movement and organized activity. *Object permanence* (the knowledge that objects continue to exist when not seen) and object recognition are attained.

Stage 2: Preoperational Skills (2 to 7 Years) Highly egocentric, the child is able to view the world only from an individual perspective. The new ability to use mental symbols develops. The child's thinking now incorporates past events and anticipations of the future.

Stage 3: Concrete Operations (7 to 11 Years) During this time period, the child develops symbolic functioning. Symbolic functioning is the ability to make one thing represent a different thing that is not present. The child is able to consider another point of view. Thinking is more logical and systematic.

Stage 4: Formal Operations (11 to Adulthood) The child uses rational thinking and deductive reasoning. Thinking in abstract terms is possible. The child is able to deal with hypothetical situations and make logical conclusions after reviewing evidence.

Psychoanalytic Theory

Sigmund Freud was an early theorist whose concepts of personality development provided the foundation for the development of many other theories. Freud believed that people are constantly adjusting to environmental changes, and that this adjustment creates conflict between outside forces (environment) and inner forces (instincts). The type of conflict varies with an individual's developmental stage, and personality develops through conflict resolution.

Psychoanalytic theory defines the structure of personality as consisting of three parts: the id, the ego, and the superego. The personality at birth consists primarily of the *id,* which is the source of instinctive and unconscious urges. The *ego* is the seat of consciousness and mediates between the inner instinctual desires of the id and the outer world. The ego, a minor nucleus at birth, expands and gains mastery over the id. In addition, it is the receiving center for the senses and forms the mechanisms of defense. The *superego* is the conscience of the personality, acting as a censor of thoughts, feelings, and behavior. The superego begins to form after age 3 or 4 years.

According to Freud's theory, children pass through five stages of psychosexual development, with each phase blending into the next without clear separation. Individuals may become fixated at a particular stage if their needs are not met or if they are overindulged. Fixation implies a neurotic attachment and interferes with normal development.

1. The *oral phase* occurs during the first year of life when the mouth is the center of pleasure. Sucking and swallowing give pleasure by relieving hunger and reducing tension.

2. The *anal phase* follows the oral phase and continues through about 3 years of age. The anus becomes the focus of gratification, and the functions of elimination take on new importance. Conflict occurs during the toilet-training process as the child is required to conform to societal expectations.

3. The *phallic phase* occurs during years 4 to 5 or 6, when the focus of pleasure shifts to the genital area. Conflict occurs as the child feels possessive toward the parent of the opposite sex and rivalry toward the parent of the same sex. These conflicts are referred to as the Oedipus and Electra complexes.

4. The *latency phase* occurs from 5 or 6 years of age to puberty. This is a time of relative quiet as previous conflicts are resolved and aggressiveness becomes latent. The child focuses energy on intellectual and physical pursuits and derives pleasure from peer and adult relationships and school.

5. The *genital stage* covers the period from puberty through adulthood. Sexual urges reawaken as hormonal influences stimulate sexual development. The individual focuses on finding mature love relationships outside the family.

Psychosocial Theory

Erikson's psychosocial theory describes eight stages of ego development, but, unlike Freud, Erikson believed the ego is the conscious core of the personality. Erikson's **psychosocial theory** states that culture and society influence development across the entire life span. Erikson viewed life as a sequence of tasks that must be achieved with each stage presenting a crisis that must be resolved. Each crisis may have a positive or negative outcome depending on environmental influences and the choices that the individual makes. Crisis resolution may be positive, incomplete, or negative. Task achievement and positive conflict resolution are supportive to the person's ego. Negative resolution adversely influences the individual's ability to achieve the next task.

Stage 1: (Birth to 1 Year) presents the crisis of trust versus mistrust. The child who develops trust develops hope and drive. Mistrust results in fear, withdrawal, and estrangement.

Stage 2: (1 to 2 Years) is the crisis of autonomy versus shame and doubt. The child who achieves autonomy develops self-control and willpower. A negative resolution of the crisis results in self-doubt.

Stage 3: (2 to 6 Years) challenges the child to develop initiative versus guilt. Initiative leads to purpose and direction, whereas guilt results in lack of self-confidence, pessimism, and feelings of unworthiness.

Stage 4: (6 to 12 Years) is the crisis of industry versus inferiority. Industry results in the development of competency, creativity, and perseverance. Inferiority creates feelings of hopelessness and a sense of being mediocre or incompetent. Withdrawal from school and peers may result.

Stage 5: (12 to 18 Years) presents the challenge of identity versus role confusion. Achieving ego identity results in the ability to make a career choice and plan for the future. Inferiority creates confusion, uncertainty, indecisiveness, and an inability to make a career choice.

Stage 6: (19 to 40 Years) is the time of intimacy versus isolation. Successful resolution allows the individual to form an intimate relationship with another person. Isolation results in the development of impersonal relationships and the avoidance of career and lifestyle commitments.

Stage 7: (40 to 65 Years) is the time of generativity versus stagnation. Positive crisis resolution results in creativity, productivity, and concern for others. Stagnation results in selfishness and lack of interests and commitments.

Stage 8: (65 Years to Death) is the time of integrity versus despair. Individuals conclude life, either appreciating the uniqueness of their lives and accepting death, or feeling a sense of loss, despair, and contempt for others.

Stages of Development

The most common and traditional approach used by developmental theorists to describe and classify human behavior is according to chronologic age. Theorists attempt to identify meaningful relationships in complex behaviors by reducing them to core problems, tasks, or accomplishments that occur during a defined age range, or stage of life. Because theorists vary in their definitions of life stages, the following stages have been delineated to best illustrate the concepts of sequential development. It is important to remember that the ages are somewhat arbitrary. It is the sequence of growth, development, and observed behaviors that is meaningful during nursing assessment. For further information about infants and children, consult the National Center on Birth Defects and Developmental Disabilities (NCBDDD) and *Bright Futures: Guidelines for Health Supervision of Infants, Children, and Adolescents.*

Infants

An **infant** is a baby from 1 month of age to 1 year. During infancy, change is dramatic and occurs rapidly. The totally dependent newborn is transformed into an active child with a unique personality, all within the first year of life. The infant rapidly becomes mobile, often displaying a new skill each day. The developmental tasks of infancy are:

- Forming close relationships with primary caregivers
- Interacting with and relating to the environment

Physiologic Growth and Development

Height, weight, and head circumference are the measurements used to monitor infant growth. At birth, most term infants weigh 2.7 to 3.8 kg (6 to 8.5 lb). During the first few days of life, many infants lose up to 10% of their birth weight but usually regain it by 14 days of age. Infants gain weight at a rate of 5 to 7 oz (0.14 to 0.2 kg) weekly during the first 6 months. Weight gain occurs in spurts rather than in a steady, predictable manner, with birth weight usually doubled in 4 to 6 months and tripled by 1 year of age.

The average height of a normal-term infant is 50 cm (20 in.) at birth. Height increases at a rate of about 2.5 cm (1 in.) a month during the first 6 months. An infant's height increases 50% during the first year of life.

Head circumference reflects growth of the skull and brain. At birth, the average-term infant's head measures 35 cm (13.75 in.). Growth occurs at a monthly rate of 1.5 cm (0.6 in.) during the first 6 months, decreasing to 1 cm (0.45 in.) in the second 6 months. Ninety percent of head growth occurs during the first 2 years of life.

The bones of the cranium are not fused at birth. The infant's skull has openings, called fontanelles and sutures, which protect the brain during birth and allow for skull and brain growth during infancy. The **posterior fontanelle** is located in the superior occiput and may not be palpable at birth. It is usually 1 to 2 cm in diameter and closes by 2 months of age. The **anterior fontanelle** is a 2- to 4-cm diamond-shaped opening, also known as a "soft spot," located at the top of the skull. The skin covering the anterior fontanelle should be even with the skull surface. The anterior fontanelle normally closes between 9 and 18 months of age. Children with premature or delayed fontanelle closure require further evaluation and assessment. Fontanelles are usually soft and flat to the touch and must be assessed while the infant is calm. Bulging can be caused by increased intracranial pressure or crying. A sunken fontanelle may suggest dehydration.

Newborns who are large for gestational age, those born vaginally, and those with birth histories of cephalopelvic disproportion or prolonged or difficult labors often have misshaped skulls from trauma or compression during labor and delivery. **Caput succedaneum** is characterized by edema that results from a collection of fluid in the tissue at the top of the skull. The swelling associated with caput succedaneum crosses the cranial suture lines. **Cephalohematomas** are blood collections inside of the skull's periosteum and do not cross suture lines. Children with cephalohematomas are at increased risk of developing jaundice during the first week of life.

The head is the largest body surface area in infants. Heat loss and cold stress can result from leaving a newborn's head uncovered in cool environments. The head remains disproportionately large in comparison to the body until approximately 5 years of age. As a result, young children are top heavy and prone to minor head injury from falls.

Dramatic changes occur within the organ systems of infants during the first year. The brain stem, which controls functions such as respiration, digestion, and heartbeat, is relatively well developed but lacks maturity at birth. As a result, these vital functions tend to be irregular during the early months of infancy, becoming regular with brain stem maturation by 1 year. The infant's nervous system is extremely immature at birth. Tremors of the extremities or chin are normal, reflecting immature myelinization. Much of the infant's physical behavior is reflexive (see Table 26.3). These reflexes, or infant automatisms, disappear as myelinization of the efferent pathways matures. Myelinization of the efferent nerve fibers follows the cephalocaudal and proximodistal principles discussed earlier.

At birth, the infant's heart lies in an almost horizontal position and is large in relation to body size. With growth, the heart gradually shifts to a more vertical position. Although the ventricles are of equal size at birth, by 2 months of age the left ventricle develops better muscularity than the right. As the heart grows larger and the left ventricle becomes stronger, the low systolic blood pressure seen in the newborn rises, and the rapid heart rate of infants becomes slower.

Prenatally, the blood shunts away from the heart and liver through the **ductus venosus,** the **ductus arteriosus,** and the **foramen ovale.**

When newborns take their first breath, increased thoracic pressure closes these shunts, although the ductus venosus may remain open for 12 to 72 hours after birth.

At birth, the lungs are filled with fluid, which is quickly eliminated and absorbed as the lungs fill with air. The full complement of conducting airways is present, and the airway branching pattern is complete. The airways increase in size and length as the infant grows. Alveoli and respiratory bronchioles continue to grow after birth. The infant's thoracic cage is relatively soft, allowing it to pull in during labored breathing. Less tissue and cartilage in the trachea and bronchi also allow these structures to collapse more easily. Infants are obligatory nose breathers until 6 months of age. They gradually learn to breathe through their mouths by 3 or 4 months of age. Children use abdominal muscles more than thoracic muscles in respiration until 6 years of age.

Development of the eyes and visual acuity occurs rapidly during infancy. The inability of the infant to fixate consistently on an object, or not always being able to fixate the eyes together, is a result of immature eye muscles, which usually develop by 4 to 6 months of age. Infants see best at a distance of about 19.05 cm (7.5 in.) and have a visual acuity of about 20/150. Visual acuity rapidly develops to 20/40 by 2 years of age.

The ears and hearing are well developed at birth. The auditory (eustachian) tube, which connects the middle ear to the back of the throat in the nasopharynx, is shorter, wider, and more horizontal during infancy than during adult years. The size and position of the auditory tube gradually change with head growth.

Taste buds are present but immature at birth. Refined taste discrimination does not appear to develop until the infant is about 3 months old. Although the sense of smell is not refined in infancy, newborns are able to discriminate among distinctive odors and to recognize the smell of their mother's milk. The sense of touch is well developed at birth. Newborn infants show discriminating response to varied tactile stimuli.

Bone development, which begins before birth, continues during infancy. Ossification, the formation of bone, gradually occurs in the bony structures. Ossification is not complete until 14 years of age. While ossification is occurring, bones grow in length and width. Muscular growth occurs about twice as fast as that of bone from 5 months through 3 years. As muscle size increases, strength increases in response to appropriate stimulation.

Motor Development

Gross and fine motor skills develop in a predictable sequence, following the direction of maturation in the nervous system. Motor skill attainment in infancy provides milestones that mark normal development. Delay of early milestones may be an early indication of a developmental or neurologic abnormality. Table 2.1 shows how gross and fine motor skills develop during infancy. The age

---

TABLE 2.1 **Motor Skill Development in Infancy**

AGE	GROSS MOTOR SKILLS	FINE MOTOR SKILLS
1 Month	Lifts head unsteadily when prone. Turns head from side to side. "Stepping" reflex when held upright. Symmetrical Moro reflex.	Hands held in fists. Tight hand grasp. Head and eyes move together. Positive Babinski reflex.
2 Months	Holds head erect in midposition. Turns from side to back. Can raise head and chest when prone.	Holds a toy placed in hand. Follows objects with eyes. Smiles.
3 Months	Holds head erect and steady. Holds head at 45- to 90-degree angle when prone. Stepping reflex absent. Sits with rounded back with support. May turn from front to back.	Plays with fingers and hands. Able to place objects in mouth.
4 Months	When prone, uses arms to support self at a 90-degree angle. Can turn from back to side and abdomen to back. Sits with support.	Spreads fingers to grasp. Hands held predominantly open. Brings hands to midline.
5 Months	Head does not lag and back is straight when pulled to sitting position. Reaches for objects. Moro reflex disappearing. Rolls from back to abdomen.	Grasps objects with whole hand. Transfers object from hand to hand.
6 Months	Sits briefly without support. May crawl on abdomen.	Bangs object held in hand. Can release an object from hand. Reaches, grasps, and carries object to mouth. Uses all fingers in opposition to thumb for grasping.
7 Months	Sits briefly with arms forward for support. Bears weight when held in a standing position.	Uses tips of all fingers against the thumb. May grasp feet and suck on toes.
8 Months	Sits well alone.	Uses index and middle fingers against the thumb to grasp.
9 Months	Creeps and crawls. Pulls to standing position.	Uses pincer grasp (thumb and forefinger). Sucks, chews, and bites objects. Holds bottle and places it in mouth.
10 Months	Stands, cruises (walks sideways holding onto something).	Can clap, wave, and bring hands together to play "peek-a-boo."
11 Months	Tries to walk alone.	Puts objects into container. Very precise pincer grasp.
12 Months	Walks alone.	Positive Babinski reflex beginning to fade. Can hold a cup.

TABLE 2.2   **Major Developmental Milestones of Early Childhood**

MILESTONE	AGE ATTAINED
Visually tracks objects	Birth to 2 months
Smiles socially	2 months
Places objects in mouth	3 to 4 months
Babbles and coos	4 months
Extends forearms to support upper body when prone	4 to 5 months
Rolls from front to back	4 to 5 months
Rolls from back to front	5 to 6 months
Sits with support	6 to 7 months
Transfers objects from one hand to another	6 to 7 months
Sits without support	7 to 8 months
Supports weight when stands	7 to 8 months
Pulls self to standing position	8 months
Creeps or crawls	8 to 9 months
Attains pincer grasp	9 months
Cruises (walks holding on to furniture/objects)	9 to 12 months
Plays "peekaboo" and "pat-a-cake"	10 months
Says one word	11 months
Walks independently	12 to 15 months
Runs/climbs	14 to 18 months
Goes up and down stairs two feet per step	2 years
Goes up and down stairs alternating feet	3 years
Pedals tricycle	3 years
Copies circle	3 years
Prints name	5 years

of skill attainment is an average, with some infants acquiring the skill somewhat earlier, some later. Table 2.2 discusses the major developmental milestones of early childhood. The Denver II is often used to assess the development of infants and children up to 6 years of age.

Language Development

Undifferentiated crying in early infancy communicates infants' needs. By 1 month of age, crying becomes differentiated as the pitch and intensity of the cry communicates various needs such as hunger, discomfort, anger, or pain. Infants are cooing with pleasure by about 6 weeks and babbling by 4 months. They begin to imitate the sounds of others by 9 to 10 months, although infants do not necessarily understand the meaning of their sounds. By 1 year, most infants say two to five words with meaning.

Cognitive Development

According to Piaget, infants are in the sensorimotor phase of cognitive development, during which the infant changes from a primarily reflexive response to being able to organize sensorimotor activities in relation to the environment. At birth, the infant responds to the environment with automatic reflexes. From 1 to 4 months, the infant perceives events as centered on the body and objects as an extension of self. By 4 to 8 months, infants gradually acknowledge the external environment (see Figure 2.2 ■). They begin to develop the notion of *object permanence*, the concept that objects and people continue to exist even though they are no longer in sight. The infant first learns to search for a partially hidden object but does not search for one completely out of sight. By 9 to 10 months, the infant learns to search behind a screen for an object if it was seen to be placed there.

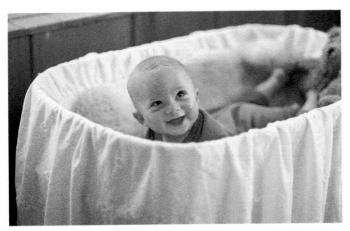

Figure 2.2 An infant begins to notice the external environment by the age of 4 to 8 months.

Psychosocial Development

According to Freud's psychoanalytic theory of personality, the id is present at birth. The unconscious source of motive and desires, the id operates on the "pleasure principle" and strives for immediate gratification. Infants are egocentric and do not differentiate themselves from the outside world. The id motivates infants, and infants view the world as existing solely for their gratification. When gratification is delayed, the ego develops as infants begin to differentiate themselves from the environment.

Infants are in what Freud called the oral stage of psychosexual development until 12 months of age. Most of their gratification is obtained from sucking nipples, hands, and objects, which satisfies the id's need for immediate gratification. Nonnutrient sucking on a pacifier, fingers, or thumb helps satisfy infants' need for oral gratification.

Erikson believed that the quality of care infants receive during the early months determines the degree to which they learn to trust themselves, other people, and the world in general. Erikson defined the primary task of infancy as developing a sense of trust or a sense of mistrust. Trust develops as the infant's basic needs are met through sucking, feeding, warmth, comfort, sensory stimulation, and other activities that convey the sense of love and security. In contrast, mistrust may stem from experiences such as rejection or inconsistent patterns of care.

Development of trust or mistrust is also a component of each successive psychosocial stage. A basically trusting child may later develop a sense of mistrust when lied to by someone the child respects. However, the foundation for all later psychosocial development is laid in infancy because, according to Erikson, the consistency and quality of the parent-infant interaction directly affect the infant's development of ego identity, or self-concept.

All theorists of infant psychosocial development acknowledge the significance of the manner in which infants' needs are met. Although the concept of infant needs and the best way to meet them varies from theorist to theorist, it is clear that infants' needs extend beyond the physiologic domain. Infants who lack sufficient social and cognitive stimulation exhibit signs of physical and affective imbalance. Children who receive adequate social and cognitive stimuli progress through sequentially more complex affective and social behaviors.

According to *attachment theory* (Bretherton, 1992), a focused, enduring relationship between the infant and the primary caregiver is imperative for the healthy attainment of infant goals and is a precursor for relating appropriately to others in the future. Occurring over a period of months, attachment requires consistent, intimate interaction between the infant and primary caregiver. Many factors affect attachment. The infant and the primary caregiver each bring a unique temperament, personality, and style to the relationship. In addition, the primary caregiver's previous life experiences and preconceived expectations of the infant and parenting experience influence the attachment process.

The quality of attachment depends on what is often referred to as the goodness of fit of the infant and primary caregiver. Goodness of fit refers to the concept that both the infant and primary caregiver must receive positive feedback and evoke a positive response in the relationship in order for attachment to develop. The crying infant who quiets in response to being held by the primary caregiver makes the primary caregiver feel successful. The infant who is difficult to console gives negative feedback with continued crying, making the primary caregiver feel unsuccessful and perhaps unloved. The primary caregiver transmits anxiety about parenting abilities to the infant, increasing the crying. By smiling and cooing in response to the primary caregiver's vocalizations, the infant encourages the caregiver to continue vocalizations, providing the infant with environmental stimulation.

By 3 months, the infant and the primary caregiver achieve social synchrony, which is apparent in reciprocal vocal and affective exchanges. This mutually satisfying synchrony signals the end of the early adjustment period. The next step in attachment occurs at 3 to 5 months when the infant develops a clear preference for primary caregivers. As memory for absent objects emerges between 7 and 9 months, the infant's preference for primary caregivers creates the reaction of stranger anxiety.

Throughout the first year of life, the infant's crying serves as the signal of the need for comfort. Research has shown that infants whose mothers respond promptly to their cries in the first months of life cry less at 1 year. It is now well accepted that responding promptly to infants' cries helps establish a sense of internal security that fosters later independence. Concern over "spoiling" infants by promptly responding to their cries is no longer an accepted concept. Chronically inconsistent nurturing of infants may result in infants and toddlers uninterested in exploring, even in the presence of the caregiver. Some such children appear unusually clingy; others appear actively angry and distrustful, ignoring or resisting caregivers' efforts to comfort them.

Assessment of Infants

Frequent assessments during the first year provide opportunities to monitor the infant's rate of growth and development as well as to compare the infant with the norm for age. Height, weight, and head circumference measurements are plotted on an appropriate growth chart at each assessment. The three measurements should fall within two standard deviations of each other. More important, each measurement should follow the expected rate of growth, following the same percentile throughout infancy.

Accurate assessment combining information obtained by history, physical assessment, and knowledgeable observation allows early identification of common problems that may easily be resolved with early intervention. Often basic parent education and support remedy problems that, left untreated, could result in significant health problems or disturbed parent–child interactions later.

Overnutrition and undernutrition are identified by weight that crosses percentiles. In *overnutrition*, the rate of weight gain is accelerated; in *undernutrition*, the rate of weight gain diminishes. Overnutrition may occur when caregivers do not learn to read infants' cues and instead assume that every cry signals hunger. Cultural beliefs that a fat baby is a healthy baby may also lead caregivers to overfeed infants.

Undernutrition may be caused by inadequate caloric intake resulting from lack of knowledge of normal infant feeding, a lack of financial resources to obtain formula, or inappropriate mixing of formula. Some quiet or passive infants do not demand feedings, and caregivers may misinterpret this passivity as lack of hunger. (See chapter 12. ∞)

Head growth that crosses percentiles requires evaluation as it may indicate *hydrocephalus* (enlargement of the head caused by inadequate drainage of cerebrospinal fluid). Early diagnosis and intervention for rapid head growth prevents or diminishes serious neurologic sequelae.

Parents and caregivers generally enjoy relaying infants' new developmental milestones and can accurately describe infants' abilities. An infant who seems to be lagging behind on milestones may not be receiving appropriate stimulation. Assessing caregivers' expectations and knowledge of infant development may reveal a knowledge deficit. Suggesting specific activities for caregivers to do with their infants may be the only intervention required. Infants who continue to lag further behind and are not achieving normal milestones require evaluation.

Healthy attachment is observed as a caregiver holds the infant closely in a manner that encourages eye contact. The caregiver looks at the infant, smiles, talks, and interacts with the infant. The infant responds by fixing on the caregiver's face, smiling, and cooing. The caregiver stays close to the infant, providing support and reassurance during examinations or procedures.

Failure to engage the infant through eye contact or to talk or smile limits available opportunities for the caregiver to receive positive feedback from the infant. The infant, in turn, finds efforts to engage the parent frustrating, resulting in decreased attempts to interact. A negative pattern is quickly established, requiring more extensive intervention the longer it persists.

Toddlers

The **toddler** (1 to 3 years of age) is a busy, active explorer who recognizes no boundaries. Maturing muscles and developing language increase the toddler's ability to interact with the environment, allowing the child to gather information and learn with every experience. The major developmental tasks of being a toddler include the following:

- Differentiating self from others
- Tolerating separation from primary caregivers
- Controlling body functions
- Acquiring verbal communication

Physiologic Growth and Development

The rate of growth decreases during the second year. The expected weight gain is about 2.5 kg (5.5 lb) between 1 and 2 years, and about 1 to 2 kg (2.2 to 4.5 lb) between 2 and 3 years. The average 3-year-old child weighs about 13.6 kg (30 lb).

Height growth is about 10 to 12 cm (4 to 5 in.) between 1 and 2 years, slowing to 6 to 8 cm (2.5 to 3.5 in.) between 2 and 3 years. Two-year-olds are approximately half of their adult size.

The head circumference of the toddler increases about 3 cm (1.25 in.) between the ages of 1 and 3 years. By 2 years the head is four fifths of the average adult size and the brain is 70% of the average adult size.

Alterations in the toddler's body proportions create striking changes in appearance as the child develops. Young toddlers appear chubby with relatively short legs and large heads. After the second year, the toddler's head becomes better proportioned, and the extremities grow faster than the trunk. Young toddlers have pronounced *lordosis* and protruding abdomens. With growth and walking, the abdominal muscles gradually develop, and the abdomen flattens.

Neurologic advances during the toddler years enable the toddler to progress developmentally. The increasing maturation of the brain contributes greatly to the child's emerging cognitive abilities. Myelinization in the spinal cord is almost complete by 2 years, corresponding to the increase in gross motor skills.

The toddler's cardiovascular system continues gradual growth. The gradual decrease in heart rate is related to the increasing size of the heart. The larger heart can pump blood more forcefully and efficiently. In addition, the toddler's capillaries constrict more efficiently to conserve body heat.

As the lungs grow in size, their volume and capacity for oxygenation also increase. This increased productivity of the lungs results in a decreased respiratory rate.

Visual acuity is close to 20/40 at 2 years and close to 20/30 by 3 years. Accommodation to near and far objects becomes fairly well developed in toddlers and continues with age. Taste and smell are well developed; taste and odor preferences and aversions are clearly communicated.

The toddler's changing body proportions are the direct result of musculoskeletal growth. Muscle grows faster than bone during the toddler years as muscle fibers increase in size and strength in response to increased use. Ossification slows after infancy but continues until maturation is complete. Long-shafted bones contain red marrow, which produces blood cells. The legs and feet of toddlers grow more rapidly than their trunks. The bowlegged appearance of young toddlers diminishes between 18 months and 2 years as the small-shafted bones rotate and gradually straighten the legs.

Motor Development

Gross and fine motor development continues at a rapid pace during the toddler years. The major accomplishments are listed below.

- *Fifteen months:* Walks independently, creeps upstairs, and is able to build a tower of two to three blocks.
- *Eighteen months:* Runs, climbs, pulls toys, and throws. Puts a block in large holes, scribbles, and builds a tower of four to five blocks.

- *Two years:* Tries to jump and can walk up and down stairs. Can turn doorknobs, imitates a vertical stroke with crayon, uses a spoon without spilling, turns pages of a book, unbuttons a large button, and builds a tower of six to seven blocks.

- *Two and a half years:* Can stand on one foot for at least 1 second, can walk on tiptoe, jumps in place, goes up and down stairs using alternating feet, and catches a ball with arms and body. Is able to make a tower of nine large blocks, likes to fill containers with objects, will take things apart, can take off some clothing, buttons a large button, twists caps off bottles, and places simple shapes in correct holes.

- *Three years:* Pedals a tricycle, jumps from a low step, is toilet trained, can undress, puts own coat on, and catches an object with both arms. Begins to use blunt scissors, strings large beads, can copy a circle, can help with simple household tasks, can wash and dry hands, and can pull pants up and down for toileting.

Language Development

Language skills develop rapidly, progressing from a few single words at 1 year to hundreds of words used in sentences by 3 years. At 1 year, children express entire thoughts by one word, saying, for instance, "out" to express "I want to go out." Simple phrases are characteristic of the speech of 2-year-olds, such as "go car." Although their speech is simple, these children understand most of what is said to them. By 3 years, sentences are more complex and include more parts of speech.

Cognitive Development

The toddler continues in Piaget's sensorimotor stage until the age of 2 years, when the preoperational stage begins. Object permanence is fully developed by 18 to 24 months. The toddler is then able to conduct a search in many places for objects hidden from sight. As object permanence develops, toddlers develop the understanding that they are separate from the environment.

By age 2 the toddler acquires the ability to think of an external event without actually experiencing it. This is called mental representation. As a result, the toddler is now able to think through plans to reach a goal, rather than proceeding by trial and error.

With the preoperational stage, the child enters into the use of symbolic function. Instead of tying thoughts to the actual, the present, or the concrete, the child is able to think back to past events, think forward to anticipate the future, and think about what might be happening elsewhere in the present. Symbolic function enables the child to demonstrate delayed imitation: The child witnesses an event, forms a mental image of it, and later imitates it. In symbolic play, the child makes one object stand for something else, such as pretending that a laundry basket is a hat (see Figure 2.3 ■).

Psychosocial Development

According to Freud, the ego, which represents reason or common sense, continues to develop as the toddler experiences increased delays in gratification. The toddler years correspond to Freud's anal stage, during which the child takes great pleasure from expelling urine and, especially, feces. Toddlers may hold their stool, not wanting to give it up, or they may consider it a gift and object to its disposal. Toilet training takes on great significance as parents

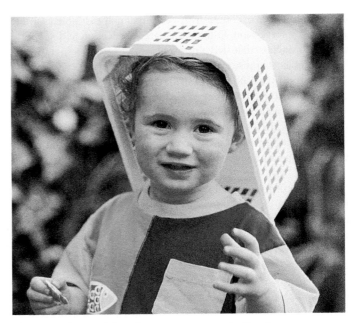

Figure 2.3 A toddler demonstrates symbolic play.

urge socially acceptable toileting while the child learns self-control and delayed gratification. Freud believed that the approach to toilet training and the child's reaction to it greatly influence the adult personality.

Toddlers' sense of trust developed during infancy leads them to a realization of their own sense of self. Realizing they have a will, they assert themselves in a quest for autonomy during Erikson's stage of autonomy versus shame and doubt. Parents are challenged to provide an environment in which toddlers may explore, while protecting them from danger and frustration above their level of tolerance. Parents provide a safe haven, with safe limits, from which the child can set out and discover the world, and keep coming back to them for support.

Erikson believed that toddlers who are not provided with safe limits by adults develop a sense of shame, or rage turned against themselves. Children who fail to develop a sense of autonomy, as a result of an overly controlling or permissive environment, may become compulsive about controlling themselves. Fear of losing self-control may inhibit their self-expression, make them doubt themselves, and make them feel ashamed.

Toddlers who have developed a firm attachment during infancy continue attachment behaviors during the toddler stage. Their repertoire of attachment behaviors becomes increasingly elaborate as they no longer seek prolonged body-to-body contact. Toddlers are sustained by only brief visual or physical contact with caregivers and can happily investigate new people and places. A secure attachment relationship in the first 2 years is characterized by the child's ability to seek and obtain comfort from familiar caregivers and by the child's willingness to explore and master the environment when supported by a caregiver's presence.

Assessment of Toddlers

Although the rate of growth of toddlers decreases, it proceeds in an expected manner. Height and weight continue to follow a percentile, although slight variations are often seen. Assessing caloric intake by obtaining a 24-hour recall gives clues to inappropriate feeding patterns. Toddlers generally feed themselves and begin to interact with the family at meals. A favorite food one week may be refused the next, causing frustration and confusion in caregivers. Concern for the toddler's health may precipitate a power struggle as parents try to force the toddler to eat. Poor weight gain may result as the toddler exerts a newfound independence by refusing to eat. Excessive weight gain occurs when caregivers use food to quiet or bribe their toddlers. Discussing appropriate eating expectations and weight gain helps parents resolve eating problems.

Since cooperation of the young toddler is unlikely, a health history is often the best way to assess development. Older toddlers are more willing to play with developmental testing materials or explore the environment while in proximity to a caregiver, enabling direct observations of development. Toddlers may not speak in a strange or threatening environment, making language assessment difficult. Listening to the child talk in a playroom or waiting room increases the probability of assessing the toddler's language.

The toddler wanders a short distance from a caregiver to explore, returning periodically to "touch base." After receiving reassurance and encouragement, the child is ready for further exploration. Exploration provides learning opportunities but also places the toddler at risk for accidental injury or poisoning.

Tantrums are a frequent occurrence. They are the result of unwanted limits or frustration. An attitude of calm understanding limits the duration of tantrums and keeps tantrums from becoming power struggles or attention-getting behavior.

Toddlers quickly turn to caregivers for comfort or when confronted with a stranger. Observing the adult-child interaction and listening to how the adult speaks to the child provides information on the quality of the relationship.

Continuous clinging of a toddler to a caregiver in a nonthreatening situation is unusual. Failure of the child to look to a caregiver for comfort and support may indicate that trust did not develop during infancy. Inappropriate caregiver expectations, such as expecting a toddler to sit quietly in a chair, may interfere with the normal progression of the toddler's development. Caregiver inattention to the activities of the child and failure to set limits result in the child's inability to develop self-control.

Preschool Children

The busy, curious **preschooler** (3 to 5 years of age) has an appearance and proportions closer to those of adults. The preschooler's world expands as relationships include other children and adults in settings outside the home. Developmental tasks during the preschool period include the following:

- Identifying sex role
- Developing a conscience
- Developing a sense of initiative
- Interacting with others in socially acceptable ways
- Learning to use language for social interaction

Physiologic Growth and Development

Preschoolers tend to grow more in height than weight and appear taller and thinner than toddlers. Weight gain is generally slow at a rate of about 2 kg (4.5 lb) per year. The rate of height growth is about 7 cm (2.75 in.) per year.

The preschooler's brain reaches almost its adult size by 5 years. Myelinization of the central nervous system continues, resulting in refinement of movement. Most physiologic systems continue to grow and are nearing maturity. Visual acuity remains approximately 20/30 throughout the preschool years. The musculoskeletal system continues to develop. Muscles are growing, and cartilage is changing to bone at a faster rate than previously. From 4 to 7 years, the active red bone marrow of earlier ages is gradually replaced by fatty tissue.

Motor Development

Gross and fine motor skills continue to be refined during the preschool years.

- *Three and a half years:* Skips on one foot, hops forward on both feet, kicks a large ball, and catches an object with hands. Cuts straight lines with scissors, manipulates large puzzle pieces into position, places small pegs in a pegboard, copies a circle, and unbuttons small buttons.
- *Four years:* Jumps well, hops forward on one foot, walks backward, and catches an object with one hand. Cuts around pictures with scissors, can copy a square, and can button small buttons.
- *Five years:* Can jump rope, and alternates feet to skip. May be able to print own name, copies a triangle, dresses without assistance, threads small beads on a string, and eats with a fork.

Language Development

Language becomes a tool for social interaction. As the preschooler's vocabulary increases, sentence structure becomes more complex, and the child becomes better able to understand another's point of view and share ideas. Speech should be 80% to 90% understandable by age 4. Sentences evolve from three or four words between 3 and 4 years to six to eight words in grammatically correct sentences by 5 to 6 years.

Cognitive Development

Preschoolers are in the middle of Piaget's preoperational stage. Although symbolic thought is an immense milestone begun as a toddler, the preschooler's thinking continues to be rudimentary. Preschoolers continue to be egocentric and unable to see another's point of view. In addition, they feel no need to defend their point of view, because they assume that everyone else sees things as they do. Preschoolers demonstrate centration; they focus on one aspect of a situation and ignore others, leading to illogical reasoning. In addition, preschoolers believe that their wishes, thoughts, and gestures command the universe. The child believes that these "magical" powers of thought are the cause of all events.

Preschoolers enter Piaget's stage of intuitive thought at about 4 years. While egocentricity continues, older preschoolers are developing the ability to give reasons for their beliefs and actions and to form some concepts. They are limited by their inability to consider more than one idea at a time, making it impossible for them to make

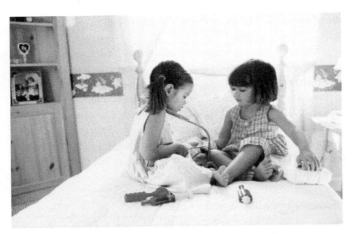

Figure 2.4 Preschoolers imitate reality in their play.
Source: Rick Gomez/Corbis.

comparisons. Fantasy play begins to give way to play that imitates reality (see Figure 2.4 ■).

Psychosocial Development

The superego, or conscience, develops as the preschooler becomes more aware of other people's interests, needs, and values. The child learns right from wrong, developing an understanding of the consequences of actions. At this stage, the child's conscience is rigid and often unrealistic. With maturity, the conscience becomes more realistic and flexible.

As preschoolers become further aware of their separateness, gender awareness develops. They learn what makes girls different from boys during what Freud called the phallic phase. At this time, Freud believed that children have a romantic attraction to the parent of the opposite sex, making them rivals with their same-sex parent. The resulting fear and guilt are resolved as children identify with the same-sex parent, realizing that they are unable to compete with the bigger, powerful parent. According to Freud, sexual urges are repressed, and the sex-related behaviors, attitudes, and beliefs of the same-sex parent are imitated.

Erikson believed that children's primary conflict at this stage is between initiative, which enables them to plan and carry out activities, and guilt over what they want to do. Their high level of energy, eagerness to try new things, and ability to work cooperatively characterize preschoolers. Children who are encouraged, reassured, and cheered on in their pursuits learn self-assertion, self-sufficiency, direction, and purpose. They develop initiative. Children who are ridiculed, punished, or prevented from accomplishing initiative develop guilt.

Preschoolers turn from a total attachment to their caregivers and begin to identify with them. A firm attachment during the early years allows preschoolers to detach from caregivers at this stage. This ability to detach enables children to explore new territory, learn new games, and form new relationships with peers.

Assessment of Preschool Children

Preschoolers' slowed rate of growth is often of concern to caregivers. The nurse can allay anxiety by showing the preschooler's growth chart and discussing eating expectations.

Preschoolers are generally pleasant, cooperative, and talkative. They continue to need the reassurance of a caregiver in view

but do not need to return to the caregiver for comfort except in threatening situations. Talking with preschoolers about favorite activities allows the nurse to assess language ability, cognitive ability, and development. The nurse evaluates the child's use of language to express thoughts, sentence structure, and vocabulary. It may be possible to identify centration, magical thinking, and reality imitation as the child relays play activities. Lack of appropriate environmental stimulation may become evident, and the nurse may need to educate caregivers about age-appropriate activities for their children.

A clinging, frightened preschooler in a nonthreatening situation may be a child who lacks trust. Lack of trust between caregiver and child limits the child's ability to learn appropriate social interaction. In addition, the child does not have the opportunity to practice language skills or to obtain information by having questions answered. See Box 2.1 for a listing of recommended preventive services across the age span.

School-age Children

School age begins about the age of 6 years, when deciduous teeth are shed, and ends with the onset of puberty at about 12 years. Tasks of the school-age child include the following:

- Mastering physical skills
- Building self-esteem and a positive self-concept
- Fitting into a peer group
- Developing logical reasoning

Physiologic Growth and Development

Most children during the years from 6 to 10 reach a relative plateau, with growth occurring in a slow but steady manner. The average child gains about 3 kg (6.5 lb) and grows about 5.5 cm (2 in.) per year. Growth accelerates again at the onset of puberty, which occurs about age 10 for girls and age 12 for boys. During preadolescence (10 to 12 or 13 years), the growth of boys and girls differs. Growth in boys is generally slow and steady and rapid in girls. Growth is variable, especially among girls at this age. Some girls of 11 years look like children, while others are starting to look like adolescents. By 12 years, some boys are beginning their growth spurt and demonstrating the onset of secondary sexual characteristics.

The body proportions of the school-age child are different from those of the preschooler. Children often appear gangly and awkward because of their proportionately longer legs, diminishing body fat, and a lower center of gravity. As increases in organ maturity and size occur, the child responds physiologically to illness in a more adult manner. The continuing maturation of the central nervous system (CNS) allows the child to perform increasingly complex gross and fine motor skills. Brain growth is slowed, with 95% of growth achieved by 9 years of age. Myelinization continues and is partly responsible for the transformation of the clumsy 6-year-old into the coordinated 12-year-old.

The prevalence of childhood obesity and risk for being overweight are a significant public health concern. Overweight and obesity in children is defined as body mass index (BMI) for age greater than the 85th percentile and the 95th percentile after adjusting for gender and age, respectively (Centers for Disease Control and Prevention [CDC], 2014).

Box 2.1 Section 1. Preventive Services Recommended by the USPSTF

The U.S. Preventive Services Task Force (USPSTF) recommends that clinicians discuss these preventive services with eligible patients and offer them as a priority. All these services have received an "A" or a "B" (recommended) grade from the Task Force.

For definitions of all grades used by the USPSTF, go to *http://www.epss.ahrq.gov.*

RECOMMENDATION	ADULTS		SPECIAL POPULATIONS	
	MEN	WOMEN	PREGNANT WOMEN	CHILDREN
Abdominal Aortic Aneurysm, Screening[1]	X			
Alcohol Misuse Screening and Behavioral Counseling Interventions	X	X	X	
Aspirin for the Prevention of Cardiovascular Disease[2]	X	X		
Asymptomatic Bacteriuria in Adults, Screening[3]			X	
Breast Cancer, Screening[4]		X		
Breast and Ovarian Cancer Susceptibility, Genetic Risk Assessment and BRCA Mutation Testing[5]		X		
Breastfeeding, Behavioral Interventions to Promote[6]		X	X	
Cervical Cancer, Screening[7]		X		
Chlamydial Infection, Screening[8]		X	X	
Colorectal Cancer, Screening[9]	X	X		
Congenital Hypothyroidism, Screening[10]				X
Dental Caries in Preschool Children, Prevention[11]				X
Depression (Adults), Screening[12]	X	X		
Diet, Behavioral Counseling in Primary Care to Promote a Healthy[13]	X	X		
Gonorrhea, Screening[14]		X	X	
Gonorrhea, Prophylactic Medication[15]				X
Hearing Loss in Newborns, Screening[16]				X
Hepatitis B Virus Infection, Screening[17]			X	
High Blood Pressure, Screening	X	X		
HIV, Screening[18]	X	X	X	X
Iron Deficiency Anemia, Prevention[19]				X
Iron Deficiency Anemia, Screening[20]			X	
Lipid Disorders in Adults, Screening[21]	X	X		
Major Depressive Disorder in Children and Adolescents, Screening[22]				X
Obesity in Adults, Screening[23]	X	X		
Osteoporosis in Postmenopausal Women, Screening[24]		X		
Phenylketonuria, Screening[25]				X
Rh (D) Incompatibility, Screening[26]			X	
Sexually Transmitted Infections, Counseling[27]	X	X		X
Sickle Cell Disease, Screening[28]				X
Syphilis Infection, Screening[29]	X	X	X	
Tobacco Use and Tobacco-Caused Disease, Counseling[30]	X	X	X	
Type 2 Diabetes Mellitus in Adults, Screening[31]	X	X		
Visual Impairment in Children Younger Than Age 5 Years, Screening[32]				X

[1] One-time screening by ultrasonography in men aged 65 to 75 who have ever smoked.
[2] When the potential harm of an increase in gastrointestinal hemorrhage is outweighed by a potential benefit of a reduction in myocardial infarctions (men aged 45–79 years) or in ischemic strokes (women aged 55–79 years).
[3] Pregnant women at 12–16 weeks gestation or at first prenatal visit, if later.
[4] Mammography every 1–2 years for women 40 and older.
[5] Refer women whose family history is associated with an increased risk for deleterious mutations in *BRCA1* or *BRCA2* genes for genetic counseling and evaluation for BRCA testing.
[6] Interventions during pregnancy and after birth to promote and support breastfeeding.
[7] Women aged 21–65 who have been sexually active and have a cervix.
[8] Sexually active women 24 and younger and other asymptomatic women at increased risk for infection. Asymptomatic pregnant women 24 and younger and others at increased risk.
[9] Adults aged 50–75 using fecal occult blood testing, sigmoidoscopy, or colonoscopy.
[10] Newborns.
[11] Prescribe oral fluoride supplementation at currently recommended doses to preschool children older than 6 months whose primary water source is deficient in fluoride.
[12] In clinical practices with systems to assure accurate diagnoses, effective treatment, and follow-up.
[13] Adults with hyperlipidemia and other known risk factors for cardiovascular and diet-related chronic disease.
[14] Sexually active women, including pregnant women 25 and younger, or at increased risk for infection.
[15] Prophylactic ocular topical medication for all newborns against gonococcal ophthalmia neonatorum.
[16] Newborns.
[17] Pregnant women at first prenatal visit.
[18] All adolescents and adults at increased risk for HIV infection and all pregnant women.
[19] Routine iron supplementation for asymptomatic children aged 6 to 12 months who are at increased risk for iron deficiency anemia.
[20] Routine screening in asymptomatic pregnant women.
[21] Men aged 20–35 and women over age 20 who are at increased risk for coronary heart disease; all men aged 35 and older.
[22] Adolescents (age 12–18) when systems are in place to ensure accurate diagnosis, psychotherapy, and follow-up.
[23] Intensive counseling and behavioral interventions to promote sustained weight loss for obese adults.
[24] Women 65 and older and women 60 and older at increased risk for osteoporotic fractures.
[25] Newborns.
[26] Blood typing and antibody testing at first pregnancy-related visit. Repeated antibody testing for unsensitized Rh (D)-negative women at 24–28 weeks gestation unless biological father is known to be Rh (D) negative.
[27] All sexually active adolescents and adults at increased risk for STIs.
[28] Newborns.
[29] Persons at increased risk and all pregnant women.
[30] Tobacco cessation interventions for those who use tobacco. Augmented pregnancy-tailored counseling to pregnant women who smoke.
[31] Asymptomatic adults with sustained blood pressure greater than 135/80 mm Hg.
[32] To detect amblyopia, strabismus, and defects in visual acuity.

Source: Agency for Healthcare Research and Quality (AHRQ), U.S. Preventive Services Task Force (USPSTF). (2012). *Guide to Clinical Preventive Services.*

Data from the 1999–2000 National Health and Nutrition Examination Survey (NHANES) indicates that the prevalence of overweight was 10.4% for 2- to 5-year-olds, 15.3% in 6- through 11-year-olds, and 15.5% in 12- through 19-year-olds (CDC, 2014; Ogden, Flegal, Carroll, & Johnson, 2002). By 2004, that number increased to 13.9% for 2- to 5-year-olds, 18.8% for 6- to 11-year-olds, and 17.4% for 12- to 19-year-olds (CDC, 2014). By 2009–2010, the prevalence of overweight was still on the rise, increasing to 12.1% for 2- to 5-year-olds, 18% in 6- to 11-year-olds, and 18.4% in 12- to 19-year-olds (Ogden, Carroll, Kit, & Flegal, 2012).

The prevalence of childhood overweight has significant ethnic and racial factors. Non-Hispanic males are more likely to be overweight than their African American and Mexican American peers, and African American females have higher rates of overweight than Mexican American and non-Hispanic white girls (CDC, 2014). As a result, assessment of a child's nutritional status and determination of complications of overweight and obesity is a significant part of childhood physical assessment.

As cardiac growth continues, the diaphragm descends, allowing more room for cardiac action and respiratory expansion. The respiratory tissues achieve adult maturity, with lung capacity proportional to body size.

Most children achieve 20/20 vision by age 5 or 6 years. Visual maturity, including fully developed peripheral vision, is usually achieved by 6 or 7 years.

The most rapid growth during the school-age years occurs in the skeletal system. Ossification continues at a steady pace. Muscle mass gradually increases in size and strength, and the body appears leaner as "baby fat" decreases. As muscle tone increases, the loose movements, "knock-knees," and lordosis of early childhood disappear.

Motor Development

The gross motor skills of the 6- to 7-year-old are far better developed than fine motor coordination. Children of this age greatly enjoy gross motor activity such as hopping, roller-skating, bike riding, running, and climbing. The child seems to be in perpetual motion. Balance and eye-hand coordination gradually improve. The 6-year-old is able to hammer, paste, tie shoes, and fasten clothes. Right- or left-hand dominance is firmly established by age 6. By age 7, the child's hands become steadier. Printing becomes smaller, and reversal of letters during writing is less common. Many children have sufficient finger coordination to begin music lessons.

Less restlessness is seen in 7- and 8-year-old children, although they retain their high energy level. Increased attention span and cognitive skills enhance their enjoyment of board games. Improved reaction time increases sports ability.

Children between 8 and 10 years of age gradually develop greater rhythm, smoothness, and gracefulness of movements. They are able to participate in physical activities that require more concentrated attention and effort. They have sufficient coordination to write rather than print words, and they may begin sewing, building models, and playing musical instruments.

Energy levels remain high in children between 10 and 12 years of age, but activity is well directed and controlled. Physical skills are almost equal to those of the adult. Manipulative skills are also comparable to the precision exhibited by adults. Complex, intricate, and rapid movements are mastered with practice.

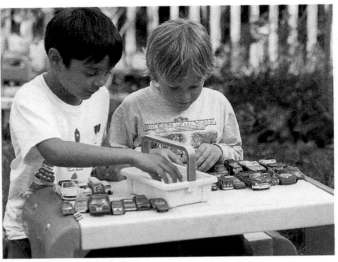

Figure 2.5 School-age children enjoy classifying objects.

Language Development

The school-age child uses appropriate sentence structure and continues to develop the ability to express thoughts in words. Comprehension of language continues to exceed the school-age child's ability of expression. Vocabulary increases as the child is exposed to a wider range of reading materials and ideas in school and through association with peers.

Cognitive Development

Sometime around 6 or 7 years of age, children become what Piaget called "operational." They are now able to use symbols to carry out operations, or mental activities, enabling them to perform activities such as reading and using numbers. The child becomes able to serialize, that is, order objects according to size or weight. In addition, the child begins to understand how to classify objects by something they have in common. Children commonly practice this new skill by collecting and frequently sorting collections of rocks, sports cards, shells, or dolls (see Figure 2.5 ■).

The school-age child develops an understanding of the principle of conservation, the ability to tell the difference between how things seem and how they really are. The child is able to see that transformation of shape or position does not change the mass or quantity of a substance. For instance, the child understands that two equal balls of clay remain equal when one ball is rolled into a "hot dog." In contrast, a younger child who has not mastered the principle of conservation believes that the cylindrical shape is bigger because it is longer.

School-age children develop logical reasoning and understand cause-and-effect relationships. They can consider various sides of a situation and form a conclusion. Egocentrism decreases as the child becomes able to consider another's point of view. Although able to reason, the child is still somewhat limited by the inability to deal with abstract ideas.

Psychosocial Development

School-age children have accepted their sex roles and are now able to turn their energies to acquiring new facts, mastering skills, and learning cultural attitudes. Freud termed this the latency stage, considering it a time of relative sexual quiet. Curiosity about sex and the use of sexual and bathroom jokes demonstrate the ongoing sexual awareness of school-age children; however, the sexual turbulence of earlier and later stages is absent.

Erikson described the crises of this stage as industry versus inferiority. If children are motivated by activities that provide a sense of worth, they focus their attention on mastering skills in school, sports, the arts, and social interaction. Approval and recognition for their achievements result in feelings of confidence, competence, and industry. When children feel that they cannot meet the expectations of family or of society, they lose confidence, lack the drive to achieve, and develop feelings of inferiority and incompetence. The challenge of caregivers and teachers is to praise accomplishments and encourage skill development while avoiding criticism in areas in which children fail to excel. Providing successful experiences and positive reinforcement for children increases their opportunities to achieve.

Belonging to groups and being accepted by peers take on a new significance for school-age children. Children form clubs and gather in groups, often implementing strict rules or secret codes. They gradually become less self-centered and selfish as they learn to cooperate as part of a group. With this increased social exposure, children begin to question parental values and ideas. The family, however, remains the major influence on behavior and decisions.

As children enter the late school-age or preadolescent years (10 to 12 or 13 years), the caregiver-child relationship becomes strained as children begin to drift away from the family. Preadolescent children increasingly challenge parental authority and reject family standards as they discover that the family is "not perfect and does not know everything." Identification with a peer group increases, and children form a close relationship with a best friend. Some children begin to show an interest in others of the opposite sex. Preadolescents continue to want and need some restrictions, because their immaturity makes determining their own rules too frightening.

Assessment of School-age Children

The slow, steady growth and changing body proportions of school-age children make them appear thin and gangly. Assessing children's intake of nutrients and calories and reviewing their growth charts reassures parents that their children are not too thin. The nurse can relieve family stress resulting from parents pushing their children to eat by educating parents to evaluate objectively their children's diets during the early school-age years. Older school-age children have an increase in appetite as they enter the prepubertal growth spurt. During the growth spurt, height and weight increase and may normally cross percentiles.

School-age children are eager to talk about their hobbies, friends, school, and accomplishments. Increasing neurologic maturity allows them to master activities requiring gross and fine motor control such as sports, dancing, playing a musical instrument, artistic pursuits, or building things. School-age children enjoy showing off newly acquired skills, and the family displays pride in their children's accomplishments.

School-age children frequently sort and classify collections of rocks, sports cards, dolls, coins, stamps, or almost anything. They are industrious in school, feeling pride in their accomplishments as they master difficult concepts and skills. The family provides positive feedback and encouragement to their children and speaks of their children's successes with pride.

Adult family members and school-age children communicate openly, with adults setting needed limits. Although peer relationships are becoming more important, the family remains the major influence during most of the school-age years. As children approach adolescence, the relationship with family may become strained as the children are drawn closer to peer groups and seek greater independence.

Children who lack hobbies or cannot think of any accomplishments may be environmentally deprived. Caregivers who are unable to think of anything positive to say about their children or who speak of them as a burden likely have a disturbed parent–child relationship. Assessment of school-age children and elderly adults should also include signs of possible abuse, which are discussed more in chapter 6. ∞ Children who lack encouragement and positive reinforcement at home for their achievements are at risk for gang recruitment. Gangs provide the "family" support children lack at home, increasing children's risk for violence, drug use, and illegal activity.

Problems in school may evolve at this time with conflicts over grades and study time. The nurse can encourage the caregiver to help the child set a consistent place and time for homework. Caregivers should also be encouraged to communicate actively with the child's teacher. Teachers, adults, family members, and healthcare providers may identify learning disabilities at this time by careful observation.

Adolescents

Adolescence marks the transition from childhood to adulthood (12 to 19 or 20 years). Although all children undergo this transformation, passing through the stages of growth and development in a predictable sequence, the age and rate at which it occurs are highly variable. In a group of children of the same age, some look and act like children and some look and act like young adults. Adolescence is divided into three phases: early (10 to 13 years), middle (14 to 17 years), and late (17 to 21 years). The search for one's unique self or identity is the foundation of the tasks of this stage. Tasks of this period include the following:

- Searching for identity
- Increasing independence from parents
- Forming close relationships with peers
- Developing analytic thinking
- Forming a value system
- Developing a sexual identity
- Choosing a career

Physiologic Growth and Development

An increase in physical size is a universal event during puberty, with maximum growth occurring prior to the onset of discernible sexual development. Pubertal weight gain accounts for about 50% of an individual's ideal adult body weight. While the percentage of body fat increases in females during puberty, it decreases in adolescent males. Pubertal height growth accounts for 20% to 25% of final adult height. The growth spurt generally begins between the ages of 12 and 14 in girls, and between 12 and 16 in boys, and lasts 24 to 30 months.

Girls experience their fastest rate of growth at about 12 years, gaining 4.6 kg (10 lb) to 10.6 kg (23.5 lb) and growing 5.4 cm (2 in.) to 11.2 cm (4.5 in.). Boys experience their fastest rate of growth at about 14 years, gaining 5.7 kg (12.5 lb) to 13.2 kg (29 lb) and growing 5.8 cm (2.25 in.) to 13.1 cm (5.25 in.).

During puberty, the period of maturation of the reproductive system, primary and secondary sexual characteristics develop in response to endocrine changes. Primary sexual development includes the changes that occur in the organs directly related to reproduction, such as the ovaries, uterus, breasts, penis, and testes. Secondary sexual development includes the changes that occur in other parts of the body in response to hormonal changes, such as development of facial and pubic hair, voice changes, and fat deposits. Some changes such as increased activity in sebaceous and sweat glands occur as early as 9 1/2 years of age in girls and at 10 1/2 years of age in boys. Further information about changes in secondary sex characteristics as well as pertinent prevention measures is included in chapters 22 and 23 of this text. ∞

Brain tissue appears to reach maturity with puberty, and myelinization continues until the middle adult years. Because growth of the cerebrum, cerebellum, and brain stem is essentially complete by the end of the tenth year, the CNS does not experience substantial growth during the pubertal period.

A cardiac growth spurt occurs during the prepubertal growth period, increasing cardiac strength, elevating the blood pressure, and stabilizing the pulse at a lower rate. Cardiac output becomes more dependent on stroke volume than heart rate.

During the growth spurt, rapid growth of the hands and feet occurs first, then growth of the long bones of the arms and legs, followed by trunk growth. Skull and facial bones change proportions as the forehead becomes more prominent and the jawbones develop. The growth rate slows after the onset of the external signs of puberty as ossification slows, and the epiphyseal maturation of the long bones occurs in response to hormonal influences. Since androgen influences bone density, the bones of males become more dense than those of females. Androgen also appears to be directly related to the significant increase in male muscle mass.

Cognitive Development

The period of adolescence corresponds to Piaget's stage of formal operations in which abstract thinking develops. Adolescents develop the ability to integrate past learning and present problems to plan for the future. They learn to use logic and solve problems by methodically analyzing each possibility. They use this new ability in scientific reasoning, and they create hypotheses and test them by setting up experiments. Analytic thinking extends to the adolescent's development of values. No longer content to accept what others say in an unquestioning manner, the adolescent can reason through inconsistencies and consider value options.

Psychosocial Development

According to Freud, sexual urges repressed during latency reawaken as adolescents enter the genital stage. Sexual gratification comes with finding a partner outside of the family.

Erikson described the conflict of adolescence as ego identity versus role confusion. Homogeneous cliques support adolescents through the difficult search for their identity. They become very concerned with their bodies, their appearances, and their abilities,

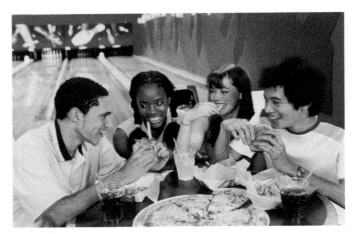

Figure 2.6 Peer group activity of adolescents.
Source: Nancy Ney/Corbis.

avoiding anything that would make them appear different. According to Erikson, the intolerance of others outside the clique displayed by adolescents is a temporary defense against identity confusion.

Adolescents' search for identity is stressful for adolescents and their families. The peer group becomes even more important than during the school-age years, providing a sense of belonging. Peer group participation allows adolescents to develop comfort in social participation (see Figure 2.6 ■). Peer group influence on clothing and hairstyles, beliefs, values, and actions may create tension between adolescents and their families. As personal identity evolves, adolescents begin to plan for a future career and prepare to enter adulthood.

Assessment of Adolescents

Caregivers rarely express concern that their adolescents are not eating. The pubertal growth spurt requires adolescents to increase their caloric intake dramatically, causing parents concern that they eat constantly but never seem full. Adolescents (particularly females) are at risk for developing eating disorders; feelings surrounding changes in the body should be explored.

Adolescents often communicate better with peers and adults outside of the family than with family members. Assessing adolescents with their parents and then one-on-one affords a more complete picture of their relationship and provides adolescents with an opportunity to freely express themselves and discuss concerns.

Adolescents are able to hold an adult conversation and are often happy to discuss school, friends, activities, and plans for the future. They tend to be anxious about their bodies and the rapid changes occurring. Often adolescents are unsure if what is happening to them is normal, and they frequently express somatic complaints.

As adolescents become more independent, adult family members become anxious over their evolving lack of control. Parents may be uncomfortable with adolescents' sexuality; rebellious dress and hairstyles; and developing values, which may differ from those of the parents. Communication between parents and adolescents is often challenging at this stage.

Severely restricting the activities and freedom of adolescents inhibits their ability to progress toward independence. Adolescents who lack social contacts and tend to spend much time alone may be depressed and at high risk for suicide. Acting out and risk-taking behaviors place adolescents at risk for serious injury from accidents or drug or alcohol use. Alliance with gangs places adolescents at risk for violence and participation in illegal activities. See Box 2.1 for a listing of recommended preventive services across the age span.

Young Adults

The **young adult** (20 to 40 years) establishes a new life on a chosen career path and in a lifestyle independent of parents. Tasks of this period include the following:

- Leaving the family home
- Establishing a career or vocation
- Choosing a mate and forming an intimate relationship
- Managing one's own household
- Establishing a social group
- Beginning a parenting role
- Developing a meaningful philosophy of life

Physiologic Development

During young adulthood, the body reaches its maximum potential for growth and development, and all systems function at peak efficiency. Skeletal system growth is completed around 25 years of age with the final fusion of the epiphyses of the long bones. The vertebral column continues to grow until about 30 years, adding perhaps 3 to 5 mm to an individual's height. Adult distribution of red bone marrow is achieved at about 25 years of age. Muscular efficiency reaches its peak performance between 20 and 30 years and declines at a variable rate thereafter.

Cognitive Development

According to Piaget, by young adulthood, cognitive structures have been completed. During the formal operations stage in adolescence, abstract thinking has been achieved. Formal operations characterize thinking throughout adulthood. Young adults continue to develop, however, as egocentrism diminishes and thinking evolves in a more realistic and objective manner.

Psychosocial Development

According to Erikson, the central task of young adults in their early 20s is intimacy versus isolation. During this stage, the young adult forms one or more intimate relationships. A secure self-identity must be established before a mutually satisfying and mature relationship can be formed with another person. The mature relationship requires the ability to establish mutual trust, cooperate with another, share feelings and goals, and completely accept the other person.

Other theorists believe that young adulthood consists of several stages. The 20s are generally accepted as the time of establishing oneself in adult society by choosing a mate, friends, an occupation, values, and a lifestyle. Around the age of 30, life is reassessed and the person either reaffirms past choices or deliberates changes. During the 30s, life again settles down, with the adult striving to build a better life in all aspects. It is a time of financial and emotional investment, and career advancement (see Figure 2.7 ■).

The decision whether to have children usually is made sometime during the young adult years. The addition of children

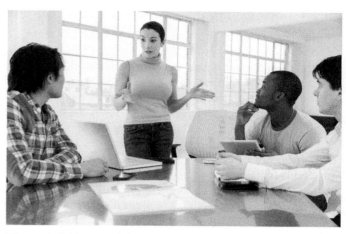

Figure 2.7 Young adults strive to advance their careers.
Source: Igor Emmerich/Corbis.

requires major role adjustment and causes readjustment in a couple's relationship.

Assessment of Young Adults

Young adults are busy, productive, and healthy. At their maximum physical potential, young adults actively pursue sports and physical fitness activities. They refine their creative talents and enjoy activities with peers.

Young adults form an intimate partnership with another in a mature, cooperative relationship. Traditionally, this intimate relationship involved marriage. Increasingly, the relationship is formed and maintained without a formal marriage or between two people of the same sex. Developmentally, the important concept is the formation of the mature, intimate relationship.

People deciding to have children have many more choices than previously: surrogate motherhood, artificial insemination, in vitro fertilization, and other technologic innovations. Deciding not to have children or delaying having children is increasingly accepted, as is the decision of single women to have children.

Young adults have chosen an occupation, established their values, and adopted a lifestyle. Career advancement, financial stability, and emotional investment characterize the young adult years.

The young adult without a steady job may lack direction and self-confidence. Marital discord may trigger feelings of failure and insecurity. Failing to achieve intimacy may place the young adult at risk for depression, alcoholism, or drug abuse. See Box 2.1 for a listing of recommended preventive services across the age span.

Middle-aged Adults

Middle adulthood (40 to 65 years) signals a halfway point, with as many years behind an individual as potentially ahead. This is a time of evaluation and adjustment, and its tasks include the following:

- Accepting and adjusting to physical changes
- Reviewing and redirecting career goals
- Developing hobbies and leisure activities
- Adjusting to aging parents
- Coping with children leaving home

Physiologic Development

Functioning of the CNS during the early years of middle adulthood is normally maintained at the same high level achieved in young adulthood. Some individuals may experience a gradual decline in mental or reflex functioning as age advances past 50 because of changes in enzyme function, hormones, and motor and sensory functions. Decreased CNS integration may result in a slower, more prolonged, and more pronounced response to stressors.

Both men and women experience decreasing hormonal production during middle adulthood. During menopause, which usually occurs between ages 40 and 55, the ovaries decrease in size, and the uterus becomes smaller and firmer. Progesterone is not produced, and estrogen levels fall, resulting in the atrophy of the reproductive organs, vasomotor disturbances, and mood swings. Men experience a gradual decrease in testosterone, causing decreased sperm and semen production and less intense orgasms.

In individuals who become more sedentary over time, the heart begins to lose tone, and rate and rhythm changes become evident. Blood vessels lose elasticity and become thicker. Degeneration of cardiovascular tissues becomes a leading cause of death in individuals over age 45.

Lung tissues become thicker, stiffer, and less elastic with age, resulting in gradually decreased breathing capacity by age 55 or 60. Respiratory rates increase in response to decreasing pulmonary function.

Visual acuity declines, especially for near vision, and auditory acuity for high-frequency sounds decreases. Skin turgor, elasticity, and moisture decrease, resulting in wrinkles. Hair thins, and gray hair appears. Fatty tissue is redistributed in the abdominal area.

Bone mass decreases from age 40 until the end of middle adulthood. Calcium loss from bone tissues becomes pronounced in females. Muscle mass and strength are maintained in individuals who continue active muscle use. In those who lead a sedentary lifestyle, muscles decline in mass, structure, and strength. Muscle loss may also result from changes in collagen fiber, which becomes thicker and less elastic.

Cognitive Development

The middle adult's cognitive and intellectual abilities remain constant, continuing the abilities characteristic in Piaget's stage of formal operations. Memory and problem solving are maintained, and learning continues, often enhanced by increased motivation at this time of life. Life experiences tend to enhance cognitive abilities as the middle adult builds on past experiences.

Psychosocial Development

Erikson defined the developmental task of middle adulthood as generativity versus stagnation. He defined generativity as the concern for establishing and guiding the next generation. People turn from the self- and family-centered focus of young adulthood toward more altruistic activities such as community involvement; charitable work; and political, social, and cultural endeavors. Erikson believed that stagnation results if the need for sharing, giving, and contributing to the growth of others is not met. Stagnation refers to feelings of boredom and emptiness, which lead individuals to become inactive, self-absorbed, self-indulgent, and chronic complainers.

Some theorists believe that the middle adult years begin with a transition during which a major reassessment of life accomplishments occurs. Typically the middle adult asks the question, "What have I done with my life?" People confront reality, accept that they

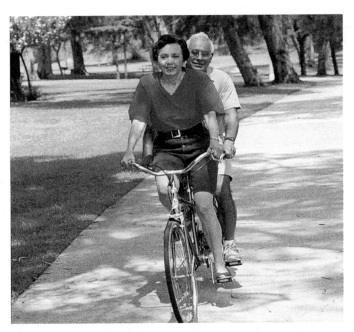

Figure 2.8 Middle adults usually have more time to focus attention on their relationships.
Source: Tony Freeman/PhotoEdit, Inc.

cannot meet some goals, and emerge with redirected goals. Reassessment involves areas of career, personal identity, and family. The middle adult may reorder career goals or choose a new career path. Adjusting in a positive manner to children leaving home helps parents to focus attention on other relationships, find satisfying leisure activities, or pursue intellectual activities (see Figure 2.8 ■). But as the economic and social landscapes change, many children are choosing to stay at home both during and after graduating high school and college. This social change in norms has prompted federal legislation, which now provides health care coverage under their parents insurance for children until they are 26 years old ("Health Insurance Coverage for Children and Young Adults under 26," n.d.). With the average life span of elderly adults increasing, many families are caring for their children and their parents in the same household, thus instigating the term "Sandwich Generation" (DeRigne & Ferrante, 2012). Coping successfully with the death of a parent helps people in middle adulthood come to terms with their own aging and death. Making financial plans and preparing for productive use of leisure time in retirement strengthen effective adaptation to retirement.

Assessment of Middle-aged Adults

The adult in the middle years of life is satisfied with past accomplishments and involved in activities outside the family. Adjusting to the physical changes of aging, individuals develop appropriate leisure activities in preparation for an active retirement. Good financial planning during the middle adult years ensures financial security during retirement.

The middle adult years signal the end of childbearing and, most often, the end of child rearing. Individuals adjust to never having had children or to children leaving home. Couples renew their relationships or sometimes find they have little in common and separate. Some women choose to delay childbearing until their late 30s or early 40s, after establishing their careers. They begin their child-rearing years as many of their peers are completing this phase of life. Older mothers must make the transition from career women to mothers, even if they continue their careers.

The dissatisfied middle adult is unhappy with the past and expresses no hope for the future. Sedentary and isolated, the individual complains about life, avoids involvement, and fails to plan appropriately for retirement.

Older Adults

Individuals in **older adulthood** (65 years and older) vary greatly in their physical and psychosocial adaptation to aging. Developmental tasks of older adults include the following:

- Adjusting to declining physical strength and health
- Forming relationships within one's peer group
- Adjusting to retirement
- Developing postretirement activities that maintain self-worth and usefulness
- Adjusting to the death of spouse, family members, and friends
- Conducting a life review
- Preparing for death

Physiologic Development

During the later years, there is an inevitable decline in body functions. The body becomes less efficient in receiving, processing, and responding to stimuli. The CNS experiences a decrease in electrical activity, resulting in slowed or altered sensory reception and decreases in reaction time and movement.

The cardiovascular system demonstrates degenerative effects in old age. Fatty plaques are deposited in the lining of blood vessels, decreasing their ability to supply blood to tissues. Systolic blood pressure increases as a result of the inelasticity of the arteries and an increase in peripheral resistance. Endocardial thickening and hardening throughout the heart decrease the efficiency of its pumping action. The valves become more rigid and less pliable, leading to reduced filling and emptying abilities. Cardiac output and reserve diminish, resulting in an inability to react to sudden stress efficiently.

Efficiency of the lungs decreases with age, increasing the respiratory effort required to obtain adequate oxygen. Vital capacity decreases, and residual air increases with age. The bronchopulmonary tree becomes more rigid, reducing bronchopulmonary movements. Ciliary activity decreases, allowing mucous secretions to collect more readily in the respiratory tree. As a result of diminished muscle tone and decreased sensitivity to stimuli, the ability to cough decreases.

Visual changes include loss of visual acuity, decreased adaptation to darkness and dim light, loss of peripheral vision, and difficulty in discriminating similar colors. Gradual loss of hearing is the result of changes in nerve tissues in the inner ear and a thickening of the eardrum. The senses of taste and smell decrease, and older adults are less stimulated by food than before. The gradual loss of skin receptors increases the threshold for sensations of pain and touch in the elderly.

Renal function is slowed by structural and functional changes associated with aging. Arteriosclerotic changes can reduce blood

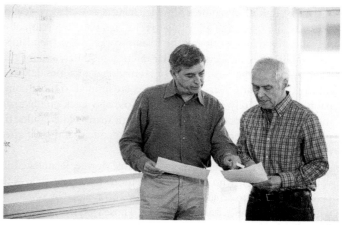

Figure 2.9 The ability to solve problems may be highly efficient in the older adult.
Source: Rana Faure/Corbis.

flow, impairing renal function. The kidney's filtering abilities become impaired as the number of functioning nephrons decreases with age. An enlarged prostate gland causes urinary urgency and frequency in men, and in women the same complaints are often due to weakened muscles supporting the bladder or weakness of the urethral sphincter. The capacity of the bladder and its ability to empty completely diminish with age in both men and women.

All bones are affected by a decrease in skeletal mass. Decreased density causes bones to become brittle and fracture more easily. Range of motion decreases as the tissues of the joints and bones stiffen.

Cognitive Development

Research continues into the effects of aging on cognitive abilities. Different kinds of cognitive functions seem to undergo different types, amounts, and rates of change in individual older adults. Functions dependent on perception rely on the acuity of the senses. When senses become impaired with aging, the ability to perceive the environment and react appropriately is diminished. Changes in the aging nervous system may also affect perceptual ability. Impaired perceptual ability diminishes the aging adult's cognitive capability.

Studies suggest that people who live in a varied environment that provides for continued use of intellectual function are often the ones who maintain or even strengthen these skills throughout life. Conversely, those who live in a static environment that lacks intellectual challenge may be the ones who most likely show some decline in intellectual ability with aging. Although learning and problem solving may not be as efficient in old age as in youth, both processes still occur to a greater extent than is often portrayed in stereotypes of older adults (see Figure 2.9 ■).

Psychosocial Development

The developmental task of late adulthood, according to Erikson, is ego integrity versus self-despair. When a review of life events, experiences, and relationships makes the adult content with life, the person attains ego integrity. Failure to resolve this last developmental crisis results in a sense of despair, resentment, futility, hopelessness, and fear of death.

Late adulthood requires lifestyle changes as well as review of one's past life. The adult adjusting to retirement must develop new activities to replace work and the role of worker. New friendships are established with peers of similar interests, abilities, and means. The person may pursue projects or recreational activities deferred during the working years, but activities are limited to those compatible with the physical limitations of old age. Lack of adequate income limits the activities and lifestyle of many older adults; financial resources enable them to be independent and look after themselves.

The lifestyle of later years is, to a large degree, formulated in youth. The person who was once gregarious and spent time with people continues to do so, and the person who avoided involvement with others continues toward isolation. Those who learned early in life to live well-balanced and fulfilling lives are generally more successful in retirement. The later years can foster a sense of integrity and continuity, or they can be years of despair.

Through the late adult years, the deaths of friends, siblings, and partner occur with increasing frequency. Reminded of the limited time left, the older adult comes to terms with the past and views death as an acceptable completion of life.

Several theories have been developed to explain the psychosocial aspects of aging. Developmental psychologists, including Erikson and Jung, discussed lifespan developmental changes ending in evaluation of life accomplishments or adaptation to change and loss. Sociologic theories address activity, dependence, and social conditions as influential in successful adjustment to age-related changes. Additionally, nursing theories, such as the Functional Consequences Theory (Miller, 1990; Miller, 2009) and the Theory of Thriving (Haight, Barba, Tesh, & Courts, 2002) explore psychosocial aspects of aging to consider in assessment of and provision of care for older adults. Table 2.3 includes an overview of psychosocial and nursing theories of aging.

Assessment of Older Adults

Comprehensive assessment of the older adult must include psychosocial factors. These factors are the ability to function, cognition, lifestyle changes, culture, and spirituality. Grossman and Lange (2006) explored biologic and psychosocial theories of aging. They developed an adult assessment tool that represents a comprehensive approach to assessment. Use of the assessment tool enables the nurse to plan care for older adults in response to the needs of this population

TABLE 2.3 Developmental, Sociologic, and Nursing Theories of Aging

DEVELOPMENTAL THEORIES		
Erikson	Stages of Personality Development	Successful aging requires achievement of the task of ego-integrity versus despair. Life is viewed as satisfying, death as completion of life.
Jung	Theory of Individualism	Successful aging encompasses acceptance of the past and adjustment to loss accompanying functional decline.
Buhler	Lifespan Development Paradigm	Life stages are structured according to roles, connections, values, and goals. Successful aging requires adjustment to changes in roles, relationships, and goals.
SOCIOLOGIC THEORIES		
Havighurst	Activity Theory	Successful adjustment to aging requires the individual to remain physically active and socially involved.
Cummings and Henry	Disengagement Theory	Aging is characterized by mutual withdrawal or disengagement between the aging individual and others in the individual's environment.
Achley	Continuity Theory	In old age the personality is stable. Personality patterns predict responses to the changes of age including health, socioeconomic status, and the activities in which one participates. Differing and varied responses to aging result from individual personality differences.
Riley	Age Stratification Theory	Different responses to aging are a result of varied experiences of different generations. Historic context and life experiences influence beliefs, roles, response to stressors, and perception of health.
NURSING THEORIES		
Haight	Theory of Thriving	Based on the concept of failure to thrive. Thriving or successful aging occurs when harmony exists among the aging individual, the physical environment, and the individual's relationships.
Miller	Functional Consequences Theory	Functioning in aging is impacted by psychobiologic, sociocultural, and environmental factors. The impact of the factors creates changes in the individual and increased risk for functional limitations.

I. Psychological

Developmental Stage Adjustment
- Assess the relationship of chronological age to corresponding developmental tasks.
- Is person a good historian?

Perceive Need Prioritization/Optimization
- Assess person's perceived priority needs.
- Is family in agreement?

Role Relationship
- Identify changes in role with family, community, and other settings significant to patient. May need more time to assess.

II. Sociological

Activity Involvement
- Identify the older adult's typical daily routine. Is there a pattern indicating the person is starting to disengage?
- Does the degree of activity involvement match what the patient desires?
- What limits are imposed by disease?

Personality
- Describe the person's general coping ability.
- Is spirituality aiding coping?
- What pattern has the patient displayed previously in managing stess?

Generation Cohort
- Identify person's work ethic and hardiness or ability to cope with multiple problems.
- What is the person's history of life?
- What is the person's belief about caring for self?
- Is the person motivated to be independent?
- How is the diagnosis perceived?
- How do cohort experiences influence health perceptions and choices?

III. Biological

Normal Aging Changes
- Identify age-related changes from a comprehensive system assessment (sensory, cognitive, physical, functional).
- Are there accelerated or abnormal changes?
- Is communication affected?

Pathophysiological Changes
- Are abnormal changes compensated?
- Is referral for treatment needed? Is the patient's life threatened?
- Is wear and tear responsible? Attempt to determine the etiology of injury/disease.

Genetic Risk Factors
- Assess the family and individual for present and potential manifestations of genetic diseases.
- Are symptoms reflective of genetic mutations?
- Are there wellness/disease patterns emerging within the family?

Impact From Pharmacologic, Surgical, or Other Health Promotion/ Disease Prevention Treatments
- Assess over-the-counter, herbal, and prescribed drugs, alternative therapy use, recent surgeries, and other treatments.
- Assimilate possible interactions and plan for prioritized needs.

Figure 2.10 Adult assessment tool.

to adapt to chronic illness, to maintain independent function, and to promote well-being (see Figure 2.10 ■).

Well-adjusted older adults maintain an active lifestyle and involvement with others and often do not appear their age. Lifestyle changes occur in response to declining physical abilities and retirement. Participation in activities that promote the older adult's sense of self-worth and usefulness also provides opportunities for developing new friendships with others of similar abilities and interests. See Box 2.2 for the Geriatric Depression Scale, which can help nurses assess negative symptomology of the elderly. Intellectual function is maintained through continued intellectual pursuits. Content with their life review, elderly adults enjoy their retirement years and accept death as the inevitable end of a productive life.

The older adult who has not successfully resolved developmental crises may feel that life has been unfair. Despair and hopelessness may be evident in the individual's lack of activity and bitter complaining. Refer to Box 2.1 on page 33 for a listing of recommended preventive services across the age span.

Box 2.2 Geriatric Depression Scale

Choose the best answer for how you have felt over the past week:

1. Are you basically satisfied with your life? YES / **NO**
2. Have you dropped many of your activities and interests? **YES** / NO
3. Do you feel that your life is empty? **YES** / NO
4. Do you often get bored? **YES** / NO
5. Are you in good spirits most of the time? YES / **NO**
6. Are you afraid that something bad is going to happen to you? **YES** / NO
7. Do you feel happy most of the time? YES / **NO**
8. Do you often feel helpless? **YES** / NO
9. Do you prefer to stay at home, rather than going out and doing new things? **YES** / NO
10. Do you feel you have more problems with memory than most? **YES** / NO

11. Do you think it is wonderful to be alive now? YES / **NO**
12. Do you feel pretty worthless the way you are now? **YES** / NO
13. Do you feel full of energy? YES / **NO**
14. Do you feel that your situation is hopeless? **YES** / NO
15. Do you think that most people are better off than you are? **YES** / NO

Answers in **bold** indicate depression. Although differing sensitivities and specificities have been obtained across studies, for clinical purposes a score > 5 points is suggestive of depression and should warrant a follow-up interview. Scores > 10 are almost always depression.

Source: Geriatric Depression Scale. (n.d.). Retrieved from http://web.stanford.edu/~yesavage/GDS.html

Growth and Development in Health Assessment

Health assessment includes gathering objective and subjective data, which are used to develop plans to maintain health or address health needs in patients of all ages. A comprehensive assessment includes data about physical, cognitive, and emotional growth and development. When conducting health assessments, the professional nurse must be able to obtain accurate data and interpret findings in relation to expectations and predicted norms and ranges for patients at various stages of physical and emotional development. Knowledge of anatomic and physiologic changes as well as theoretic information about cognitive, psychoanalytic, and psychosocial events and expectations at each stage of human development are invaluable resources for the nurse.

Physical growth and development change across the age span. Stages from infancy through adolescence are marked by spurts of rapid growth and development. Health assessment includes the use of clinical growth charts to index individual patient measurements of height and weight (and head circumference in infants) as expected normal values for age and gender. Additional indicators for normal growth and development throughout these stages are eating, sleeping, elimination, and activity patterns. Neurologic and sensory functions are assessed by monitoring development of speech and language, muscular growth, strength and coordination, and tactile sensibility.

Puberty is a period of rapid physiologic growth and development. It occurs between the ages of 10 and 14 years in females and is marked by menarche, breast development, presence of pubic hair, and a spurt in height. In males, puberty occurs between the ages of 12 and 16 years and is characterized by a spurt in height, development of the penis and testicles, and presence of pubic hair. Young adulthood is the stage marked by completed growth in physical and mental structures. Physical development continues to be assessed by comparing individual findings to clinical growth charts and by assessing eating, sleeping, and activity patterns.

Middle age, occurring between the ages of 45 and 60 years, is another period in which dramatic changes in physical development occur. Primary changes are related to hormonal changes of the male and female climacteric. In addition, changes occur in all systems and include decreases in basal metabolic rate, muscle size, nerve conduction, lung capacity, glomerular filtration, and cardiac output. There are increased adipose tissue deposit; skeletal changes leading to decreases in height; and changes in tactile sensibility, vision, and hearing. The physical changes continue into the stage of older adulthood. The middle and older adult is at risk for obesity and health problems associated with it. Therefore, health assessment will include use of the body mass index (BMI) to assess weight and risk for disease. Information about calculation of BMI is included in chapter 12 of this text. ∞ In addition, assessment will include checking the ability to carry out activities of daily living (ADLs), and regular testing of vision and hearing.

In addition to expectations about physical growth and development, there are also expectations about cognitive, psychosocial, and emotional development across the age span. For example, attachment is an essential element in infant development. Attachment refers to the tie between the infant and caregivers that promotes physical and psychosocial well-being. Assessment of attachment includes observation of interactions between the infant and caregivers for eye contact, apparent interest in the child, talking or cooing to the child, response to infant needs, and so on. Children are expected to develop language and cognitive abilities that enable them to learn and over time become independent beings. Young adults are expected to develop relationships with others and to become productive members of society. Maturity and aging lead individuals to contribute to the well-being of communities and their families and often to adapt to change and loss. Developmental milestones and crises occur in all stages of development and must be assessed. A variety of instruments and scales can be used to identify developmental delays, behavioral patterns, and responses that indicate potential or actual problems with emotional, cognitive, and psychosocial development and adaptation in children and adults of all ages. Table 2.4 includes a list and description

TABLE 2.4	Instruments to Measure Growth and Development
Ages & Stages Questionnaire	This parent-completed questionnaire covers developmental areas of communication, gross motor, fine motor, problem solving, and personal-social.[1]
Battelle Developmental Inventory	This tests developmental domains of cognition, motor, adaptive, communication, and personal-social skills in children from 21–90 months.[1]
Brigance Screen	This assesses academics/pre-academics; expressive language; receptive language; social-emotional skills; and gross motor, fine motor, and self-help skills. Used from birth through 1st grade.[1]
Eyberg Child Behavior Inventory	The ECBI is a 5-minute parent report behavioral screening test for conduct aggression and attention in children ages 2.5 to 4 years.[1]
Family Psychosocial Screening	A clinic intake form identifies parent risk factors for child behavior problems, including parent history of physical abuse as a child, parent substance abuse, and maternal depression.[1]
Hassles and Uplifts Scale	This measures adult attitudes about daily situations defined as "hassles" and "uplifts." It focuses on evaluation of positive and negative events in daily life rather than on life events.[3]
Life Experiences Survey	This self-administered questionnaire reviews life-changing events of a given year. Ratings are used to evaluate the level of stress one is experiencing.[4]
McCarthy Scales of Children's Ability	The McCarthy scale evaluates the general intelligence level of children ages 2.5 to 8.5. The scale identifies strengths and weaknesses in cognitive ability and gross and fine motor skills.[1]
Neonatal Behavioral Assessment Scale	This scale is used to assess newborns and infants up to 2 months of age. It measures 28 behavioral and 18 reflex items. It provides information about the baby's strengths, adaptive responses, and potential vulnerabilities.[5]
Pediatric Symptom Checklist	This checklist of short statements identifies conduct behaviors and behaviors associated with depression, anxiety, and adjustment in children from 4 to 16 years of age. Item patterns determine the need for behavioral or mental health referrals.[1]
Stanford-Binet Intelligence Scale	This test measures general intelligence. The areas of verbal reasoning, quantitative reasoning, abstract/visual reasoning, and short-term memory can be tested from age 2 to 23 years.[1]
The Child Development Inventory	This scale measures social, self-help, gross motor, fine motor, expressive language, language comprehension, letters, numbers, and general development in children from 15 months to 6 years of age.[1]
Denver II	This screening is administered to well children between birth and 6 years of age. The Denver II is designed to test 20 simple tasks and items in four sectors: personal-social, fine motor–adaptive, language, and gross motor.[1]
The Mini-Mental Status Examination (MMSE)	This brief, quantitative measure of cognitive status in adults can be used to screen for cognitive impairment, to estimate the severity of cognitive impairment at a given point in time, to follow the course of cognitive changes in an individual over time, and to document an individual's response to treatment.[2]
Wechsler Preschool and Primary Scale of Intelligence—Revised (WPPSI-R)	This is a standardized test of language and perception for children ages 3 to 7.

[1.] (Moses, "Pediatrics," 2014)
[2.] (Moses, "Mini-mental," 2014)
[3.] (Kanner, Coyne, Schaefer, & Lazarus, 1981)
[4.] (Sarasson, Johnson, & Seigel, 1978)
[5.] ("Understanding the baby's language," 2013)

of some of the instruments available to measure aspects of growth and development.

Factors That Influence Growth and Development

Factors that influence growth and development include nutrition, family, culture, race, and socioeconomic status. The following discussion provides examples of ways in which these factors impact growth and development.

Nutrition

Nutrition is essential to physical and mental development. Growth patterns, in large part, are genetically determined. However, malnutrition can delay or prevent growth and development. Healthcare professionals routinely use measures of height and weight in comparison to clinical growth charts to identify slowed growth in children. Slowed growth is an early indicator of inadequate nutrition. The body is made up of water, fat, protein, and minerals, and nutritional intake determines the amounts of each of these essential components. Alteration in one or more of the components affects development and health. Balanced nutrition promotes brain development in children and has been reported to prevent some forms of dementia in older adults. Further discussion of these concepts is included in chapter 12 of this text. ∞

Family

Family refers to a social system made up of two or more individuals living together, who are related by blood, marriage, or agreement. Families today may be identified as nuclear families, extended families, same-sex families, single-parent families, stepfamilies, or single-state families. Families share bonds of affection or love, loyalty, commitment of an emotional or financial nature, continuity, and common shared values and rituals. Families help members to develop physically and emotionally by providing for the economic and safety needs of one another. Included in safety needs would be provision of appropriate nutrition to foster physical growth and development as well as objects, interactions, and activities that promote cognitive and emotional well-being. Family members provide support for each other during physical and emotional crises, and serve as models for social interaction, all of which impact individual members as they move through the stages of development from infancy to old age.

Culture

Growth and development are influenced by cultural factors. For example, perceptions of family roles, in particular those in child rearing, differ among cultures. Attachment is considered an essential element in psychosocial development. Among Caucasian parents the trend is to have both paternal and maternal attachment occur early in the neonatal period. This differs among cultures. For example, among Latin Americans, the extended family, including older siblings, is employed for childcare. This increases the number of attachments by the child while decreasing each family member's influence on the child. European Americans adhere to a more nuclear model in rearing infants, thus decreasing the number of attachments, but increasing each family member's influence on the child (Sherry, Adelman, Farwell, & Linton, 2013). Culture influences the training and discipline of children; the value placed on developing cognitive skills; social interactions outside of the home that promote development; and attitudes toward change, including illness and aging. In addition, for immigrants to the United States,

language differences may impact their ability to communicate, to form social bonds outside of the cultural community, and to identify and utilize resources that foster development and provide support for individuals and families experiencing developmental and situational crises.

Differences in measures of growth and development have been noted between and among various ethnic groups. For example, newborn infants of African American, Indian, and Asian American populations have been reported to have lower birth weights than Caucasians. Females are generally smaller than males in all ethnic groups. Differences in weight, length, and head circumference have been noted in Mexican American and Caucasian children at 48 to 56 weeks of age. Mexican American children have shorter stature and greater weight than Caucasian children, while head circumference has been found to be greater in Caucasian children. In other reports, African American toddlers were found to have increased motor skills and earlier walking than did Caucasian toddlers.

Socioeconomic Status

Socioeconomic status is a major influence on growth and development. Overall, school-age children of low socioeconomic status have been found to have lower height and weight than those in other economic groups. Poverty impacts the ability to meet nutritional needs at all stages of development and increases exposure to environmental elements that influence health status and physical well-being. Socioeconomic status influences values and role expectations and behaviors regarding marriage; family; and gender responsibilities in parenting, education, and occupation. Income, values, and role expectations impact physical and psychosocial development across the age span. Further information about culture and psychosocial development is included in chapters 4 and 5 of this text. ∞

Planning care for individuals is dependent upon comprehensive health assessment of health status and all of the factors that impact health. Accurate interpretation of data requires one to use knowledge and resources in formulating judgments about findings. The previous discussion provided information about measures that assist in health assessment of physical and psychosocial growth and development across the life span. The U.S. Preventive Services Task Force has developed guidelines for health examination and recommendations for preventive strategies. These are available through the National Library of Medicine.

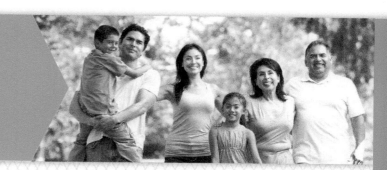

Application Through Critical Thinking

▶ Case Study

Casey is a 2-year-old girl whose mother brought her in for a checkup. Her mother reports that Casey was born at 40 weeks' gestation after an uncomplicated pregnancy and vaginal delivery. She is pretty sure that Casey has met each developmental milestone at the normal age and does not have any problems that she has identified. Casey has no history of medical problems or diseases other than an occasional "cold" and her immunizations are up-to-date. Casey is a very energetic child and is often running around in the back yard and loves to play in the sandbox and with their dog Max. The mother states that she is very careful with what she feeds her family and that Casey has good eating habits although sometimes she throws her food at the dog and laughs. Casey's parents have some good friends whose youngest child is being carefully followed by his pediatrician because of what is thought to be "significant developmental delays." Consequently, Casey's mother is very concerned about developmental milestones and wants her daughter "checked to make sure everything is all right." The mother states that she has read a lot of information on the Internet on child development but asks many questions regarding the care and needs of her child. Mom seems very anxious during the visit and very concerned that she may have missed something in Casey's development.

▶ Critical Thinking Questions

1. What are the expectations regarding the physical development for a 2-year-old child such as Casey?

2. What level of language development is expected for a toddler?

3. Identify at least two standardized tools that are used to assess physical and psychosocial development across the age span.

4. What are the expectations for cognitive development for a 2-year-old child?

5. How might you validate mom's assessment that Casey has good eating habits?

▶ References

Adolescent and school health. (2013, December 24). *Centers for Disease Control and Prevention*. Retrieved February 21, 2014, from http://www.cdc.gov/HealthyYouth

Anthony, D. (Ed.). (2011). Adolescence: An age of opportunity. *The state of the world's children 2011. United Nations Children's Fund (UNICEF)*. Retrieved February 21, 2014, from http://www.unicef.org/sowc2011/pdfs/SOWC-2011-Main-Report_EN_02092011.pdf

Berman, A.J., & Snyder, S. (2011). *Kozier and Erb's fundamentals of nursing: Concepts, process and practices* (9th ed.). Upper Saddle River, NJ: Prentice Hall.

Body mass index table 1. (2014). *National Heart, Lung, and Blood Institute*. Retrieved February 21, 2014, from https://www.nhlbi.nih.gov/guidelines/obesity/bmitbl.htm

Bretherton, I. (1992). The origins of attachment theory: John Bowlby and Mary Ainsworth, *Developmental Psychology, 28*, 759–775.

Centers for Disease Control and Prevention (CDC). (2014). *About BMI for children and teens*. Retrieved from http://www.cdc.gov/healthyweight/assessing/bmi/childrens_bmi/about_childrens_bmi.html

DeRigne, L., & Ferrante, S. (2012). The sandwich generation: A review of the literature. *Florida Public Health Review, 9*, 95–104. Retrieved from http://health.usf.edu/publichealth/fphr/index.htm

Family practice notebook. (2014). Retrieved from http://www.fpnotebook.com/Peds/Neuro/index.htm

Grossman, S., & Lange, J. (2006). Theories of aging as basis for assessment. *Medsurg Nursing, 15*(2), 77–83.

Growth charts. (2010, September 9). *Centers for Disease Control and Prevention*. Retrieved from http://www.cdc.gov/growthcharts

Haight, B. K., Barba, B. E., Tesh, A. S., & Courts, N. F. (2002). Thriving: A life span theory. *Journal of Gerontological Nursing, 28*(3), 14–22.

Health insurance coverage for children and young adults under 26. (n.d.). Retrieved from https://www.healthcare.gov/can-i-keep-my-child-on-my-insurance-until-age-26/

Kanner, A. D., Coyne, J. C., Schaefer, C., & Lazarus, R. S. (1981). Comparison of two modes of stress measurement: Daily hassles and uplifts versus major life events. *Journal of Behavioral Medicine, 4*(1), 1–39.

Liu, W. M. (2013). The Impact of social class on parenting and attachment. In *The Oxford handbook of social class in counseling* (p. 284). New York, NY: Oxford University Press.

Lutz, C. A., & Prztulski, K.R. (2010). *Nutrition and diet therapy: Evidence-based applications* (4th ed.). Philadelphia: F.A. Davis.

Miller, C. A. (1990). *Nursing care of older adults: Theory and practice* (3rd ed.). Glenview, IL: Scott/Forsman/Little Brown Higher Education.

Miller, C. A. (2009). *Nursing for wellness in older adults* (6th ed.). Philadelphia, PA: Wolters Kluwer Health.

Moses, S. (2014, February 16). Mini-mental state exam. *Family Practice Notebook.* Retrieved from http://www.fpnotebook.com/Neuro/Exam/MnMntlStExm.htm

Moses, S. (2014, February 16). Pediatrics: Neurology chapter. *Family Practice Notebook.* Retrieved from http://www.fpnotebook.com/Peds/Neuro/index.htm

Murray, R. B., Zentner, J. P., and Yakimo, R. (2009). *Health promotion strategie, through the life span* (8th ed.). Upper Saddle River, NJ: Prentice Hall.

National adolescent and young adult health information center. (2012). Retrieved from http://nahic.ucsf.edu/

Ogden, C. L., Carroll, M. D., Kit, B. K., & Flegal, K. M. (2012). Prevalence of obesity in the United States, 2009–2010. *NCHS Data Brief, No. 82.* Hyattsville, MD: National Center for Health Statistics.

Ogden, C. L., Flegal, K. M., Carroll, M. D., & Johnson, C. L. (2002). Prevalence and trends in overweight among US children and adolescents, 1999–2000. *Journal of the American Medical Association, 288,* 1728–1732.

Purnell, L. D. (2008). *Transcultural health care: A culturally competent approach* (4rd ed.). Philadelphia: F.A. Davis.

Sarasson, I. G., Johnson, J. H., & Seigel, J. M. (1978). Assessing the impact of life changes: Development of the life experiences survey. *Journal of Consulting and Clinical Psychology, 46*(5), 932–946.

Sherry, A., Adelman, A., Farwell, L., & Linton, B. (2013). The impact of social class on parenting and attachment. In W. M. Liu (Ed.), *The Oxford handbook of social class in counseling* (p. 284). New York, NY: Oxford University Press.

Understanding the baby's language. (2013). *The Brazleton Institute.* Retrieved from http://www.brazelton-institute.com/intro.html

Valdivia, R. (1999). The implications of culture on developmental delay. *The ERIC Clearinghouse on Disabilities and Gifted Children.* Retrieved February 21, 2014, from http://www.ericdigests.org/2000-4/delay.htm

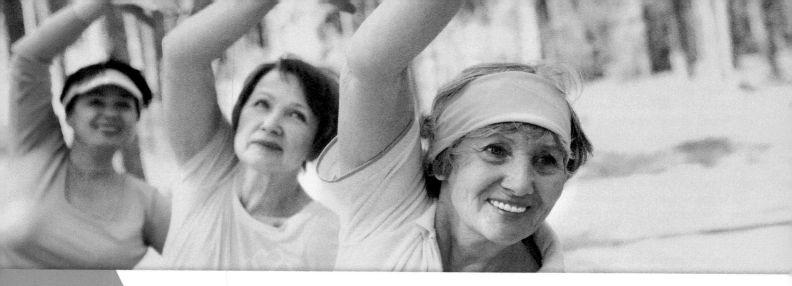

Wellness and Health Promotion

▶ Learning Outcomes

Upon completion of this chapter, you will be able to:

1. Distinguish between concepts of wellness and health promotion.

2. Compare and contrast selected theories of wellness.

3. Relate perspectives of health promotion to the individual, family, and community.

4. Apply the goals and objectives for each topic area in *Healthy People 2020* to nursing practice.

5. Demonstrate how to use the nursing process to encourage health promotion.

Key Terms

aerobic exercise, 63
anaerobic exercise, 63
health promotion, 49
Healthy People 2020, 54
primary prevention, 48
secondary prevention, 48
tertiary prevention, 48
wellness, 48

In the modern world, wellness, health promotion, and health maintenance have become concerns to all. The patient, the consumer of health care, is more active in the decision-making process related to healthcare issues. The patient now has more control regarding the planning, implementation, and evaluation of strategies and outcomes of his or her health. As the healthcare delivery system has changed and become more complex, the roles of the healthcare providers, including the nurse, have expanded.

Individuals are currently more conscious of health and wellness. People have become more proactive regarding health and healthcare practices. This places a stronger emphasis on wellness, health promotion, and disease prevention. The *Healthy People 2020* agenda describes factors that influence individual and community health and wellness. The goals, topic areas, and objectives of this important initiative that are related to wellness and health promotion are discussed in this chapter. Factors influencing health, identified in *Healthy People 2020*, are described in unit I of this text. ∞ Strategies that have been developed to promote wellness are then described and discussed in relation to health assessment in unit III. ∞

Wellness

Wellness describes a state of life that is balanced, personally satisfying, and characterized by the ability to adapt and to participate in activities that enhance quality of life. Concepts basic to wellness include self-responsibility and decision making regarding nutrition, physical fitness, stress management, emotional growth and well-being, personal safety, and health care.

Wellness Theories

Perceptions of wellness influence the nurse's approach to patient care. When using a wellness perspective, the nurse focuses on the patient's personal strengths and abilities to enhance health. The goals of nursing care are to assist the patient to participate in health-promoting activities, prevent illness, and seek help for needs and problems. Additionally, the nurse focuses on the wellness concerns of the patient and supports the patient's spiritual and end-of-life needs. Theories regarding wellness have been developed and can assist nurses to clarify their perceptions of wellness. The theories of Dunn; Leavell and Clark; and Hattie, Myers, and Sweeney are presented in the following section.

Dunn

Dunn defined wellness for the individual as an integrated method of functioning that is oriented toward maximizing the potential of which the individual is capable. It requires the individual to maintain a continuum of balance and purposeful direction within the environment where he or she is functioning (Dunn, 1973). This theory is seen as a grid with two intersecting axes. Health intersects with environment, creating four quadrants (see Figure 3.1 ■). The health axis extends from peak wellness to death, creating various degrees of health and illness. The environmental axis moves from a very favorable environment to a very unfavorable environment. This model takes into consideration the uniqueness of the individual and the influence of family and community regarding healthcare practices.

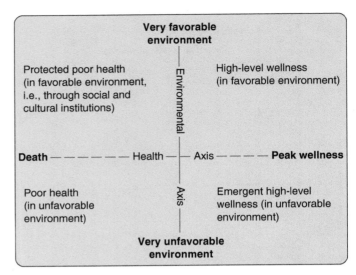

Figure 3.1 Dunn's model of wellness.

Leavell and Clark

Leavell and Clark (1965) described primary, secondary, and tertiary levels of prevention in the healthcare system. In their model, actions are taken to maintain health, prevent illness, provide early detection of a disease, and restore the individual to the highest level of optimum functioning (see Figure 3.2 ■). The key word to emphasize as the focus of primary prevention is *prepathogenic*, that is, before the development of disease or pathology. Actions are taken to prevent disease, illness, or injury. **Primary prevention** implies health and a high level of wellness for the individual. Immunizations, a healthy diet, health teaching, genetic counseling, and the correct use of safety equipment at work are examples of primary prevention strategies.

Early diagnosis of health problems, and prompt treatment with the restoration of health, is the focus of **secondary prevention.** Emphasis is on resolving health problems and preventing serious consequences. Screenings, blood tests, x-rays, surgery, and dental care are strategies utilized at this level of prevention.

Tertiary prevention is activity aimed to restore the individual to the highest possible level of health and functioning. Rehabilitation is the focus for tertiary prevention. Strategies include use of rehabilitation centers for orthopedic and neurologic problems. Teaching the patient and family members interventions to improve coping with a chronic illness and recognition of complications are examples of tertiary prevention strategies. Table 3.1 provides examples of nursing considerations in relation to the levels of prevention.

Hattie, Myers, and Sweeney

According to Hattie, Myers, and Sweeney (2004), a holistic model of wellness and prevention incorporates an awareness of the many

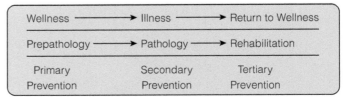

Figure 3.2 Levels of prevention.

TABLE 3.1	Levels of Prevention	
LEVEL OF PREVENTION	**FOCUS**	**EXAMPLES**
Primary	Improving overall health	Education about diet, exercise, environmental hazards, accident protection
	Health promotion	Immunization
	Prevention of illness, injury	Assessment of risks for injury, illness
Secondary	Early identification of illness	Health screening and diagnostic procedures
		Promotion of regular healthcare examinations across the life span
	Treatment for existing health problems	Regimens for treatment of illness
Tertiary	Return to optimum level of wellness after an illness or injury has occurred	Education to reduce or prevent complications of disease
	Prevention of recurrence of problems	Referral to rehabilitation services

factors that influence individuals, including global events, family and community, religion, media and the government, education, and business. These outside forces are viewed through the lens of five life tasks, including work and leisure, friendship, love, self-direction, and spirituality. The life task of self-direction is influenced by personal choices about nutrition, exercise, self-care, stress management, gender identity, cultural identity, sense of worth, sense of control, realistic beliefs, emotional awareness and coping, problem solving and creativity, and sense of humor. These tasks must be in balance for individuals to attain wellness (Hattie et al., 2004).

Health Promotion

Health promotion refers to those actions used to increase health or well-being and the improvement of the health of individuals, families, and communities. Health promotion includes the prevention of disease and primary prevention measures, such as immunization.

Definition

Pender, Murdaugh, and Parsons (2011) define **health promotion** as "behavior motivated by the desire to increase well-being and actualize human health potential" (p. 5). Examples of health promotion activities include but are not limited to weight-control measures, exercise, management of stress, and coping with life experiences.

Perspectives on Health Promotion

An individual's health status or level of wellness is determined by risk factors, physical fitness, nutrition, health behaviors, and lifestyle. Certain risk factors cannot be controlled and these include age, genetic factors, biologic characteristics, and family history. Individual health promotion includes the identification of lifestyle and environmental risks that influence the level of wellness as well as promoting efforts to reduce or eliminate those risks.

A variety of models have been developed to explain health promotion behaviors. These models assist in understanding individual health behaviors and in guiding interventions. They can also be used in research related to health promotion. These models include but are not limited to the health belief model, the theory of reasoned action/planned behavior, and the health promotion model.

Health Belief Model

The health belief model (Rosenstock, 1974) was developed to predict who would participate in health screenings or obtain vaccinations (see Figure 3.3 ■). According to the health belief model, the following individual perceptions influence the decision to act to prevent illness:

- One is vulnerable to an illness.
- The effects of the illness are serious.
- The behavior prevents the illness.
- The benefit of reducing a risk is greater than the cost of the preventive behavior.

Mediating variables influence individual perceptions. The first of the variables is perceived susceptibility, that is, the belief about the likelihood of developing an illness. Perceived severity is the second variable and refers to the individual's determination of how serious an illness would be. The severity includes the physical, psychological, and social effects of illness. Another variable is the perceived cost of the health-promoting behavior. This refers to factors that interfere with the performance of a behavior. The individual must weigh the physical and psychological costs versus the benefit.

The health belief model includes two constructs. These are cues to action and self-efficacy. Cues to action are internal and external stimuli that affect the individual's motivation to participate in health-promoting activities. For example, heart disease in a family member or the Great American Smokeout, a mass media campaign by the American Cancer Society, may motivate one to stop smoking. Self-efficacy refers to the level of confidence an individual has about the ability to perform the activity.

Last, mediating factors affect the health-promoting behaviors by influencing the perceptions of vulnerability, severity, effectiveness, and cost. Mediating factors include age, gender, ethnicity, education, and economic status.

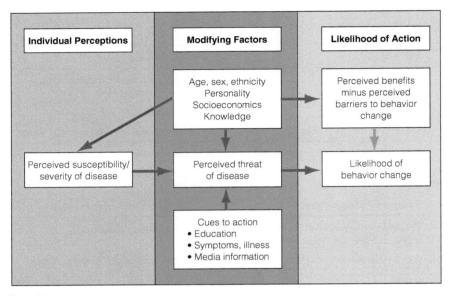

Figure 3.3 Health belief model.

Theory of Reasoned Action/Planned Behavior

The theory of reasoned action/planned behavior is a prediction theory representing a sociopsychologic method for predicting health behavior (see Figure 3.4 ■). The theory of reasoned action/planned behavior is based on the assumptions that behavior is under volitional control and that people are rational beings. The theory holds that the intention to perform a behavior is a determinant in performance of the behavior.

Three variables affect the intention to perform a behavior: subjective norms, attitudes, and self-efficacy. *Subjective norms* refer to the individual's perception of what significant others believe or expect in relation to the individual's performance of a behavior. For example, whether one intends to begin a daily exercise program would be influenced by what one believes a spouse's opinion of the activity would be. *Attitudes* refer to value ascribed to a behavior. An attitude may be that eating a low-fat diet is a good way to prevent heart disease. *Self-efficacy* refers to the level of confidence in one's ability to perform a behavior (for example, feeling confident that a low-fat diet can be followed). According to the theory of reasoned action/planned behavior, an individual is likely to engage in health-promoting behavior when the individual believes that the benefit outweighs the cost.

Health Promotion Model

The health promotion model (Pender et al., 2011) is a competence model. This model describes "the multidimensional nature of persons interacting with their interpersonal and physical environments

as they pursue health" (p. 44). Along with emphasizing individual characteristics and behaviors, the health promotion model focuses on variables that impact motivation and behavioral outcomes (see Figure 3.5 ■). The health promotion model provides a framework through which nurses can develop strategies to assist individuals to engage in health-promoting activities. Each aspect of the model is discussed in the following sections of this chapter.

INDIVIDUAL CHARACTERISTICS AND BEHAVIORS According to the health promotion model, prior related behaviors and personal factors have an effect on future behaviors. Prior related behaviors include knowledge, skill, and experience with health-promoting activities. Prior behavior can have a positive or negative effect on health promotion. When one has engaged in health promotion and recognized the benefit, it is likely that health-promoting behavior will occur in the future. Conversely, when health-promoting activities have been difficult or when barriers to participation arose, one is less likely to participate in health promotion in the future.

Personal factors that can influence behavior are biologic, psychologic, and sociologic. Biologic factors include age, gender, body mass index, strength, agility, and balance. Psychologic factors refer to self-esteem, motivation, and perceptions of one's health status. Socioeconomic status, education, race, and ethnicity are among the sociologic factors considered within the health promotion model.

BEHAVIOR-SPECIFIC COGNITION AND AFFECT Behavior-specific cognition and affect are variables that impact motivation to begin and continue activities to promote health. These variables

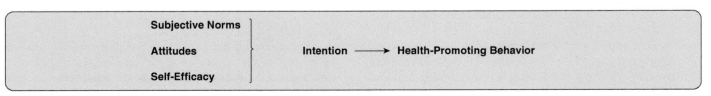

Figure 3.4 Theory of reasoned action/planned behavior.

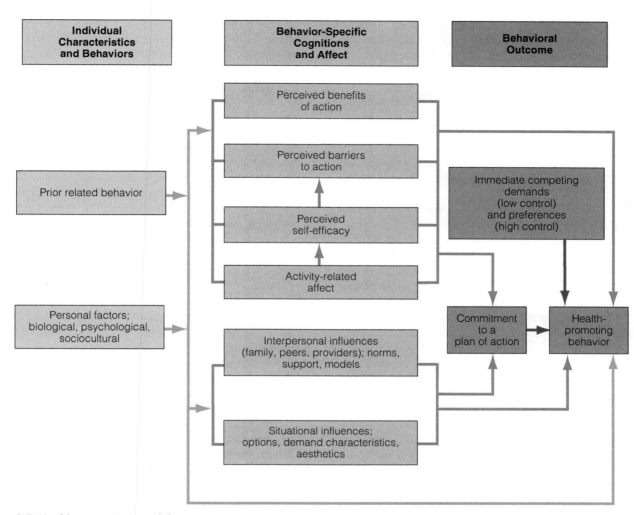

Figure 3.5 Health promotion model.

include perceived benefit of action, perceived barriers to action, perceived self-efficacy, activity-related affect, interpersonal influences, and situational influences. Each of these variables is described in the following sections with appropriate examples.

PERCEIVED BENEFITS OF ACTION Engagement in a particular behavior is determined by the belief that the behavior is beneficial or results in a positive outcome. Benefits may be intrinsic, such as stress reduction, or extrinsic, such as financial reward. Perceived benefits of actions motivate the individual to participate in health-promoting activities.

PERCEIVED BARRIERS TO ACTION Barriers to participation in health-promoting activities may be real or imagined. The barriers include perceptions about the availability, expense, convenience, difficulty, and time required for an activity. Barriers are seen as hurdles and personal costs of participating in a behavior.

PERCEIVED SELF-EFFICACY Perceived self-efficacy is a judgment of one's ability to successfully participate in a health-promoting activity to achieve a desired outcome. Individuals with high self-efficacy are more likely to overcome barriers and commit to health-promoting activity. Those with low self-efficacy have diminished efforts or cease participation in activities.

ACTIVITY-RELATED AFFECT Activity-related affect refers to subjective feelings before, during, and after an activity. The positive or negative feelings influence whether a behavior will be repeated or avoided.

INTERPERSONAL INFLUENCES Interpersonal influences are the individual's perceptions of the behaviors, beliefs, or attitudes of others. The family, peers, and health professionals are interpersonal influences on health-promoting behaviors. These influences also include expectations of others, social support, and modeling the behaviors of others.

SITUATIONAL INFLUENCES Situational influences include perceptions and ideas about situations or contexts. Situational influences on health-promoting activities include perceptions of available options, demand characteristics, and aesthetics of an environment. Access to a cafeteria offering healthy foods at work or having a gym nearby are examples of available options that promote health. Demand characteristics include policies and procedures in employment and public environments. No-smoking policies in public buildings and work environments are demand characteristics that promote health. Aesthetics refers to the physical and interpersonal characteristics of environments. Environments that are safe and interesting and that promote comfort and acceptance versus alienation are factors that facilitate health promotion.

Situational influences may be direct or indirect. For example, the requirement to wear protective eyewear and gloves in a microbiology laboratory creates a direct demand characteristic; that is, employees must comply with the regulation.

COMMITMENT TO A PLAN OF ACTION Commitment to a plan of action includes two components: The first component is commitment to carry out a specific activity. The second component is identification of strategies for carrying out and reinforcing the activity. Commitment without strategies often leads to "good intentions" but results in failure to actually carry out the activity.

IMMEDIATE COMPETING DEMANDS AND PREFERENCES Competing demands are alternative activities over which the individual has little control. These demands include family or work responsibilities. Neglect of competing demands may have a more negative impact on health than nonparticipation in a planned health-promoting activity. Competing preferences are alternative behaviors over which the individual has high control. The control is dependent on the ability to self-regulate. Choosing to have lunch with a friend at the health club rather than participating in the aerobics class is an example of choosing the competing preference over the health-promoting activity. Unless an individual can recognize, address, or overcome competing demands and preferences, a plan for health promotion may unravel.

BEHAVIORAL OUTCOMES Health-promoting behavior is the expected outcome in the health promotion model. Health-promoting behaviors can lead to improved health, better functional ability, and improved quality of life across the age span. An example of application of each of the models is presented in Figures 3.6 ■, 3.7 ■, and 3.8 ■. The information is derived from the following case study.

Mrs. Lucia Alvarado is a 34-year-old Hispanic American. She has been a heavy smoker for the past 21 years. Both of her parents and two of her siblings also have a history of smoking. Her father died at age 57 from lung cancer, her mother was recently diagnosed

with early stage lung cancer, her older sister suffers from asthma, and her younger brother often struggles with shortness of breath. Mrs. Alvarado is married and the mother of a 13-year-old boy and a 5-year-old girl. She is currently pregnant with her third child. She was able to quit smoking while she was pregnant with her first two children and plans to do the same during her current pregnancy. However, after her second pregnancy, she started smoking again. Mrs. Alvarado works as an hourly employee at a local hotel, and she often has a hard time catching her breath during repeated bending, lifting, and walking. Mrs. Alvarado realizes that her smoking habit can create physical, emotional, family, and economic problems. She frequently sees anti-smoking commercials on TV, and she knows the dangers of smoking during pregnancy, the effects of secondhand smoke on her children's health, and the reality that her children are likely to smoke if they see her smoking. She wants to use her pregnancy as a stimulus to quit smoking for good. Mrs. Alvarado will start a smoking cessation program with the support of her physician and family.

As stated earlier, the models for health promotion guide intervention. Nurses promote positive health-promoting behaviors by emphasizing the benefits of the behaviors, assisting the patient to overcome barriers, and providing positive feedback for success. Personal factors influence health behaviors. Some of the factors such as age, gender, and family history cannot be changed. Nursing interventions will generally focus on factors that can be modified. However, it is also important to develop interventions to address factors that cannot be changed. For example, a patient with a family history of colon cancer may avoid screening programs because of fear or a belief that the development of colon cancer is inevitable. Nurses can provide support for these patients and emphasize the importance of early detection in improved outcomes in colon cancer.

Health assessment and screening provides a rich database from which the nurse can assist the patient, family, or community to identify the current health status, risks for illness or injury, strengths and weaknesses, and resources required to begin or continue appropriate

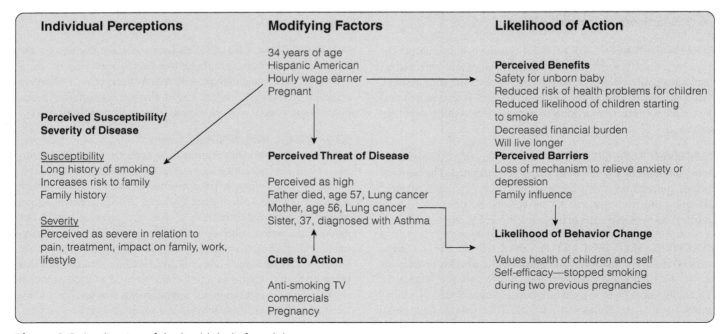

Figure 3.6 Application of the health belief model.

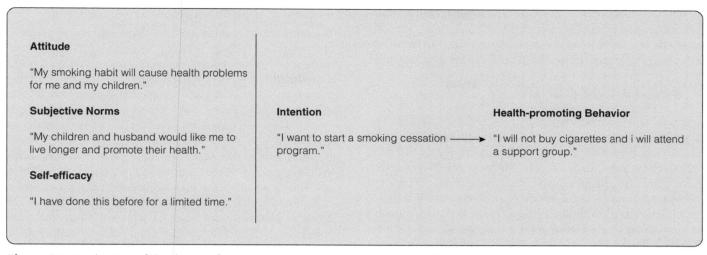

Figure 3.7 Application of the theory of reasoned actions/planned behavior model.

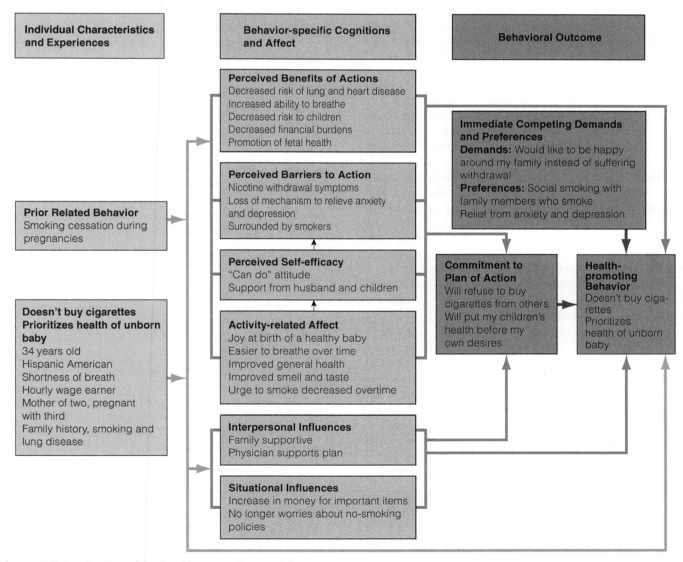

Figure 3.8 Application of the health promotion model.

health promotion activities. A variety of strategies including education, support, and modeling are used in health promotion. The nurse assists the individual to develop a plan of action and serves as a resource to guide the activity, monitor progress, and evaluate outcomes.

Healthy People 2020

Improvement in the health of every person in the United States is the focus of the agenda set forth in *Healthy People 2020* (United States Department of Health and Human Services [USDHHS], 2013). The goals of *Healthy People 2020* are to attain high-quality, longer lives free of preventable disease, disability, injury, and premature death; achieve health equity, eliminate disparities, and improve the health of all groups; create social and physical environments that promote good health for all; and promote quality of life, healthy development, and healthy behaviors across all life stages.

The goals of *Healthy People 2020* redirect attention from health care to health determinants. Health determinants include personal, social, economic, and environmental factors that influence individual and population health. Social determinants include but are not limited to family, community, income, education, sex, race/ethnicity, place of residence, and access to health care. Physical determinants include both natural environments and built environments. Natural environments are locations or systems that have not been significantly modified by humans with regard to ecological processes or landscape. Protected natural areas, such as national parks, are examples of natural environments (Newsome, Moore, & Dowling, 2013). Built environments comprise structures and systems that are designed or modified by humans such as water and sanitation systems, housing structures, residential developments, urban landscapes, roadways, and even food sources (Glanz & Kegler, n.d.).

Healthy People 2020 is intended to differ from past versions in that it will not be distributed in a printed, static format accessible through chapter headings, but rather through a Web interface in which users would access the broad categories of interventions, determinations, and outcomes. The mission of *Healthy People 2020* is to offer practical guidance on using information, education, and other interventions to improve health.

Healthy People 2020 objectives guide interventions and allow for monitoring of achievement. Topic areas were identified in developing the objectives for *Healthy People 2020*. Topic areas related to wellness and health promotion include but are not limited to access to health services, education and community-based programs, immunization and infectious diseases, injury and violence prevention, nutrition and weight status, physical activity, sexually transmitted diseases and HIV, environmental health, sleep health, substance abuse, and tobacco use. Table 3.2 provides an overview of the concerns, factors, and recommendations for health promotion related to each of these topic areas. For more information about *Healthy People 2020*, contact the USDHHS.

Topic Areas

Each of the topic areas and the associated factors is discussed in the following sections.

Access to Health Services

To maintain good health, people must have easy and affordable access to quality healthcare services. Access to health care depends on the ability of individuals to gain entry into a healthcare system, access healthcare services at a convenient location and in a timely fashion, and find a healthcare provider that they can trust. If health services are accessible and used appropriately, they have the opportunity to improve the overall physical, social, and mental health status of individuals. People with convenient access to health services are more likely to take advantage of preventative services such as wellness checkups; immunizations; and eye, teeth, and ear checkups. This allows early detection and treatment of diseases, leading to decreased healthcare expenses, increased quality of life and life expectancy, and decreased incidence of preventable deaths. In contrast, individuals who do not have good access to health care because of location, cost, or lack of insurance may suffer from unmet health needs, delays in care, lack of preventative care, and unnecessary hospitalizations.

With the implementation of the Affordable Care Act in 2014, the already overwhelmed healthcare system may feel an even greater burden as a higher percentage of Americans have health insurance (Anderson, 2014). To face these challenges, the healthcare system will need a greater influx of primary care physicians, nurses, and other healthcare professionals. Individuals will need access to providers with whom they can communicate, emphasizing the need for bilingual skills in the healthcare workforce. They will also need providers who show cultural sensitivity for the diverse American population, including foreign immigrants and lesbian, gay, bisexual, and transgender individuals.

Education and Community-based Programs

Achieving health and wellness is greatly enhanced by successful implementation of health education programs. As education programs are implemented at multiple levels, including personal education and educational programs at schools, worksites, healthcare facilities, and communities, individuals begin to understand the importance of maintaining good health. These programs can play a role in improving health, preventing disease and injury, and enhancing the overall quality of life. Educational programs that are successfully implemented in one setting can often be easily adapted for other settings, increasing the number of people who are influenced by the healthcare recommendations provided in the program.

Healthy People 2020 is encouraging the implementation of educational and community-based programs in chronic diseases, injury and violence prevention, mental illness, unintended pregnancy, oral health, tobacco use, substance abuse, nutrition, and physical activity. These programs may be influential in initiating new policies and practices; changing organizational infrastructures; and changing community attitudes, beliefs, and social norms. Physicians, nurses, and other healthcare professionals can participate in this topic area by helping implement educational programs in their own community.

Immunization and Infectious Diseases

Immunizations can prevent disease, disability, and the spread of infection and are largely responsible for improvements in child

| TABLE 3.2 | Topic Areas and Recommendations for Prevention of Disease and Health Promotion |

TOPIC	CONCERN	INFLUENCING FACTORS/ DETERMINANTS	RECOMMENDATIONS FOR HEALTH PROMOTION
Access to Health Services	Lack of access to health services results in unmet health needs, delays in care, more advanced disease at time of detection, and unnecessary hospitalization and death.	Individuals who live in rural areas are further from needed health services. Individuals in low-income families have reduced access to health care because of cost and lack of insurance. Foreign immigrants have communication barriers when seeking health care.	Increase the availability of affordable health insurance. Increase the number of primary care providers and the percentage of individuals with a primary care provider. Increase the use of preventative services. Provide efficient access to emergency medical services. Reduce wait times in doctors' offices and emergency departments. Decrease time between tests and receiving needed treatments.
Education and Community-Based Programs	Individuals without proper health education are more likely to engage in risky behavior and less likely to participate in preventative services.	People who have restricted access to healthcare services because of location or cost may be more likely to receive health education if they are provided with multiple opportunities in community settings.	Increase health education and community-based programs in multiple settings. Use nontraditional settings for education to improve sharing between peers. Increase education programs in Head Start settings; elementary, middle, and senior high schools; and colleges and universities. Increase access to employee health promotion programs at worksites. Increase the number of community-based organizations providing prevention services. Increase prevention content in medical, dental, pharmacy, and nursing schools.
Immunization and Infectious Diseases	Individuals who do not receive immunizations are at increased risk for illness and death from preventable diseases.	Children have a higher rate of immunization than adults. Adults with influencing factors such as age or chronic diseases are more susceptible to infectious diseases.	When recommendations in immunization schedules are followed, the incidence of many childhood illnesses is reduced. Immunization decreases the incidence of death or complications of infectious disease in older adults.
Injury and Violence Prevention	Serious injuries can occur from motor vehicle accidents, falls, drowning, fires, poisons, and shootings.	Death associated with vehicular accidents occurs with the greatest frequency among those between 18 and 24 years of age. Alcohol use is associated with one-third of the vehicular fatalities in the United States. In the United States, injuries are the leading cause of disability and death for those between 1 and 44 years of age.	Education about the use of safety equipment can reduce injuries from accidents. Reduction in distracted driving and in driving under the influence of alcohol or drugs can reduce accident-related injuries.
Nutrition and Weight Status	Poor nutrition contributes to many health conditions, including overweight and obesity, heart disease, high blood pressure, diabetes, osteoporosis, and some cancers.	More than one-third of U.S. adults are obese, and these individuals have higher medical costs than normal-weight individuals. Obesity is higher in African Americans and Hispanics than in Caucasians (CDC, 2013d). Approximately 17% of children aged 2–19 years are obese (CDC, 2014a).	Nutrition and exercise are important in maintaining or attaining healthy weight. Dietary guidelines recommend consuming a variety of foods including vegetables, fruits, whole grains, fat-free dairy products, lean meats, and foods low in sugar and saturated fat. Sensible portions are recommended.
Physical Activity	Important to all ages. Promotes physical health and emotional well-being. Increases strength, decreases body fat. In children: Promotes and maintains skeletal development and mass. In older adults: Needed to maintain agility, reduce safety risks, and maintain independence in ADLs.	Men are more active than women. Higher income or education in individuals is related to higher levels of physical activity. Individuals with convenient access to exercise facilities and safe neighborhoods are more likely to exercise than those without access. Individuals over 75 years are less active than younger people.	Children and adolescents: 1 hour of physical activity daily. Adults: At least 2 hours 30 minutes of activity per week. Muscle strengthening exercises.

(continued)

TABLE 3.2 **Topic Areas and Recommendations for Prevention of Disease and Health Promotion** (continued)

TOPIC	CONCERN	INFLUENCING FACTORS/ DETERMINANTS	RECOMMENDATIONS FOR HEALTH PROMOTION
Sexually Transmitted Diseases (STDs) and HIV	Unprotected sexual activity increases the risk for pregnancy, STDs, and HIV infection.	Half of new STD cases are in people aged 15 to 24. New cases of HIV are highest in gay and bisexual men and African Americans. Biological, social, economic, and behavioral factors all contribute to STD transmission.	Detection, early treatment, and prevention of STDs and HIV are essential to reducing transmission, preventing complications, and changing behavior associated with STDs.
Environmental Health	Bioterrorism remains an increasingly significant threat to national and international health.	Areas of concern include outdoor air quality, water quality, and indoor allergens (including rodent- and insect-related), all of which are linked to numerous health problems.	Education about health hazards associated with exposure to pollutants, as well as teaching about the importance of maintaining a sanitary living environment.
Sleep Health	Poor sleep health contributes to fatigue, irritability, decreased performance, increased risk of accidents and injuries, and increased risk of chronic diseases and infection.	Children and adolescents with poor sleep health have decreased performance at school. Older adults with chronic diseases are at higher risk of developing sleep disorders because of chronic diseases and medications. Sleep disorders such as sleep disordered breathing, including sleep apnea, are common in middle-aged and older adults, especially obese adults.	Education about proper sleep health, including avoiding caffeine and alcohol, exercising regularly, and establishing a relaxing bedtime routine. Increase the detection of obstructive sleep apnea in adults. Decrease the number of vehicle crashes due to drowsy driving.
Substance Abuse	Alcohol and substance abuse are associated with health problems that include accidents, sexually transmitted diseases (STDs), violence, and family problems. Alcohol use can increase the risk for heart and liver diseases. Alcohol use in pregnancy has been linked with low birth weight and fetal alcohol syndrome.	Drug and alcohol use in adolescents depends on age and drug type. Up to 6.5% of middle and high school students use marijuana daily. In the United States, 17 million adults have alcohol use disorder. Adults aged 18 to 25 have the highest rate of drug, alcohol, and tobacco use among individuals aged 12 and older.	Education about the risks associated with drugs and alcohol is warranted for children and adolescents. Use the CAGE-AID questionnaire to screen for alcohol and other drug abuse in adults. Counseling, therapy, and rehabilitation are among the options for drug users. Families may benefit from support groups.
Tobacco Use	Tobacco use is responsible for approximately 443,000 deaths per year in the United States, and almost 9 million people suffer from tobacco-related illnesses. Smoking is a risk factor for heart disease, breathing disorders, and lung cancer. Secondary smoke increases the incidence of asthma and bronchitis in children. Smoking during pregnancy increases the risk for premature birth, miscarriage, and sudden infant death syndrome (SIDS). Use of chewing tobacco and cigars increases the risk of oral and gastrointestinal cancers.	Individuals with low income and education are more likely to smoke than are those with higher income and education. Men have slightly higher rates of smoking than women. Native Americans, Alaska Natives, and military personnel have the highest smoking rates. Smoking habits most frequently begin in adolescence.	Cessation of smoking and never starting to smoke are the only methods to prevent associated risks and problems. Education of adolescents and children about the hazards may decrease the numbers who start smoking.

survival in the 20th century. In spite of available vaccines to prevent them, viral hepatitis, influenza, and tuberculosis are still among the leading causes of illness and death in the United States. Recommendations for childhood and adult immunizations have been developed and, when followed, reduce the incidence of many illnesses. Table 3.3 includes recommended schedules for childhood and adult immunizations. For further information, contact the Centers for Disease Control and Prevention (CDC).

In addition to immunizations, *Healthy People 2020* goals for preventing the spread of infectious diseases include investing in technological advances, helping government and local health departments work together to control the spread of infectious diseases, and increasing surveillance of infectious diseases for earlier detection. Other areas of focus are preventing the spread of infectious diseases due to international travel, decreasing inappropriate use of antibiotics, and more rapidly detecting new infectious agents and diseases.

Injury and Violence Prevention

Serious injuries can occur from motor vehicle accidents, falls, drowning, fires, poison, and shootings. Table 3.4 on page 62 describes the application of the levels of prevention for specific aspects of this focus area. In the United States, injuries are the leading cause of death for those between the ages of 1 and 44 years and the leading cause of disability for all ages. Death as a result of motor vehicle accidents occurs with greatest frequency among those between 18 and 24 years of age. Alcohol has been associated with almost one third of the traffic fatalities in the United States. The incidence of injury related to distracted driving has also increased recently with the advent of texting and smartphones. Increased use of appropriate safety equipment, especially for children; increased road awareness; and decreased driving after consumption of alcohol are considered the best ways to reduce motor vehicle–related injuries and deaths.

According to the CDC (2014b), violence is a public health problem in the United States. Violence resulting in death and disability affects people across the age span. Violence occurs in many forms—from child maltreatment to abuse of the elderly—and occurs in intimate relationships, sexual encounters, schools, and communities. Among youth populations, emerging issues related to violence include bullying, dating violence, and sexual violence. Among elderly populations, elder maltreatment is a rising problem and needs continued research to help quantify and understand the cause. For more information about injury and violence, contact the CDC.

Nutrition and Weight Status

Good nutrition helps reduce the risk of many health conditions, including overweight and obesity, heart disease, high blood pressure, diabetes, osteoporosis, and some cancers. More than one third of U.S. adults are considered obese, and these individuals incur medical costs that are 37% higher than those who are normal weight. Non-Hispanic blacks have the highest rates of obesity, followed by Mexican Americans, all Hispanics, and non-Hispanic whites. In addition, approximately 17% of children aged 2–19 years are obese. Physiologic, genetic, cultural, environmental, and social factors contribute to obesity.

One common link to childhood overweight and obesity concerns the type of feeding received by the child. Specifically, recent research suggests that formula feedings significantly increase a child's likelihood for developing overweight and obesity, while breastfeeding decreases the risk for these conditions. Along with weight-related benefits, breastfeeding also affords children immunological benefits. Mothers who breastfeed benefit, too: for these women, the positive effects include a decreased risk for developing breast cancer. Based on the health benefits for both mother and child, the U.S. Surgeon General has issued a call to action for mothers to breastfeed their infants (USDHHS, 2011).

Nutrition and exercise are important in attaining or maintaining a healthy weight. *Healthy People 2020* objectives focus not only on individual behaviors but also on developing policies and environments that support healthy eating behaviors in schools, worksites, and communities. Dietary guidelines have been established for individuals ages 2 and older. Refer to chapter 12 for an in-depth discussion of nutrition. ∞ The guidelines stress eating sensible portions of an assortment of nutrient-dense foods across the food groups—such as vegetables and fruits, whole grains, fat-free dairy products, and lean meats—as well as limiting foods that contain saturated and trans fats, cholesterol, added sugars, sodium, and alcohol. Dietary guidelines also include the recommendation for exercise for adults and children when involved in maintaining or losing weight.

Physical Activity

Physical activity is important at all ages to maintain physical health; promote psychological well-being; and reduce the incidence of cardiovascular diseases, diabetes, and some forms of cancer. Physical activity increases skeletal and muscular strength, helps decrease body fat, is important in weight control, is indicated for reduction of depression, and improves emotional well-being. Regular physical activity is required in children to promote and maintain skeletal development and mass. In older adults, maintenance of agility through exercise reduces safety risks and enables individuals to continue independent activities of daily living (ADLs). Data indicate that in general men are more active than women, individuals of higher income and education are more physically active than those of low income and education, and individuals with convenient access to exercise facilities or safe neighborhoods are more likely to exercise than those without access.

Regular physical activity reduces the risk for developing or dying from some of the leading causes of illness in the United States. Regular physical activity results in the following:

- Reduced risk of premature death
- Reduced risk of death from coronary heart disease and stroke
- Reduced risk of development of type 2 diabetes
- Reduced risk of development of hypertension
- Reduced risk of development of breast and colon cancer
- Reduced risk of falls
- Reduction in depression and anxiety
- Weight reduction or control

TABLE 3.3 **Immunizations**

Recommended Immunization Schedules for Persons Aged 0 Through 18 Years—UNITED STATES, 2014

This schedule includes recommendations in effect as of January 1, 2014. Any dose not administered at the recommended age should be administered at a subsequent visit, when indicated and feasible. The use of a combination vaccine generally is preferred over separate injections of its equivalent component vaccines. Vaccination providers should consult the relevant Advisory Committee on Immunization Practices (ACIP) statement for detailed recommendations, available online at http://www.cdc.gov/vaccines/hcp/acip-recs/index.html. Clinically significant adverse events that follow vaccination should be reported to the Vaccine Adverse Event Reporting System (VAERS) online (http://www.vaers.hhs.gov) or by telephone (800-822-7967).

The Recommended Immunization Schedules for
Persons Aged 0 Through 18 Years are approved by the

Advisory Committee on Immunization Practices
(http://www.cdc.gov/vaccines/acip)

American Academy of Pediatrics
(http://www.aap.org)

American Academy of Family Physicians
(http://www.aafp.org)

American College of Obstetricians and Gynecologists
(http://www.acog.org)

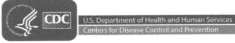

U.S. Department of Health and Human Services
Centers for Disease Control and Prevention

Figure 1. Recommended immunization schedule for persons aged 0 through 18 years – United States, 2014.
(FOR THOSE WHO FALL BEHIND OR START LATE, SEE THE CATCH-UP SCHEDULE [FIGURE 2]).
These recommendations must be read with the footnotes that follow. For those who fall behind or start late, provide catch-up vaccination at the earliest opportunity as indicated by the green bars in Figure 1. To determine minimum intervals between doses, see the catch-up schedule (Figure 2). School entry and adolescent vaccine age groups are in bold.

Vaccine	Birth	1 mo	2 mos	4 mos	6 mos	9 mos	12 mos	15 mos	18 mos	19–23 mos	2-3 yrs	4-6 yrs	7-10 yrs	11-12 yrs	13-15 yrs	16-18 yrs
Hepatitis B¹ (HepB)	1st dose	←— 2nd dose —→			←————————— 3rd dose —————————→											
Rotavirus² (RV) RV1 (2-dose series); RV5 (3-dose series)			1st dose	2nd dose	See footnote 2											
Diphtheria, tetanus, & acellular pertussis³ (DTaP: <7 yrs)			1st dose	2nd dose	3rd dose		←——— 4th dose ———→					5th dose				
Tetanus, diphtheria, & acellular pertussis⁴ (Tdap: ≥7 yrs)														(Tdap)		
Haemophilus influenzae type b⁵ (Hib)			1st dose	2nd dose	See footnote 5		←— 3rd or 4th dose, See footnote 5 —→									
Pneumococcal conjugate⁶ (PCV13)			1st dose	2nd dose	3rd dose		←— 4th dose —→									
Pneumococcal polysaccharide⁶ (PPSV23)																
Inactivated poliovirus⁷ (IPV) (<18 yrs)			1st dose	2nd dose	←————————— 3rd dose —————————→							4th dose				
Influenza⁸ (IIV; LAIV) 2 doses for some: See footnote 8					←——————— Annual vaccination (IIV only) ———————→							←—— Annual vaccination (IIV or LAIV) ——→				
Measles, mumps, rubella⁹ (MMR)							←— 1st dose —→					2nd dose				
Varicella¹⁰ (VAR)							←— 1st dose —→					2nd dose				
Hepatitis A¹¹ (HepA)							←———— 2-dose series, See footnote 11 ————→									
Human papillomavirus¹² (HPV2: females only; HPV4: males and females)														(3-dose series)		
Meningococcal¹³ (Hib-MenCY ≥ 6 weeks; MenACWY-D≥9 mos; MenACWY-CRM ≥ 2 mos)					←——————————— See footnote 13 ———————————→									1st dose		Booster

Range of recommended ages for all children · Range of recommended ages for catch-up immunization · Range of recommended ages for certain high-risk groups · Range of recommended ages during which catch-up is encouraged and for certain high-risk groups · Not routinely recommended

This schedule includes recommendations in effect as of January 1, 2014. Any dose not administered at the recommended age should be administered at a subsequent visit, when indicated and feasible. The use of a combination vaccine generally is preferred over separate injections of its equivalent component vaccines. Vaccination providers should consult the relevant Advisory Committee on Immunization Practices (ACIP) statement for detailed recommendations, available online at http://www.cdc.gov/vaccines/hcp/acip-recs/index.html. Clinically significant adverse events that follow vaccination should be reported to the Vaccine Adverse Event Reporting System (VAERS) online (http://www.vaers.hhs.gov) or by telephone (800-822-7967).Suspected cases of vaccine-preventable diseases should be reported to the state or local health department. Additional information, including precautions and contraindications for vaccination, is available from CDC online (http://www.cdc.gov/vaccines/recs/vac-admin/contraindications.htm) or by telephone (800-CDC-INFO [800-232-4636]).

This schedule is approved by the Advisory Committee on Immunization Practices (http://www.cdc.gov/vaccines/acip), the American Academy of Pediatrics (http://www.aap.org), the American Academy of Family Physicians (http://www.aafp.org), and the American College of Obstetricians and Gynecologists (http://www.acog.org).

NOTE: The above recommendations must be read along with the footnotes of this schedule.

FIGURE 2. Catch-up immunization schedule for persons aged 4 months through 18 years who start late or who are more than 1 month behind —United States, 2014.
The figure below provides catch-up schedules and minimum intervals between doses for children whose vaccinations have been delayed. A vaccine series does not need to be restarted, regardless of the time that has elapsed between doses. Use the section appropriate for the child's age. Always use this table in conjunction with Figure 1 and the footnotes that follow.

Vaccine	Minimum Age for Dose 1	Dose 1 to dose 2	Dose 2 to dose 3	Dose 3 to dose 4	Dose 4 to dose 5
			Minimum Interval Between Doses		
Persons aged 4 months through 6 years					
Hepatitis B¹	Birth	4 weeks	8 weeks and at least 16 weeks after first dose; minimum age for the final dose is 24 weeks		
Rotavirus²	6 weeks	4 weeks	4 weeks²		
Diphtheria, tetanus, & acellular pertussis³	6 weeks	4 weeks	4 weeks	6 months	6 months³
Haemophilus influenzae type b⁵	6 weeks	4 weeks if first dose administered at younger than age 12 months / 8 weeks (as final dose) if first dose administered at age 12 through 14 months / No further doses needed if first dose administered at age 15 months or older	4 weeks⁵ if current age is younger than 12 months and first dose administered at < 7 months old / 8 weeks and age 12 months through 59 months (as final dose)⁵ if current age is younger than 12 months and first dose administered between 7 through 11 months (regardless of Hib vaccine [PRP-T or PRP-OMP] used for first dose); OR if current age is 12 through 59 months and first dose administered at younger than age 12 months; OR first 2 doses were PRP-OMP and administered at younger than 12 months. No further doses needed if previous dose administered at age 15 months or older	8 weeks (as final dose) This dose only necessary for children aged 12 through 59 months who received 3 (PRP-T) doses before age 12 months and started the primary series before age 7 months	
Pneumococcal⁶	6 weeks	4 weeks if first dose administered at younger than age 12 months / 8 weeks (as final dose for healthy children) if first dose administered at age 12 months or older / No further doses needed for healthy children if first dose administered at age 24 months or older	4 weeks if current age is younger than 12 months / 8 weeks (as final dose for healthy children) if current age is 12 months or older / No further doses needed for healthy children if previous dose administered at age 24 months or older	8 weeks (as final dose) This dose only necessary for children aged 12 through 59 months who received 3 doses before age 12 months or for children at high risk who received 3 doses at any age	
Inactivated poliovirus⁷	6 weeks	4 weeks⁷	4 weeks⁷	6 months⁷ minimum age 4 years for final dose	
Meningococcal¹³	6 weeks	8 weeks¹³	See footnote 13	See footnote 13	
Measles, mumps, rubella⁹	12 months	4 weeks			
Varicella¹⁰	12 months	3 months			
Hepatitis A¹¹	12 months	6 months			
Persons aged 7 through 18 years					
Tetanus, diphtheria; tetanus, diphtheria, & acellular pertussis⁴	7 years⁴	4 weeks	4 weeks if first dose of DTaP/DT administered at younger than age 12 months / 6 months if first dose of DTaP/DT administered at age 12 months or older and then no further doses needed for catch-up	6 months if first dose of DTaP/DT administered at younger than age 12 months	
Human papillomavirus¹²	9 years	Routine dosing intervals are recommended¹²			
Hepatitis A¹¹	12 months	6 months			
Hepatitis B¹	Birth	4 weeks	8 weeks (and at least 16 weeks after first dose)		
Inactivated poliovirus⁷	6 weeks	4 weeks	4 weeks⁷	6 months⁷	
Meningococcal¹³	6 weeks	8 weeks¹³			
Measles, mumps, rubella⁹	12 months	4 weeks			
Varicella¹⁰	12 months	3 months if person is younger than age 13 years / 4 weeks if person is aged 13 years or older			

NOTE: The above recommendations must be read along with the footnotes of this schedule.

Footnotes — Recommended immunization schedule for persons aged 0 through 18 years—United States, 2014

For further guidance on the use of the vaccines mentioned below, see: http://www.cdc.gov/vaccines/hcp/acip-recs/index.html. For vaccine recommendations for persons 19 years of age and older, see the adult immunization schedule.

Additional information

- For contraindications and precautions to use of a vaccine and for additional information regarding that vaccine, vaccination providers should consult the relevant ACIP statement available online at http://www.cdc.gov/vaccines/hcp/acip-recs/index.html.
- For purposes of calculating intervals between doses, 4 weeks = 28 days. Intervals of 4 months or greater are determined by calendar months.
- Vaccine doses administered 4 days or less before the minimum interval are considered valid. Doses of any vaccine administered ≥5 days earlier than the minimum interval or minimum age should not be counted as valid doses and should be repeated as age-appropriate. The repeat dose should be spaced after the invalid dose by the recommended minimum interval. For further details, see *MMWR, General Recommendations on Immunization and Reports* / Vol. 60 / No. 2; Table 1. *Recommended and minimum ages and intervals between vaccine doses* available online at http://www.cdc.gov/mmwr/pdf/rr/rr6002.pdf.
- Information on travel vaccine requirements and recommendations is available at http://wwwnc.cdc.gov/travel/destinations/list.
- For vaccination of persons with primary and secondary immunodeficiencies, see Table 13, "*Vaccination of persons with primary and secondary immunodeficiencies,*" in General Recommendations on Immunization (ACIP), available at http://www.cdc.gov/mmwr/pdf/rr/rr6002.pdf.; and American Academy of Pediatrics. Immunization in Special Clinical Circumstances, in Pickering LK, Baker CJ, Kimberlin DW, Long SS eds. *Red Book: 2012 report of the Committee on Infectious Diseases. 29th ed.* Elk Grove Village, IL: American Academy of Pediatrics.

1. **Hepatitis B (HepB) vaccine. (Minimum age: birth)**

Routine vaccination:

At birth:

- Administer monovalent HepB vaccine to all newborns before hospital discharge.
- For infants born to hepatitis B surface antigen (HBsAg)-positive mothers, administer HepB vaccine and 0.5 mL of hepatitis B immune globulin (HBIG) within 12 hours of birth. These infants should be tested for HBsAg and antibody to HBsAg (anti-HBs) 1 to 2 months after completion of the HepB series, at age 9 through 18 months (preferably at the next well-child visit).
- If mother's HBsAg status is unknown, within 12 hours of birth administer HepB vaccine regardless of birth weight. For infants weighing less than 2,000 grams, administer HBIG in addition to HepB vaccine within 12 hours of birth. Determine mother's HBsAg status as soon as possible and, if mother is HBsAg-positive, also administer HBIG for infants weighing 2,000 grams or more as soon as possible, but no later than age 7 days.

Doses following the birth dose:

- The second dose should be administered at age 1 or 2 months. Monovalent HepB vaccine should be used for doses administered before age 6 weeks.
- Infants who did not receive a birth dose should receive 3 doses of a HepB-containing vaccine on a schedule of 0, 1 to 2 months, and 6 months starting as soon as feasible. See Figure 2.
- Administer the second dose 1 to 2 months after the first dose (minimum interval of 4 weeks), administer the third dose at least 8 weeks after the second dose AND at least 16 weeks after the **first** dose. The final (third or fourth) dose in the HepB vaccine series should be administered no earlier than age 24 weeks.
- Administration of a total of 4 doses of HepB vaccine is permitted when a combination vaccine containing HepB is administered after the birth dose.

Catch-up vaccination:

- Unvaccinated persons should complete a 3-dose series.
- A 2-dose series (doses separated by at least 4 months) of adult formulation Recombivax HB is licensed for use in children aged 11 through 15 years.
- For other catch-up guidance, see Figure 2.

2. **Rotavirus (RV) vaccines. (Minimum age: 6 weeks for both RV1 [Rotarix] and RV5 [RotaTeq])**

Routine vaccination:

Administer a series of RV vaccine to all infants as follows:

1. If Rotarix is used, administer a 2-dose series at 2 and 4 months of age.
2. If RotaTeq is used, administer a 3-dose series at ages 2, 4, and 6 months.
3. If any dose in the series was RotaTeq or vaccine product is unknown for any dose in the series, a total of 3 doses of RV vaccine should be administered.

Catch-up vaccination:

- The maximum age for the first dose in the series is 14 weeks, 6 days; vaccination should not be initiated for infants aged 15 weeks, 0 days or older.
- The maximum age for the final dose in the series is 8 months, 0 days.
- For other catch-up guidance, see Figure 2.

3. **Diphtheria and tetanus toxoids and acellular pertussis (DTaP) vaccine. (Minimum age: 6 weeks. Exception: DTaP-IPV [Kinrix]: 4 years)**

Routine vaccination:

- Administer a 5-dose series of DTaP vaccine at ages 2, 4, 6, 15 through 18 months, and 4 through 6 years. The fourth dose may be administered as early as age 12 months, provided at least 6 months have elapsed since the third dose.

Catch-up vaccination:

- The fifth dose of DTaP vaccine is not necessary if the fourth dose was administered at age 4 years or older.
- For other catch-up guidance, see Figure 2.

4. **Tetanus and diphtheria toxoids and acellular pertussis (Tdap) vaccine. (Minimum age: 10 years for Boostrix, 11 years for Adacel)**

Routine vaccination:

- Administer 1 dose of Tdap vaccine to all adolescents aged 11 through 12 years.
- Tdap may be administered regardless of the interval since the last tetanus and diphtheria toxoid-containing vaccine.
- Administer 1 dose of Tdap vaccine to pregnant adolescents during each pregnancy (preferred during 27 through 36 weeks gestation) regardless of time since prior Td or Tdap vaccination.

Catch-up vaccination:

- Persons aged 7 years and older who are not fully immunized with DTaP vaccine should receive Tdap vaccine as 1 (preferably the first) dose in the catch-up series; if additional doses are needed, use Td vaccine. For children 7 through 10 years who receive a dose of Tdap as part of the catch-up series, an adolescent Tdap vaccine dose at age 11 through 12 years should NOT be administered. Td should be administered instead 10 years after the Tdap dose.
- Persons aged 11 through 18 years who have not received Tdap vaccine should receive a dose followed by tetanus and diphtheria toxoids (Td) booster doses every 10 years thereafter.
- Inadvertent doses of DTaP vaccine:
  - If administered inadvertently to a child aged 7 through 10 years may count as part of the catch-up series. This dose may count as the adolescent Tdap dose, or the child can later receive a Tdap booster dose at age 11 through 12 years.
  - If administered inadvertently to an adolescent aged 11 through 18 years, the dose should be counted as the adolescent Tdap booster.
- For other catch-up guidance, see Figure 2.

5. ***Haemophilus influenzae*** **type b (Hib) conjugate vaccine. (Minimum age: 6 weeks for PRP-T [ACTHIB, DTaP-IPV/Hib (Pentacel) and Hib-MenCY (MenHibrix)], PRP-OMP [PedvaxHIB or COMVAX], 12 months for PRP-T [Hiberix])**

Routine vaccination:

- Administer a 2- or 3-dose Hib vaccine primary series and a booster dose (dose 3 or 4 depending on vaccine used in primary series) at age 12 through 15 months to complete a full Hib vaccine series.
- The primary series with ActHIB, MenHibrix, or Pentacel consists of 3 doses and should be administered at 2, 4, and 6 months of age. The primary series with PedvaxHib or COMVAX consists of 2 doses and should be administered at 2 and 4 months of age; a dose at age 6 months is not indicated.
- One booster dose (dose 3 or 4 depending on vaccine used in primary series) of any Hib vaccine should be administered at age 12 through 15 months. An exception is Hiberix vaccine. Hiberix should only be used for the booster (final) dose in children aged 12 months through 4 years who have received at least 1 prior dose of Hib-containing vaccine.
- For recommendations on the use of MenHibrix in patients at increased risk for meningococcal disease, please refer to the meningococcal vaccine footnotes and also to *MMWR* March 22, 2013; 62(RR02);1-22, available at http://www.cdc.gov/mmwr/pdf/rr/rr6202.pdf.

Catch-up vaccination:

- If dose 1 was administered at ages 12 through 14 months, administer a second (final) dose at least 8 weeks after dose 1, regardless of Hib vaccine used in the primary series.
- If the first 2 doses were PRP-OMP (PedvaxHIB or COMVAX), and were administered at age 11 months or younger, the third (and final) dose should be administered at age 12 through 15 months and at least 8 weeks after the second dose.
- If the first dose was administered at age 7 through 11 months, administer the second dose at least 4 weeks later and a third (and final) dose at age 12 through 15 months or 8 weeks after second dose, whichever is later, regardless of Hib vaccine used for first dose.
- If first dose is administered at younger than 12 months of age and second dose is given between 12 through 14 months of age, a third (and final) dose should be given 8 weeks later.
- For unvaccinated children aged 15 months or older, administer only 1 dose.
- For other catch-up guidance, see Figure 2. For catch-up guidance related to MenHibrix, please see the meningococcal vaccine footnotes and also *MMWR* March 22, 2013; 62(RR02);1-22, available at http://www.cdc.gov/mmwr/pdf/rr/rr6202.pdf.

Vaccination of persons with high-risk conditions:

- Children aged 12 through 59 months who are at increased risk for Hib disease, including chemotherapy recipients and those with anatomic or functional asplenia (including sickle cell disease), human immunodeficiency virus (HIV) infection, immunoglobulin deficiency, or early component complement deficiency, who have received either no doses or only 1 dose of Hib vaccine before 12 months of age, should receive 2 additional doses of Hib vaccine 8 weeks apart; children who received 2 or more doses of Hib vaccine before 12 months of age should receive 1 additional dose.
- For patients younger than 5 years of age undergoing chemotherapy or radiation treatment who received a Hib vaccine dose(s) within 14 days of starting therapy or during therapy, repeat the dose(s) at least 3 months following therapy completion.

5. ***Haemophilus influenzae*** **type b (Hib) conjugate vaccine (cont'd)**

- Recipients of hematopoietic stem cell transplant (HSCT) should be revaccinated with a 3-dose regimen of Hib vaccine starting 6 to 12 months after successful transplant, regardless of vaccination history; doses should be administered at least 4 weeks apart.
- A single dose of any Hib-containing vaccine should be administered to unimmunized* children and adolescents 15 months of age and older undergoing an elective splenectomy; if possible, vaccine should be administered at least 14 days before procedure.
- Hib vaccine is not routinely recommended for patients 5 years or older. However, 1 dose of Hib vaccine should be administered to unimmunized* persons aged 5 years or older who have anatomic or functional asplenia (including sickle cell disease) and unvaccinated persons 5 through 18 years of age with human immunodeficiency virus (HIV) infection.

* *Patients who have not received a primary series and booster dose or at least 1 dose of Hib vaccine after 14 months of age are considered unimmunized.*

6. **Pneumococcal vaccines. (Minimum age: 6 weeks for PCV13, 2 years for PPSV23)**

Routine vaccination with PCV13:

- Administer a 4-dose series of PCV13 vaccine at ages 2, 4, and 6 months and at age 12 through 15 months.
- For children aged 14 through 59 months who have received an age-appropriate series of 7-valent PCV (PCV7), administer a single supplemental dose of 13-valent PCV (PCV13).

Catch-up vaccination with PCV13:

- Administer 1 dose of PCV13 to all healthy children aged 24 through 59 months who are not completely vaccinated for their age.
- For other catch-up guidance, see Figure 2.

Vaccination of persons with high-risk conditions with PCV13 and PPSV23:

- All recommended PCV13 doses should be administered prior to PPSV23 vaccination if possible.
- For children 2 through 5 years of age with any of the following conditions: chronic heart disease (particularly cyanotic congenital heart disease and cardiac failure); chronic lung disease (including asthma if treated with high-dose oral corticosteroid therapy); diabetes mellitus; cerebrospinal fluid leak; cochlear implant; sickle cell disease and other hemoglobinopathies; anatomic or functional asplenia; HIV infection; chronic renal failure; nephrotic syndrome; diseases associated with treatment with immunosuppressive drugs or radiation therapy, including malignant neoplasms, leukemias, lymphomas, and Hodgkin disease; solid organ transplantation; or congenital immunodeficiency:
  1. Administer 1 dose of PCV13 if 3 doses of PCV (PCV7 and/or PCV13) were received previously.
  2. Administer 2 doses of PCV13 at least 8 weeks apart if fewer than 3 doses of PCV (PCV7 and/or PCV13) were received previously.
  3. Administer 1 supplemental dose of PCV13 if 4 doses of PCV7 or other age-appropriate complete PCV7 series was received previously.
  4. The minimum interval between doses of PCV (PCV7 or PCV13) is 8 weeks.
  5. For children with no history of PPSV23 vaccination, administer PPSV23 at least 8 weeks after the most recent dose of PCV13.
- For children aged 6 through 18 years who have cerebrospinal fluid leak; cochlear implant; sickle cell disease and other hemoglobinopathies; anatomic or functional asplenia; congenital or acquired immunodeficiencies; HIV infection; chronic renal failure; nephrotic syndrome; diseases associated with treatment with immunosuppressive drugs or radiation therapy, including malignant neoplasms, leukemias, lymphomas, and Hodgkin disease; generalized malignancy; solid organ transplantation; or multiple myeloma:
  1. If neither PCV13 nor PPSV23 has been received previously, administer 1 dose of PCV13 now and 1 dose of PPSV23 at least 8 weeks later.
  2. If PCV13 has been received previously but PPSV23 has not, administer 1 dose of PPSV23 at least 8 weeks after the most recent dose of PCV13.
  3. If PPSV23 has been received but PCV13 has not, administer 1 dose of PCV13 at least 8 weeks after the most recent dose of PPSV23.
- For children aged 6 through 18 years with chronic heart disease (particularly cyanotic congenital heart disease and cardiac failure), chronic lung disease (including asthma if treated with high-dose oral corticosteroid therapy), diabetes mellitus, alcoholism, or chronic liver disease, who have not received PPSV23, administer 1 dose of PPSV23. If PCV13 has been received previously, then PPSV23 should be administered at least 8 weeks after any prior PCV13 dose.
- A single revaccination with PPSV23 should be administered 5 years after the first dose to children with sickle cell disease or other hemoglobinopathies; anatomic or functional asplenia; congenital or acquired immunodeficiencies; HIV infection; chronic renal failure; nephrotic syndrome; diseases associated with treatment with immunosuppressive drugs or radiation therapy, including malignant neoplasms, leukemias, lymphomas, and Hodgkin disease; generalized malignancy; solid organ transplantation; or multiple myeloma.

7. **Inactivated poliovirus vaccine (IPV). (Minimum age: 6 weeks)**

Routine vaccination:

- Administer a 4-dose series of IPV at ages 2, 4, 6 through 18 months, and 4 through 6 years. The final dose in the series should be administered on or after the fourth birthday and at least 6 months after the previous dose.

Catch-up vaccination:

- In the first 6 months of life, minimum age and minimum intervals are only recommended if the person is at risk for imminent exposure to circulating poliovirus (i.e., travel to a polio-endemic region or during an outbreak).
- If 4 or more doses are administered before age 4 years, an additional dose should be administered at age 4 through 6 years and at least 6 months after the previous dose.
- A fourth dose is not necessary if the third dose was administered at age 4 years or older and at least 6 months after the previous dose.
- If both OPV and IPV were administered as part of a series, a total of 4 doses should be administered, regardless of the child's current age. IPV is not routinely recommended for U.S. residents aged 18 years or older.
- For other catch-up guidance, see Figure 2.

8. **Influenza vaccines. (Minimum age: 6 months for inactivated influenza vaccine [IIV], 2 years for live, attenuated influenza vaccine [LAIV])**

Routine vaccination:

- Administer influenza vaccine annually to all children beginning at age 6 months. For most healthy, nonpregnant persons aged 2 through 49 years, either LAIV or IIV may be used. However, LAIV should NOT be administered to some persons, including 1) those with asthma, 2) children 2 through 4 years who had wheezing in the past 12 months, or 3) those who have any other underlying medical conditions that predispose them to influenza complications. For all other contraindications to use of LAIV, see *MMWR* 2013; 62 (No. RR-7):1-43, available at http://www.cdc.gov/mmwr/pdf/rr/rr6207.pdf.

For children aged 6 months through 8 years:

- For the 2013–14 season, administer 2 doses (separated by at least 4 weeks) to children who are receiving influenza vaccine for the first time. Some children in this age group who have been vaccinated previously will also need 2 doses. For additional guidance, follow dosing guidelines in the 2013-14 ACIP influenza vaccine recommendations, *MMWR* 2013; 62 (No. RR-7):1-43, available at http://www.cdc.gov/mmwr/pdf/rr/rr6207.pdf.
- For the 2014–15 season, follow dosing guidelines in the 2014 ACIP influenza vaccine recommendations.

For persons aged 9 years and older:

- Administer 1 dose.

9. **Measles, mumps, and rubella (MMR) vaccine. (Minimum age: 12 months for routine vaccination)**

Routine vaccination:

- Administer a 2-dose series of MMR vaccine at ages12 through 15 months and 4 through 6 years. The second dose may be administered before age 4 years, provided at least 4 weeks have elapsed since the first dose.
- Administer 1 dose of MMR vaccine to infants aged 6 through 11 months before departure from the United States for international travel. These children should be revaccinated with 2 doses of MMR vaccine, the first at age 12 through 15 months (12 months if the child remains in an area where disease risk is high), and the second dose at least 4 weeks later.
- Administer 2 doses of MMR vaccine to children aged 12 months and older before departure from the United States for international travel. The first dose should be administered on or after age 12 months and the second dose at least 4 weeks later.

9. **Measles, mumps, and rubella (MMR) vaccine. (cont'd)**

Catch-up vaccination:

- Ensure that all school-aged children and adolescents have had 2 doses of MMR vaccine; the minimum interval between the 2 doses is 4 weeks.

10. **Varicella (VAR) vaccine. (Minimum age: 12 months)**

Routine vaccination:

- Administer a 2-dose series of VAR vaccine at ages 12 through 15 months and 4 through 6 years. The second dose may be administered before age 4 years, provided at least 3 months have elapsed since the first dose. If the second dose was administered at least 4 weeks after the first dose, it can be accepted as valid.

Catch-up vaccination:

- Ensure that all persons aged 7 through 18 years without evidence of immunity (see *MMWR* 2007; 56 [No. RR-4], available at http://www.cdc.gov/mmwr/pdf/rr/rr5604.pdf) have 2 doses of varicella vaccine. For children aged 7 through 12 years, the recommended minimum interval between doses is 3 months (if the second dose was administered at least 4 weeks after the first dose, it can be accepted as valid); for persons aged 13 years and older, the minimum interval between doses is 4 weeks.

11. **Hepatitis A (HepA) vaccine. (Minimum age: 12 months)**

Routine vaccination:

- Initiate the 2-dose HepA vaccine series at 12 through 23 months; separate the 2 doses by 6 to 18 months.
- Children who have received 1 dose of HepA vaccine before age 24 months should receive a second dose 6 to 18 months after the first dose.
- For any person aged 2 years and older who has not already received the HepA vaccine series, 2 doses of HepA vaccine separated by 6 to 18 months may be administered if immunity against hepatitis A virus infection is desired.

Catch-up vaccination:

- The minimum interval between the two doses is 6 months.

Special populations:

- Administer 2 doses of HepA vaccine at least 6 months apart to previously unvaccinated persons who live in areas where vaccination programs target older children, or who are at increased risk for infection. This includes persons traveling to or working in countries that have high or intermediate endemicity of infection; men having sex with men; users of injection and non-injection illicit drugs; persons who work with HAV-infected primates or with HAV in a research laboratory; persons with clotting-factor disorders; persons with chronic liver disease; and persons who anticipate close, personal contact (e.g., household or regular babysitting) with an international adoptee during the first 60 days after arrival in the United States from a country with high or intermediate endemicity. The first dose should be administered as soon as the adoption is planned, ideally 2 or more weeks before the arrival of the adoptee.

12. **Human papillomavirus (HPV) vaccines. (Minimum age: 9 years for HPV2 [Cervarix] and HPV4 [Gardasil])**

Routine vaccination:

- Administer a 3-dose series of HPV vaccine on a schedule of 0, 1-2, and 6 months to all adolescents aged 11 through 12 years. Either HPV4 or HPV2 may be used for females, and only HPV4 may be used for males.
- The vaccine series may be started at age 9 years.
- Administer the second dose 1 to 2 months after the first dose (minimum interval of 4 weeks), administer the third dose 24 weeks after the first dose and 16 weeks after the second dose (minimum interval of 12 weeks).

Catch-up vaccination:

- Administer the vaccine series to females (either HPV2 or HPV4) and males (HPV4) at age 13 through 18 years if not previously vaccinated.
- Use recommended routine dosing intervals (see above) for vaccine series catch-up.

13. **Meningococcal conjugate vaccines. (Minimum age: 6 weeks for Hib-MenCY [MenHibrix], 9 months for MenACWY-D [Menactra], 2 months for MenACWY-CRM [Menveo])**

Routine vaccination:

- Administer a single dose of Menactra or Menveo vaccine at age 11 through 12 years, with a booster dose at age 16 years.
- Adolescents aged 11 through 18 years with human immunodeficiency virus (HIV) infection should receive a 2-dose primary series of Menactra or Menveo with at least 8 weeks between doses.
- For children aged 2 months through 18 years with high-risk conditions, see below.

Catch-up vaccination:

- Administer Menactra or Menveo vaccine at age 13 through 18 years if not previously vaccinated.
- If the first dose is administered at age 13 through 15 years, a booster dose should be administered at age 16 through 18 years with a minimum interval of at least 8 weeks between doses.
- If the first dose is administered at age 16 years or older, a booster dose is not needed.
- For other catch-up guidance, see Figure 2.

Vaccination of persons with high-risk conditions and other persons at increased risk of disease:

- Children with anatomic or functional asplenia (including sickle cell disease):
  1. For children younger than 19 months of age, administer a 4-dose infant series of MenHibrix or Menveo at 2, 4, 6, and 12 through 15 months of age.
  2. For children aged 19 through 23 months who have not completed a series of MenHibrix or Menveo, administer 2 primary doses of Menveo at least 3 months apart.
  3. For children aged 24 months and older who have not received a complete series of MenHibrix or Menveo or Menactra, administer 2 primary doses of either Menactra or Menveo at least 2 months apart. If Menactra is administered to a child with asplenia (including sickle cell disease), do not administer Menactra until 2 years of age and at least 4 weeks after the completion of all PCV13 doses.
- Children with persistent complement component deficiency:
  1. For children younger than 19 months of age, administer a 4-dose infant series of either MenHibrix or Menveo at 2, 4, 6, and 12 through 15 months of age.
  2. For children 7 through 23 months who have not initiated vaccination, two options exist depending on age and vaccine brand:
     a. For children who initiate vaccination with Menveo at 7 months through 23 months of age, a 2-dose series should be administered with the second dose after 12 months of age and at least 3 months after the first dose.
     b. For children who initiate vaccination with Menactra at 9 months through 23 months of age, a 2-dose series of Menactra should be administered at least 3 months apart.
     c. For children aged 24 months and older who have not received a complete series of MenHibrix, Menveo, or Menactra, administer 2 primary doses of either Menactra or Menveo at least 2 months apart.
- For children who travel to or reside in countries in which meningococcal disease is hyperendemic or epidemic, including countries in the African meningitis belt or the Hajj, administer an age- appropriate formulation and series of Menactra or Menveo for protection against serogroups A and W meningococcal disease. Prior receipt of MenHibrix is not sufficient for children traveling to the meningitis belt or the Hajj because it does not contain serogroups A or W.
- For children at risk during a community outbreak attributable to a vaccine serogroup, administer or complete an age- and formulation-appropriate series of MenHibrix, Menactra, or Menveo.
- For booster doses among persons with high-risk conditions, refer to *MMWR* 2013; 62(RR02);1-22, available at http://www.cdc.gov/mmwr/preview/mmwrhtml/rr6202a1.htm.

Catch-up recommendations for persons with high-risk conditions:

1. If MenHibrix is administered to achieve protection against meningococcal disease, a complete age-appropriate series of MenHibrix should be administered.
2. If the first dose of MenHibrix is given at or after 12 months of age, a total of 2 doses should be given at least 8 weeks apart to ensure protection against serogroups C and Y meningococcal disease.
3. For children who initiate vaccination with Menveo at 7 months through 9 months of age, a 2-dose series should be administered with the second dose after 12 months of age and at least 3 months after the first dose.
4. For other catch-up recommendations for these persons, refer to *MMWR* 2013; 62(RR02);1-22, available at http://www.cdc.gov/mmwr/preview/mmwrhtml/rr6202a1.htm.

For complete information on use of meningococcal vaccines, including guidance related to vaccination of persons at increased risk of infection, see *MMWR* March 22, 2013; 62(RR02);1-22, available at http://www.cdc.gov/mmwr/pdf/rr/rr6202.pdf.

(continued)

| TABLE 3.3 | Immunizations (continued) |

Recommended Adult Immunization Schedule—United States - 2014

Note: These recommendations must be read with the footnotes that follow containing number of doses, intervals between doses, and other important information.

Figure 1. Recommended adult immunization schedule, by vaccine and age group[1]

VACCINE ▼ AGE GROUP ▶	19-21 years	22-26 years	27-49 years	50-59 years	60-64 years	≥ 65 years
Influenza [2,*]	1 dose annually					
Tetanus, diphtheria, pertussis (Td/Tdap) [3,*]	Substitute 1-time dose of Tdap for Td booster; then boost with Td every 10 yrs					
Varicella [4,*]	2 doses					
Human papillomavirus (HPV) Female [5,*]	3 doses					
Human papillomavirus (HPV) Male [5,*]	3 doses					
Zoster [6]					1 dose	
Measles, mumps, rubella (MMR) [7,*]	1 or 2 doses					
Pneumococcal 13-valent conjugate (PCV13) [8,*]	1 dose					
Pneumococcal polysaccharide (PPSV23) [9,10]	1 or 2 doses					1 dose
Meningococcal [11,*]	1 or more doses					
Hepatitis A [12,*]	2 doses					
Hepatitis B [13,*]	3 doses					
Haemophilus influenzae type b (Hib) [14,*]	1 or 3 doses					

*Covered by the Vaccine Injury Compensation Program

[ ] For all persons in this category who meet the age requirements and who lack documentation of vaccination or have no evidence of previous infection; zoster vaccine recommended regardless of prior episode of zoster

[ ] Recommended if some other risk factor is present (e.g., on the basis of medical, occupational, lifestyle, or other indication)

[ ] No recommendation

Report all clinically significant postvaccination reactions to the Vaccine Adverse Event Reporting System (VAERS). Reporting forms and instructions on filing a VAERS report are available at www.vaers.hhs.gov or by telephone, 800-822-7967.

Information on how to file a Vaccine Injury Compensation Program claim is available at www.hrsa.gov/vaccinecompensation or by telephone, 800-338-2382. To file a claim for vaccine injury, contact the U.S. Court of Federal Claims, 717 Madison Place, N.W., Washington, D.C. 20005; telephone, 202-357-6400.

Additional information about the vaccines in this schedule, extent of available data, and contraindications for vaccination is also available at www.cdc.gov/vaccines or from the CDC-INFO Contact Center at 800-CDC-INFO (800-232-4636) in English and Spanish, 8:00 a.m. - 8:00 p.m. Eastern Time, Monday - Friday, excluding holidays.

Use of trade names and commercial sources is for identification only and does not imply endorsement by the U.S. Department of Health and Human Services.

The recommendations in this schedule were approved by the Centers for Disease Control and Prevention's (CDC) Advisory Committee on Immunization Practices (ACIP), the American Academy of Family Physicians (AAFP), the American College of Physicians (ACP), American College of Obstetricians and Gynecologists (ACOG) and American College of Nurse-Midwives (ACNM).

Figure 2. Vaccines that might be indicated for adults based on medical and other indications[1]

VACCINE ▼ INDICATION ▶	Pregnancy	Immunocompromising conditions (excluding human immunodeficiency virus [HIV])[4,6,7,8,15]	HIV infection CD4+ T lymphocyte count [4,6,7,8,15] < 200 cells/μL	HIV infection CD4+ T lymphocyte count ≥ 200 cells/μL	Men who have sex with men (MSM)	Kidney failure, end-stage renal disease, receipt of hemodialysi	Heart disease, chronic lung disease, chronic alcoholism	Asplenia (including elective splenectomy and persistent complement component deficiencies) [6,14]	Chronic liver disease	Diabetes	Healthcare personnel
Influenza [2,*]	1 dose IIV annually				1 dose IIV or LAIV annually	1 dose IIV annually					1 dose IIV or LAIV annually
Tetanus, diphtheria, pertussis (Td/Tdap) [3,*]	1 dose Tdap each pregnancy	Substitute 1-time dose of Tdap for Td booster; then boost with Td every 10 yrs									
Varicella [4,*]	Contraindicated			2 doses							
Human papillomavirus (HPV) Female [5,*]	3 doses through age 26 yrs				3 doses through age 26 yrs						
Human papillomavirus (HPV) Male [5,*]	3 doses through age 26yrs				3 doses through age 21 yrs						
Zoster [6]	Contraindicated			1 dose							
Measles, mumps, rubella (MMR) [7,*]	Contraindicated			1 or 2 doses							
Pneumococcal 13-valent conjugate (PCV13) [8,*]	1 dose										
Pneumococcal polysaccharide (PPSV23) [9,10]	1 or 2 doses										
Meningococcal [11,*]	1 or more doses										
Hepatitis A [12,*]	2 doses										
Hepatitis B [13,*]	3 doses										
Haemophilus influenzae type b (Hib) [14,*]	post-HSCT recipients only	1 or 3 doses									

*Covered by the Vaccine Injury Compensation Program

[ ] For all persons in this category who meet the age requirements and who lack documentation of vaccination or have no evidence of previous infection; zoster vaccine recommended regardless of prior episode of zoster

[ ] Recommended if some other risk factor is present (e.g., on the basis of medical, occupational, lifestyle, or other indications)

[ ] No recommendation

These schedules indicate the recommended age groups and medical indications for which administration of currently licensed vaccines is commonly indicated for adults ages 19 years and older, as of February 1, 2014. For all vaccines being recommended on the Adult Immunization Schedule: a vaccine series does not need to be restarted, regardless of the time that has elapsed between doses. Licensed combination vaccines may be used whenever any components of the combination are indicated and when the vaccine's other components are not contraindicated. For detailed recommendations on all vaccines, including those used primarily for travelers or that are issued during the year, consult the manufacturers' package inserts and the complete statements from the Advisory Committee on Immunization Practices (www.cdc.gov/vaccines/hcp/acip-recs/index.html). Use of trade names and commercial sources is for identification only and does not imply endorsement by the U.S. Department of Health and Human Services.

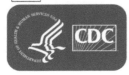

U.S. Department of Health and Human Services
Centers for Disease Control and Prevention

TABLE 3.3 Immunizations (continued)

Footnotes

Recommended Immunization Schedule for Adults Aged 19 Years or Older: United States, 2014

1. **Additional information**
   - Additional guidance for the use of the vaccines described in this supplement is available at www.cdc.gov/vaccines/hcp/acip-recs/index.html.
   - Information on vaccination recommendations when vaccination status is unknown and other general immunization information can be found in the General Recommendations on Immunization at www.cdc.gov/mmwr/preview/mmwrhtml/rr6002a1.htm.
   - Information on travel vaccine requirements and recommendations (e.g., for hepatitis A and B, meningococcal, and other vaccines) is available at http://wwwnc.cdc.gov/travel/destinations/list.
   - Additional information and resources regarding vaccination of pregnant women can be found at http://www.cdc.gov/vaccines/adults/rec-vac/pregnant.html.
2. **Influenza vaccination**
   - Annual vaccination against influenza is recommended for all persons aged 6 months or older.
   - Persons aged 6 months or older, including pregnant women and persons with hives-only allergy to eggs, can receive the inactivated influenza vaccine (IIV). An age-appropriate IIV formulation should be used.
   - Adults aged 18 to 49 years can receive the recombinant influenza vaccine (RIV) (FluBlok). RIV does not contain any egg protein.
   - Healthy, nonpregnant persons aged 2 to 49 years without high-risk medical conditions can receive either intranasally administered live, attenuated influenza vaccine (LAIV) (FluMist), or IIV. Health care personnel who care for severely immunocompromised persons (i.e., those who require care in a protected environment) should receive IIV or RIV rather than LAIV.
   - The intramuscularly or intradermally administered IIV are options for adults aged 18 to 64 years.
   - Adults aged 65 years or older can receive the standard-dose IIV or the high-dose IIV (Fluzone High-Dose).
3. **Tetanus, diphtheria, and acellular pertussis (Td/Tdap) vaccination**
   - Administer 1 dose of Tdap vaccine to pregnant women during each pregnancy (preferred during 27 to 36 weeks' gestation) regardless of interval since prior Td or Tdap vaccination.
   - Persons aged 11 years or older who have not received Tdap vaccine or for whom vaccine status is unknown should receive a dose of Tdap followed by tetanus and diphtheria toxoids (Td) booster doses every 10 years thereafter. Tdap can be administered regardless of interval since the most recent tetanus or diphtheria-toxoid containing vaccine.
   - Adults with an unknown or incomplete history of completing a 3-dose primary vaccination series with Td-containing vaccines should begin or complete a primary vaccination series including a Tdap dose.
   - For unvaccinated adults, administer the first 2 doses at least 4 weeks apart and the third dose 6 to 12 months after the second.
   - For incompletely vaccinated (i.e., less than 3 doses) adults, administer remaining doses.
   - Refer to the ACIP statement for recommendations for administering Td/Tdap as prophylaxis in wound management (see footnote 1).
4. **Varicella vaccination**
   - All adults without evidence of immunity to varicella (as defined below) should receive 2 doses of single-antigen varicella vaccine or a second dose if they have received only 1 dose.
   - Vaccination should be emphasized for those who have close contact with persons at high risk for severe disease (e.g., health care personnel and family contacts of persons with immunocompromising conditions) or are at high risk for exposure or transmission (e.g., teachers; child care employees; residents and staff members of institutional settings, including correctional institutions; college students; military personnel; adolescents and adults living in households with children; nonpregnant women of childbearing age; and international travelers).
   - Pregnant women should be assessed for evidence of varicella immunity. Women who do not have evidence of immunity should receive the first dose of varicella vaccine upon completion or termination of pregnancy and before discharge from the health care facility. The second dose should be administered 4 to 8 weeks after the first dose.
   - Evidence of immunity to varicella in adults includes any of the following:
     — documentation of 2 doses of varicella vaccine at least 4 weeks apart;
     — U.S.-born before 1980, except health care personnel and pregnant women;
     — history of varicella based on diagnosis or verification of varicella disease by a health care provider;
     — history of herpes zoster based on diagnosis or verification of herpes zoster disease by a health care provider; or
     — laboratory evidence of immunity or laboratory confirmation of disease.
5. **Human papillomavirus (HPV) vaccination**
   - Two vaccines are licensed for use in females, bivalent HPV vaccine (HPV2) and quadrivalent HPV vaccine (HPV4), and one HPV vaccine for use in males (HPV4).
   - For females, either HPV4 or HPV2 is recommended in a 3-dose series for routine vaccination at age 11 or 12 years and for those aged 13 through 26 years, if not previously vaccinated.
   - For males, HPV4 is recommended in a 3-dose series for routine vaccination at age 11 or 12 years and for those aged 13 through 21 years, if not previously vaccinated. Males aged 22 through 26 years may be vaccinated.
   - HPV4 is recommended for men who have sex with men through age 26 years for those who did not get any or all doses when they were younger.
   - Vaccination is recommended for immunocompromised persons (including those with HIV infection) through age 26 years for those who did not get any or all doses when they were younger.
   - A complete series for either HPV4 or HPV2 consists of 3 doses. The second dose should be administered 4 to 8 weeks (minimum interval of 4 weeks) after the first dose; the third dose should be administered 24 weeks after the first dose and 16 weeks after the second dose (minimum interval of at least 12 weeks).
   - HPV vaccines are not recommended for use in pregnant women. However, pregnancy testing is not needed before vaccination. If a woman is found to be pregnant after initiating the vaccination series, no intervention is needed; the remainder of the 3-dose series should be delayed until completion of pregnancy.
6. **Zoster vaccination**
   - A single dose of zoster vaccine is recommended for adults aged 60 years or older regardless of whether they report a prior episode of herpes zoster. Although the vaccine is licensed by the U.S. Food and Drug Administration for use among and can be administered to persons aged 50 years or older, ACIP recommends that vaccination begin at age 60 years.
   - Persons aged 60 years or older with chronic medical conditions may be vaccinated unless their condition constitutes a contraindication, such as pregnancy or severe immunodeficiency.
7. **Measles, mumps, rubella (MMR) vaccination**
   - Adults born before 1957 are generally considered immune to measles and mumps. All adults born in 1957 or later should have documentation of 1 or more doses of MMR vaccine unless they have a medical contraindication to the vaccine or laboratory evidence of immunity to each of the three diseases. Documentation of provider-diagnosed disease is not considered acceptable evidence of immunity for measles, mumps, or rubella.

   Measles component:
   - A routine second dose of MMR vaccine, administered a minimum of 28 days after the first dose, is recommended for adults who:
     — are students in postsecondary educational institutions;
     — work in a health care facility; or
     — plan to travel internationally.
   - Persons who received inactivated (killed) measles vaccine or measles vaccine of unknown type during 1963–1967 should be revaccinated with 2 doses of MMR vaccine.

   Mumps component:
   - A routine second dose of MMR vaccine, administered a minimum of 28 days after the first dose, is recommended for adults who:
     — are students in a postsecondary educational institution;
     — work in a health care facility; or
     — plan to travel internationally.
   - Persons vaccinated before 1979 with either killed mumps vaccine or mumps vaccine of unknown type who are at high risk for mumps infection (e.g., persons who are working in a health care facility) should be considered for revaccination with 2 doses of MMR vaccine.

   Rubella component:
   - For women of childbearing age, regardless of birth year, rubella immunity should be determined. If there is no evidence of immunity, women who are not pregnant should be vaccinated. Pregnant women who do not have evidence of immunity should receive MMR vaccine upon completion or termination of pregnancy and before discharge from the health care facility.

   Health care personnel born before 1957:
   - For unvaccinated health care personnel born before 1957 who lack laboratory evidence of measles, mumps, and/or rubella immunity or laboratory confirmation of disease, health care facilities should consider vaccinating personnel with 2 doses of MMR vaccine at the appropriate interval for measles and mumps or 1 dose of MMR vaccine for rubella.
8. **Pneumococcal conjugate (PCV13) vaccination**
   - Adults aged 19 years or older with immunocompromising conditions (including chronic renal failure and nephrotic syndrome), functional or anatomic asplenia, cerebrospinal fluid leaks, or cochlear implants who have not previously received PCV13 or PPSV23 should receive a single dose of PCV13 followed by a dose of PPSV23 at least 8 weeks later.
   - Adults aged 19 years or older with the aforementioned conditions who have previously received 1 or more doses of PPSV23 should receive a dose of PCV13 one or more years after the last PPSV23 dose was received. For adults who require additional doses of PPSV23, the first such dose should be given no sooner than 8 weeks after PCV13 and at least 5 years after the most recent dose of PPSV23.
   - When indicated, PCV13 should be administered to patients who are uncertain of their vaccination status history and have no record of previous vaccination.
   - Although PCV13 is licensed by the U.S. Food and Drug Administration for use among and can be administered to persons aged 50 years or older, ACIP recommends PCV13 for adults aged 19 years or older with the specific medical conditions noted above.
9. **Pneumococcal polysaccharide (PPSV23) vaccination**
   - When PCV13 is also indicated, PCV13 should be given first (see footnote 8).
   - Vaccinate all persons with the following indications:
     — all adults aged 65 years or older;
     — adults younger than 65 years with chronic lung disease (including chronic obstructive pulmonary disease, emphysema, and asthma), chronic cardiovascular diseases, diabetes mellitus, chronic renal failure, nephrotic syndrome, chronic liver disease (including cirrhosis), alcoholism, cochlear implants, cerebrospinal fluid leaks, immunocompromising conditions, and functional or anatomic asplenia (e.g., sickle cell disease and other hemoglobinopathies, congenital or acquired asplenia, splenic dysfunction, or splenectomy [if elective splenectomy is planned, vaccinate at least 2 weeks before surgery]);
     — residents of nursing homes or long-term care facilities; and
     — adults who smoke cigarettes.
   - Persons with immunocompromising conditions and other selected conditions are recommended to receive PCV13 and PPSV23 vaccines. See footnote 8 for information on timing of PCV13 and PPSV23 vaccinations.
   - Persons with asymptomatic or symptomatic HIV infection should be vaccinated as soon as possible after their diagnosis.
   - When cancer chemotherapy or other immunosuppressive therapy is being considered, the interval between vaccination and initiation of immunosuppressive therapy should be at least 2 weeks. Vaccination during chemotherapy or radiation therapy should be avoided.
   - Routine use of PPSV23 vaccine is not recommended for American Indians/Alaska Natives or other persons younger than 65 years unless they have underlying medical conditions that are PPSV23 indications. However, public health authorities may consider recommending PPSV23 for American Indians/Alaska Natives who are living in areas where the risk for invasive pneumococcal disease is increased.
   - When indicated, PPSV23 vaccine should be administered to patients who are uncertain of their vaccination status and have no record of vaccination.
10. **Revaccination with PPSV23**
    - One-time revaccination 5 years after the first dose of PPSV23 is recommended for persons aged 19 through 64 years with chronic renal failure or nephrotic syndrome, functional or anatomic asplenia (e.g., sickle cell disease or splenectomy), or immunocompromising conditions.
    - Persons who received 1 or 2 doses of PPSV23 before age 65 years for any indication should receive another dose of the vaccine at age 65 years or later if at least 5 years have passed since their previous dose.
    - No further doses of PPSV23 are needed for persons vaccinated with PPSV23 at or after age 65 years.
11. **Meningococcal vaccination**
    - Administer 2 doses of quadrivalent meningococcal conjugate vaccine (MenACWY [Menactra, Menveo]) at least 2 months apart to adults of all ages with functional asplenia or persistent complement component deficiencies. HIV infection is not an indication for routine vaccination with MenACWY. If an HIV-infected person of any age is vaccinated, 2 doses of MenACWY should be administered at least 2 months apart.
    - Administer a single dose of meningococcal vaccine to microbiologists routinely exposed to isolates of *Neisseria meningitidis*, military recruits, persons at risk during an outbreak attributable to a vaccine serogroup, and persons who travel to or live in countries in which meningococcal disease is hyperendemic or epidemic.
    - First-year college students up through age 21 years who are living in residence halls should be vaccinated if they have not received a dose on or after their 16th birthday.
    - MenACWY is preferred for adults with any of the preceding indications who are aged 55 years or younger as well as for adults aged 56 years or older who a) were vaccinated previously with MenACWY and are recommended for revaccination, or b) for whom multiple doses are anticipated. Meningococcal polysaccharide vaccine (MPSV4 [Menomune]) is preferred for adults aged 56 years or older who have not received MenACWY previously and who require a single dose only (e.g., travelers).
    - Revaccination with MenACWY every 5 years is recommended for adults previously vaccinated with MenACWY or MPSV4 who remain at increased risk for infection (e.g., adults with anatomic or functional asplenia, persistent complement component deficiencies, or microbiologists).
12. **Hepatitis A vaccination**
    - Vaccinate any person seeking protection from hepatitis A virus (HAV) infection and persons with any of the following indications:
      — men who have sex with men and persons who use injection or non-injection illicit drugs;
      — persons working with HAV-infected primates or with HAV in a research laboratory setting;
      — persons with chronic liver disease and persons who receive clotting factor concentrates;
      — persons traveling to or working in countries that have high or intermediate endemicity of hepatitis A; and
      — unvaccinated persons who anticipate close personal contact (e.g., household or regular babysitting) with an international adoptee during the first 60 days after arrival in the United States from a country with high or intermediate endemicity. (See footnote 1 for more information on travel recommendations.) The first dose of the 2-dose hepatitis A vaccine series should be administered as soon as adoption is planned, ideally 2 or more weeks before the arrival of the adoptee.
    - Single-antigen vaccine formulations should be administered in a 2-dose schedule at either 0 and 6 to 12 months (Havrix), or 0 and 6 to 18 months (Vaqta). If the combined hepatitis A and hepatitis B vaccine (Twinrix) is used, administer 3 doses at 0, 1, and 6 months; alternatively, a 4-dose schedule may be used, administered on days 0, 7, and 21 to 30 followed by a booster dose at month 12.
13. **Hepatitis B vaccination**
    - Vaccinate persons with any of the following indications and any person seeking protection from hepatitis B virus (HBV) infection:
      — sexually active persons who are not in a long-term, mutually monogamous relationship (e.g., persons with more than 1 sex partner during the previous 6 months); persons seeking evaluation or treatment for a sexually transmitted disease (STD); current or recent injection drug users; and men who have sex with men;
      — health care personnel and public safety workers who are potentially exposed to blood or other infectious body fluids;
      — persons with diabetes who are younger than age 60 years as soon as feasible after diagnosis; persons with diabetes who are age 60 years or older at the discretion of the treating clinician based on the likelihood of acquiring HBV infection, including the risk posed by an increased need for assisted blood glucose monitoring in long-term care facilities, the likelihood of experiencing chronic sequelae if infected with HBV, and the likelihood of immune response to vaccination;
      — persons with end-stage renal disease, including patients receiving hemodialysis, persons with HIV infection, and persons with chronic liver disease;
      — household contacts and sex partners of hepatitis B surface antigen–positive persons, clients and staff members of institutions for persons with developmental disabilities, and international travelers to countries with high or intermediate prevalence of chronic HBV infection; and
      — all adults in the following settings: STD treatment facilities, HIV testing and treatment facilities, facilities providing drug abuse treatment and prevention services, health care settings targeting services to injection drug users or men who have sex with men, correctional facilities, end-stage renal disease programs and facilities for chronic hemodialysis patients, and institutions and nonresidential day care facilities for persons with developmental disabilities.
    - Administer missing doses to complete a 3-dose series of hepatitis B vaccine to those persons not vaccinated or not completely vaccinated. The second dose should be administered 1 month after the first dose; the third dose should be given at least 2 months after the second dose (and at least 4 months after the first dose). If the combined hepatitis A and hepatitis B vaccine (Twinrix) is used, give 3 doses at 0, 1, and 6 months; alternatively, a 4-dose Twinrix schedule, administered on days 0, 7, and 21 to 30 followed by a booster dose at month 12 may be used.
    - Adult patients receiving hemodialysis or with other immunocompromising conditions should receive 1 dose of 40 mcg/mL (Recombivax HB) administered on a 3-dose schedule at 0, 1, and 6 months or 2 doses of 20 mcg/mL (Engerix-B) administered simultaneously on a 4-dose schedule at 0, 1, 2, and 6 months.
14. ***Haemophilus influenzae* type b (Hib) vaccination**
    - One dose of Hib vaccine should be administered to persons who have functional or anatomic asplenia or sickle cell disease or are undergoing elective splenectomy if they have not previously received Hib vaccine. Hib vaccination 14 or more days before splenectomy is suggested.
    - Recipients of a hematopoietic stem cell transplant should be vaccinated with a 3-dose regimen 6 to 12 months after a successful transplant, regardless of vaccination history; at least 4 weeks should separate doses.
    - Hib vaccine is not recommended for adults with HIV infection since their risk for Hib infection is low.
15. **Immunocompromising conditions**
    - Inactivated vaccines generally are acceptable (e.g., pneumococcal, meningococcal, and inactivated influenza vaccine) and live vaccines generally are avoided in persons with immune deficiencies or immunocompromising conditions. Information on specific conditions is available at http://www.cdc.gov/vaccines/hcp/acip-recs/index.html.

TABLE 3.4	Levels of Prevention in Action		
	PRIMARY PREVENTION	**SECONDARY PREVENTION**	**TERTIARY PREVENTION**
Childhood	Educate parents about the use of bicycle safety helmets. Educate parents about recognition of the signs of head injury that require health care. In 2012, at least 65% of bicycle deaths were for individuals who were not wearing helmets (IIHS, 2014).	Diagnostic procedures in head injury. X-ray, magnetic resonance imaging (MRI). Treatment of severe head injury. Head injuries are the most serious injury in pedacyclists and are the most frequent cause of death in bicycle crashes (IIHS, 2014).	Rehabilitation following head injuries. May require physical, cognitive, or emotional therapy. Emotional support for the child and family dealing with disability.
Adulthood	Educate adults about the dangers of drinking and driving. Almost one third of traffic-related deaths were caused by alcohol use (CDC, 2013c). Educate adults about the health-related consequences of chronic alcohol, tobacco, and drug use. Educate adults about the importance of using proper safety equipment.	Diagnostic procedures to identify injuries after accidents, such as fractured bones or internal injuries. X-ray, magnetic resonance imaging (MRI). Treatment of injuries by surgical or non-surgical methods. Diagnostic procedures to identify liver or lung diseases, including blood tests, biopsies, and others.	Rehabilitation following major injuries, including physical and occupational therapy. Detoxification methods and smoking cessation programs. Counseling and support groups to prevent relapse.
Older Adulthood	Educate older adults regarding the following: importance of exercise to increase strength and balance; review of medications to determine side effects and interactions; improving home safety, including removal of throw rugs, improved lighting, installation of rails and grab bars; vision examination; importance of continued care for chronic conditions. These actions can reduce or modify risks for falls (CDC, 2013a).	Diagnostic procedures for hip fracture. Treatment of hip fracture. The majority of fractures in older adults are a result of falls, and falls are the leading cause of traumatic brain injury (CDC, 2013a). More than 95% of hip fractures are caused by falls, and one out of five patients dies within a year of their injury (CDC, 2013b).	Rehabilitation following treatment for hip fracture. Education regarding measures to prevent further injury or disability.

The *2008 Physical Activity Guidelines for Americans*, published by the U.S. Department of Health and Human Services (2008), is the first publication of national guidelines for physical activity. Guidelines for physical activity are as follows:

Adults should:

- Engage in moderate intensity physical activities for at least 2 hours and 30 minutes per week or 1 hour and 15 minutes of vigorous intensity aerobic physical activity per week or an equivalent combination of moderate and vigorous intensity aerobic activity. Aerobic activity should occur for at least 10-minute episodes throughout the week.

Children and adolescents (aged 6 to 17) should:

- Do 1 hour or more of physical activity every day.
- Most of the 1 hour or more per day should be either moderate or vigorous intensity aerobic physical activity.
- As part of their 60 or more minutes of daily physical activity, children and adolescents should include muscle-strengthening physical activity on at least 3 days of the week.
- As part of their 60 or more minutes of daily physical activity, children and adolescents should include bone-strengthening physical activity on at least 3 days of the week.

Older adults should:

- Follow the adult guidelines.
- If chronic conditions cause limitations, older adults should be as physically active as abilities allow.
- Avoid inactivity.
- Perform exercises to maintain or improve balance if they are at risk for falls.

The level of intensity of exercise may be measured by use of the metabolic equivalent level (MET). The MET is used to estimate the amount of energy expenditure used during activity. One MET is the amount of energy required for a light intensity activity such as sitting quietly, reading a book, or talking on the phone. The MET increases when the body has to work harder. Moderate intensity activities require 3.0 to 5.9 METs, and vigorous intensity activity requires 6.0 METs or more.

The intensity of an activity can be measured by determining the percent of aerobic capacity reserve being used. In moderate intensity exercise, aerobic capacity reserve is between 45 percent and 64 percent. In vigorous intensity activity, aerobic capacity reserve is between 65 percent and 84 percent. Table 3.5 provides examples of moderate and vigorous intensity activities.

TABLE 3.5	Physical Activities According to Level of Intensity	
MODERATE INTENSITY		**VIGOROUS INTENSITY**

MODERATE INTENSITY

- Walking briskly (3 mph or more)
- Water aerobics
- Bicycling at 5 to 9 mph
- Stationary cycling
- Ballroom dancing
- Tennis doubles
- Golf
- Softball
- Gymnastics
- Calisthenics
- Recreational swimming
- Playing on playground equipment
- Skateboarding
- Dodgeball
- Gardening
- Shoveling light snow
- Moderate housework
- Occupations that require periods of walking, pushing, pulling objects weighing less than 75 lb (maid service, waiting tables, patient care, farming, home building)

VIGOROUS INTENSITY

- Racewalking and aerobic walking at 5 mph or faster
- Jogging
- Running
- Backpacking
- Mountain climbing
- Rollerblading at a brisk pace
- Bicycling at 10 mph or faster
- High-impact aerobic dancing
- Step aerobics
- Boxing in the ring
- Tennis singles
- Karate, tae kwon do
- Competitive sports
- Handball
- Synchronized swimming
- Swimming paced laps
- Skipping
- Jumping rope
- Jumping jacks
- Shoveling heavy snow
- Heavy housework
- Carrying heavy bags of groceries (25 lb or more) up stairs
- Vigorous play with children
- Occupations such as firefighting, masonry, mining, aerobics instructor, professional mover

Exercise may be categorized according to the type of muscle activity and source of energy. Muscle activities are classified as isotonic, isometric, or resistive. Isotonic exercise is also called dynamic exercise. In isotonic exercise, the muscle shortens, producing contraction and active movement. Isotonic exercises increase the tone, strength, and mass of muscles; maintain joint flexibility; and improve circulation. Running, walking, cycling, and ADLs are examples of isotonic exercises.

Isometric exercises include those that affect muscle tension but do not result in muscle or joint movement. Isometric exercise is useful for strengthening abdominal, gluteal, and quadriceps muscles; for maintaining strength of immobilized muscles (for example, following a sprain or fracture); and for endurance training. Isometric exercise refers to exertion of pressure against a solid object. Examples of isometric exercise would include tensing of thigh muscles and extending the arms and pushing against a wall.

Resistive exercise refers to muscle contraction against resistance. Resistive exercise can be isotonic (movement against resistance) or isometric (tension against resistance). An example of resistive exercise is lifting weights to increase the size and strength of pectoral muscles.

Exercises classified according to the source of energy include aerobic and anaerobic. **Aerobic exercise** refers to activity in which oxygen is metabolized to produce energy. Examples of aerobic activity include walking, jogging, swimming, and skating. Aerobic exercise can result in improved cardiovascular function and physical fitness. Guidelines for aerobic activity include exercise of 30 minutes or more on 3 to 5 days of the week at an intensity that produces a heart rate of 220 beats per minute minus the age of the individual. **Anaerobic exercise** refers to activities in which the energy required is provided without using inspired oxygen. Anaerobic activity includes non-endurance training and is generally limited to short periods of vigorous activity, such as weightlifting or sprinting.

Individuals may use two simple methods to assess the intensity of aerobic activity: absolute intensity and relative intensity. Absolute intensity is measured by the amount of energy expended per minute of activity. Light intensity activity requires between 1.1 and 2.9 times the energy expended when at rest. Moderate intensity activity requires between 3.0 and 5.9 times the energy used at rest. Vigorous intensity activity requires 6.0 or more times the energy used at rest.

In contrast, relative intensity measures the amount of effort required to complete an activity. This measure is relative because less fit individuals will require more effort to do the same activity than more fit individuals. The relative intensity scale measures between 0 and 10, with 0 corresponding to sitting still and 10 corresponding to maximum effort. Using this scale, moderate activity is between 5 and 6 whereas vigorous activity is a 7 or higher.

Sexually Transmitted Diseases and HIV

Unprotected sexual activity increases the risk for pregnancy, sexually transmitted diseases (STDs), and infection with the human immunodeficiency virus (HIV). There are more than 25 infectious organisms that are transmitted through sexual activity, including chlamydia, gonorrhea, and syphilis. HIV can be transmitted through sexual activity or injection drug use. STDs diseases can lead to reproductive health problems, fetal and perinatal health problems, cancer, and continued facilitation of disease transmission.

An estimated 19 million new cases of STDs are contracted each year, and this estimate may be low because many cases of STDs go undiagnosed. Almost half of these new cases are in young people aged 15 to 24. Among the new cases of HIV, almost 75 percent occur in men, more than half are in gay and bisexual men, and forty-five percent occur in African Americans. In addition, almost 20 percent of individuals with HIV do not know they have it. Abstinence can ensure complete protection from infection and pregnancy. Correct use of condoms can reduce the incidence of risks associated with sexual activity.

In order to prevent the spread of STDs, *Healthy People 2020* is attempting to understand factors that contribute to the STD transmission. The following factors impact the rate of infection in a population:

- Biological factors such as the asymptomatic nature of STDs, gender and age disparities, and lag time between infection and complications
- Social factors such as racial and ethnic disparities
- Economic factors such as poverty, marginalization, and access to health care
- Behavioral factors such as substance abuse, secrecy associated with sexuality, and connection to risky sexual networks

Objectives of *Healthy People 2020* include reducing the proportion of individuals with chlamydia, human papillomavirus, and genital herpes; increasing chlamydia screenings; reducing the number of females who need treatment for pelvic inflammatory disease; and reducing the transmission of syphilis. For HIV, objectives include reducing HIV transmission among adolescents and adults; reducing new AIDS cases among heterosexuals, homosexuals, and injection drug users; reducing perinatal transmission of HIV; detecting HIV infections before progression to AIDS; increasing survival after AIDS diagnosis; increasing HIV testing for susceptible individuals; and implementing education and prevention programs.

Primary healthcare providers have an active role in screening for behaviors that increase the risk for STDs. Examples of questions to be asked during a health assessment include the following:

- Are you sexually active?
- When was the last time you had sexual activity (oral, vaginal, anal)?
- When you had sexual activity, did you use a condom?

- Do you now have or have you had more than one sexual partner?
- Have you ever been treated for an STD?
- Have you had sexual activity with a partner who uses intravenous drugs?

Healthcare providers are expected to screen for symptoms of STDs during all aspects of health assessment, including the physical assessment. When risks or disease are identified, interventions are developed to treat the illness and to counsel individuals about methods to reduce the transmission of the disease. Additional information about reproductive health is provided in chapters 23 and 24 of this text. ∞ For further information, contact the National Center for HIV/AIDS, Viral Hepatitis, STD, and TB Prevention (NCHHSTP).

Environmental Health

Environmental health is of global significance. Throughout the world, environmental factors contribute to an estimated 24 percent of the disease burden and are a factor in approximately 23 percent of all deaths (Prüss-Üstün & Corvalán, 2006, p. 59).

In the context of health, the World Health Organization (WHO) defines environment as encompassing all of the external biological, chemical, and physical factors that affect an individual, as well as the related behaviors (Prüss-Üstün & Corvalán, 2006, p. 21). *Healthy People 2020* describes environmental health as involving the control or prevention of disease, disability, and injury related to interactions between individuals and their environment. *Healthy People 2020* objectives related to environmental health include (USDHHS, 2013):

- Outdoor air quality
- Surface and ground water quality
- Hazardous wastes and toxic materials
- Residences and communities
- Surveillance and infrastructure
- Global environmental health.

Sleep Health

Sleep is critical to the health and development of infants, toddlers, children, and adolescents. Adults also need adequate sleep to maintain health and wellness, including the ability to fight off infection. Fatigue, irritability, difficulty concentrating, and impatience can all occur when an individual experiences sleeping difficulties or lack of sleep. Poor sleep health is associated with reduced productivity at work or school, increased risk of accidents and injuries, and increased risk for diseases such as heart diseases and diabetes. Requirements for sleep vary across the age span, but recommendations for sleep needs have been developed. These recommendations appear in Table 3.6.

Sleep is affected by aging, lifestyle changes, behavior, and illness. For example, middle-aged and older adults experience sleep disorders including sleep apnea, restless legs syndrome, and nocturia more than younger people. Illnesses such as arthritis, heart disease, respiratory disease, heartburn, and osteoporosis may interrupt or delay sleep. Untreated sleep disorders can decrease the quality of life and contribute to a loss of independence. Medications may affect

TABLE 3.6	**Minimum Sleep Requirements Across the Age Span**

AGE/STAGE	HOURS OF SLEEP*
Infants/Babies	
Newborns	16 to 18 hours
1 to 2 months	10.5 to 18 hours
3 to 11 months	9.5 to 16 hours
Toddlers/Children	
1 to 3 years	12 to 14 hours
3 to 5 years	11 to 13 hours
5 to 10 years	10 to 11 hours
Adolescents	At least 10 hours
Teens	9 to 10 hours
Adults	7 to 9 hours

*Includes naps

Sources: Adapted from National Sleep Foundation. (n.d.a). *Children and sleep.* Retrieved from http://sleepfoundation.org/sleep-topics/children-and-sleep; National Sleep Foundation. (n.d.b). *How much sleep do we really need?* Retrieved from http://www.sleepfoundation.org/article/how-sleep-works/how-much-sleep-do-we-really-need; and Centers for Disease Control and Prevention (CDC). (2013e). *How much sleep do I need?* Retrieved from http://www.cdc.gov/sleep/about_sleep/how_much_sleep.htm

sleep, and mental disorders including depression and anxiety may result in sleep difficulties.

Nurses can use a variety of tools to assist patients to identify sleep problems. These include asking the patient to record a sleep diary and using a list of questions to identify sleep difficulties. These questions include the following:

- Do you snore loudly?
- Have you observed that you stop breathing or gasp for breath during sleep?
- Do you feel drowsy or fall asleep while reading, when watching TV, while driving, or in other daily activities?
- Do you have unpleasant feelings in your legs when trying to sleep?
- Are there interruptions to your sleep (pain, dreams, light, or temperature)?
- Do you have some trouble with sleep on three or more nights a week?

Recommendations for improving sleep include establishing a sleep routine with a regular bedtime and waking time. Other recommendations include (National Sleep Foundation, n.d.b):

- Avoid caffeine.
- Avoid alcohol.
- Get regular exercise.
- Establish a bedtime relaxation routine.
- Create a sleep-conducive environment.

Substance Abuse

The use of alcohol and illicit drugs has been linked with a variety of health problems including accidents, STDs, violence, injury from accidents, and disruptions in families. Alcohol use can also increase the risk of heart and liver diseases. During pregnancy, alcohol use can result in fetal alcohol syndrome. Alcohol abuse is found in individuals of both genders and in all races and nationalities. Approximately 17 million Americans have an alcohol use disorder, which includes both alcoholism and harmful drinking without dependence. In addition, nearly 80,000 people die from alcohol-related causes each year in the United States (National Institute on Alcohol Abuse and Alcoholism, 2014).

The National Institute of Drug Abuse is conducting an ongoing study called *Monitoring the Future* that tracks trends in the prevalence of drug use for 8th-, 10th-, and 12th-graders. For drugs other than marijuana, alcohol, and tobacco, 0.7 to 7.1 percent of 8th to 12th graders have used illicit drugs in their lifetime, 0.4 to 4.0 percent have used some form of drugs in the past year, and 0.1 to 1.5 percent have used some form of drugs in the past month. This includes drugs such as cocaine, heroin, and methamphetamines. Marijuana has the highest percentage of use in young people, with 1.1 to 6.5 percent of 8th to 12th graders using marijuana daily and 16.5 to 45.5 percent using marijuana at least once in their lifetime. In addition, between 10.2 and 39.2 percent of middle and high school students have drunk alcohol in the past month. In general, lifetime, past year, and past month use increases with age for this group of young people (Johnston, O'Malley, Miech, Bachman, & Schulenberg, 2014).

A similar study was performed for individuals aged 12 and older. For drugs other than marijuana, alcohol, and tobacco, individuals aged 18–25 were most likely to have used drugs, with a past-month use ranging from 0.1 to 1.1 percent, depending on the drug. Use of illicit drugs at least once in their life ranged from 1.8 to 14.5 percent, depending on the drug, for all age ranges combined. Similar to middle and high school students, marijuana was the most-used drug for adults, with use in the past month of 18.7 percent for adults aged 18 to 25 and 7.3 percent for all age groups combined. Alcohol use is also prevalent in all age ranges, with 52.1 percent drinking alcohol in the past month (Johnston et al., 2014).

Adolescent abuse of prescription drugs continues to increase (National Institute on Drug Abuse, 2011). Prevention and identification of prescription drug abuse includes screening for abuse and the symptoms associated with substance abuse. Screening for prescription drug abuse is part of the health history in which one asks the patient about prescription and over-the-counter medication use. Specific symptoms of prescription drug abuse can be identified during the health assessment. Healthcare providers must be alert to requests for increasing amounts of medication to relieve symptoms or for frequent refills of prescriptions. Ewing (1984) developed the CAGE questionnaire, which is a useful tool for assessment of alcohol and substance abuse. CAGE is a mnemonic for questions about **C**utting down on drinking, **A**nnoyance with criticism about drinking, **G**uilt about drinking, and using alcohol as an "**E**ye-opener."

Healthy People 2020 goals for the topic of Substance Abuse including reducing the number of adolescents who have ridden with a drunk driver; increasing adolescent disapproval of substance abuse; increasing treatment programs for injection drug use; and reducing complications, injuries, and deaths resulting from drug and alcohol use.

Tobacco Use

Tobacco use is responsible for approximately 443,000 deaths per year in the United States, and almost 9 million people suffer from tobacco-related illnesses. Smoking is a risk factor for heart disease, breathing disorders, and lung cancer. Secondary smoke increases the incidence of asthma and bronchitis in children and heart and lung diseases in adults. Smoking during pregnancy increases the risk for miscarriage, prematurity, and sudden infant death syndrome (SIDS). Use of chewing tobacco and cigar smoking also increase the risk for cancer of the mouth. Adolescent use of tobacco has decreased over the past several years, but between 1.8 and 8.5 percent of 8th to 12th graders still smoke cigarettes daily. Almost half of these smoke at least half a pack of cigarettes per day. In addition, more than 20 percent of individuals aged 12 and over have smoked a cigarette in the past month.

Making a choice to never start smoking and cessation of the use of tobacco products are the only means to prevent the associated risks and problems. Individuals with low income and education are more likely to smoke than those with higher income and education. Men have slightly higher rates of smoking than women. In the United States, Native Americans, Alaska Natives, and military personnel have the highest smoking rates.

Smoking cessation will result in immediate and long-term improvements in health. Assisting patients to stop smoking is a role of the healthcare professional to promote wellness. Guidelines for clinicians have been developed and recommend assessment in relation to smoking and the desire to stop smoking. For smokers willing to stop, the guidelines include five A's for use by healthcare providers: ask, advise, assess, assist, and arrange. These five A's are implemented as follows:

1. Ask about smoking at every health visit.
2. Advise (that is, urge) all smokers to stop.
3. Assess the patient's willingness to stop.
4. Assist or aid the patient in quitting. Work with the patient to develop a plan to quit while providing counseling, recommending pharmacotherapy, and providing resource materials.
5. Arrange for follow-up to determine progress or the need for further assistance (Agency for Healthcare Research and Quality [AHRQ], 2012).

Consumer information about nicotine addiction, difficulties involved with smoking cessation, benefits of smoking cessation, and steps for quitting are provided through the BeTobaccoFree.gov website, which was launched by the USDHHS in 2012 (USDHHS, 2014a). The guidelines include the key steps of preparing, obtaining support, acquiring new skills and behaviors, obtaining and using medications correctly, and preparing for difficulties. Information about clinician and consumer guidelines for smoking cessation and about tobacco use is available through the USDHHS.

Health Promotion and the Nursing Process

The nurse works with the patient as the nursing process is applied in problem identification. The process continues through the development and implementation of the plans for care and is completed when the nurse and patient evaluate the outcomes.

Box 3.1 Areas of Assessment in Health Risk Appraisal

- Demographic information (age, gender, height, weight)
- Type and amount of exercise
- Occupation
- Smoking
- Twenty-four-hour dietary history
- Family history of heart disease, diabetes, cancer
- History of screening tests according to gender and age (mammography, prostatic specific antigen [PSA] test)
- Oral hygiene and dental care history
- Immunization history
- Personal history of illness
- Safety measures (seat belt, sunscreen, condom)
- Sexual activity and reproductive history
- Use of alcohol, illicit drugs, prescription drugs
- Emotional state or mood

Assessment

Comprehensive assessment is essential to health promotion. Through the health history and physical assessment, the nurse gathers information about the patient's current health status, risk factors, and predisposing factors associated with specific diseases. These risk factors are revealed through data about age, gender, race, and family history. The physical findings yield information including height, weight, and vital signs, and data about behaviors and practices. Additional assessments are conducted in relation to health promotion. These include physical fitness, nutritional status, a health risk appraisal, lifestyle inventories, assessment of current stressors, and stress management strategies. Social structure assessments include family and support systems, level of education, income, roles, and other activities. Areas included in most health risk appraisals are presented in Box 3.1. Information about health assessment tools is available through the National Center for Chronic Disease Prevention and Health Promotion (NCCD-PHP). Instructions for patient self-assessment are available in written form, in English and Spanish, and online through organizations such as the American Diabetes Association and the American Heart Association. The CDC has established the Behavioral Risk Factor Surveillance System Survey. Tools to assess risk, lifestyle, and stress include Lifescan, Health Risk Appraisal, Live Well, Wellness Appraisal, and Stress Assess.

Plan Development

Once data are gathered, the professional nurse works with the patient to identify current, ongoing, or potential problems. Diagnoses are established and include problems and strengths. For example, problems may include obesity and smoking. A patient's strength could be identified as physical fitness. Then goals and priorities are established to develop a plan to meet the needs of the patient.

Roles of the Professional Nurse

In implementing the plan, the nurse takes on the roles of educator, counselor, facilitator, nurturer, and role model. As educator, the nurse interprets and informs the patient of the significance of findings from all of the completed assessments. Education then may consist of one-on-one sessions related to specific aspects of care or preventive measures as dictated by need. The nurse provides education about specific problems, risks, treatments, or behaviors and may have to provide education about resources available to meet the needs of the patient and family.

As a counselor, the nurse creates and plans opportunities to discuss the implementation of specific activities and to review progress in behavior change or in goal attainment. The counseling role can occur in one-on-one sessions or with groups of patients involved in the same treatment, prevention, or promotion activity. In the facilitator role, the nurse may meet with the patient's family to provide information, to encourage their participation with the patient in health-related activities, or to promote family support for the patient. As a facilitator, the nurse helps the patient and family gain access to services and facilities required to meet the identified health needs.

The nurturing role of the nurse includes providing the types and amounts of support and encouragement that will assist patients to meet their health-related goals. The nurturing role is particularly important when a patient is attempting to change or modify a behavior. Lastly, the nurse models wellness and health-promoting behaviors and is willing to share experiences and difficulties in developing plans or meeting goals for healthy behaviors and lifestyles. Additionally, the nurse will identify individuals within the same culture or community who have experienced similar problems or have similar goals in relation to health promotion and wellness with whom the patient can interact and relate to as a model.

The nurse and patient are involved in continual evaluation of progress in meeting goals. The evaluation process provides opportunities to address concerns. During evaluation, the patient has the opportunity to modify, continue, or discontinue the plan. As a result of evaluation, priorities may be reordered or the methods and tactics may be changed.

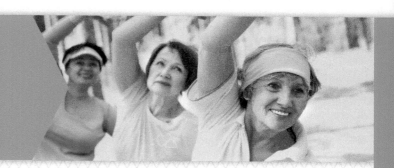

Application Through Critical Thinking

▌ Case Study

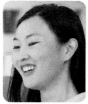

You are participating in a health fair performing wellness screening. Gina Clark, a 22-year-old female, approaches your table. She states that she is interested in seeing how healthy her habits are and wants to learn what suggestions you have to help her feel better about her health. Your screening findings show a blood pressure of 132/83, pulse 88, respirations 18, temperature 98.2°F, height 5 ft 4 in., and weight 190.

Gina reports that she drinks a lot of soda and eats fast food several times each week. She does not like vegetables and tends to "snack" a lot rather than sitting down for prepared meals. She states that she would like to eat better and exercise, but she never seems to find the time. She had joined a gym with a friend about a month ago but stopped going after 2 weeks when she became frustrated with sore muscles and lack of results. She would like to lose about 60 pounds and is interested in information on how to accomplish this goal. She tells you that because she is self-conscious about her weight, she does not socialize much or go out with friends. Her weight, she says, makes her feel uncomfortable. She slowly leans forward and quietly tells you that she is "repulsed" by her body and does not ever want to look in a mirror or have a picture taken. She indicates that whenever she is stressed about something, she tends to eat even more. "It is like a vicious cycle. I don't know what to do."

▌ Critical Thinking Questions

1. Describe the importance of wellness in comprehensive health assessment.

2. Where does the patient see herself on the health-illness continuum?

3. What information is appropriate to share with Gina regarding healthy weight loss?

4. What guidelines around physical activity should you share with Gina?

5. How does the Theory of Reasoned Action/Planned Behavior relate to Gina's situation and her intent to exercise?

References

Agency for Healthcare Research and Quality (AHRQ). (2012). *Five major steps to intervention (The "5 A's")*. Retrieved from http://www.ahrq.gov/professionals/clinicians-providers/guidelines-recommendations/tobacco/5steps.html

Anderson, A. (2014). *The impact of the Affordable Care Act on the health care work force*. Retrieved from http://www.heritage.org/research/reports/2014/03/the-impact-of-the-affordable-care-act-on-the-health-care-workforce

Becker, M. H. (Ed.). (1974). *Historical origins of the health belief model. The health belief model and personal health behavior*. Thorofare, NJ: Charles B. Slack.

Berman, A., Snyder, S. J., Kozier, B., & Erb, G. (2011). *Kozier and Erb's fundamentals of nursing: Concepts, process and practice* (9th ed.). Upper Saddle River, NJ: Prentice Hall.

Centers for Disease Control and Prevention (CDC). (2009). Cigarette smoking among adults and trends in smoking cessation—United States, 2008. *MMWR Weekly, 58*(44), 1227–1232.

Centers for Disease Control and Prevention (CDC). (2013a). *Home and recreational safety. Falls among older adults: An overview*. Retrieved from http://www.cdc.gov/homeandrecreationalsafety/falls/adultfalls.html

Centers for Disease Control and Prevention (CDC). (2013b). *Home and recreational safety. Hip fractures among older adults*. Retrieved from http://www.cdc.gov/HomeandRecreationalSafety/Falls/adulthipfx.html

Centers for Disease Control and Prevention (CDC). (2013c). *Impaired driving: Get the facts*. Retrieved from http://www.cdc.gov/motorvehiclesafety/impaired_driving/impaired-drv_factsheet.html

Centers for Disease Control and Prevention (CDC). (2013d). *Overweight and obesity: Adult obesity facts*. Retrieved from http://www.cdc.gov/obesity/data/adult.html

Centers for Disease Control and Prevention (CDC). (2013e). *How much sleep do I need?* Retrieved from http://www.cdc.gov/sleep/about_sleep/how_much_sleep.htm

Centers for Disease Control and Prevention (CDC). (2014a). *Overweight and obesity: Childhood obesity facts*. Retrieved from http://www.cdc.gov/obesity/data/childhood.html

Centers for Disease Control and Prevention (CDC). (2014b). *Violence prevention*. Retrieved from http://www.cdc.gov/violenceprevention/

Dunn, H. (1973). *High level wellness*. Arlington, VA: R. W. Beatty.

Edelman, C. L., Mandel, C. L., & Kudzma, E. C. (2014). *Health promotion throughout the life span* (8th ed.). St. Louis, MO: Mosby.

Ewing, J. A. (1984). Detecting alcoholism: The CAGE questionnaire. *Journal of the American Medical Association, 252*, 1905–1907.

Glanz, K., & Kegler, M. C. (n.d.). *Environments: Theory, research and measures of the built environment*. Retrieved from http://cancercontrol.cancer.gov/BRP/constructs/environment/environment.pdf

Hattie, J. A., Myers, J. E., & Sweeney, T. J. (2004). A factor structure of wellness: Theory, assessment, analysis, and practice. *Journal of Counseling & Development, 82*(3), 354–364.

Health promotion models [Special issue]. (2000). *International Electronic Journal of Health Education, 3*, 180–193.

Hyner, G. C., Peterson, K. W., Travis, J. W., Dewey, J. E., Foerster, J. J., & Framer, E. M. (Eds.). (1999). *SPM handbook of health assessment tools*. Pittsburgh, PA: The Society of Prospective Medicine & The Institute for Health and Productivity Management.

Insurance Institute for Highway Safety (IIHS). (2014). *Pedestrians and bicyclists*. Retrieved from http://www.iihs.org/iihs/topics/t/pedestrians-and-bicyclists/fatalityfacts/bicycles

Johnston, L. D., O'Malley, P. M., Miech, R. A., Bachman, J. G., & Schulenberg, J. E. (2014). *Monitoring the future—National survey results on drug use 1975–2013: Overview, key findings on adolescent drug use*. Ann Arbor, MI: Institute for Social Research, University of Michigan.

Leavell, H. C., & Clark, E. G. (1965). *Preventive medicine for the doctor in his community* (3rd ed.). New York: McGraw-Hill.

Murray, R. B., & Zentner, J. P. (2009). *Health assessment and promotion strategies through the life span* (8th ed.). Upper Saddle River, NJ: Prentice Hall.

National Cancer Institute. (2013). *Prevention and cessation of cigarette smoking: Control of tobacco use*. Retrieved February 24, 2014, from http://www.cancer.gov/cancertopics/pdq/prevention/control-of-tobacco-use/HealthProfessional

National Center for Health Statistics. (2013). *Health United States, 2012*. Retrieved February 24, 2014, from http://www.cdc.gov/nchs/hus.htm

National Institute on Alcohol Abuse and Alcoholism. (2014). *Alcohol facts and statistics*. Retrieved from http://www.niaaa.nih.gov/alcohol-health/overview-alcohol-consumption/alcohol-facts-and-statistics

National Institute on Drug Abuse. (2011). *Research report series—Prescription drugs: Abuse and addiction*. Retrieved from http://www.drugabuse.gov/publications/research-reports/prescription-drugs#Trends

National Sleep Foundation. (n.d.a). *Children and sleep*. Retrieved from http://sleepfoundation.org/sleep-topics/children-and-sleep

National Sleep Foundation. (n.d.b). *How much sleep do we really need?* Retrieved from http://www.sleepfoundation.org/article/how-sleep-works/how-much-sleep-do-we-really-need

Newsome, D., Moore, S. A., & Dowling, R. K. (2013). *Natural area tourism: Ecology, impacts and management* (2nd ed.). Ontario, Canada: Channel View Publications.

Pender, N. J., Murdaugh, C. L., & Parsons, M. A. (2011). *Health promotion in nursing practice* (6th ed.). Upper Saddle River, NJ: Prentice Hall.

Prüss-Üstün, A., & Corvalán, C. (2006). *Preventing disease through healthy environments: Towards an estimate of the environmental burdens of disease*. Geneva, Switzerland: World Health Organization (WHO).

Rosenstock, I. M. (1974). Historical origins of the health belief model. In M. H. Becker (Ed.), *The health belief model and personal health behavior*. Thorofare, NJ: Charles B. Slack.

United States Department of Health and Human Services (USDHHS). (2008). *2008 Physical Activity Guidelines for Americans*. Retrieved from http://www.health.gov/paguidelines/pdf/paguide.pdf

United States Department of Health and Human Services (USDHHS). (2011). *The Surgeon General's Call to Action to Support Breastfeeding*. Rockville, MD: U.S. Department of Health and Human Services, Office of the Surgeon General.

United States Department of Health and Human Services (USDHHS). (2013). *Healthy people 2020*. Retrieved from http://www.healthypeople.gov/2020/default.aspx

United States Department of Health and Human Services (USDHHS). (2014a). *BeTobaccoFree.gov*. Retrieved from http://betobaccofree.hhs.gov/index.html

United States Department of Health and Human Services (USDHHS). (2014b). *smokefree.gov*. Retrieved February 24, 2014, from http://smokefree.gov/

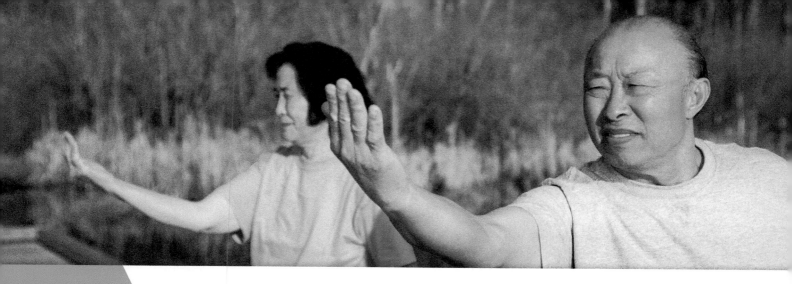

Cultural Considerations

▶ Learning Outcomes

Upon completion of this chapter, you will be able to:

1. Examine the components included in the definition of culture.

2. Practice using terms related to culture.

3. Describe the impact of cultural phenomena on health and wellness.

4. Demonstrate culturally sensitive methods of communication when interacting with patients.

5. Formulate strategies to promote cultural competence when assessing patients from specific cultural groups.

Key Terms

The United States is made up of people of many races, ethnicities, religions, and heritages. It is expected that the diversity in the United States will continue to expand throughout this century. In 2012, the United States Census Bureau predicted that by 2060 the Asian population will have increased from 5% to 8%, African Americans from 13% to 15%, and the Hispanic groups from 17% to 31% of the total U.S. population (U.S. Census Bureau, 2012).

An individual's culture, race, and ethnicity impact beliefs about health and illness and the practices related to both. The nurse must gain knowledge of several cultures, although it is not possible to completely understand all of them. The nurse must continue to learn about other cultures and bring acknowledgment of personal cultural beliefs and values to each nurse-patient encounter.

According to the American Nurses Association (ANA) (1991), knowledge of cultural diversity is vital in all areas of practice. This knowledge can strengthen the delivery of health care. Nurses need to understand how cultural groups perceive life processes, define health and illness, maintain health, determine the causes of illness, and provide care and cure. It is also important to understand the ways in which the nurse's cultural background influences care. When nurses understand cultural diversity, apply cultural knowledge, and act in culturally competent ways, they can be more effective in assessing patients, developing culturally sensitive interventions, and influencing healthcare policy and practice.

Culture

The National Institutes of Health (NIH) describes **culture** as a combination of knowledge, beliefs, and behaviors that often are specific to racial, ethnic, geographic, social, or religious groups (NIH, 2013). Culture includes a variety of nonphysical traits that are learned from families by way of socialization (Spector, 2013). Examples of cultural elements may include the following:

- Personal identification
- Language
- Communications
- Thoughts
- Actions
- Beliefs
- Customs
- Values
- Institutions (NIH, 2013)

Culture frames an individual's perception of health and illness. Culture also influences how healthcare information is received, how rights and protections are exercised, what is considered to be a health problem, how symptoms are perceived, and the type of treatment to be provided. Culture is learned generally within the family group, is shared by the majority within the culture, and changes in response to interactions with events in the external environment (see Figure 4.1 ■). Culture has also been identified as the way a population or group finds a shared meaning for information.

Culture may be divided into material and nonmaterial culture. Objects such as dress, art, utensils, and tools and the ways they are used are components of the *material culture. Nonmaterial culture* is composed of the verbal and nonverbal language, beliefs, customs, and

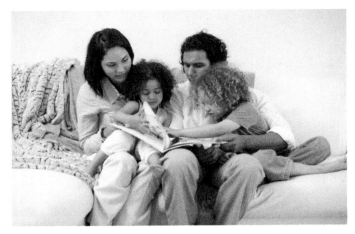

Figure 4.1 Nuclear family interaction.
Source: Wavebrakmedia/Shutterstock.

social structures. Cultures may be further defined as *macrocultures*, that is, national, racial, or ethnic groups within which *microcultures* exist based on age, gender, or religious affiliation. **Subcultures** exist within larger cultural groups. Subcultures are composed of individuals who have a distinct identity based on occupation, membership in a social group, or heritage. For example, professional nurses are a subculture within the larger culture of healthcare professionals and further are part of the larger American culture (see Figure 4.2 ■). Many individuals refer to themselves according to an ethnic origin, such as Italian American, Greek American, or Arab American. These individuals form associations with others of the same ethnic origin to form a subculture within the larger American culture.

Generational subcultures also exist. At present, the impact of this phenomenon is highlighted in the workplace setting as, for the first time in United States history, individuals from four generations are working side-by-side. While diversity in knowledge and experience can be beneficial, generational differences also may create significant sources of miscommunication and conflict. The four generations are categorized as follows:

- Veterans: Born before 1946
- Baby boomers: Born 1946–1964
- Generation X: Born 1965–1981
- Generation Y: Born 1982–2000 (Reynolds, Bush, & Geist, 2008).

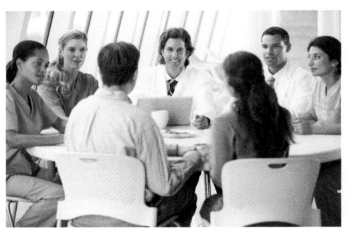

Figure 4.2 Diversity within the subculture of nursing.
Source: Monkey Business/Fotalia.

Each generation differs with regard to numerous aspects of workplace behaviors and attitudes, including views about authority, preferences regarding communication style, and knowledge of computer technology (Reynolds et al., 2008). For the nurse, the dynamic of generational subcultures is relevant both to interactions with other healthcare team members and to nurse-patient relationships.

Terms Related to Culture

The terms *culture, race,* and *ethnicity* are often used synonymously. However, these terms refer to different aspects and characteristics of populations and groups of people. These terms and others related to culture are defined in the following sections.

Race

Race refers to the identification of an individual or group by shared genetic heritage and biologic or physical characteristics. Members of a given race have similarities in skin color, skeletal structure, texture of the hair, and facial features. Knowledge of the differences in racial characteristics is significant in health assessment since findings are interpreted according to norms for age, gender, and race. However, gene pools are becoming increasingly diverse. Skin color is not always a clear indication of racial identity. For example, dark-skinned individuals from Pakistan, Bangladesh, and parts of India are Caucasian by race. Additionally, racial blending is increasingly common in the United States. Many individuals identify themselves as biracial or multiracial. Definitions of minority racial and ethnic populations in the United States are provided by the Office of Minority Health (OMH). In 2010, the United States Census Bureau identified the following categories of race:

- Hispanic, Latino, or Spanish origin
- Black or African American
- American Indian and Alaska Native
- Asian
- Native Hawaiian and Other Pacific Islander
- White (Humes, Jones, & Ramirez, 2011)

Heritage

According to the UMass Amherst Center for Heritage and Society (n.d.), **heritage** is defined as "the full range of our inherited traditions, monuments, objects, and culture. Most important, it is the range of contemporary activities, meanings, and behaviors that we draw from them." **Heritage consistency** describes the extent to which one's lifestyle reflects one's traditional heritage, as well as the degree to which the individual identifies with his traditional heritage. **Heritage inconsistency** describes the adoption and implementation of beliefs and practices obtained by way of acculturation into a dominant or host culture (Spector, 2013; Berman & Snyder, 2012). See Box 4.1 for an example of a heritage assessment tool.

Ethnicity

The term *ethnic* refers to a group of people who share a common culture and who belong to a specific group. Ethnic groups are those with common social and cultural values over generations. **Ethnicity** is the awareness of belonging to a group in which certain characteristics or aspects such as culture and biology differentiate the members of one group from another. Ethnicity is defined by shared interest, ethnic heritage, religion, food, politics, or geography and nationality.

Ethnicity incorporates internal and external identification with a group. Internal identification means that one considers oneself a member of an ethnic group. For example, one may identify oneself as Arab, African, French, Irish, Italian, or Jamaican American. External identification means that those outside of the group perceive the person as a group member.

However, while "Asian American" is a recognized ethnic group, one must be aware that national origin is often a more important component of ethnicity. As a result, Asian Americans are likely to identify themselves, for example, as Japanese, Filipino, Vietnamese, Chinese, or Samoan.

In the United States, ethnicity is often demonstrated by participation in groups that promote the heritage or traditions of the group. For example, Emerald Societies exist to promote Irish heritage; Italian American social groups promote bonds for those of Italian ancestry.

Ethnicity refers to the degree of attachment with ancestral groups, heritage, or place of birth. Some ethnic identities such as Polish or Syrian are traced to locations in which ancestors were born outside of the United States. Ethnic groups such as Cajuns or Pennsylvania Dutch evolved from geographic regions within the United States.

Ethnocentrism is the tendency to believe that one's own beliefs, way of life, values, and customs are superior to those of others. Ethnocentrism creates the belief that one's own customs and values are the standard for judging the values, customs, and practices of others. Ethnocentrism can interfere with collection and interpretation of data as well as the development of plans of care to meet patient needs. Awareness of one's own cultural beliefs, values, and biases can reduce ethnocentrism and foster culturally competent care.

Diversity

Diversity is defined as the state of being different. Diversity occurs between and within cultural groups. Characteristics of diversity include nationality, race, color, gender, age, and religion. In addition, diversity is established by socioeconomic status, education, occupation, residence in urban versus suburban or rural areas, marital status, parental status, sexual orientation, and the time spent away from one's country of origin.

For example, Arab Americans are considered a cultural group in the United States. They share tradition as descendants of tribes of the Arabian Peninsula and share Arabic as a common language. However, diversity within this group is characterized by differences in religion, occupation, geography, and period of immigration to the United States. Many of the early Arab immigrants were from Libya and Syria, and identified themselves as Christians. However, because Muslims were forbidden to emigrate, fear of deportation may have influenced their recorded statement of religious faith. These immigrants came to the United States seeking economic opportunity (Abdelhady, 2014). Later immigrants settled in urban areas of the northeastern United States and for the most part were self-employed or in managerial and professional occupations. In contrast, Arab immigrants after World War II were and continue to be predominantly refugees from nations undergoing political strife.

Box 4.1 Heritage Assessment

1. Where was your mother born? _____
2. Where was your father born? _____
3. Where were your grandparents born? _____
   A. Your mother's mother? _____
   B. Your mother's father? _____
   C. Your father's mother? _____
   D. Your father's father? _____
4. How many brothers _____ and sisters _____ do you have?
5. What setting did you grow up in? Urban _____ Rural _____
6. What country did your parents grow up in?
   Father _____
   Mother _____
7. How old were you when you came to the United States? _____
8. How old were your parents when they came to the United States?
   Mother _____
   Father _____
9. When you were growing up, who lived with you? _____
10. Have you maintained contact with
    A. Aunts, uncles, cousins? (1) Yes _____ (2) No _____
    B. Brothers and sisters? (1) Yes _____ (2) No _____
    C. Parents? (1) Yes _____ (2) No _____
    D. Your own children? (1) Yes _____ (2) No _____
11. Did most of your aunts, uncles, and cousins live near your home?
    1. Yes _____
    2. No _____
12. Approximately how often did you visit family members who lived outside of your home?
    1. Daily _____
    2. Weekly _____
    3. Monthly _____
    4. Once a year or less _____
    5. Never _____
13. Was your original family name changed?
    1. Yes _____
    2. No _____
14. What is your religious preference?
    1. Catholic _____
    2. Jewish _____
    3. Protestant _____ Denomination _____
    4. Other _____
    5. None _____
15. Is your spouse the same religion as you?
    1. Yes _____
    2. No _____

16. Is your spouse the same ethnic background as you?
    1. Yes _____
    2. No _____
17. What kind of school did you go to?
    1. Public _____
    2. Private _____
    3. Parochial _____
18. As an adult, do you live in a neighborhood where the neighbors are the same religion and ethnic background as you?
    1. Yes _____
    2. No _____
19. Do you belong to a religious institution?
    1. Yes _____
    2. No _____
20. Would you describe yourself as an active member?
    1. Yes _____
    2. No _____
21. How often do you attend your religious institution?
    1. More than once a week _____
    2. Weekly _____
    3. Monthly _____
    4. Special holidays only _____
    5. Never _____
22. Do you practice religion in your home?
    1. Yes _____ (if yes, please specify by checking activities below)
    2. No _____
    3. Praying _____
    4. Bible reading _____
    5. Diet _____
    6. Celebrating religious holidays _____
    7. Other _____
23. Do you prepare foods special to your ethnic background?
    1. Yes _____
    2. No _____
24. Do you participate in ethnic activities?
    1. Yes _____ (if yes, please specify by checking activities below)
    2. No _____
    3. Singing _____
    4. Holiday celebrations _____
    5. Dancing _____
    6. Festivals _____
    7. Costumes _____
    8. Other _____
25. Are your friends from the same religious background as you?
    1. Yes _____
    2. No _____

Box 4.1 Heritage Assessment (continued)

26. Are your friends from the same ethnic background as you?

    1. Yes _____

    2. No _____

27. What is your native language other than English?

    _____

28. Do you speak this language?

    1. Prefer _____

    2. Occasionally _____

    3. Rarely _____

29. Do you read your native language?

    1. Yes _____

    2. No _____

Source: Spector, R. E. (2013). *Cultural diversity in health and illness* (8th ed.). Upper Saddle River, NJ: Prentice Hall.

These were mainly followers of the Islamic religion who settled in the Midwestern and western United States and maintained strong ethnic ties to the nations from which they emigrated, including Palestine, Iraq, Lebanon, and Egypt. Many Arab immigrants sought educational degrees or were professionals who remained in the United States.

Acculturation

Acculturation refers to the process of adaptation and change that occurs when members of different cultures are exposed to one another (Berry, 2003). When the host group has the most power, the host group usually applies its power to influence change among incoming cultural groups (Spector, 2013). In contrast to this unidirectional change, acculturation also may produce bidirectional change, in which the dominant and nondominant cultural groups effect changes on one another (Smokowski, David-Ferdon, & Stroupe, 2009).

Assimilation

Assimilation refers to the adoption and incorporation of characteristics, customs, and values of the dominant culture by those new to that culture. Assimilation is unidirectional in nature (Smokowski et al., 2009). For example, immigrants to the United States may assimilate over time and adopt the values of one culture over another. The assimilation process occurs more easily for those who have willingly emigrated from their native land.

Assimilation is affected by several factors including beliefs, language, age, and geography. Those who hold similar values and speak the language of the adopted country more easily assimilate. Assimilation occurs more easily in second-generation immigrants. For example, children born to Chinese parents in Western countries adopt Western culture easily, while parents tend to maintain the traditional culture. Chinese Americans living in "Chinatown" districts in cities on the East and West Coasts of the United States are more likely to maintain much of their traditional Chinese cultural practices and beliefs.

Slow assimilation has occurred in the Cuban American population. Cuban Americans have established enclaves in Miami, Florida, and Union City, New Jersey. In these enclaves, Spanish remains the predominant language in the home and in many of the workplaces. The slow assimilation to English, as well as the isolation within Cuban communities, results in strong ethnic identity and some degree of insulation from the prevailing American culture.

Cultural Competence

Cultural competence refers to the capacity of nurses or health service delivery systems to effectively understand and plan for the needs of a culturally diverse patient or group. Spector (2013) views cultural competence as a complex combination of knowledge, attitudes, and skills used by the healthcare provider to deliver services that attend to the total context of the patient's situation across cultural boundaries. The development of cultural competence is essential to nursing. Because cultural competence develops over time through knowledge acquisition and experience, the key to developing cultural competence is to be sensitive to each patient's culture even if you are initially unfamiliar with their specific cultural beliefs. Incorporating the patient's cultural values, beliefs, customs, and practices improves the nurse's ability to gather and interpret data and to plan care appropriate to meet the needs of diverse patients.

A key goal in the *Healthy People* initiatives is to eliminate health disparities. Objectives related to improving access to health care include increasing the number of individuals who have health insurance, increasing the number of available healthcare providers, and improving access to pre-hospital medical services for all individuals in the United States (U.S. Department of Health and Human Services [USDHHS], 2010). See Table 4.1.

Another effort to eliminate disparities is the development of culturally and linguistically appropriate standards (CLAS). First published in 2000 by the Office of Minority Health (OMH), the CLAS standards were updated in 2010. As described in Box 4.2, the CLAS standards are intended to correct current inequities and promote cultural competence in meeting the needs of racial, ethnic, and linguistic populations that experience unequal access to health care.

TABLE 4.1 **Examples of *Healthy People 2020* Objectives Related to Access to Health Services**

OBJECTIVE NUMBER	DESCRIPTION
AHS-1	Increase the proportion of persons with health insurance
AHS-2	(Developmental) Increase the proportion of insured persons with coverage for clinical preventive services
AHS-3	Increase the proportion of persons with a usual primary care provider
AHS-4	(Developmental) Increase the number of practicing primary care providers
AHS-5	Increase the proportion of persons who have a specific source of ongoing care
AHS-6	Reduce the proportion of persons who are unable to obtain or delay in obtaining necessary medical care, dental care, or prescription medicines
AHS-7	(Developmental) Increase the proportion of persons who receive appropriate evidence-based clinical preventive services
AHS-8	(Developmental) Increase the proportion of persons who have access to rapidly responding prehospital emergency medical services
AHS-9	(Developmental) Reduce the proportion of hospital emergency department visits in which the wait time to see an emergency department clinician exceeds the recommended time frame

Source: U.S. Department of Health and Human Services (USDHHS). (2014). *Healthy People 2020*. Retrieved from http://www.healthypeople.gov/2020/default.aspx

---

Box 4.2 National Standards for Culturally and Linguistically Appropriate Services in Health Care

Principal Standard

1. Provide effective, equitable, understandable, and respectful quality care and services that are responsive to diverse cultural health beliefs and practices, preferred languages, health literacy, and other communication needs.

Governance, Leadership and Workforce:

2. Advance and sustain organizational governance and leadership that promotes CLAS and health equity through policy, practices, and allocated resources.

3. Recruit, promote, and support a culturally and linguistically diverse governance, leadership, and workforce that are responsive to the population in the service area.

4. Educate and train governance, leadership, and workforce in culturally and linguistically appropriate policies and practices on an ongoing basis.

Communication and Language Assistance:

5. Offer language assistance to individuals who have limited English proficiency and/or other communication needs, at no cost to them, to facilitate timely access to all health care and services.

6. Inform all individuals of the availability of language assistance services clearly and in their preferred language, verbally and in writing.

7. Ensure the competence of individuals providing language assistance, recognizing that the use of untrained individuals and/or minors as interpreters should be avoided.

8. Provide easy-to-understand print and multimedia materials and signage in the languages commonly used by the populations in the service area.

Engagement, Continuous Improvement and Accountability:

9. Establish culturally and linguistically appropriate goals, policies, and management accountability, and infuse them throughout the organization's planning and operations.

10. Conduct ongoing assessments of the organization's CLAS-related activities and integrate CLAS-related measures into measurement and continuous quality improvement activities.

11. Collect and maintain accurate and reliable demographic data to monitor and evaluate the impact of CLAS on health equity and outcomes and to inform service delivery.

12. Conduct regular assessments of community health assets and needs and use the results to plan and implement services that respond to the cultural and linguistic diversity of populations in the service area.

13. Partner with the community to design, implement, and evaluate policies, practices, and services to ensure cultural and linguistic appropriateness.

14. Create conflict and grievance resolution processes that are culturally and linguistically appropriate to identify, prevent, and resolve conflicts or complaints.

15. Communicate the organization's progress in implementing and sustaining CLAS to all stakeholders, constituents, and the general public.

Source: Office of Minority Health (OMH). (2013). *The National CLAS standards.* Retrieved from http://minorityhealth.hhs.gov/templates/browse.aspx?lvl=2&lvlID=15

Cultural Phenomena That Impact Health Care

Culture and heritage influence an individual's perceptions about internal and external factors that contribute to health or cause illness as well as the practices the individual follows to prevent and treat health problems. For example, Mexicans believe that health is largely God's will and is maintained by practices that keep the body in balance. Mexicans also believe that many diseases are caused by disturbance in the hot and cold balance of the body (Spector, 2013). Navajo Indians believe that health is related to achieving harmony with nature. Illness is explained as disruption in harmony, which is caused by some acts on the part of the ill person or by having a curse placed on the person. Navajos seek the care of a healer or "medicine man" to determine what the individual has done to disrupt harmony and to restore harmony through a healing ceremony (Spector, 2013). Mexicans may eat foods that oppose the diseases associated with hot and cold imbalances (Spector, 2013). Cold foods such as fruit, barley, fish, and vegetables are eaten to combat hot diseases that include infections and kidney diseases.

In the United States and in many Westernized countries, beliefs about health and illness are derived from a scientific approach. The scientific approach includes "germ theory" as applied in infectious diseases; knowledge of changes in body structures and functions associated with aging including arthritis, menopause, and vision changes; and the understanding that diet and lifestyle choices influence health and illness. Health practices include seeking health care from healthcare providers who use scientific methods to diagnose and treat illness. Healthcare practices include following recommendations for disease prevention such as screening for risks, screening for early detection of problems, and immunization.

Two factors have influenced perceptions of health and healthcare practices in the United States. The first factor is that people of all nations continue to immigrate to the United States. As a result, the beliefs and practices of these individuals, families, and groups influence the ways in which individual health care is managed. Many of the immigrant populations have adapted to and use the healthcare system in the United States but retain cultural practices. For example, patients with an Irish heritage believe that eating a healthy diet, getting proper sleep, and not going to bed with wet hair promote health. These patients are likely to use home remedies for colds and headaches. These remedies include the use of honey for a sore throat and applying a wet rag to the head for headaches (Spector, 2013). Cuban Americans are accustomed to Westernized approaches to all aspects of health care, yet many consult an elder or use a *botanica* for herbal treatments before seeking care and continue the use of herbs while receiving prescribed treatments (Purnell, 2013). The adoption of Westernized or scientific beliefs and practices is influenced by the length of time from immigration and often by the age of the patient. Conversely, the exposure to and knowledge of a variety of cultural beliefs and healthcare practices has promoted the adoption of many treatments, remedies, and therapies from those cultures by healthcare practitioners in the United States. For example, acupuncture, which is part of traditional Chinese medicine, has become a widely accepted therapy and is now used in many modern health care settings, including some hospitals, for pain relief, although it has many other traditional uses as well (Spector, 2013).

Culture influences the patient's perceptions of healthcare providers as well. For example, African Americans recognize the doctor as the head of the healthcare team. Arab Americans, Jewish Americans, and Chinese Americans hold physicians in high regard. Mexican Americans respect healthcare professionals but fear seeking care because of concerns about confidentiality (Purnell, 2013).

The view of nurses is often dependent on the cultural view of women's roles in society and a lack of respect for those viewed as subservient to the physician. In many cultures, the assistance of a family member or cultural healer is sought before that of a healthcare professional. Furthermore, health-seeking behaviors are influenced by the type of illness, language barriers, and concerns that family and cultural rituals surrounding care of the sick and dying will not be respected or permitted.

From a broad standpoint, categories of cultural phenomena that impact the provision of health care include communication, temporal relationships, family patterns, dietary patterns, health beliefs, and health practices. Understanding these phenomena is essential to comprehensive health assessment and to the delivery of safe and effective nursing care. Selected examples of each of the phenomena are described in the following sections. Table 4.2 provides an overview of characteristics considered as representative of health beliefs and practices of certain cultural groups, as well as implications for nursing care. It is important to note that expertise with regard to every culture is neither expected nor needed in order to develop cultural competence. Ideally, the nurse should be familiar with the cultural beliefs of the groups who are most often served by a given institution or organization, while using reliable resources to obtain information about cultural groups with whom the nurse is not familiar.

Likewise, it is important to note that differences in language, beliefs, values, and customs exist within cultural groups. As such, cultural beliefs and behaviors are patient specific and may or may not include attributes that are generalized to a given culture. To avoid stereotyping, assessment of an individual's beliefs is essential. In every case, the patient—and the patient's beliefs—should be treated with respect.

Communication

Communication refers to the verbal and nonverbal methods with which individuals and groups transmit information. Communication occurs between and among individuals for a variety of purposes. For example, cultural beliefs, customs, values, and morals are passed from generation to generation within a specific culture by communication. Communication provides information about a culture to those outside of the culture. Communication is the mechanism through which individuals establish relationships. How a sender encodes a message and how a receiver decodes it depend on a combination of factors such as culture, ethnicity, religion, nationality, education, health status, and level of intelligence. When two people differ in any of these ways, each must be more open to the other person's way of thinking and foster mutual understanding.

Of central importance to all communication is the concept of linguistic competence. According to the National Center for Cultural Competence (NCCC), **linguistic competence** is the ability of an organization and its members to effectively communicate and to convey information in such a way that diverse audiences

TABLE 4.2	**Selected Culturally Based Beliefs and Practices and Nursing Implications**	
CULTURAL GROUP	**EXAMPLES OF BELIEFS AND PRACTICES**	**NURSING IMPLICATIONS**
Jehovah's Witnesses	• Blood transfusion is biblically prohibited • Blood fractions, such as clotting factors and immune globulin, are not absolutely prohibited	• Recognize that acceptance of blood administration may vary based upon the individual • Maintain open lines of communication between the patient and all members of the healthcare team • Anticipate potential for implementing bloodless interventions in certain cases, such as administering iron supplements and erythropoietin-stimulating agents (ESAs) when caring for anemic patients.
Muslims	• Muslims are followers of the religion of Islam • Islamic beliefs require followers to offer prayer five times each day • Prayer must be performed while facing Mecca (the holiest city in Islam, located in Saudi Arabia); although popular belief suggests Muslim prayer is always directed toward the east, this is true only if the individual is west of Mecca	• Facilitate prayer by scheduling care and activities around designated prayer times • Be prepared to assist the patient with identifying the cardinal direction (i.e., north, south, east, or west) of Mecca in relationship to the hospital or institution.
Mexican/Latino	• Supernatural forces are believed to cause illness • *Mal de ojo*, or the evil eye, is caused by an individual enviously admiring another individual's child • *Mal puesto* occurs when one individual uses witchcraft to cause disease in another individual • Diseases caused by supernatural forces are not cured by non-supernatural remedies	• Understand that poor compliance may be rooted in a belief that a non-supernatural remedy will not cure an illness that is supernatural in origin • Respectfully educate the patient about the natural cause of the illness and explain the benefits of the prescribed treatment.
Vietnamese	• Avoidance of eye contact is reflective of respect • Slightly bowing one's head when communicating conveys respect for an individual • Modesty is highly valued	• Understand that making direct eye contact may be viewed as disrespectful • Mirror the patient's behaviors and, if appropriate, avoid direct eye contact when speaking to the patient or family members • Whenever possible, allow adults and older children to remain fully clothed (rather than changing into a gown) during assessment or treatment.

Sources: Panico, M. L., Jenq, G. Y., & Brewster, U. C. (2011). When a patient refuses life-saving care: Issues raised when treating a Jehovah's Witness. *American Journal of Kidney Diseases, 58*(4), 647–653; Loma Linda University Health System. (n.d.). *Health care and religious beliefs.* Retrieved from http://www.lomalindahealth.org/media/medical-center/departments/employee-wholeness/healthcare-religious-beliefs.pdf; and Caplan, S., Escobar, J., Paris, M., Alvidrez, J., Dixon, J. K., Desai, M. M.,... Whittemore, R. (2013). Cultural influences on causal beliefs about depression among Latino immigrants. *Journal of Transcultural Nursing, 24*(1), 68–77.

may easily comprehend the intended meaning (NCCC, 2009). Diverse audiences include individuals who demonstrate the following characteristics:

• Limited English proficiency
• Limited literacy skills
• Disabilities
• Deafness or other hearing impairments (NCCC, 2009)

The nurse is careful not to bring cultural stereotypes to the communication process. Each individual, whether patient or nurse, has some degree of ethnocentrism; that is, the individual sees a culturally specific way of life as being the "normal" way. Nurses must not impose their own culturally specific values on patients. Avoiding cultural bias requires effort because these values may be so ingrained that they may surface unconsciously during communication. All people have a right to have their cultural heritage recognized as valuable. No one culture is better than another. The nurse who works in a community with patients from many cultures and nationalities should learn as much as possible about the cultures, values, and belief systems of the patients who present for health care. The best way to learn is by asking and observing the "cultural experts," patients, and patients' families.

In the United States, many individuals are often uncomfortable with silence and speak constantly to avoid any lag in the conversation. In Vietnam, a talkative individual could be perceived as impatient, inconsiderate, and superficial. The nurse who makes a lot of small talk while interviewing a patient of Vietnamese descent may find it difficult to obtain information from the patient. A Cantonese patient using English as a second language may misplace stress on syllables and use short vowels. A nurse from a different cultural background may think this patient is angry, curt, impatient, or rude, resulting in miscommunication.

Consider the following situation: Mrs. Pearl Robinson, a 76-year-old African American who has lived most of her life in the rural South, had her blood pressure checked at the local senior

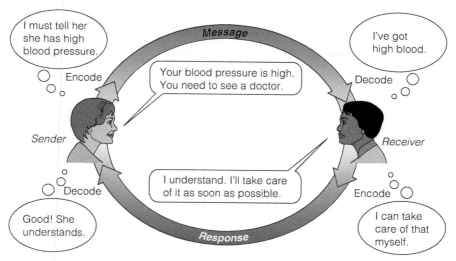

Figure 4.3 Differences in cultural or regional background may become barriers to effective nurse-patient communication.

citizen center while visiting her daughter in Detroit. The nurse who checked Mrs. Robinson told her that her blood pressure was high and suggested that she see her healthcare provider as soon as possible. Mrs. Robinson interpreted the nurse's statement to mean that she had "high blood," a simple condition the "old folks talked about." Mrs. Robinson believed she could treat "high blood" by drinking vinegar and water and eating salty foods. In this situation, the difference in cultural and regional background between Mrs. Robinson and the nurse contributed to the difference in the way each one encoded and decoded the term "high blood pressure" (see Figure 4.3 ■).

Verbal Communication

Verbal communication includes spoken and written language. Diversity in language, word usage, and meaning has become an unavoidable part of life in the United States. According to the U.S. Census Bureau report, languages spoken at home by at least 20% of the population included Spanish, French, Creole, German, Italian, Chinese, and/or Pacific Island languages (Ryan, 2013). In addition, differences in word use and pronunciation exist in regions of the United States among English-speaking populations.

Verbal communication is essential to the provision of health care. The nurse must communicate with the patient or family to:

- Obtain assessment data about physical and emotional health.
- Work with patients to identify strengths and weaknesses.
- Guide the pursuit of care to address problems and needs.
- Provide instruction regarding aspects of care.
- Evaluate progress toward health-related goals.

The tone of voice as well as the words spoken is of significance in many cultures. Loud tones of voice, for example, denote anger to Chinese Americans and are considered rude by Navajo Indians.

Linguistic differences can inhibit the communication that is essential to health care. Language differences can create barriers to initiating or maintaining contact with healthcare agencies or providers. Difficulties associated with language differences include the inability to make telephone contact and misunderstanding of dates, times, and locations for appointments. Language differences affect the amount and type of information that can be obtained during an

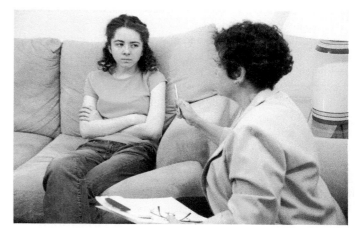

Figure 4.4 Nonverbal communication.
Source: Lisa F. Young/Shutterstock.

interview and physical examination as well as interfere with instruction regarding diagnostic testing and healthcare maintenance.

Nonverbal Communication

Nonverbal communication incorporates the gestures, facial expressions, and mannerisms that inform others of emotions, feelings, and responses that occur in interactions with others. Nonverbal behaviors include silence, touch, eye contact, lack of eye contact, distancing from others during communication, and posture (see Figure 4.4 ■). The nurse must recognize that each of these behaviors has personal and cultural significance and then interpret behaviors appropriately. In some cultures, silence is used to demonstrate respect for another person. In other cultures, silence indicates agreement. For example, in the Navajo culture, periods of silence are common. The silence indicates interest in what another is saying. The silence allows time for information processing. Not allowing this time can result in inaccurate responses or no response. Filipino Americans are comfortable with silence as well. They often use nodding of the head during communication, which may appear to indicate agreement or understanding but may simply mean "I hear you." In some cultures, casual touch is forbidden, and in many cultures the appropriate types of touch between members of the opposite sex are clearly delineated. Egyptian Americans are accustomed to close personal space, yet touch between individuals of different gender is limited to family members and in private. Personal space is greater for Navajos than for European Americans and so great in Appalachian American culture that members will stand at some distance from one another during social and healthcare situations.

Body Language

Body language is extremely important when developing the nurse-patient relationship. If the nurse and the patient are from different cultures, body language is an even more critical part of the communication process. Simple body movements such as eye contact, handshakes, or posture may carry different messages in different cultures. For example, some Native American communities consider direct eye contact an invasion of privacy and a firm handshake aggressive. The nurse of Northern European descent might believe that a patient who avoids direct eye contact is suspicious and cannot be trusted and that a weak handshake translates into a weak personality. The nurse of Asian descent might believe that the outgoing and talkative patient of Italian descent is being rude.

The differences in verbal and nonverbal communication and body language among individuals in a group are often greater than the differences between the groups themselves. Therefore, although nurses should attempt to individualize communication styles to ethnic groups, they must not make assumptions about the patient's ethnicity. For example, a patient or nurse of Japanese descent who is a fourth-generation American differs little in communication style from an American of European descent. As another example, consider the reverse of the earlier situation with Mrs. Robinson. The patient, Mrs. Robinson, is a well-educated, urban woman, but the nurse assumes that, simply because Mrs. Robinson is of African American descent, she must believe in the concept of "high blood." The potential for miscommunication in this situation is even greater than in the first example. Nurses must never stereotype patients because they are of a different culture, are from a different country, or practice a different religion. Rather, it is the nurse's responsibility to learn about a patient's culture and use this knowledge as a basis for developing a meaningful nurse-patient relationship.

Communicating with Language Differences

Communication is challenged if the patient does not speak the same language as the nurse or uses the language of the dominant culture, such as English, as a second language. If the patient does not speak the same language, the nurse should bring in a translator to assist with the interview (see Figure 4.5 ■). It is helpful to meet with the translator before approaching the patient to discuss the purpose of the interview, the terms the nurse needs to use, the kinds of information the nurse needs to collect, and the confidentiality of the subject matter. Learning a few key health-related terms in the patient's language contributes to developing trust and establishing an effective nurse-patient relationship.

During the interview, the seating should be arranged so that the patient can see the nurse and the translator at the same time without turning the head from side to side. The nurse looks at the patient, not the translator, as the interview progresses. It is important to avoid discussing the patient with the translator, leaving the patient out of the conversation. Throughout the interview, the nurse asks questions

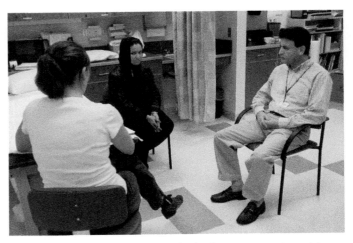

Figure 4.5 A translator may help facilitate interaction with a patient who does not speak English.
Source: Portland Press Herald/Getty Images.

one at a time using clear, concise terms. Even patients who are not bilingual may understand some of the words that are used. Although some patients speak English extremely well as a second language, they may have some difficulty communicating their thoughts when overcome by extreme stress. It is not uncommon for patients who speak fluent English to revert back to their native language during times of stress. If this is the case, the nurse should follow the recommendations for patients who do not speak English. A translator is usually not needed unless the patient is extremely stressed or in severe pain. Some patients communicate better in writing or understand the written word better than the spoken word, so it is a good idea to have a pencil and paper readily available. Box 4.3 provides guidelines for interviewing patients who do not speak English.

Temporal Relationships

Temporal relationships refer to an individual or group's orientation in terms of past, present, or future as well as time orientation. There are cultural variations in temporal orientation. For example, the temporal orientation of the Cherokee is past oriented. Their actions are based on tradition and respect for ancestral practices. The European American culture is future oriented as demonstrated by the propensity to invest in the future and "save for tomorrow." Individuals from Hispanic or Chinese cultures are more likely to be "present," that is, concerned about the here and now. Another trait of European Americans is concern with time in terms of abiding by the clock, schedules, and punctuality. In other cultures and groups such as Cuban Americans, Mexican Americans, and Native Americans, time is not regarded to be as important.

Family Patterns

Family patterns refer to the roles and relationships that exist within families. These roles and relationships include patterns for responsibilities, values, inclusion, and decision making. The roles and responsibilities of family members are often culturally specific in terms of age and gender. For example, patriarchal households, in which the male is responsible for all decisions, including those related to health care, are common in Appalachian, Italian, and Filipino groups. African American groups are more likely to follow matriarchal patterns.

Box 4.3 Guidelines for Interviewing Patients Who Do Not Speak English

- Be open to ways you can communicate effectively. Imagine yourself entering a care setting where few people speak your language. Your sensitivity to your patient's fear and unease will be your greatest strength in providing quality care for your patient.

- Determine what language your patient speaks. Your first assumption may not be correct. For example, South American immigrants may speak one of a variety of Native American dialects, Portuguese, or Spanish.

- Make sure the patient can read and write, as well as speak, in the native language. Be alert for any confusion.

- Learn key foreign phrases that will help you communicate with the patient.

- Use language assistive services that healthcare agencies must provide at all points of contact during all hours of operation.

- Family and friends should not be used to provide interpretive services except on request by the patient.

- Look at your *patient* while telling the translator what to say. This helps your patient feel connected to you and conveys meaning through body language and facial expression.

- Use clear, simple language. For example, do not tell the translator to ask for a clean-catch specimen; rather, explain what you mean, step by step.

- Pause frequently for the translator.

- Ask the translator to provide the proper context for any colloquial expressions your patient may use.

If You Cannot Find a Translator

- Develop cards with phrases or illustrations to aid communication. Have several translators review the cards before using them.

- Use written handouts for patient teaching. These can be developed or purchased. Look for handouts with plenty of diagrams.

Dietary Patterns

Nutritional intake has an impact on health from infancy through old age. The types and amounts of foods that individuals include in the diet are often culturally determined. In addition, certain foods and beverages as well as mealtimes are part of cultural rituals or accepted practices. For example, Americans are known for morning coffee or coffee break rituals, and those from Hispanic cultures are known to eat "dinner" late in the evening. Eating practices are also associated with culturally determined events or holidays. Muslims fast (no food or drink) from dawn to sunset during the month of Ramadan. Lent is a period during which Roman Catholics fast by eating just one full meal and two small meals on Ash Wednesday and Good Friday, and abstain from meat on Ash Wednesday and all Fridays until Easter. In the United States, turkey is a traditional Thanksgiving meal. Certain foods are prohibited in some religious or cultural groups. For example, Muslims and Jews both prohibit the eating of pork. In most cultures, there are theories about nutrition and health. Different types of foods are selected, and food preparation practices vary according to needs in relation to health and illness. In Mexican, Iranian, Chinese, and Vietnamese cultures, a balance is sought between hot and cold foods to prevent illness and as one of the aids for cure in certain illnesses. When a culture adheres to guidelines from the Western healthcare perspective, foods high in fat and salt are avoided as a way to prevent heart disease and some cancers.

Health Beliefs and Health Practices

There are three general categories of health beliefs: the magico-religious, the biomedical, and the holistic health belief groups. In a magico-religious belief system, health and illness are believed to be controlled supernaturally or are seen as "God's will." This type of belief system is found in Hispanic and West Indian cultures in which illness may be attributed to the "evil eye" or "voodoo."

Those who hold biomedical health beliefs consider illness to be caused by germs, viruses, or a breakdown in body processes and functions, and they believe that physiologic human processes can be affected by human intervention. Individuals who follow traditional Western medical practice hold this belief.

In a holistic health belief system, one holds that human life must be in harmony with nature and that illness results from disharmony between the two. The holistic belief system is consistent with the concepts of yin and yang in the Chinese culture, the hot and cold theory of illness in some Hispanic cultures, and the dimensions of the medicine wheel as accepted by some Native Americans.

Health practices are influenced by one's health beliefs as well as economics, geography, knowledge, and culture. In some geographic regions and areas where there is limited access to Westernized health care, people often rely on folk healing or folk medicine. Folk healing is generally derived from cultural traditions and includes the use of teas, herbs, and other natural remedies to treat or cure illness. Seeking health care for illness and disease is one health practice that is influenced by culture. In many cultures, care is sought only when all other remedies have been exhausted or when the symptoms have become severe. This custom often results in complications and prolonged illness or hospitalization. This practice may be a result of stoicism exhibited in Appalachians and older European Americans, or it may be a result of lack of knowledge and understanding of the healthcare system or language barriers that can occur in other cultural groups who have immigrated to the United States.

Access to health care impacts one's health practices as well. Those in lower socioeconomic groups or without insurance are more likely to self-medicate, use folk or family remedies, and seek episodic acute care than are those who have higher income levels and health insurance.

Culture and Obesity

Obesity has become a global healthcare concern. According to the World Health Organization (WHO), in 2008 there were 300 million obese adults and 1 billion overweight adults worldwide (WHO, 2013). Obesity or overweight occurs in 69% of the adults in the United States (CDC, 2013). Worldwide, as many as 40 million children under age 5 are estimated to be overweight (WHO, 2013). In the United States in the past 30 years, the number of overweight children has doubled and the number of overweight adolescents has quadrupled (CDC, 2014).

Several causative factors for obesity have been discussed in the literature. Many of these factors are tied to cultural influences, including dietary habits, lack of exercise, and psychosocial factors. Cultural dietary habits contributing to obesity include greater fat intake; increased consumption of fast foods, soda, and snacks; and lower intake of fiber and whole grains. In the United States, food options have broadened to include prepackaged foods, fast foods, and foods marketed as low in fat or fat free, but many foods labeled as healthy in relation to fat content actually increase calorie intake.

Weight gain has also been consistently linked with a decrease in physical activity. In mainstream American culture, both sedentary lifestyles and, in particular, an increase in television watching, increase the risk for obesity. Poverty and low education levels have been suggested as social factors influencing obesity. However, the link has not been conclusively established. Further, research indicates that obesity is increasing in high income groups (Hurley, Cross, & Hughes, 2011).

The increased prevalence of obesity and overweight in the United States has been observed across racial and ethnic groups. However, Mexican American and black (non-Hispanic) adults are more obese than adults who are white (non-Hispanic) adults. The prevalence of obesity and overweight are high in the American Indian population as well. Overall, females have higher rates of obesity and overweight than males (Ogden, Carroll, Kit, & Flegal, 2013).

Culture in Comprehensive Health Assessment

Comprehensive health assessment refers to obtaining subjective and objective data that are used to identify patient needs. The data are then used to develop and implement plans to meet those needs. Cultural data are essential to this process, because they inform the nurse about a variety of factors and practices that impact the current and future health status of the patient. Cultural data in comprehensive assessment would include all of the cultural phenomena described in the previous section.

When conducting the assessment of culture, the nurse must be careful to avoid stereotyping. That is, the nurse must not assume that, because a patient looks a certain way or has a certain name, he or she belongs to or identifies with a certain cultural or religious group. For example, Mexico is considered a Catholic country, but not all Mexican people are Catholics. In addition, even if the nurse is of the same cultural or ethnic background as the patient, it cannot be assumed that the nurse's beliefs and practices are the same. The nurse and the patient may identify themselves as Hispanic. However, if the nurse relates to a Colombian culture while the patient is from Cuba, the nurse must recognize that aspects of the Latin or Hispanic cultures from those areas can be quite different. A nurse who was born and raised in the United States must avoid assuming that a patient who states, "I'm all American" shares the same beliefs and values. The nurse should ask patients to describe what identification with a specific culture means to them. The use of open-ended

questions helps to obtain information about the meaning of the patient's statements about ethnic or cultural identity. Often the follow-up question about the family's cultural or ethnic identity can reveal areas to explore in relation to beliefs about illness or disease, about diet, and about relationships. For example, a patient who states, "I'm all American," may reveal links with ethnic groups after further questioning by saying, "My parents are from Germany, and we eat lots of German foods, but I'm like all of my American friends."

Ethnic Identity and Culture

Information about ethnicity and culture is gathered because it enables the nurse to determine physical and social characteristics that influence healthcare decisions. Ethnicity and culture may influence a number of health-related factors for the patient. These factors include health beliefs; health practices; verbal and nonverbal methods of communication; roles and relationships in the family and society; perceptions of healthcare professionals; diet; dress and rituals; and rites associated with birth, marriage, child rearing, and death.

Information about the patient's ethnicity and culture is obtained by asking the following questions:

- Do you identify with a specific ethnic group?
- How strong would you say that identity is?
- What language do you speak at home?
- Do you or members of your family speak a second language?
- Are you comfortable receiving information about your health in English?
- Would you like an interpreter during this interview?
- Would you like to have an interpreter during the physical examination?
- Are there rules in your culture about the ways an examination must be carried out?
- Are there rules about the gender of the person who is examining you?
- Do you need to have someone in your family participate in the interview or examination?

Information about health beliefs and practices, family, roles and relationships, cultural influences on diet, activity, emotional health, and other topics are included in other components of the health history, including the review of systems. For example, when asking about the patient's health patterns, the nurse will gather information about cultural healing or rituals associated with health and health maintenance. Further, when asking about nutrition, the nurse will gather information about cultural influences on food selection, preparation, and consumption.

Information about ethnicity and culture can be obtained by conducting a complete cultural assessment at this point in the health history. Box 4.4 includes the information to be obtained in a complete cultural assessment. Box 4.5 includes a "mini" cultural assessment with generalized questions and information on how to ask these questions.

Spirituality refers to the individual's sense of self in relation to others and a higher being and what one believes gives meaning

Box 4.4 Cultural Assessment

1. What racial group do you identify with?
2. What is your ethnic group?
3. How closely do you identify with that ethnic group?
4. What cultural group does your family identify with?
5. What language do you speak?
6. What language is spoken in your home?
7. Do you need an interpreter to participate in this interview?
8. Would you like an interpreter to be with you when health issues are discussed?
9. Are there customs in your culture about talking and listening, such as the amount of distance one should maintain between individuals, or making eye contact?
10. How much touching is allowed during communication between members of your culture and between you and members of other cultures?
11. How do members of your culture demonstrate respect for another?
12. What are the most important beliefs in your culture?
13. What does your culture believe about health?
14. What does your culture believe about illness or the causes of illness?
15. What are the attitudes about health care in your culture?
16. How do members of your culture relate to healthcare professionals?
17. What are the rules about the sex of the person who conducts a health examination in your culture?
18. What are the rules about exposure of body parts in your culture?
19. What are the restrictions about discussing sexual relationships or family relationships in your culture?
20. Do you have a preference for your healthcare provider to be a member of your culture?
21. What do members of your culture believe about mental illness?
22. Does your culture prefer certain ways to discuss topics such as birth, illness, dying, and death?
23. Are there topics that members of your culture would not discuss with a nurse or doctor?
24. Are there rituals or practices that are performed by members of your culture when someone is ill or dying or when they die?
25. Who is the head of the family in your culture?
26. Who makes decisions about health care?
27. Do you or members of your culture use cultural healers or remedies?
28. What are the common remedies used in your culture?
29. What religion do you belong to?
30. Do most members of your culture belong to that religion?
31. Does that religion provide rules or guides related to health care?
32. Does your culture or religion influence your diet?
33. Does your culture or religion influence the ways children are brought up?
34. Are there common spiritual beliefs in your culture?
35. How do those spiritual beliefs influence your health?
36. Are there cultural groups in your community that provide support for you and your family?
37. What supports do those groups provide?

to life. Assessment of spirituality may include asking the following questions:

- How do you meet your spiritual needs?
- Do you have special objects of a religious or spiritual nature that you carry with you or are in your home?
- Are there any religious or spiritual objects that you would want with you if you were ill or hospitalized?
- Is there a member of the clergy you would want to contact if you were ill or hospitalized?
- Is there a person who you would want to contact to help you with prayer or spiritual practices if you were ill or hospitalized?
- Do you use spiritual healers?
- Are there rituals that are important to you when you are ill or have a health problem?
- Tell me about the rituals you use when you are ill or need health care.

Chapter 5 of this text provides information about spirituality and spiritual assessment. ∞

The nurse has an obligation to prioritize meeting the needs of all patients. Therefore, knowledge of cultural and language differences is essential in current practice. The nurse must examine his or her own cultural values and beliefs and reflect on their significance to encounters and interactions with patients of diverse cultures. The nurse must continue to learn about a variety of cultures and languages. The NCCC provides a self-assessment checklist for healthcare personnel that includes examples of the beliefs, attitudes, and practices that promote cultural competence. When language differences exist, the nurse must use all resources possible to ensure that decisions are based on accurate information. These resources include the use of translators and written materials provided in the language of the patient. Last, the nurse must seek information about community resources to meet the needs of the diverse cultural groups for whom care is provided.

Box 4.5 Mini Cultural Assessment

The mini cultural assessment provides a starting point for asking patients about any cultural beliefs that would affect how you provide health care. Before beginning the cultural assessment, inform the patient that you will be asking them questions about their cultural beliefs. When asking the questions, provide examples to explain the type of information you are looking for. If the patient gives a positive answer to any of these questions, a more thorough cultural assessment should be conducted. Recording the patient's answers to these questions will be vital to providing ongoing culturally sensitive care, especially for patients who are in the hospital for multiple shifts.

1. What is your preferred language? Would you feel more comfortable with an interpreter present?

2. Do you identify with a specific ethnic or other group? For example, Mexican, Black, Chinese, LGBT?

3. Do you follow any cultural rules about how an examination should be carried out? For example, would you prefer a provider of the same sex? Are there rules about exposure of certain body parts?

4. Do you follow any cultural or spiritual practices that would affect your health care? For example, do you have any dietary restrictions? Do you have rituals that must be performed at certain times of the day? Do you have a spiritual leader you would like us to contact?

5. Do you prefer to have a family member present during exams or discussions about your health and treatment?

Application Through Critical Thinking

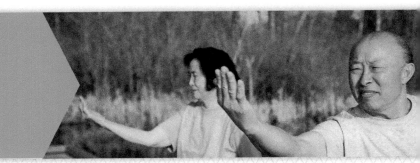

▶ Case Study

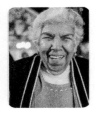

Rachel Wood is a nursing student doing her rotation at a clinic that provides care to patients who do not have health insurance. Today they are seeing an elderly Hispanic woman from Mexico, Mrs. Reyes, who is here visiting her granddaughter and became ill. Her granddaughter Antonia brought her to the clinic because she does not have any health insurance. Mrs. Reyes, whose native language is Spanish, does not speak English. Antonia speaks both English and Spanish, was born in the United States, and is a citizen. Her parents came here when they were in their twenties and are very happy here in the United States. Antonia lives with her parents and brother. Her grandmother wants to see a *curandero* (a traditional Latin American healer that she normally sees in Mexico), but her granddaughter is explaining to her that there are none in this area and they need to see the nurse practitioner in the free clinic. Antonia says to her grandma, "That is so old fashioned grandma, no one does that here." The nurse practitioner requests a translator and then proceeds to interview the patient.

▶ Critical Thinking Questions

1. What is important for the nurse to understand about the culture as it relates to Mrs. Reyes?

2. Mrs. Reyes will need discharge educational materials. What standards support ensuring that these are available in Spanish?

3. Antonia's comment to her grandmother about "no one does that (sees a curandero) here" could be an example of assimilation. Why would that be true?

4. How should the nurse approach Mrs. Reyes's request for a curandero?

5. How should the nurse interact with the translator during the patient interview?

▶ References

Abdelhady, D. (2014). The sociopolitical history of Arabs in the United States: Assimilation, ethnicity, and global citizenship. In S C. Nassar-McMillan, K. J. Ajrouch, & J. Hakim-Larson (Eds.), *Biopsychosocial perspectives on Arab Americans: Culture, development, and health* (17–43). New York, NY: Springer.

American Nurses Association. (1991). *Cultural diversity in nursing practice. Position Statement: Ethics and human rights.* Retrieved from http://www.nursingworld.org/MainMenuCategories/EthicsStandards/Ethics-Position-Statements/prtetcldv14444.html

Berman, A., & Snyder, S. J. (2012). *Kozier and Erb's fundamentals of nursing: Concepts, process and practice* (9th ed.). Upper Saddle River, NJ: Prentice Hall.

Berry, J. W. (2003). Conceptual approaches to acculturation. In K. M. Chun, P. Balls-Organista, & G. Marin (Eds.). *Acculturation: Advances in theory, measurement, and applied research* (pp. 17–37). Washington, DC: American Psychological Association.

Caplan, S., Escobar, J., Paris, M., Alvidrez, J., Dixon, J. K., Desai, M. M., . . . Whittemore, R. (2013). Cultural influences on causal beliefs about depression among Latino immigrants. *Journal of Transcultural Nursing, 24*(1), 68–77

Centers for Disease Control and Prevention (CDC). (2013). *Obesity and overweight.* Retrieved from http://www.cdc.gov/nchs/fastats/overwt.htm

Centers for Disease Control and Prevention (CDC). (2014). *CDC Childhood obesity facts.* Retrieved from http://www.cdc.gov/healthyyouth/obesity/facts.htm

Diederichs, C., Berger, K., & Bartels, D. B. (2011). The measurement of multiple chronic diseases—a systematic review on existing multimorbidity indices. *The Journals of Gerontology Series A: Biological Sciences and Medical Sciences, 66*(3), 301–311.

Humes, K., Jones, N. A., & Ramirez, R. R. (2011). *Overview of race and Hispanic origin, 2010.* (C2010BR-02). Retrieved from http://www.census.gov/prod/cen2010/briefs/c2010br-02.pdf

Hurley, K. M., Cross, M. B., & Hughes, S. O. (2011). A systematic review of responsive feeding and child obesity in high-income countries. *The Journal of Nutrition, 141*(3), 495–501.

Leininger, M., & McFarland, M. (2002). *Transcultural nursing: Concepts, theories, research and practice* (3rd ed.). New York: McGraw-Hill.

Loma Linda University Health System. (n.d.) *Health care and religious beliefs.* Retrieved from http://www.lomalindahealth.org/media/medical-center/departments/employee-wholeness/healthcare-religious-beliefs.pdf

Murray, R. B., & Zentner, J. P. (2008). *Health promotion strategies through the lifespan* (8th ed.). Upper Saddle River, NJ: Prentice Hall.

National Center for Cultural Competence. (2009). *Linguistic competence.* Retrieved from http://nccc.georgetown.edu/documents/Definition%20of%20Linguistic%20Competence.pdf

National Institutes of Health (NIH). (2013). *Clear communication: Cultural competency.* Retrieved from http://www.nih.gov/clearcommunication/culturalcompetency.htm

Office of Minority Health (OMH). (2013). *The national CLAS standards.* Retrieved from http://minorityhealth.hhs.gov/templates/browse.aspx?lvl=2&lvlID=15

Ogden, C. L., Carroll, M. D., Kit, B. K., & Flegal, K. M. (2013). Prevalence of obesity among adults: United States, 2011–2012. *NCHS Data Brief,* (131), 1–8.

Panico, M. L., Jenq, G. Y., & Brewster, U. C. (2011). When a patient refuses life-saving care: Issues raised when treating a Jehovah's Witness. *American Journal of Kidney Diseases, 58*(4), 647–653.

Pender, N. J., Murdough, C. L., & Parsons, M. A. (2011). *Health promotion in nursing practice* (6th ed.). Upper Saddle River, NJ: Prentice Hall.

Purnell, L. D. (2013). *Transcultural health care: A culturally competent approach* (4th ed.). Philadelphia: F.A. Davis.

Reynolds, L., Bush, E. C., & Geist, R. (2008). The Gen Y imperative. *Communication World, 25*(2), 19–22.

Ryan, C. (2013). *Language use in the United States: 2011–American community survey reports.* Retrieved from http://www.census.gov/prod/2013pubs/acs-22.pdf

Smokowski, P. R., David-Ferdon, C., & Stroupe, N. (2009). Acculturation and violence in minority adolescents: A review of the empirical literature. *The Journal of Primary Prevention, 30*(3–4), 215–263.

Spector, R. E. (2013). *Cultural diversity in health and illness* (8th ed.). Upper Saddle River, NJ: Prentice Hall.

U.S. Census Bureau. (2012). *U.S. Census Bureau projections show a slower growing, older, more diverse nation a half century from now* [Press release]. Retrieved from http://www.census.gov/newsroom/releases/archives/population/cb12-243.html

U.S. Department of Health and Human Services (USDHHS). (2014). *Healthy people 2020.* Retrieved from http://www.healthypeople.gov/2020/default.aspx

UMass Amherst Center for Heritage and Society. (n.d.) *What is heritage?* Retrieved from http://www.umass.edu/chs/about/whatisheritage.html

Wells, J. C. (2012). The evolution of human adiposity and obesity: where did it all go wrong? *Disease Models & Mechanisms, 5*(5), 595–607.

World Health Organization. (2008). *Global strategy on diet, physical activity and health: Obesity and overweight.* Retrieved February 17, 2008, from http://www.who.int/dietphysicalactivity/publications/facts/obesity/en/

World Health Organization (WHO). (2013). *Obesity and overweight.* Retrieved from http://www.who.int/mediacentre/factsheets/fs311/en/

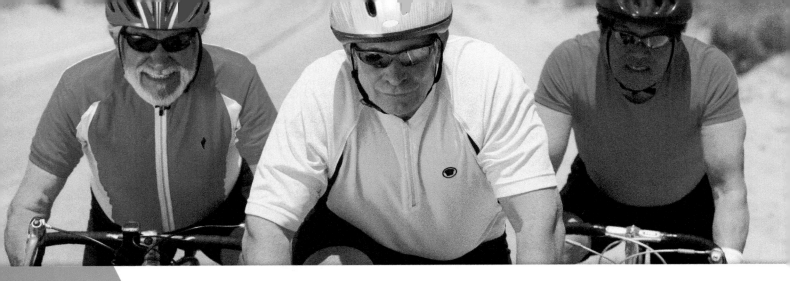

Psychosocial Assessment

▶ Learning Outcomes

Upon completion of the chapter, you will be able to:

1. Categorize the major components of psychosocial health.

2. Apply knowledge of psychosocial functioning to assessment of overall health and wellness.

3. Examine factors that affect psychosocial health in patients across the life span.

4. Describe application of the nursing process in the assessment of psychosocial health.

5. Formulate patient-specific strategies for assessment of psychosocial health in patients across the life span.

Key Terms

Psychosocial functioning includes the way a person thinks, feels, acts, and relates to self and others. It is the ability to cope and tolerate stress and the capacity for developing a value and belief system. Psychosocial functioning is part of an intricate set of subsystems making up the human organism. These subsystems are interrelated components that make up an individual who is greater than a sum of parts. Assessment of the patient must consider the interaction of body, mind, and spirit in their entirety rather than as separate body systems. When one part is missing or dysfunctional, all other parts of the individual are affected. Illness, developmental changes, or life crises may bring about changes in psychosocial functioning. The patient may become stressed, may lose self-esteem, or may experience positive changes such as greater closeness with family. Changes in psychosocial functioning may, in turn, affect the patient's physical health or response to treatment. For example, a patient who is extremely stressed may not be able to understand or remember instructions for self-care, and a patient who is socially isolated may not be able to get needed help at home. There is increasing evidence supporting the theory that mind-body interactions play a key role in both health and illness. No matter what the source of the patient's concern, a psychosocial assessment can provide significant insights that help to individualize patient care.

Psychosocial Health

Psychosocial health can be defined as being mentally, emotionally, socially, and spiritually well (see Figure 5.1 ■). Psychosocial health includes mental, emotional, social, and spiritual dimensions. The mental dimension refers to an individual's ability to reason, to find meaning in and make judgments from information, to demonstrate rational thinking, and to perceive realistically. The emotional dimension is subjective and includes one's feelings. Social functioning refers to the individual's ability to form relationships with others. Included in the spiritual dimension are beliefs and values that give meaning to life.

Factors That Influence Psychosocial Health

Psychosocial health is influenced by internal and external factors. Internal factors consist of one's genetic makeup, physical health, and physical fitness. External factors include the influence of those

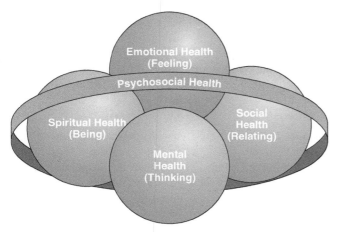

Figure 5.1 Psychosocial health.

responsible for one's upbringing and experiences in the social environment, in which culture, geography, and economic status are contributory aspects. Additional factors to consider when addressing psychosocial health are self-concept; role development; interdependent relationships; and the abilities to manage stress, to cope with and adapt to change, and to develop a belief and values system.

Internal Factors

Internal factors that affect psychosocial health include hereditary characteristics or those related to genetic makeup. In addition, the individual's physical health, developmental stage, and level of fitness influence psychosocial health.

Genetics

The majority of health disorders have a basis in genetics (National Human Genome Research Institute, 2012). With the completion of the Human Genome Project, gene-based testing and treatment are expected to be incorporated into health care with the goal of promoting public health. The Office of Public Health Genomics (OPHG), which is a division of the Centers for Disease Control and Prevention (CDC), is evaluating strategies for responsibly incorporating genomic advances into public health programs (OPHG, 2013).

An individual's genetic makeup influences physical and psychosocial health throughout life. Research indicates that certain forms of hypertension are inherited, that children of parents who are manic-depressive have a slightly higher risk of experiencing that illness, and that shyness is reportedly an inherited personality trait. Parents with attention deficit/hyperactivity disorder (ADHD) have an increased likelihood of having offspring with the disorder, and there appears to be a genetic link to conditions such as obesity, alcoholism, and hypoglycemia. Some studies of identical twins reveal that they often have the same habits, mannerisms, and perceptions of anxiety, even when raised separately.

Hereditary differences impact one's development in two ways: First, experiences impact a hereditary predisposition for certain health problems. For example, an individual with a genetic predisposition to develop schizophrenia would likely develop the disease in a particular environment. Second, genetic characteristics result in reactions from others that can have an impact on the developing personality. Consider the fact that body structure, appearance, and overall physical attractiveness are inherited. Most people respond more positively to children who are physically attractive than to those who are not. Repeated responses of a positive or negative nature can impact one's developing self-concept and self-esteem as well as one's overall behavior and interaction with others. Positive responses result in feelings of self-worth and confidence. Negative responses lead to low self-concept and may result in unmanageable levels of stress, resulting in unacceptable behavior or mental illness. Furthermore, cognitive processes, including the abilities to think, perceive, remember, and make judgments, are dependent on one's innate or inherited capacity and are enhanced or diminished in response to environmental and educational factors.

Physical Health

Physical health is associated with satisfaction of basic needs, quality of life, and psychosocial well-being. Research indicates that there is a mind-body-spirit connection. Physical health enables an individual to respond to stressors and, therefore, to adapt, cope with change, and grow as a functioning individual capable of personal and social interaction. Conversely, problems with health, particularly chronic illness, can negatively impact coping, adaptation, and personal and emotional fulfillment.

The mind-body-spirit connection is further explained as the body's response to thoughts and feelings. Positive and negative stress and anxiety may result in physical symptoms. Situations of positive and negative stress include marriage, childbirth, success in school or job performance, financial difficulties, the death of a friend or family member, or loss of a job. Physical symptoms that indicate a problem related to emotional stress or distress include the following:

- Back pain
- Chest pain
- Breathlessness
- Constipation
- Fatigue
- Hypertension
- Palpitations
- Dry mouth
- Nausea
- Weight loss or gain

Emotional **stress** affects health in several ways: First, stress affects the immune system, resulting in increased susceptibility to infection. Second, during periods of stress or change, individuals are less likely to attend to habits that promote health such as eating nutritious meals or following an exercise routine. Third, research points to a molecular link between prolonged stress and obesity. Researchers describe the use of comfort foods, which result in the deposit of fat in the abdomen, as a way to alter the stress response and the anxiety that accompanies it (Tomiyama, Dallman, & Epel, 2011). Last, some individuals use alcohol, tobacco, or drugs to "feel better."

Measures to deal with stress and reduce the negative impact on physical and emotional health include talking openly about feelings; thinking about positive aspects of life; using relaxation techniques such as meditation, yoga, prayer, or positive imagery; and following a regimen to promote health that includes healthy eating, exercise, and sleep.

Developmental Stage

The patient's developmental stage greatly influences psychosocial health. For example, even at the most basic level, children and adults have different understandings of health and illness. It is common for children to believe they are ill because of bad thoughts or behaviors. The belief that illness is a punishment for wrongdoing is common. Young children cannot identify or modify health risks. Children do not have the cognitive ability to understand cause-and-effect relationships until late school age or early adolescence. Parents and guardians function as proxies for their children in most healthcare decisions.

Nurses should use a caring and supportive yet firm approach with children. Whenever possible, play should be incorporated into nursing procedures. It is helpful to allow children to touch and manipulate equipment. Adhesive bandages or empty syringes can be provided for playacting with dolls. The nurse should encourage children to talk about their fears and concerns. Painful procedures should not be performed while a child is seated on a parent's lap. Children need to know they are safe from painful experiences when they are with their parents. When possible, give the child choices about the ordering of their assessment and care.

Unique developmental and lifespan considerations significantly affect the older adult's psychosocial health, as well. For the older adult, psychosocial assessment should include functional ability, cognition, and lifestyle changes.

Functional ability refers to the ability to perform tasks required for independent living. These activities include eating, bathing, dressing, cooking, shopping, and management of finances. Strength and mobility are essential factors related to functional ability. They require the objective assessment of test administrators in observations of tasks or movements. Performance tests measure upper and lower body strength, range of motion, balance, or speed of gait. Tests of the upper body include dexterity and strength.

The maintenance and improvement of learning, memory, decision making, and planning are skills associated with cognitive health. Cognitive changes do occur with aging; however, forgetting or becoming senile (cognitive decline) is not a normal part of aging.

Physical Fitness

Physical fitness can be described as a condition that helps individuals feel, appear, and perform at an optimal level. The President's Council on Physical Fitness and Sports (2010) describes physical fitness as comprising the components of fitness that generally correlate with good health. Included among the fitness components are cardiovascular fitness, body composition, muscular endurance, strength, and flexibility.

Physical health can affect emotional and psychosocial well-being. Maintaining fitness requires fulfilling needs related to exercise, nutrition, rest, and relaxation, as well as adopting practices that promote and preserve health. Physical activity and a healthy diet are factors in the prevention of overweight and obesity. In the United States, obesity is an epidemic, including among children. Recommendations related to physical activity are described in chapter 3 of this text. ∞

External Factors

An individual's personality, sense of self, and role as a member of a larger society are influenced by a number of external factors. The manner and conditions in which a child is raised are an important influence. Additionally, the experiences during childhood and throughout life that are framed by culture, geography, and economic status contribute in great part to psychosocial well-being.

Family

Research indicates that children with consistent love, attention, and security grow into adults who are able to adapt to change and stress. Child rearing or caregiving generally occurs within a family unit. Families are considered social units of individuals who are related or live together over a period of time. Individual members in families have ongoing contact with each other; share goals, values, and concerns; and develop practices common to that specific group. Today, families involved in child rearing can be two-parent families; single parent families; heterosexual or homosexual domestic partnerships; blended or stepfamilies; adoptive families; or families in which grandparents, members of the extended family, or others provide child care in the absence of parents.

Families influence psychosocial health because they are expected to provide for physical safety and economic needs; to help members develop physically, emotionally, and spiritually; and to help each individual develop an identity as self and member of the family. Families foster the development of social skills, spiritual beliefs, and a value system. Families promote adaptive and coping skills and assist members to become part of the greater society. The ability to provide these basic needs is dependent on the maturity of the caregivers and the support system available to them from the family, community, and society.

Culture

Culture is a complex system that includes knowledge, beliefs, morals, and customs that provide a pattern for living. Cultures may be composed of individuals from the same ethnic or racial group or background, in the same socioeconomic group, from the same geographic region, who practice a certain religion, or who share common values and beliefs. Culture influences the roles and relationships within families and groups that may be gender specific or determined by age. Culture dictates child rearing and health practices. Overall, behavior is defined by culture. The cultural norms affect physical, social, and mental well-being. An individual's experience and the ways in which one responds to stress, coping, and life situations are determined in great part by culture. Recall the details about the relationship of cultures and health described in chapter 4. ∞

Geography

Geography refers to the country, region, section, community, or neighborhood in which one was born and raised or in which one currently resides or works. The geography of an area affects family life and the development of individuals within families. Psychosocial health is influenced by the climate, terrain, resources, and aesthetics in varied locations. Community resources including schools, churches, healthcare facilities, transportation systems, support services, and safety systems affect the social development and emotional well-being of individuals within the community. Individuals in urban areas are subjected to stressors associated with crowded conditions, congestion, and crime rates higher than in other areas. Residents of rural areas may experience the stressors of limited resources and isolation.

In addition, in the United States one must consider the geographic impacts on psychosocial health that accompany regional characteristics, immigration, and the increased mobility of individuals and families. Some regions in the United States have a highly ethnic character. This character shapes the individual's self-concept and the ways one appraises, is appraised, and interacts with others from within and without the regional/ethnic norm. Immigrants face the stress of adapting to new geographic characteristics and cultural norms. Communities into which immigrants settle and the individuals within them must adapt to the differences in language, customs, morals, values, and roles of the immigrant population. Children of immigrants face the difficulty of being raised in a family with "old-world" values and norms, while growing and developing as members of their adopted community and culture. Because of economic demand or opportunity, families tend to move more frequently today than in the past. Adults and children then must adjust to the culture of the new location, the loss of the familiar, and the stress of separation from family and friends.

Additionally, geography, or one's local environment, influences health-related habits including access to healthy foods and places to walk and exercise. It has been suggested that the increase in obesity in the United States is a result of increasing numbers of people living where driving to work is required; residing in neighborhoods that are unsafe for walking or exercise; and eating convenient, readily available, high-fat "fast foods" rather than healthy foods.

Economic Status

Economic status affects the formation of values and attitudes. Values and role expectations related to marriage, gender roles, family roles, sex, parenting, education, housing, leisure activities, clothing, occupation, and religious practice are influenced by an individual's or family's economic status. In the United States, the higher the income the more likely it is that individuals and families will have achieved higher levels of education or provide for higher levels of education for their children. Better education leads to greater occupational opportunity, better housing, and the ability to participate in a variety of leisure activities. These advantages contribute to the development of high self-worth and self-esteem and result in individuals and families better equipped to manage and adapt to life changes. Those in lower economic groups or in poverty are focused on the present, that is, the immediate needs of self or family including the basic needs of food, clothing, and shelter. Self-esteem and self-image are often lower in poor individuals and families. Continual confrontation with the results of the disparities in income may result in anger, frustration, difficulty in coping, family disturbances, abnormal behaviors, and mental illness. Many times these individuals lack any form of health insurance and do not know how to access the healthcare delivery system.

Additional Factors in Psychosocial Health

Additional factors to consider in psychosocial health are self-concept; role development; sexuality; interdependent relationships; and the abilities to manage stress, to cope and adapt to change, and to develop a belief and value system.

Self-concept

Self-concept refers to the beliefs and feelings one holds about oneself. A positive self-concept is essential to a person's mental and physical health. Individuals with a positive self-concept are better able to develop and maintain interpersonal relationships and resist psychologic and physical illness.

Self-concept develops over time as a person reacts to and learns from interactions with others. As an individual develops across the life span, the interactions move from the immediacy of contact with caregivers as children to contact with individuals in the greater environment.

Body image and self-esteem are components of self-concept. Body image is the way one thinks about physical appearance, size, and body functioning. Self-esteem refers to the sense of worth or

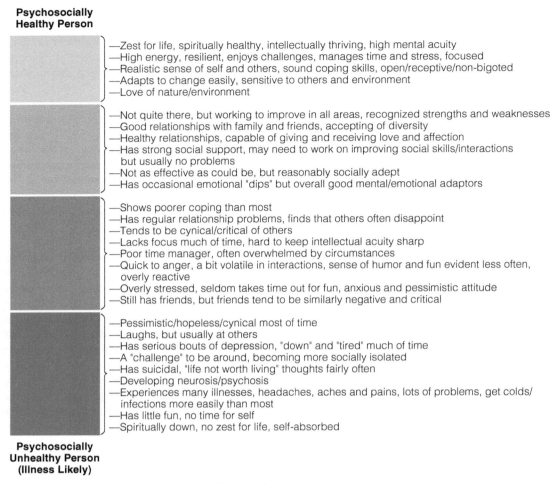

Figure 5.2 Psychosocially healthy person versus psychosocially unhealthy person.

self-respect of an individual. All aspects of self-concept affect psychosocial health. Psychosocially healthy people have a realistic sense of self, adapt to change, develop ways to cope with problems, and form relationships that promote growth and development. In contrast, psychosocially unhealthy individuals often have problems with self-concept, which manifest as pessimism, social isolation, feelings of worthlessness, neglect of physical health, depression, anxiety, substance abuse, or suicidal thoughts (see Figure 5.2 ■).

Body image is affected by a variety of factors, including the individual's size and weight. Among children and adolescents, being overweight or obese can result in physical problems later in life. For example, overweight and obesity in childhood is linked to an increased risk for illness and premature death in adulthood (Reilly & Kelly, 2011).

Likewise, overweight children are subject to bias and stereotyping from peers, teachers, and even parents. Overweight and obese children are prone to low self-esteem, depression, and suicidal thoughts. The long-term effects of cruel treatment and social isolation in overweight children include physical health problems, interference with the development of significant relationships, and problems with employment (Puhl & Latner, 2007; Puhl & Heuer, 2010). The incidence of overweight and obesity is more prevalent in people of low economic status. Causative factors include the use of less expensive, high-calorie processed foods; unsafe conditions

for exercise; and differing perceptions about body weight in relation to health.

FEEDING AND EATING DISORDERS An eating disorder is a condition in which a person's current intake of food differs significantly from that person's normal intake. Eating disorders typically result from an attempt to lose weight; however, the attempt to lose weight may be a misguided response to psychosocial problems.

Anorexia nervosa is a complex psychosocial problem characterized by a severely restricted intake of nutrients and a low body weight. Subjective findings associated with anorexia nervosa include:

- Intense fear of gaining weight or becoming fat
- Perception of being overweight even when in an emaciated state
- Refusal to maintain body weight over a minimal normal weight for age and height
- Constipation and gastrointestinal bloating
- Abdominal pain

Objective manifestations associated with anorexia nervosa may include:

- Emaciation or extreme weight loss
- Refusal to consume food or nutritional supplements

- Electrolyte imbalances due to fluid loss through vomiting or abuse of laxatives

- Damage to teeth enamel due to overexposure to gastric acid if purging behaviors include vomiting

- Esophageal and stomach injury if purging behaviors include vomiting

- Irregular or absent menses (NAMI, 2013a)

Bulimia nervosa is an eating disorder characterized by binge eating and purging or another compensatory mechanism to prevent weight gain. Typically, the bulimic consumes large portions of high-calorie food, typically up to 4,000 calories at one time. The individual then tries to force the food out of the body by vomiting or using laxatives, enemas, diuretics, or diet pills. Subjective manifestations associated with bulimia nervosa may include:

- Obsession with physical appearance

- Periods of excessive food consumption followed by purging activities (for example, vomiting, diuretic or laxative abuse, or extreme exercise)

Objective manifestations associated with bulimia nervosa may include:

- Normal weight or slightly overweight

- Electrolyte imbalances due to fluid loss through vomiting or abuse of laxatives

- Esophageal and stomach injury

- Damage to teeth enamel due to overexposure to gastric acid if purging through vomiting (NAMI, 2013b)

Role Development

Role development refers to the individual's capacity to identify and fulfill the social expectations related to the variety of roles assumed in a lifetime. Roles are reciprocal relationships in which expectations exist for each participant. Examples of reciprocal roles are child-parent, student-teacher, and employee-employer, as well as the reciprocal roles of spouse, sibling, friend, and neighbor. Roles are learned through socialization. The earliest learning generally occurs within the family when children observe and model adult behavior. When role development is healthy and occurs in a supportive environment, self-concept and psychosocial well-being are enhanced as the individual gains confidence in the ability to interact with others according to societal norms. However, nonsupportive, violent, or abusive family relationships are stressful and can lead to unsuccessful role relationships. Individuals who receive support and understand role expectations are able to meet the challenges of changing roles as they develop and mature. Individuals who have experienced family stress have conflicting views of role expectations or are unclear regarding social norms. They often experience frustration or a sense of inadequacy associated with fear or negative judgment from others if their performance is not in accordance with expectations for new or changing roles.

Sexuality

Sexuality and sexual development also greatly influence an individual's health, both physically and psychosocially. Key components of sexuality include sexual identity, sexual orientation, and sexual orientation label.

Sexual identity is self-assigned and comprises the most significant aspects of an individual's sexual life, including sexual attractions, behaviors, desires, and fantasies (Savin-Williams, 2011). **Sexual orientation** refers to an individual's innate predisposition toward affiliation, affection, bonding, thoughts, or sexual fantasies in relationship to members of the same sex, the other sex, both sexes, or neither sex (Savin-Williams, 2011). A **sexual orientation label** is sometimes used to simplify and describe an individual's sexual orientation. Examples of sexual orientation labels include straight (or heterosexual), gay, lesbian, and bisexual (Savin-Williams, 2011). **Transgender,** or gender nonconforming, individuals identify themselves and live as the gender that is not associated with their birth gender (Forbes, 2014). Transgender identity is not associated with any specific sexual orientation label. As such, an individual who is transgender may be heterosexual, gay, lesbian, or bisexual (Morrow & Messinger, 2013).

Historically and at present, members of the lesbian, gay, bisexual, and transgender (LGBT) community have been subject to discrimination, intolerance, and violence. When caring for lesbian, gay, bisexual, and transgender individuals, the nurse should be sensitive to the patient's potential fear of being stereotyped, judged, or discriminated against due to sexuality-related issues. As with all patients, respectful, compassionate care helps build trust, which is the foundation of the nurse-patient relationship. Once trust is established, if the patient so desires, the nursing assessment should include a professional and sensitive discussion about health-related aspects of the patient's sexuality.

Interdependent Relationships

Interdependent relationships are those in which the individual establishes bonds with others based on trust. Interdependent relationships are characterized by mutual reliance and support. According to Roy and Andrews (1999), these relationships are based on the human needs of love, respect, and value for another. These important relationships include the individuals that one identifies as the significant other and one's support system. The ability to form, maintain, and adapt to changes in interdependent relationships is impacted by the individual's self-esteem. Individuals generally choose loving and close relationships with those who have similar levels of self-esteem. For example, when two people with high self-esteem form a loving and caring relationship, the high self-esteem is reinforced. Conversely, individuals with low self-esteem choose relationships with others with low self-esteem. As a result, feelings of negative self-worth are reinforced. Positive self-esteem enhances psychosocial health and enables the individual to grow and develop, adapt to change, solve problems, make decisions, maintain physical well-being, and seek help when needed for physical or emotional difficulties. Further, quality of life and length of life, which are measures of psychosocial health, have been linked to positive interdependent relationships.

Stress and Coping

Stress and coping are the individual's physical and emotional response to psychosocial or physical threats called stressors. An automobile accident, a failing grade, an illness, obesity, and loss of a job are examples of stressors. However, stress is not the event itself but rather the individual's response to it. Events that are highly stressful for one individual may not be stressful for another. The stress response may include familiar physical symptoms such as sweaty palms or a pounding heart. The immediate physical reaction to stress is also referred to as the fight-or-flight response. Physical response to long-term stress may include symptoms such as habitually cold hands or suppression of immune function. The emotional reactions to stress may include difficulty sleeping, inability to concentrate, or anxiety. Positive as well as negative events may produce stress. The physical signs of stress include the following:

- Increased heart rate
- Decreased blood clotting time
- Increased rate and depth of respirations
- Dilated pupils
- Elevated glucose levels
- Dilated skeletal blood vessels
- Elevated blood pressure
- Dilated bronchi
- Increased blood volume
- Contraction of the spleen
- Increased blood supply to vital organs
- Release of T lymphocytes

Stress, in itself, is not bad. In fact, stress can sometimes motivate or enhance performance. Coping mechanisms are what an individual uses to deal with threats to physical and mental well-being. Like other patterns of behavior, patterns of coping with stress stem from early development when the child models the ways significant people in his or her life have coped with and dealt with stress.

Spiritual and Belief Patterns

Spiritual and belief patterns reflect an individual's relationship with a higher power or with something, such as an ideal, a group, or humanity itself, that the person sees as larger than self and that gives meaning to life. The outward demonstration of spirituality may be reflected in religious practice, lifestyle, or relationships with others. A moral code is often included in one's belief patterns. A moral code is the internalized values, virtues, and rules one learns from significant others. It is developed by the individual to distinguish right from wrong. An individual's spiritual beliefs and moral code are affected by culture and ethnic background.

Assessment of spiritual and belief patterns may incorporate a variety of approaches. As an overview, Box 5.1 describes sample components of a general spiritual assessment. In addition, numerous researchers have designed formal spiritual assessment tools, including the following well-known frameworks:

- Stoll (1979) introduced direct questioning as a method to assess spirituality. Stoll incorporated four basic areas for questioning: the patient's concept of God, sources of hope and strength, religious practices, and the relationship between spiritual beliefs and health.
- McSherry and Ross (2002) described methods for assessment of spirituality and spiritual needs as including direct questioning, indicator tools, and values clarification tools.

Box 5.1 Sample Components of a Spiritual Assessment

- Desire to discuss spirituality or religious beliefs
- Choice of individual with whom discussion of spirituality or region is preferred (for example, nurse, hospital chaplain, physician, or another individual)
- Life philosophy or beliefs about life
- Affiliation with religion or particular spiritual beliefs
- Importance of spirituality or religion in daily life
- Significant spiritual rituals or practices, including prayer or meditation
- Conflicts between religious or spiritual beliefs and health-related treatments

Sources: Adapted from WebMD (2011). *Spiritual assessment.* Retrieved from http://www.webmd.com/balance/tc/ncicdr0000301599-spiritual-assessment; Williams, J.A., Meltzer, D., Arora, V., Chung, G., & Curlin, F. A. (2012). Attention to inpatients' religious and spiritual concerns: Predictors and association with patient satisfaction. *Journal of General Internal Medicine, 26*(11), 1265–1271; and Hodge, D. R. & Horvath, V. E. (2010). Spiritual needs in health care settings: A qualitative meta-synthesis of patients' perspectives. *Social Work, 56*(4), 306–316.

- Anadarajah and Hight (2001) developed the use of HOPE questions as a formal spiritual assessment in the patient interview. The mnemonic *HOPE* is explained as follows: *H* refers to questions about the patient's spiritual resources. These include sources of hope, meaning, love, and comfort. *O* refers to participation in or association with organized religion. *P* includes personal spiritual practices. *E* refers to the effects of healthcare and end-of-life issues.
- Hodge (2001) described a narrative framework for spiritual assessment. This qualitative instrument incorporates a spiritual history and a framework to identify spiritual strengths as summarized in Table 5.1.

The Nursing Process in Psychosocial Assessment

The professional nurse uses knowledge, effective communication skills, and critical thinking in applying the nursing process in psychosocial assessment. In conducting psychosocial assessment, the professional nurse uses a holistic approach in assessing the patient's responses to life experiences and the environment. The information is used to formulate nursing diagnoses and to plan care for the patient.

Assessment

When assessing psychosocial health, the nurse gathers data related to several important areas. These include psychosocial concerns, self-concept and beliefs, stress and coping mechanisms, and reasoning ability.

Psychosocial assessment begins before the initial interview when the nurse gathers information from the medical record relating to past emotional or psychiatric problems as well as physiologic

TABLE 5.1	**Narrative Spiritual Assessment**

Part I. Narrative Framework—Spiritual History

Sample Interview

1. Describe your personal and family religious traditions. (Include importance of religion and religious practices.)

2. What practices were important to you in youth? How have those experiences influenced your life?

3. How would you describe your religiosity or spirituality today? Do you believe your spirituality provides strength? How?

Part II. Interpretive Framework—Evokes Spiritual Strengths

1. Affect: How does spirituality affect joy, sorrow, coping? What part does spirituality play in providing hope?

2. Behavior: What rites or rituals do you use or follow? Do you have a relationship with a religious community or leader?

3. Cognition: Describe your current beliefs. Do your beliefs affect the ways you deal with difficulties or impact healthcare decisions?

4. Communion: What is your relationship with God? How do you communicate? Does your relationship help you in difficult times?

5. Conscience: Describe your values. How do you determine right and wrong?

6. Intuition: Have you experienced spiritual hunches, premonitions, or insights?

Source: Adapted from Hodge, D. R. (2001). Spiritual assessment: A review of major qualitative methods and a new framework for assessing spirituality. *Social Work, 46*(3), 203–214.

illnesses that may have affected the patient's psychologic or social functioning. For example, psychosocial problems may be related to brain tumors, multiple sclerosis, or bipolar disorder.

During the initial interview, the nurse gathers more information about the patient's social history (for example, marital status and occupation), history of growth and development, past emotional problems, response to crises and illnesses, and family history of emotional or psychiatric illness. If an area of heightened concern is discovered, the nurse may focus on that area during the initial interview and may also conduct a focused interview at a later time during the course of the patient's care. During the focused interview, the nurse uses information obtained from the medical history, the initial interview, and subsequent patient interactions to help the patient conduct a careful inventory of past and current psychosocial health status.

Psychosocial Well-being

The nurse conducts an interview focused on psychosocial well-being when:

- The patient presents with multiple complaints.
- The information collected during the health history indicates psychosocial dysfunction.
- The patient's behavior during the initial interview is anxious, depressed, erratic, or bizarre.
- More information is needed to determine if any relationships exist between past disease processes and potential emotional or psychiatric concerns.

CASE STUDY

Mrs. Ada Sweeney, a 54-year-old grandmother, was admitted to intensive care with gastrointestinal bleeding. Over the next few days, Mrs. Sweeney was diagnosed with severe ulcerative colitis, anemia, and dehydration. Although the physician initiated an aggressive therapeutic medical regimen, Mrs. Sweeney failed to respond to therapy and continued to experience diarrhea accompanied by gastrointestinal bleeding, elevated temperatures, and severe abdominal pain. One evening the nurse on duty, Indira Singh, discovered Mrs. Sweeney crying in her room. Ms. Singh then used a focused interview to gather information regarding the behavior Mrs. Sweeney was demonstrating. "I'm worried about my grandson," Mrs. Sweeney told the nurse. "I'm raising him and his sisters until their mother is able to come back for them." Mrs. Sweeney went on to tell Ms. Singh that her daughter had been sent to prison on drug charges and there was no one else to care for her four children. "I do the best I can, but there's never enough money to go around, and I'm terrified the authorities will take the children away from me." Ms. Singh questioned Mrs. Sweeney about her immediate and extended family, income, job, and available support systems. After Ms. Singh reviewed the data she gathered during the focused interview, it became clear that Mrs. Sweeney's anxiety and fear over the future of her grandchildren was interfering with her recovery.

Within the next few days the social service department at the hospital found a state program that provided a homemaker for the children until their grandmother recovered, assisted the family in obtaining food stamps, and began a search for better housing. Mrs. Sweeney immediately began to show a response to her nursing and medical treatment and was able to leave the hospital within 2 weeks.

Figure 5.3 Case study.

In some situations a psychosocial concern is not apparent at the time of the initial interview but becomes apparent at a later time, such as when a patient learns of a negative prognosis or undergoes disfiguring surgical procedures. In these cases, the nurse should seek a focused psychosocial interview whenever the emotional problem becomes apparent. The case study (see Figure 5.3 ■) describes a situation where anxiety and fear impeded a patient's recovery from a physical illness. Only after the nurse focused on the emotional impact of the illness was the patient able to respond to therapy.

In some situations the patient's primary health concern is psychosocial in nature. Patients with substance abuse, depression, neurosis, or psychosis fall into this category. In these situations, the nurse should integrate the questions outlined here as part of the focused interview into the initial interview during the first contact with the patient, family, or friends.

The focused interview should be structured to obtain the most information with the fewest questions. Patients may feel uncomfortable answering questions about themselves, making it difficult for the nurse to gather accurate and detailed data regarding the psychosocial aspects of the patient's life. The following sections include a variety of questions to use as a guide for collecting information about the patient's past history of psychosocial and physiologic problems as well as the five areas of psychosocial functioning.

History of Psychosocial Concerns

Some psychosocial concerns begin early in life and reappear whenever a patient faces a major stressor or life crisis. The way the patient coped with problems and treatment modalities in the past can be useful information for planning for the patient's current problems. The following questions are helpful in eliciting this information:

1. Describe any emotions you find yourself frequently experiencing both currently and in the past.
   When the nurse assesses patients, a complete psychosocial history is helpful in determining whether the current health problem is related to previous psychosocial dysfunction.

2. If you have had an emotional problem in the past, were you treated for it? What kind of treatment did you have? Was the treatment successful? Who gave you the treatment? When? Do you still have the problem?
   This information is helpful in developing the current nursing care plan if previous methods of treatment were successful.

3. Do you use alcohol or drugs? If so, what do you use, how much, and how often? Have you had any treatment for substance abuse? What kind of treatment? Where?
   Substance abuse may be the underlying cause of physiologic or psychosocial health problems or may be the result of some other underlying problem.

4. Have you had any eating problems such as anorexia, bulimia, or binge eating? Were you treated? How? By whom? When?
   A patient who has an eating disorder may be in denial and unable to give accurate information on this question. If an eating disorder is suspected, the nurse should look for the diagnostic cues during the physical assessment.

History of Physiologic Alterations or Diseases

When being treated for medical-surgical conditions, patients and their families may be unaware that the physical problems may be related to or caused by an underlying psychosocial problem. An understanding of the body-mind interaction, both positive and negative, can help nurses and patients realize when covert cognitive, perceptual, or affective problems are related to the overt signs and symptoms. Sometimes the underlying problem does not surface immediately but becomes apparent only after several days of nursing care.

The following questions are helpful for uncovering additional information:

1. Describe any chronic illnesses you have had.
   Patients with recent onset of chronic illnesses often have problems complying with treatment or adjusting to living with the condition.

2. How has your illness changed your mood or feelings? When you are nervous or anxious, how does your body feel?
   A physiologic condition may be an underlying cause of anxiety, nervousness, or other abnormal behavior. Conversely, abnormal psychosocial behavior may aggravate or cause a physiologic condition.

3. Have you had any of the following health problems: arthritis? asthma? bowel disorders? heart problems? glandular problems? headaches? stomach ulcer? skin disorders? If so, describe how the condition has affected your life.
   These conditions sometimes have both a psychologic and physiologic component. The presence of the condition may signal an underlying psychosocial disturbance.

Self-concept

It is difficult to gather significant data about self-concept, because most patients find it embarrassing to answer questions about themselves. Patients feel more comfortable divulging this information after a positive nurse-patient relationship has been established and when the nurse integrates questions into general conversation.

The following questions are helpful in obtaining additional information about self-concept:

1. How would you describe yourself to others?
   Asking patients to describe themselves is an excellent technique for determining how they perceive themselves.

2. What are your best characteristics? What do you like about yourself?

3. What would you change about yourself if you could?
   This is a positive way of asking a patient to talk about negative self-perceptions.

4. Would you describe yourself as shy or outgoing?

5. Do you consider yourself attractive? Sexually appealing? If no, why not?
   The patient's self-perception of attractiveness and sex appeal may reveal problems with self-image.

6. Have your feelings about your appearance changed with this illness? If so, how?
   Self-image may change if the illness or treatment has caused a change in appearance.

7. Who comes first in your life: your spouse, children, friends, parents, or yourself?

8. Do you have difficulty saying "no" to others?
   Patients who are depressed, feel hopeless, or feel powerless have difficulty with assertiveness.

9. Do you like to be alone?
   Patients with positive self-concept enjoy spending time by themselves, but those who indicate that they would rather be alone most of the time may be experiencing emotional problems.

10. Describe your social life. What do you do for fun?
    Patients who are unable to answer this question may be depressed or out of touch with reality.

11. What are your hobbies or interests? Do you spend much time pursuing them?

12. For heterosexuals only. Are you comfortable relating to the opposite sex? If no, why not?
    Persons with self-concept or self-image problems may experience difficulty relating to the opposite sex.

13. Are you comfortable with your sexual preference? If not, why not?
    Patients who are homosexual and have not learned to accept their sexuality may experience a self-image problem.

14. Do you have any concerns about your sexual function? If so, what?

Family History

The nurse should explore this area more fully if the health history indicates a family history of psychosocial dysfunction. Although no member of the family may have been diagnosed as being mentally ill, the nurse should explore individual as well as family dysfunction.

The nurse should ask the following questions in relation to the patient's parents, siblings, and extended family in the case of a child, and also in relation to the patient's current family if an adult.

1. Describe any problems your family may have had with mental disorders.
   Some mental disorders such as schizophrenia are familial, that is, the illness recurs in the same family over several generations.

2. What were your major responsibilities in your family?

3. Describe your relationships with your parents and extended family.
   The nurse should look for family dysfunction problems such as schisms (families in chronic controversy), disengagement (detached relationships), or enmeshment (family interactions that are intense and focus on power conflicts rather than affections) as the patient describes his or her family life.

4. What is your birth order in your family? How many brothers and sisters do you have? Are your sisters and brothers older or younger?
   Age and gender birth order influence how an individual relates to other men and women throughout life.

5. Describe your relationship with your siblings growing up at home. Did you and your siblings have problems getting along? If so, how did you solve them?
   The way a patient learned to handle stress and conflict with siblings as a child influences the way the patient handles these issues throughout life.

6. What members of your extended family (grandparents, aunts, uncles, cousins) were important to you as you grew up? How did they influence you?
   Significant others shape an individual's self-concept and self-esteem. Descriptions of significant others help the nurse understand why patients feel and act as they do.

7. Did you have death or losses in your family as you grew up? How did your parents teach you to cope with the loss? How did they cope with the loss?
   Patients who are depressed may not have learned how to deal with loss as a child and may have difficulty dealing with the loss of a loved one or with their own or a significant other's declining health status.

8. Were your parents divorced or remarried during your childhood? If so, whom did you live with? Describe your life growing up with a single parent or stepparent.

Children who are products of a divorce may carry emotional scars into adulthood, affecting their psychosocial health and indirectly affecting their physical health status.

9. Describe how your parents raised you. How did it affect you?
   Patients who were raised by parents who had serious emotional problems, or who were abused by their parents, are more likely to have emotional problems as adults.

10. How did your family deal with adversity and conflict?
    Patients learn to deal with problems from their family. Knowing how the patient learned to deal with problems as a child helps the nurse understand how the patient might deal with the present health problem.

11. When disagreement arose in your family, how was it solved? Who sided with whom?
    In dysfunctional families, schisms result, causing family members to align themselves into coalitions against other family members such as parents against children, father and sons against mother and daughters, and sisters against brothers.

Other Roles and Relationships

It is also important for the nurse to ask questions about other roles and relationships in the patient's life.

1. Describe your relationships with your friends, neighbors, and coworkers.

2. Do you belong to any social groups? Community groups?

3. Who is your closest friend? How do you maintain your friendship?
   An individual's ability to form close relationships indicates a healthy self-concept. An individual who consistently fails to form close relationships may have a self-concept problem.

4. Is your closest friend the most important person in your life? If not, who is the most important person in your life? Explain why.

Stress and Coping

A person learns coping mechanisms from significant others during early childhood and throughout life. The ability to cope is also greatly affected by the number and severity of stressors that have occurred in a person's life. One method for assessing stress in a patient's life is to administer the Holmes Social Readjustment Rating Scale (SRRS). Developed by psychiatrists Thomas Holmes and Richard Rahe in 1967, the SRRS—and modifications of this tool—are still used today. The SRRS lists a series of life stressors that require the individual to change established norms and patterns, along with an assigned point value for each stressor (Holmes & Rahe, 1967). Since stress is a response to events—not the events themselves—not all people are equally stressed by these events. However, on average, the higher the patient's score, the more likely it is that the individual has responded with stress. As a result, the individual is more likely to experience stress-related disorders (such as headaches, asthma, skin rashes, back pain, frequent colds, and anxiety). Because positive life events also evoke a stress response, they should also be part of a psychosocial assessment. For example, the death of a spouse has a relative point value of 100; marriage has a relative point value of 50, and a vacation has a relative point value of 13 (Holmes & Rahe, 1967).

(The complete SRRS is available at the American Institute of Stress website.)

As a baseline assessement, the following questions are helpful to gather additional information about the patient's stress and coping mechanisms.

1. What do you do for relaxation? For recreation?

2. What is your greatest source of comfort when you are feeling upset?
   This question identifies the patient's coping mechanisms.

3. Who do you call when you need help?
   This question identifies important persons in the patient's support system.

4. What is the greatest source of stress in your life at the present time? How have you coped with similar situations in the past?
   A person who has successfully coped with stress in the past may be able to call upon these coping skills to deal with current problems.

5. Describe how you are dealing with your illness. Have you had difficulty adjusting to: changes in your appearance, your ability to carry out activities of daily living, or your relationships? If so, describe how you feel.
   Patients who have undergone severe, sudden changes that are apparent to others frequently have difficulty adjusting to these changes.

6. Do you take any drugs, medications, or alcohol to cope with your stress? If so, describe what you are taking.
   Patients who are experiencing stress are at risk for becoming addicted to these substances, especially if there is a family history of drug or alcohol abuse.

7. Do you use comfort foods, or do you overeat when you are feeling stressed?
   A link between prolonged stress, eating comfort foods, and obesity has been described.

8. Are you experiencing any of the following: sadness? crying spells? insomnia? lack of appetite? weight loss? weight gain? loss of sex drive? constipation? fatigue? hopelessness? irritability? indecisiveness? confusion? pounding heart or pulse? trouble concentrating?
   These may indicate a high level of stress or major depression.

9. Have you ever considered taking your life? If so, describe what you would do.
   Patients who are suicidal often admit their intentions if questioned directly. Patients are at high risk for suicide if they can describe a method for committing the suicide and have the necessary means at their disposal.

Ineffective coping may lead to a variety of maladaptaptive behaviors, including self-directed violence (SDV). **Self-directed violence (SDV)** is behavior committed by and aimed at oneself that results in deliberate actual or potential self-harm (Crosby, Ortega, & Melanson, 2011). Forms of SDV include self-injury (such as self-mutilation) and suicide. **Suicidal ideation**—which is considering, planning, or thinking about committing suicide— also is considered a form of SDV. SDV does not include risky behaviors and lifestyle choices, such as speeding in motor vehicles, using tobacco, or using drugs without the intent to inflict self-harm (Crosby et al., 2011).

Suicide remains a major health concern in the United States. In 2009, the number of suicide-related deaths exceeded the number of deaths due to motor vehicle crashes (CDC, 2013). Although traditional suicide prevention efforts have focused on adolescents and older adults, current research suggests that individuals of all ages are at risk for suicide (CDC, 2013).

For the nurse, awareness of the widespread problem of suicide and knowledge of the factors that may increase an individual's risk for SDV, including one or more previous suicide attempt, are keys to identifying at-risk patients (see Box 5.2 for an overview of factors associated with an increased risk for attempting suicide.)

In addition to being familiar with risk factors for suicide, the nurse also should be aware of the warning signs of an impending potential suicide attempt. Warning signs of an impending suicide attempt vary among individuals. However, certain behaviors—such as researching methods of suicide or giving away prized personal belongings—are critical indicators that should be immediately reported to the patient's primary care provider. See Box 5.3 for examples of warning signs that may signal an impending suicide attempt.

Should analysis of nursing assessment data suggest that a patient is at risk for attempting suicide or committing any other form of SDV, the nurse should immediately notify the patient's primary care provider. Patients who are known or believed to be at risk for SDV should be continually monitored and care of these patients should include immediate implementation of the hospital's or organization's safety protocols.

Sensory Perception and Cognition

Patients who are out of contact with reality may display illusional, delusional, and hallucinatory speech and behaviors, such as talking to themselves (auditory hallucinations); reacting to objects, noises, or other people in strange ways (illusions); or discussing false beliefs (delusions). Direct questioning may increase the patient's anxiety and escalate the abnormal behavior or cause confusion. The nurse should use direct questioning only when the patient appears to be in control and in touch with reality.

The following questions are helpful to gather additional information. The nurse should preface these questions by first explaining to the patient that some of the questions may seem silly or unimportant, but they are helpful in assessing memory.

1. What is your name?

2. How old are you?

3. Where were you born?

4. Where are you right now?

5. What day of the week is it? What is the date?
   Questions 1 through 5 determine whether the patient is oriented to person, place, and time.

6. What would you take with you if a fire broke out?
   The patient's ability to make a judgment is tested here.

7. Count backward from 10 to 1.
   Tests cognitive function.

8. What did you have for breakfast?
   Tests recent memory.

9. Who were the last two presidents?
   Tests remote memory.

Box 5.2 Factors That Increase an Individual's Risk for Attempting Suicide

- History of suicide attempt(s)
- Age (with highest risk among older adults)
- Lower socioeconomic status
- Limited education
- Single/unmarried status
- Unemployment
- History of drug or alcohol abuse
- History of childhood adversities (including physical or sexual abuse)
- History of mental illness/psychiatric disorder
- Physiologic disorders such as cancer, HIV, or a terminal illness
- Recent legal/criminal problems
- Chaotic or troubled interpersonal relationships

Sources: Adapted from Borges, G., Nock, M. K., Haro, J. M., Hwang, I., Sampson, N. A., Alonso, J., . . . Kessler, R. C. (2010). Twelve-month prevalence of and risk factors for suicide attempts in the World Health Organization World Mental Health Surveys. *Journal of Clinical Psychiatry, 71*(12), 1617–1628; Haw, C., Hawton, K., Niedzwiedz, C., & Platt, S. (2013). Suicide clusters: A review of risk factors and mechanisms. *Suicide and Life-Threatening Behavior, 43*(1), 97–108; Logan, J., Hall, J., & Karch, D. (2011). Suicide categories by patterns of known risk factors: A latent class analysis. *Archives of General Psychiatry, 68*(9), 935–941; and Valente, S. M. (2010). Assessing patients for suicide risk. *Nursing 2014, 40*(5), 36–40.

Box 5.3 Potential Warning Signs of an Impending Suicide Attempt

- Reckless behavior
- Increased incidence of alcohol and/or drug abuse
- Seeking out information on suicide methods or purchasing a weapon
- Changes in sleep patterns
- Panic attacks, anxiety, or agitation
- Giving away treasured personal belongings
- Expression of feelings of worthlessness or hopelessness
- Contacting people to say goodbye
- Social withdrawal
- Dramatic changes in mood.

Sources: Adapted from American Foundation for Suicide Prevention. (n.d.). Risk factors and warning signs. Retrieved from http://www.afsp .org/understanding-suicide/risk-factors-and-warning-signs; Valente, S. M. (2010). Assessing patients for suicide risk. *Nursing 2014, 40*(5), 36–40; and McDowell, A. K., Lineberry, T. W., & Bostwick, J. M. (2011). Practical suicide-risk management for the busy primary care physician. *Mayo Clinic Proceedings, 86*(8), 792–800.

10. Describe what the following statement means: People who live in glass houses should not throw stones.
    Tests the patient's ability to do abstract or symbolic thinking.

11. Are you having any problems thinking? If so, describe what happens.
    The patient may not be able to answer this question if a thought disorder is present. Patients with bipolar disorders and who are manic describe their thoughts as "racing."

12. Do you have trouble making decisions? Describe what happens when you have to make a decision.
    The inability to make decisions may indicate depression or low self-esteem.

13. Do you ever hear voices, see objects, or experience other sensations that do not make sense? If so, describe your experiences.
    The patient who is out of touch with reality may experience auditory, visual, gustatory, somatic, and olfactory hallucinations (hearing, seeing, tasting, feeling, and smelling stimuli that are not real). Discussing hallucinatory experiences in detail may reinforce them for the patient; therefore, it is important not to dwell on these symptoms with the patient.

14. If you hear voices, do they tell you what you must do?
    The nurse asks this question to determine if the patient is experiencing command hallucinations. These are dangerous hallucinations that may lead the patient to self-destructive behavior or to harm others.

15. Do you ever misinterpret objects, sounds, or smells? If so, please describe.
    Patients who are very anxious or out of contact with reality may experience illusions (misinterpretation of environmental stimuli).

In order to provide for the patient's safety and the safety of others, it is important to assess the content of a patient's hallucinations and delusions. Command hallucinations tell patients to carry out acts against themselves or others that are usually harmful. The command hallucinations may be part of an elaborate delusional system in which patients feel persecuted or in danger. In some cases, patients are disturbed by these thoughts and share them with others. In other situations, however, patients keep their thoughts to themselves, and these thoughts do not become apparent until they commit some violent act. A patient who demonstrates these symptoms should be referred to a psychiatric/mental health nurse or clinical specialist who has the skill and expertise needed to uncover hallucinatory and delusional thinking without exacerbating the symptoms.

Spiritual and Belief Systems

The questions in this section determine how patients' ethical, moral, and religious values affect their health status. Often the patient's statements about values play an important role in how the nurse should implement care. It is important to be sensitive to the patient's reaction to these questions when assessing this area, because the patient's spiritual life and belief systems may be very personal.

The nurse should also be careful about querying a patient who is hallucinating or is delusional, because the questions can exacerbate delusional or hallucinatory behavior.

The spiritual and belief systems of patients usually derive from their culture and ethnic background. A patient may have beliefs about health and illness, God, or the supernatural that are culturally derived. The nurse needs to understand that these issues play an important role in the patient's ability to cope with a psychosocial health concern or illness.

The following questions are used to assess the patient's spiritual and belief systems and the cultural and ethnic considerations surrounding them. While collecting this information, the nurse should observe the patient's verbal and nonverbal behavior, interpersonal relationships, and immediate environment.

1. Describe your ethnic and cultural background.
   Patients from some ethnic and cultural groups are more likely to have health-related beliefs and practices that have an impact on nursing care (see chapter 4 ∞).

2. To whom do you go for help regarding your health (doctor, nurse, practitioner, folk healer, medicine man, or other healer)?
   The nurse is more likely to gain the patient's compliance if the patient's folk healer is included in the planning stage.

3. What are your beliefs about life, health, illness, and death?
   The nurse needs this knowledge about the patient's health-related beliefs to develop an individualized plan of care.

4. Does religion or God play a part in your life? If so, what is it?
   The nurse should incorporate the patient's religion and faith in God in the plan of care if they are important to the patient.

5. What part do hope and faith play in your life? Is your faith helpful to you during times of stress? If so, describe how.

6. Has your present health concern affected your spiritual life? If so, describe how.

7. Do your spiritual beliefs help you cope with illness or stress? If so, describe how.

8. Have you experienced any anger with God or a higher being or force because of things that have happened to you? If so, describe how you feel.
   Patients who feel anger toward God or a higher force may project this anger toward family, friends, and healthcare providers.

9. Do you believe your illness is a punishment for past sins or wrongdoing?
   Patients who feel they are being punished may feel guilty and lose the ability to cope with the illness.

10. If you use prayer, describe how you use it to cope with life or stress.
    The nurse should incorporate the patient's use of prayer in the plan of care if it is meaningful to the patient.

11. Are you affiliated with any religion?

12. Describe any religion-related nutrition or health practices that you must follow.

13. Are you concerned about the morality or ethical implications of any of the treatments planned for you?

Physical Observation

During the initial or focused interview, the nurse should also observe the patient's general appearance, posture, gait, body language, and speech patterns. The patient's general appearance includes the manner of dress, personal hygiene, and grooming.

- The patient should be clean and well groomed. The clothes should be clean, worn properly, and appropriate for the patient's age and the time and place. The nurse must be careful not to impose his or her own standards when judging the dress of another.

Box 5.4 Abnormal Speech Patterns Associated with Altered Thought Processes

- Loud, rapid, pressured, and high-pitched
- Circumlocution (inability to communicate an idea due to numerous digressions)
- Flight of ideas (jumping from one subject to another)
- Word salad (a conglomeration of multiple words without apparent meaning)
- Neologisms (coining new words that have symbolic meaning to the patient)
- Clanging (rhyming conversation)
- Echolalia (constant repetition of words or phrases that the patient hears others say)

- Abnormal speech patterns may indicate anxiety, fear, or altered thought processes (see Box 5.4). The nurse should observe the coherence and organization of the patient's speech. The patient's speech should be logical and sequential.

- Patients may demonstrate the following: talking to themselves (auditory hallucinations); reacting to objects, noises, or other people in strange ways (illusions); or manifesting erratic beliefs (delusions). The patient may appear to be aphasic or incoherent. These patients may be experiencing altered communication, altered thought processes, and ineffective coping.

- The patient who is dirty, disheveled, or unshaven or who has a body odor may have an altered body image caused by a low self-esteem. The nurse should further assess the patient for changes in skin integrity due to unclean conditions and should look for signs of ringworm, pediculosis, or other skin problems (see chapter 13 ∞).

The nurse should next observe the patient's posture, gait, and general body language.

- The patient's posture should be erect and relaxed. The body language should be open with direct eye contact unless inappropriate for the patient's ethnic group. Movements should be fluid, relaxed, and spontaneous. A closed, guarded posture with poor eye contact may indicate fear, anxiety, or defense mechanisms. The patient who paces, wrings hands, appears restless, or exhibits tics (involuntary movements) may also be experiencing anxiety. A slow, shuffling gait may indicate depression or poor contact with reality.

The nurse must also observe the facial expression and affect. The expression and affect should be appropriate for the conversation and circumstances.

- An unusually sad (depressed) or extremely happy (euphoric) demeanor that is inappropriate for the circumstances, labile (rapid) mood swings, or flat affect (absence of emotional expression) may indicate difficulty coping.

Box 5.5 Healthy Days Measures

The CDC uses a set of questions called the "Healthy Days Measures." These questions include the following:

1. Would you say that in general your health is
   A. Excellent
   B. Very good
   C. Good
   D. Fair
   E. Poor

2. Now thinking about your physical health, which includes physical illness and injury, for how many days during the past 30 days was your physical health not good?

3. Now thinking about your mental health, which includes stress, depression, and problems with emotions, for how many days during the past 30 days was your mental health not good?

4. During the past 30 days, for about how many days did poor physical or mental health keep you from doing your usual activities, such as self-care, work, or recreation?

Source: Adapted from Centers for Disease Control and Prevention (CDC). (2011). *Health-related quality of life (HRQOL): CDC HRQOL–14 "Healthy Days Measure."* Retrieved from http://www.cdc.gov/hrqol/hrqol14_measure.htm

Finally, the nurse should notice the content and manner of speech. The content, tone, pace, and volume of the speech should be appropriate for the situation.

Measures, scales, and instruments are available to assess particular aspects of psychosocial health including quality of life, social support, stress, and psychosocial well-being. For example, the CDC uses "Healthy Days Measures" to assess quality of life in populations. Box 5.5 includes questions used in healthy days measures.

Several instruments have been developed to assess factors related to body image. These include the Multidimensional Body Self-Relations Questionnaire, Body Image Ideals Questionnaire, Body Image Quality of Life Inventory, and the Body Exposure During Sexual Activities Questionnaire. The Body Image Assessment for Obesity (BIA-O) was developed to examine body image disturbances in men and women who are obese (Williamson et al., 2000).

Other measures to assess particular aspects of psychosocial health include the Multidimensional Health Profile–Psychosocial (MHP–P). An instrument designed to screen for psychosocial problems, the MHP–P assesses life stress, coping, social supports, and mental health. One may also use the Duke Social Support and Stress Scale (DUSOCS). This is a 24-item self- and interviewer-administered instrument to measure family and nonfamily support and stress. Psychologic well-being may be assessed with a variety of scales including the delighted–terrible scale, the faces scale, the ladder scale, and the life satisfaction index. Each of these scales provides a system to rank the patient's perceptions of well-being.

Organizing the Data

Once the nurse has collected the data from all of the various sources, the information is sorted, grouped, and categorized. Each diagnostic cue falls under one of the psychosocial functioning groups

mentioned earlier in this chapter: self-concept, roles and relationships, stress and coping, the senses and cognition, and spiritual and belief systems. After the diagnostic cues have been grouped and clustered under one of the psychosocial groups, the nurse determines the final nursing diagnoses.

The following case study demonstrates how diagnostic cues obtained during the assessment lead to nursing diagnoses related to psychosocial well-being and function.

Mr. Abe Johnson, a transient passing through town, was admitted to the local hospital emergency department after being arrested for disturbing the peace and possession of heroin. The guards at the jail had brought him to the hospital after they were unable to control his violent behavior. When approached by the admitting nurse, Ms. Quan, Mr. Johnson shouted, "Don't come near me with that gas machine! The High Lord has told me that I control the secret of life and death, and if you touch me you must die!" The nurse recognized that Mr. Johnson had seen the stethoscope she carried as a "gas machine." After observing Mr. Johnson's manner and tone for a few minutes, she also noted that he was hearing voices. Ms. Quan knew that Mr. Johnson's behavior could become violent if he continued to experience command hallucinations. She removed the stethoscope from around her neck and showed it to Mr. Johnson. She said, speaking in a quiet calm voice, "This is the stethoscope that I use to listen to a patient's heart. Sometimes I use it to take blood pressures. Would you like to look at it?" As Mr. Johnson doubtfully held the stethoscope and rapidly and repeatedly turned it over, she said, "Most stethoscopes are black and silver but mine is white and gold. I think it's a pretty color, don't you?" Mr. Johnson threw the stethoscope back at Ms. Quan, mumbling "OK." After a few minutes she said, "You've been brought to the hospital, Mr. Johnson. I'm Ms. Quan, your nurse, and I'm here to take care of you. Have you noticed that even though I've been helping you remove your clothes, nothing has happened to me?"

In this clinical situation, the nurse showed Mr. Johnson respect and concern for his feelings and well-being. She did not, however, validate his perceptions about the stethoscope or acknowledge the voices he heard. Instead, she reinforced reality for him by describing the white and gold stethoscope and pointing out that he had no special power to harm her.

The nurse then clustered the information gained from the assessment and identified the significant cues demonstrated by Mr. Johnson:

- Hallucinations
- Delusions
- Illusions
- Fearful thoughts
- Irritability
- Inaccurate interpretation of environment

Ms. Quan reviewed all the data and saw the following factors as contributing to Mr. Johnson's problems:

- Substance abuse
- Transient lifestyle

Then, after reviewing the assessment data, identifying contributing factors, and clustering the information, Ms. Quan formulated diagnoses and a plan of care.

The holistic approach to nursing holds that the individual must be viewed as a total being, by which body, mind, and spirit continuously interact with self and with the environment. The psychosocial assessment is a key component that must be integrated into the nurse's holistic approach to data collection. This assessment guides the nurse toward a true and accurate picture of the patient as a total human being.

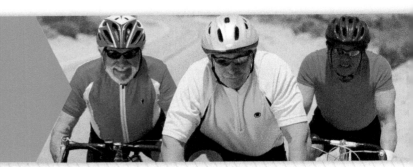

Application Through Critical Thinking

▶ Case Study

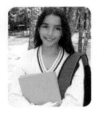

Crystal is a 15-year-old Hispanic female who has come to the women's clinic for birth control. During her interview you find out she has been abusing prescription drugs for the past 3 years. This began shortly after her father passed away from a long battle with colon cancer. She was very close to her father, and when he died she was feeling very sad and she took some of his pain medication to help her sleep. She began to use the drugs and eventually became addicted. Her father was the main support in the home and when he was alive he kept the family together. He worked in the restaurant industry and did not have any death benefits other than Social Security and a small life insurance policy. Her mother suffers from depression and has been unable to work since her father died and has periods where she is so depressed she is unable to get out of bed. She refuses to get any help. Crystal is left to care for herself and her mom and says she uses drugs just to escape from her life. She does not attend school regularly and has poor grades. She has a part time job at a restaurant to pay for her drugs and to buy food. She and her mom live in an apartment in a low-income housing area after they lost their home due to foreclosure. Crystal shares with you that she is sexually active and does not want to become pregnant.

▶ Critical Thinking Questions

1. What external/internal factors contributed to Crystal's current situation?
2. What additional factors are applicable in psychosocial health?
3. What questions might you ask to understand Crystal's self-concept?
4. What questions might you ask to find out more information about Crystal's relationship with her mother?
5. What suicide risk factors does Crystal have?

▶ References

American Foundation for Suicide Prevention. (n.d.). *Risk factors and warning signs*. Retrieved from http://www.afsp.org/understanding-suicide/risk-factors-and-warning-signs

Anadarajah, G., & Hight, E. (2001). *Spirituality and medical practice: Using the HOPE questions as a practical tool for spiritual assessment*. Retrieved from http://www.aafp.org/afp/2001/0101/p81.html

Berman, A., & Snyder, S. (2012). *Kozier and Erb's fundamentals of nursing: Concepts, process and practice* (9th ed.). Upper Saddle River, NJ: Prentice Hall.

Borges, G., Nock, M. K., Haro, J. M., Hwang, I., Sampson, N. A., Alonso, J., . . . Kessler, R. C. (2010). Twelve-month prevalaence of and risk factors for suicide attempts in the WHO World Health Organization mental health surveys. *Journal of Clinical Psychiatry, 71*(12), 1617–1628.

Centers for Disease Control and Prevention (CDC). (2011) *Health-related quality of life (HRQOL): CDC HRQOL–14 "Healthy Days Measure."* Retrieved from http://www.cdc.gov/hrqol/hrqol14_measure.htm

Centers for Disease Control and Prevention (CDC). (2013). Suicide among adults aged 35–64 years—United States, 1999–2010. *Morbidity and Mortality Weekly Report (MMWR), 62*(17), 321–325.

Clark, M. (2008). *Community health nursing: Advocacy for populations health* (5th ed.). Upper Saddle River, NJ: Prentice Hall.

Crosby, A. E., Ortega, L., & Melanson, C. (2011). *Self-directed violence surveillance: Uniform definitions and recommended data elements*. Atlanta, GA: Centers for Disease Control and Prevention, National Center for Injury Prevention and Control, Division of Violence Prevention.

Donatelle, R. J. (2012). *Health: The basics* (10th ed.). San Francisco: Benjamin Cummings.

Forbes, A. (2014). Define "Sex": Legal outcomes for transgender individuals in the United States. In D. Peterson & V. Panfil (Eds.), *Handbook of LGBT Communities, Crime, and Justice* (pp. 387–403). New York: Springer.

Haw, C., Hawton, K., Niedzwiedz, C., & Platt, S. (2013). Suicide clusters: A review of risk factors and mechanisms. *Suicide and Life-Threatening Behavior, 43*(1), 97–108.

Hodge, D. R. (2001). Spiritual assessment: A review of major qualitative methods and a new framework for assessing spirituality. *Social Work, 46*(3), 203–214.

Hodge, D. R., & Horvath, V. E. (2010). Spiritual needs in health care settings: A qualitative meta-synthesis of patients' perspectives. *Social Work, 56*(4), 306–316.

Holmes, T., & Rahe, R. J. (1967). Social Readjustment Rating Scale. *Journal of Psychosomatic Research, 11*(2), 213–218.

Logan, J., Hall, J., & Karch, D. (2011). Suicide categories by patterns of known risk factors: A latent class analysis. *Archives of General Psychiatry, 68*(9), 935–941.

McDowell, A. K., Lineberry, T. W., & Bostwick, J. M. (2011). Practical suicide-risk management for the busy primary care physician. *Mayo Clinic Proceedings, 86*(8), 792–800.

McSherry, W., & Ross, L. (2002). Dilemmas of spiritual assessment: Considerations for nursing practice. *Journal of Advanced Nursing, 38*(5), 479–488.

Morrow, D. F., & Messinger, L. (Eds.). (2013). *Sexual orientation and gender expression in social work practice: Working with gay, lesbian, bisexual, and transgender people.* New York: Columbia University Press.

National Alliance on Mental Illness (NAMI). (2013a). *Anorexia nervosa.* Retrieved from http://www.nami.org/Template.cfm?Section=By_Illness&Template=/ContentManagement/ContentDisplay.cfm&ContentID=149438

National Alliance on Mental Illness (NAMI). (2013b). *Bulimia nervosa.* Retrieved from http://www.nami.org/Content/ContentGroups/Helpline1/Bulimia.htm

National Association of Mental Illness (NAMI). (2013a). *Anorexia nervosa.* Retrieved from http://www.nami.org/Template.cfm?Section=By_Illness&Template=/ContentManagement/ContentDisplay.cfm&ContentID=149438

National Association of Mental Illness (NAMI). (2013b). *Bulimia nervosa.* Retrieved from http://www.nami.org/Template.cfm?Section=By_Illness&Template=/ContentManagement/ContentDisplay.cfm&ContentID=149448

National Human Genome Research Institute. (2012). *Frequently asked questions about genetic disorders: What are genetic disorders?* Retrieved from https://www.genome.gov/19016930

Office of Public Health and Genomics (OPHG). (2013). *Identifying opportunities to improve health and transform healthcare.* Retrieved from http://www.genome.gov/Pages/Health/PatientsPublicInfo/GeneticTestingWhatItMeansForYourHealth.pdf

Osborn K. S., Wraa, C. E., Watson, A., & Holleran, R. S. (2013). *Medical-surgical nursing: Preparation for practice.* (2nd ed.). Upper Saddle River, NJ: Pearson.

President's Council on Physical Fitness and Sports. (2010). *Fitness fundamentals: Guidelines for personal exercise programs.* Washington, DC: U.S. Department of Health and Human Services.

Puhl, R. M., & Heuer, C. A. (2010). Obesity stigma: Important considerations for public health. *American Journal of Public Health, 100*(6), 1019–1028.

Puhl, R. M., & Latner, J. D. (2007). Stigma, obesity, and the health of the nation's children. *Psychological Bulletin, 133*(4), 557–580.

Reilly, J. J., & Kelly, J. (2011). Long-term impact of overweight and obesity in childhood and adolescence on morbidity and premature mortality in adulthood: Systematic review. *International Journal of Obesity, 35*(7), 891–898.

Roy, C., & Andrews, H. (1999). *The Roy adaptation model* (2nd ed.). Stamford, CT: Appleton & Lange.

Savin-Williams, R. C. (2011). Identity development among sexual-minority youth. In S. Schwartz, K. Luyckx, & V. Vignoles (Eds.), *Handbook of identity theory and research* (pp. 671–689). New York: Springer.

Stoll, R. I. (1979). Guidelines for spiritual assessment. *American Journal of Nursing, 79*(9), 1574–1577.

Tomiyama, A. J., Dallman, M. F., & Epel, E. S. (2011). Comfort food is comforting to those most stressed: Evidence of the chronic stress response network in high stress women. *Psychoneuroendocrinology, 36*(10), 1513–1519.

Valente, S. M. (2010). Assessing patients for suicide risk. *Nursing2014, 40*(5), 36–40.

WebMD. (2011). *Spiritual assessment.* Retrieved from http://www.webmd.com/balance/tc/ncicdr0000301599-spiritual-assessment

Williams, J. A., Meltzer, D., Arora, V., Chung, G., & Curlin, F. A. (2012). Attention to inpatients' religious and spiritual concerns: Predictors and association with patient satisfaction. *Journal of General Internal Medicine, 26*(11), 1265–1271.

Williamson, D. A., Womble, L. G., Zucker, N. L., Reas, D. L., White, M. A., Blouin, D. C., & Greenway, F. (2000). Body image assessment for obesity (BIA-O): Development of a new procedure. *International Journal of Obesity, 24*(10), 1326–1332. Retrieved from http://www.nature.com/ijo/journal/v24/n10/full/0801363a.html

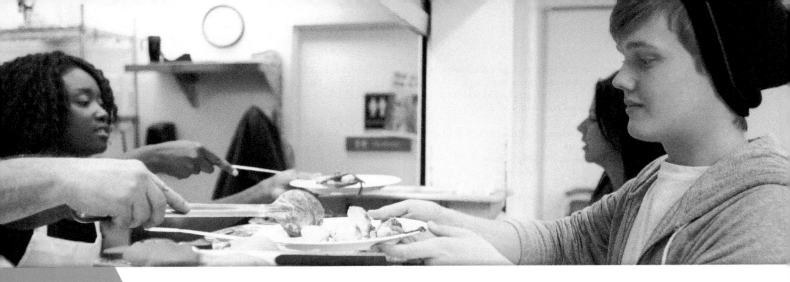

Assessment of Vulnerable Populations

▶ Learning Outcomes

Upon completion of the chapter, you will be able to:

1. Identify vulnerable patient groups.

2. Identify the factors that influence each of the vulnerable populations.

3. Discuss the nursing role in relation to assessment of a person from a vulnerable population.

4. Describe types of abuse and recognize associated signs and symptoms.

5. Discuss the goals for eliminating health disparities for vulnerable populations.

6. Describe the physical and social determinants of vulnerable populations.

Key Terms

disabilities, 107
elder abuse, 104
geography, 106
health disparities, 101
intimate partner violence, 104
metabolic syndrome, 106
mixed-status family, 108
social determinants of health, 108
vulnerable populations, 101

Vulnerable populations are groups that are not well integrated into the U.S. healthcare system because of racial, ethnic, cultural, economic, geographic, or health characteristics. This isolation places members of these groups at risk for not obtaining necessary preventive or medical care, and thus constitutes a potential threat to their health. Significant health disparities continue for vulnerable populations in the United States. Vulnerable populations include the economically disadvantaged, racial and ethnic minorities, the uninsured, low-income children, and the elderly.

Some people in the United States face more barriers to health care because of health disparities. In particular, racial and ethnic contrasts have been identified between African Americans, Hispanics, Asians, American Indians, and Caucasians. Socioeconomic contrasts between poor and high-income people have been identified as well. According to the National Institutes of Health (NIH, 2013), **health disparities** are gaps in the quality of health and health care that mirror differences in socioeconomic status, racial and ethnic background, and levels of education. Such gaps include factors such as accessibility of health care, increased risk of disease from occupational or environmental exposure, and increased risk of disease from genetic, environmental, or familial factors. For example, approximately two million Hispanics/Latinos in the United States have asthma; Puerto Rican Americans have asthma at almost three times the rate of the overall Hispanic population; and African Americans are diagnosed with asthma at a 28% higher rate than Caucasians. The nurse's awareness of the patient's racial and ethnic background as well as any related health disparities—such as in the diagnosis of asthma—benefits both the nurse and the patient.

The Centers for Disease Control and Prevention (CDC), in partnership with other organizations, continues to identify and address the different factors that may lead to health disparities among racial, ethnic, geographic, socioeconomic, and other groups. It assesses vulnerable populations as defined by:

- Race/ethnicity
- Socioeconomic status
- Geography
- Gender
- Age
- Disability status
- Risk status related to sex and gender

In addition to this list, the CDC (2014d) also includes the following groups in its list of at risk/vulnerable populations:

- Cancer survivors
- Immigrants and refugees
- Incarcerated men and women
- Persons who use drugs (PWUD)
- Pregnant women
- Veterans

In addition, *Healthy People 2020* describes health disparities based on race, ethnicity, gender, sexual identity, age, disability, socioeconomic status, and geographic location. The goal of *Healthy People 2020* is to eliminate health disparities by improving access, quality, and care among identified vulnerable populations.

A focus on improving the availability and quality of care among persons who are experiencing health disparities—including patient history-taking, physical examination, and assessment—allows clinical interventions to become opportunities for each individual to attain his or her full health potential. For example, the Omaha System was developed for use in diverse practice settings such as public health, home health, and nurse-managed centers. It is a system that documents patient assessment and nurse interventions directed toward wellness, support systems, and coping skills. Using this system identifies and categorizes teaching needs, guidance and counseling, treatments and procedures, case management, and surveillance to address health disparities of vulnerable populations (Thompson, Monsen, Wanamaker, Augustyniak, & Thompson, 2012).

This chapter will review the factors that influence at-risk vulnerable populations.

Factors That Influence Vulnerable Populations

Nurses provide care for patients from vulnerable populations in all healthcare settings. The nurse performs a crucial role when performing health assessments for these patients. Assessment determines the patient's current and ongoing health status, predicts risk, and identifies health promotion activities. As is true with all patients, in assessing a patient from a vulnerable population, nurses must be aware of the patient's social factors that are linked to his or her cultural identity. Cultural competence in nursing is more than an understanding of race and ethnicity. Cultural competence is described as the integration and transformation of knowledge and skills about persons or a group in a community regarding their practices, beliefs, values, attitudes, or policies to increase the quality of healthcare services with the goal of providing better health outcomes. The process of cultural awareness, knowledge, skills, and comfort in patient care encounters begins with the nurse (Mareno & Hart, 2014). Nurses working with vulnerable populations need to be aware of their own cultural heritage before they can be sensitive to others' vulnerabilities and be able to demonstrate competence in understanding and caring for vulnerable populations (see chapter 4 ∞). Identification, assessment, intervention, and evaluation through the nursing process are thought to be an integral part of nursing practice to protect vulnerable populations.

Race and Ethnicity

According to the 2010 U.S. Census, over 36 percent of the U.S. population identifies as belonging to a racial or ethnic minority group. Awareness of the nation's changing racial and ethnic diversity will guide healthcare professionals to identify areas in which certain groups may need special services; plan and implement education; and provide housing, health needs, and health programs.

The following sections describe the factors that can influence vulnerable populations that are identified by race and ethnicity: Asian American, Black or African American, Hispanic or Latino, Native Hawaiian and Other Pacific Islander, American Indian and Alaska Native, White or Caucasian, and Multiracial (see Table 6.1).

TABLE 6.1	**Summary of Racial Groups**
Asian American	Origins in Far East, Southeast Asia, or the Indian subcontinent including Cambodia, China, India, Japan, Korea, Malaysia, Pakistan, Philippine Islands, Thailand, and Vietnam
Black or African American	Origins in United States, and immigrants from Africa, the Caribbean, and the West Indies
Hispanic or Latino	Origins in Cuba, Mexico, Puerto Rico, South or Central America, or other Spanish culture regardless of race.
Native Hawaiian and Other Pacific Islander	Origins in any of the original peoples of Hawaii, Guam, Samoa, or other Pacific Islands
American Indian and Alaska Native	Origins in any of the original peoples of North and South America who maintain a tribal affiliation or community attachment.
White or Caucasian	Origins in any of the original peoples of Europe, the Middle East, or North Africa
Multiracial	People who belong to two or more racial categories

Asian American

Asians are people having origins in any of the original peoples of the Far East, Southeast Asia, or the Indian subcontinent including Cambodia, China, India, Indonesia, Japan, Korea, Malaysia, Myanmar, Pakistan, Philippine Islands, Thailand, and Vietnam. The ten leading causes of death for Asian Americans in order of prevalence are cancer; heart disease; stroke; unintentional injuries; diabetes; influenza and pneumonia; chronic lower respiratory diseases; nephritis, nephrotic syndrome, and nephrosis; Alzheimer's disease; and suicide (National Center for Health Statistics, 2014a).

Asian Americans can represent the extremes of both health outcomes and socioeconomic status. For example, Asian American women experience higher rates of nephrotic syndrome and nephrosis, chronic lower respiratory disease, homicide, septicemia, and Alzheimer's disease as compared to other populations, yet they have the longest life expectancy (85.8 years) of any ethnic group in the United States. Asian Americans may contend with infrequent medical visits due to fear of deportation, language and cultural barriers, and lack of health insurance (U.S. Census Bureau, 2012).

Black or African American

Most African Americans have a long history in the United States, some for many generations, while others are recent immigrants from Africa, the Caribbean, and the West Indies. The ten leading causes of death for African Americans in order of prevalence are heart disease; cancer; stroke; diabetes; unintentional injuries; nephritis, nephrotic syndrome, and nephrosis; chronic lower respiratory disease; homicide; septicemia; and Alzheimer's disease (CDC, 2011).

Health disparities between African Americans and other racial and ethnic populations include life expectancy, death rates, infant mortality, and other measures of health and risk behaviors. For example, African Americans have the highest death rates from heart disease and stroke; the highest prevalence of hypertension, diabetes, and peritonitis; the largest HIV infection rate; and the highest death rate from homicide (National Institutes of Health, 2013). Factors contributing to poor health outcomes among some members of this population include discrimination, cultural barriers, and lack of healthcare access (CDC, 2010).

Hispanic or Latino

Hispanic or Latino origin, as used in the U.S. Census, refers to a person of Cuban, Mexican, Puerto Rican, South or Central American, or other Spanish culture or origin regardless of race. The U.S. Census (2010) estimated that 52 million Hispanics live in the United States, representing 16.7% of the population. It is predicted that by 2050, the Hispanic population will increase to 30% of the total U.S. population. Mexican represents the largest subgroup of Hispanics at 63%, followed by Puerto Rican at 9.2%, Cuban at 3.5%, Salvadoran at 3.3%, and Dominicans at 2.8%; the remaining 18.2% were people of other Hispanic or Latino origins. The ten leading causes of death among this population in order of prevalence are cancer; heart disease; unintentional injuries; stroke; diabetes; chronic liver disease and cirrhosis; chronic lower respiratory diseases; influenza and pneumonia; homicide; and nephritis, nephrotic syndrome, and nephrosis (CDC, 2011). Some Hispanic and Latino patients face disparities in income, education level, and housing quality.

Native Hawaiian and Other Pacific Islander

Native Hawaiians and Other Pacific Islanders are individuals who have origins in any of the original peoples of Hawaii, Guam, Samoa, or other Pacific Islands. States with the largest population concentrations are Hawaii and California. The ten leading causes of death among this population in order of prevalence are cancer; heart disease; stroke; unintentional injuries; diabetes; influenza and pneumonia; chronic lower respiratory diseases; nephritis, nephrotic syndrome, and nephrosis; Alzheimer's disease; and suicide (National Center for Health Statistics, 2014a). Native Hawaiians and Other Pacific Islanders have higher cancer rates than other racial or ethnic minority groups, and their five-year cancer survival rate for all cancers is lower than the rates of other racial and ethnic populations. Native Hawaiian and Other Pacific Islanders have higher rates of smoking, alcohol consumption, and obesity. Major causes of premature death are obesity, cardiovascular disease, cancer, and diabetes. Compared to the rest of the U.S. population, Native Hawaiians and other Pacific Islanders are more likely to live in poverty.

American Indian and Alaska Native

American Indians and Alaska Natives are people who have origins in any of the original peoples of North and South America and who maintain a tribal affiliation or community attachment (CDC, 2011). There are 565 federally recognized tribes representing approximately 1.7% of the total U.S. population. This number is projected to increase to 2% by 2050. The state with the largest population is California, followed by Oklahoma and then Arizona. The ten leading causes of death among this population in order of prevalence are heart disease; cancer; unintentional injuries; diabetes; chronic liver disease and cirrhosis; chronic lower respiratory disease; stroke; suicide; influenza and pneumonia; and nephritis, nephrotic syndrome, and nephrosis (CDC, 2011).

Although the Indian Health Service (IHS) typically serves the health needs of this population, more than half of the people in this group do not permanently reside on reservations and have limited or no access to IHS services. Factors that may contribute to poorer health outcomes among this population are cultural barriers, geographic isolation, inadequate sewage disposal, and economic factors. American Indian infants are second to African American infants in infant death rates. This population also experiences high rates of death related to motor vehicle accidents and suicide. It also experiences the highest rates of binge drinking and has a high rate of smoking. The percentage of adults of this population living in poverty was among the largest as compared with other racial/ethnic groups (CDC, 2011).

White or Caucasian

Whites, or Caucasians, are people having origins in any of the original peoples of Europe, the Middle East, or North Africa and comprise 70% of the total U.S. population. It is estimated that by 2060, white Americans will decrease to 50% of the total U.S. population. The ten leading causes of death among this group in order of prevalence are heart disease; cancer; chronic lower respiratory disease; stroke; unintentional injuries; Alzheimer's disease; diabetes; influenza and pneumonia; nephritis, nephrotic syndrome, and nephrosis; and suicide (CDC, 2011). Factors that may contribute to poor health outcomes among this population include lack of access to health care and lack of health insurance.

Multiracial

Multiracial Americans are those people who belong to two or more racial categories. According to the U.S. Census, 2.4% of the U.S. population self-identify with two or more racial categories. The highest concentration of multiracial Americans lives in Alaska, California, Hawaii, and Washington. The ten leading causes of death among this group in order of prevalence are heart disease; cancer; stroke; chronic lower respiratory disease; unintentional injuries; Alzheimer's disease; diabetes; influenza and pneumonia; nephritis, nephrotic syndrome, and nephrosis; and septicemia (CDC, 2011).

Racial and Ethnic Approaches to Community Health (REACH)

Racial and Ethnic Approaches to Community Health (REACH) is a national initiative of the CDC to eliminate racial and ethnic disparities in health. The CDC supports community-based programs and culturally tailored interventions to eliminate health disparities among African Americans, American Indians, Hispanic/Latinos, Asian Americans, Alaska Natives, and Pacific Islanders. The goal is to eliminate barriers to healthcare access faced by racial and ethnic minority populations. Heart disease, obesity, and diabetes are the most common health issues that are experienced among most ethnicities that have been identified by REACH. REACH partners use community-based participatory approaches to develop effective strategies for addressing health disparities. The complexities of the racial and ethnic health disparities include the individual, community, societal, cultural, and environmental factors for the identified health concerns. For example, the Community Health Council, an advocacy program to eliminate health disparities serving communities in Los Angeles and across California and the United States, is working with Los Angeles County to develop and implement policies, systems, and environmental improvements to reduce disparities in obesity rates and hypertension among African American and Hispanic/Latino residents. REACH's Obesity and Hypertension Project is being implemented in Boston to focus on five neighborhoods with the largest population of Black and Latino residents. This project includes both children and adults. In addition, another resident-driven Boston coalition has executed programs to address the health disparities in cancer and chronic diseases (CDC, 2014e).

Age

When performing a health assessment on a patient from a vulnerable population perspective, the nurse considers health issues that occur across the life span. Considering a patient's cognitive and emotional development through the lens of vulnerable populations is imperative.

Abuse

Age discrimination across the life span can result in different forms of abuse. Abuse can occur in all age groups and has been identified as physical, sexual, psychological, neglect, acts of omission, discriminatory, and financial.

Physical abuse may present in a variety of ways, from hitting, punching, slapping, burning, choking, shaking, or otherwise harming another person. Patients of all ages can present with signs and symptoms such as bruising at different stages of healing, unexplained injuries, fractures, malnourishment, and marks associated with physical restraint. It is important to note that some cultural practices use treatments that may cause petechiae that imitate physical signs of child abuse. Coining (rubbing the skin with a coin in a symmetric pattern) and cupping (placing heated cups on the skin to create a vacuum) are cultural practices used to treat illness by bringing a source of illness to the surface of the skin. Providers' knowledge of these cultural practices along with its incidence history can avoid accusations of physical abuse.

Sexual abuse may present as rape, sexual assault, molestation, or sexual contact to which the individual has not consented. It also includes incest, sexual exploitation, and prostitution. Research indicates that sexual abuse is underreported and under-identified in part because of societal taboos and perceptions about the gender roles of the offenders and victims. The unfortunate psychological and behavioral effects of sexual abuse such as stigmatization, betrayal, and powerlessness may enhance the victim's increasing vulnerability to health problems, illness, disease, and socioeconomic challenges.

Psychological abuse can result from humiliation, intimidation, and forced isolation. This type of abuse can be manifested by depression, withdrawal, low self-esteem, attention-seeking behavior, and change in personality or behavior. Neglect refers to the failure or refusal to provide food, shelter, protection, or health care for a child or older adult. Self-neglect refers to behaviors of older adults that threaten their own health and safety.

Discriminatory abuse related to a person's disability, age, gender, race, sexuality, religion, or cultural background can be difficult for the nurse to identify. Lastly, financial abuse is related to theft, fraud, exploitation of inheritance, unexplained bank account withdrawals and unusual bank account activities, and loss of valuables. Financial abuse is often a serious issue for elderly patients who may be dependent on caregivers or others for assistance with bill-paying or other financial matters.

Childhood Maltreatment

The Federal Child Abuse Prevention and Treatment Act (CAPTA), (USDHHS, 2010) defines child abuse and neglect at a minimum as any recent act or failure to act on the part of a parent or caretaker that results in death, serious physical or emotional harm, or sexual abuse or exploitation, or an act or failure to act that presents an imminent risk of a serious harm.

Elder Abuse

According to the United States Department of Health and Human Services (USDHHS), Administration on Aging (USDHHS, 2007), hundreds of thousands of older persons are abused, neglected, and exploited by family members and others annually. Elder victims are often frail and vulnerable and depend on others to meet basic needs. **Elder abuse** is a term referring to a knowing, intentional, or negligent act that causes harm or risk of harm to an older adult. The acts may be committed by a caregiver or any other person. As our society ages, it is anticipated that the number of people that experience abuse will increase. People with dementia require an increased amount of care and are looked after by family members, often with little support. Family caregivers are at risk for increased stress and burden, and therefore are at risk for becoming perpetrators of abuse.

Many cases of elder abuse are not reported because the vulnerable elders are afraid to inform the police, friends, or family about the violence. Types of abuse include physical, sexual, emotional, and financial abuse; neglect; and abandonment. The vulnerable older adult with increased disabilities, low income, and poor health is at greatest risk for abuse and violence (CDC, 2013b).

Intimate Partner Violence

Intimate partner violence (IPV) is a serious, preventable, public health problem that affects millions of Americans. IPV can be described as physical, sexual, or psychological harm by a current or former partner or spouse that can occur among heterosexual or same-sex couples and does not require sexual intimacy. According to the National Intimate Partner Sexual Violence Survey conducted in 2010, on average 24 people per minute are victims of rape, physical violence, or stalking by an intimate partner (CDC, 2010). IPV can have a lasting harmful effect on individuals, families, and communities. The goal is to stop it from happening in the first place by using prevention efforts including promoting healthy, respectful, nonviolent relationships to reduce known risk factors (CDC, 2014c). The United States Preventive Services Task Force (2013) issued recommendations to screen women ages 18 to 46 for IPV with referral to appropriate interventions services. The assessment should be routinely conducted on all adolescent and adult women at each patient encounter. The assessment should take place in private, as part of routine practice, using neutral terms such as "hit" or "forced to have sex," rather than "abuse" or "rape." Ask questions such as "Tell me about your relationship with your partner," or ask "Has your partner ever hit, slapped, kicked, or otherwise hurt you?" These are initial questions that are broad and nonthreatening and help to progress toward more sensitive ones if IPV is disclosed.

Assessment also includes observation for possible IPV-related injuries. Once IPV is disclosed, the nurse's validation that no one deserves to be hurt is followed by assessment of the patient's immediate safety, such as asking, "Is it safe for you to go home?" or, "Is your partner here with you now?" The emphasis should be on appropriate concern for safety and on offering information that would include appropriate resources and referrals (Davila, Mendias, & Juneau, 2013).

Infant, Child, and Adolescent Health

Infants and children who live in poverty and belong to certain minority groups as described previously in this chapter are at a higher risk for illness and death than infants and children in the broader population. Miller and Chen (2013) reported that childhood poverty rates in the United States have climbed steadily since the 2008 recession. Lower socioeconomic–status children may experience household crowding, inadequate nutrition, and more exposure to secondhand smoke. These and similar social and physical conditions may result in a pro-inflammatory phenotype that results in both rats and humans from injuries and poor infection care. Because of frequent exposure to events that are uncontrollable and unpredictable, as the child matures the social difficulties encountered and unhealthy lifestyle circumstances exacerbate the pro-inflammatory tendencies. Inflammatory response is essential for survival; however, if persistent it can lead to various diseases. Research on resilience suggests that parental nurturance plays a role in the family's emotional climate and provides protective factors (Miller & Chen, 2013). If mothers and infants in these groups were as healthy as their non-vulnerable counterparts, infant death rates would decrease tremendously.

As children transition to adolescence their choices are influenced more by friends, community, school, and work environments than by family. The CDC identifies six critical types of adolescent behavior that contribute to death and disability among youths and adults; these include:

- Alcohol or other drug use
- Injury and violence, including suicide
- Tobacco use
- Unhealthy dietary behaviors
- Physical inactivity
- Sexual risk behaviors

These types of behaviors increase in the vulnerable population that the child and adolescent find themselves in. For example, adolescent alcohol and drug use or experimentation is an important health concern for those who participate in this high-risk behavior. The healthcare provider's role is to identify early signs of health risks while taking into consideration the impact of social context (Thompson, Connelly, Thomas-Jones, & Eggert, 2013).

Adults and Older Adults

Due to longer life spans and aging baby boomers, the growth in the number and proportion of older adults is unprecedented in the history of the United States. It is estimated that by 2030 older adults will account for 20% of the U.S. population. As a group, older adults are managing multiple chronic conditions and degenerative illnesses. The National Report Card on Healthy Aging (CDC, 2013a) reports on 15 indicators of older adult health, eight of which are listed in *Healthy People 2020*. The 15 indicators are grouped into four areas: Health Status, Health Behaviors, Preventative Care and Screening, and Injuries. The vulnerable older adult experiences many challenges and barriers to obtaining health care. Challenges may include geographical location, fixed retirement income, and management of multiple chronic conditions.

Nursing Assessment: Age

Knowledge of the aging process is essential when caring for vulnerable populations. Milestones occur along the life span, from newborn to infant, toddler, preschooler, school-age, adolescent, young adult, middle age, and elderly. Nurses need to be cognizant of the patient's developmental stage when performing an evaluation. Abusive behavior often occurs because of a combination of complex and varied factors (Selwood & Cooper, 2009). The nurse must recognize that abuse frequently goes unreported and undetected; therefore, he or she must be aware of a person's age and vulnerability; be aware of the best way of detecting verbal, psychological, and less severe abuse; and know how to ask, in a nonjudgmental way, what is happening. In addition, the nurse must observe and assess for signs of abuse such as changes in behavior, unexplained injuries, evidence of neglect, other indicators of distress, and previous history of allegations. The nurse must know how to recognize abuse and how to report it. Box 6.1 lists signs of sexual abuse in children.

Elder abuse is underreported for a variety of reasons, including fear of repercussions by the abuser. The nurse must observe the patient for cues related to abuse including appearance and affect and must be prepared to use direct questions regarding harm or threats by others; limitations imposed by others on activities, leaving the home, or using the phone; and problems with basic needs.

Comprehensive assessment of the older adult would include screening for abuse in any of the types previously described. In addition, a reliable tool called the Elder Assessment Instrument (EAI) is an easy-to-use scale for assessment of elder abuse.

A summary of factors associated with abuse includes the following:

- *Caregiver Factors:* Living with care recipient, such as caring for a spouse, and factors such as social isolation, undertaking more caregiving tasks, and reporting higher burden. Depression, anxiety, and low self-esteem may be experienced.

Box 6.1 Signs of Sexual Abuse in Children

- Presence of vaginal foreign body (exception: retained toilet paper)
- Presence of condyloma acuminata (genital warts)
- Genital bruises, lacerations, or abrasions without plausible history of trauma
- Absence of hymenal tissue between the 3 o'clock and 9 o'clock positions
- Presence of perianal lacerations that extend to the anal sphincter
- Presence of purulent genital discharge (may indicate the presence of a sexually transmitted disease)
- Incidence of urinary tract infections

- *Care Recipient Factors:* More disruptive and abusive behavior and abusiveness toward caregiver, due to cognitive and functional impairment that are experienced from progression of disease.

Each state in the United States has policies in place for protecting and reporting abuse situations. Nurses have a key role in the protection of vulnerable people at any age and a duty to report to authorities when a patient is experiencing abuse of any type.

Gender

Health care, illness prevention, and health promotion are challenges within vulnerable populations when considering the issue of gender as it relates to men and women in general, gay men, lesbians, bisexual men and women, and transgender people. The sexual orientation section later in this chapter will discuss lesbian, gay, bisexual, and transgender issues. The following sections will discuss women's and men's health.

Women's Health

When power relationships are uneven, dependency can play a major role in women's vulnerability. Primarily it's the unequal status and role in the family in certain cultures that contributes to perceived vulnerability that can lead to victimization and poor health outcomes.

The National Breast and Cervical Cancer Early Detection Program (NBCCEDP) supports women's health by promoting cancer prevention, including early detection and treatment for breast and cervical cancer. The NBCCEDP helps low-income, uninsured, and underinsured women ages 40 to 64 gain access to breast and cervical cancer screenings and diagnostic services. Another program, Well-Integrated Screening and Evaluation for Women Across the Nation (WISEWOMEN), provides low-income, under- or uninsured women with the knowledge, skills, and opportunities to improve their diets, physical activities, and other lifestyle behaviors to prevent, delay, and control cardiovascular and other chronic diseases. These programs stem from women seeking preventive health care more than men.

Men's Health

Men generally seek care when there is a problem and they do not seek preventative screenings. According to the National Center for Health Statistics (2012), 12% of men ages 18 years and over are in fair-to-poor health. The risk factors for this group include lack of physical activity, alcohol consumption, cigarette smoking, obesity, and hypertension. For example, 21% of males currently smoke cigarettes, 34.6% are obese, and 31.6% have hypertension. Leading causes of death are heart disease, cancer, and unintentional injuries. Older male veterans are more likely than nonveterans to have two or more chronic conditions.

Sexual Orientation

As with many vulnerable populations, in order to ensure sensitivity to lesbian, gay, bisexual, and transgender (LGBT) individuals, nurses must possess an awareness and understanding of the terms and definitions that are specific to the LGBT population. Researchers in the field of gender identity development have raised awareness that gender is not exclusively determined by an assigned sex at birth, but rather is determined by a person's sense, belief, and ultimate expression of self (U.S. Department of Health and Human Services, 2012).

LGBT youth and those perceived as LGBT are at increased risk of being bullied. Creating a safe environment is an intervention to ensure that all youth can thrive when they feel supported. Parents, schools, and communities can all play a role in helping LGBT youth feel physically and emotionally safe. Building strong connections and effective communication, establishing a safe environment at school, and protecting privacy are ways to create a safe environment and minimize bullying for LGBT youth.

Physical health issues for LGBT individuals include heart disease, cancers, fitness, obesity, and injury/violence. Behavioral health issues for LGBT individuals include emotional health, depression, anxiety, smoking status, alcohol use, mental health, suicide, and substance abuse. And lastly, sexual health issues for LGBT individuals include sexually transmitted diseases such as HIV/AIDS, syphilis, gonorrhea, chlamydia, pubic lice, and anal papilloma; hepatitis A, B, and C; human papillomavirus–caused anal and genital warts; and an increased incidence of anal cancer, particularly for gay men.

Nursing Assessment: Gender, Sexual Orientation

Nurses must understand the concept of gender in regard to distinguishing the biologically founded sexual differences between women and men from the culturally determined differences between the roles accepted or undertaken by women and men in society. Gender roles are affected by a number of factors such as age, class, race, ethnicity, religion, and ideologies, in addition to geographical, economic, and political environments. When caring for vulnerable people, it is important for the nurse to be aware of the different roles women and men perform, their different responsibilities, and their often unequal status. Performing a gender assessment from a gender perspective addresses the gender dynamic and potential inequalities in healthcare practice and policies. Understanding women's health and men's health and the differences between them is important. Women have unique health issues such as pregnancy and menopause. They usually keep regular appointments during their childbearing years. Compared to women, men are more likely to smoke and drink, make unhealthy or risky

choices, and put off regular checkups. Prostate cancer and low testosterone are health issues specific to males (MedlinePlus, 2014a).

When assessing LGBT patients, the nurse should always ask how they identify and/or how they wish to be addressed. Beliefs around gender will touch upon many aspects of life and can be manifested by the healthcare provider's reactions toward clothing and words used in conversation; therefore, it is important that they demonstrate sensitivity to all patients regardless of perceived gender (USDHHS, Substance Abuse and Mental Health Services Administration [SAMHSA], 2012). Table 6.2 lists terms and definitions related to gender identity.

Geography

The CDC considers **geography** as one of the issues for populations being identified as at-risk for health disparities. Geography refers to the country, region, section, community, or neighborhood in which one was born and raised or in which one currently resides or works. Residing in a metropolitan (urban) area or residing in a rural area both have their geographic challenges for some individuals seeking healthcare. Metropolitan and urban areas are usually thought of as convenient when a person needs to access care. However, vulnerable patient populations may not live in close proximity to providers, and the cost of in-city transportation may pose a barrier to access to healthcare services. According to Papachristos and Wildeman (2014), more than 10,000 people are killed by firearms each year and another 40,000 are hospitalized or treated for gunshot injuries. In the urban setting, reluctance to leave living areas due to fear of violence may be one of the complex factors of increasing obesity and risk for **metabolic syndrome**. In addition, although African Americans, Hispanics, and Native Americans comprise more than one-third of the total U.S. population, they account for only 9% of physicians, 7% of dentists, 10% of pharmacists, and 6% of registered nurses (Urban Universities for Health, n.d.).

Patients who live in rural regions can be disproportionately affected by the physical locations of healthcare services. For example, hospitals may be farther away, the number of providers may be limited, and specialists may be unavailable. Patients with limited financial resources may be unable or reluctant to travel long distances for routine preventative care. This means health conditions may go undiagnosed and become more serious.

Depending on where a person resides in the United States, emergencies and disasters can strike quickly and without warning. For example, being prepared for a hurricane in south Florida, for tornados in the Midwest, or for earthquakes in California is common knowledge. However, it is the disaster that strikes with unpredictability and without warning that can force people to leave or be confined to their homes. People with disabilities are disproportionately affected by these disasters both during the event and during the aftermath. For example, people on dialysis require special preparations; thus they often panic and arrive at emergency departments for fear of loss of electricity for their lifesaving treatment. In theory, living close to a hospital with a generator is good practice; however, in the face of a disaster the people requiring dialysis can be an unintentional hindrance to the emergency department and emergency medical system services. An assessment of social and physical determinants based on the geography of the community is essential to having an effective preparedness plan in place.

TABLE 6.2	Terms and Definitions Specific to Gender Identity

TERM	DEFINITION
Bigender	A person whose gender identity encompasses both male and female genders. Some may feel that one identity is stronger, but both are present.
FTM	A person who transitions from female to male, meaning a person who was assigned the female sex at birth but identifies and lives as a male. *Note: Also known as a transgender man.*
Gender Identity	A person's internal sense of being male, female, or something else. Since gender identity is internal, one's gender identity is not necessarily visible to others.
Gender Nonconforming	A person whose gender expression is different from societal expectations related to their perceived gender.
Genderqueer	A term used by persons who may not entirely identify as either male or female.
MTF	A person who transitions from male to female, meaning a person who was assigned the male sex at birth but identifies and lives as a female. *Note: Also known as a transgender woman.*
Transgender	A person whose gender identity and/or expression are different from that typically associated with their assigned sex at birth. *Note: The term* transgender *has been used to describe a number of gender minorities including, but not limited to, transsexuals, cross-dressers, androgynous people, genderqueers, and gender non-conforming people. "Trans" is shorthand for "transgender."*
Transgender Man	A transgender person who currently identifies as a male (see also "FTM").
Transgender Woman	A transgender person who currently identifies as a female (see also "MTF").
Transsexual	A person whose gender identity differs from their assigned sex at birth.
Two-Spirit (2-S)	A contemporary term that references historical multiple-gender traditions in many First Nations cultures. Many Native/First Nations people who are lesbian, gay, bisexual, transgender, or gender non-conforming identify as Two-Spirit. In many First Nations, Two-Spirit status carries great respect and leads to additional commitments and responsibilities to one's community.

Nursing Assessment: Geography

The assessment of the vulnerable population's physical environment and social environment as related to geography includes housing and where it is located, transportation, land use, and water safety as well as risks associated with stress, violence, and injury. An awareness of the patient's geographical surroundings is beneficial in the context of the psychosocial component of the comprehensive health assessment. The social determinants of a vulnerable population include where the person lives, where the person works, and whether there is access to healthcare services.

Disabilities

Vulnerable populations who have **disabilities** are people who may be in need of healthcare services by reason of mental health, physical, sensory, developmental, age, or illness concerns. Also, persons with disabilities are people who may be unable to take care of themselves or protect themselves against harm or exploitation. Examples of vulnerable persons with disabilities are those with mental health problems, learning disabilities, and physical disabilities or illnesses that result in a degree of dependence on others. Several chronic disorders—such as asthma, congestive heart failure, chronic obstructive pulmonary disease, diabetes, and inflammatory bowel disease—can also be reasons for a person to become disabled, especially as the

disease progresses (CDC, 2014a). The following sections will discuss both physical and social determinants of health.

Physical Determinants of Health

The World Health Organization defines health as a state of complete physical, mental, and social well-being and not simply the absence of disease or infirmity. The context in which a person lives is important for both health status and quality of life. The main determinants of health include the physical, social, and economic environments. People with physical challenges can be referred to as persons with disabilities. Many types of disabilities can affect a person, including those involving hearing, vision, movement, thinking, remembering, learning, communicating, mental health, and social relationships.

Nursing Assessment: Disabilities

Some disabilities can be hidden or are not easy to see. The International Classification of Functioning, Disability and Health (ICF) provides a standard language for classifying changes in body function and structure, activity, participation levels, and environmental factors that influence health. The ICF can help assess the health and functioning activities and factors that can help or create barriers for a person to fully participate in society (WHO, 2001).

The World Health Organization Disability Assessment Schedule 2.0 (WHODAS 2.0) demonstrates advantages over other assessment instruments for health and disability; this assessment is short, simple to administer, and applicable across cultures and clinical and general population settings. The instrument covers cognition, mobility, self-care, getting along with others, life activities, and participation.

The Disability and Health Data System (DHDS) is an innovative disability and health data tool that is used to identify disparities in health between adults with and without disabilities. The DHDS allows for comparing answers to questions on a state-by-state basis for the percentage of disabilities by age, sex, race/ethnicity, and veteran status; percentage of those who smoke; obesity; vaccine coverage; and preventive services (CDC, 2014b). Access this comprehensive data tool for the 50 United States by using this link: www.dhds.cdc.gov/help/gettingStarted.

Socioeconomic Status

Social determinants of health are the situations in which a person is born, lives, works, and ages as well as the systems in place to deal with illness. Social and economic conditions and their effects on people's lives determine a population's risk of illness and the actions taken to prevent illness or treat illness when it occurs. Health inequities arise from inequalities within and between societies; examples are infant mortality, maternal death during or shortly after pregnancy, education levels, and degrees of wealth. The poorest of the poor around the world have the worst health. This is a global phenomenon of a social gradient in that it runs from top to bottom of the socioeconomic spectrum (WHO, 2001).

The CDC (2010) outlined a strategy for reducing health disparities and promoting health equity related to the following conditions: HIV/AIDS, viral hepatitis, sexually transmitted diseases (STDs), and tuberculosis (TB) prevention. The goal is to provide a holistic approach for public health programs to advance the health of communities and increase opportunities for healthy living.

Health Insurance

The Affordable Care Act (ACA) puts patients in charge of their own health care. Under the ACA law a new Patient's Bill of Rights gives Americans the stability and flexibility needed to make informed choices about their health care. The hallmarks of the ACA are the end of pre-existing condition exclusions; increasing the age to 26 that a child can be covered under a parent's insurance plan; ending lifetime limits on coverage; ensuring that premium dollars are spent on health care, not administrative costs; and providing preventive care coverage at no cost to the individual. Preventive healthcare services such as screenings, vaccinations, and healthy pregnancy counseling are thought to improve the health and well-being of pregnant woman, promote the healthy delivery of babies, and enhance overall population health (U.S. Department of Health and Human Services, 2014).

Immigrants and Refugees

Current immigrant family characteristics differ from those in the past in that today's immigrant families are more likely to be from Latin America or the Caribbean rather than from Europe. According to the U.S. Census Bureau, the majority of current immigrants are from Latin America (Latinos), and they represent the largest group of foreign-born immigrants and the largest minority group in the United States today

(U.S. Census Bureau, 2010). This immigration includes an unprecedented number of unauthorized immigrants who are settling in different regions of the United States that are unaccustomed to an influx of undocumented immigrants. Within the immigrant family, having "unauthorized status" may cause stress and uncertainty, may negatively affect health outcomes and educational attainment, and may result in increased social isolation for immigrant children (Chavez, Lopez, Englebrecht, & Anguiano, 2012; U.S. Census Bureau, 2010).

The U.S. Department of Homeland Security reports that 11.5 million undocumented immigrants currently live in the United States. Among undocumented immigrants, 47% are men, 41% are women, and 12% are children. As of 2011, 24.3% of all children living in the United States who are under the age of 18 have at least one foreign-born parent. U.S.-born children of immigrants are 81% of all children living in immigrant families. With increasing numbers of children growing up in families in the United States where one or both parents are foreign born, it becomes more important that healthcare providers understand the impact of this trend on immigrants and refugees, as recognized in the relatively new term "mixed-status families" (Hoefer, Rytina, & Baker, 2011).

The term **mixed-status family** has been defined as a family in which one or more family members are undocumented immigrants and other family members are citizens, lawful permanent residents, or immigrants with another form of temporary legal immigration status. Belonging to a mixed-status family where at least one parent is a non-U.S. citizen has its disadvantages in regard to health care and health insurance. Illegal immigrants often are wary of applying for public health benefits for their children because they fear doing so will alert authorities about their own legal status. In addition, these families may not seek health care because of fear of deportation. Immigration status can also exacerbate the level of violence in an abusive relationship when the batterer uses the threat of deportation and release of information about the victim's legal status.

Nursing Assessment: Immigrants

Nurses should conduct a comprehensive heritage assessment to determine a patient's ethnic, cultural, and religious heritage and background as well as how the patient's relationship to personal and healthcare traditions is associated with how the patient identifies with his or her race and ethnicity. The nurse should ask where the person was born, where the parents and grandparents were born, and whether the patient lives in an urban or rural area setting. Continuing the assessment with questions about past and current spiritual and religious practices is helpful in determining how patients experience health within their own cultures.

Since October, 2013, about 52,000 unaccompanied children from Latin America have been apprehended at the U.S.–Mexico border. Factors such as gang violence, enduring poverty, and drug trafficking have been identified as reasons why these child immigrants made the greater-than-1,500-mile journey from Guatemala, El Salvador, and Honduras to the United States. The Office of the United Nations High Commissioner for Refugees (UNHCR) agency found that of 404 children who left Latin America, at least 59 cited international protection needs from homicide, rape, poverty, police corruption, and gang violence as reasons for crossing the border. Upon entering the United States, the unaccompanied children remain vulnerable due to language barriers, health risks such as dehydration, and no parental presence or guidance (Yu-Hsi Lee, 2014).

Incarcerated Men and Women

Once incarcerated, men and women will most likely be diagnosed with a chronic disease, mental health problem, substance abuse problem, or infectious disease over the course of their confinement. The correctional population has expanded more than 4.5-fold as a result of tougher sentencing laws, the "war on drugs," and the closure of large mental institutions across the country, resulting in prisons serving as the new mental illness asylums. Prisoners suffer higher rates of communicable diseases than the general population. Chronic diseases such as HIV/AIDS, MRSA, STDs, hepatitis, and communicable diseases such as tuberculosis are on the rise. Among the growing older population of prisoners, hypertension, diabetes, and lower-lung disease are also on the rise (Gostin, Vanchieri, & Pope, 2007).

Incarcerated men far outnumber incarcerated women. However, the female prisoner population has been steadily increasing at a faster rate than the rate of male prisoners. Not only is the female prison population becoming larger, it is also becoming more diverse. Women prisoners are older, more likely to be minorities, and more likely to be drug users. Female prisoners are also more likely than male prisoners to report medical problems on admission to prison (Gostin et al., 2007). Women prisoners have needs that are different from those of men. These different and diverse needs, such as breast health and reproductive health, are often neglected by the prison system (Gostin et al., 2007).

Lastly, race and ethnicity disparities are noted within the prisoner population, with African Americans and Hispanics comprising a disproportionate number of the incarcerated. With felony laws known as "three strikes and you're out," and the increase in sentencing for life, male and female prisoners will age in prison and chronic diseases will impact their healthcare needs (Gostin et al., 2007).

Nursing Assessment for a Person Who Is Incarcerated

Oftentimes people in the justice system who are in prison for a crime have higher risk health concerns and illnesses. Nurses work in prisons in the correctional healthcare system and often prisoners will require services of the nearby hospital. Once an incarcerated person who seeks care is in the hospital, nurses may reflect on their personal beliefs and feelings about how an incarcerated person might experience non-judgmental caring.

Veterans

The Veterans Administration (VA) cares for a disproportionate number of disadvantaged, low-income, and vulnerable individuals. Due to their propensity for premature morbidities and mortality, vulnerable veterans experience challenges when accessing the healthcare system, especially within the VA system itself.

As World War II and Korean War veterans age and require more comprehensive care and caregiver support, older veterans, especially those with cognitive impairment, increased fragility, and limited social support, make up the fastest growing segment of the VA's patients.

Women veterans represent a growing population within the VA system, and have specific needs and challenges related to accessing care in a previously male-oriented and dominated system. This subgroup is associated with greater healthcare needs and use of urgent and emergent levels of health services. O'Toole et al. (2011) conducted a quasi-experimental study examining homeless veterans, cognitively impaired elderly veterans, women veterans, and patients with serious mental illness. They measured primary care, emergency department, and inpatient care use and chronic disease management both in a general internal medicine clinic and in a medical home. The study revealed a significant increase in primary care use and improvement in monitoring chronic diseases such as diabetes control. There was an increase in emergency department use and hospitalizations for a subgroup; however, health improved when the primary care model was utilized. The researchers concluded that utilization of a medical home model for the veteran population can increase primary care utilization and improve chronic disease monitoring and diabetes management.

Nursing Assessment: Veterans

Male and female veterans who experience VA health care will be useful in assessing the overall general health status of veterans. The VA has been effective in collecting data on specific behavioral risk factors, such as physical activity levels, smoking, and alcohol use. The information will assist both state and federal health officials in developing strategies for preventing and controlling health problems for the estimated 25.6 million veterans and 1.8 million active duty, reserve, and National Guard personnel in the United States. Each war has had a specific impact on the health of servicemen and servicewomen and their families. For example, health research on the Vietnam War has described the illnesses and diseases related to Agent Orange, including depression, anxiety, and PTSD. The utilization of advances in body protection during the recent warfare in Iraq and Afghanistan has yielded more injured soldiers coming home alive, but with traumatic brain injury (TBI) as well as loss of limb or limbs. According to O'Neil et al. (2014), a history of mild traumatic brain injury (mTBI) is common among military members who served in Operations Enduring Freedom, Iraqi Freedom, and New Dawn (OEF/OIF/OND). Cognitive, physical, and mental health symptoms were commonly reported by veterans and military members with a history of mTBI. The findings of the study suggest that appropriate reintegration services are needed for treatment of PTSD, substance-use disorders, headaches, and other difficulties veterans experienced after deployment regardless of mTBI history. The fact is, the veterans who provided service to our country require the nurse's recognition that they are an especially vulnerable population during wartime.

Homelessness

Despite signs of improvement, in the United States and throughout the world, homelessness remains a serious problem. Statistics suggest the prevalence of homelessness is steadily declining. Since 2005, the U.S. homeless population has decreased by approximately 16 percent. More recently, between 2012 and 2014, homelessness decreased by 3.7 percent (National Alliance to End Homelessness, 2014). However, statistics must be considered in the context of the bigger picture; for example, deaths account for a portion of the decrease in homelessness.

The U.S. Department of Housing and Urban Development (HUD) recognizes four primary categories of homelessness for individuals and families:

- Literally homeless
- At imminent risk for homelessness
- Homeless as defined by other federal statues
- Fleeing or attempting to flee domestic violence (HUD, n.d.).

According to the National Alliance to End Homelessness (2014), more than 610,000 people were homeless in 2013. For the majority of this population, shelters and transitional housing units served as temporary residences. However, an estimated 35 percent (215,344) of homeless people lived on the streets or in another location that was not intended for used as a residence (National Alliance to End Homelessness, 2014). In 2013, of the total homeless population, more than 58,000 (9.5 percent) were veterans and nearly 50,000 (almost 8 percent) were unaccompanied homeless youth (National Alliance to End Homelessness, 2014).

The high incidence of homelessness can be attributed to a number of factors, including increased unemployment rates, decreased incomes, and lack of affordable health care. In general, over the past 25 years, two simultaneous trends have been significantly affected the incidence of homelessness in the U.S.: decreased availability of affordable housing and increased poverty rates (National Coalition for the Homeless [NCH], 2011).

Populations who are at increased risk for homelessness include victims of domestic violence, many of whom are forced to choose between being abused and becoming homeless. Individuals with mental illness or substance abuse disorders are at increased risk for becoming homeless, as well (NCH, 2011).

Nursing Assessment for Homeless Individuals and Families

Assessment of the homeless individual or family begins with establishing trust. A nonjudgmental attitude is essential to developing rapport with all patients, including members of the homeless population. For these individuals, actual and perceived powerlessness can affect every aspect of life, including physical and mental health. For women and children, the risk for physical and emotional trauma is compounded. Homeless women are at increased risk for sexual or domestic abuse. In turn, often as a result of witnessing abuse, emotional and behavioral problems are common among homeless children (National Institutes of Health [NIH], 2014).

For homeless individuals, the combination of increased physical and psychosocial stress plus poor nutrition contributes to a variety of health issues. While each individual has unique needs, people who are homeless are at increased risk for numerous chronic and acute health disorders, including:

- Mental health issues
- Addiction and substance abuse
- Respiratory illness, including bronchitis and pneumonia
- Skin and wound infections (NIH, 2014).

Along with physical assessment, psychosocial assessment is essential to effectively caring for members of this population. In addition to ensuring that the individual's or family's physical health needs are met, the nurse should conduct a thorough psychosocial assessment (see chapter 5 ∞). Collaboration with other members of the healthcare team should include facilitating referrals to social services, mental health professionals, community assistance programs, and other organizations that may be able to offer assistance.

Application Through Critical Thinking

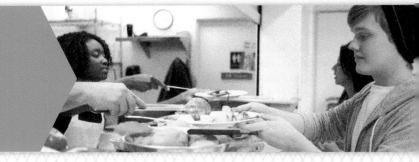

▌ Case Study

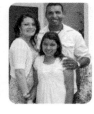

The Molina family immigrated to the United States three years ago when Roberto and Rita started a family. Roberto and Rita met and married in El Salvador and are undocumented citizens. They have one female child, Vanessa, who was born in the United States three years ago. Rita is pregnant with her second child and is seeking health care for her growing family and pre-school for Vanessa. Roberto works in the fields picking lettuce and has a handyman business to support his family.

▌ Critical Thinking Questions

1. Discuss how the Molina family is at risk and vulnerable.
2. What factors must be considered when performing a health history and assessment for Rita?
3. Identify health promotion activities.
4. How would you see Rita as vulnerable?
5. What would be the predictors of health for the Molina family?

▶ References

Centers for Disease Control and Prevention (CDC). (2010). *Establishing a holistic framework to reduce inequities in HIV, viral hepatitis, STD, and tuberculosis in the United States.* Retrieved from http://www.cdc.gov/socialdeterminants

Centers for Disease Control and Prevention (CDC). (2011). *Racial and ethnic minority populations: 10 leading causes of death.* Retrieved from http://www.cdc.gov/minorityhealth/populations/remp.html

Centers for Disease Control and Prevention (CDC), National Center for Chronic Disease Prevention and Health Promotion, Division of Population Health. (2013a). *The state of aging & health in America.* Retrieved from http://www.cdc.gov/aging/pdf/state-aging-health-in-america-2013.pdf

Centers for Disease Control and Prevention (CDC). (2013b). *Understanding elder abuse fact sheet.* Retrieved from http://www.cdc.gov/violenceprevention/pdf/em-factsheet-a.pdf

Centers for Disease Control and Prevention (CDC). (2014a). *Disability and health.* Retrieved from http://www.cdc.gov/ncbddd/disabilityandhealth/index.html

Centers for Disease Control and Prevention (CDC). (2014b). *Disability and health data system.* Retrieved from http://www.cdc.gov/ncbddd/disabilityandhealth/dhds.html

Centers for Disease Control and Prevention (CDC). (2014c). *Injury prevention & control: Intimate partner violence.* Retrieved from www.cdc.gov/viollenceprevention/intimatepartnerviolence/

Centers for Disease Control and Prevention (CDC). (2014d). *Minority Health: Other At Risk Populations.* Retrieved from www.cdc.gov/minorityhealth/populations/atrisk.html#Other

Centers for Disease Control and Prevention (CDC). (2014e). *New REACH Demonstration Projects.* Retrieved from http://www.cdc.gov/nccdphp/dch/programs/reach/new_reach/reach-demo.htm

Chavez, J. M., Lopez, A., Englebrecht, C. M., & Anguiano, R. P. V. (2012). Exploring the impact of unauthorized immigration status on children's well-being. *Family Court Review 50*(4), 638–649.

Davila, Y. R., Mendias, E. P., & Juneau, C. (2013). Under the RADAR: Assessing and intervening for intimate partner violence. *The Journal of Nurse Practitioners 9*(9), 594–599.

Find Youth Info. (2013). *Safe schools/healthy students toolkit.* Retrieved from http://www.findyouthinfo.gov/federal-link/3-bold-steps-school-community-change

Gostin, L. O., Vanchieri, C., & Pope, A. (Eds.). (2007). *Ethical considerations for research involving prisoners.* IOM: National Academies Press.

Healthy People. (n.d.). *Access to health services.* Retrieved from http://www.healthypeople.gov/2020/topicsobjectives2020/overview.aspx?topicid=1

Healthy People. (n.d.). *Disparities.* Retrieved from http://www.healthypeople.gov/2020/about/disparitiesAbout.aspx

Healthy People. (n.d.). *Lesbian, gay, bisexual, and transgender health.* Retrieved from http://www.healthypeople.gov2020/topicsobjectives2020/overview.aspx?topicId=25

Healthy People. (n.d.). *Social determinants of health.* Retrieved from http://www.healthypeople.gov/2020/topicsobjectives2020/overview.aspx?topicid=39

Heron, M. (2013, December). Deaths: Leading causes for 2010. *National Vital Statistics Reports, 62*(6), Table 1, p. 31. Retrieved from http://www.cdc.gov/nchs/data/nvsr/nvsr62/nvsr62_06.pdf

Hoefer, M., Rytina, N., & Baker, B. (2011). *Estimates of unauthorized immigrant population residing in the United States: January 2011.* Retrieved from Department of Homeland Security website: http://www.dhs.gov/xlibrary/assets/statistics/publications/oi%5Fill%5F2011.pdf

Mareno, N., & Hart, P. L. (2014). Cultural competency among nurses with undergraduate and graduate degrees: Implications for nursing education. *Nursing Education Perspectives 35*(2), 83–88.

MedlinePlus. (2014a). *Men's health.* Retrieved from http://www.nlm.nih.gov/medlineplus/menshealth.html

MedlinePlus. (2014b). *Women's health.* Retrieved from http://www.nlm.nih.gov/medlineplus/womenshealth.html

Miller, G. E., & Chen, E. (2013). The biological residue of childhood poverty. *Child Development Perspectives, 7*(2), 67–73.

National Alliance to End Homelessness. (2014). *The state of homelessness in America 2014.* Retrieved from http://www.endhomelessness.org/page/-/files/2014_State_Of_Homelessness_final.pdf

National Center for Health Statistics. (2012). *Men's health.* Retrieved from http://www.cdc.gov/nchs/fastats/mens-health.htm

National Center for Health Statistics. (2014a). *FastStats, Health of Asian or Pacific Islander population.* Retrieved from http://www.cdc.gov/nchs/fastats/asian-health.htm

National Center for Health Statistics. (2014b). *Minority health: Black or African American populations.* Retrieved from http://www.cdc.gov/minorityhealth/populations/remp/black.html

National Coalition for the Homeless (NCH). (2011). *Why are people homeless?* Retrieved from http://www.nationalhomeless.org/factsheets/why.html

National Institutes of Health (NIH). (2014). *Homeless health concerns.* Retrieved from http://www.nlm.nih.gov/medlineplus/homelesshealthconcerns.html

National Institutes of Health (NIH). (2013). *What are health disparities?* Retrieved from http://www.niaid.nih.gov/topics/minorityhealth/pages/disparities.aspx

O'Neil, M. E., Carlson, K. F., Storzbach, D., Brenner, L. A., Freeman, M., Quinones, A. R., . . . & Kansagara, D. (2014). Factors associated with mild traumatic brain injury in veterans and military personnel: A systematic review. *Journal of the International Neuropsychological Society 20,* 249–261.

O'Toole, T. P., Pirraglia, P.A., Dosa, D., Bourgault, C., Redihan, S., O'Toole, M. B., & Blumen, J. (2011). Building care systems to improve access for high-risk and vulnerable veteran populations. *Journal of General Internal Medicine, 26*(2), 683–688. doi: 10.1007/s11606-011-1818-2

Papachristos, A. V., & Wildeman, C. (2014). Network exposure and homicide victimization in an African American community. *American Journal of Public Health, 104*(1), 143–147.

Selwood, A., & Cooper, C. (2009). Abuse of people with dementia. *Reviews in Clinical Gerontology, 19,* 35–43.

The National Intimate Partner and Violence Survey. (2010). *NISVS: An overview of 2010 findings on victimization by sexual orientation.* Retrieved from http://www.cdc.gov/violenceprevention/pdf/cdc_nisvs_victimization_final-a.pdf

Thompson, C. W., Monsen, K. A., Wanamaker, K., Augustyniak, K., & Thompson, S. L. (2012). Using the Omaha System as a framework to demonstrate the value of nurse managed wellness center services for vulnerable populations. *Journal of Community Health Nursing, 29,* 1–11.

Thompson, E. A., Connelly, C. D., Thomas-Jones, D., & Eggert, L. L. (2013). School difficulties and co-occurring health risk factors: Substance use, aggression, depression, and suicidal behaviors. *Journal of Child and Adolescent Psychiatric Nursing, 26,* 74–84.

U.S. Census Bureau. (2010). *The foreign-born population in the United States: 2010.* Retrieved from http://www.census.gov/prod/2012pubs/acs-19.pdf

U.S. Census Bureau. (2012). *The Asian population: 2010.* Retrieved from http://www.census.gov/prod/cen2010/briefs/c2010br-11.pdf

U.S. Department of Health and Human Services, Administration on Aging. (2007). *What is elder abuse?* Retrieved from http://www.aoa.gov/AoARoot/AoA_Programs/Elder_Rights/EA_Prevention/whatIsEA.aspx

U.S. Department of Health and Human Services (USDHHS), Administration for Children and Families. (2010). *The child abuse prevention and treatment act: As amended by PL 111-320, The CAPTA Reauthorization Act of 2010.* Retrieved from http://www.acf.hhs.gov/sites/default/files/cb/capta2010.pdf

U.S. Department of Health and Human Services, Substance Abuse and Mental Health Services Administration, Center for Substance Abuse Prevention. (2012). *Top health issues for LGBT populations information & resource kit.* Retrieved from http://www.samhsa.gov

U.S. Department of Health and Human Services (2014). *About the law.* Retrieved from health http://www.hhs.gov/healthcare/rights/

U.S. Department of Housing and Urban Development (HUD). (n.d.). *Homeless assistance.* Retrieved from http://portal.hud.gov/hudportal/HUD?src=/program_offices/comm_planning/homeless

United States Preventive Services Task Force. (2013). *Screening for intimate partner violence and abuse of elderly and vulnerable adults.* Retrieved from http://www.uspreventiveservicestaskforce.org/uspstf/uspsipv.htm

Urban Universities for Health. (n.d.). *Fact Sheet on health disparities and the urban health workforce.* Retrieved from http://urbanuniversitiesforhealth.org/knowledge-base/data

World Health Organization (WHO). (2001). *World Health Organization disability assessment Schedule 2.0.* Retrieved from http://www.who.int/classifications/icf/whodasii/en/

Yu-Hsi Lee, E. (2014). *Why kids are crossing the desert alone to get to America.* Retrieved from http://www.thinkprogress.org/immigration/2014/07/02/3453051/push-factors-el-slavador-honduras-and-guatemala/

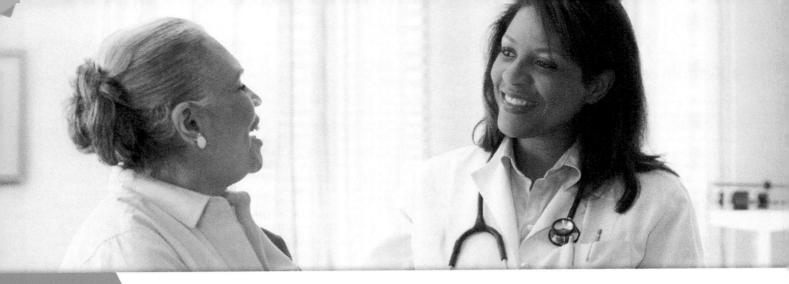

Interviewing and Communication Techniques

▶ Learning Outcomes

Upon completion of this chapter, you will be able to:

1. Identify strategies that promote effective communication when conducting a health history.

2. Analyze barriers to effective nurse-patient communication.

3. Outline the professional characteristics used in establishing a nurse-patient relationship.

4. Explain the potential effects of cultural and lifespan influences on communication between the nurse and the patient.

5. Implement effective interviewing and communication techniques throughout each phase of the patient interview.

Key Terms

attending, 113
communication, 113
concreteness, 117
empathy, 117
encoding, 113
false reassurance, 115
focused interview, 120
genuineness, 117
health history, 113
interactional skills, 113
listening, 113
paraphrasing, 115
positive regard, 117
preinteraction, 118
primary source, 117
reflecting, 115
secondary source, 118
summarizing, 115

ffective communication skills play an essential role in developing a healthy nurse-patient relationship. Communication is vital to building trust, which serves as the foundation of a therapeutic relationship. Effective communication also is needed for the nurse to conduct the health assessment interview and collect data for the health history. The **health history,** which is a comprehensive record of the patient's past and current health, is discussed in detail in chapter 8. ∞

Communication provides the means for educating, guiding, facilitating, directing, and counseling the patient. The nurse cannot develop trust, establish rapport, or carry out nursing interventions for patients without application of effective communication techniques. For example, nurses may need to modify their communication skills when dealing with younger or older patients. The younger nurse teaching the elderly patient about ways to add fiber to the diet may need to use a serious and respectful communication technique. Conversely, an older nurse counseling a teenage patient regarding safe and responsible sexual practices may need to make special efforts to create an informal atmosphere that allows the teenager to open up and speak freely.

Communication Skills

Communication is the exchange of information between individuals. During the communication process an individual, sometimes called the sender, develops an idea and transmits it in the form of a message to another person, or receiver. The receiver perceives the message (the sender's transmitted idea) and interprets it. Once the receiver interprets the meaning, the receiver formulates a response and transmits it back to the sender as feedback. **Encoding** is the process of formulating a message for transmission to another person. To encode an idea, the sender has to choose the words, body language, signs, or symbols that will be used to convey the message. Decoding is the process of searching through one's memory, experience, and knowledge base to determine the meaning of the intended message (see Figure 7.1 ■).

To communicate successfully, the patient must be able to accurately decode the messages the nurse sends. For example, communication may break down if the nurse uses words the patient does not understand or behaves in a manner that is frightening to the patient.

Communication may also break down if the nurse fails to decode the patient's messages accurately by not listening actively and attentively.

Interactional Skills

Interactional skills are actions that are used during the encoding/decoding process to obtain and disseminate information, develop relationships, and promote understanding of self and others. Nurses use a variety of interactional skills during the communication process to gather assessment data from the patient, family, significant others, and other healthcare personnel. The interactional skills that are helpful during an interview include listening, attending, paraphrasing, leading, questioning, reflecting, and summarizing (see Table 7.1). The nurse uses these interactional techniques to help the patient communicate information thoroughly and also to confirm that the nurse has understood the patient's communication correctly.

Listening

Listening is paying undivided attention to what the patient says and does. It involves interpretation of what has been said. Listening is a basic part of the communication process and is the most important interactional skill. People who have not developed listening skills have problems relating to others and difficulty attaining their goals. Successful listening involves taking in the patient's whole message by hearing the words as well as interpreting body language. Successful listening is an active process requiring effort and attention on the part of the nurse. While listening to a patient, it is important to push thoughts about the day's schedule or the next patient from one's mind and to give full attention to the patient, so as not to miss some of the message. The nurse should note not only the words the patient speaks, but also the tone of voice and even what the patient does not say. Attentive listening skills also include encouraging the patient to speak by making comments such as "I see" and "Go on." The woman who states, "My mother died last week" and immediately moves on to another topic of discussion has told the nurse a lot about how she is dealing with a death in her family.

Attending

Giving full attention to verbal and nonverbal messages is called **attending.** Body language may be as much as 93% of the message a patient sends. Body language, or nonverbal messages, also provides

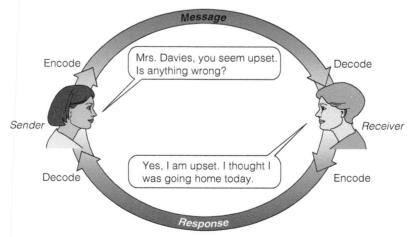

Figure 7.1 The communication process.

TABLE 7.1	Interactional Skills	
SKILL/DEFINITION	**TECHNIQUE**	**EXAMPLES**
Attending Giving the patient undivided attention.	• Use direct eye contact if appropriate for culture. Look at the patient during the conversation. • Lean toward the patient slightly. • Select quiet area with no distractions for interview. • Convey unhurried manner; avoid fidgeting and looking at watch.	Nurse arranges with peers for no interruptions during interview. Nurse sits facing patient, remains alert, and focuses on what patient is saying.
Paraphrasing/Clarification Restating the patient's basic message to test whether it was understood.	• Listen for the patient's basic message. • Restate the patient's message in your own words. • Ask the patient if your words are an accurate restatement of the message.	*Patient:* "I toss and turn all night. Sometimes I can't get to sleep at all. I don't know why this is happening. I've always been a deep sleeper." *Nurse:* "It sounds like you're not getting enough sleep. Is that right?"
Direct Leading Directing the patient in order to obtain specific information or to begin an interaction.	• Decide what area you want to explore. • Tell the patient what you want to discuss. • Encourage the patient to follow your lead.	"Let's discuss the pain in your back." "When did your symptoms begin?"
Focusing Helping the patient zero in on a subject or get in touch with feelings.	• Use focusing when the patient strays from the topic or uses tangential speech. • Listen for themes, issues, or feelings in the patient's rambling conversation. • Ask the patient to give more information about a specific theme, issue, or feeling. • Encourage the patient to emphasize feelings when giving this information.	"Describe how you feel when you can't sleep." "Did you say you were angry and frustrated before you went to bed? Go over that again."
Questioning Gathering specific information on a topic through the process of inquiry.	• Use open-ended questions whenever possible. Avoid using questions that can be answered with "yes," "no," "maybe," or "sometimes." • Ask the patient to express feelings about what is being discussed. • Ask questions that help the patient gain insight.	"What did you mean when you said your back was breaking?" "How did you feel after you talked to your boss?"
Reflecting Letting the patient know that the nurse empathizes with the thoughts, feelings, or experiences expressed.	• Take in the patient's feelings from verbal and nonverbal body language. • Determine which combination of "cues" you should reflect back to the patient. • Reflect the "cues" back to the patient. • Observe the patient's response to the reflected feelings, experience, or content.	*Feelings:* "It sounds like you're feeling lonely." "It must really be frustrating not to be able to get enough sleep." *Experience:* "You're yawning. You must be tired." "You act as if you're in pain." *Content:* "You think you're going to die." "You believe the medication is helping."
Summarizing Tying together the various messages that the patient has communicated throughout the interview.	• Listen to verbal and nonverbal content during the interview. • Summarize feelings, issues, and themes in broad statements. • Repeat them to the patient, or ask the patient to repeat them to you.	"Let's review the health problems you've identified today."

significant information that the nurse might otherwise overlook. Body language signals information that the patient may have omitted intentionally or unintentionally. For example, a male patient who feels expressing pain is a weakness may deny that he is in pain. However, his facial expression, guarded reaction to abdominal palpation, and drawn position in bed send a message of severe pain. Because body language can send messages such as hostility, defensiveness, or confusion, the nurse must tune in to the patient's nonverbal as well as verbal messages. Nonverbal cues such as posture, eye contact, makeup, dress, accessories, and items in the patient's environment

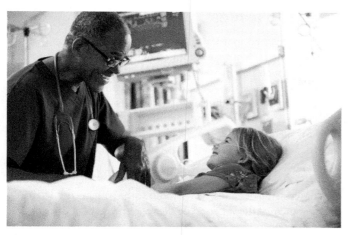

Figure 7.2 The nurse conveys attentive listening through a posture of involvement.
Source: Monkey Business/Fotolia.

(books, a rosary, or photographs) tell a significant story and add more depth to the intended message.

For the nurse, attending includes maintaining consistent, appropriate eye contact with the patient as well as using proper body positioning to demonstrate attentiveness (see Figure 7.2 ■). For example, after establishing rapport with the patient, the nurse should use body posture to reflect involvement by slightly leaning forward toward the patient (Berman & Snyder, 2012).

Paraphrasing

Communication skills include checking to make sure that the nurse has understood the patient accurately by paraphrasing. **Paraphrasing**, or clarification, means that the nurse restates the patient's basic message. For example, the patient may say, "I don't really know if I should have this test." The nurse would paraphrase by saying, "You haven't received enough information yet to make a decision."

Leading

Nurses use leading skills to encourage open communication. These skills are most effective when starting an interaction or when trying to get the patient to discuss specific health concerns. Leading skills are especially helpful in getting patients to explore their feelings and to elaborate on areas already introduced in the discussion. The leading techniques nurses commonly use when interviewing a patient include direct leading, focusing, and questioning.

Questioning

Questioning is a very direct way of speaking with patients to obtain subjective data for decision making and planning care. Questioning techniques include open-ended and closed questions. *Closed questions* limit the patient's response to "yes," "no," or one-word answers ("Were you feeling angry when your mother said that?"). *Open-ended questions* are purposely general and encourage the patient to provide additional information. Examples of open-ended questions include "Tell me what brought you here today" or "You said that your ankle hurts. Tell me more about that."

Reflecting

Reflecting is repeating the patient's verbal or nonverbal message for the patient's benefit. It is a way of showing the patient that the nurse empathizes or is in tune with the patient's thoughts, feelings, and experiences. For example, Mr. Bates, a 60-year-old with diabetes, is admitted to an outpatient clinic to be evaluated for a possible amputation of his right lower leg because of gangrene. During the clinic visit, Mr. Bates sits in a chair in the examination room with his head in his hands. When the nurse begins to question him, he looks up and says, "Leave me alone. Nothing you can do will help. I might as well be dead." The nurse's response might be, "Mr. Bates, may I sit here for awhile? I can see that you are upset" (reflecting feeling). "You must feel angry that this is happening to you" (reflecting content). This example demonstrates that thoughts, feelings, and experiences are reflected at the same time. Silence is also a form of therapeutic communication. By remaining with the patient and allowing several seconds—or even minutes—to pass without speaking, the nurse demonstrates caring while allowing the patient time to process and potentially verbalize emotions (Berman & Snyder, 2012).

Summarizing

Summarizing is the process of gathering the ideas, feelings, and themes that patients have discussed throughout the interview and restating them in several general statements. Summarizing is a useful tool because it shows patients that the nurse has listened and understood their concerns. It also allows patients to know that progress is being made in resolving their health concerns and signals closure of the interview. One strategy is to read back to the patient what has been documented and then ask, "Is that correct?"

Barriers to Effective Patient Interaction

In some situations the nurse may unknowingly hinder the flow of information by using nontherapeutic interactions (interactions that are harmful rather than helpful). Nontherapeutic interactions interfere with the communication process by making the patient uncomfortable, anxious, or insecure. Some interactions that can be most harmful if used during the health assessment interview are false reassurance, interrupting or changing the subject, passing judgment, cross-examination, avoidance language, unwanted advice, use of technical terms, and insensitivity. Euphemisms or the use of terms thought to be less harsh can also create barriers by misleading or confusing the patient and family. One such example is the use of "passed away" when speaking of a patient's death (Reid, 2011).

False Reassurance

False reassurance occurs when the nurse assures the patient of a positive outcome with no basis for believing in it. False reassurance deprives patients of the right to communicate their feelings. Examples include "Everything will be all right" or "Don't worry about not being able to sleep at night. You'll be fine." False reassurance can be implied by the tone of voice used by the nurse in the communication process.

Interrupting or Changing the Subject

Interrupting the patient or changing the subject shows insensitivity to the patient's thoughts and feelings. In most cases this happens when the nurse is ill at ease with the patient's comments and is unable to deal with their content. Patients who show extreme emotion (e.g., anger, weeping) during the interview, who ask intimate questions about the nurse's personal life, or who are sexually aggressive in the presence of the nurse may make the nurse uncomfortable during the interview. In these instances, the nurse must recognize what it is about the patient's behavior that is making him or her uncomfortable and deal with the situation at hand in a professional manner rather than changing the subject. For example, "Your questions about my personal life are making me feel uncomfortable. We need to talk about what is concerning you today instead."

Passing Judgment

Judgmental statements convey a strong message that the patient must live up to the nurse's value system to be accepted. These statements imply nonacceptance and discourage further interaction. Examples include "Abortion is the same as murder" or "You're not following your diet."

Cross-Examination

Asking question after question during an assessment interview may cause the patient to feel threatened, and the patient may seek refuge by revealing less information. Because all interviews include many questions, the nurse should be careful not to make patients feel that they are being cross-examined with an endless barrage of questions. It is helpful to pause between questions and ask how the patient is tolerating the interview to this point. Encouraging patients to express their feelings about the pace and nature of the interview makes them feel more at ease.

Unwanted Advice

Even when advice is well-intentioned, if it is unsolicited or unwanted, the patient may feel imposed upon. This is especially true when offering casual advice that pertains to the patient's personal life (Berman & Snyder, 2012). Rather than offering unwanted casual advice, the nurse's role includes offering expert guidance based on therapeutic principles that are intended to promote health and wellness. For example, when teaching a patient regarding smoking cessation, the nurse should focus on the facts about smoking and its physiological effects on the patient's body rather than on its negative social stigma, which can be understood as passing judgment.

Technical Terms

Whenever possible, the nurse should use lay rather than technical terms and avoid jargon, slang, or clichés. Terms such as *anterior* and *posterior* are useful for nursing and medical personnel but are more confusing to the patient than the terms *front* and *back*. It is best to avoid the use of initials and acronyms unless they are commonly accepted as everyday language. For instance, most patients will understand the term *urinate* but not the term *void* when asked about urinary elimination.

Sensitive Issues

Nurses often need to ask patients questions that are sensitive and personal. The patient may feel uncomfortable providing information about such concerns as abuse, homelessness, emotional and psychological problems, use of drugs and alcohol, self-image, sexuality, or religion. Discomfort with these issues may cause the patient to lapse into silence. It is important to be sensitive to the patient's need for silence. The patient may need to reflect on what was said or to come to grips with emotions the question has evoked before proceeding.

The nurse also watches for nonverbal signs, such as tear-filled eyes or wringing of hands, which indicate the patient's need to pause for a moment. After a period of silence, if the patient does not resume the conversation, the nurse may need to prompt the patient by saying, "After that, what happened?" or "You were saying. . . ." Certain questions may cause a patient to cry. The nurse should offer tissues, let the patient cry, and wait until the patient is ready to proceed before asking additional questions. Some patients may feel that they need permission to cry. A nurse who sees that the patient is holding back tears can give the patient permission to cry by saying, "I know that you are upset. It is all right to cry." If the patient reacts to questions about sensitive issues with anger, the nurse should acknowledge what the patient is feeling: "I can see that you are angry. Please tell me why." If the patient becomes angry, the nurse should acknowledge the anger, apologize, and wait to resume the interview until the patient's anger dissipates.

Asking the patient sensitive questions may make the nurse uncomfortable. A nurse who anticipates being uncomfortable with certain questions should take time to reflect on and come to terms with these feelings before beginning the interview. Role-playing the situation with another nurse as the patient or mentally visualizing how to react in the anticipated situation will help avoid uncomfortable feelings during the interview. When asking sensitive questions, it is best to be direct and honest with the patient: "I feel uncomfortable asking you such personal questions, but I need the information to complete your plan of care." Communication strategies like these will help the nurse conduct a thorough and effective interview in these sensitive situations.

The Influence of Culture on Nurse-Patient Interactions

Differences in culture and the ways in which they are demonstrated have a significant impact on the interactions that occur in the nurse-patient relationship. The professional nurse must be prepared to recognize and adapt the interactional processes to cultural differences. Further, nurses must not allow their own cultural values and practices to bias the impressions of the patient nor to impair the interaction.

For example, while silence or a lag in conversation may be viewed as awkward or uncomfortable in some societies, this practice varies widely based on several factors, including those related to cultural background. For example, among American Indians, nonverbal communication is prioritized and healthcare providers may be expected to identify a health-related problem through instinctive reasoning, as opposed to asking the American Indian patient a series of questions. In addition, note taking is considered taboo among some members of the American Indian culture. For generations, history has been passed down by way of oral storytelling. As such, it may be preferable for the nurse who is gathering the American Indian patient's history to refrain from taking notes during the interview and to instead rely on memory while with the patient (Spector, 2013).

Again, it is critical that the nurse avoid stereotyping the patient based on cultural background. However, equally important is maintaining an awareness of the influence of cultural background on the patient's beliefs and behaviors and seeking to recognize those potential influences for each patient. See chapter 4 ∞ for discussion of culturally-competent communication in nursing.

Professional Characteristics to Enhance the Nurse-Patient Interaction

Patients are more willing to discuss their health issues if they perceive that they are in a trusting, helping relationship and have developed a sense of rapport or mutual trust and understanding with the interviewing nurse. Carl Rogers, founder of the humanities psychology movement, developed patient-centered therapy. Rogers defined the helping relationship as one "in which at least one of the parties has the intent of promoting the growth, development, maturity, improved functioning, and improved coping with life of the other" (1957, pp. 27–32). Nurses who establish helping relationships with their patients believe that the positive aspects of the helping relationship are shared by the nurse as well as the patient.

The nurse interviewer's attitude plays an important role in the success of the interview. The patient is more likely to cooperate if the nurse conveys a willingness to help and assist the patient. According to Rogers (1957); Brammer, Abrego, and Shostrum (1993); Carkhuff (2000); and other social psychologists, a helping person possesses the characteristics of positive regard, empathy, genuineness, and concreteness.

Positive Regard

Positive regard is the ability to appreciate and respect another person's worth and dignity with a nonjudgmental attitude. Nurses who respect their patients value their individuality and accept them regardless of race, religion, culture, ethnic background, or country of origin. Patients sense positive regard in nurses by their demeanor, attitudes, and verbal and nonverbal communication.

Empathy

Empathy is "the capacity to respond to another's feelings and experiences as if they were your own" (Cormier, Cormier, & Weiser, 1984). Nurses demonstrate empathy by showing their understanding and support of the patient's experience or feelings through actions and words. Empathy allows the nurse to see the issues through the patient's eyes, fostering understanding of the patient's health concerns.

Genuineness

Genuineness is the ability to present oneself honestly and spontaneously. People who are genuine present themselves as down-to-earth and real. To be genuine, nurses must convey interest in, and focus on, the situation at hand, giving the patient their full attention. They use direct eye contact, facial expressions appropriate to the situation, and open body language. Facing the patient, leaning forward during conversation, and sitting with arms and legs uncrossed are examples of open body language. A genuine person communicates in a congruent manner, making sure that verbal and nonverbal messages are consistent. The nurse who tells a patient to "take your time" during the interview, but constantly looks at the clock, gives a mixed or incongruent message. Genuineness and congruent communication promote rapport and trust with the patient.

Concreteness

For the nurse, **concreteness** means speaking to the patient in specific terms rather than in vague generalities. For instance, saying "I need this information to help you to plan a diet to lower your cholesterol level" is more specific than "I need this information to plan your nursing care." The more specific statement promotes understanding and a sense of security in the patient. Speaking to the patient in concrete terms implies that the nurse respects the patient's ability to understand and recognizes the patient's right to know the details of the plan of care.

The Health History Interview

The health history interview is the exchange of information between the nurse and the patient. This information, along with the data from the physical assessment, is used to develop nursing diagnoses and design the nursing care plan. Unlike other types of interviews nurses conduct, the health history interview is a formal, planned interaction to inquire about the patient's health patterns, ADLs, past health history, current health issues, self-care activities, wellness concerns, and other aspects of the patient's health status. In most situations, nurses use a special health history tool to collect assessment data. The health history is a critical component of the comprehensive health interview.

Sources of Information

A variety of sources of information are included in a comprehensive health assessment. In the health history portion, subjective data are gathered. Therefore, the professional nurse will seek to obtain information from the most reliable source.

The Primary Source

The patient is the best and **primary source** of information for the health assessment interview. The patient is the only one who can describe personal symptoms, experiences, and factors leading to the current health concern. In some situations, the patient may be unable or unwilling to provide information. For example, a patient who has had a cerebral vascular accident (brain attack) may not be able to understand what is being said or verbalize a response. The nurse carefully evaluates the patient who is unable to give accurate and reliable information and uses another source of information if indicated. The following patients may be unable to provide accurate and reliable information:

- Infants or children
- Patients who are seriously ill, comatose, sedated, or in substantial pain
- Patients who are developmentally disabled
- Patients disoriented to person, place, or time
- Patients with psychosocial concerns
- Patients who cannot speak the common language
- Patients with aphasia

In some situations an adult patient is able but unwilling to provide certain types of information because of fear, anxiety, embarrassment, or distrust. Some reasons why patients may be hesitant to share information include:

- *Fear of a terminal diagnosis:* A patient may not be ready to cope with the stress of a terminal illness and deny its possibility.
- *Fear of undergoing further physical examination:* A patient with claustrophobia may deny problems because of fear of a magnetic resonance imaging (MRI) scan.
- *Embarrassment:* A male patient may refuse to discuss urinary problems because he fears catheterization or rectal examination.
- *Fear of legal implications:* A patient who is an alcoholic involved in a car accident may fear revealing the addiction to alcohol.
- *Fear of losing a job:* An airline pilot may be reluctant to admit visual problems or hearing loss.
- *Lack of trust:* A patient with AIDS who wishes the diagnosis to remain private may fear a breach in confidentiality.

Secondary Sources

A **secondary source** is a person or record that provides additional information about the patient. The nurse uses secondary sources when the patient is unable or unwilling to communicate. For example, the parent or caregiver is the source of information for a child who cannot communicate. Secondary sources are used to augment and validate previously obtained data. The most commonly used secondary sources are significant others to whom the patient has expressed thoughts and feelings about lifestyle or health status and medical and other records containing descriptions of the patient's subjective experience. The interviewing nurse should not overlook the attending physician and other healthcare personnel who have cared for the patient as excellent secondary sources of information.

Patients often share their personal experiences, feelings, and emotions with significant others. A significant other is a person who has won the patient's respect and who holds a position of importance in the patient's life. A significant other may be a family member, lover, cohabitant, legal guardian (if the patient is a minor or legally incompetent), close friend, coworker, pastor, teacher, or health professional. These individuals often provide a different viewpoint or perspective about the patient's stresses and thoughts, attitudes, and concerns about daily life and illness. The significant other who has the closest relationship with the patient is usually the most accurate source of information when the patient is unable or unwilling to speak.

Whenever possible, the nurse should obtain the patient's permission before requesting information from another person. Patient privacy is protected under the Health Insurance Portability and Accountability Act (HIPAA). HIPAA regulations expressly permit the use of professional judgment and experience in solicitation of information from secondary sources under emergency circumstances or when the patient is incapacitated.

The nurse must be cautious when collecting patient data from another person. This information may be prejudiced by that person's own bias, life experience, and values and may not be a true reflection of the patient's own thinking. Every attempt must be made to validate secondary information by verifying it with the patient, by observation, or by confirming the information with at least one other source. The nurse does not seek secondary information if the patient is competent but unwilling to provide personal information and has not granted the nurse permission to explore information with secondary sources. The nurse should respect the wishes and confidentiality of the patient and attempt to obtain the information at a later time.

The medical record is an excellent source of accurate subjective and objective data about the patient. The subjective statements made by the patient and recorded in the nursing progress notes provide insight about the patient's symptoms and feelings. Nursing progress notes, descriptions of patient responses to treatment, physicians' progress notes, treatment plans, medical histories, laboratory results, and vital signs are examples of excellent secondary resources the nurse can use to develop the nursing care plan. The nurse also investigates medical records from previous hospitalizations or clinic visits. If the medical record is available, it should be reviewed before the health assessment interview because it provides cues to actual and potential health problems to explore. During the interview, one should always validate any information from a secondary source, especially if it conflicts with the patient's statements during the interview.

Phases of the Health Assessment Interview

The health assessment interview is divided into three phases: preinteraction, the initial or formal interview, and the focused interview. The first two phases provide information the nurse uses along with information from the physical assessment to develop the total patient database, formulate nursing diagnoses, and initiate the nursing care plan. The third phase, the focused interview, occurs throughout all stages of the nursing process. Its purpose is to gather, clarify, and update additional patient data as they become available.

The focused interview is used to validate probable or hypothetical nursing or collaborative diagnoses. After the initial interview, the nurse develops several hypothetical nursing diagnoses. Before making a final diagnosis, the nurse conducts a focused interview along with a physical assessment to gather additional data. These additional data are then compared with defining characteristics of the probable diagnoses to determine the most appropriate nursing diagnosis for the patient. The chapters in unit III contain focused interview questions for each body region or system. ∞

Phase I: Preinteraction

The **preinteraction** phase is the period before first meeting with the patient. During this time, the nurse collects data from the medical record; previous health risk appraisals; health screenings; therapists;

dietitians; and other healthcare professionals who have cared for, taught, or counseled the patient; and family members or friends. The nurse reviews the patient's name, age, sex, nationality, medical and social history, and current health concern. If necessary, the nurse also reviews literature describing recent research, new treatments, medication, prevention strategies, and self-care interventions that might have a bearing on the patient's care.

The nurse uses information obtained during the preinteraction phase to plan and guide the direction of the initial interview. Nurses are more likely to conduct a successful interview if they know in advance, for example, that the patient has an emotional problem, is deaf, speaks a foreign language, or is a triathlete.

Information about the patient is not the nurse's only consideration during the preinteraction stage. During this phase, the nurse reflects on his or her own strengths and limitations. For example, a nurse opposed to abortion may have difficulty interviewing a patient who is considering an abortion. In this situation, the nurse's anxiety could interfere with the collection of data and the provision of nursing care. Nurses should be aware of their own feelings and prejudices and plan how to interact with the patient. For instance, a nurse who has had an experience similar to the patient's would need to decide whether to reveal that to the patient.

Environment

The nurse chooses the setting and time before the initial interview takes place. A quiet, private place where few distractions or interruptions will occur is most conducive to a successful interview. The patient will feel more relaxed and comfortable if the area has subdued lighting, moderate temperature, and comfortable seating. More chairs should be provided if family members or an interpreter will be present. A glass of water and tissues should be available for the patient's use. The most ideal setting is one that is private because the presence of another person might hinder the patient's ability to be free and open. If the patient is hospitalized, the nurse should hold the interview in a private conference room if one is available. The nurse can also hold the interview in the patient's room, preferably with no roommates present. If this is not possible, the nurse should select a quiet time of day for the interview, draw bedside curtains or place a screen for privacy, and use a subdued level of speech. In the home setting, a quiet room or even the backyard may be used as long as the patient is comfortable and no distractions are present.

The nurse should sit facing the patient at a comfortable distance without using a table, a desk, or any other barrier that might make communication difficult. When possible, the nurse and the patient should be on the same level. If the nurse sits in a chair that is higher than the patient's or stands at the bedside, it places the patient in an inferior position that might make the patient uncomfortable. A distance of approximately 1.5 to 4 ft between the nurse and the patient is most likely to make the patient feel at ease. Moving closer than 1.5 ft may invade the patient's intimate space, and patients from some cultures may consider this impingement on private space aggressive or seductive. Although 1.5 to 4 ft is the average distance, each person's personal space differs slightly. If the patient moves back in the chair, suddenly crosses arms and legs, or seems anxious, the nurse may be invading the patient's intimate space. If so, the nurse should move back until the patient seems more relaxed. A translator or family member who is present to assist with the interview should sit on one side of the patient so that conversation flows easily (see chapter 4 ∞).

The interview should be scheduled at a time that is convenient for the nurse and the patient. The interview should not interfere with cooking dinner, picking up the children after school, or work. If the patient is hospitalized, the nurse takes care not to schedule the interview at the same time diagnostic tests or treatments are scheduled, during mealtimes, or during visiting hours. The interview should be postponed if the patient is in pain, has been sedated recently, is upset, or is confused.

Phase II: The Initial Interview

The initial interview is a planned meeting in which the nurse interviewer gathers information from the patient. In most cases, the nurse uses a health history form to collect the data to avoid overlooking any area of information. The nurse gathers information about every facet of the patient's health status and state of wellness at this time. These data will be used to develop tentative nursing diagnoses. In addition to providing data, the initial interview also helps establish a nurse-patient relationship based on mutual trust and communication and gives the nurse insight into the patient's lifestyle; values; and feelings about wellness, health, and illness. The health assessment interview is an anxiety-producing situation for most patients. In few other situations is a person required to tell a stranger such intimate details about his or her personal history, health habits, or physical and emotional problems. The nurse has a great responsibility to allay these fears and anxieties so that the patient can communicate as effectively as possible. One way to make patients feel at ease is to address them by their title (Dr., Mrs., Mr., Ms.) and family name (last name) rather than given name (first name). It is important to ask permission to use the patient's given name, since some patients may feel that the nurse is being overly familiar or inappropriate. In this case, the patient will be reluctant to divulge personal information.

The nurse begins by describing the interviewing process, explaining its importance, and telling the patient what to expect. The nurse might say something like this: "Good morning, Mrs. Jentzen. I'm Eric Hernandez, the nurse who will be taking care of you today. To plan your care, I need some additional information. For about the next 45 minutes I would like to find out as much as possible about you and why you are here. Since we will be talking about a variety of things, I'll be jotting down some notes as we speak. Please stop me at any time if you don't understand a question or need more information about something. Some questions have to do with personal and private areas such as your beliefs, family, income, emotions, and sexual activity. Everything we discuss will be held in strict confidence. However, you may choose not to disclose some information."

Notice several things about these introductory remarks. First, the nurse introduced himself and described the purpose of the interview in a friendly, caring tone intended to make the patient feel at ease. Second, the nurse gave the patient a time frame and said notes would be taken during the interview. This advance notice is important, because some patients become threatened or anxious when the nurse writes down information. Third, the nurse encouraged the patient to interrupt or ask questions at any point during the interview. Finally, the nurse reinforced the privacy and confidentiality of the interview.

After making the introductory comments, the nurse will begin to seek information about the patient's health status. The opening questions are purposely broad and vague to let the patient adjust to the questioning nature of the interview. For instance, "What led up to your seeking assistance with your health?" If the nurse begins the interview with a series of very specific personal questions, the patient may begin to "shut down," giving less and less information, until no exchange takes place. The nurse continuously assesses the patient's anxiety level as the interview continues. Restlessness, distraction, and anger are signs that the patient perceives the interview as threatening. The nurse will elicit the best information from patients by asking carefully thought-out and clearly stated, open-ended questions throughout the interview.

After gathering sufficient information, the nurse proceeds with closure of the interview. The nurse indicates that the interview is almost at an end and gives the patient an opportunity to express any final questions or concerns. For example, "Is there anything else you would like to discuss or ask about, since our time is just about at an end?" It is important to take a few minutes to summarize the information gathered in the interview and to identify key health strengths as well as concerns. The nurse should review what the patient can expect next with regard to nursing care. A final step is to thank the patient: "I've appreciated your time and cooperation during the interview."

Phase III: The Focused Interview

The nurse uses the **focused interview** throughout the physical assessment, during treatment, and while caring for the patient. The purpose of the focused interview is to clarify previously obtained assessment data, gather missing information about a specific health concern, update and identify new diagnostic cues as they occur, guide the direction of a physical assessment as it is being conducted, and identify or validate probable nursing diagnoses.

Consider the following situation: Mr. Geoffrey Tripton is a 28-year-old stockbroker who is a new patient at the outpatient clinic. He told the nurse during the initial interview that he experiences severe abdominal pain, nausea, and bloating after eating spicy foods and that this is why he has decided to seek help. After establishing rapport with Mr. Tripton, the nurse used a focused interview to elicit the following additional information: The patient drinks at least 8 cups of coffee and smokes one pack of cigarettes a day, tends to forget to eat when feeling stressed, uses over-the-counter medication to treat his heartburn, and recently lost a large amount of money in the stock market. When questioned further, Mr. Tripton confirmed that his pain sometimes occurs at times when he has not eaten spicy food. He further stated that his smoking recently had doubled to two packs of cigarettes daily. By using a focused interview, the nurse clarified information that had been previously obtained (the patient's abdominal pain is not associated with spicy food), included additional needed information, and identified several new cues not observed before (caffeine and nicotine intake, stress, and anxiety). It is not unusual for patients like Mr. Tripton to fail to give complete information during the initial interview because of anxiety, distrust, discomfort, or confusion.

Nurses use the focused interview continuously to update diagnostic cues because signs, symptoms, and patient health concerns often change from moment to moment or day to day. Nurses perform most focused interviews during routine nursing care. For example, while bathing a patient who recently had surgery, the nurse focuses on the patient's discomfort by asking pertinent questions about his pain. Examples of focusing questions or statements a nurse might use in this situation to update information include: "Is the pain as severe as it was yesterday?" or "Describe the pain you are experiencing now."

In some cases, the information that the nurse learns during the focused interview plays an important part in how physical assessment is performed. For example, if the patient states that he is experiencing severe pain in the upper right quadrant of the abdomen, the nurse would examine this area last. Beginning the assessment with the nontender areas permits the nurse to establish the borders of the affected area. Examination of a painful area can exacerbate symptoms, increase the pain, and force termination of the assessment process.

In Mr. Tripton's situation, the nurse's initial hypothetical nursing diagnosis was pain related to consumption of spicy foods, as evidenced by abdominal discomfort, nausea, and abdominal distention. However, with the additional information obtained during the focused interview, the nurse changed the nursing diagnosis to *Pain related to nicotine and caffeine intake, stress, and missed meals, as evidenced by abdominal discomfort, nausea, and abdominal distention*. In view of the new information, the nurse added the following nursing diagnosis: *Anxiety related to financial losses, as evidenced by chain smoking, forgetting meals, increased intake of coffee, and agitation* (NANDA-I, © 2014).

When obtaining subjective data about patient symptoms, many nurses find it helpful to use an acronym to guide the interview. One acronym is OLDCART & ICE. When using the acronym, the nurse will elicit information about the onset, location, duration, characteristics, aggravating factors, relieving factors, and treatment of symptoms, as well as the impact of symptoms on ADLs, the coping strategies used to deal with symptoms, and the emotional responses to the symptoms. An explanation of the acronym appears in Figure 7.3 ■. Consider the following situation: Mrs. Jennifer Dellarsini, a 54-year-old computer engineer, has come to an urgent care center for cough and discomfort lasting over a week. The nurse used the OLDCART & ICE acronym to guide information gathering about Mrs. Dellarsini's symptom of a cough. The chart in Figure 7.4 ■ is an example of the documentation of Mrs. Dellarsini's responses during the interview.

The example demonstrates that use of the OLDCART & ICE acronym yields important information about Mrs. Dellarsini, her cough, and her responses to this symptom. Follow-up questions in several areas will expand the database and guide the physical assessment. For example, it would be important to determine whether

---

OLDCART & ICE Acronym

O = Onset
L = Location
D = Duration
C = Characteristics
A = Aggravating Factors
R = Relieving Factors
T = Treatment
&
I = Impact on ADLs
C = Coping Strategies
E = Emotional Response

Figure 7.3 OLDCART & ICE acronym.

OLDCART & ICE Acronym	
Symptom: Cough	
Onset	8 days ago.
Location	Mostly in my throat.
Duration	Every day, and coughing jags last 4 or 5 minutes at various times during the day and night.
Characteristics	Wet and painful, mucous comes up, it is clear, it comes on when my throat feels like it has mucous from my nose running down.
Aggravating Factors	It is worse in the morning and at night, if I exert myself too much, like rushing around to get dressed or cook.
Relieving Factors	It quiets if I sit still and drink a cup of tea.
Treatment	I have just been using cough drops and tea or warm water with lemon juice. I have taken ibuprofen for the pain.
Impact on ADLs	I am exhausted, that's why I came. I'm worried this may be more than a virus. I have not been able to do all of the things I need to do. I go to work and that's about it. I really need to do some grocery shopping and laundry, but I don't feel up to it.
Coping Strategies	I'm trying to deal with it by resting when I can. My friends encouraged me to come here.
Emotional Response	Well, I am a little worried that this could be really serious. I have to admit that the worry has not helped me relax and rest.

Figure 7.4 Documentation of the Symptom—Cough, with OLDCART & ICE.

Mrs. Dellarsini had experienced similar symptoms in the past. The statement about the cough being induced by mucus running down her throat would lead to questions about a history of allergy or an environmental exposure to irritants or allergens prior to the onset of the cough. Mrs. Dellarsini indicated that she was worried about the seriousness of her problem. This may indicate that she is experiencing anxiety. Information about the root of the anxiety would be helpful. Specific questions about risk factors and family history of serious respiratory problems may be indicated. In addition, the anxiety may contribute to her exhaustion and further limit her ability to carry out some ADLs. This patient stated that her friends encouraged her to visit the urgent care center. This indicates the presence of a support system. Further information about family may be warranted. The nurse will decide whether it is necessary to address each symptom separately (for example, pain and exhaustion were described by Mrs. Dellarsini when questioned about treatment and the impact on ADLs) and whether to consider additional symptoms during follow-up questioning in the interview or as part of the physical assessment.

Mrs. Dellarsini's visit to the urgent care center was related to her cough and discomfort. The data from the interview regarding the characteristics of the cough guide the physical assessment to include the upper and lower respiratory systems. In addition, the information about exhaustion and disrupted activity indicates the need for assessment of oxygenation, tissue perfusion, and nutrition. Follow-up in response to patient cues throughout the physical assessment will enable the nurse to develop appropriate nursing diagnoses to guide the care for this patient.

Lifespan Considerations

The basic components of a health history are the same whether the nurse works with children or adults. However, for pediatric patients and older adult patients, a number of variations must be incorporated into the health history. The following sections explore unique lifespan considerations related to each of these patient populations.

Focused Interview for Pediatric Patients

With pediatric patients, the nurse must determine the relationship between the child who seeks health care and the adult who presents with the child. One must never assume legal or family ties between children and the adults who accompany them. Nannies, babysitters, friends, siblings, and stepparents often transport children to healthcare appointments. State law determines which individuals can legally consent to medical treatment of a minor child. Federal privacy laws limit access to protected health information. Direct questions of relationships are the easiest way to ensure compliance with the legal and ethical concerns regarding the medical treatment of children. See Table 7.2 for information on potential secondary sources of patient data.

Many children are nonverbal or possess limited language ability; therefore, nurses depend on parents and guardians for health history information. This can limit the specificity of the history information. However, it is important to ask preschoolers and older children about their chief complaint and symptoms even though the information they provide may not be as detailed as the information provided by their parents or guardians. This chapter uses the phrase *primary caregiver* to represent parents, caregivers, or guardians.

The nurse should determine whether the primary caregiver is stressed or distracted prior to the health interview. Many primary caregivers of ill children are sleep deprived because of their child's altered sleep patterns. Sleep deprivation can result in altered recall,

TABLE 7.2	Potential Secondary Sources for Patient Data Related to Infants, Children, and Adolescents	

LABORATORY TESTS	NORMAL VALUES	
Neonate		
Hemoglobin (Hgb) Screen	Hgb 14–20 g/dL	
	No hemoglobinopathies	
Screening for:		
Congenital Adrenal Hyperplasia	Cord Blood: 1,000–3,000 ng/dL of 17-OH progesterone, decreasing to < 100 ng/dL after 24 hours	
Galactosemia	<6 mg/dL	
Congenital Hypothyroidism	T_3 80–100 ng/dL	
Maple Syrup Urine Disease (MSUD)		
Phenylketonuria (PKU)	<2 mg/dL	
Biotinidase Deficiency	Negative	
Toxoplasmosis	Negative	
HIV	Negative	
Tyrosinemia	Tyrosine < 148 micromol/L	
Homocystinuria	<1 mg/dL	
Infant		
Blood Lead Level	<5 mcg/dL	
Hemoglobin and Hematocrit	Hgb > 11 g/dL, Hct > 30%	
Toddler		
Blood Lead Level	<5 mcg/dL	
Urinalysis	Color	Yellow–straw
	Specific Gravity	1.005–1.030
	pH	5–8
	Glucose	Negative
	Sodium	10–40 mEq/L
	Potassium	<8 mEq/L
	Chloride	<8 mEq/L
	Protein	negative–trace
	Osmolality	500–800 mOsm/L
School Age	(As above)	
Urinalysis		
Adolescent Female		
Pap Smear	Negative	
Chlamydia Screen	Negative	
Hemoglobin and Hematocrit	Hgb 12–16 g/dL, HCT 38%–47%	
DIAGNOSTIC TESTS		
Hearing Evaluation		
Height and Weight		
Tuberculosis Screening (PPD)		
Vision Examination		

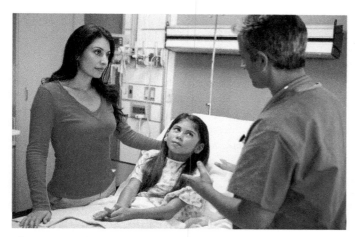

Figure 7.5 The nurse should use open-ended questions to elicit information from the pediatric patient's primary caregiver.
Source: Monkey Business/Fotolia.

limited ability to follow complex questions, and diminished ability to remember verbal instructions. The presence of other children can be distracting, especially if the children are loud, active, or irritable. Nurses can distract energetic or fussy children with books, crayons, or toys.

The nurse should listen carefully to the primary caregiver and use open-ended questions to elicit health information (see Figure 7.5 ■). Primary caregivers usually develop an accurate understanding of the child's regular pattern of behavior as well as the child's baseline physical attributes. They are able to detect subtle differences in their child's behavior and physical appearance. It is essential to pay special attention to the chief complaints that primary caregivers provide. A thorough physical assessment is based on the issues and concerns raised in the health history.

Focused Interview for Older Adult Patients

Comprehensive health assessment of the older adult includes the interview and physical assessment. Subjective data are gathered during the focused interview, in which the patient's own words and perceptions are recorded. Objective data are collected during the physical assessment, from patient records, laboratory results, and other diagnostic studies.

It is important to respect the older adult patient's worth and individuality (see Figure 7.6 ■). He or she should initially be interviewed alone and considered to be mentally competent unless a different mental status is previously known. If caregivers or family members remain in the room for the interview, the patient may not feel comfortable telling the "whole truth." When the patient is very frail, the nurse may tend to address the spouse or adult child of the patient rather than the patient. This may happen unconsciously when the patient is slow to answer or does not interact as quickly as the nurse would wish. Frailness does not necessarily mean an inability to respond appropriately; however, ignoring the patient at the beginning of the interview may serve as a barrier to gaining trust, as well as to gathering information. If the patient is

unable to communicate sufficiently during the initial private interview to supply the nurse with all of the needed information, then it is appropriate to meet later with family or other caregivers. The nurse should consider cultural differences when asking about the patient's state of health and functional abilities and save sensitive subjects, such as sexual and cognitive function, until rapport has been established.

The temperature of the room should be in a comfortable range, with the patient dressed appropriately for that temperature. A robe, blanket, or slippers may be necessary if the patient is not wearing street clothes. Thin paper or cotton examining gowns often make the older adult patient feel uncomfortably chilly and less able to attend to the health history questions.

In order to facilitate older adult patients' abilities to see and hear clearly, the nurse should ensure that the patient is wearing assistive devices, such as glasses or hearing aids, as indicated. The nurse also should minimize background noise, turn off background music, and shut the door or screen the area. Once both participants are seated, the patient should have his or her back to the window or strong light source. Thus, glare is reduced, and the light falls on the face of the examiner. If the older adult patient is known to have vision impairment, additional lighting may be needed. Eye contact should be maintained at eye level, which requires the interviewer to sit if the patient is seated or supine, and to be sure that the patient has a back support.

The nurse should address the patient by the appropriate title (e.g., Mr. or Mrs.) and his or her last name. Other titles, such as Colonel or Doctor, should also be retained. As rapport is established, a more informal approach can develop.

Once comfort, seating, lighting, and environmental distractions are cared for, it is important to know whether the patient is in pain and whether pharmaceutical or alternative pain therapies should be considered before conducting the interview. It is also important to consider sleepiness and the effects of any recent medication.

The interview precedes the physical assessment; this allows the patient and nurse time to become comfortable with each other. After the initial questions and fact-finding are done, and rapport is established, the physical assessment may be started. The nurse continues the interview during the physical assessment by asking questions about the function of each body system as it is assessed.

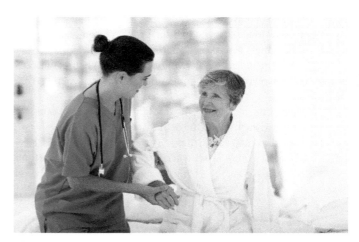

Figure 7.6 Establishing rapport with the older adult patient.
Source: Michael Jung/Fotolia.

Nursing Considerations

The nurse must consider the ability of the patient to participate in the interview process. As stated previously, culture and language are important considerations in establishing a positive relationship. Additional factors that can affect the interview process are alterations in the senses, such as blindness or hearing deficits; developmental level; and pain. The nurse may have to develop written questions for use with patients with hearing deficits to overcome that difficulty.

It is important to consider the patient's developmental level when conducting an interview. Word usage and overall communication will differ when interviewing children and adolescents. In addition, one may find that the developmental level of a patient differs from that expected for a stated age. Patients who have experienced neurologic problems congenitally, or as a result of injury or aging, may not be able to participate effectively in an interview. Last, when a patient is experiencing unrelieved acute or chronic pain, the ability to participate in a lengthy interview is diminished. The nurse must then focus on the immediacy of the problem and gather in-depth information at another time.

Application Through Critical Thinking

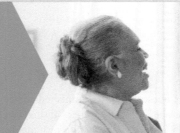
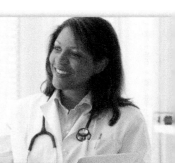

▶ Case Study

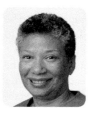

The nurse conducts a health history interview with Mrs. Martha Washburn, a 67-year-old African American. The following are excerpts from the health history:

"Mrs. Washburn, I am going to ask you a lot of questions before the physical assessment. I need to have correct responses and I have to tell you, there will be a lot of them if we are to get to the root of your problem. I will use the information to develop a plan of care.

"What are you here for? Did someone come with you? I see on your chart that you have some problems with urination; are you incontinent? How long have you had the problem? You really should use the adult diapers when you go out."

The nurse includes the following questions: "What is your economic status? Do you go to church? What do you do when you are ill?"

"We need information about your family, so let's start out with your parents. Are they alive? Do you have siblings?"

During the interview, Mrs. Washburn seems very anxious. She becomes quite upset when the nurse asks her about her incontinence. She tries to deny it at first and then admits it when the nurse makes reference to her medical record documentation of the problem.

The nurse completes a review of symptoms and prepares the patient for the physical examination by showing her a room and telling her to get undressed.

▶ Critical Thinking Questions

1. Critique the nurse's actions in the initial interview phase of the case study.

2. Identify the types of information sought in the questions in the case study.

3. Create alternative approaches to the interview and questioning techniques in the case study.

4. Describe your own preparation for an interview of Mrs. Washburn.

5. If Mrs. Washburn did not speak English, how would you modify the health history exam?

▶ References

Barkauskas, V., Baumann, L., & Darling-Fischer, C. (2002). *Health and physical assessment* (3rd ed.). Philadelphia: Mosby.

Berman, A., & Snyder, S. (2012). *Kozier and Erb's fundamentals of nursing: Concepts, process, and practice* (9th ed.). Upper Saddle River, NJ: Prentice Hall.

Bikley, L. S. (2012). *Bates guide to physical examination and history taking* (11th ed.). Philadelphia: Lippincott.

Brammer, L. M., Abrego, P., & Shostrum, E. (1993). *Therapeutic counseling and psychotherapy* (6th ed.). Upper Saddle River, NJ: Prentice Hall.

Carkhuff, R. R. (2000). *The art of helping in the 21st century* (8th ed.). Amherst, MA: Human Resources Development Press.

Cormier, L. S., Cormier, W. H., & Weiser, R. J. (1984). *Interviewing and helping skills for health professionals.* Belmont, CA: Wadsworth.

Doenges, M. A., Moorhouse, M. F., & Murr, A. C. (2008). *Nurse's pocket guide: Diagnoses, prioritized interventions, and rationales.* (11th ed.). Philadelphia: F.A. Davis.

Lutz, C., & Przytulski, K. (2010). *Nutrition and diet therapy: Evidence-based applications* (4th ed.). Philadelphia: F.A. Davis.

Murray, R. B., Zentner, J. P., & Yakimo, R. (2008). *Health promotion strategies through the life span* (8th ed.). Upper Saddle River, NJ: Prentice Hall.

Nursing Diagnoses - Definitions and Classification 2015–2017. Copyright © 2014, 1994–2014 by NANDA International. Used by arrangement with John Wiley & Sons Limited. In order to make safe and effective judgments using NANDA-I nursing diagnoses it is essential that nurses refer to the definitions and defining characteristics of the diagnoses listed in this work.

Orem, D. E. (2001). *Nursing: Concepts of practice* (5th ed.). St. Louis, MO: Mosby.

Reid, M. (2011). Breaking news of death to relatives. *Nursing Times: Ethical and Compassionate Nursing Supplement, 107*(5), 27–30.

Rogers, C. R. (1946). Significant aspects of patient-centered therapy. First published in *American Psychologist, 1,* 415–422. Retrieved from http://psychclassics.yorku.ca/Rogers/therapy.htm

Rogers, C. R. (1957). The necessary and sufficient conditions of therapeutic personality change. *Journal of Consulting Psychology, 21,* 95–103.

Spector, R. E. (2013). *Cultural diversity in health and illness* (8th ed.). Upper Saddle River, NJ: Pearson.

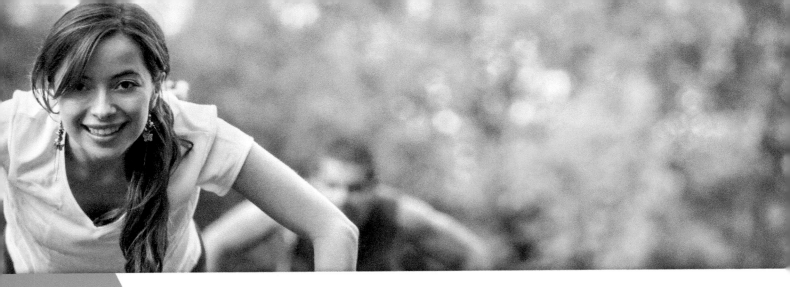

▶ Learning Outcomes

Upon completion of this chapter, you will be able to:

1. Discuss the purpose of the nursing health history.

2. Summarize components of the nursing health history for patients across the life span.

3. Explain the importance of combining each component of the nursing health history to provide holistic patient care.

4. Collect a nursing health history that incorporates patient-specific findings related to health, illness, and wellness.

5. Develop a pedigree.

Key Terms

communication, 127
consanguinity, 135
health history, 127
health pattern, 132
Healthy People 2020, 127
pedigree, 135
primary source, 131
proband, 135
sexual orientation, 130
sexual orientation label, 130
transgender, 130

The health assessment interview provides an opportunity to gather detailed information about events and experiences that have contributed to a patient's current state of health. The **health history** is a comprehensive record of the patient's past and current health. The health history is gathered during the initial health assessment interview, which usually occurs at the patient's first visit to a healthcare facility. This database is updated with each visit. The purpose of the health history is to document the responses of the patient to actual and potential health concerns. Thus, the health history includes a wellness assessment covering questions on how the patient optimizes health and well-being in such areas as nutrition, stress management, and social interaction.

The health history performed by the nurse has a different focus from the medical history performed by the physician. Although both consist of subjective data, the focus of the medical history is to gather data about the cause and course of disease. Thus, the medical history focuses on the disease rather than on the patient and the patient's lifestyle practices. For example, the physician may ask a patient to relate the details of the range of motion in the left hip to determine the cause of abnormal movement and to prescribe a specific treatment. The nurse obtains the same information but uses it to determine the extent to which the patient will need support and teaching regarding ambulation and performance of activities of daily living (ADLs), such as getting dressed independently at home. The nurse and the physician gather the same information for different purposes. The nursing health history may produce information about a medical diagnosis, but the focus is on patient-centered care or on the patient's response to the health concern as a whole person, not just on one or two body parts or systems.

The nursing health history also emphasizes collection of data that can be used to promote wellness through teaching about topics such as nutrition, self-examination (for example, of the breasts or testicles), and health screenings. Wellness promotion is a primary focus in nursing and in health care. Improvement the health status of every person in the United States is the focus of the agenda set forth in *Healthy People 2020* (United States Department of Health and Human Services [USDHHS], 2014). *Healthy People 2020* is a government-designed plan that describes objectives and goals intended to help individuals attain high-quality, longer lives free of preventable disease, disability, injury, and premature death. The desired time frame for achieving goals and objectives is set at 10-year intervals. Examples of additional goals of *Healthy People 2020* include the following:

- Achieving health equity
- Eliminating disparities and improving the health of all groups
- Creating social and physical environments that promote good health for all
- Promoting quality of life, healthy development, and healthy behaviors across all life stages.

Healthy People 2020 is discussed in greater detail in chapter 3. ∞ In application to health assessment and wellness promotion, selected goals and objectives outlined in *Healthy People 2020* are incorporated throughout the chapters contained in units III and IV of this text. ∞

The Health History

The goal of the interview process is to obtain a health history containing information about the patient's health status. In many healthcare settings, including both inpatient and outpatient settings, the nurse and physician complete separate health histories regarding the patient. The nursing health history focuses on the patient's physical status, patterns of daily living, wellness practices, and self-care activities as well as psychosocial, cultural, environmental, and other factors that influence health status. As nurses gather information during the nursing history, they allow patients an opportunity to express their expectations of the healthcare staff as well as the agency or institution. The information in a nursing health history is used along with the subsequent data from the physical assessment to develop a set of nursing diagnoses that reflect the patient's health concerns.

A medical history, by contrast, focuses on the patient's past and present illnesses, medical problems, hospitalizations, and family history. The major aim of the medical history is to determine a medical diagnosis that accounts for the patient's physiologic alteration.

Although nursing and medical histories tend to overlap in some areas, neither format alone presents a true picture of the patient's total health status and health needs. Combining the nursing and medical history into one format, the complete health history, provides the most comprehensive source of information for assessing the patient's total health needs. Integrating the salient features from the nursing and medical history has distinct advantages for both the patient and the caregivers. The information in the health history directs coordinated or collaborative medical and nursing treatment plans that complement one another. The health history saves both the staff and the patient time and energy, because the patient has to provide significant information only once.

Communication is the exchange of information between individuals. Using a health history fosters communication among members of the healthcare team, because they all share its contents. The health history, therefore, fosters effective communication, teamwork, and collaboration between and among the nurse, physician, and other healthcare providers. Principles of communication are discussed in detail in chapter 7. ∞

Components of the Health History

Most healthcare settings have implemented electronic systems for collecting the data, organizing it, and ensuring that the interviewer does not omit any information. A variety of terms may be used to describe the electronic system of documentation, including the following:

- Electronic health record (EHR)
- Electronic medical record (EMR)
- Computerized patient record (CPR)
- Computerized medical record (CMR)
- Electronic health records system (EHRS)
- Patient medical records software (PMRS)
- Personal health record (PHR)

Of the terms used to describe electronic systems of documentation, EHR and EMR are the most commonly used. While these

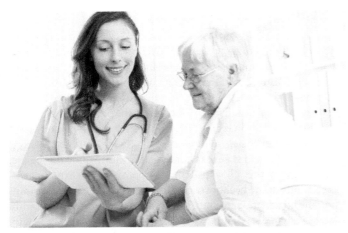

Figure 8.1 Healthcare provider using a tablet to document assessment data.
Source: vgajic/Getty Images.

two terms are sometimes used interchangeably, they are not synonymous. The EMR is focused on treatment and diagnosis, and is not necessarily portable. In comparison, the EHR is designed to be portable and is broader in scope; it incorporates multidisciplinary aspects of the patient's assessment, care, and treatment. While this text will primarily describe use of the EHR, the type of electronic documentation system used will vary depending on the facility, agency, or institution. Devices used for electronic documentation will also vary, and may include laptop computers, tablets, or other devices (see Figure 8.1 ■).

The format, sequencing, and organization of the nursing health history data collection also will vary in different institutions, agencies, or facilities. That organization often reflects the conceptual framework or nursing model used by that facility. The required information remains constant regardless of which framework or nursing model is used, how the information is labeled, or how the data are categorized. For instance, Orem's model is organized according to self-care deficits (Orem, 2001); Gordon's model according to 11 functional health patterns (Gordon, 1990, 2010); and Doenges's model according to 13 diagnostic divisions (Doenges, Moorhouse, & Murr, 2008; Doenges & Moorhouse, 2013). Nonetheless, all models focus on the current health concerns along with an additional broad focus on all aspects of the patient's lifestyle and response to the environment.

In general, health histories (see Table 8.1) include the following groups of information:

- Biographic Data
- Present Health or Illness
- Past History
- Family History
- Psychosocial History
- Review of Body Systems

The information gathered for each of the components of the health history serves a purpose in health assessment and in application of the nursing process for each patient. Responses to the questions asked in the health history provide specific information about

TABLE 8.1	**Health History Format**	
I. Biographic Data	**III. Past History**	Family
Name	Medical	Social Structure/Emotional Concerns
Address	Surgical	Self-Concept
Age	Hospitalization	**VI. Review of Body Systems**
Date of Birth	Outpatient Care	Skin, Hair, and Nails
Birthplace	Childhood Illnesses	Head, Neck, and Lymphatics
Gender	Immunizations	Eyes
Marital Status	Mental and Emotional Health	Ears, Nose, Mouth, and Throat
Race	Allergies	Respiratory
Ethnic Identity/Culture	Substance Use	Breasts and Axillae
Religion and Spirituality	**IV. Family History**	Cardiovascular
Occupation	Immediate Family	Peripheral Vascular
Health Insurance	Extended Family	Abdomen
Source of Information/Reliability	Pedigree	Urinary
II. Present Health or Illness	**V. Psychosocial History**	Male Reproductive
Reason for Seeking Care	Occupational History	Female Reproductive
Health Beliefs and Practices	Education	Musculoskeletal
Health Patterns	Financial Background	Neurologic
Medications, Prescription and Over the Counter	Roles and Relationships	

the individual. The nurse will use professional judgment in determining the significance of the responses, the need for follow-up questioning, and the relevance of information to meeting the health needs of the patient.

Biographic Data

The biographic data include the patient's name and address, age and date of birth, birthplace, gender, marital or relationship status, sexual orientation label, race, religion, occupation, health insurance information, and the reliability of the source of information. When possible, the patient completes a paper form or an online document that elicits these data. Otherwise, the interviewing nurse documents it.

Ideally, to allow for a holistic approach to assessing and caring for the patient, biographic data should include information related to sexual health, including sexual orientation label. However, discussion of sensitive information, including that related to sexual health and practices, requires the nurse to first establish trust and a rapport with the patient. As such, this information is best discussed in person, as opposed to collecting the data by way of paper, telephonic, or online questionnaire.

Biographic data provide a data set from which the nurse can begin to make clinical judgments. The biographic data will be used to relate and compare individual characteristics to established expectations and norms for physical and emotional health. Furthermore, the biographic data provide information about social and environmental characteristics that impact physical and emotional health.

A thorough discussion of each of the pieces of information in the biographic data section of the health history is presented in the following sections.

NAME AND ADDRESS The patient's name and address are generally the first pieces of biographic data to be collected. Listening to the patient state his or her name and address provides the first opportunity to assess the patient's ability to hear and speak. The patient's address reveals information about the patient's environment. The nurse will associate the environment with known health benefits and risks. For example, individuals living in crowded urban environments are at risk for problems associated with heavy vehicular traffic, including respiratory problems from exhaust. Conversely, access to a variety of healthcare facilities and services is usually greater in urban areas than in rural areas.

AGE AND DATE OF BIRTH The patient's age and date of birth are requested in the biographic data. Establishing the age of the patient permits the nurse to begin evaluation of individual characteristics in relation to norms and expectations of physical and social characteristics across the age span. For example, the skin of a 20-year-old is expected to be smooth and elastic, while the skin of a 70-year-old would be expected to have wrinkles and decreased elasticity. The patient's age also influences behavior, communication, and dress. For example, one would expect that the vocabulary of an 18-year-old would be greater than that of a 6-year-old. It is expected that adolescent clothing and appearance will be influenced by trends more frequently than will that of older adults.

BIRTHPLACE The biographic data include identification of the patient's birthplace. Identification of the birthplace allows the nurse to determine the environmental and cultural factors that impacted or contributed to the patient's current state of health and well-being. For example, in the United States, individuals who are born and live in areas where coal mining accounts for much of the industry are at greater risk for respiratory diseases such as black lung, emphysema, and tuberculosis than are individuals who are born in coastal areas or mountain areas of the western United States. Further, individuals born in tropical areas outside of the United States are more likely to have been exposed to parasitic diseases than are those born within the United States.

It is important to determine the length of time the patient spent in and near the place of birth and the places in which the patient lived before locating to the current residence. Cultural, environmental, and geographic characteristics of regions and nations influence the health and well-being of the inhabitants. For example, there is an increase in the number of Chinese women who smoke, particularly among those who immigrate to the United States. Further, geographic moves force individuals to adapt and adjust to new cultural norms. Problems in development may result when frequent moves prohibit individuals from forming and maintaining attachments to family and friends. It is important to understand the characteristics of the areas in which patients were born and where they resided throughout their lives. Knowledge of the characteristics of cities, communities, and regions beyond one's own experience is difficult. For example, a nurse who was born and lived in or near New York City can describe an urban and suburban environment that encompasses a highly developed area in terms of industry, business, and entertainment, with a transportation and highway system that permits rapid travel and access to business and leisure activities, schools, and a variety of healthcare facilities. That nurse will understand that there are communities within New York City that reflect ethnic, cultural, economic, and social differences. Yet, that same nurse may not be able to describe the characteristics of locations beyond New York City. Immigrants in the United States may have knowledge about their location of origin and the region in which they now reside. However, they may not be able to describe the physical environment of regions beyond their experience. All nurses encounter patients who were born or lived in cities, regions, or countries with which they have little specific knowledge. Therefore, nurses must ask patients to describe the locations in which they were born or resided over time, using questions or statements such as the following:

- Is the place you were born in a city?
- Is the region in which you lived close to a large city?
- Tell me about the place where you were born.

To find out about the physical and environmental characteristics of each location, the nurse will include questions such as these:

- Was the area you grew up in an industrial area?
- Was the place where you were born a farming area?
- How far did you have to travel to shop or go to school or get to a healthcare facility?
- How many people reside in that city?

GENDER The patient's gender is an element of the biographic data. There are differences according to gender in terms of physical development, secondary sex characteristics, and reproduction. For example, males have greater muscle mass than do females.

Fat distribution in the thighs, hips, and buttocks is seen in females in greater amounts than in males. Males develop coarse facial hair as a beard while females do not. Moreover, there are health risks associated with sexual differences. For example, although breast cancer can occur in males, it occurs more frequently in females. Osteoporosis occurs in both sexes; however, postmenopausal females are at greater risk. Adolescent males are at greater risk for injury from motor vehicle accidents than are females; however, adolescent females have a higher incidence of eating disorders than do adolescent males.

The nurse should be aware that gender extends beyond sex characteristics. In particular, **transgender,** or gender nonconforming, individuals identify themselves and live as the gender that is not associated with their birth gender (Forbes, 2014).

MARITAL STATUS Marital status is another element of the biographic data. Marital status indicates whether the patient is single, married, widowed, or divorced. To include all sexual orientations and potential relationship statuses, the nurse should ask the patient if he or she is in a partnership (or partnered) with another person. It is helpful to determine the length of marriage, relationship, partnership, widowhood, and divorced status.

The patient's marital or relationship status provides initial information about the presence of significant others who may provide physical or emotional support for the patient. In addition, when a patient relates the loss of a significant other through death or divorce, the nurse begins to evaluate emotional responses and coping ability expected in relation to the event and length of time from the event. The nurse also considers the information in relation to expectations for development. Developmental theorists such as Erikson, discussed in chapter 2 of this text, have described stages across the life span, which include the establishment of intimate relationships. ∞

SEXUAL ORIENTATION Although the terms *sexual orientation* and *sexual orientation label* often are used interchangeably, current literature encourages individuals to consider the two terms as separate from one another. According to Savin-Williams (2011), **sexual orientation** refers to an individual's innate predisposition toward affiliation, affection, bonding, thoughts, or sexual fantasies in relationship to members of the same sex, the other sex, both sexes, or neither sex. However, a **sexual orientation label** is sometimes used to simplify and describe an individual's sexual orientation. For example, sexual orientation labels include straight (or heterosexual), gay, lesbian, and bisexual (Savin-Williams, 2011). Because transgender identity is not associated with any specific sexual orientation label, an individual who identifies as transgender may be heterosexual, gay, lesbian, or bisexual (Morrow & Messinger, 2013).

Due in part to fear of discrimination, certain patients may be hesitant to discuss with healthcare providers issues related to sexual orientation or sexual orientation labels (Pettinato, 2012). To provide holistic care, the nurse should seek to build trust and to create an environment that promotes discussion of all health-related issues, including those related to sexual health. Sexual practices and an individual's self-identified sexual orientation label may provide insight about a number of potential health risks. For example, members of the lesbian, gay, bisexual, and transgender (LGBT) community

are at increased risk for numerous health alterations, including the following:

- Illness due to cardiovascular disease; compared to heterosexual men, gay, bisexual and transgender men are 2.0 to 2.5 times more likely to smoke, and compared to heterosexual women, lesbian, bisexual and transgender women are 1.5 to 2.0 times more likely to smoke (American Lung Association, 2010).
- Complications related to obesity, which is more prevalent among bisexual and lesbian individuals (Strubel, Lindley, Montgomery, Hardin, & Burcin, 2010).
- Issues related to use of anabolic steroids or club drugs, as well as complications associated with human immunodeficiency virus (HIV) infection, especially among homosexual men (Brennan, Barnsteiner, Siantz, Cotter, & Everett, 2012).

RACE Race refers to classification of people according to shared biologic and genetic characteristics. The nurse can begin to identify characteristics of the patient in relation to expectations, norms, and risk factors associated with race. For example, skin coloration is an important health indicator in relation to oxygenation and in identification of jaundice. Assessment of African Americans, Asians, and Caucasians differs because of the levels of melanin, which alters the coloration of the skin across racial lines. Low levels of hemoglobin (as in anemia) in Caucasians and Asians can be assessed as pallor, but in African Americans are best assessed by examining the oral mucosa and assessing capillary refill. Jaundice is best assessed by examination of the sclera of the eye in Asians, who ordinarily have a yellowish skin color or tone. Further, the bone density of African Americans is higher than that of Caucasians or Asians. The following are some health problems associated with racial differences:

- African Americans have a higher incidence of hypertension than Caucasians (Yoon, Burt, Louis, & Carroll, 2012).
- Caucasians and Asians are at highest risk for developing osteoporosis (Mayo Clinic, 2013).
- African Americans are at greater risk for peripheral arterial disease (CDC, 2013).

It is important to note that there has been and continues to be a blending of racial distinctions in the United States. Many individuals identify themselves as biracial or as having mixed racial origins. Families can consist of members of any given cultural background (see Figure 8.2 ■) Therefore, expectations, norms, and risks are not as clearly delineated as they have been in the past. Assessment requires careful history taking.

RELIGION Religion generally refers to an organizing framework for beliefs and practices and is associated with rites, rituals, and ceremonies that mark specific life passages such as birth, adulthood, marriage, and death. Religious beliefs often influence perceptions about health and illness. Religions can impose certain restrictions that impact health, such as not eating pork in the Jewish and Muslim religions.

The nurse will ask the patient the following questions or use the following statements to elicit information:

- What is your religion or religious preference?
- Have you ever belonged to a religious group?

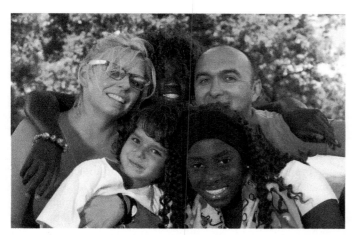

Figure 8.2 Families can consist of individuals with a variety of cultural backgrounds.
Source: DNF-Style/Fotolia.

- How long have you followed the religion?
- Do you adhere to all of the rules of the religion?
- Tell me how your religion influences your health.
- Are there beliefs that govern your life?
- Tell me how your beliefs affect your relationships with others.

Additional information about the role of religion in the patient's life is obtained when asking about health practices, when asking about family history, and when obtaining psychosocial information (see chapter 4 for a detailed discussion of cultural assessment; see chapter 5 for information about psychosocial assessment). ∞

OCCUPATION The patient's occupation is part of the biographic data. Information about the patient's occupation is important in determining whether physical, psychological, or environmental factors associated with work impact the patient's health. For example, coal mining is associated with black lung disease. Those employed in law enforcement and safety are at risk for physical injury and experience psychological stresses associated with ensuring one's own safety and that of the community. An occupational history or profile provides information about previous, current, or potential health-related risks and problems associated with occupations and workplace environments. The following are some questions to elicit information about work-related health concerns:

- What type of work is performed?
- Where does the work take place?
- How many hours are spent at work?
- How much time is involved in commuting to work?
- Does the workplace have safety guidelines in place?
- Are health services available in the workplace?
- Are health promotion programs available in the workplace?
- Does health screening occur in the workplace?
- What types of safety equipment is used in the workplace?
- Does the work environment contribute to stress?
- Does the type of work or the work schedule contribute to conflicts in family or other relationships?

- Are there risks for crime victimization or violence in the workplace?
- Is childcare available at the workplace?
- Does the workplace have disaster and emergency plans?
- Does the work situation provide social support?

HEALTH INSURANCE Health prevention, health seeking, and health maintenance behaviors are influenced by the ability to pay for services. While health insurance information usually is collected by administrative staff, it may be appropriate for the nurse to ask the patient questions regarding access to health insurance.

Health insurance alone does not indicate the patient's inclination to participate in health care. For example, uninsured individuals seek and receive health care in clinics and through other low- or no-cost means, and others are private payers for health services. Recent changes in national health insurance policy have significantly impacted the ability to obtain health insurance in the United States. In 2010, the Patient Protection and Affordable Care Act (PPACA or ACA) was passed by Congress and signed into law by President Barack Obama. The ACA, which includes thousands of pages of regulations, seeks to allow all Americans access to affordable health care. Healthcare system changes outlined in the ACA will be implemented through 2020. Among the most significant changes enacted by the ACA is the availability of insurance premiums at a reduced price for families whose incomes are between 100% and 400% of the federal poverty level (USDHHS, n.d.).

SOURCE OF INFORMATION The biographic data must identify the source of the information for the health history. The usual source of information is the patient, who is the **primary source** (see Figure 8.3 ■). Secondary sources of information include family members, friends, healthcare professionals, and others who can provide information about the patient's health status. The use of translators or interpreters must be indicated when recording the source of information. Whenever possible, a professional interpreter should be used rather than asking the patient's family member or friend to serve as an interpreter.

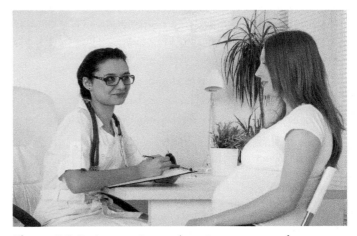

Figure 8.3 Patient serving as the primary source of assessment data.
Sourcce: Dmitriy Melnikov/Fotolia.

RELIABILITY OF THE SOURCE Reliability of the source means that the person providing information for the health history is able to provide a clear and accurate account of present health, past health, family history, psychosocial information, and information related to each of the body systems. The patient is considered to be the most reliable source. Determining reliability of the patient includes assessing the ability to hear and speak and the ability to accurately recall health-related past events. However, parents or guardians must serve as the source of information for children. Secondary sources are used when the patient cannot participate in the interview because of physical or emotional problems. Secondary sources are selected when their knowledge of the patient is sufficient to provide thorough and accurate information. A complete health history may be impossible, for example, when a person has no living relatives or friends who can provide information, when the patient is unable to provide information because of a language barrier and no translator is available, and in an emergency when the patient is unable to respond and sources of information cannot be identified.

Present Health or Illness

The history of present health or illness includes information about all of the patient's current health-related issues, concerns, and problems. The history includes determination of the reason for seeking care as well as identification of health beliefs and practices, health patterns, health goals, and information about medication and therapies.

REASON FOR SEEKING CARE The patient usually gives the reason for seeking care when the nurse asks, "Why are you seeking help today?" or "What is bothering you?" The reason for seeking care, which may be described as the chief complaint, is an important part of the health history picture. The reason for seeking care also may be stated as the presenting problem or reason for encounter (RFE). The nurse explores the reason for seeking care because it provides the first indicators for possible nursing diagnoses and sets the direction of the rest of the health history interview. It is not appropriate, however, to attempt to develop nursing diagnoses at this point. The patient has given minimal information, and no physical assessment or diagnostic testing has been performed. Instead, the nurse develops a list of statements that reflect the patient's major reasons for seeking care. Each statement is a brief, concise, and time-oriented description of the patient's concern. Here are some examples of statements describing the reason for seeking care:

- Substernal chest pain since 9:00 a.m.
- Swelling in lower legs and feet for the past 2 weeks
- Physical examination needed for football team by next Tuesday
- Weight gain of 10 lb since discontinuing daily walking regimen

The patient's own words should be used to document the reason for contact whenever possible: "I've lost 15 pounds in the last 3 weeks" or "I've lost the feeling in my right arm and hand." The nurse explores the onset and progression of each behavior, symptom, or concern the patient relates. Also, the nurse asks patients how their concern has affected their lives and what expectations they have for recovery and subsequent self-care. The answers to these questions provide valuable information about the patients' ability to tolerate and cope with the stress brought on by their health concern and health care.

HEALTH BELIEFS AND PRACTICES A person's beliefs about health and illness are influenced by numerous factors, including exposure to information and personal experiences. Culture and heritage, which have a profound influence on the patient's beliefs about health and illness, are discussed in chapter 4. ∞

Healthcare information is widely available in all forms of media, through educational programs, and in literature provided by healthcare and community organizations. The Internet is responsible for dissemination of healthcare information to a growing number of computer owners and users. Increased information about preventive and treatment services has promoted a different approach to health care. Patients who use a variety of information sources are more likely to be informed about recommendations for screening and preventive measures for themselves or family members according to age. Informed patients are more likely to seek therapies they have read or heard about, to question recommended therapies, or to seek many opinions about therapy. There are risks associated with the use of the Internet for healthcare information. Patients may not be able to judge the reliability of the source. In addition, healthcare products are available for purchase through the Internet. Patients may purchase and use products that interfere with current therapies or are harmful. The nurse's role includes evaluating the patient's health-related knowledge base in terms of both the amount and the accuracy of the information. In addition, the nurse should encourage the patient to use authoritative, evidence-based online resources when seeking educational health information. During any discussion about the patient's use of online health resources, the nurse should reinforce the importance of speaking with a primary care provider prior to making health decisions.

HEALTH PATTERNS A **health pattern** is a set of related traits, habits, or acts that affect a patient's health. The description of the patient's health patterns plays a key role in the patient's total health history because it is the "lifestyle thread" that, woven throughout the fabric of the health history, gives it depth, detail, and definition. For example, the number of hours a patient sleeps, the time a patient awakens and falls asleep, the number of times a patient awakens during the night, and any dream activity are the behaviors that define a patient's sleep patterns. Inadequate sleep can contribute to patient stress, which in turn can be related to gastrointestinal symptoms, such as upset stomach.

The nurse compares a patient's health behavior to predetermined standard health patterns. For example, most people sleep 7 to 9 hours per night, seldom awaken once asleep, and can recall some dream activity. When assessing a patient's rest and sleep patterns, the nurse compares the patient's behavior to the health pattern standard. Assessment of sleep-related health patterns as well as sleep requirements across the life span are discussed in chapter 3. ∞

Health pattern assessment includes information about diet and nutrition. Chapter 12 of this text provides details about nutritional assessment. ∞ The nurse usually collects information about a patient's health patterns as the system or section of the body with which the health pattern is associated is assessed. For example, the nurse might collect information on patterns related to rest and sleep as the neurologic system is assessed, on activity and exercise as the musculoskeletal system is assessed, and on sexuality as the reproductive system is assessed.

Health patterns also refer to the types and frequency of health care in which a patient participates. The nurse will ask questions related to the frequency of healthcare visits and preventive and screening measures used by the patient including laboratory and other diagnostic testing, and the results if known. For example, the nurse will ask the patient to give the dates of the last physical, dental, hearing, and eye examinations. In addition, the nurse will inquire about preventive measures such as flu or hepatitis immunization and will ask the patient about screening for health problems (e.g., mammography for breast cancer, stool examination for bleeding as a sign of rectal cancer, and laboratory screening of cholesterol and glucose levels because of their links with heart disease and diabetes, respectively).

MEDICATIONS Information about the use of medications is obtained during this part of the health history. The information should include the use of prescription and over-the-counter (OTC) medications. The nurse should determine the name, dose, purpose, duration, frequency, and desired or undesired effects of each of the medications. When the patient provides information about medications, the nurse is able to determine the patient's level of knowledge about the medication regimen, whether the patient has an understanding of the problem for which the medication has been prescribed, and whether the patient has noted or received information about the therapeutic effects of the medication. The source of the medication must be identified as well. For example: Has the medication been obtained from another country? Has a cultural healer prepared the medication? Is the patient using medication that was prescribed for someone else? Sharing of medication is common in some cultures, but this practice can have harmful effects. In an acute illness, such as a respiratory infection, medication is prescribed according to dose and duration (length of time the drug will be taken) to reduce symptoms and, ultimately, to cure the illness. When medication is shared, the appropriate dose for the intended duration cannot be achieved. As a result, the illness is ineffectively treated and may become worse. In addition, the medication shared with another may interact or interfere with drugs that the other individual is currently using.

The medication history includes the use of home remedies, folk remedies, herbs, teas, vitamins, dietary supplements, or other substances. The use of folk remedies and herbs is common among immigrant groups in the United States, and the use of vitamins is increasing in the nonimmigrant population (Osborne & Osborne, 2014; Gahche et al., 2011). The use of herbal remedies, teas, vitamins, and folk remedies can interfere with the action of some prescribed medications and can, in some instances, be harmful. For example, exceeding the recommended daily allowance (RDA) of vitamins can result in side effects and toxicity. Large doses of vitamin E can result in increased levels of cholesterol, produce headaches or blurred vision, and increase the risk of bleeding in patients who are taking Coumadin ("Vitamin E," 2013). The nurse uses the medication reconciliation and history to identify any potential drug interactions and to determine if the patient requires education about medications, dosing, side effects, and interactions.

When gathering information about medications, it is helpful to ask whether the patient has the container. Reading the name and dosage is called medication reconciliation, and it provides the specific information the nurse needs to make judgments about patient data. It is also helpful to ask patients about categories of OTC medications. Categories may include laxatives; vitamins; herbs; pain relievers, including aspirin and nonsteroidal anti-inflammatory drugs (NSAIDs); dietary supplements; cold remedies; drops for the eyes, nose, or ears; enemas; allergy preparations; appetite stimulants or suppressants; sleeping aids; and medicated lotions, creams, or unguents. Asking about each category is an efficient method to obtain a comprehensive assessment of medication use.

Past History

The past history includes information about childhood diseases; immunizations; allergies; blood transfusions; major illnesses; injuries; hospitalizations; labor and deliveries; surgical procedures; mental, emotional, or psychiatric health problems; and the use of alcohol, tobacco, and other substances. Many health history forms include a checklist of the most commonly occurring illnesses or surgical procedures to help the patient recall information. The nurse asks the patient to recall all childhood diseases. A history of German measles, polio, chickenpox, streptococcal throat infections, or rheumatic fever is especially significant because these diseases have sequelae that may affect the patient's health status and health concerns in adulthood. Also, the nurse ascertains a history of the patient's immunizations. If the patient is a child, the nurse checks whether the immunizations are up to date. If possible, the immunization data should be verified through immunization records. The nurse questions adult patients concerning the administration of recent tetanus immunizations or boosters, flu shots, or immunizations required for foreign travel. The complete immunization history includes the name of the immunization, the number of doses, and the date of each dose. Chapter 3 provides information about recommended immunization schedules across the age span. ∞

The nurse elicits information about any history of major illnesses, injuries, surgical procedures, hospitalizations, major outpatient care, or therapies. The patient should describe each incident, including the date, treatment, healthcare provider, and any other pertinent information. If the patient has had a surgical procedure, the nurse elicits specific information concerning the type of surgery and postoperative course. Complicated labor and deliveries are recorded here as well as in the reproductive section of the review of the systems.

It is important to obtain a thorough history of any chronic illness and major health concerns. Disease processes such as diabetes, heart disease, or asthma are examples of illnesses in this category. The nurse records the onset, frequency, precipitating factors, signs and symptoms, method of treatment, and long-term effects so that this information can be used to meet the learning needs of the patient and develop appropriate nursing interventions in the nursing care plan.

Information about the patient's emotional, mental, or psychiatric health should include the description of the problem. The nurse asks the patient to identify whether care was received through a healthcare provider, through a support group, from a clergyperson or pastor, or within the family or community. The information should include a description of the therapy or remedy as well as the outcome of treatment. The nurse's questioning must reflect sensitivity to individual and cultural reluctance to describe problems of an emotional or psychiatric dimension. For example, mental or emotional illness is considered as a disgrace by many Asian cultures and as a stigma by those of Arab heritage (Dalky, 2012).

The following questions or statements are used to obtain information about emotional and mental health:

- Have you ever had an emotionally upsetting experience?
- Tell me about any emotional upsets you have experienced.
- Have you ever sought assistance for an emotional problem?
- Where did you go to get assistance?
- Did the assistance help you with the problem?
- Have you ever been told that you have a mental illness or psychiatric disorder?
- What were the circumstances that led to the mental or psychiatric problem?
- What care did you receive for the mental or psychiatric problem?
- Has the care helped the problem?
- Do you take any medication for a mental or psychiatric problem?
- Are you experiencing problems now?
- What kind of help would you like to receive for the emotional, mental, or psychiatric problem?

Information about allergies and the use of illicit drugs, caffeine, alcohol, and tobacco is included in the health history. Information about allergies should include determination of the allergy as food, drug, or environmentally occurring as well as the symptoms, treatment, and personal adaptation. It is important to determine the extent of the patient's knowledge about allergens, especially when exposure to allergens can result in anaphylactic reactions. The nurse should ask the patient to describe the ways allergies are managed. The information should indicate whether a patient's allergies have been identified through testing, through confirmation of a cause by a healthcare professional, or by informal means. Eliciting information about adaptation includes identification of patient practices such as avoidance of allergens; the use of environmental controls (e.g., filters, air conditioners, or other devices) in the home or work environment; and the use of ingested remedies or medications. The information enables the nurse to begin to identify educational needs about allergies. The learning needs may include general or specific details about avoidance of allergens, methods to manage allergy symptoms, and measures to employ in severe allergic reactions. For example, the nurse may suggest that a patient obtain and wear a medic alert bracelet when an allergy to medications is identified.

When gathering information about the use of alcohol, tobacco, caffeine, and illicit drugs, the nurse will want to know the type, amount, duration, and frequency of use of each substance. The information is elicited whether the patient is currently using any substances or reports that he or she has stopped using the products. Tobacco use includes cigarettes, cigars, and products that are chewed or inhaled as snuff. Use of any of these products has an impact on the physical and emotional health of the patient and family. Smoking is a causative factor in lung cancer and emphysema. Family members of smokers are at risk for asthma, emphysema, and cancer from secondhand smoke. Alcohol abuse promotes liver disease, increases risk of injury or death in accidents, and is associated with disruptions in families.

Family History

The family history is a review of the patient's family to determine if any genetic or familial patterns of health or illness might shed light on the patient's current health status. For example, if the patient has a family history of type 1 diabetes, the nurse will question the patient closely about signs of the disease. These signs include increased appetite, frequent urination, and weight loss. The family history begins with a review of the immediate family, parents, siblings, children, grandparents, aunts, uncles, and cousins. The nurse should encourage the patient to recall as many generations as possible to develop a complete picture. If the patient provides data about a genetic or familial disease, it is helpful to interview older members of the family for additional information. Adopted children, spouses, and other individuals living with the patient may not be related by blood; however, their health history should be reviewed because the patient's concern may have an environmental basis. For example, illnesses in the spouse or child of a smoker may be associated with secondhand smoke, or illness may be associated with exposure to toxins or fumes carried into the home on the clothing of a spouse or family member.

Collecting a family history has always been part of health assessment. Traditionally, family history focused on inherited conditions caused by a defect in a single gene or a variation in the number or structure of a particular chromosome. For years, an important focus of family history was to inform reproductive decision making in families affected by inherited conditions such as Down syndrome, muscular dystrophy, cystic fibrosis, and rare inherited disorders. In recent years, however, family health history has taken on a new importance and an expanded role. In 2003, successful completion of the Human Genome Project revealed the total human DNA sequence—the order of the nucleotides A, T, C, and G that make up the human genome. That significant feat, which was the result of international collaboration, marked the beginning of the genome era of health care and has led to rapid advances in genetic research.

Comparing DNA sequences between people with and without specific diseases has revealed that virtually all diseases and health conditions have a genetic component. This new understanding has expanded the usefulness of family history to assess risk for common conditions that contribute to most of the global health burden. No longer is family history limited to rare inherited diseases. Instead, the greatest benefit may come from establishing a basis to predict risk (or susceptibility) for common diseases such as diabetes, cancer, and heart disease. Knowing an individual's disease risk can be used to personalize health care, targeting interventions to those who will benefit most. If a person is found to have a strong family history of diabetes, for example, a personalized strategy for diabetes prevention and screening can be recommended. A patient with a strong family history of colorectal cancer may be advised to have a first colonoscopy at age 30, rather than the standard recommendation of age 50. Including common diseases in family history assessment means that many more people at increased risk will be identified in time to tailor disease prevention and screening. Evidence-based recommendations based on family history are rapidly being implemented, and family history is now considered to be a critical tool for improving the public's health (Valdez, Yoon, Qureshi, Green, & Khoury, 2010). *Healthy People 2020* objectives include a new goal of using genomic tools, including family history, to improve health and prevent harm. Family history plays a key role among emerging genomic tools (USDHHS, 2014).

Family history has been described as "the first genetic test" (Pyeritz, 2012), and all professional nurses, regardless of academic preparation, practice setting, role, or specialty, are expected to elicit family history information, depict that information in a pedigree, and identify patients who may benefit from specific genetic information or services (Consensus Panel, 2009). In fact, all health professions are encouraged to achieve competency in collecting family history information and in identifying patients who would benefit from genetic services (NCHPEG, 2007). Several barriers to routine application of family history information have been identified; among these are limited training of health professionals, the considerable time required to elicit and document family history, and medical record systems that do not support pedigree information.

Beginning about 2004, national awareness campaigns were launched by multiple governmental and professional organizations to highlight the importance of family history information and provide resources for people to collect their own family health histories. One of these, the Surgeon General's Family Health History Initiative, provides a web-based tool that allows people to organize their family history, save it on their own computer, share it with relatives, and even print a pedigree to give to their own health providers. When the website was launched, the Surgeon General declared Thanksgiving to be National Family History Day, suggesting families make use of holiday gatherings to discuss and record health problems and create their own family health history.

Family history is part of the subjective nursing assessment; as such, its accuracy and completeness rely on patients having a certain level of health literacy, knowing pertinent details about the health of their relatives, and being willing and able to share that information with health professionals. Sharing family history information may raise issues of privacy and fear of discrimination. The nurse should remember that a pedigree is different from a personal health history in that it reflects information about multiple individuals, which greatly increases the risk for harm if confidentiality is broken. In addition, a pedigree may reveal sensitive details about reproduction (such as infertility or pregnancy termination), health conditions (e.g., suicide or alcoholism), or relationships (e.g., misassigned paternity or same-sex relationships). Therapeutic communication skills are particularly important when eliciting information that can be sensitive.

Nurses and other health professionals should know how to elicit a multigenerational family history; document the history in the form of a **pedigree;** and identify "red flags," or information that indicates a patient may benefit from referral to a genetic specialist. Although the process entails three steps, the first two steps are often combined, creating the pedigree as information is elicited. A pedigree is a graphic representation or diagram that depicts both medical history and genetic relationships. In a pedigree, each family member is represented by a symbol, using a circle for females and a square for males. Figure 8.4 ■ shows standardized symbols used in pedigrees. Individuals are connected by lines to represent genetic relationships (see Figure 8.5 ■). Each family member's health information is coded and printed below their symbol. The result is a visual representation of a family's health information in the context of genetic relationships, allowing easy identification of disease incidence and patterns of inheritance.

A family history should include at least three generations; if the **proband** (the person around whom the pedigree is created) has

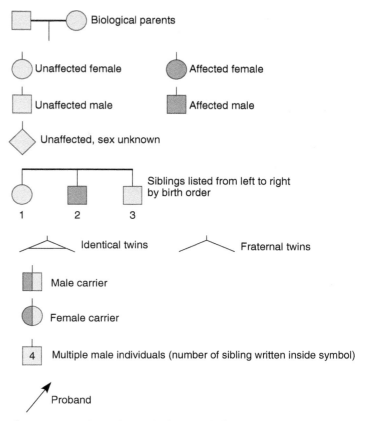

Figure 8.4 Selected standard symbols for use in drawing a pedigree.

children, often four generations are depicted. It is useful to begin with the proband and then "build" the pedigree by adding the most closely-related family members. Include first, second, and third-degree relatives (i.e., parents, siblings and children, aunts, uncles, and grandparents, and first cousins). Depict members of each generation along the same horizontal plane. Record coded health information under each individual's symbol. Information to document includes:

- First name of each family member with age or year of birth
- Any medical conditions or diseases, including age at diagnosis
- Age and cause of death
- Infertility or no children by choice
- Pregnancy complications with gestational age indicated
- Adoption status
- Ancestry
- **Consanguinity** (union between closely related individuals)

At the top of the pedigree, indicate the ancestry (country of origin) of individuals in the originating generation. Be sure to date the pedigree to facilitate future updates.

The last step in utilizing family history is interpreting the pedigree to inform care planning. Formal risk assessments may be conducted by genetic specialists or nurses with specialized training to quantify the risk of having a child with a particular condition or to

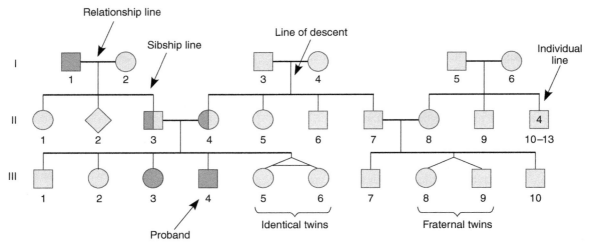

Figure 8.5 Sample three-generation pedigree.

calculate cancer susceptibility. More commonly, pedigrees are examined for genetic red flags, conditions that indicate an individual may benefit from specific genetic information or services. Nurses should be able to evaluate a pedigree for red flags, which include:

- Known genetic conditions
- Multiple family members with the same condition or related conditions (e.g., colon and endometrial cancer)
- Condition in the less-often affected sex (e.g., breast cancer in a male)
- Early age of disease onset (e.g., dementia before age 60)
- Sudden death
- Multiple pregnancy losses
- Birth defects, neurodevelopmental delay, or regression

Upon identifying a genetic red flag, the nurse should discuss the finding with the patient and explore options for follow-up or referral. The follow-up may be casual or formal. For example, about 40% of people who have one parent with type 2 diabetes go on to develop the disease themselves (Ali, 2013). Upon identifying such a case, the nurse might simply mention that general risk to a patient, perhaps creating a "teachable moment" to review diabetes prevention strategies. In contrast, a nurse who identifies a family that has several members with early-onset cancer may suggest a referral for formal cancer risk assessment.

In order to deliver competent care in the genome era, nurses must remember to "think genetic" and thoughtfully elicit, document, and interpret family history information. By following the suggestions outlined in this chapter, nurses can help ensure patients receive maximal benefit from recent advances in genome science.

Psychosocial History

The psychosocial history includes information about the patient's occupational history, educational level, financial background, roles and relationships, ethnicity and culture, family, spirituality, and self-concept. The information about occupation, education, and finances provides the nurse with cues about previous experiences that may impact current or future health. A patient's occupational history can reveal risk factors for a variety of problems. For example, coal

mining increases the risk for respiratory diseases, truck driving is associated with kidney disease, and exposure to asbestos in the shipbuilding and construction industries is associated with lung cancer. Determining the patient's level of education establishes expectations related to the ability to comprehend verbal and written language. These abilities are significant during the assessment process, in discussion of health problems or needs, and in education of the patient. The types of words that will be used and the choice of educational approaches and materials are influenced by the patient's abilities to read, write, and in some cases perform calculations. The patient's financial situation, that is, the ability to obtain health insurance or pay for health services, has an impact on health, health practices, and health-seeking behaviors. Low income is associated with a lowered health status and predisposition to illness. A patient may report that he now enjoys a secure financial situation. However, he may have been born and raised in poverty. Poverty in youth is associated with poor nutrition and lack of regular medical and dental care. These deficiencies can have long-term consequences for the patient.

The nurse will also gather information about the patient's roles and relationships, family, ethnicity and culture, spirituality, and self-concept. The nurse will ask the patient to identify a significant other and support systems. Support systems include family members, friends, neighbors, club members, clergy and church members, and members of the healthcare team. The information provides an initial impression of the family dynamics and informs the nurse of religious and spiritual needs of the patient. Remember that culture influences roles and relationships within families and society. For example, the head of the Cuban household is the male. In Filipino households, the authority in the family is egalitarian, yet the decisions related to health care are made mostly by the women. In many Native American groups, mothers and grandmothers are the decision makers. Determination of roles and relationships is important when planning health care and assisting the patient to make healthcare decisions. The nurse must respect the practices of the patient and prepare to include recognized decision makers in the planning process.

The following are questions and statements to elicit information about roles and relationships, family, and self-concept:

- Tell me about your family.
- How many people are in your family?

- Who is the head of the family?
- What is your role in the family?
- Who makes decisions about health care in your family?
- Who is involved in discussing health or emotional problems in your family?
- Are there certain roles for children in the family?
- Who is your significant other?
- Tell me about your support system.
- Tell me how you feel about yourself.
- How would you describe yourself to someone else?
- Tell me about your body image.

Chapter 4 provides a thorough discussion of cultural considerations related to assessment. Principles of psychosocial assessment, including spirituality, are described in chapter 5. ∞

Review of Body Systems

The focus of this portion of the health history is to uncover current and past information about each body system and its organs. The nurse asks the patient about system function and any abnormal signs or symptoms, paying special attention to gathering information about the functional patterns of each system. For example, when assessing the gastrointestinal system, the nurse should ask the patient to describe digestive and elimination patterns ("How many bowel movements do you have each day?") as well as function ("Are your bowel movements usually hard or soft?"). Open-ended questions or statements are best for eliciting information about abnormal signs or symptoms: "Describe the abdominal pain you've been experiencing. What other symptoms are associated with the pain?" The nurse carefully explores the characteristics and quality of each subjective symptom the patient identifies to obtain a total picture of each system.

Some health history formats use a cephalocaudal or head-to-toe approach for collecting data. In this approach, one considers regions of the body rather than systems. Other formats use an approach related to a nursing theory. Regardless of the method, each area of the body must be reviewed until all systems are covered in each region.

Unit III of this text provides information related to the systems of the body. ∞ Each chapter provides suggestions for questions to gather data about a particular system. Focused interview questions are included and follow-up information is provided to elicit details when symptoms are reported. Examples of the types of information required for a comprehensive system review are included in the sample documentation of the health history. Box 8.1 lists the systems included in this part of the health history.

Documentation

The data collected during the interview are recorded in the nurse's health history. The type of recording is often influenced by the agency or facility in which the interview is carried out. Forms for documentation are varied and include checklists, fill-in forms, and narrative records. The nurse's health history becomes part of the patient record and is a legal document. Principles of documentation must be applied.

Box 8.1 Review of Body Systems

- Skin, Hair, and Nails
- Head, Neck, and Related Lymphatics
- Eyes
- Ears, Nose, Mouth, and Throat
- Respiratory System
- Breasts and Axillae
- Cardiovascular System
- Peripheral Vascular System
- Abdomen
- Urinary System
- Reproductive System
- Musculoskeletal System
- Neurologic System

The subjective data are recorded using quotes. The nurse uses communication skills to elicit as much detail as possible about each area and topic within the health history. The nurse should ask the patient to explain his or her meaning of words such as "good," "average," "okay," "normal," and "adequate." The nurse must be sure to record what the patient intended by use of such terms.

When recording data, the information must be presented in a clear and concise manner. For example, the nurse would use dates and write them in descending order from present to past when providing details about events. Sample documentation of the health history is included in Boxes 8.2 and 8.3. As previously noted, the formats of data collection tools, including those used as part of an electronic documentation system, may vary depending on the facility, agency, or institution. Box 8.2 is a case study presented in narrative form. Box 8.3 represents a fill-in form for documentation of the health history. As shown in the example, quotation marks are not used because all entries are stated by the patient.

Nursing Considerations

The nurse must consider the ability of the patient to participate in the interview process. As stated previously, culture and language are important considerations in establishing a positive relationship. Additional factors that can affect the interview process are alterations in the senses, such as blindness or hearing deficits; developmental level; and pain. The nurse may have to develop written questions for use with patients with hearing deficits to overcome that difficulty.

It is important to consider the patient's developmental level when conducting an interview. Word usage and overall communication will differ when interviewing children and adolescents. In addition, one may find that the developmental level of a patient differs from that expected for a stated age. Patients who have experienced neurologic problems congenitally or as a result of injury or aging may not be able to participate effectively in an interview. Last, when a patient is experiencing unrelieved acute or chronic pain, the ability to participate in a lengthy interview is diminished. The nurse must then focus on the immediacy of the problem and gather in-depth information at another time.

Box 8.2 Narrative Recording of the Health History

Biographic Data Mrs. Corrina Soto, age 33, comes to the health center for a health assessment. She is employed as a graphic designer for a community-based financial institution. Mrs. Soto has insurance through Corporate Insurance Company, through her employer. It covers medical, dental, and vision care. She lives in a single-family residence at 22 Highland Avenue, Midland Park, New Jersey. Mrs. Soto lives with her husband, who she names as her emergency contact. Mrs. Soto was born on July 20, 1981, in Santa Clara, Cuba. She immigrated to the United States 9 years ago. She speaks English with an accent. Mrs. Soto can read and write in English and Spanish. Aside from her husband and in-laws, Mrs. Soto has no immediate family in the United States. She completed 16 years of schooling in Cuba, including earning a university degree in graphic design. She has no formal religious affiliations, because religious practice was not permitted in Cuba when she was there. Some of her family were "hidden" Catholics. She states, "I am happy with my life. I have made adjustments to being in the United States. I have many Cuban friends and have a close relationship with my husband's family. I like my job, except when it gets really stressful."

Present Health Status: Reason for Seeking Health Care Mrs. Soto has no complaints except "weight gain and occasional headaches relieved with aspirin." The weight gain has occurred "over 3 years since I started dating my husband and more since we got married last year." The headaches occur "when I'm tired, stressed, or spending too much time on my computer."

Health Beliefs and Practices Mrs. Soto has no current health problems, except as stated above. She believes "health is important and you need to take care of yourself, but sometimes it's out of your control." When she was a child her mother used to tell her things like "no bathing when you have your period, no water at all" and she "prepared certain foods for certain illnesses and sometimes got medicines from a botanica for ailments." Since she has been covered by health insurance and encouraged by her husband, she has had regular physical, gynecologic, dental, and eye examinations, all of which have been completed annually for 3 years.

Mrs. Soto states she "sleeps well most nights about 8 hours, unless I stay up and read." She "feels rested most mornings."
She tries to exercise but finds it hard "after work and when it's cold out."

Mrs. Soto would like to lose weight. She would "feel healthier, my clothes would fit and I'd feel good about myself." People in Cuba would not have a problem with this weight, but "I don't like it." Eating patterns include "fast foods at lunch, bread at every meal, and dessert or snacks at night."

Medications Mrs. Soto uses oral contraceptives "for 4 years," without problems, and takes a multivitamin and a fish oil capsule every day. She is not undergoing any therapy and "really have never needed any specific care."

Past History, Surgeries, and Illnesses Mrs. Soto had measles as a child. She received smallpox, polio, mumps, tetanus, and other "vaccines" as a child. She has had no major illnesses. She has never been hospitalized, received a blood transfusion, been pregnant, or had allergies. Mrs. Soto cut her lower left leg on glass as a child and had sutures, and a scar remains. She had four wisdom teeth extracted 2 years ago with no complications, "no other surgery."

Emotional History Mrs. Soto states, "I miss my family and get sad when I can't see them. I get frustrated when I don't understand some American ways. I'm pretty emotional. I cry over books and movies, but I haven't had a mental problem." She doesn't smoke, but her whole family smoked when she was in Cuba. "I drink some one or two glasses of wine on weekends or at dinner with my in-laws. I have never used drugs or anything like that."

Family History Mrs. Soto's father died at age 56 from "some type of cancer. He didn't live with us, so I don't know for sure and my mother doesn't talk about him." Her mother is 49 and has no known illnesses. She has a brother, 30, and a sister, 27. Both are "well." Her grandparents were not really known to her but were "old when they died."

Psychosocial History-Occupation Mrs. Soto held jobs in restaurants as a teenager in Cuba. "Since coming to America, I have worked as a graphic designer for two different employers." She states, "I have not been poor but just okay almost all my life until the last 4 or 5 years. My current employer pays very well and I have a good retirement plan now. At home in Cuba, things are really bad, no proper food or medicine. They were better when I was there, but not like here."

Roles and Relationships She states, "I love my family, but I can't see them. I have friends here that are like my family. My friends were a big part of my wedding. One walked me down the aisle. I call home to Cuba, but it's hard to be far away. My husband was born and raised in the United States, but his family is originally from Mexico. We dated for 2 years before we got engaged. He helped me a lot and we love each other very much. His family is like my new family. We see them a lot, they help us, and they treat me like a daughter, so it's very good."

Ethnicity and Culture Mrs. Soto says she will always consider herself Cuban, but "I am an American citizen now, and am so much more of a gringo than my friends. I have come to like American food, especially pasta, but still make my beans and rice and other Cuban foods. My husband likes it too, but not every day. I laugh sometimes when I call my mother in Cuba and speak English sometimes."

Spirituality Mrs. Soto states, "I have no real religion; family and honesty are important to me. I believe in God and sometimes pray, but really believe your family helps you when you are in need."

Self-Concept Mrs. Soto says of herself, "I am a good person. I worry about others. I want to have a family, with children who embrace their Cuban and Mexican heritage, but who know America is their home. I take care of myself and other than some extra pounds think I look pretty good."

Review of Systems

Skin, Hair, and Nails

Denies problems. "I use sunscreen, shower daily, use conditioner on my hair and lotion to prevent dry skin. I would like to have a professional manicure more often, but I keep my nails looking nice."

Head and Neck

Denies problems except "occasional headache relieved by acetaminophen."

Eyes

Annual eye exam for 3 years. Reading glasses for "computer work."

Ears, Nose, Mouth, and Throat

Denies problems with hearing, has "never had an official exam."
Regular dental exams. Wisdom teeth extracted with no problems. No trouble eating or swallowing.

Respiratory

Denies problems. "A cold once a year."
No exposure to pollutants. No history of tobacco use. Exposure to secondhand smoke from birth to 24 years of age at home. Denies cough, difficulty breathing.

Breasts and Axillae

"I have large breasts and have since I was 12. I don't like to examine my breasts; I get scared I might find something. I do get them checked every year by the doctor." No changes, discharge, discomfort.

Cardiac

Denies problems. No history of heart disease. Never has palpitations.

Peripheral Vascular

Denies problems. "The doctor says my blood pressure is fine. I have two veiny spots on my legs, but they don't hurt. They are flat and stringy."

Gastrointestinal

Denies problems. "My bowels move every day with no problem. I get diarrhea when I'm nervous sometimes."

Box 8.2 Narrative Recording of the Health History (continued)

Urinary

Denies problems. "I pass urine five or six times a day and more if I drink more water or coffee."

Reproductive

Onset of menses age 11. "Regular every 28 days for 3 or 4 days. I take birth control pills." Denies pregnancy, abortion.

Sexuality

"I'm heterosexual." "Relations are good with my husband."

Musculoskeletal

Denies problems. "I don't get enough exercise."

Neurologic

No history of head injury, seizure, tremor, loss of consciousness. "Other than headache, I'm okay."

Box 8.3 Documentation of a Health History

Health History

Date: June 30th

Name:	*Corrina Soto*
Address:	*22 Highland Avenue*
	Midland Park, NJ 07432
Telephone:	*201-555-0000*
Age:	*33*
Date of birth:	*July 20, 1981*
Birthplace:	*Santa Clara, Cuba.*
	(Sixth largest city in Cuba, hospital,
	university, manufacturing. Three hours
	from Havana. Historic significance:
	Last battle site of Revolution,
	memorial to Che Guevara.)
	Came to the United States 9 years ago.
Gender:	*Female*
Marital status:	*Married (Chris, age 34, emergency contact)*
Race:	*Cuban*
Religion:	*None really, religious practice was forbidden in Cuba.*
	Some family are hidden Catholics.
Occupation:	*Graphic designer, Financial institution.*
Health insurance:	*Corporate insurance. Medical, dental, eye care.*
Source:	*Patient*
Reliability:	*Reliable, alert, oriented, recall of information*
	intact (nursing assessment).

Present Health/Illness

Reason for seeking care

Scheduled health assessment. No complaints except weight gain and occasional headaches, relieved with aspirin. Weight gain of 20 pounds over 3 years since I started dating my husband, most since we got married last year. I get headaches when I'm stressed, tired, or read too much.

Height/Weight

5'6"/157 lbs. (71.36 kg)

Vital signs

B/P: 128/64 HR: 72 RR: 20 T: 97.9 F

Health beliefs and practices

Health is important and you need to take care of yourself, but sometimes it's out of your control. When I was younger, my mother would tell me no bathing when you have your period, no water at all. My mother prepared certain foods for certain illnesses and sometimes got medicine from a botanica for ailments. All medical care was done well because it was all free.

Health patterns

At first in America I didn't see doctors. Since I have health insurance and my husband reminds me to make appointments, I have medical, dentist, gynecologist, and eye doctor exams. I have had them all every year for the last 3 years. I don't examine my breasts but the doctor does it each year. I haven't had any vaccines since I came here and I think my blood tests are okay. I sleep well most nights for about 8 hours, unless I stay up and read. I try to exercise but it is so hard after work and when it's cold out. Diet is crazy sometimes. I have coffee and toast in the morning. Lunch depends on my schedule, sometimes a sandwich, sometimes a salad. Dinner is probably pizza or fast food three or four times a week. I have a sweet at night.
I like all kinds of foods and I still like Cuban foods like beans, pork, and rice. I eat all kinds of American foods. I especially like pasta and I like bread, I have it at almost all meals.

Medications

I take birth control pills.
I have been on them for 4 years.
I have not had a problem.
I take a vitamin "one-a-day" every day and fish oil, my doctor told me to.
I take acetaminophen for headaches but that's all.
I don't use stuff like my mother did in Cuba and that some of my friends do.

Health goals

To lose weight so my clothes fit and I feel better about myself. In Cuba people would not have a problem with this weight, but I don't like it.

Past History

Childhood illnesses

Measles when I was little. I don't remember other illnesses.

(continued)

Box 8.3 Documentation of a Health History (continued)

Immunizations

Smallpox, polio, and other vaccines like tetanus as a child. I don't remember other specifically.

Medical illnesses

A cold every year—but really no serious illnesses.

Hospitalization

I've never been in the hospital.

Surgery

Never had any except wisdom teeth. All four out 2 years ago because the dentist said they were packed in. I did okay.

Injury

Cut on my leg on glass, had stitches and have a scar by my knee.

Blood transfusion

Never had one.

Emotional/psychiatric problems

I miss my family and get sad when I can't see them. I get frustrated when I don't understand some American ways and I'm pretty emotional. I cry over books and movies, but I haven't had a mental problem.

Allergies

Food: None I know of. Medication: I don't know of any. Environment: No, I don't have a problem.

Use of tobacco?

I don't smoke, never have, but my family smoked when I was in Cuba.

Use of alcohol

I have one or two glasses of wine on weekends or at dinner with my in-laws. I don't like beer or liquor.

Use of illicit drugs

I have never used drugs or anything like that.

Family History

Father

He died at age 56 from "some cancer." He didn't live with us, so I don't know for sure and my mother doesn't say.

Mother

Her mother is 49 and well.

Siblings

She has a brother, 33, and a sister, 27. Both are "well."

Grandparents

Her grandparents were not really known to her but were "old" when they died.

Psychosocial History

Occupational history

Jobs in restaurants as teenager in Cuba. In America—graphic designer for two employers over the past 9 years, most recently for a financial institution.

Educational level

Completed 16 years in Cuba, including a college degree in graphic design. Speaks: English, Spanish Reads: English, Spanish

Financial background

I have not been poor but just okay for all my life until the last 4 or 5 years. My current employer pays well and I have a good retirement plan now. Things are really bad in Cuba. No food or medicine. They were better when I was there but not like here.

Roles and relationships

I love my family but I can't see them. I have friends here that are like my family. My friends were a big part of my wedding. One walked me down the aisle. I call home to Cuba but it's hard to be far away.

Ethnicity and culture

I will always consider myself Cuban but I am an American citizen now and am comfortable with American culture. I like all American things, especially food. I still make beans and rice and other Cuban foods. My husband likes Cuban and Mexican food, but not every day.

Family

My family is in Cuba. I miss them a lot. Would like them to come here someday. My husband was born and raised here, but his parents are from Mexico. We dated for 2 years before we got married. He helped me a lot and we love each other very much. His family is my new family. We see them a lot, they help us out, they treat me like a daughter so it's very good.

Spirituality

I have no real religion. Family and honesty are important to me. I believe in God and sometimes pray but I really believe your family helps you when you are in need.

Self-concept

I am a good person. I worry about others. I want to have a family with children who understand being Cuban but who believe America is a good place. I take care of myself and except for a few pounds I think I look pretty good.

Review of Systems

Skin, hair, nails

No changes, rashes, lesions, color changes, sweating. No birthmarks. Scar left knee. Shower daily, hair shampoo every other day. No use of hair dyes for 2 years. Would like professional manicure more often but keeps nails trimmed and polished.

Box 8.3 **Documentation of a Health History** (continued)

Head, neck, related lymphatics

Occasional headaches relieved by acetaminophen. No history of injury, seizure, tremor, dizziness. No neck swelling.

Eyes

Annual exam—no change in 2 years. Glasses for distance. Next exam—3 months. Pupils equal and reactive to light.

Ears, nose, mouth, and throat

Denies hearing problems, never had specific exam. Nose patent, no injury, sense of smell intact, clear drainage with cold. No trouble eating or swallowing. Dental exam annually, last exam 1 month ago. Brushes and flosses twice daily.

Respiratory

Denies respiratory problems. A cold once a year. No exposure to pollutants. No history of tobacco use. Exposure to secondhand smoke birth to 24 years. Denies cough, difficult breathing. No history of respiratory problems. Unsure of TB screening. Respirations regular and non-labored. Lungs clear to auscultation in all fields bilaterally.

Breasts and axillae

Annual exam by physician. No SBE. Large breasts with no masses, lumps, or discharge.

Cardiovascular

No history of heart disease. Never has palpitations. No edema or cyanosis. Apical pulse regular to auscultation with normal S1 S2 noted. Capillary refill *** 2 seconds.

Peripheral vascular

The doctor says my blood pressure is fine. I have two veiny spots on my legs but they don't hurt. No peripheral edema noted. Pedal pulses palpable.

Abdomen

Denies problems. My bowels move every day with no problem. I get diarrhea when I'm nervous sometimes. Active bowel sounds present in all quadrants. Abdomen soft and non-tender to palpation.

Urinary

Denies problems. No history of UTI. I pass urine five or six times a day and more if I drink more.

Reproductive

On oral contraceptives. Onset menses age 11. Regular every 28 days for 3 to 4 days. Para 0
Gravida 0

Sexual

Self-described as heterosexual. Relations are good with my husband.

Musculoskeletal

Denies problems. I don't get enough exercise. Range of motion—normal. Denies problems with strength.

Neurologic

Other than headache, I'm okay. Denies falls, balance problems, memory problems. Right-handed. Alert and oriented. Can sense touch and temperature.

The nurse uses the health history and interview in various healthcare settings to create a comprehensive account of the patient's past and present health. The completed health history is a compilation of all the patient data collected by the nurse, and it is combined with information obtained during the nursing physical assessment to form the total health database for the patient. The nurse can use this database, which provides a total picture of the patient's past and present physical, psychological, social, cultural, and spiritual health, to formulate nursing diagnoses and plan the patient's care.

The process of interviewing to obtain a complete picture of the patient can be uncomfortable. To obtain the required information the nurse will be asking patients to provide information about their physical and psychosocial well-being, family, personal habits, body functions, and lifestyle. The nurse may believe that patients will perceive questions about religion, culture, economic status, body functions, and sexuality as intrusive. The nurse may feel that he or she is prying or being nosy by asking certain questions. Remember that the nurse-patient interaction is different from social interaction experienced in the nurse's past. When acting in the role of the nurse, the questions asked are intended to guide healthcare decisions. It is helpful to practice the communication techniques that are discussed

in chapter 7. ∞ The nurse will also find it helpful to prepare a list of questions or statements for each category of the health history before conducting the interview. For example, when asking about the financial status of the patient, the nurse may say, "Tell me about your financial situation" or "How would you classify your economic situation?" The nurse may want to use a list of categories in the following way. "Of the following economic levels—low, middle, or high income—how would you rate your current situation?" The nurse could add actual dollar amounts to be more specific.

The nurse should be prepared to address areas concerned with the patient's self-esteem and emotional state. For example, patients may be asked to describe their image in a mirror. The nurse could ask each patient to describe the following in a few sentences: self-perception of strengths and weaknesses, personality, or how a friend or loved one would describe him or her. Often, when addressing sensitive areas such as mental and emotional health, a straightforward question is the best approach. For example, "Have you ever experienced an emotional upset?" If the response is yes, the nurse should ask the patient to describe it. The nurse might ask the patient, "Have you ever had a strong emotional response to a person or situation?" If the response is yes, the nurse would ask the patient to describe it. The nurse may also list a number of emotional behaviors and ask the patient to respond yes or no to each item on the list. Examples of emotional behaviors include anxiety, depression, fear, grief, loneliness, or joy.

Asking questions about body functions, habits, adaptation, and lifestyle may be difficult for a novice in nursing. It is helpful to use the words and terms associated with parts of the body, body functions, and habits regularly when speaking and writing. The focused interview questions provided in each chapter of unit III of this text are intended to guide the nurse in eliciting information about functions, practices, and behaviors associated with each of the body systems. ∞ One should refer to these frequently and use them in preparation for patient interviews.

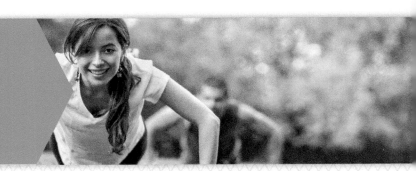

Application Through Critical Thinking

▌ Case Study

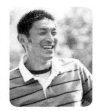

Thomas Lee is a 32-year-old Japanese American marketing executive who is being seen in the clinic for headaches. He tells you that he has been having headaches for several years, that they are getting worse and more frequent, and that the medications he takes are just not helping anymore. Thomas does not have a regular primary care provider, so you tell him you are going to do a complete health history including a pedigree. You are now reviewing that pedigree with Thomas as part of his visit. You note the following items in his pedigree that are of particular importance:

- His parents are both of Japanese descent but born here in American. His mother (age 55) has a history of migraines and depression and his father (age 56) has heart disease and has had one MI.

- His paternal grandparents were born in Japan and moved to the United States. His grandfather died at age 85 from heart disease, and his grandmother committed suicide at age 65. It is thought she had depression but no one in the family will discuss it because they are ashamed.

- His maternal grandparents are both alive. His grandmother is 78 and has had a stroke. His grandfather is 82 and has lung cancer and is only expected to live about 6 months.

- His sister is 34 and suffers from migraines and depression.

- His mother's sister also has migraines and depression.

▌ Critical Thinking Questions

1. Why did the nurse do an extensive health history when Thomas came in with a specific complaint?

2. What types of information should be included in the health history?

3. What cultural considerations are there in this case?

4. How does the pedigree help the nurse?

5. What area would the nurse want to focus on based on the information found in the pedigree?

▶ References

Ali, O. (2013). Genetics of type 2 diabetes. *World Journal of Diabetes, 49*(4), 114–123.

American Lung Association. (2010). *Smoking out a deadly threat: Tobacco use in the LGBT community.* Retrieved from http://www.lung.org/about-us/our-impact/top-stories/smoking-out.html

Barkauskas, V., Baumann, L., & Darling-Fischer, C. (2002). *Health and physical assessment* (3rd ed.). Philadelphia: Mosby.

Bikley, L. S., & Szilagyi, P. G. (2013). *Bates guide to physical examination and history taking* (11th ed.). Philadelphia: Lippincott.

Brammer, L. M., Abrego, P., & Shostrum, E. (1993). *Therapeutic counseling and psychotherapy* (6th ed.). Upper Saddle River, NJ: Prentice Hall.

Brennan, A. M., Barnsteiner, J., Siantz, M. L., Cotter, V. T., & Everett, J. (2012). Lesbian, gay, bisexual, transgendered, or intersexed content for nursing curricula. *Journal of Professional Nursing, 28*(2), 96–104.

Carkhuff, R. R. (2009). *The art of helping in the 21st century* (9th ed.). Amherst, MA: Human Resources Development Press.

Centers for Disease Control and Prevention (CDC). (2013). *Peripheral arterial disease (PAD) fact sheet.* Retrieved from http://www.cdc.gov/dhdsp/data_statistics/fact_sheets/fs_pad.htm

Consensus Panel on Genetic/Genomic Nursing Competencies (2009). *Essentials of genetic and genomic nursing: Competencies, curricula guidelines, and outcome indicators.* Silver Spring, MD: American Nurses Association.

Dalky, H. F. (2012). Perception and coping with stigma of mental illness: Arab families' perspectives. *Issues in Mental Health Nursing, 33*(7), 486–491. doi: 10.3109/01612840.2012.676720

Doenges, M. A., & Moorhouse, M. F. (2013). *Application of nursing process and nursing diagnosis: An interactive text for diagnostic reasoning.* (13th ed.). Philadelphia, PA: F.A. Davis.

Doenges, M. A., Moorhouse, M. F., & Murr, A. C. (2008). *Nurse's pocket guide: Diagnoses, prioritized interventions, and rationales.* (11th ed.). Philadelphia: F.A. Davis.

Forbes, A. (2014). Define "Sex": Legal outcomes for transgender individuals in the United States. In *Handbook of LGBT Communities, Crime, and Justice* (pp. 387–403). New York: Springer.

Gahche, J., Bailey, R., Burt, V., Hughes, J., Yetley, E., Dwyer, J., . . . & Sempos, C. (2011). Dietary supplement use among U.S. adults has increased since NHANES III (1988–1994) *NCHS Data Brief, 61*, 1–8.

Gordon, M. (1990). Toward theory-based diagnostic categories. *International Journal of Nursing Terminologies and Classifications, 1*(1), 5–11.

Gordon, M. (2010). *Manual of nursing diagnosis.* (12th ed.). Sudbury, MA: Jones & Bartlett.

Lutz, C., & Przytulski, K. (2010). *Nutrition and diet therapy: Evidence-based application* (4th ed.). Philadelphia: F.A. Davis.

Mayo Clinic. (2013). *Osteoporosis: Risk factors.* Retrieved from http://www.mayoclinic.org/diseases-conditions/osteoporosis/basics/risk-factors/con-20019924

Morrow, D. F., & Messinger, L. (Eds.). (2013). *Sexual orientation and gender expression in social work practice: Working with gay, lesbian, bisexual, and transgender people.* New York: Columbia University Press.

Murray, R. B., Zentner, J. P., & Yakimo, R. (2008). *Health promotion strategies through the life span* (8th ed.). Upper Saddle River, NJ: Prentice Hall.

National Coalition for Health Professional Education in Genetics (NCHPEG). (2007). *Core competencies in genetics essential for all health care professionals* (3rd ed.). Lutherville, MD: Author.

Orem, D. E. (2001). *Nursing: Concepts of practice* (6th ed.). St. Louis, MO: Mosby.

Osborn, K. S., & Osborn, K. S. (2014). Health Assessment. In *Medical-surgical nursing: Preparation for practice* (p. 125). Boston: Pearson.

Pettinato, M. (2012). Providing care for GLBTQ patients. *Nursing 2012, 42*(12), 22–27.

Pyeritz, R. (2012). The family history: the first genetic test, and still useful after all those years? *Genetics in Medicine, 14*(1), 2–9.

Savin-Williams, R. C. (2011). Identity development among sexual-minority youth. In *Handbook of identity theory and research* (pp. 671–689). New York: Springer.

Struble, C. B., Lindley, L. L., Montgomery, K., Hardin, J., & Burcin, M. (2010). Overweight and obesity in lesbian and bisexual college women. *Journal of American College Health, 59*(1), 51–56.

United States Department of Health and Human Services (USDHHS). (n.d.) *Key features of the Affordable Care Act by year.* Retrieved from http://www.hhs.gov/healthcare/facts/timeline/timeline-text.html

United States Department of Health and Human Services (USDHHS). (2014). *Healthy people 2020.* Retrieved from http://www.healthypeople.gov/2020/default.aspx

Valdez, R., Yoon, P. W., Qureshi, N., Green, R. F., & Khoury, M. J. (2010). Family history in public health practice: A genomic tool for disease prevention and health promotion. *Annual Review of Public Health, 31*, 69-87.

Vitamin E. (2013, November 1). Retrieved from http://www.mayoclinic.org/drugs-supplements/vitamin-e/safety/hrb-20060476

Yoon, S. S., Burt, V., Louis, T., & Carroll, M. D. (2012). Hypertension among adults in the United States, 2009–2010. *NCHS Data Brief, 107*, 1–8.

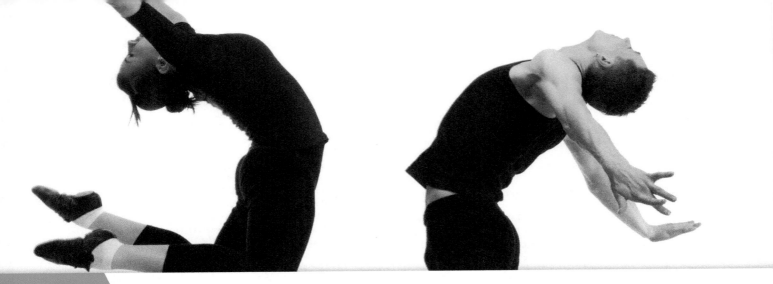

Techniques and Equipment

▶ Learning Outcomes

Upon completion of this chapter, you will be able to:

1. Differentiate between the four basic techniques used by the professional nurse when performing physical assessment.

2. Compare and contrast the purpose of equipment required to perform a complete physical assessment.

3. Demonstrate patient safety and comfort measures that should be implemented when performing a physical assessment.

4. Apply critical thinking when using the four basic techniques of physical assessment.

5. Apply the principles of Standard Precautions in practice.

Key Terms

Unit I of this book identifies and discusses many concepts to be considered when assessing the overall health status of the patient. ∞ These concepts include but are not limited to health, wellness, growth and development, culture, and psychosocial considerations. Much of the data gathered in relation to these concepts are subjective and are obtained through patient interviews during the health history and focused interview sessions. For example, when a patient reports feeling "pins and needles" in his left foot, or feelings of "nausea" after drinking cold water, subjective data are being reported and collected.

Objective data must be gathered as part of the **database.** This is accomplished through the physical assessment of the patient. Objective data are obtained by using the four basic or cardinal techniques of physical assessment: inspection, palpation, percussion, and auscultation. Special equipment and the senses of the nurse are used to measure, observe, touch, and listen to sounds of the body. A safe, comfortable environment conducive to patient comfort, dignity, and privacy is essential. Individual patients will react differently to each situation. The nurse must obtain patient permission to proceed, make the patient feel comfortable, and communicate with the patient throughout the physical assessment.

Basic Techniques of Physical Assessment

When performing physical assessment, the nurse will utilize four basic techniques to obtain objective and measurable data. These techniques are inspection, palpation, percussion, and auscultation, and they are performed in an organized manner. This pattern of organization varies when assessing the abdomen. The sequence for abdominal assessment is inspection, auscultation, percussion, and palpation. Percussion and palpation could alter the natural sounds of the abdomen; therefore, it is important to auscultate before performing palpation and percussion. This sequence is further discussed in chapter 21 of this text. ∞

Inspection

Inspection is the skill of observing the patient in a deliberate, systematic manner. It begins the moment the nurse meets the patient and continues until the end of the patient-nurse interaction (see Figure 9.1 ■). Inspection always precedes the other assessment skills and is never rushed. Most novice nurses feel uncomfortable staring at the patient; nevertheless, careful scrutiny provides critical assessment data. The nurse should talk to the patient, help the patient relax before proceeding with inspection, and avoid the temptation to touch the patient. It is important to complete inspection of the patient before using any of the other techniques. However, if the patient is a child, the nurse may need to vary the approach to secure the child's attention and cooperation.

Inspection begins with a survey of the patient's appearance and a comparison of the right and left sides of the patient's body, which should be nearly symmetric. As the nurse assesses each body system or region, he or she inspects for color, size, shape, contour, symmetry, movement, or drainage. When inspecting a large body region, the nurse should proceed from general overview to specific detail. For example, when inspecting the leg, the nurse surveys the entire leg

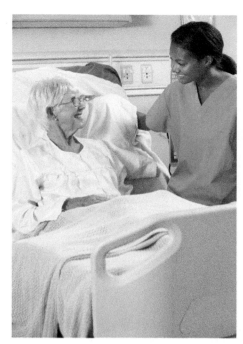

Figure 9.1 Inspection of patient.
Source: Monkey Business Images/Shutterstock.

first and then focuses on each part, including the thigh, knee, calf, ankle, foot, and toes in succession. One should remember to look at the patient, listen for natural sounds, and use the sense of smell to detect odors. Use of each of the senses enhances the findings.

Throughout inspection, the nurse applies the skills of critical thinking to analyze the observations and determine the significance of the findings to the general health of the patient. The nurse must know the anticipated findings regarding inspection of a body part. The nurse asks: Are the findings considered to be within normal parameters, or are they unexpected? Are the findings consistent with other diagnostic cues? What other information is needed to support this finding?

Although the nurse will perform most of the inspection without the help of instruments, some special tools for visualizing certain body organs or regions are important. For example, the ophthalmoscope is used to inspect the inner aspect of the eye. This and other instruments used to enhance inspection are discussed later in this chapter.

Palpation

Palpation is the skill of assessing the patient through the sense of touch to determine specific characteristics of the body. These characteristics include size, shape, location, mobility of a part, position, vibrations, temperature, texture, moisture, tenderness, and edema. The approach used by the nurse to obtain these data is important. The nurse must be gentle and obtain the confidence of the patient. The hand of the nurse must be moved slowly and intentionally. The nurse must learn how much pressure to use with the examination hand during palpation. Too much pressure may produce pain for the patient. Too little pressure may not permit the nurse to perceive the data accurately. This is a skill that requires practice and is developed over time.

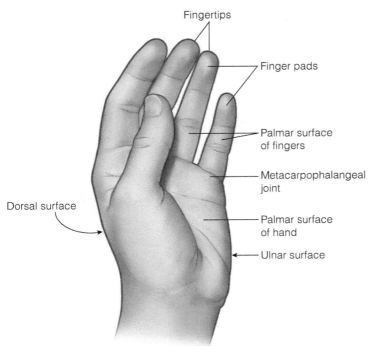

Figure 9.2 Sensitive areas of the hand.

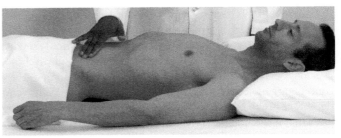

Figure 9.3 Light palpation.

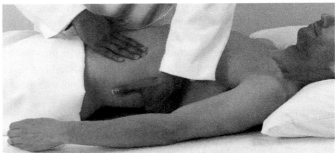

Figure 9.4 Moderate palpation.

The hand has several sensitive areas; therefore, it is important to use the part of the hand most responsive to body structures and functions. The nurse will use the fingertips, finger pads, base of the fingers, palmar surface of the fingers, and the dorsal and ulnar surfaces of the hand (see Figure 9.2 ■).

The finger pads are used for discrimination of underlying structures and functions such as pulses, superficial lymph nodes, or crepitus. Vibratory tremors felt through the chest wall are known as **fremitus.** Fremitus can be vocal, when the patient speaks, or tussive, during coughing. Vibrations are best perceived by the examiner when using the base of the fingers (metacarpophalangeal joints). The palmar aspect of the fingers is used to determine position, consistency, texture, size of structures, pain, and tenderness. The dorsal surface of the fingers is most sensitive to temperature. The ulnar surface of the hand, including the finger, is most sensitive to vibrations such as fremitus. Remember, the dominant hand is always more sensitive than the nondominant hand. The fingertips are used in percussion and are discussed later in this chapter. During palpation, the nurse should use light, moderate, or deep pressure, depending on the depth of the structure being assessed and the thickness of the layers of tissue overlying the structure.

Light Palpation

One must always begin with light palpation. This is the safest, least uncomfortable method and allows the patient to become accustomed to the nurse's touch. Light palpation is used to assess surface characteristics, such as skin texture; pulse; or a tender, inflamed area near the surface of the skin. For light palpation, the finger pads of the dominant hand are placed on the surface of the area to be examined. The hand is moved slowly, and the finger pads, at a depth of 1 cm (0.39 in.), form circles on the skin during assessment, as demonstrated in Figure 9.3 ■.

Moderate Palpation

Moderate palpation is used to assess most of the other structures of the body. For moderate palpation, the nurse uses moderate pressure, places the palmar surface of the fingers of the dominant hand over the structure to be assessed, and presses downward approximately 1 to 2 cm (approximately 0.4 to 0.75 in.), rotating the fingers in a circular motion. Now the nurse can determine the depth, size, shape, consistency, and mobility of organs as well as any pain, tenderness, or pulsations that might be present (see Figure 9.4 ■).

Deep Palpation

Deep palpation is used to palpate an organ that lies deep within a body cavity such as the kidney, liver, or spleen, or when overlying musculature is thick, tense, or rigid such as in obesity or with abdominal guarding. The nurse should use more than moderate pressure by placing the palmar surface of the fingers of the dominant hand on the skin surface. The extended fingers of the nondominant hand are placed over the fingers of the dominant hand, pressing and guiding the fingers downward. This technique provides extra support and pressure and allows the nurse to palpate at a deeper level from 2 to 4 cm (approximately 0.75 to 1.5 in.). All palpation must be used with caution; however, greatest caution must be used with deep palpation (see Figure 9.5 ■). When associated with pain, involuntary guarding or rigidity, especially in the abdomen, may be a sign of pathology. Deep palpation is contraindicated if one suspects that the rigidity is caused by inflammation or alterations in underlying organs and structures due to conditions such as dissecting aneurysms, peritonitis, or ectopic pregnancy.

Before beginning the technique of palpation, the nurse should explain to the patient what will occur. It is difficult to feel underlying structures if there is rigidity in the area to be palpated. Voluntary guarding or rigidity may occur if the patient is tense or frightened. Therefore,

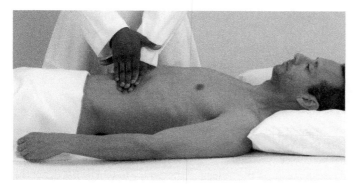

Figure 9.5 Deep palpation.

it is important to help the patient relax and become comfortable before proceeding. To help prevent discomfort, the nurse should warm the hands; keep fingernails short, smooth, and trimmed; and not wear jewelry. Nonsterile gloves should be used if open skin areas or drainage were noted during inspection. Gloves may be latex or nonlatex materials depending on the latex allergy of the nurse or the patient.

The nurse should proceed slowly, using smooth, deliberate movements and avoiding abrupt changes. Most patients will be more relaxed if the nurse talks to them during the examination, explaining each movement in advance. For example, during an abdominal assessment, the nurse might say, "I'm going to place my hand on your abdomen next. Tell me if you feel any discomfort and I will stop right away. How does it feel when I press down in this area?" It is a good idea to touch each area before palpating it. This touch informs the patient that the examination of the area is about to begin and may prevent a startled reaction. Known painful areas of the body are usually the last areas to be palpated.

Through palpation, the nurse perceives data from the assessment and applies critical thinking. The nurse must be able to anticipate the findings regarding palpation of a body structure. Examples of critical thinking questions include: Should light, moderate, or deep pressure be used? If so, why? Are the findings consistent with normative parameters or are they unexpected findings? Does the patient report any discomfort or pain during the process of palpation? Is there voluntary or involuntary guarding? Are the findings consistent with other diagnostic cues? What other information is needed to support this finding?

Percussion

Percussion is the third technique used by the nurse to obtain data when performing physical assessment. **Percussion** comes from the Latin word *percutire,* meaning "to strike through." Therefore, the nurse strikes through a body part with an object, fingers, or reflex hammer, ultimately producing a measurable sound. The striking or tapping of the body produces sound waves. As these waves travel toward underlying structures, they are heard as characteristic tones. The procedure is similar to a musician striking a drum, creating a vibration heard as a musical tone. Percussion is used to determine the size and shape of organs and masses and whether underlying tissue is solid or filled with fluid or air.

Three methods of percussion can be used: direct percussion, blunt percussion, and indirect percussion. The part of the body to be percussed indicates the method to be used.

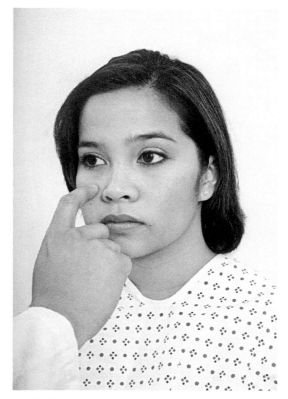

Figure 9.6 Direct percussion.

Direct Percussion

Direct percussion is the technique of tapping the body with the fingertips of the dominant hand. It is used to examine the thorax of an infant and to assess the sinuses of an adult, as illustrated in Figure 9.6 ■.

Blunt Percussion

Blunt percussion involves placing the palm of the nondominant hand flat against the body surface and striking the nondominant hand with the dominant hand. A closed fist of the dominant hand is used to deliver the blow. This method is used for assessing pain and tenderness in the gallbladder, liver, and kidneys, as shown in Figure 9.7 ■.

Indirect Percussion

Indirect percussion is the technique most commonly used because it produces sounds that are clearer and more easily interpreted. A hammer or tapping finger used to strike an object is called a **plexor,** derived from the Greek word *plexis.* **Pleximeter,** from the Greek word *metron,* meaning "measure," refers to the device that accepts the tap or blow from a hammer (see Figure 9.8 ■).

To perform indirect percussion, the hyperextended middle finger of the nondominant hand is placed firmly over the area being examined. This finger is the pleximeter. It is important to keep the other fingers and the palm of this hand raised in order to avoid contact with the body surface. Pressure from the other fingers and palm on the adjacent surface muffles tones being produced. Using only wrist action of the dominant hand to generate motion, the nurse delivers two sharp blows with the plexor. The plexor is the fingertip of the flexed middle finger of the dominant hand.

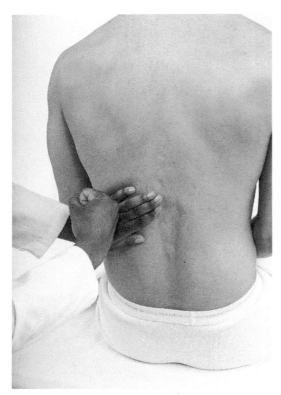

Figure 9.7 Blunt percussion.

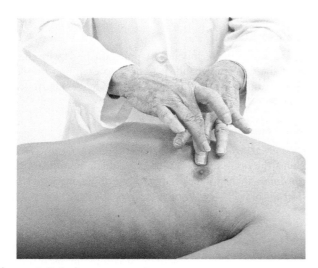

Figure 9.8 Indirect percussion.

The plexor makes contact with the distal phalanx of the pleximeter and is immediately removed. When the plexor maintains contact with the distal phalanx, the sound waves are muffled. Enough force should be used to generate vibrations, and ultimately a sound, without causing injury to the patient or self. Some helpful percussion hints are:

- Ensure that motion is from the wrist, not the forearm or plexor finger.
- Release the plexor finger immediately after the delivery of two sharp strikes.
- Ensure that only the pleximeter makes contact with the body.

- Use the tip of the plexor finger, **NOT** the finger pad, to deliver the blow.
- Use two strikes and then reposition the pleximeter. Delivery of more than two rapid consecutive strikes creates the "woodpecker syndrome" and sounds are muffled.

Sounds

Interpreting a percussion tone is an art that takes time and experience to develop. The amount of air in the underlying structure being percussed is responsible for the tone being produced. The more dense the tissue is, the softer and shorter the tone. The less dense the tissue is, the louder and longer the tone. The five percussion sounds are classified as follows:

1. **Tympany** is a loud, high-pitched, drumlike tone of medium duration characteristic of an organ that is filled with air. It is heard commonly over the gastric bubble in the stomach or over air-filled intestines.
2. **Resonance** is a loud, low-pitched, hollow tone of long duration. It is the normal finding over the lungs.
3. **Hyperresonance** is an abnormally loud, low tone of longer duration than resonance. It is heard when air is trapped in the lungs.
4. **Dullness** is a high-pitched tone that is soft and of short duration. It is usually heard over solid body organs such as the liver or a stool-filled colon.
5. **Flatness** is a high-pitched tone, very soft, and of very short duration. It occurs over solid tissue such as muscle or bone.

Percussion sounds have characteristic features the nurse learns to interpret. These features include intensity, pitch, duration, and quality.

Intensity or *amplitude* of a sound refers to the softness or loudness of the sound. The louder the sound is, the greater the intensity or amplitude of the sound. This is influenced by the amount of air in the structure and the ability of the structure to vibrate.

Pitch or *frequency* of the sound refers to the number of vibrations of sound per second. Slow vibrations produce a low-pitched sound, while a high-pitched sound comes from more rapid vibrations.

Duration refers to the length of time of the produced sound. This time frame ranges from very short to very long, with variation in between.

Quality refers to the recognizable overtones produced by the vibration. This will be described as clear, hollow, muffled, or dull.

Like other assessment skills, the nurse perceives data from the assessment of the patient and applies critical thinking. The nurse must be able to anticipate and identify the produced sound. Is this sound the expected sound? Is this sound considered to be within the normative range for this body part? Does the patient report any discomfort or pain during percussion? Are the findings consistent with other diagnostic cues? What other information is needed to support this finding?

Auscultation

Auscultation is the skill of listening to the sounds produced by the body. When auscultating, one uses both the unassisted sense of hearing and special instruments such as a stethoscope. Body sounds that can be heard with the ears alone include speech, coughing, respirations, and percussion tones. Many body sounds are extremely soft, and a stethoscope is needed to hear them. Stethoscopes work not by amplifying sounds but by blocking out other noises in the environment. Use of the stethoscope is described later in this chapter.

Auscultating body sounds requires a quiet environment in which the nurse can listen not just for the presence or absence of sounds, but also for the characteristics of each sound. External distractions such as radios, televisions, and loud equipment should be eliminated whenever possible. The nurse should avoid rubbing against patients' clothes or drapes or touching the stethoscope tubing, because these actions produce sounds that will obscure the sounds of the body. The nurse should place the diaphragm of the stethoscope firmly over the area to be auscultated. Movement of the stethoscope over thick or coarse hair on the chest or back may alter or obscure sounds. It is important to keep the patient warm, because shivering is uncomfortable and also obscures body sounds.

Sounds are described in terms of intensity, pitch, duration, and quality. For example, the nurse might note that a patient's respirations are loud, high-pitched, long, and raspy. Many times the nurse will hear more than one sound at a time. It is important to focus on each sound and identify the characteristics of each sound. Closing the eyes and concentrating on each sound might help the nurse focus on the sound.

The nurse uses critical thinking with the technique of auscultation. The nurse must know the expected sound in the body region being auscultated. Is this sound considered to be within the normative range for this body region? Are unusual sounds heard? Are these findings consistent with other diagnostic cues? What other information is needed to support this finding?

Equipment

Throughout physical assessment, the nurse will use various instruments and pieces of equipment. These will help in visualizing, hearing, and measuring data. It is the responsibility of the nurse to know how to operate and when to use all equipment in order to comply with patient safety regulations. Before beginning the physical assessment, the nurse should gather all the equipment, organize it, and place it within easy reach. Table 9.1 gives a complete list of the equipment needed for a typical screening exam. Some of the more complex items on the list are discussed in greater detail within this section or in later chapters.

TABLE 9.1 Equipment Used During the Physical Assessment

EQUIPMENT	USED BY THE NURSE TO
Computer, laptop, or tablet	Record data from the exam
Cotton balls or wisps	Test the sense of touch
Cotton-tipped applicators	Obtain specimens
Culture media	Obtain cultures of body fluids and drainage
Dental mirror	Visualize mouth and throat structures
Doppler ultrasonic stethoscope	Obtain readings of blood pressure, pulse, and fetal heart rate
Flashlight	Provide a direct source of light to view parts of the body
Gauze squares	Obtain specimens; collect drainage
Gloves	Protect the nurse and patient from contamination
Goggles	Protect the nurse's eyes from contamination by body fluids
Lubricant	Provide lubrication for vaginal or rectal examinations
Nasal speculum	Dilate nares for inspection of the nose
Ophthalmoscope	Inspect the interior structures of the eye
Otoscope	Inspect the tympanic membrane and external ear canal
Penlight	Provide a direct light source and test pupillary reaction
Reflex hammer	Test deep tendon reflexes
Ruler, marked in centimeters	Measure organs, masses, growths, and lesions
Scale	Measure the weight of the patient
Skin-marking pen	Outline masses or enlarged organs
Slides	Make smears of body fluids or drainage
Specimen containers	Collect specimens of body fluids, drainage, or tissue
Sphygmomanometer	Measure systolic and diastolic blood pressure
Stadiometer	Measure the height of the patient
Stethoscope	Auscultate body sounds
Tape measure, flexible, marked in centimeters	Measure the circumference of the head, abdomen, and extremities
Test tubes	Collect specimens

(continued)

TABLE 9.1 **Equipment Used During the Physical Assessment** (continued)

EQUIPMENT	USED BY THE NURSE TO
Thermometer	Measure body temperature
Tongue blade	Depress the tongue during assessment of the mouth and throat
Tuning fork	Test auditory function and vibratory sensation
Vaginal speculum	Dilate the vaginal canal for inspection of the cervix
Vision charts	Test near and far vision
Watch with second hand	Time heart rate, fetal pulse, or bowel sounds when counting

SPECIAL EQUIPMENT	USE/DESCRIPTION
Goniometer 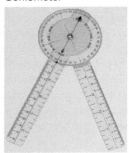	Measures the degree of joint flexion and extension. Consists of two straight arms of clear plastic usually marked in both inches and centimeters. The arms intersect and can be angled and rotated around a protractor marked with degrees. The nurse places the center of the protractor over a joint and aligns the straight arms with the extremity. The degree of flexion or extension is indicated on the protractor.
Skinfold calipers 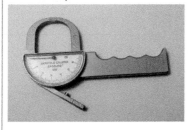	Measures the thickness of subcutaneous tissue. The nurse grasps a fold of skin, usually on the upper arm at the triceps area, waist, or thigh, keeping the sides of the skin parallel. The edges of the caliper are placed at the base of the fold and the calipers tightened until they grasp the fold without compressing it.
Transilluminator 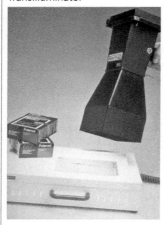	Detects blood, fluid, or masses in body cavities. Instruments manufactured for transillumination are available, or a flashlight with a rubber adapter may be used. In either case, the light beam produced is strong but narrow. When directed through a body cavity, the beam produces a red glow that reveals the presence of air or fluid. Solid material such as blood or masses will obstruct the beam of light, thus producing no glow or passage of the light beam.
Wood's lamp 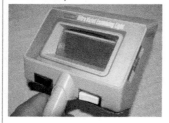	Detects fungal infections of the skin. The Wood's lamp produces a black light, which the nurse shines on the skin in a darkened room. If a fungal infection is present, a characteristic yellow-green fluorescence appears on the skin surface.

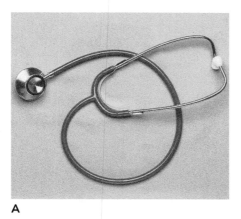 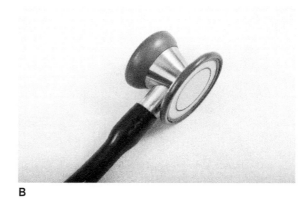

A **B**

Figure 9.9 A. Stethoscope with both a bell-shaped and flat-disc amplifier. B. Close-up of flat disc amplifier (bottom) and a bell amplifier (top).

Stethoscope

The stethoscope is used to auscultate body sounds such as blood pressure, heart sounds, respirations, and bowel sounds. The stethoscope has three parts: the binaurals (earpieces), the flexible tubing, and the end piece. The end piece contains the diaphragm and the bell (see Figure 9.9 ■). To be effective in blocking out environmental noise, the binaurals should fit snugly but comfortably, sloping forward, toward the nose, to match the natural slope of the ear canals. (Most manufacturers supply different binaurals from which to choose.)

The tubing that joins the binaurals to the diaphragm and bell is thick, flexible, and as short as possible (approximately 30 to 36 cm, or 12 to 14 in.). Longer tubing may distort the sound.

The flat end piece, called the diaphragm, screens out low-pitched sounds and, therefore, is best for transmitting high-pitched sounds such as lung sounds and normal heart sounds (see Figure 9.10 ■). The nurse should place the diaphragm evenly and firmly over the patient's exposed skin. The deep, hollow end piece, called the bell, detects low-frequency sounds such as heart murmurs. It is placed lightly against the patient's skin so that it forms a seal but does not flatten to a diaphragm. Either end piece may be held against the patient's skin between the index and middle fingers of the examiner (see Figure 9.11 ■). Friction on the diaphragm or bell from coarse body hair may cause a crackling sound easily confused with abnormal breath sounds. This problem can be avoided by wetting the hair before auscultating the area. Stethoscopes usually include an assortment of interchangeable diaphragms and bells in different sizes for different purposes; for example, smaller diaphragm pieces are used for examining children.

Doppler Ultrasonic Stethoscope

A Doppler ultrasonic stethoscope uses ultrasonic waves to detect sounds that are difficult to hear with a regular stethoscope, such as fetal heart sounds and peripheral pulses that cannot be easily palpated (see Figure 9.12 ■). It operates on a principle discovered in the 19th century by Johannes Doppler, the Austrian physicist who found that the pitch of a sound varies in relation to the distance between the source and the listener. To the listener, the pitch sounds higher when the distance from the source is small and lower when the distance from the source is great.

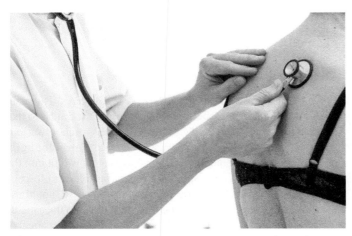

Figure 9.10 Nurse using a stethoscope to auscultate the patient's lungs. The nurse should place the diaphragm of the stethoscope evenly and firmly over the patient's exposed skin.
Source: © Photographee.eu.

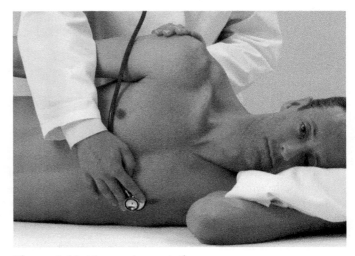

Figure 9.11 Nurse using a stethoscope.

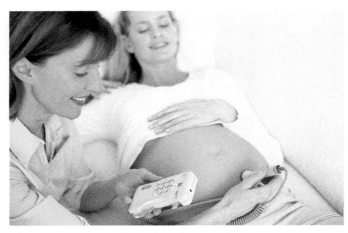

Figure 9.12 Using a Doppler ultrasound.
Source: Ian Hooton/Science Photo Library.

The way to eliminate interference is to apply a small amount of gel to the end of the Doppler probe (the transducer), which may resemble a wand or a disk. When using the Doppler ultrasonic stethoscope to assess the pulse, the nurse turns it on and places the probe gently against the patient's skin over the artery to be auscultated. It is important to avoid heavy pressure, because it may impede blood flow. The probe sends a low-energy, high-pitched sound wave toward the underlying blood vessel. As the blood ebbs and flows, the probe picks up and amplifies the subtle changes in pitch, and the nurse will hear a pulsing beat.

Ophthalmoscope

An ophthalmoscope is used to inspect internal eye structures. Its main components are the handle, which holds the battery, and the head, which houses the aperture selector, viewing aperture, lens selector disk, lens indicator, lenses of varying powers of magnification, and mirrors (see Figure 9.13 ■).

The light source shines light through the viewing aperture, which is adjusted to select one of five apertures (see Figure 9.14 ■).

1. The large aperture is used most often. It emits a large, full spot for viewing dilated pupils.
2. The small aperture is used for undilated pupils.
3. The red-free filter shines a green beam used to examine the optic disc for pallor or hemorrhaging, which appears black with this filter.
4. The grid allows the examiner to assess the size, location, and pattern of any lesions.
5. The slit allows for examination of the anterior eye and aids in assessing the elevation or depression of lesions.

The lens selector dial must be rotated to bring the inner eye structures into focus. While looking through the viewing aperture, one rotates the lens selection dial to adjust the convergence or divergence of the light. At the zero setting, the lens neither converges nor diverges the light. The lens dial is moved clockwise to access the numbers in black, which range from +1 to +40. These lenses improve visualization in a patient who is farsighted. The lens dial is moved counterclockwise to access the red numbers, which range from –1 to –20. These lenses improve visualization if the patient is nearsighted. See chapter 15 for a more detailed discussion of assessment of the eye. ∞

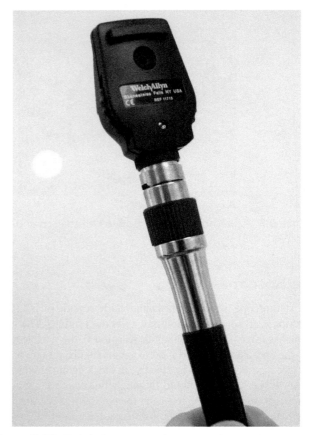

Figure 9.13 Ophthalmoscope demonstrating aperture.

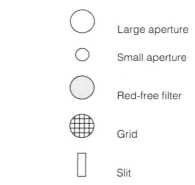

Large aperture

Small aperture

Red-free filter

Grid

Slit

Figure 9.14 Apertures of ophthalmoscope.

Otoscope

The otoscope is used to inspect external ear structures. The main components of the otoscope are the handle, which is similar to that of the ophthalmoscope, the light, the lens, and specula of various sizes (see Figure 9.15 ■). The specula are used to narrow the beam of light. The nurse should select the largest one that will fit into the patient's ear canal. If a nasal speculum is not available, the otoscope can be used to inspect the nose. In this case, the nurse should use the shortest, broadest speculum and insert it gently into the patient's naris. See chapter 16 for a more detailed discussion of assessment of the ears and nose. ∞

Special equipment is required for assessment of several body systems. For example, the reflex hammer is used in the neurologic assessment and the vaginal speculum in assessment of the female reproductive system. Each chapter in unit III of this text provides

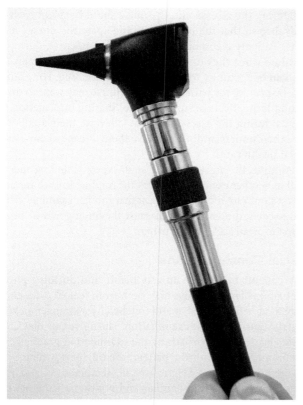

Figure 9.15 Otoscope.

a discussion of specialized equipment and how it is used in physical assessment of a particular system. ∞

Professional Responsibilities

Throughout all aspects of the assessment process, the nurse must apply critical thinking while providing a safe and comfortable environment for the patient. The nurse must identify cues presented by the patient and apply critical thinking to determine the relevance of these data. The safe external environment created by the nurse includes comfort, warmth, privacy, and the use of Standard Precautions, which will be discussed later in this chapter.

Cues

In addition to developing the skills of inspection, palpation, percussion, and auscultation, the nurse must be able to recognize the relative significance of the many visual, palpable, or auditory cues that may be present during an assessment. **Cues** are bits of information that hint at the possibility of a health problem. In other words, the nurse needs to know what to look for. To become skilled at cue recognition, nurses should cultivate their senses until they readily perceive even slight cues. For example, some things that are noticed during an initial survey or inspection of the patient may hint at an underlying health problem. Swelling (edema) of the legs provides a cue to assess for heart problems. Bruising (ecchymosis) of the skin is a cue to ask the patient about recent falls, trauma, injury, anticoagulant medication, or a bleeding problem. Grimacing, guarding (protective posture), or wincing when a patient moves or when a body part is moved during assessment are cues to examine the underlying joint and muscles for problems or masses. Cues that suggest hearing loss include not following directions, looking at the examiner's lips during conversation, or speaking in a loud voice. Asymmetry of facial expression is a cue to assess function of the cranial nerves. Odors are cues to suggest a problem with hygiene or drainage from an orifice or wound. Cue recognition develops with practice, but beginners can acquire the skill by observing an experienced nurse, by practicing on partners, and by studying the visual aids in this text.

Critical Thinking

Throughout the assessment process, the nurse gathers subjective and objective data. Recall that subjective data are reported by the patient during the interviews, and the objective data come from the physical assessment and the application of the four techniques of inspection, palpation, percussion, and auscultation. These data form the database reflecting the health status of the patient. During this process, the presented cues must be interpreted.

The interpretation of cues and other collected data utilizes the process of critical thinking. The nurse should be organized when collecting data; this allows the nurse to look for inconsistencies and check to be sure the data are accurate. The data are compared to normative values and ranges. Data are clustered and patterns are identified. Missing information is identified and, after the database is completed, valid conclusions are drawn. At this time, the nurse establishes priorities of care. In collaboration with the patient, the nurse identifies desired patient outcomes and develops the patient's nursing care plan. Evaluation follows implementation of each nursing intervention.

Once cues are recognized and data are collected, the nurse must be able to interpret the findings. Is a particular finding normal, or does it indicate an alteration in the patient's health? Normal data are assessment findings that fall within an accepted standard range for a specific type of data. For example, the normal range for the adult pulse rate is 60 to 100 beats per minute. A pulse of 76 is, therefore, considered normal. Some healthy individuals exhibit characteristics that are outside the standard range for a specific type of data. Such findings are considered variations from the norm. For example, a long-distance runner with a pulse of 48 resulting from regular cardiovascular conditioning exhibits a variation from the norm for pulse rate. Findings that are outside the range for a specific type of data and that may indicate a threat to the patient's health are considered unexpected findings or deviations from the norm. For example, an irregular, thready pulse rate of 120 is an unexpected finding that could indicate the presence of a harmful condition. It is important to note that not all unexpected findings indicate the presence of a disease or disorder. For example, fatigue in a 20-year-old student may indicate anemia or infection, or it may be caused simply by a lack of sleep.

Providing a Safe and Comfortable Environment

Patients are more likely to discuss health problems and consent to a physical assessment if they feel they are in a safe and comfortable environment. The nurse plays a vital role in developing this environment by providing an examination space that is appropriate for the setting, ensuring privacy for the patient, and noting special considerations for each patient. These special considerations may include personal preferences, cultural differences, or health status.

Setting

The physical assessment may be performed in a variety of settings, including a clinic, a hospital room, a school nurse's office, a corporate health services office, or a patient's home. No matter where the location, the nurse is responsible for preparing a setting that is conducive to the patient's comfort and privacy. The examination room should be warm, private, and free from distractions and interruptions. Overhead lighting must ensure good visibility and be free of distortion. A portable lamp to highlight body surfaces and contours may be needed.

Preparation

Before beginning the assessment, the nurse should thoroughly explain to the patient what is to follow and encourage the patient to ask questions. If the patient does not speak the nurse's language, it is important to secure the assistance of a translator. If the patient's hearing is impaired, the nurse must determine the best method for communication, which may include the use of sign language.

In many healthcare institutions, the patient is asked to sign a consent form for the physical assessment, especially if invasive procedures such as a vaginal or rectal examination or blood studies are to be performed. It is the nurse's responsibility to ensure that the patient understands the procedures to be performed and that all necessary consent forms are signed.

In most cases, patients should empty their bladder prior to the examination. Voiding helps patients feel more comfortable and relaxed and facilitates palpation of the abdomen and pubic area. If urinalysis is to be done, the patient should be instructed in obtaining a clean-catch specimen and be given a container for the urine sample.

Privacy

After ensuring that the examination room is warm, the nurse shows the patient how to put on the examination gown and leaves the patient to undress in privacy. It may be helpful to assure the patient that it is all right to leave underpants on until just before the genital assessment. Before reentering the examination room, the nurse should knock to alert the patient.

Drapes are used to preserve the patient's privacy and to provide warmth. When invasive procedures such as vaginal or rectal assessments are performed, drapes provide an aseptic field. When used properly, a drape exposes only the part of the body being examined and covers the surrounding area. Drapes are available in a variety of shapes and materials ranging from simple rectangular sheets made of linen to disposable drapes made of paper lined with waterproof plastic (see chapter 24). ∞

Examination Considerations

To begin the assessment, the patient should be positioned on a sturdy examination table with a firm surface that is covered with a clean sheet or paper cover. Though not as efficient, a firm bed will suffice if an examination table is not available. The table must be placed to allow the nurse easy access to both sides of the patient's body. The table's height should allow the nurse to perform the examination without stooping. The nurse should also have a stool to sit on during certain parts of the examination and a small table or stand to hold the examination equipment.

During the assessment, the nurse should explain each step in advance so that the patient can anticipate the nurse's movements. Patients are more relaxed and cooperative during the procedure when they understand what is about to happen. This is also an opportunity to provide patient teaching. For example, while inspecting the patient's skin, the nurse may want to discuss the long-term effects of sun exposure. Sharing information with patients during the assessment may alleviate their anxiety, enhance their understanding, and give them a sense of partnership in their health care.

At times, the nurse may note an unexpected finding and want to call in another examiner to check the finding. In such instances, it is best simply to inform the patient that another examiner is being asked to check the assessment. Because the finding may be normal, it is best to avoid alarming the patient.

Special Considerations

Many patients experience anxiety before and during a physical examination. These feelings may stem from fear of pain, embarrassment at being looked at and touched by a stranger, or worry about the outcome of the examination. The nurse can alleviate the patient's anxiety by approaching the examination gradually, first by communicating with the patient, then by performing simple measurements such as height, weight, temperature, and pulse, which most patients find familiar and nonthreatening. As these measurements are taken, the patient will have the opportunity to ask additional questions and to become accustomed to the nurse's presence.

The examination should be individualized according to the patient's personal values and beliefs. Some patients, for example, may request that a family member be present during the examination. Some may ask for a nurse of the same sex. Some female patients may object to breast and vaginal examinations, regardless of the gender of the examiner, and some male patients may refuse penile, scrotal, and rectal examinations. A thorough assessment of the patient's culture, religious beliefs, and environment, as described in previous chapters, may help the nurse to anticipate these needs. Although explaining the reason for a certain procedure may help the patient understand its benefit, a nurse must never attempt to influence or coerce the patient to agree to any procedure. In all cases, the nurse must document which procedures took place and any that were refused.

The physical assessment may be an exhausting experience for a patient who is elderly, debilitated, frail, or suffering from a chronic illness, because the nurse must examine every part of the body and the patient must make frequent changes in position. Consequently, the nurse should consider the patient's age, health status, level of functioning, and severity of illness at all times and adapt the examination accordingly. In addition, the nurse can conserve the patient's energy by moving around the patient during the examination, rather than asking the patient to move, and by carrying out the examination as quickly and efficiently as possible. The techniques and approaches for physical assessment vary for children, pregnant females, and older adults. Lifespan considerations are included in each assessment chapter in unit III, while the chapters in unit IV discuss health assessment of pregnant women and hospitalized patients. ∞

Techniques and Equipment in Assessment of the Obese Patient

Since the prevalence of obesity in the United States is rising, nurses must be prepared to address the special needs of the obese patient during a comprehensive assessment. Equipment used for assessment must be appropriate for accurate data collection and to ensure patient safety.

To ensure both comfort and safety, chairs in the waiting and examination areas and wheelchairs used for transport must be wide and sturdy. Examination tables should be wide and sturdy with hand bars or footstools to help the patient move onto the table. Examination tables should be bolted to the floor to avoid tipping. If the patient needs helps stepping up or sitting on the exam table, use a gait belt or other assistive device to provide stability and support. If necessary, ask a second person to assist in moving the patient to avoid injury to both the patient and nurse.

Because of the weight of the chest wall and fat in the intercostal muscles, respiratory muscles can be exausted quickly when obese patients are placed in a supine position. Nurses should keep the head of the examination table elevated as much as possible during the examination. If the patient's head must be lowered, the nurse should continually monitor the patient's respiratory status, and the head of the bed should be raised as soon as possible after the exam is complete (Muir & Archer-Heese, 2009).

Extra-large examination gowns should be available. Scales with a capacity of greater than 350 pounds are required. Blood pressure cuffs must have a bladder width of 40% to 50% of the circumference of the arm and a length of 80% of the circumference of the arm. A large adult-sized cuff, a thigh cuff, or special cuffs designed for the obese patient must be considered for accurate measurement of the blood pressure.

Comprehensive assessment of the obese patient requires adjustments in the use and selection of equipment and techniques. The special considerations related to assessment of each of the body systems in an obese patient are discussed in each chapter of unit III. ∞

Standard Precautions

Throughout the physical assessment, the professional nurse is required to apply the principles of asepsis. The Centers for Disease Control and Prevention (CDC) and the Occupational Safety and Health Administration (OSHA) have provided guidelines to protect the patients and healthcare workers. Hand washing, use of gloves, use of protective barriers, disposal of sharps, cleaning of equipment after use, handling of specimens, and proper disposal of body wastes are included in the guidelines. Each healthcare agency has created agency policies based on these guidelines. A nurse working at an agency is responsible for knowing the policies and following the guidelines. Refer to appendix A to review Standard Precautions. ∞

Hand Hygiene

Before beginning the physical assessment, the nurse should wash his or her hands in the presence of the patient. Hand hygiene not only protects the nurse and the patient, but also signals that the nurse is providing for the patient's safety. According to World Health Organization (2009) recommendations, nurses should scrub and rinse hands with soap for 40–60 seconds when the hands are visibly soiled, after using the restroom, after removing gloves, and before and after contact with medical equipment. In addition, alcohol-based antiseptic hand rubs in the form of rinses, gels, or foams should be used before and after direct patient contact. Nonsterile examination gloves should be available and used appropriately during the assessment. The bell and diaphragm of the stethoscope should be cleaned after the assessment of each patient to prevent the spread of infection.

Healthcare-associated infections (HAIs) are a common cause for prolonged hospital stays and complications of both simple and complex procedures. Using safety precautions to prevent the spread of infections is particularly important for high-risk patients such as patients with compromised immune systems or older patients. Hand washing and the use of antiseptic hand rubs are the most effective ways to prevent transfer of infection from one patient to another in both clinical and hospital settings.

Use and Care of Medical Equipment

To decrease the risk of infection transfer between patients, medical staff should ensure the proper cleaning, use, and disposal of medical equipment that is used during the physical assessment. For noncritical surfaces such as bed rails, blood pressure cuffs, stethoscope surfaces, and other equipment that touches the patient's intact skin but not open sores or mucous membranes, a light disinfectant should be used to cleanse the surface between use on different patients. Equipment that touches non-intact skin or mucous membranes should be cleaned with a high-level disinfectant between every patient. Equipment that enters normally sterile areas or the bloodstream should be cleaned and sterilized between every use. In addition, nurses should use sterile disposable equipment when possible, especially for procedures that require contact with mucous membranes, non-intact skin, or sterile tissues.

When using medical equipment during a physical examination, the nurse should prepare all the needed instruments and tools in a clean area. The clean area should be draped with a sterile cloth or paper liner, and clean or sterile instruments should be placed on the clean surface. After use, the dirty instruments should be placed either directly in a regular or biohazard trash can as appropriate or in a separate area reserved for dirty equipment. Dirty equipment should be separated from clean equipment to prevent potential cross-contamination of infectious agents between different areas of the body.

Patient Hazards

Some situations that arise during a physical assessment pose a potential hazard for the patient. For example, a patient might become light-headed and dizzy from taking deep breaths during a respiratory assessment or fall when asked to touch the toes during a musculoskeletal assessment. A patient who is frail, weak, debilitated, or suffering from a chronic illness is at greatest risk. Throughout the procedure, it is necessary to anticipate potential hazards and modify the assessment to prevent them. In addition, some assessment techniques may injure the patient if used indiscriminately. For example, vigorous, deep palpation of a throbbing mass might lead to a ruptured abdominal aneurysm.

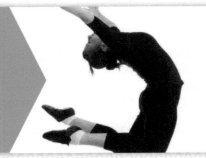
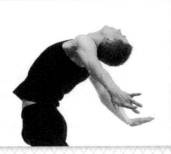

Application Through Critical Thinking

▶ Case Study

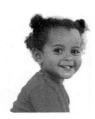

As part of a comprehensive health assessment course, Jose Espero, a student nurse, must conduct a physical assessment of a child between the ages of 2 and 5 years. Jose contacts the parents of a 3-year-old African American female named Kelsey for consent to carry out the assessment. The parents have asked Jose to meet with them. Kelsey is an active 3-year-old who attends pre-school and has an older brother, Randall. She has received regular childhood care including well-child visits and is up to date on her immunizations. She recently was seen in the emergency room for an accident in which she fell off her bike and cut her arm and had to have stitches placed. Her parents tell Jose she had a very traumatic experience and they are concerned how she might react to the exam, so they would like Jose to meet with them and explain in detail what he will be doing prior to their giving consent.

▶ Critical Thinking Questions

1. What should be included in the explanation of the assessment procedures to the parents?

2. How will the the physical assessment techniques need to be adapted for a pediatric patient?

3. Identify the equipment Jose must prepare for the physical assessment.

4. What safety and comfort issues must be addressed when conducting the assessment for the child?

5. What particular issues must Jose be concerned with considering Kelsey's recent experience?

▶ References

Berman, A., Snyder, S. J., Kozier, B., & Erb, G. (2011). *Kozier and Erb's fundamentals of nursing: Concepts, process, and practice* (9th ed.). Upper Saddle River, NJ: Prentice Hall.

Centers for Disease Control and Prevention. (2009). *Guideline for disinfection and sterilization in healthcare facilities, 2008*. Retrieved from http://www.cdc.gov/hicpac/Disinfection_Sterilization/17_00Recommendations.html

Lewis, S., Dirksen, S., Heitkemper, M., Bucher, L., & Camera, I. (2010). *Medical-surgical nursing: Assessment and management of clinical problems* (8th ed.). St. Louis, MO: Mosby.

Muir, M., & Archer-Heese, G. (2009). Essentials of a bariatric patient handling program. *The Online Journal of Issues in Nursing, 14*(1), Manuscript 5.

National Institute for Occupational Safety and Health (NIOSH). (1998). *Preventing allergic reactions to natural rubber latex in the workplace*. Retrieved from http://www.cdc.gov/niosh/docs/97-135/

United States Department of Health and Human Services (USDHHS). (1999). *Latex allergy: A prevention guide*. Retrieved from http://www.cdc.gov/niosh/docs/98-113/

United States Department of Health and Human Services. National Institutes of Health. Weight Control Information Network. (2013). *Medical care for patients with obesity*. Retrieved from http://win.niddk.nih.gov/publications/medical.htm

Wilson, S., & Giddens, J. (2013). *Health assessment for nursing practice* (5th ed.). St. Louis, MO: Mosby.

Winningham, M., & Preusser, B. (2004). *Critical thinking in medical-surgical settings* (3rd ed.). St. Louis, MO: Mosby.

World Health Organization. (2009). *WHO guidelines on hand hygiene in health care*. Geneva, Switzerland: WHO Press.

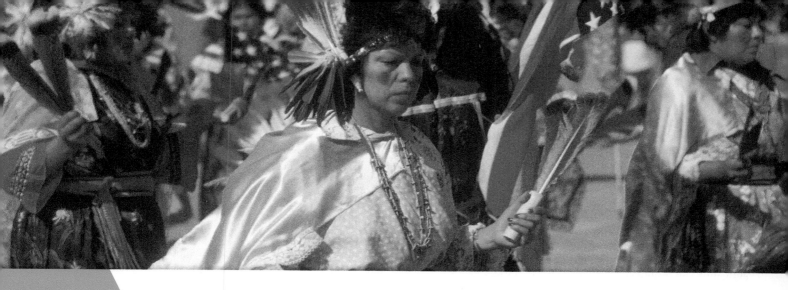

10 General Survey

◗ Learning Outcomes

Upon completion of this chapter, you will be able to:

1. Identify the components of the general survey.

2. Apply the general survey to the comprehensive health assessment.

3. Explain techniques used in the measurement of vital signs.

4. Differentiate the physiologic and psychosocial factors that affect vital signs.

5. Apply critical thinking during the initial nurse-patient encounter.

Key Terms

blood pressure, 161
diastolic pressure, 166
functional assessment, 169
general survey, 158
hyperthermia, 162
hypothermia, 162
oxygen saturation, 165
pain, 161
pulse, 161
respiratory rate, 161
sinus arrhythmia, 168
sphygmomanometer, 167
systolic pressure, 166
temperature, 161
vital signs, 161

The **general survey** begins during the interview phase of a comprehensive health assessment (see Figure 10.1 ■). While collecting subjective data, the nurse is observing the patient, developing initial impressions about the individual's health and formulating strategies for the physical assessment. The initial impression should include what is seen, heard, or smelled during the initial phase of assessment. Data collected during the general survey will guide the nurse during later assessment of body regions and systems. Additionally, this information will help to determine the patient's ability to participate in all aspects of the assessment process. Should assessment reveal urgent or emergent problems, the patient will require treatment prior to proceeding. For example, the patient having chest pain or difficulty breathing (dyspnea) will need appropriate evaluation and treatment before conducting a full assessment.

Upon completion of the general survey, the nurse will assess height, weight, and vital signs. Information about each of these important phases of comprehensive health assessment is discussed in the following sections.

Components of the General Survey

The general survey is composed of four major categories of observation: physical appearance, mental status, mobility, and patient behavior. Lifespan considerations also must be taken into account for each patient. Specific observations are required in the general survey. The following sections identify these required observations. During the general survey, the nurse will determine if the observed behaviors fall within an expected range for the patient's gender, age, race or ethnic background, and culture. The nurse must also determine the patient's ability to participate in all aspects of the process before proceeding.

Physical Appearance

The patient's physical appearance provides immediate and important cues to the level of individual wellness. Thus, beginning with the initial meeting, the nurse notes any factors about the patient's physical appearance that are in any way unexpected. For example, the nurse might note that a patient appears undernourished; seems

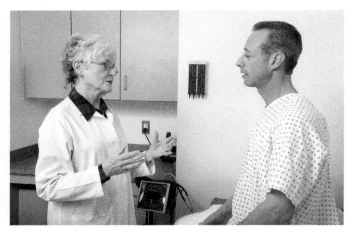

Figure 10.1 The nurse begins the general survey.

older than his or her stated age; has a frown; is smiling; or has skin color that is pale, flushed, ruddy, or cyanotic.

Body shape and build may indicate the patient's general level of wellness. The patient's height and weight should be within normal ranges for age and body build. Extreme thinness or obesity may indicate an eating disorder. The nurse must consider the patient's lifestyle, socioeconomic level, and environment.

Mental Status

The nurse assesses the patient's mental status while the patient is responding to questions and giving information about health history. The nurse notes the patient's affect and mood, level of anxiety, orientation, and speech. Findings in these areas may be evaluated further during the assessment of the patient's psychosocial status and neurologic system.

The nurse assesses patients for orientation to person, place, and time. Patients should typically be able to state their name, location, the date, month, season, and time of day. In most cases, the nurse will be able to sense a patient's orientation during the initial interview. If the patient appears confused, the nurse should ask him or her to respond to the following: "Tell me your name." "Where are you now?" "What is today's date?" and "What time is it?" If the patient cannot respond or responds incorrectly, a more detailed assessment of mental status must be performed. Tools for assessment of mental status in adults are discussed in chapter 26. ∞

Mobility

The nurse observes the patient's gait, posture, and range of motion (the complete movement possible for a joint). Normally, the patient walks in a rhythmic, straight, upright position with arms swinging at each side of the body. The shoulders are level and straight. Difficulty with gait and posture, such as stumbling, shuffling, limping, or the inability to stand erect, calls for further evaluation. Range of motion should be fluid and appropriate to the age of the patient. The nurse will observe for deviations from the normal that include weakness; stiffness; involuntary motor activity; or limitations in movement related to trauma, deformity, or those associated with obesity. See chapter 25 for information on assessing the musculoskeletal system and range of motion. ∞

Patient Behavior

An assessment of the patient's behavior includes information about the following factors: dress and grooming, body odors, facial expression, mood and affect, ability to make eye contact, and level of anxiety. The way in which patients dress may provide clues to their sense of self-esteem and body image. However, the nurse must consider many factors before drawing conclusions based on a patient's appearance. For example, a patient who wears clothing that is inappropriate for the situation or weather may be blind, mentally ill, experiencing situational grief or anxiety, or mentally fit but unable to buy other clothes due to financial constraints.

The nurse observes the patient for cleanliness and personal hygiene. The patient who is dirty or has a strong body odor or poor dental hygiene may be depressed, have poor self-concept, lack knowledge about personal hygiene practices, or have difficulty managing hygiene because of obesity. However, one must consider the patient's environment, habits, and cultural background before drawing conclusions. For example, a patient who is dirty may have just come from working on a construction site.

The nurse assesses the patient's emotional state by noting what the patient says, the patient's body language, facial expression, and the appropriateness of the patient's behavior in relation to the situation and circumstances. The patient should exhibit comfort in talking with the examiner. Giggling when answering questions about bowel movements may simply indicate embarrassment, whereas giggling when describing the death of a loved one may be an example of inappropriate affect.

The nurse also assesses the patient for apprehension, fear, and nervousness. Like affect and mood, the patient's level of anxiety is revealed through speech, body language, and facial expression. During the health assessment, the patient may exhibit anxiety due to embarrassment, fear of pain, or worry about the outcome of the examination. If the patient's anxiety seems to have no cause, the patient must be evaluated further. To obtain a relative impression of the level of anxiety, patients may be asked to rate their feelings of anxiety on a scale of 0 to 10. The nurse uses the patient's response as an indicator of the need for further assessment and as a baseline for future assessment of anxiety levels.

The nurse assesses the patient's speech for quantity, volume, content, articulation, and rhythm. The patient should speak easily and fluently to the nurse or to an interpreter. Disorganized speech patterns, silence, or constant talking may indicate normal nervousness or shyness or may signal a speech defect, neurologic deficit, depression, or another disorder.

Lifespan Considerations

For pediatric patients, instead of assessing mental status based on orientation, nursing assessment includes comparing the patient's developmental stage to the expected findings based on age. Just as the brain is not fully mature at birth, all of the major organ systems are immature and develop throughout childhood. The most dramatic development changes occur primarily in infancy and adolescence, although each stage of childhood is marked by unique changes.

Newborns are children between birth and 1 month of age. Infants are children between 1 and 12 months of age. Infancy is characterized by dramatic changes in height and weight and the development of gross physical and social skills. Young children have cephalocaudal physical growth. That is, their development progresses in a head-to-toe fashion. Development and growth begin proximally before developing distally. For example, fine motor skills follow gross motor skills, and the ability to grasp precedes the ability to stand or walk. Toddlers are children who are at least 1 year old but who have not yet reached 3 years of age. Toddlerhood is marked by slower, steadier growth, fine motor skill improvement, and language development. Preschoolers are children between 3 and 5 years of age. The preschool years are characterized by motor and language skill refinement and beginning social skill development. School-age children are between 6 and 10 years old. The major developmental tasks of school-age children involve cognitive and social growth. Adolescence is characterized by periods of rapid growth, sexual maturation, and cognitive refinement. Adolescence is the period between 11 and 21 years of age. For additional discussion of developmental stages throughout the life span, see chapter 2. ∞

For patients across the life span, general appearance can provide very useful assessment data. For example, the appearance of the younger child reveals a great deal of information about the child's parents or caretakers, and the appearance of an older child gives clues about self-care. In other words, a child 3 years of age whose skin and clothes are dirty may be a victim of neglect, while a 13-year-old in the same condition may lack knowledge about proper hygiene.

The nurse should note the child's interaction with the parents or caretakers. Their relationship should exhibit mutual warmth and caring. Signs of child abuse include clinging to a parent or strong attachment to a parent because of fear of parental anger; absence of separation anxiety in a child who, because of developmental stage, would ordinarily demonstrate it; avoidance of eye contact between caretaker and child; a caretaker's demonstration of disgust with a child's behavior, illness, odor, or stool; flinching when people move toward the child; and regression to infantile behavior.

Assessment of general appearance also offers insight into the older adult's overall health status. The dress, grooming, and personal hygiene of an older adult may be affected by limitations in mobility from arthritis, cardiovascular disease, and other disorders, or by a lack of funds.

The gait of an older adult is often slower and the steps shorter. To maintain balance, older adults may hold their arms away from the body or use a cane. The posture of an older adult may look slightly stooped because of a generalized flexion, which also causes the older adult to appear shorter. A loss in height may also be due to thinning or compression of the intervertebral disks.

The behavior of the older adult may be affected by various disorders common to this age group, such as vascular insufficiency and diabetes. In addition, medications may affect the patient's behavior. Some medications may cause the patient to feel anxious, and others may affect the patient's alertness, orientation, or speech. Older adults are likely to have one or more chronic conditions associated with age, such as arthritis, hypertension, or diabetes. As a result, older adults must consume several prescription medications. Overmedication may occur because older adults seek care from multiple healthcare providers without collaboration regarding treatment. Multiple medications may combine to produce dangerous side effects. Additionally, the schedules for multiple medications may be confusing and result in overmedication, forgotten doses, negative side effects, or ineffectiveness of medication. Therefore, the nurse must conduct a thorough assessment of the patient's medication schedule and history.

Measuring Height and Weight

The nurse measures the patient's height and weight to establish baseline data and to help determine health status. The patient should be asked about height and weight before taking any measurements. Large discrepancies between the stated height and weight and the actual measurements may provide clues to the patient's self-image. Alternatively, discrepancies in weight may indicate the patient's lack of awareness of a sudden loss or gain in weight that may be due to illness.

Height

To measure height, the nurse uses a measuring stick attached to a platform scale or to a wall. The patient should look straight ahead while standing as straight as possible with heels together and shoulders back. When using a platform scale, the nurse raises the height attachment rod above the patient's head, then extends and lowers the right-angled arm until it rests on the crown of the head. The measurement is read from the height attachment rod (see Figure 10.2 ■). When using a measuring stick, the nurse should place an L-shaped level on the crown of the patient's head at a right angle to the measuring stick (see Figure 10.3 ■).

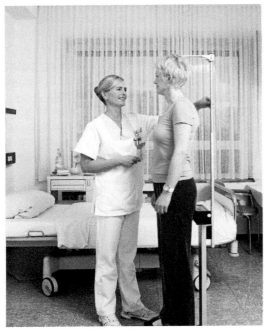

Figure 10.2 Measuring the patient's height with a platform scale.
Source: Joos Mind/Stone/Getty Images.

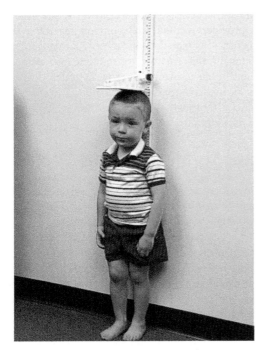

Figure 10.3 Measuring a child's height with a measuring stick.

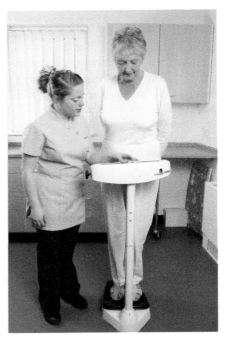

Figure 10.4 Measuring the patient's weight with a standard platform scale.
Source: Jim Varney/Science Source.

Weight

A standard platform scale or digital scale (see Figure 10.4 ■) is used to measure the weight of older children and adults. It is best to use the same scale at each visit and to weigh the patient at the same time of day in the same kind of clothing (e.g., the examination gown) and without shoes. If using a digital scale, the nurse simply reads the weight from the lighted display panel. Otherwise, the scale is calibrated by moving both weights to 0 and turning the knob until the balance beam is level. The nurse moves the large and small weights to the right and takes the reading when the balance beam returns to level. Special bed and chair scales are available for patients who cannot stand. Obese patients require scales that have a capacity of greater than 159 kg (350 lb).

Average height and weight for adult men and women are available in charts prepared by governmental agencies and insurers. Table 10.1 illustrates average acceptable weights for adults. The body mass index (BMI) is considered a more reliable indicator of healthy weight. The BMI and other measures in relation to weight are discussed in chapter 12 of this text. ∞

Lifespan Considerations

Children who are able to stand on their own at full height should be measured for height in a standing position rather than length in a laying position. However, length should be used to measure infants who are unable to stand independently. To measure an infant's length, the nurse places the child in a supine position on an examining table that is equipped with a ruler, headboard, and adjustable footboard. The nurse positions the head against the headboard, extends the infant's leg nearest the ruler, and adjusts the footboard until it touches the infant's foot. The space between the headboard and footboard represents the length of the infant. Alternatively, the nurse

TABLE 10.1	Guidelines for Ideal Weight Based on Height
HEIGHT	**IDEAL WEIGHT**
4'10"	91–115 lbs.
4'11"	94–119 lbs.
5'0"	97–123 lbs.
5'1"	100–127 lbs.
5'2"	104–131 lbs.
5'3"	107–135 lbs.
5'4"	110–140 lbs.
5'5"	114–144 lbs.
5'6"	118–148 lbs.
5'7"	121–153 lbs.
5'8"	125–158 lbs.
5'9"	128–162 lbs.
5'10"	132–167 lbs.
5'11"	136–172 lbs.
6'0"	140–177 lbs.
6'1"	144–182 lbs.
6'2"	148–186 lbs.
6'3"	152–192 lbs.
6'4"	156–197 lbs.

Source: U.S. Department of Health and Human Services, National Institutes of Health. (1998). *Clinical guidelines on the identification, evaluation, and treatment of overweight and obesity in adults* (NIH Publication No. 98-4083).

places the infant on a standard examination table, extends the infant's leg, marks the paper covering at the infant's head and foot, and measures the distance between the markings (see Figure 10.5 ■). Another common length measurement for children under 3 years old is head circumference. The infant or toddler's head circumference should be measured at the widest point, usually around the most prominent part of the occiput and above the eyebrows, and the measurement

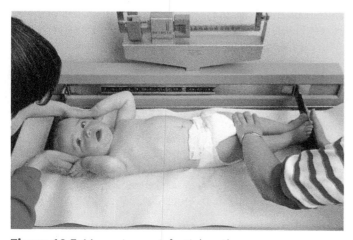

Figure 10.5 Measuring an infant's length.

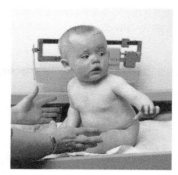

Figure 10.6 Weighing an infant.

should be taken with flexible, non-stretchable measuring tape. Normal head circumference ranges from 34 to 37 cm (approximately 13 to 14.5 in.) in newborns up to 47 to 51 cm (approximately 18.5 to 20 in.) at 3 years of age (CDC, 2001).

Infants are weighed on a modified platform scale with curved sides to prevent injury. The scale measures weight in grams and in ounces. The nurse places the unclothed baby on the scale on a paper drape and watches the baby to prevent a fall (see Figure 10.6 ■). Measurements are taken to the nearest 10 g (0.5 oz).

Children over the age of 2 or 3 years may be weighed on the upright scale or seated on the infant scale. The child's underpants should be left on. To measure height, the nurse uses the platform scale or a measuring stick attached to the wall, as for an adult. By the age of 4, most children enjoy being weighed and measured and finding out how much they have grown. Growth and development are discussed in chapter 2 of this text. ∞

The height of older adults may decline somewhat as a result of thinning or compression of the intervertebral disks and a general flexion of the hips and knees. Body weight may decrease because of muscle shrinkage. The older patient may appear thinner, even when properly nourished, because of loss of subcutaneous fat deposits from the face, forearms, and lower legs. At the same time, fat deposits on the abdomen and hips may increase.

Measuring Vital Signs

Vital signs include body **temperature**, **pulse**, **respiratory rate**, **blood pressure**, and **pain**. Measurement of oxygen saturation may be included when taking vital signs. The nurse measures vital signs to obtain baseline data, to detect or monitor a change in the patient's health status, and to monitor patients at risk for alterations in health.

Measuring Body Temperature

The body's surface temperature—the temperature of the skin, subcutaneous tissues, and fat—fluctuates in response to environmental factors and is, therefore, unreliable for monitoring a patient's health status. Instead, the nurse should measure the patient's core temperature, or the temperature of the deep tissues of the body (e.g., the thorax and abdominal cavity). This temperature remains relatively constant at about 37°C, or 98.6°F.

Sensors in the hypothalamus regulate the body's core temperature. When these hypothalamic sensors detect heat, they signal the body to decrease heat production and increase heat loss (e.g., by vasodilation and sweating). When sensors in the hypothalamus detect cold, they signal the body to increase heat production and decrease heat loss (e.g., by shivering, vasoconstriction, and inhibition of sweating).

Factors That Influence Body Temperature

A variety of factors may influence normal core body temperature. These include:

- *Age.* The core temperature of infants is highly responsive to changes in the external environment; therefore, infants need extra protection from even mild variations in temperature. Indicators for assessing rectal temperature in children rather than tympanic temperature include recent exposure to extreme temperatures (cold winters or hot summers) and illness, especially otitis media. The core body temperature of children is more stable than that of infants but less so than that of adolescents or adults. However, older adults are more sensitive than middle adults to variations in external environmental temperature. This increased sensitivity may be due to the decreased thermoregulatory control and loss of subcutaneous fat common in older adults, or it may be due to environmental factors such as lack of activity, inadequate diet, or lack of central heating.

- *Diurnal variations.* Core body temperature is usually highest between 8:00 p.m. and midnight and lowest between 4:00 and 6:00 a.m. Normal body temperature may vary by as much as 1°C, or 1.8°F, between these times. Some individuals have more than one complete cycle in a day.

- *Exercise.* Strenuous exercise can increase core body temperature by as much as 2°C, or 5°F.

- *Hormones.* A variety of hormones affect core body temperature. For example, in women, progesterone secretion at the time of ovulation raises core body temperature by about 0.35°C, or 0.5°F.

- *Stress.* The temperature of a highly stressed patient may be elevated as a result of increased production of epinephrine and norepinephrine, which increase metabolic activity and heat production.

- *Illness.* Illness or a central nervous system disorder may impair the thermostatic function of the hypothalamus. **Hyperthermia**, also called fever, may occur in response to viral or bacterial infections or from tissue breakdown following myocardial infarction, malignancy, surgery, or trauma. **Hypothermia** is usually a response to prolonged exposure to cold.

Routes for Measuring Body Temperature

Core body temperature was once typically measured with a mercury-in-glass thermometer. However, because of the toxicity associated with mercury, most glass thermometers now use alcohol and galinstan, and even these are being replaced. For more information, visit the U.S. Environmental Protection Agency Web site. Today, nurses are more likely to use an electronic thermometer (see Figure 10.7 ■), which gives a highly accurate reading in only 2 to 60 seconds. These portable, battery-operated devices consist of an electronic display unit, a probe, and disposable probe sheaths. The nurse attaches the appropriate probe to the unit, covers it with a sheath, and inserts it into the body orifice. The probe is left in place

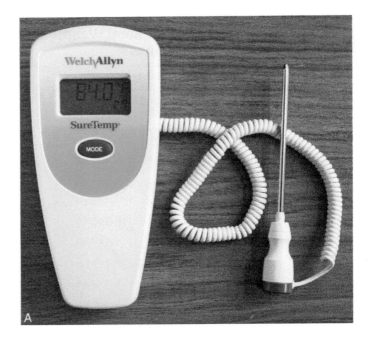

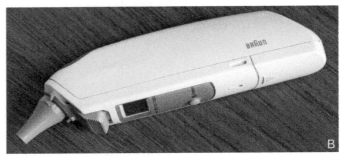

Figure 10.7 Electronic thermometers. A. This device may be used to measure oral rectal, or axillary temperature. B. This device is used to measure tympanic temperature.

until the temperature appears on the liquid crystal display (LCD) screen. There are five routes for measuring core body temperature: oral, rectal, axillary, tympanic, and temporal artery.

ORAL Measuring the oral temperature is the most accessible, accurate, and convenient method. Due to safety concerns, the U.S. Environmental Protection Agency (EPA) is working to phase out the manufacture, sale, and use of mercury thermometers. In several states, the sale of mercury thermometers is prohibited (EPA, 2014). Mercury thermometers are no longer used in the clinical setting because of the possibility of breaking and mercury exposure. Oral temperatures may be evaluated by using an electronic or digital probe device. Place the covered probe, usually blue in color, at the base of the tongue in either of the sublingual pockets to the right or left of the frenulum (see Figure 10.8 ■), and instruct the patient to keep the lips tightly closed around the thermometer. The thermometer is left in place until the device beeps or shows indication that the measurement is completed. After removing the thermometer, the nurse either discards the disposable sheath or cleans the device. The temperature reading will be in the display window.

RECTAL A rectal temperature is taken if the patient is comatose, confused, having seizures, or unable to close the mouth. It is

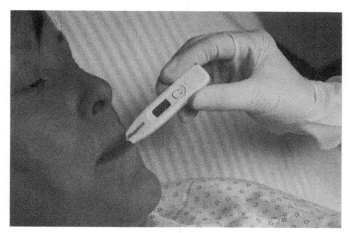

Figure 10.8 Placement of the thermometer for an oral temperature.

important to use prelubricated thermometer covers and put on disposable examination gloves. The patient should be in a side-lying position. The nurse then inserts the thermometer from 1.5 to 4 cm (approximately 0.6 to 1.6 in.) into the anus, being careful not to force insertion of the thermometer. The probe, usually red in color, is left in place until there is a beep or the device indicates that the reading is completed. Remove the probe, dispose of the disposable sheath, and obtain the reading in the display window.

AXILLARY Occasionally, the nurse needs to take an axillary temperature. This is the safest method and is less invasive than the oral or rectal routes, especially for infants and young children. Because of the variability of probe positioning, many authorities consider the axillary route to be least accurate. For an axillary temperature, the nurse places the thermometer in the patient's axilla and assists the patient in placing the arm tightly across the chest to keep the thermometer in place.

TYMPANIC The tympanic temperature can be taken only with an electronic thermometer. Using infrared technology, it measures a patient's core body temperature quickly and accurately. This method is comfortable and noninvasive for the patient. The measuring probe resembles an otoscope. The nurse gently places the covered tip of the

probe at the opening of the ear canal, being careful not to force the probe into the ear canal or occlude the canal opening. After about 2 seconds, the patient's temperature reading will appear on the LCD screen.

TEMPORAL ARTERY The temporal artery thermometer is a noninvasive device to measure temperature with a scan of the forehead across the temporal artery. The temperature reading appears on an LCD screen in seconds. Research has shown a high correlation between temperatures taken using temporal artery thermometers and those taken using other methods of body temperature measurement, such as rectal temperature measurement (Kemp, 2013).

Measuring the Pulse Rate

The heart is a muscular pump. The left ventricle of the heart contracts with every beat, forcing blood from the heart into the systemic arteries. The amount of blood pumped from the heart with each heartbeat is called the *stroke volume.* The force of the blood against the walls of the arteries generates a wave of pressure that is felt at various points in the body as a pulse. The ability of the arteries to contract and expand is called *compliance.* When compliance is reduced, the heart must exert more pressure to pump blood throughout the body.

Location of Pulse Points

The apical pulse is felt at the apex of the heart. Figure 10.9 ■ illustrates the location of the apical pulse for a child under 4 years, a child 4 to 6 years, and an adult. The peripheral pulse is the pulse as felt in the body's periphery, for example, in the neck, wrist, or foot. Figure 10.10 ■ shows eight sites where the peripheral pulse is most easily palpated. In a healthy patient, the peripheral pulse rate is equivalent to the heartbeat. Assessment of the peripheral pulse is an important component of a thorough health assessment.

Alterations in the patient's health can weaken the peripheral pulse, making it difficult to detect. In obese patients, the radial pulse is the most accessible and palpable of peripheral pulses. The carotid pulse is difficult to assess due the short thick neck in morbidly obese patients. The use of a Doppler device may be required to assess peripheral pulses in obese patients. More detailed information related to assessment of peripheral pulses is located in chapters 19 and 20. ∞

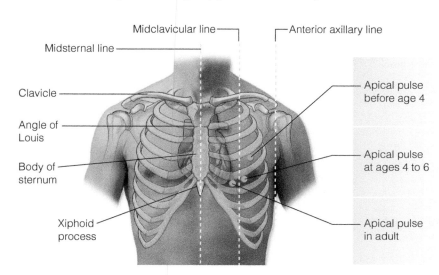

Figure 10.9 Location of the apical pulse in a child under age 4, a child ages 4 to 6, and an adult.

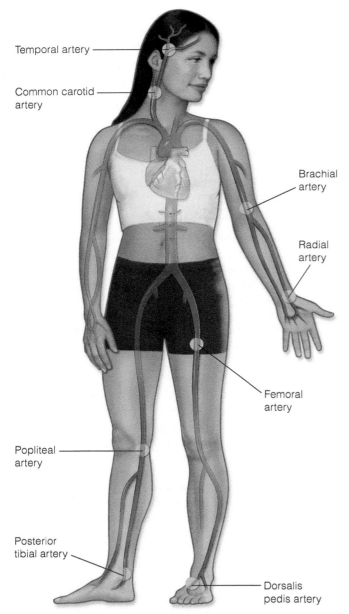

Figure 10.10 Body sites where the peripheral pulse is most easily palpated.

Factors That Influence Pulse Rate

A variety of factors may influence the normal pulse rate. These include:

- *Age.* The average pulse rate of infants and children is higher than that of teens and adults. After age 16, the pulse stabilizes to an average of about 70 beats per minute (beats/min) in males and 75 beats/min in females.

- *Gender.* As previously noted, the average pulse rate of the adult male is slightly lower than that of the adult female.

- *Exercise.* The pulse rate normally increases with exercise.

- *Stress.* In response to stress, fear, and anxiety, the heart rate and the force of the heartbeat increase.

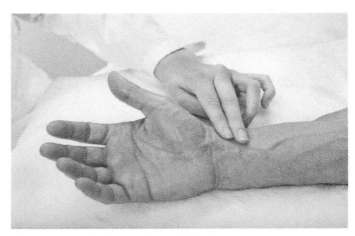

Figure 10.11 Palpating the radial pulse.

- *Fever.* The peripheral vasodilation that accompanies an elevated body temperature lowers systemic blood pressure, in turn causing an increase in pulse rate.

- *Hemorrhage.* Pulse rate increases in response to significant loss of blood from the vascular system.

- *Medications.* A variety of medications may either increase or decrease the heart rate.

- *Position changes.* When patients sit or stand for long periods, blood may pool in the veins, resulting in a temporary decrease in venous blood return to the heart and, consequently, reduced blood pressure and lowered pulse rate.

Palpation of the Radial Pulse

The radial pulse is the most commonly measured peripheral pulse. The radial pulse is palpated by placing the pads of the first two or three fingers on the anterior wrist along the radius bone (see Figure 10.11 ■). If the pulse is regular, the nurse counts the beats for 30 seconds and multiplies by 2 to obtain the total beats per minute. If the pulse is irregular, the nurse counts the beats for a full minute.

Four factors are considered when assessing the pulse: rate, rhythm, force, and elasticity. A pulse rate of less than 60 beats/min, called *bradycardia*, may be found in a healthy, well-trained athlete. A pulse rate over 100 beats/min, called *tachycardia*, may also be found in the healthy patient who is anxious or has just finished exercising.

The pulse of a healthy adult has a relatively constant rhythm; that is, the intervals between beats are regular. Irregularities in heart rhythm are discussed fully in chapter 19 of this text. ∞

The nurse assesses the force of a pulse, or its stroke volume, by noting the pressure that must be exerted before the pulse is felt. A "full, bounding" pulse is difficult to obliterate. It may be caused by fear, anxiety, exercise, or a variety of alterations in health. A "weak, thready pulse" is easy to obliterate. It also may indicate alterations in health such as hemorrhage. The nurse palpates along the radial artery in a proximal-to-distal direction to assess the elasticity of the artery. A normal artery feels smooth, straight, and resilient. See Table 10.2 for expected pulse rates across the life span.

TABLE 10.2 Variations in Normal Ranges of Vital Signs by Age

AGE	PULSE	RESPIRATIONS	BLOOD PRESSURE	
			SYSTOLIC	DIASTOLIC
Newborn	100–205 (awake) 90–160 (asleep)	30–80	60–76	31–45
Infant (1–12 months)	100–180 (awake) 90–160 (asleep)	30–53	72–104	37–56
1–2 years	98–140 (awake) 80–120 (asleep)	22–37	86–106	42–63
3–5 years	98–140 (awake) 80–120 (asleep)	22–34	89–112	46–72
6–12 years	70–120 (awake) 50–90 (asleep)	18–25	97–120	57–80
Teen years	60–100	12–18	110–135	75–85
Adult	60–100	12–20	Less than 120	Less than 80
Older adult	60–100	15–20	Less than 120	Less than 80

Classification of Blood Pressure for Adults 18 Years and Older

CLASSIFICATION	SYSTOLIC		DIASTOLIC
Normal	Less than 120	and	Less than 80
Prehypertension	120–139	or	80–89
Hypertension (Stage 1)	140–159	or	90–99
Hypertension (Stage 2)	160 or higher	or	100 or higher
Hypertensive Crisis	Higher than 180	or	Higher than 110

Source: Based on American Heart Association (AHA). (2012). *Understanding blood pressure readings.* Retrieved from http://www.heart.org/HEARTORG/Conditions/HighBloodPressure/AboutHighBloodPressure/Understanding-Blood-Pressure-Readings_UCM_301764_Article.jsp; Madhur, M. S., Riaz, K., Dreisbach, A. W., & Harrison, D. G. (2014). *Hypertension treatment & management: Approach considerations.* Retrieved from http://emedicine.medscape.com/article/241381-treatment; Hazinski, M. F. (2012). *Nursing care of the critically ill child* (3rd ed.). St. Louis, MO: Mosby; and Kliegman, R. M., Stanton, B. M. D., St. Geme, J., Schor, N., & Behrman, R. E. (2011). *Nelson textbook of pediatrics* (19th ed.). Philadelphia: Saunders Elsevier.

Measuring Respiratory Rate

The human body continuously exchanges oxygen and carbon dioxide through the act of respiration. Normal respiratory rates are dependent on age.

Assessment of Respiratory Rate

Counting the number of respirations per minute assesses respiratory rate. The nurse observes the full respiratory cycle (one inspiration and one expiration) for rate and pattern of breathing. The patient's respiratory rate is assessed by counting the number of breaths for 30 seconds and then multiplying by 2. If the nurse detects irregularities or difficulty breathing, the respirations are counted for one full minute.

Factors That Influence Respiratory Rate

The respiratory rate may increase in some patients if they become aware that their breaths are being counted. For this reason, while counting breaths per minute, the nurse should maintain the posture of counting the radial pulse. Other factors that may increase respiratory rate include exercise, stress, increased temperature, and increased altitude. Some medications may either increase or decrease respiratory rate. Table 10.2 lists normal respiratory rates for newborns through older adults. Obese patients have difficulty with respiration as a result of increased fatty tissue in the chest wall and abdomen. These patients are most comfortable in a sitting position for all assessment. Exertion from moving onto an examination table may cause an increased respiratory rate. Allow time for the patient to adjust to a change in position and to recover from movement before counting respirations. See chapter 17 for a more detailed discussion of respiration. ∞

Oxygen Saturation

Oxygen saturation of the hemoglobin is measured using a pulse oximeter. The pulse oximeter uses a sensor and a photodetector to determine the light sent and absorbed by the hemoglobin. The reported percentage represents the light absorbed by oxygenated and deoxygenated hemoglobin. In a healthy individual, a value of 97% to 99% is considered normal (Osborn, Wraa, Watson, & Holleran, 2013), and an oxygen saturation of less than 90% should be investigated further. This noninvasive procedure allows oxygen saturation values to be easily obtained and rapidly updated.

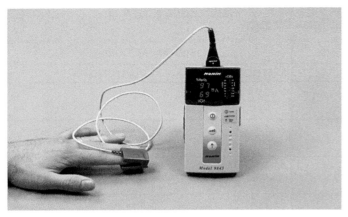

Figure 10.12 Pulse oximeter.

The sensor is usually placed on the finger of the patient. In obese patients and patients with vascular disease, and in patients with thickened nails or heavy nail polish, placement of the sensor on the earlobe promotes more accurate findings. Pulse oximetry can detect hypoxemia before symptoms such as cyanosis (blue color) of the skin appear (see Figure 10.12 ■). Pulse oximetry readings can be altered by conditions such as low hemoglobin and low body temperature (hypothermia), especially in children (Ross, Newth, & Khemani, 2014).

Lifespan Considerations

Lung development is complete in healthy full-term newborns; however, there are significant differences between child and adult respiratory tracts. Infants have thinner, less muscular chest walls with a more noticeable xiphoid process. Breath sounds are louder and harsher. Referred sounds from the upper airways are common. The anterior-posterior chest diameter is approximately equal in infants, and the ribs appear more horizontal. Infants are obligate nose breathers until 6 months of age; they cannot breathe through their mouths. The nurse should carefully assess children under the age of 6 months with nasal congestion for signs of respiratory distress. Abdominal breathing is common until age 6 years. Thoracic breathing begins in the school-age years. For additional discussion of lifespan considerations related to the pediatric respiratory system, see chapter 17. ∞

Measuring Blood Pressure

Blood ebbs and flows within the systemic arteries in waves, causing two types of pressure. The **systolic pressure** is the pressure of the blood at the height of the wave, when the left ventricle contracts. This is the first number recorded in a blood pressure measurement. The **diastolic pressure** is the pressure between the ventricular contractions, when the heart is at rest. This is the second number recorded in a blood pressure measurement.

To measure blood pressure, the bladder of the blood pressure cuff must fit the length and width of the patient's limb. The cuff should cover two-thirds of the upper arm from shoulder to elbow, and the lower edge of the cuff should be positioned approximately one inch above the elbow. In addition, the inflatable portion of the cuff should cover 80% of the arm width (Mayo Clinic, 2013). In adults, the ideal blood pressure reading is less than 120/80 mmHg.

Circulatory Factors That Influence Blood Pressure

Factors that influence blood pressure include but are not limited to the following:

- Cardiac output is the amount of blood ejected from the heart. Cardiac output is equal to the stroke volume, or amount of blood ejected in one heartbeat (measured in milliliters per beat), multiplied by the heart rate (measured in beats per minute). Cardiac output averages about 5.5 liters per minute (L/min).

- Blood volume is the total amount of blood circulating within the entire vascular system. Blood volume averages about 5 L in adults. In children, blood volume is approximately 80 mL/kg (London et al., 2014). A sudden drop in blood pressure may signal sudden blood loss, as with internal bleeding.

- Peripheral vascular resistance is the resistance the blood encounters as it flows within the vessels. Peripheral resistance is in turn influenced by various factors, such as vessel length and diameter. Two of the most important factors influencing peripheral resistance are blood viscosity and vessel compliance.

- Blood viscosity is the ratio between the blood cells (the formed elements) and the blood plasma. When the total amount of formed elements is high, the blood is thicker, or more viscous. The molecules pass one another with greater difficulty, and more pressure is required to move the blood.

- Vessel compliance describes the elasticity of the smooth muscle in the arterial walls. Highly elastic arteries respond readily and fully to each heartbeat. Rigid, hardened arteries, as are found with arteriosclerosis, are less responsive, and greater force is required to move the blood along.

Note that blood in the systemic circulation flows along a pressure gradient from central to peripheral; in other words, pressure is higher in the arterioles than in the capillaries and higher still in the aorta. The average blood pressure of a healthy adult is 120/80 mmHg.

Additional Factors Affecting Blood Pressure

Additional factors that influence blood pressure include but are not limited to the following:

- *Age.* Systolic blood pressure in newborns averages about 78 mmHg. Blood pressure rates tend to rise with increasing age through age 18 and then tend to stabilize. In older adults, blood pressure rates tend to rise again as elasticity of the arteries decreases.

- *Gender.* After puberty, females tend to have lower blood pressure than males of the same age. Reproductive hormones may influence this difference because blood pressure in women usually increases after menopause.

- *Race.* American individuals of African ancestry over the age of 35 tend to have higher blood pressures than American individuals of European descent (Go et al., 2013).

- *Obesity.* Blood pressure tends to be higher in people who are overweight and obese than in people of normal weight of the same age.

- *Physical activity.* Physical activity (including crying in infants and children) increases cardiac output and, therefore, increases blood pressure.

- *Stress.* Stress increases cardiac output and arterial vasoconstriction, resulting in increased blood pressure.
- *Diurnal variations.* Blood pressure is usually lowest in the early morning and rises steadily throughout the day, peaking in the late afternoon or early evening.
- *Medications.* A variety of medications may increase or decrease blood pressure.

Blood pressure is also affected by alterations in health. Any condition that affects the cardiac output, peripheral vascular resistance, blood volume, blood viscosity, or vessel compliance can affect blood pressure. See Table 10.2 for information related to blood pressure values across the life span.

Assessment of Blood Pressure

An accurate measurement of blood pressure is an essential part of any complete health assessment.

PATIENT PREPARATION It is important to reassure the patient that the procedure for taking blood pressure is generally quick and painless. The patient should be at rest for at least 5 minutes before taking a blood pressure measurement and up to 20 minutes if the patient has been engaging in heavy physical activity. Patient anxiety may also cause a temporary elevation of blood pressure.

EQUIPMENT The nurse measures blood pressure with a blood pressure cuff, a **sphygmomanometer,** and a stethoscope. There are various cuff sizes as shown in Figure 10.13 ■. The cuff consists of an inflatable bladder, which is covered by cloth and has two tubes attached to it. One of these tubes ends in a rubber bulb with which to inflate the bladder. A small valve on the side of the bulb regulates air in the bladder. When the valve is loosened, air in the bladder is released. After the valve is tightened, pumped air remains in the bladder. The second tube attached to the bladder ends in a sphygmomanometer, a device that measures the air pressure in the bladder. Blood pressure is measured with an aneroid sphygmomanometer.

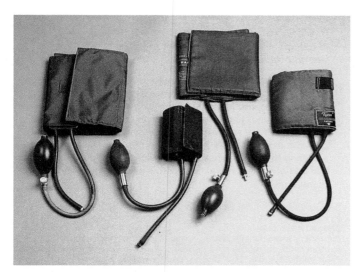

Figure 10.13 A variety of cuff sizes: a pediatric small cuff for a child; a small adult cuff for a frail adult or large child; a normal adult-size cuff; and a large cuff for use on the arm of an obese adult or the leg of an average-size adult.

The aneroid sphygmomanometer has a small, calibrated dial with a needle. The bladder of the blood pressure cuff must fit the length and width of the patient's limb. If the bladder is too narrow, the blood pressure reading will be falsely high. Conversely, if the bladder is too wide the blood pressure reading will be falsely low. The width of the bladder should equal 40% of the circumference of the limb. The length of the bladder should equal 80% of the circumference of the limb. This is important in accurate measurement of blood pressure in obese patients, who may require special cuffs. Note that the circumference of the patient's limb, and not the age of the patient, determines the cuff used. Automatic monitors can be used to measure blood pressure. These devices include a cuff attached to an electronic monitor. Application of the cuff is the same as in the manual method. The monitor provides a reading on an LCD screen of the systolic, diastolic, and mean blood pressures.

THE PROCEDURE Blood pressure measurements are usually taken by placing the cuff on the patient's arm and auscultating the pulse in the brachial artery. The nurse must use common sense when choosing which arm to use for the measurement. For example, blood pressure should not be measured in an arm on the same side as a mastectomy or in an arm with a shunt. If blood pressure cannot be measured in either arm because of disease or trauma, a thigh blood pressure may be taken, using the popliteal artery, or a leg blood pressure may be taken, using the posterior tibial or dorsalis pedis arteries.

To measure the blood pressure in the patient's arm, the nurse follows these steps:

1. Place the patient in a comfortable position in a quiet room.
2. Confirm that the blood pressure cuff is the appropriate size for the patient's arm.
3. Remove any clothing from the patient's arm.
4. Slightly flex the arm and hold it at the level of the heart with the palm upward.
5. Palpate the brachial pulse.
6. Place the cuff on the arm with the lower border 1 inch above the antecubital area, making sure that the cuff is smooth and snug. One finger should fit between the cuff and the patient's arm. Be sure that the center of the bladder is over the brachial artery. Many cuffs have an arrow to indicate the center of the bladder, thus the part of the cuff to be over the artery.
7. Palpate the radial pulse.
8. Close the release valve on the pump.
9. Inflate the cuff until the radial pulse is no longer palpable and note the reading on the sphygmomanometer. Release the valve and rapidly deflate the cuff. Wait 15 to 30 seconds before proceeding to the next step. This is the palpatory systolic blood pressure.
10. Place the diaphragm of the stethoscope over the brachial pulse (see Figure 10.14 ■).
11. Pump up the cuff until the sphygmomanometer registers 30 mmHg above the palpatory systolic blood pressure (the point at which the radial pulse disappeared).
12. Release the valve on the cuff carefully so that the pressure decreases at the rate of 2 to 3 mmHg per second.

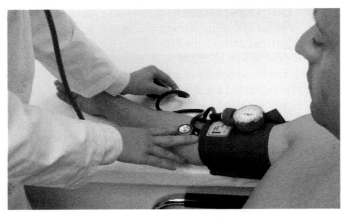

Figure 10.14 Measuring the patient's blood pressure.

13. Note the manometer reading at each of the five Korotkoff phases (see Box 10.1). The first sound is recorded as the systolic blood pressure and the last sound is recorded as the diastolic blood pressure.

14. Deflate the cuff rapidly and completely.

15. Remove the cuff from the patient's arm.

Lifespan Considerations

The patient's age can impact the methods and equipment used to assess vital signs. The following sections address considerations the nurse should take into account when caring for patients throughout the life span. See Table 10.2 for an overview of normal ranges of vital signs based on age.

Temperature

Respirations and pulse rate are assessed before measuring rectal temperature in infants because taking a rectal temperature may cause an infant to cry. Holding the infant in a lateral position with the knees flexed onto the abdomen, or prone on the nurse's lap, the nurse separates the infant's buttocks with the nondominant hand and inserts the thermometer with the dominant gloved hand. The nurse should use a blunt-tipped thermometer, insert it no more than 2.5 cm, or 1 in., and hold on to the exposed end. To avoid the risk of rectal perforation, an axillary temperature may be taken rather than a rectal temperature in newborns. The nurse should take the axillary temperature also in toddlers and older children whenever possible to eliminate their anxiety over the invasive rectal procedure. An oral route may be used as early as age 5 if the child is able to keep his or her mouth closed. Electronic thermometers, which are unbreakable and register quickly, are particularly useful with children.

Body temperature in the older adult may be reduced because of decreased thermoregulatory control and loss of subcutaneous fat. Older adults are more sensitive to environmental changes in temperature, possibly because of lack of physical activity, inadequate diet, or inability to afford adequate heating.

Pulse

The apical site is used for children younger than age 2. In preschool children, the nurse uses the brachial site and counts the pulse for a full minute. It is important to pay attention to any irregularities in rhythm, such as **sinus arrhythmia**, which is not uncommon in children. The pulse rate of the healthy older adult is in a range from 60 to 100 beats/min. The radial artery may feel rigid if there is loss of elasticity in the arterial walls.

Respirations

The nurse should count respirations for one full minute in infants, because the breathing pattern may show considerable variation. Infants have irregular breathing patterns characterized by frequent brief rate accelerations or decelerations. This is a normal variant that disappears during the first few months of life. The respiratory rate

---

Box 10.1 Korotkoff Sounds

When measuring blood pressure, auscultate to identify five phases in a series of sounds called Korotkoff sounds, named after the Russian surgeon who first described them. These five phases are:

Phase 1: The period initiated by the first faint, clear, tapping sounds. These sounds gradually increase in intensity. Sounds heard during this phase correspond to appearance of a palpable pulse. To verify that they are not extraneous sounds, identify at least two consecutive tapping sounds.

Phase 2: The period during which the sounds become softer and longer; murmuring or swishing sounds are reflective of turbulent blood flow.

Phase 3: The period during which the sounds are crisper and louder; sounds have a rhythmic pattern.

Phase 4: Rhythmic sounds become muffled and have a soft, blowing quality.

Phase 5: The point at which the sounds disappear. The silence reflects the absence of pressure in the cuff. Normal blood flow is inaudible.

Document the blood pressure measurements as follows:

- The systolic pressure is the point at which the first tapping sound is heard (Phase 1).

- In adults, the diastolic pressure is the point at which the sounds become inaudible (Phase 5).

- In children, the diastolic pressure is the point at which the sounds become muffled (Phase 4).

- Older patients may have a wide pulse pressure. A pulse pressure is calculated by finding the difference between the systolic and diastolic pressures. In older patients with a wide pulse pressure, Korotkoff sounds may become inaudible between systolic and diastolic pressure and reappear as cuff deflation continues. This is known as auscultatory gap. This can often be eliminated by elevating the arm overhead for 30 seconds before inflating the cuff and bringing the arm to the usual position for continued measurement.

Sources: Pickering, T. G., Hall, J, E., Appel, L. J., Falkner, B. E., Graves, J., Hill, M. N., . . . & Roccella, E. J. (2005). Recommendations for blood pressure measurement in humans and experimental animals: Part 1: Blood pressure measurement in humans: A statement for professionals from the Subcommittee of Professional and Public Education of the American Heart Association Council on High Blood Pressure Research. *Hypertension, 45,* 142–161; Burton, M. A., & Ludwig, L. J. M. (2010). *Fundamentals of nursing care: Concepts, connections & skills.* Philadelphia, PA: F.A. Davis; and Portman, H., & Sheppard, S. (2011). Vital information about a vital sign: BP. *Nursing2014, 41*(2), 66.

in older adults may be increased to accommodate a decrease in vital capacity and inspiratory reserve volume.

Blood Pressure

An ultrasonic Doppler flow detector is the preferred instrument for measuring blood pressure in infants and in children under the age of 2. However, traditional electronic sphygmomanometers may also be used. In children over the age of 2, it is imperative that the nurse use both the correct size cuff and a small diaphragm for the stethoscope. The American Heart Association recommends that, in children, diastolic pressure be read at the beginning of Korotkoff phase 4, when the sounds become muffled. In adults, the heart pumps against increased resistance, and systolic blood pressure increases as the systemic arteries lose elasticity with increasing age.

Blood pressure accuracy depends on the selection of an appropriately sized cuff. Blood pressure cuffs must be wide enough to cover at least two-thirds of the upper arm (from the acromion process to the olecranon process). The blood pressure cuff should be long enough for the bladder of the cuff to encircle 80 to 100% of the arm's circumference. Like adult blood pressure cuffs, pediatric blood pressure cuffs also are available in various sizes as shown in Figure 10.13. If the cuff is too narrow, the reading will be falsely high. If the cuff is too wide, it will be falsely low. Blood pressure readings should be done with the child's arm supported at the heart level. The diastolic pressure is recorded as the point when the Korotkoff sounds disappear. See Table 10.2 for a range of the normal pediatric vital signs. Blood pressure should be measured in all four extremities of neonates before discharge from the nursery. Higher readings in upper extremities indicate possible cardiac anomaly needing further medical assessment.

Pain—The Fifth Vital Sign

Assessment of pain is essential in comprehensive health assessment. Pain is an entirely subjective and personal experience. When pain is present, it impacts every aspect of an individual's health and well-being. Pain can be acute and chronic, or severe or mild, but overall it is an experience unique to the individual. The perception of pain and the ways in which the individual responds to pain vary according to age, gender, culture, and developmental level. When conducting a pain assessment, the nurse must consider all factors influencing the individual's experience with pain. Refer to chapter 11 of this text for a thorough discussion of pain. ∞

The Functional Assessment as Part of the General Survey

Nurses use their observational skills in many situations. When making observations, nurses are continually thinking about the data and using their knowledge of the physical, behavioral, and social sciences to interpret the findings. The findings are interpreted according to the expected norms for patients in relation to age, gender, race, development, and culture.

Functional Assessment Defined

The **functional assessment** is an observation to gather data while the patient is performing common or routine activities.

Functional Assessment During the General Survey

During the general survey of a healthy patient, the nurse will observe the patient while performing the following common activities: walking into the examination room, taking a seat for the interview, and moving the arms and hands to arrange clothing or to shake hands as an introduction. The nurse will also observe the facial expression while these acts occur. From this brief encounter, the nurse applies knowledge to begin to gather and interpret data about the patient's mobility and strength as well as the symmetry of the face and parts of the body.

Critical Thinking

When applying the critical thinking process, the professional nurse uses a variety of skills that culminate in assisting patients to make healthcare decisions.

The following case study and analysis is presented to demonstrate the application of critical thinking in the functional assessment of a patient as part of the general survey.

The nurse conducted a comprehensive health assessment of a 21-year-old African American male who was new to the clinic. The interaction began when the nurse went to the waiting area to bring the patient to the interview area. The following occurred: As the nurse entered the waiting area, all of the patients looked up. The nurse called out "Jason C." and looked about the room. An African American male wearing a local college football jersey said, "That's me." The man rose quickly, pushing himself up with his hands placed on the arms of the chair. Upon standing, he grimaced slightly. The patient demonstrated a slight limp and appeared to be bearing only partial weight on his right leg. As the patient approached, the nurse noted that he had smooth skin on his face and hands. He was approximately 6′2″ and muscular. As he moved through the door, he stated, "Just tell me I didn't tear anything in my knee that's going to need surgery."

As stated early in this chapter, the general survey begins with the initial encounter with the patient and provides cues about the patient. The observations from the brief case study include the following:

- All of the patients looked up when the nurse entered the waiting area.
- When a name was called, a young adult African American male wearing a local college football jersey responded.
- The young man rose quickly.
- The young man used his arms to push himself out of the chair.
- The young man grimaced slightly upon standing.
- The young man had smooth skin on his face and hands.
- The young man was approximately 6′2″ tall and was muscular.
- He walked with a slight limp.
- He appeared to be bearing only partial weight on his right leg.
- As he entered the exam area, he stated, "Just tell me I didn't tear anything in my knee that's going to need surgery."

In applying critical thinking, the nurse will begin to sort information and determine an approach to continue data gathering. The nurse considers each of the observations in terms of normal and abnormal findings in relation to the age, gender, race, and culture of the patient. Interpretations of the nurse's observations in the preceding case study are as follows:

- All the patients looked up when the nurse entered the room.
  The patient was aware that someone entered the room; this indicates that his vision and hearing are intact. This is considered a normal finding.

- The patient responded when his name was called.
  This is further indication that hearing is intact. This is a normal finding.

- The patient rose quickly.
  This is an expected finding in a young adult because of good muscle tone and strength.

- The patient used his arms to push herself out of the chair.
  This is an indication of diminished strength or mobility in one or both lower extremities. This is an unexpected finding in a young adult because of increased muscle tone and strength. This requires follow-up to determine the actual muscle strength of the patient.

- The patient grimaced upon standing.
  This indicates discomfort. This is initially interpreted as an abnormal finding. Discomfort is indicative of an underlying problem. In this case, the problem may be musculoskeletal.

- The patient had smooth skin on his face and hands.
  This finding suggests that the patient is in a state of fluid and nutritional balance and that he follows hygiene practices. This has the suggestion of being a normal finding. However, the nurse will consider other factors during the assessment.

- The patient was approximately 6′2″ tall and was muscular.
  Increased muscular tone may be a normal finding among young adults. Additionally, the nurse recognizes that the young man is wearing a football jersey from a local college, which suggests he may be a college athlete.

- The patient limped and appeared to be bearing only partial weight on his right leg.
  This is an abnormal finding. The nurse must explore the underlying cause. This is suggestive of a musculoskeletal problem.

- As he entered the exam area, he stated, "Just tell me I didn't tear anything in my knee that's going to need surgery."
  This response indicates the patient's concern regarding an injury. The statements are not unexpected in relation to observations about the movements and gait of the patient. This statement forces the nurse to make a rapid decision about the process of the health assessment. The nurse must quickly gather more data to determine the patient's ability to participate in all aspects of the assessment.

The preceding analyses demonstrate that a great deal of information can be obtained through observation. In this situation much information is missing. As this information is gathered, the nurse will determine the relevance of each piece of data to the overall situation. The nurse applies critical thinking throughout the comprehensive health assessment while working with the patient to meet health-related needs.

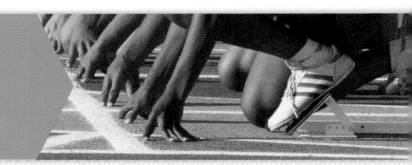

Application Through Critical Thinking

▶ Case Study

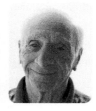

It is a Friday morning. You are the nurse who is conducting a physical examination of Joseph Miller, a 73-year-old Caucasian male. You begin with a patient interview during which the following occurs.

The patient enters the room, looks right at you, smiles, and states "How do you do?" in a clear voice. When you introduce yourself, he gives you a firm handshake, then holds both of your hands in his and comments, "Boy, you sure have cold hands." He walks steadily to the chair you indicate but holds onto the desk while getting seated. You inform the patient of the purpose of the interview. He states "no" when asked if he has any specific complaints or problems. He then shrugs his shoulders and comments, "I don't think I have anything special going on, I'm here for my 3-month check and I expect to get a clean bill of health." You ask him to sign an admission form. He puts on reading glasses, peruses the form, and signs it.

When asked about current medications, the patient states "I have them with me, let me show you." He then takes out three medicine bottles. He reads each label and comments as follows about each: "This is Pardivil, it's for my blood pressure; this one is ferrous sulfate, that's iron, I have some anemia; this last one is Digit, I take it every other day for my heart." He frowns and says, "This bottle is nearly empty." After opening the bottle and looking at the contents he says, "Yup, just as I thought, I only have three pills left so I'll have to fill it. I'll be out of pills by Thursday and the drug store is always packed just before the weekend."

You continue the interview and conclude it by telling the patient you are going to check his blood pressure, pulse, temperature, and weight before escorting him to the examination room.

▶ References

American Heart Association (AHA). (2012). *Understanding blood pressure readings*. Retrieved from http://www.heart.org/HEARTORG/Conditions/HighBloodPressure/AboutHighBloodPressure/Understanding-Blood-Pressure-Readings_UCM_301764_Article.jsp

Berk, L. E. (2010). *Development through the lifespan* (5th ed.). Boston: Pearson Education, Inc.

Berman, A., & Snyder, S. (2012). *Kozier and Erb's fundamentals of nursing: Concepts, process, and practice* (9th ed.). Upper Saddle River, NJ: Prentice Hall.

Burton, M. A., & Ludwig, L. J. M. (2010). *Fundamentals of nursing care: Concepts, connections & skills*. Philadelphia, PA: F.A. Davis.

Centers for Disease Control and Prevention (CDC). (2001). *Data table of infant head circumference-for-age charts*. Retrieved from http://www.cdc.gov/growthcharts/html_charts/hcageinf.htm

Go, A. S., Mozaffarian, D., Roger, V. L., Benjamin, E. J., Berry, J. D., Borden, W. B., . . . & Turner, M. B. (2013). Heart disease and stroke statistics—2013 update: A report from the American Heart Association. *Circulation, 127*, e6–e245.

Harkreader, H., Hogan, M., & Thobaben, M. (2008). *Fundamentals of nursing: Caring and clinical judgment* (3rd ed.). Philadelphia: W. B. Saunders.

Hazinski, M. F. (2012). *Nursing care of the critically ill child* (3rd ed.). St. Louis, MO: Mosby.

Kemp, C. (2013). Temporal artery thermometers may rival rectal thermometers in ED. *AAP News, 34*(4), 2.

Kliegman, R. M., Stanton, B. M. D., St. Geme, J., Schor, N., & Behrman, R. E. (2011). *Nelson textbook of pediatrics* (19th ed.). Philadelphia: Saunders Elsevier.

Lewis, S., Dirksen, S., Heitkemper, M., Bucher, L., & Camera, I. (2010). *Medical-surgical nursing: Assessment and management of clinical problems* (8th ed.). St. Louis, MO: Mosby.

London, M. L., Ladewig, P. A. W., Davidson, M. R., Ball, J. W., Bindler, R. C., & Cowen, K. J. (2014). *Maternal & child nursing care* (4th ed.). Upper Saddle River, NJ: Pearson.

▶ Critical Thinking Questions

1. What are the findings from the case study for Mr. Miller?

2. How would you interpret the findings in relation to the categories for observation in the general survey?

3. Which findings indicate the need for follow-up in the interview or physical assessment?

4. What factors must be considered when evaluating the vital signs assessment for Mr. Miller?

5. What psychosocial factors (if noted) would indicate further follow-up is needed?

Madhur, M. S., Riaz, K., Dreisbach, A. W., & Harrison, D. G. (2014). *Hypertension treatment & management: Approach considerations*. Retrieved from http://emedicine.medscape.com/article/241381-treatment

Mayo Clinic. (2013). Does cuff size affect blood pressure readings? Retrieved from http://www.mayoclinic.org/diseases-conditions/high-blood-pressure/expert-answers/blood-pressure-cuff/faq-20058337

Murray, R. B., & Zentner, J. P. (2008). *Health promotion strategies through the life span* (8th ed.). Upper Saddle River, NJ: Prentice Hall.

Osborn K. S., Wraa, C. E., Watson, A., & Holleran, R. S. (2013). *Medical-surgical nursing: Preparation for practice* (2nd ed.). Upper Saddle River, NJ: Pearson.

Pickering, T. G., Hall, J. E., Appel, L. J., Falkner, B. E., Graves, J., Hill, M. N., . . . & Roccella, E. J. (2005). Recommendations for blood pressure measurement in humans and experimental animals: Part 1: Blood pressure measurement in humans: A statement for professionals from the Subcommittee of Professional and Public Education of the American Heart Association Council on High Blood Pressure Research. *Hypertension, 45*, 142–161.

Portman, H., & Sheppard, S. (2011). Vital information about a vital sign: BP. *Nursing2014, 41*(2), 66.

Potter, P., Perry, A., Stockert, P., & Hall, A. (2011). *Basic nursing* (7th ed.). St. Louis, MO: Mosby.

Ross, P. A., Newth, C. J. L., & Khemani, R. G. (2014). Accuracy of pulse oximetry in children. *Pediatrics, 133*(1), 22–29.

Rush University Medical Center. (n.d.). *What is a healthy weight?* Retrieved from http://www.rush.edu/rumc/page-1108048103230.html

U.S. Environmental Protection Agency (EPA). (2014). *Phase-out of mercury thermometers used in industrial and laboratory settings*. Retrieved from http://www.epa.gov/mercury/thermometer.htm

WebMD. (2012). *Vital signs in children: Topic overview*. Retrieved from http://www.webmd.com/a-to-z-guides/vital-signs-in-children-topic-overview

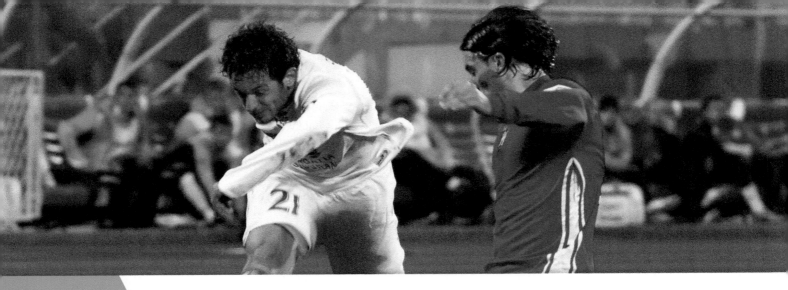

Pain Assessment

▶ Learning Outcomes

Upon completion of this chapter, you will be able to:

1. Explore the concept of pain.

2. Outline the physiologic process involved in the perception of pain.

3. Differentiate between the various types of pain.

4. Examine factors that influence pain perception and expression of pain.

5. Identify cultural and developmental influences that affect assessment of pain for patients across the life span.

6. Demonstrate techniques used for assessment of a patient having pain.

Key Terms

ain is a highly unpleasant sensation that affects a person's physical health, emotional health, and well-being. Healthcare professionals include pain as a component of vital signs assessment. Pain assessment is identified as the fifth vital sign.

Assessment of pain requires a strong knowledge base regarding the concept of pain and methods used to collect information about the pain experience. Accurate assessment of pain is essential to developing, monitoring, and evaluating the effectiveness of pain relief interventions.

Pain assessment, treatment, and relief present one of the greatest challenges to the nurse and other members of the healthcare team. The nurse has a primary role regarding the collection and analysis of data, the implementation of treatment modalities, and the evaluation of the patient regarding pain experiences.

Definition of Pain

Pain comes from the Greek word *poinē* meaning "penalty," implying the person is paying for something. An individual's perception of pain is influenced by age, culture, and previous experience with pain.

Pain has been defined as "whatever the experiencing person says it is, existing whenever he or she says it does" (McCaffery & Pasero, 1999, p. 5). Pain is a universal experience. Everyone experiences pain at some time and to some degree. It is a highly subjective, unpleasant, and personal sensation that cannot be shared with others. This sensation can be associated with actual or potential tissue damage. Pain can be the primary problem or be associated with a specific diagnosis, treatment, or procedure.

No two people experience pain in the same manner. It can occupy all of a person's thinking, force changes in the ability to function on a daily basis, and produce changes in the individual's life. For the patient, it is a difficult concept to describe, thus making pain treatment and relief most difficult.

The nurse cannot see or feel the pain being experienced by the patient; however, the effects produced by the pain will be assessed. These changes can be physiologic, psychologic, and behavioral in nature.

Physiology of Pain

Pain is a complex, subjective, multidimensional phenomenon that is not clearly understood. Theories that have been developed to explain the conceptual and physiologic aspects of pain include specific theory, pattern theory, and gate control theory.

Theories of Pain

The concept of specific theory explains the complexity of pain. This theory demonstrates that pain neurons are as specific and unique as other specific neurons (taste, smell) in the body. The special pain neurons transport the sensation to the brain for interpretation. The transport occurs in a straight line to the brain, making the pain equal to the injury. This theory does not include a consideration of any psychologic component to pain.

The pattern theory indicates that individuals will respond in a different manner to a similar stimulus. This theory implies that the pattern of the stimulus is more important than the specific stimulus.

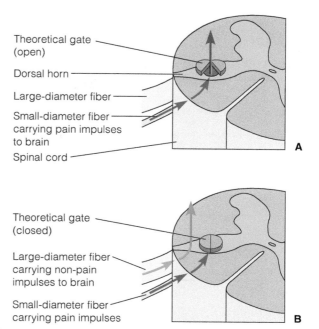

Figure 11.1 Gate control theory: A. open gate, B. closed gate.

It does not take into consideration the psychosocial component to pain.

According to Melzack and Wall's gate control theory (1965), peripheral nerve fibers carrying pain impulses to the spinal cord can have their input modified at the spinal cord level before transmission to the brain. Synapses in the dorsal horns act as gates that close to keep impulses from reaching the brain, or open to permit impulses to ascend to the brain.

In application of the gate control theory, small-diameter nerve fibers carry pain impulses through a gate and ultimately, to the brain. However, according to this theory, impulses that are simultaneously transmitted by large-diameter nerve fibers can block transmission of the pain impulses carried by the small-diameter nerve fibers—that is, close the gate (see Figure 11.1 ■). The gate mechanism is thought to be situated in the substantia gelatinosa cells in the dorsal horn of the spinal cord. Because a limited amount of sensory information can reach the brain at any given time, certain cells can interrupt the pain impulses. The brain also appears to influence whether the gate is open or closed. For example, previous experiences with pain affect the way an individual responds to pain. The involvement of the brain helps explain why painful stimuli are interpreted differently by different people. Although the gate control theory is not unanimously accepted, it does help explain why electrical and mechanical interventions as well as heat and pressure can relieve pain. For example, a back massage may stimulate impulses in large nerves, which in turn close the gate to back pain.

Nervous System

The nervous system must receive and interpret a stimulus to allow the individual to recognize the pain process. How pain is transmitted and perceived is not completely understood. Whether pain is perceived and to what degree depends on the interaction between the body's analgesia system and the nervous system's transmission and interpretation of stimuli.

TABLE 11.1	Types of Pain Stimuli	
STIMULUS TYPE	**PHYSIOLOGIC BASIS OF PAIN**	
Mechanical		
1. Trauma to body tissues (e.g., surgery)	Tissue damage; direct irritation of the pain receptors; inflammation	
2. Alterations in body tissues (e.g., edema)	Pressure on pain receptors	
3. Blockage of a body duct	Distention of the lumen of the duct	
4. Tumor	Pressure on pain receptors; irritation of nerve endings	
5. Muscle spasm	Stimulation of pain receptors (also see chemical stimuli)	
Thermal		
1. Extreme heat (e.g., burns)	Tissue destruction; stimulation of thermosensitive pain receptors	
2. Extreme cold (e.g., frostbite)		
Chemical		
1. Tissue ischemia (e.g., blocked coronary artery)	Stimulation of pain receptors because of accumulated lactic acid (and other chemicals, such as bradykinin and enzymes) in tissues	
2. Muscle spasm	Tissue ischemia secondary to mechanical stimulation (see above)	

Nociception

The peripheral nervous system includes primary sensory neurons specialized to detect tissue damage and to evoke the sensations of touch, heat, cold, pain, and pressure. The receptors that transmit pain sensation are called **nociceptors.** These pain receptors or nociceptors can be excited by mechanical, thermal, or chemical stimuli (see Table 11.1). The physiologic processes related to pain perception are described as **nociception.** The processes involved in nociception include transduction, transmission, perception, and modulation (Paice, 2002).

TRANSDUCTION During the transduction process, biochemical mediator release is triggered by injury to the tissues. These biochemical mediators—such as prostaglandins, bradykinin, serotonin, histamine, and substance P—sensitize the nociceptors. Painful or noxious stimulation also causes ions to move across cellular membranes, which leads to excitement of the nociceptors. Pain medications, or analgesics, act during the transduction process by inhibiting the synthesis of prostaglandin (e.g., nonsteroidal anti-inflammatory medications, such as ibuprofen) or by decreasing the movement of ions across the cellular membrane (e.g., local anesthetic agents) (Berman & Snyder, 2011).

TRANSMISSION Pain transmission, which is the second process involved in nociception, incorporates three phases (McCaffery & Pasero, 1999). During the first phase, the pain impulse is transmitted from the peripheral nerve fibers to the spinal cord. At this point, substance P functions as a neurotransmitter, promoting the movement of impulses across the nerve synapse from the primary afferent neuron to the second-order neuron in the dorsal horn of the spinal cord (see Figure 11.2 ■). Transmission of the pain impulse to the dorsal horn of the spinal cord involves two types of nociceptive fibers: A-delta fibers, which transmit localized, sharp pain; and C fibers, which transmit dull, aching pain. During phase two of transmission, the pain impulse travels from the spinal cord and ascends via spinothalamic tracts to the brain stem and thalamus (see Figure 11.3 ■).

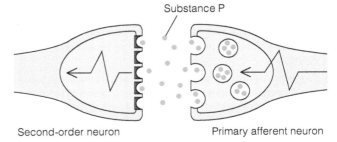

Figure 11.2 Substance P assists the transmission of impulses across the synapse from the primary afferent neuron to a second-order neuron in the spinothalamic tract.

In phase three of transmission, signals are transmitted between the thalamus and the somatic sensory cortex, which is the site of pain perception (Berman & Snyder, 2011).

Pain control can take place during the transmission process. For example, opioids (narcotic analgesics) inhibit the release of certain neurotransmitters, particularly substance P, thus blocking pain at the spinal level.

PERCEPTION During perception, which is the third process, the patient becomes aware of the pain. Pain perception is believed to occur in the cortical structures, which allows for different cognitive-behavioral strategies to be applied to reduce the sensory and affective components of pain (McCaffery & Pasero, 1999). For example, nonpharmacologic interventions such as distraction, guided imagery, and music can help direct the patient's attention away from the pain (Berman & Snyder, 2011).

MODULATION The fourth process, modulation, is commonly referred to as the "descending system." During modulation, neurons in the brain stem transmit signals back to the dorsal horn of the spinal cord (Paice, 2002, p. 75). At this point, these descending fibers

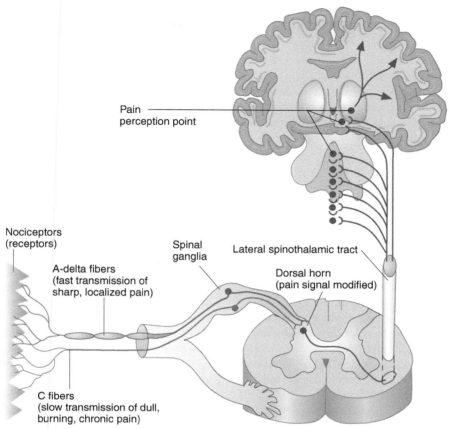

Figure 11.3 Physiology of pain perception.

release substances that can block the ascending painful impulses in the dorsal horn; for example, endogenous opioids, serotonin, and norepinephrine may be released. Because these neurotransmitters undergo reuptake, during which they are taken back by the body, their analgesic effectiveness is limited (McCaffery & Pasero, 1999). Patients with chronic pain may be prescribed tricyclic antidepressants, which inhibit the reuptake of norepinephrine and serotonin. This action increases the modulation phase that helps inhibit painful ascending stimuli (Berman & Snyder, 2011).

Responses to Pain

The pain response is complex and incorporates both physiologic and psychosocial aspects. Initially, sympathetic nervous system stimulation triggers the fight-or-flight response. Eventually, as the body adapts to the pain, the parasympathetic nervous system takes over, reversing many of the initial physiologic responses. This adaptation to pain occurs after several hours or days of pain. The actual pain receptors adapt very little and continue to transmit the pain message. The person may learn to cope through cognitive and behavioral activities, such as diversions, imagery, and excessive sleeping. The individual may seek out physical interventions to manage the pain, such as analgesics, massage, and exercise.

A proprioceptive reflex also occurs with the stimulation of pain receptors. Impulses travel along sensory pain fibers to the spinal cord. There they synapse with motor neurons, and the impulses travel back via motor fibers to a muscle near the site of the pain (see Figure 11.4 ■). The muscle then contracts in a protective action.

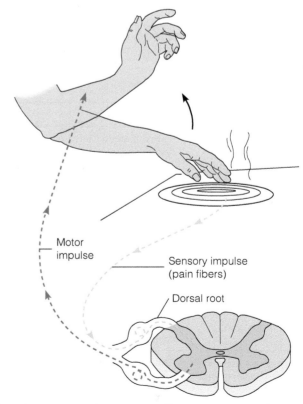

Figure 11.4 Proprioceptive reflex to a pain stimulus.

For example, when a person touches a hot stove, the hand reflexively draws back from the heat even before the person is aware of the pain.

Nature of Pain

Pain, which is a subjective and personal experience, can be described in many ways. The type of pain, the point of origin, and the duration of pain are several ways that the nurse and other members of the healthcare team may describe pain.

Types of Pain

Pain may be described in terms of duration, location, or etiology. When pain lasts only through the expected recovery period from illness, injury, or surgery, it is described as **acute pain,** whether it has a sudden or slow onset and regardless of the intensity. Depending on the patient's condition, acute pain may last for a few minutes up to several weeks, but usually not longer than 6 months. **Chronic pain** is prolonged, usually recurring or persisting over 6 months or longer, and interferes with functioning. Chronic pain can be further classified as chronic malignant pain, when associated with cancer or other life-threatening conditions, or as chronic nonmalignant pain, when the etiology is a nonprogressive disorder. Such disorders include cluster headaches, low back pain, and myofascial pain dysfunction. Acute pain and chronic pain result in different physiologic and behavioral responses, as shown in Table 11.2.

Pain may be categorized according to its origin as cutaneous, deep somatic, or visceral. **Cutaneous pain** originates in the skin or subcutaneous tissue. A paper cut causing a sharp pain with some burning is an example of cutaneous pain. **Deep somatic pain** arises from ligaments, tendons, bones, blood vessels, and nerves. It is diffuse and tends to last longer than cutaneous pain. An ankle sprain is an example of deep somatic pain. **Visceral pain** results from stimulation of pain receptors in the abdominal cavity, cranium, and thorax. It tends to appear diffuse and often feels like deep somatic pain, that is, burning, aching, or a feeling of pressure. Visceral pain is frequently caused by stretching of the tissues, ischemia, or muscle spasms. For example, an obstructed bowel will result in visceral pain.

Pain may also be described according to where it is experienced in the body. **Radiating pain** is perceived at the source of the pain and extends to nearby tissues. For example, cardiac pain may be felt not only in the chest but also along the left shoulder and down the arm. **Referred pain** is felt in a part of the body that is considerably removed from the tissues causing the pain. For example, pain from one part of the abdominal viscera may be perceived in an area of the skin remote from the organ causing the pain (see Figure 11.5 ■).

Intractable pain is highly resistant to relief. One example is the pain from an advanced malignancy. When caring for a patient experiencing intractable pain, nurses are challenged to use a number of methods, pharmacologic and nonpharmacologic, to provide pain relief.

Neuropathic pain is the result of current or past damage to the peripheral or central nervous system and may not have a stimulus, such as tissue or nerve damage, for the pain. Neuropathic pain is long lasting; is unpleasant; and can be described as burning, dull, and aching. Episodes of sharp, shooting pain can also be experienced (Sadosky, Hopper, & Parsons, 2014). Examples of this pain include trigeminal neuralgia and peripheral neuropathy.

Phantom pain, which is perceived in a body part that is missing (e.g., an amputated leg) or paralyzed by a spinal cord injury, is an example of neuropathic pain. This can be distinguished from phantom sensation, that is, the feeling that the missing body part is still present. The incidence of phantom pain can be reduced when analgesics are administered via epidural catheter prior to the amputation.

Concepts Associated with Pain

When a person perceives pain from injured tissue, the pain threshold is reached. An individual's **pain threshold** is the amount of pain stimulation the person requires to feel pain. A person's pain threshold is fairly uniform; however, it can change. For example, the same stimuli that once produced mild pain can at another time produce intense pain. Excessive sensitivity to pain is called **hyperalgesia.**

Two additional terms used in the context of pain are pain sensation and pain reaction. **Pain sensation** can be considered the same as pain threshold; **pain reaction** includes the autonomic nervous system and behavioral responses to pain. The autonomic nervous system response is the automatic reaction that often protects the individual from further harm, for example, the automatic withdrawal of the hand from a hot stove. The behavioral response is a learned response used as a method of coping with pain.

Pain tolerance is the maximum amount and duration of pain that an individual is willing to endure. Some patients are unable to tolerate even the slightest pain, whereas others are willing to endure severe pain rather than be treated for it. Pain tolerance is widely influenced by psychological and sociocultural factors. According to current research, there is not sufficient evidence to support

TABLE 11.2	Comparison of Acute and Chronic Pain	
ACUTE PAIN	**CHRONIC PAIN**
Mild to severe	Mild to severe

Sympathetic nervous system responses:
  Increased pulse rate
  Increased respiratory rate
  Elevated blood pressure
  Diaphoresis
  Dilated pupils
	Parasympathetic nervous system responses:
	  Vital signs normal
	
	Dry, warm skin
	Pupils normal or dilated

Related to tissue injury; resolves with healing	Continues beyond healing
Patient appears restless and anxious	Patient appears depressed and withdrawn
Patient reports pain	Patient often does not mention pain unless asked
Patient exhibits behavior indicative of pain: crying, rubbing area, holding area	Pain behavior often absent

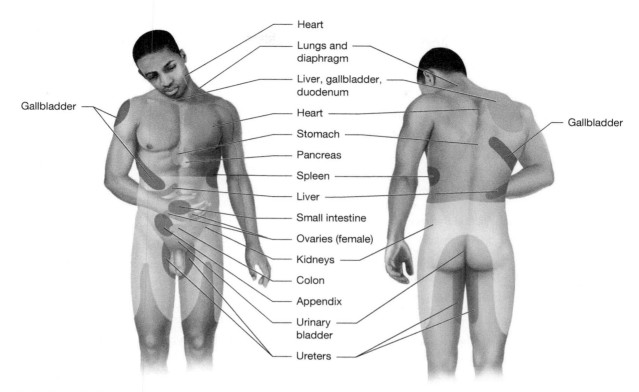

Figure 11.5 Sites of referred pain.

gender-based variations in pain sensitivity; that is, when compared strictly based on gender, men and women appear to be equally susceptible to pain perception (Racine et al., 2012). Even so, gender-based cultural influences may shape an individual's expression of pain.

Factors Influencing Pain

Factors that influence the individual's perception of and reaction to pain include lifespan considerations, cultural factors, and the environment.

Lifespan Considerations

The age and developmental stage of a patient will influence both the reaction to and the expression of pain. The expression of pain may also be influenced by past experience. Age variations and related nursing interventions are presented in Table 11.3.

The field of pain management for infants and children has grown significantly. It is now accepted that anatomic, physiologic, and biochemical elements necessary for pain transmission are present in newborns, regardless of their gestational age. The American Academy of Pediatrics and the Canadian Paediatric Society (2000) have recommended that environmental, nonpharmacologic, and pharmacologic interventions be used to prevent, reduce, or eliminate pain in neonates. This recommendation was reaffirmed in 2006 by the American Academy of Pediatrics Committee on Fetus and Newborn et al. (2006). Physiologic indicators may vary in infants, so behavioral observation is recommended for pain assessment (Ball & Bindler, 2012). Children may be less able than an adult to articulate their experience or needs related to pain, which may result in their pain being undertreated. When interpreting pediatric complaints,

the nurse should take into consideration reports from parents or caregivers, the child's developmental stage, and psychosocial factors. For example:

- Small children commonly will complain of a "tummy ache" or "my throat hurts" while parents may be concerned about fussiness or altered sleep patterns.
- Preadolescent children will complain of stomach pain when they are gassy, if they are nauseated, or if they actually feel abdominal pain.
- Children with sore throats often present with a history of normal fluid intake but decreased solid food intake.
- Anxious or frightened preschool and school-age children may complain of headache or stomachache.

Older adults constitute a major portion of the individuals within the healthcare system. The prevalence of pain in the older population is generally higher due to both acute and chronic disease conditions. Pain threshold does not appear to change with aging, although the effect of analgesics may increase due to physiologic changes related to drug metabolism and excretion (Kee, Hayes, & McCuistion, 2012).

Cultural Influences

Ethnic background and cultural heritage have long been recognized as influencing both a person's reaction to pain and the expression of that pain. Behavior related to pain is part of the socialization process. For example, individuals in one culture may learn to be expressive about pain, whereas individuals from another culture may learn to keep those feelings to themselves and not bother others. Chinese Americans and patients from other Asian cultures are usually stoic

TABLE 11.3	Lifespan Considerations Related to the Pain Experience	
AGE GROUP	**PAIN PERCEPTION AND BEHAVIOR**	**SELECTED NURSING INTERVENTIONS**
Infant	Perceives pain Responds to pain with increased sensitivity. Older infant tries to avoid pain; for example, turns away and physically resists.	Give a glucose pacifier. Use tactile stimulation. Play music or tapes of a heartbeat.
Toddler and Preschooler	Develops the ability to describe pain and its intensity and location. Often responds with crying and anger because child perceives pain as a threat to security. Reasoning with child at this stage is not always successful. May consider pain a punishment. Feels sad. May learn there are gender differences in pain expression. Tends to hold someone accountable for the pain.	Distract the child with toys, books, pictures. Involve the child in blowing bubbles as a way of "blowing away the pain." Appeal to the child's belief in magic by using a "magic" blanket or glove to take away pain. Hold the child to provide comfort. Explore misconceptions about pain.
School-age Child	Tries to be brave when facing pain. Rationalizes in an attempt to explain the pain. Responsive to explanations. Can usually identify the location and describe the pain. With persistent pain, may regress to an earlier stage of development.	Use imagery to turn off "pain switches." Provide a behavioral rehearsal of what to expect and how it will look and feel. Provide support and nurturing.
Adolescent	May be slow to acknowledge pain. Recognizing pain or "giving in" may be considered weakness. Wants to appear brave in front of peers and not report pain.	Provide opportunities to discuss pain. Provide privacy. Present choices for dealing with pain. Encourage music or TV for distraction.
Adult	Behaviors exhibited when experiencing pain may be gender-based behaviors learned as a child. May ignore pain because to admit it is perceived as a sign of weakness or failure. Fear of what pain means may prevent some adults from taking action.	Deal with any misconceptions about pain. Focus on the patient's control in dealing with the pain. Allay fears and anxiety when possible.
Older Adult	May have multiple conditions presenting with vague symptoms. May perceive pain as part of the aging process. May have decreased sensations or perceptions of the pain. Lethargy, anorexia, and fatigue may be indicators of pain. May withhold complaints of pain because of fear of the treatment, fear of any lifestyle changes that may be involved, or fear of becoming dependent. May describe pain differently, that is, as "ache," "hurt," or "discomfort." May consider it unacceptable to admit or show pain.	Thorough history and assessment is essential. Spend time with the patient and listen carefully. Clarify misconceptions. Encourage independence whenever possible.

and, therefore, may request little or no pain medication (Davidhizar & Giger, 2004). Black Americans tend to report higher levels of pain and are more verbal when experiencing pain compared to White Americans (Andrews & Boyle, 2011). Jewish and Italian patients also tend to be more vocal about pain (Davidhizar & Giger, 2004). Arab Americans believe pain is punishment, and suffering is viewed as atonement. Arab American women express pain verbally to family members, whereas the men are stoic. Women are more likely to express pain than men in many cultures (Defrin, Eli, & Pud, 2011). In addition, non-Hispanic women are more likely to ask for pain medication during childbirth than Hispanic women (Andrews & Boyle, 2011)

Cultural background can affect the level of pain that a person is willing to tolerate. In some Middle Eastern and African cultures, self-infliction of pain is a sign of mourning or grief. In other groups, pain may be anticipated as part of the ritualistic practices, and tolerance of pain may signify strength and endurance. There are significant variations in the expression of pain. Studies have shown that individuals of northern European descent tend to be more stoic and less expressive of their pain than individuals from southern European backgrounds.

The culture of health care also influences pain perception in terms of the healthcare provider's assessment of the patient's pain. In particular, nurses may have their own attitudes and expectations about pain. Andrews & Boyle (2011) pointed out that health care has been dominated by White Anglo-Saxon Protestants, and most nurses have been influenced by these values and beliefs. For example, nurses may place a higher value on silent suffering or self-control in response to pain. They may expect patients to be objective about pain and to be able to provide a detailed description of their pain. Nurses may deny or minimize the pain they observe in others. Because nurses serve a more diverse population in terms of ethnicity and cultural responses to pain than they once did, nurses must identify their own personal attitudes about pain in order to provide culturally competent care for patients in pain (Andrews & Boyle, 2011).

Environmental Considerations

Environmental factors will influence a person's ability to identify and seek relief for pain. The external environment includes a variety of stimuli for pain. Objects that may contribute to pain include restrictive clothing; ill-fitting shoes; or furniture and other objects in the work and home environments that cause pressure, strain, discomfort, or pain in healthy or already painful areas of the body. The ability to move freely influences the person's ability to avoid or control painful stimuli.

Family members and support systems, including members of the health team, are factors in the external environment that must be considered. A strange environment such as a hospital, with its noises, lights, and activity, can compound pain. The lonely person who is without a support network may perceive pain as severe, whereas the person who has supportive people around may perceive less pain. Some people prefer to withdraw when they are in pain; others prefer the distraction of people and activity around them. Family caregivers can be a significant support for a person in pain. With the increase in outpatient and home care, families are assuming an increased responsibility for pain management. Education related to the assessment and management of pain can positively affect the perceived quality of life for both patients and their caregivers (McCaffery & Pasero, 1999).

Expectations of significant others can affect a person's perceptions of and responses to pain. In some situations, girls may be permitted to express pain more openly than boys. Family role can also affect how a person perceives or responds to pain. For instance, a single mother supporting three children may ignore pain because of her need to stay on the job. The presence of support people often changes a patient's reaction to pain. For example, toddlers often tolerate pain more readily when supportive parents or nurses are nearby.

The internal environment includes individual perceptions and experiences related to pain. Previous pain experiences alter a patient's sensitivity to pain. People who have experienced pain, or who have been exposed to the suffering of someone close who experienced pain, are often more threatened by anticipated pain than people without a pain experience. The success or lack of success of pain relief measures influences a person's expectations for relief. For example, a person who has tried several pain relief measures without success may have little hope about the helpfulness of nursing interventions.

Some patients may accept pain more readily than others, depending on the circumstances. A patient who associates the pain with a positive outcome may withstand the pain amazingly well. For example, a woman giving birth to a child or an athlete undergoing knee surgery to prolong his career may tolerate pain better because of the benefit associated with it. These patients may view the pain as a temporary inconvenience rather than a potential threat or disruption to daily life.

By contrast, patients with unrelenting chronic pain may suffer more intensely. They may respond with despair, anxiety, and depression because they cannot attach a positive significance or purpose to the pain. In this situation, the pain may be looked upon as a threat to body image or lifestyle and as a sign of possible impending death.

Anxiety often accompanies pain. The threat of the unknown and the inability to control the pain or the events surrounding it often augment the pain perception. Fatigue also reduces a person's ability to cope, thereby increasing pain perception. When pain interferes with sleep, fatigue and muscle tension often result and increase the pain; thus a cycle of pain–fatigue–pain develops. People who believe that they have control of their pain have decreased fear and anxiety, which decreases their pain perception. A perception of lacking control or a sense of helplessness tends to increase pain perception. Patients who are able to express pain to an attentive listener and participate in pain management decisions can increase their sense of control and decrease pain perception.

Assessment

Accurate and timely patient assessment is imperative for effective pain management. Poorly managed or untreated pain will influence every aspect of an individual's health and well-being. Pain assessment is considered the fifth vital sign. The strategy of linking pain assessment to routine vital sign assessment and documentation ensures pain assessment for all patients. Because pain is subjective and experienced uniquely by each person, nurses need to assess all factors affecting the pain experience—physiologic, psychologic, behavioral, emotional, and sociocultural.

The extent and frequency of the pain assessment varies according to the situation. For patients experiencing acute or severe pain, the nurse may focus only on location, quality, severity, and early intervention. Patients with less severe or chronic pain can usually provide a more detailed description of the experience. Frequency of pain assessment usually depends on the pain control measures being used and the clinical circumstances. For example, in the initial postoperative period, pain is often assessed whenever vital signs are taken, which may be as often as every 15 minutes and then extended to every 2 to 4 hours. Following pain management interventions, pain intensity should be reassessed at an interval appropriate for the intervention. For example, following the intravenous administration of morphine, the severity of pain should be reassessed in 20 to 30 minutes.

Because many people will not voice their pain unless asked about it, pain assessments must be initiated by the nurse. It is also essential that nurses listen to and rely on the patient's perceptions of pain. Believing the patient who is experiencing and conveying the perceptions is crucial in establishing a sense of trust.

Pain assessments consist of two major components: (a) a pain history to obtain facts from the patient and (b) direct observation of behavioral and physiologic responses of the patient. The goal of assessment is to gain an objective understanding of a subjective experience. The nurse typically initiates pain assessment because many individuals do not discuss their pain until asked about it. Pain assessment consists of two phases. The first phase is a pain history, and the second phase is observation of behaviors and responses to pain.

Pain History

A detailed history to obtain subjective data from the patient is essential for successful treatment and relief from pain. During the history taking and focused interview, the nurse provides patients an opportunity to express in their own words how they view pain. It also gives the nurse an opportunity to observe the body language or nonverbal communication of the patient. The responses made by the patient will help the nurse understand the meaning of pain to the patient and the coping strategies being used. Each person's pain experience is unique, and the patient is the best interpreter of the pain experience.

A pain history includes collection of data about the location, intensity, quality, and pattern of pain; precipitating factors; actions aimed at relief of pain; impact on activities of daily living (ADLs); coping strategies; and emotional responses. A suggested method for assessment of physical complaints, including pain, is the acronym *OLDCART & ICE*. Figure 11.6 ■ describes the meanings of the letters in the OLDCART and ICE acronym. (Also see chapter 7. ∞) The following items discuss the factors related to each aspect of pain assessment.

Onset

The nurse asks the patient to discuss and describe when the pain began.

Location

The nurse should ask the patient to point to the specific location of pain. Charts in which body outlines are depicted are a useful method

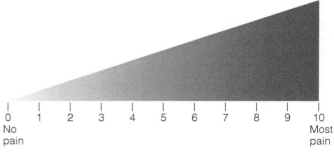

Figure 11.7 Pain rating intensity scale.

for children and adults to accurately identify the site of pain. When recording the location, the body outline charts may be used. The nurse is also expected to record locations, using appropriate terminology in relation to the proximity or distance from known landmarks (e.g., "pain in substernal area 3 cm [1.18 in.] below the xiphoid process").

Duration

The patient is asked to describe the length of time the pain lasts. Included would be a determination of the pain as constant or intermittent. If the pain is intermittent, the nurse must assess the length of time without pain or between episodes of pain.

Characteristics

The characteristics of the pain are assessed by asking the patient to apply an adjective to the pain. For example, pain may be experienced as burning, stabbing, piercing, or throbbing. Children may have difficulty describing pain; therefore, it is important to use familiar terminology, such as "boo-boo," "feel funny," or "hurt." The nurse must use quotation marks to record the description of the pain in the exact words spoken by the patient.

The intensity of pain is most accurately assessed through the use of **pain rating scales** (see Figure 11.7 ■). Most scales use a numerical rating of 0 to 5 or 0 to 10, with 0 indicating the absence of pain. Descriptors accompany the number ratings in many scales. The descriptors assist the patient to "quantify" the intensity of the pain. For children and adults who cannot read or are unable to numerically rate their pain, self-report measures may include using drawings that depict facial expressions, or visual analog scale (VAS) tools. Several variations of VAS tools are available, with one of the earliest and best-known being the Faces Pain Scale (Bieri, Reeve, Champion, Addicoat, & Ziegler, 1990). Numbers accompany each facial expression so that pain intensity can be identified. A sample pain scale that may be used to assess non–English-speaking patients and diverse populations is available at *https://ethnomed.org/clinical/end-of-life/cultural-relevance-in-end-of-life-care*.

Aggravating Factors

A variety of factors can precipitate pain. These aggravating factors include activity, exercise, turning, breathing, swallowing, urinating, and temperature or other climactic changes. Fear, anxiety, and stress can also aggravate pain.

Relieving Factors

Assessment of pain includes gathering data about the measures taken by the patient to relieve or alleviate the pain. The nurse will

---

OLDCART & ICE Acronym
O = Onset
L = Location
D = Duration
C = Characteristics
A = Aggravating Factors
R = Relieving Factors
T = Treatment
&
I = Impact on ADLs
C = Coping Strategies
E = Emotional Response

Figure 11.6 OLDCART and ICE acronym.

inquire about the use of medications; home and folk remedies; and alternative or complementary therapies, such as acupuncture, massage, and imagery. The nurse must also gather data about the effectiveness of the measures.

Treatment

This assessment includes gathering data about pharmacologic and nonpharmacologic treatments for pain.

Impact on Activities of Daily Living

Assessment of the impact of pain on ADLs enables the nurse to understand the severity of the pain and the impact of the pain on the patient's quality of life. ADLs include work, school, household and family management, mobility and transportation, leisure activities, and marital and family relationships. The nurse may ask the patient to rate the impact of the pain on each of the ADLs.

Coping Strategies

There are a variety of ways in which individuals cope with pain. Various coping strategies include but are not limited to prayer, yoga, tai chi, chi quong, support groups, distraction, relaxation techniques, or withdrawal. The strategies are often unique to the individual or reflect cultural values and beliefs. The nurse attempts to identify coping strategies employed by the patient and to determine if they are effective in pain management.

Emotional Responses

An assessment of the patient's emotional response to pain is important. Pain, especially chronic or debilitating pain, can result in depression, anxiety, and physical and emotional exhaustion. The emotional response to pain is often related to the type, intensity, and duration of pain.

Behavior and Physiologic Reponses to Pain

The observation phase of the pain assessment includes the direct observation of the patient's behavior and physiologic responses. During observation, the nurse should remember that cultural factors may significantly affect the patient's behavioral responses to pain.

Behavior

A variety of behaviors indicate the presence of pain. Many of these behaviors are nonverbal or consist of vocalizations. Behaviors indicative of pain include facial grimacing, moaning, crying or screaming, guarding or immobilization of a body part, tossing and turning, and rhythmic movements.

Physiologic Responses

The site of the pain and the duration of the pain influence physiologic responses to pain. The sympathetic nervous system is stimulated in the early stage of acute pain. The response is demonstrated in elevation of blood pressure and pulse and respiratory rates, pallor, and diaphoresis. Parasympathetic stimulation often accompanies visceral pain. This results in lowered blood pressure and pulse rate and warm, dry skin.

Focused Interview

During the focused interview, qualitative and quantitative information regarding pain will be collected. The qualitative data will include the factors under consideration when using the OLDCART & ICE acronyms described earlier in this chapter. These factors include onset, location, duration, and characteristics of the pain. The quantitative data will provide information regarding the intensity of the pain. Further questions address aggravating and relieving factors, treatments, impact on activities of daily living (ADLs), coping strategies, and emotional responses. These subjective data will be obtained using open-ended and closed questions. Follow-up questions may be needed for greater clarification regarding the pain experience. Sample questions are provided for the nurse to use to obtain the subjective data. This list of questions is not all-inclusive but does represent the types of questions required in a comprehensive focused interview. Additional questions specific to a body system are found in the assessment chapters in unit III of this text. ∞

Questions Regarding Onset

1. When did the pain begin?
2. Can you describe any circumstances associated with the onset of pain?
   Questions 1 and 2 allow the patient to describe the time frame and circumstances, both physical and emotional, that accompanied the start of the pain experience.

Questions Regarding Location

1. Where is your pain?
2. Does the pain move or is it just in one place?
3. Are you able to point to or put your finger on the painful area?
   Questions 1 to 3 give the patient the opportunity to specifically locate the pain and identify the body parts involved. An alternative method would be to give the patient a picture of the body and ask him or her to color the areas of the body affected by the pain.

Questions Regarding Duration

1. Do you have pain now?
2. Is the pain constant or intermittent?
3. How long does the pain last?
   These questions give the patient the opportunity to explain a pattern associated with pain.

Questions Regarding Characteristics of the Pain

1. How bad is the pain now?
2. Using a scale of 0 to 10, with 0 being no pain and 10 being the worst possible pain, how would you rate your present pain level?
   Questions 1 and 2 give the patient the opportunity to describe the level or intensity of the pain being experienced at the present time.
3. An alternative method would be to give the patient a pain intensity scale (refer to Figure 11.7) and ask the patient to place a mark to correspond to the pain being experienced. The nurse should be sure to use an appropriate tool for the patient. Rating scales include use of numbers and pictures, and they are language specific.

4. What does the pain feel like?

5. Describe your pain.
   Questions 4 and 5 give patients the opportunity to describe the pain using their own words.

6. An alternative method would be to list the possible descriptive terms and ask the patient to respond "yes" or "no" to each descriptor. The terms include *deep, superficial, burning, aching, pressure-like, dull, sharp, shooting, stabbing, piercing, crushing,* or *tingling. This is a comprehensive and easy way to elicit information regarding the quality of the pain.*

Questions Regarding Aggravating Factors

1. What do you think started the pain?
   This question elicits patient perceptions about the cause of pain.

2. What were you doing just before the pain started?
   This question is intended to identify triggers or factors related to the onset of pain.

3. Have you been under a great deal of stress lately?
   This is an attempt to determine a link to psychosocial factors or psychogenic sources of pain.

4. An added method to determine aggravating factors is to list common factors and ask the patient to respond "yes" or "no" when the list is read. The factors would include but are not limited to: moving, walking, turning, breathing, swallowing, and urinating.
   This permits the patient to provide specific information regarding the pain.

Questions Regarding Relieving Factors

1. What have you done to relieve the pain?

2. Did it work?

3. Have you used this before? When?

4. Why do you think it worked (or did not work) this time?
   Questions 1 to 4 provide the patient the opportunity to discuss what actions have been taken to help decrease or eliminate the pain.

Questions Regarding Treatment

1. Do you take a prescribed pain pill?

2. Do you take an over-the-counter medicine for the pain?

3. Do you change your diet in any way when you have pain?

4. Do you use an ice pack or heating pad on the pain?

5. Do you use prayer?

6. Do you or a family member perform some ritual?

7. Do you rest when you have the pain?

8. Do you do anything that has not been mentioned?
   When the patient responds "yes," the nurse must then determine the effectiveness of the strategy.

Questions Regarding Impact on Activities of Daily Living

1. Describe your daily activities.

2. How well are you able to perform these activities?

3. Does the pain in any way hinder your ability to function?
   Questions 1 to 3 encourage the patient to describe the ability to function independently on a daily basis.

4. An alternative method would be to list possible daily activities and ask the patient to respond with a "yes" or "no" if the pain hinders the ability to perform the actions.
   Examples include:
   Do you have difficulty sleeping?
   Has your appetite changed?
   Are you able to get out of bed without help?
   Do you have difficulty walking, standing, sitting, or climbing stairs?
   Are you able to perform your work activities?
   Are you able to concentrate at school, work, or home?
   Are you able to drive? To ride in a car?
   Do you have mood swings?
   Do you find yourself being short with family members and friends?

Questions Related to Coping Strategies

1. Describe how you deal or cope with the pain.

2. Are you in a support group for pain?

3. What do you do to decrease the pain so you can function and feel better?
   Questions 1 to 3 enable the patient to share his or her coping strategies. These may be unique to the individual and may reflect family values and cultural beliefs.

Questions Related to Emotional Responses

1. Emotionally, how does the pain make you feel?

2. Does your pain make you feel depressed?

3. Does your pain ever make you feel anxious, tired, or exhausted?
   Questions 1 to 3 give the nurse the opportunity to explore with the patient emotional feelings. These feelings are often related to the type, intensity, and duration of pain.

Physiologic Responses

Assessment of patient behaviors will include the collection of objective data. There are wide variations in nonverbal responses to pain. For patients who are very young, aphasic, confused, or disoriented, nonverbal expressions may be the only means of communicating pain. Facial expression is often the first indication of pain, and it may be the only one. Clenched teeth, tightly shut eyes, open somber eyes, biting of the lower lip, and other facial grimaces may be indicative of pain. Vocalizations like moaning and groaning or crying and screaming are sometimes associated with pain.

Immobilization of the body or a part of the body may also indicate pain. The patient with chest pain often holds the left arm across the chest. A person with abdominal pain may assume the position of greatest comfort, often with the knees and hips flexed, and move reluctantly.

Purposeless body movements can also indicate pain—for example, tossing and turning in bed or flinging the arms about. Involuntary movements such as a reflexive jerking away from a needle inserted through the skin indicate pain. An adult may be able to control this reflex; however, a child may be unable or unwilling to do so.

Rhythmic body movements or rubbing may indicate pain. An adult or child may assume a fetal position and rock back and forth when experiencing abdominal pain. During labor a woman may massage her abdomen rhythmically with her hands. Because behavioral responses can be controlled, they may not be very revealing. When pain is chronic, there are rarely overt behavioral responses because the individual develops personal coping styles for dealing with pain, discomfort, or suffering.

Physiologic responses vary with the origin and duration of the pain. Early in the onset of acute pain, the sympathetic nervous system is stimulated, resulting in increased blood pressure, increased pulse rate, increased respiratory rate, pallor, diaphoresis, and pupil dilation. The body does not sustain the increased sympathetic function over a prolonged period. Therefore, the sympathetic nervous system adapts, making the physiologic responses less evident or even absent. Physiologic responses are most likely to be absent in people with chronic pain because of central nervous system adaptation. Thus, it is important that the nurse assess more than the physiologic responses, because they may be poor indicators of pain.

Assessment Tools

Assessment tools have been developed to help the patient use measurable terms to describe the pain being experienced. The same tools will help the nurse obtain precise data needed to implement treatment modalities and evaluate pain relief.

The tool should be easy to use, tabulate, and score. It should be in the language of the patient, and it should be used consistently. The nurse must teach the patient, family members, and other members of the healthcare team the correct use of the tool. All tools have advantages and disadvantages. It is the responsibility of the nurse to identify these factors before implementation of the appropriate tool.

Tools used for pain assessment are designed and classified as unidimensional or multidimensional tools. A unidimensional tool will seek data regarding one aspect of pain. Many times this single element relates to the intensity of pain. Numeric rating scales, visual analogue scales, the Oucher Scale, and the Poker Chip Scale are examples of unidimensional tools (Partners Against Pain, 2013).

A multidimensional tool will seek data regarding more than one factor of pain. These tools look at intensity and other elements, including affective and sensory elements. The McGill Pain Questionnaire, short and long form, is an example of a multidimensional tool.

Unidimensional Tools

Assessment tools employed by the nurse help patients describe their pain. Unidimensional tools are used to help determine the patient's level of acute pain. The tool is called unidimensional because it assesses one aspect of pain. These tools can be used in any clinical setting across the age span. It is important for the nurse to use the tool consistently throughout the assessment, treatment, and reassessment of the patient. Because they measure just one element of the pain experience, unidimensional tools can lead to inadequate use of treatment modalities.

The Numeric Rating Scale asks the patient to describe pain intensity with a number. The selected number then equates to pain severity. The Simple Verbal Descriptive Scale is another unidimensional tool. The individual is presented with six descriptive words and is asked to select one that corresponds to the present level of intensity.

The Body Diagram tool presents an outline of the body. The individual is asked to mark the picture showing the location of the pain. Shading of the body parts by the patient will describe the intensity of the pain. As previously discussed, visual methods of rating pain have been developed that use illustrations of faces ranging from neutral to distressed. Examples of the most commonly used faces-type pain rating scales include the following:

- Faces Pain Scale (FPS) (scored 0–6)
- Faces Pain Scale–Revised (FPS-R) (scored 0–10)
- Oucher pain scale (scored 0–10)
- Wong-Baker FACES Pain Rating Scale (WBFPRS) (scored 0–10)

Research suggests that children tend to prefer the WBFPRS; however, all of the scales have proven to be useful in the clinical setting (Tomlinson, von Baeyer, Stinson, & Sung, 2010).

Multidimensional Tools

The multidimensional assessment tools assess two or more elements of pain. These tools go beyond pain intensity. They assess the nature and location of pain, the patient's mood, and the impact of pain regarding ADLs. The McGill Pain Questionnaire is available in a long and short form and is used when pain is prolonged. The long form measures intensity, location, pattern, sensory dimensions, and affective dimensions of pain. The short form measures intensity, sensory dimensions, and affective dimensions of pain.

The Brief Pain Inventory is another multidimensional scale used for assessment of pain. This tool provides information on pain and how pain interferes with the person's ability to function. Questions on this tool address medications, relief, individual beliefs, and quality of life.

Many tools are available to assist the patient and nurse to assess, treat, and evaluate pain and to measure the effectiveness of the treatment modalities. Tools must be appropriate for the age, culture, language, and cognitive abilities of the individual. Additional information about pain rating scales and tools to assess pain are available through the through authoritative online references. This chapter emphasizes pain as both physiologic and emotional. Pain perception may be increased when a patient also experiences anxiety, fatigue, or depression. The psychologic aspect of pain is a subjective and personal experience influenced by age, culture, religion, and past experience with pain.

Pain assessment requires respect for the patient's beliefs and attitudes about pain. Establishing a caring relationship, listening to the patient, and using comprehensive interview techniques are essential in the assessment of pain. Numeric scales and surveys assist the nurse in quantifying pain.

Successful management of pain is dependent on an accurate assessment of the type and degree of pain the patient is experiencing as well as the identification of underlying causes.

The assessment data are used by the nurse in interaction with the patient and other health professionals to develop a plan for pain management. The holistic approach to nursing assessment of pain permits the plan to reflect the individual beliefs, needs, and wishes of the patient.

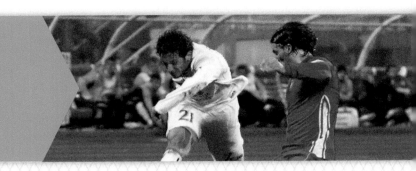

Application Through Critical Thinking

▶ Case Study

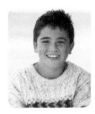

John Taylor, age 12, was hit by a car while riding his bicycle. He has several injuries and is brought to the emergency department at the local community hospital. The emergency technician informs the staff that his right leg was splinted at the scene, right pedal pulse was 56, and left pedal pulse was 76. He has a cut above his right eye that is bleeding and his right eye is swollen and partially closed. John has had no loss of consciousness; however, his respirations are 32 and shallow. He is crying and tells the nurse he has a lot of pain in his right leg, his head hurts, and he cannot seem to catch his breath. His father is at the bedside and tells him that big boys don't cry. His mom is hysterical and keeps telling John it's okay to cry.

The emergency department physician asks for a chest x-ray immediately, starts supportive oxygen therapy, and gives direction for administration of pain medication.

▶ Critical Thinking Questions

1. How and when should the nurse assess the pain in this patient?
2. What pain-scale tool, if any, would be appropriate to use?
3. What additional information regarding pain is needed?
4. What role will the parents have at this time?
5. How do cultural values and belief systems impact the perception and management of pain?

▶ References

American Academy of Pediatrics Committee on Fetus and Newborn, American Academy of Pediatrics Section on Surgery, Canadian Paediatric Society Fetus and Newborn Committee, Batton, D. G., Barrington, K. J., & Wallman, C. (2006). Prevention and management of pain in the neonate: An update. *Pediatrics, 118*(5), 2231–2241.

American Academy of Pediatrics and the Canadian Paediatric Society. (2000). Prevention and management of pain and stress in the neonate. *Pediatrics, 105*(2), 454–461.

American Pain Society. (2009). *Principles of analgesic use in the treatment of acute pain and cancer pain* (6th ed.). Glenview, IL: Author.

Andrews, M. M., & Boyle, J. S. (2011). *Transcultural concepts in nursing care* (6th ed.). Philadelphia: Lippincott Williams & Wilkins.

Ball, J. W., & Bindler, R. C. (2012). *Pediatric nursing: Caring for children* (5th ed.). Upper Saddle River, NJ: Prentice Hall.

Berman, A. J., & Snyder, S. (2011). *Kozier and Erb's fundamentals of nursing: Concepts, process, and practice* (9th ed.). Upper Saddle River, NJ: Prentice Hall.

Bieri, D., Reeve, R., Champion, G., Addicoat, L., & Ziegler, J. B. (1990). The Faces Pain Scale for the assessment of the severity of pain experienced by children: Development, initial validation, and preliminary investigation for ratio scale properties. *Pain, 41*(2), 139–150.

Bulechek, G. M., Butcher, H. K., Dochterman, J. M., & Wagner, C. (Eds.). (2013). *Nursing interventions classification (NIC)* (6th ed.). St. Louis, MO: Mosby.

Davidhizar, R. & Giger, J. N. (2004). A review of the literature on care of clients in pain who are culturally diverse. *International Nursing Review, 51*(1), 47–55.

Defrin, R., Eli, I., & Pud, D. (2011). Interactions among sex, ethnicity, religion, and gender role expectations of pain. *Gender Medicine, 8*(3), 172–183.

Hockenberry, M., & Wilson, D. (2013). *Wong's essentials of pediatric nursing* (9th ed.). St. Louis, MO: Mosby.

Kee, J., Hayes, E., & McCuistion, L. (2012). *Pharmacology: A nursing process approach* (7th ed.). St. Louis, MO: Mosby.

McCaffery, M., Ferrell, B. R., & Pasero, C. (2000). Nurses' personal opinions about patients' pain and their effect on recorded assessments and titration of opioid doses. *Pain Management Nursing, 1*(3), 79–87.

McCaffery, M., & Pasero, C. (1999). *Pain: Clinical manual* (2nd ed.). St. Louis, MO: Mosby.

Melzack, R., & Wall, P. D. (1965). Pain mechanisms: A new theory. *Science, 150,* 971–979.

Moorhead, S., Johnson, M., Maas, M., & Swanson, E. (Eds.). (2012). *Nursing outcomes classification* (5th ed.). St. Louis, MO: Mosby.

Osborn K. S., Wraa, C. E., Watson, A., & Holleran, R. S. (2013). *Medical-surgical nursing: Preparation for practice* (2nd ed.). Upper Saddle River, NJ: Pearson.

Paice, J. A. (2002). Understanding nociceptive pain. *Nursing, 32*(3), 74–75.

Partners Against Pain. (2013). *Pain assessment scales.* Stanford, CT: Purdue Pharma L. P. Retrieved from http://www.partnersagainstpain.com/measuring-pain/assessment-tool.aspx

Pasero, C., & McCaffery, M. (2002). Pain control: Monitoring sedation. *American Journal of Nursing, 102*(2), 67–68.

Racine, M., Tousignant-Laflamme, Y., Kloda, L. A., Dion, D., Dupuis, G., & Choinière, M. (2012). A systematic literature review of 10 years of research on sex/gender and experimental pain perception–Part 1: Are there really differences between women and men? *Pain, 153*(3), 602–618.

Sadosky, A., Hopper, J., & Parsons, B. (2014). Painful diabetic peripheral neuropathy: Results of a survey characterizing the perspectives and misperceptions of patients and healthcare practitioners. *The Patient-Patient-Centered Outcomes Research, 7*(1), 107-114.

Tomlinson, D., von Baeyer, C. L., Stinson, J. N., & Sung, L. (2010). A systematic review of faces scales for the self-report of pain intensity in children. *Pediatrics, 126*(5), e1168–e1198.

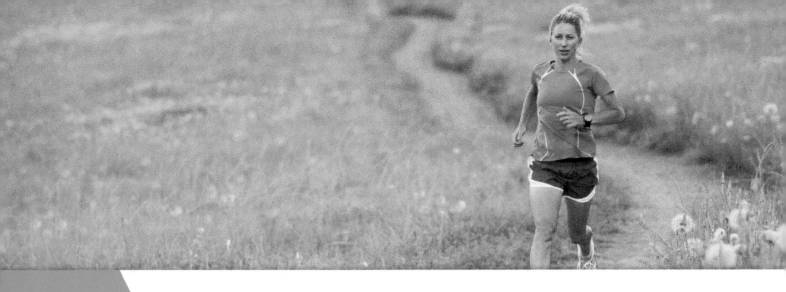

▶ Learning Outcomes

Upon completion of this chapter, you will be able to:

1. Define nutritional health.

2. Outline risk factors that affect nutritional health status.

3. Discuss the objectives described in *Healthy People 2020* that relate to nutrition.

4. Identify the physical and laboratory parameters utilized in a nutrition assessment.

5. Identify the components of a diet history and techniques for gathering diet history data.

6. Describe existing validated nutritional assessment tools.

7. Develop questions to be used when completing a focused interview.

8. Differentiate between normal and abnormal findings in a nutritional assessment.

9. Determine specific nutritional assessment techniques and tools appropriate for unique stages in the life span.

10. Discuss strategies for integrating a complete nutritional assessment into the nursing care process.

Key Terms

Nutritional health is a crucial component of overall health across the life span. The nutritional health of a pregnant female will influence pregnancy outcome. Nutritional health in growing children plays a central role in growth and development. In adults and older adults, nutritional health can be associated with the prevention or development of chronic disease in conditions involving both **undernutrition** and **overnutrition**. Undernutrition, also called **malnutrition**, describes health effects of insufficient nutrient intake or poor nutrient stores; overnutrition results from excesses in nutrient intake or stores.

The determination of an individual's nutritional status is based on the foundation of a thorough nutritional assessment. The assessment portion of the nursing care process incorporates the gathering and interpretation of data often used as part of a nutritional assessment. These data then create the base for later development of appropriate nursing and nutritional interventions aimed at preserving or improving nutritional health.

Defining Nutritional Health

Nutritional health can be defined as the physical result of the balance between nutrient intake and nutritional requirements. For example, an individual who consumes excess saturated fat may be at risk for elevated blood cholesterol and cardiovascular disease. This person may, therefore, be considered to have poor nutritional health due to overnutrition. A pregnant female who consumes less than the required amounts of folic acid may place her unborn child at risk for certain birth defects, such as neural tube defects, and could be considered in poor nutritional health due to undernutrition. A patient who consumes adequate nutrition to meet individual needs and avoids habitual excesses and insufficiencies would be considered in good nutritional health.

Many factors can influence nutritional health. When gathering data for a nutritional assessment, it is important to realize common risk factors for a poor nutritional status. Overnutrition in the form of excess dietary intake of fat, especially saturated fat, has been associated with an increased risk of atherosclerosis. **Overweight** and **obesity** are linked with increased risk of hypertension, cardiovascular disease, type 2 diabetes, some cancers, degenerative joint disease, and other conditions. Additionally, excess body weight has been shown to increase the risk of mortality from cardiovascular disease, diabetes mellitus, kidney disease, and certain cancers in adults 30 to 74 years of age. In the United States, almost 70% of males and females 20 to 74 years of age are considered overweight or obese. More than one-third of adults are obese, a statistic that has not improved over the last decade. More than one-third of children and adolescents are overweight or obese. Excess alcohol intake is associated with chronic liver disease and cirrhosis,

the 12th leading cause of death in the United States according to the National Center for Health Statistics at the Centers for Disease Control and Prevention (CDC).

Undernutrition is less common than overnutrition in the United States, but it can have devastating physical health consequences when **protein-calorie malnutrition** or other nutrient deficiencies develop. Undernutrition can lead to growth faltering, compromised immune status, poor wound healing, muscle loss, physical and functional decline, and lack of proper development. Generally, individuals at risk for undernutrition include those who have a chronic illness or are poor, elderly, hospitalized, restrictive eaters (from chronic dieting or disordered eating), or alcoholics. An individual can have both overnutrition and undernutrition, such as an overweight child who consumes no fruit or vegetables. The **obesity paradox** is a term used to denote both the presense of obesity and nutritional deficiency together. **Food deserts** contribute to the obesity paradox. Food deserts are low-income, urban or rural areas that lack access to healthy, affordable food. When food is available in a food desert, it is generally high-calorie food of poor nutritional quality, such as food that is found in fast-food restaurants and convenience stores. (USDA, n.d.b). Box 12.1 outlines additional risk factors for overnutrition and undernutrition to consider when conducting a nutrition assessment. The patient education section on page 270 offers suggestions on advice and education to reduce these risks.

Health Promotion

As discussed in previous chapters, the U.S. Department of Health and Human Services, Office of Disease Prevention and Health Promotion, has established a collaborative public health initiative called *Healthy People 2020* aimed at both increasing the quality and years of healthy life in the U.S. population and reducing health disparities. Overarching goals of *Healthy People 2020* are to promote health and prevent disease. The *Healthy People 2020* objectives are important reminders to the clinician of the central role nutrition plays in overall health across the life span. Issues related to overweight and obesity are considered to be among the areas monitored to track progress toward achievement of overall goals. The *Healthy People 2020* goals related to nutrition and weight status (NWS) and Maternal, Infant, and Child Health (MICH) are presented in Table 12.1.

The increasing prevalence of overweight and obesity in the United States, as well as the statistics on nutritional health disparities, illustrate the importance of nutritional screening and assessment as the first step toward reaching these important goals. Box 12.2 outlines the cultural and socioeconomic influences that may affect nutritional health.

Box 12.1　Risk Factors for Poor Nutritional Health

Undernutrition

- Chronic disease, acute illness, wounds, or injury—including symptoms and treatment.
- Multiple medications and medication side effects that reduce intake or alter nutrient metabolism.
- Food insecurity—lack of money or access to adequate and safe food. Includes food deserts.
- Restrictive eating due to medical conditions requiring altered diet that reduces intake of food groups or nutrients. For example, a very low-fat diet with fat malabsorption, a gluten-free diet with celiac disease, or a low potassium and protein modified diet with renal failure.
- Food allergies and intolerances. Multiple food allergies further increase risk because of broader avoidance of food groups.
- Self-diagnosed or self-prescribed diets. Avoidance of foods or food groups without demonstrated medical need leads to unnecessary elimination of foods, food groups, and accompanying nutrients. For example, eliminating gluten without celiac disease or diagnosed gluten intolerance.
- Restrictive eating due to chronic dieting, disordered eating, or food faddism such as trendy diets, cleanses, or nutritional beliefs. For example, following a vegan diet and not assuring adequate supplemental sources of vitamins B_{12} and D, which are lacking in a plant-only diet.

- Alcohol abuse, which may cause both reduced intake and altered nutrient metabolism.
- Depression, bereavement, loneliness, social isolation.
- Poor dental health.
- Chewing and swallowing difficulties including those from altered dental/oral health, decreased saliva production, medication side-effects, or a medical diagnosis.
- Alterations in sensory perception such as decreased vision, hearing, taste and smell, touch.
- Decreased functional status (e.g., dependency on others, cognitive changes).
- Decreased knowledge or skills about food preparation and recommendations.
- Extreme age—premature infants or adults over 80 years of age.

Overnutrition

- Excess intake of solid fats, added sugars, or calories.
- Excess intake of any nutrient from foods, fortified foods, or dietary supplements.
- Alcohol abuse.
- Sedentary lifestyle.
- Decreased knowledge or skills about food preparation and recommendations.

TABLE 12.1　Examples of *Healthy People 2020* Objectives Related to Nutrition and Weight Status (NWS) and Maternal, Infant, and Child Health (MICH)

OBJECTIVE NUMBER	DESCRIPTION
NWS-1/2	Increase the number of States with nutrition standards for foods and beverages provided to preschool-aged children in child care. Increase the proportion of schools that offer nutritious foods and beverages outside of school meals
NWS-3	Increase the number of States that have State-level policies that incentivize food retail outlets to provide foods that are encouraged by the Dietary Guidelines for Americans.
NWS-4	(Developmental) Increase the proportion of Americans who have access to a food retail outlet that sells a variety of foods that are encouraged by the Dietary Guidelines for Americans
NWS-5	Increase the proportion of primary care physicians who regularly measure the body mass index of their patients
NWS -6	Increase the proportion of physician office visits that include counseling or education related to nutrition or weight
NWS-7	(Developmental) Increase the proportion of worksites that offer nutrition or weight management classes or counseling
NWS-8/9/10/11	Increase the proportion of adults who are at a healthy weight. Reduce the proportion of adults who are obese. Reduce the proportion of children and adolescents who are considered obese. Prevent inappropriate weight gain in youth and adults
NWS-12/13	Eliminate very low food security among children. Reduce household food insecurity and in doing so reduce hunger

TABLE 12.1	Examples of *Healthy People 2020* Objectives Related to Nutrition and Weight Status (NWS) and Maternal, Infant, and Child Health (MICH) (continued)

OBJECTIVE NUMBER	DESCRIPTION
NWS-14/15/16/17/18/19/20	In the diet of the population aged 2 years and older: Increase the variety and contribution of vegetables Increase the contribution of whole grains Reduce the consumption of calories from solid fats and added sugars Reduce consumption of saturated fat Reduce consumption of sodium Increase consumption of calcium
NWS-21/22	Reduce iron deficiency among young children and females of childbearing age. Reduce iron deficiency among pregnant females.
MICH-8	Reduce low birth weight (LBW) and very low birth weight (VLBW)
MICH-14	Increase the proportion of women of childbearing potential with intake of at least 400 mcg of folic acid from fortified foods or dietary supplements

Source: United States Department of Health and Human Services. (2014). *Healthy People 2020.* Retrieved from http://www.healthypeople.gov/2020/topicsobjectives2020/default.aspx

Box 12.2 Cultural and Socioeconomic Influences on Nutritional Health

Overweight and Obesity

- Almost 70% of adults ages 20 to 74 years are overweight or obese. Almost 35% of adults are obese, a statistic that has not improved in the last decade.
- Over 17% of children ages 2 to 19 years are obese.
- Prevalence of obesity in males is highest among Hispanic males.
- Prevalence of obesity in females is highest among Black females.
- Hypertension, a comorbidity of overweight and obesity, affects 55.1% of adults in the United States.
- Prevalence of hypertension is highest among Mexican American and Black males.
- Adults of low socioeconomic status have almost double the rate of overweight or obesity compared to those of medium and high socioeconomic status.

Undernutrition

- Up to 60% of older adults in dependent care or hospitals are malnourished.
- Adequate folic acid and iron status are important for healthy outcomes during pregnancy. Pregnant Mexican American and Black females are more likely than other ethnic groups to have iron deficiency and low folic acid levels. Females of lower economic status and those with less education are also more likely to have inadequate folic acid or iron status.
- Black women and adolescents under age 15 years are more likely to have insufficient gestational weight gain and more likely to deliver low–birth weight babies than other populations.

Poverty and Food Insecurity

- Among Americans, the prevalence of poverty is 15%.
- Children under age 18 experience a 21.8% poverty rate.
- Prevalence of poverty is highest among Blacks (27.2%) and Hispanics (25.6%).

Sources: Centers for Disease Control and Prevention (CDC). (2014). *Health, United States, 2012.* Retrieved from http://www.cdc.gov/nchs/hus.htm; United States Department of Health and Human Services. (2013). *Healthy People 2020. 19 Nutrition and weight status.* Retrieved from http://www.healthypeople.gov/2020/topicsobjectives2020/objectiveslist.aspx?topicId=29; Ogden, C. L., Carroll, M. D., Kit, B. K., & Flegal, K. M. (2014). Prevalence of childhood and adult obesity in the United States, 2011–2012. *Journal of the American Medical Association, 311,* 806–814; U.S. Census Bureau. (2013). *Current Population Survey Annual Social and Economic Supplement (CPS ASEC): Income, poverty, and health insurance coverage in the United States, 2012.* Retrieved from http://www.census.gov/hhes/www/poverty/data/incpovhlth/2012/index.html.

Nutritional Assessment

A nutritional assessment is the foundation on which nursing diagnoses are developed and on which the implementation of goals and objectives in the nursing care process are later created. The prevention or treatment of malnutrition and overnutrition first requires a nutritional assessment. Determination of an individual's nutritional status should be accomplished while gathering data for a nursing assessment.

Nutritional assessment techniques and tools vary in their level of sophistication and depth. No one piece of data can give a complete nutritional assessment. Many parameters used to assess nutritional status can be affected by nonnutritional influences such as disease, medication, or environment. This illustrates the need to gather data from varying resources. Generally, an assessment done using multiple variables will be more valuable than an assessment made with limited data. In some healthcare situations, not all parameters or data are available. The nurse must rely on available information and sharp clinical judgment when making an assessment.

Varying medical diagnoses or issues specific to the life span will also influence pertinent parameters and techniques used in assessing a patient's nutritional status. For example, measuring waist circumference may be of use when assessing potential overnutrition in some adults, but would be of little nutritional use when assessing either a patient with ascites or a pregnant female.

A registered dietitian (RD) is generally responsible for completing a comprehensive nutritional assessment in most acute or long-term care settings; a nurse may do this as well and is most often the frontline clinician who obtains the data needed for a nutritional assessment. A nurse is ideally situated to identify nutritionally at-risk patients who need further intervention targeting nutritional health.

The components used in a nutritional assessment include the physical assessment, anthropometric measurements, laboratory values, and a nutritional history. Several validated assessment tools exist to streamline the nutritional assessment process for use in a variety of healthcare settings or with specific populations. Other tools exist that simply screen for risk factors for poor nutritional health and facilitate the necessary referrals to appropriate clinicians.

Nutritional History

A careful nutritional history is part of a comprehensive nutritional assessment and is best accomplished using more than one tool. A diet recall, a food frequency questionnaire, and a food record are components of a nutritional history that can be complemented with a focused interview for more specific information.

Diet Recall

A **diet recall**, also called a 24-hour recall, can be done quickly in most settings to obtain a snapshot assessment of dietary intake. A patient is asked to verbally recall all food, beverages, and nutritional supplements or products consumed in a set 24-hour period. Obtaining a recall for both a weekday and one weekend day will strengthen the data obtained by showing examples of more than one type of typical day. In order to appear nonjudgmental and not hint at "correct" answers to questions, the nurse should ask primarily open-ended questions. The nurse should begin the diet recall by asking, "Tell me what you ate yesterday (or on a specific day). When was the

first time you had something to eat or drink in the day?" This type of questioning avoids asking the assuming question "What did you have for breakfast?" Patients may feel judged if they admit they skip breakfast or feel too embarrassed to admit missing a meal. The result may be an inaccurate recall in which patients contrive answers they feel the nurse is seeking. Gentle prompting to obtain complete information is often needed. The nurse should ask about all food from meals and snacks; all liquids, remembering to include alcohol; and any use of nutritional supplements such as herbs, vitamins, and minerals, or diet and sports nutritional products. One must determine whether fortified versions of common foods are consumed in order to assess nutrient intake accurately. Many foods are now fortified and should not be overlooked as significant sources of vitamins and minerals. Cereals and juices are examples of fortified foods to which nutrients not normally found in the product, such as calcium, have been added. The nurse can prompt the patient to share information regarding modifications in the diet by asking "Have you ever followed a special diet for any reason such as to change your weight, treat a condition, or alter your nutritional health?" and following with "Please tell me more about that" if an affirmative answer is given. Notice that the question uses the phrase "change your weight" and does not specifically ask about weight loss or gain so as to not appear judgmental. A family member may participate in the interview with the permission of the patient or if the patient is unable to give a recall as in the case of an adult with communication difficulties or a child. Accuracy of a secondhand recall, even from a family member, has been found to be variable.

A best estimate of portion sizes will improve the accuracy of a recall. It is easy to over- and underestimate portion sizes of foods and liquids without a visual comparison. Life-size culturally appropriate food models are available. Digital photographs are less cumbersome and easily available as well. It is not always convenient to carry facsimiles to different settings where the nurse may be interviewing a patient. In such cases, use of the food analogies in Figure 12.1 ■ can be helpful.

There are drawbacks to the exclusive use of a diet recall for a obtaining a patient's nutritional history. A 24-hour recall is simply a 1-day example of intake and may not be indicative of normal habits. Other types and amounts of intake may occur on different days that were not assessed. Patients may have significant food habits that occur occasionally but not on the day recalled. The use of dietary supplements or alcohol often does not occur in the same fashion each day, yet it is crucial information to assess. Many other important data related to diet could be overlooked by relying on the recall alone. The accuracy of the recall relies heavily on the memory of the patient and good interviewing skills of the nurse. Repeated diet recalls taken during subsequent healthcare visits can be used for comparison purposes and validation of intake.

Underreporting bias can occur with all parts of a nutritional history and may become apparent during the recall. Patients seeking the social approval of the nurse or wanting to avoid disapproval for their habits may underreport. Underreporting occurs for all ages and is seen more often in smokers, the obese, and individuals with lower educational and socioeconomic levels. Additionally, alcohol and drug use are frequently underreported. A nonjudgmental approach during the nutritional history will provide an environment conducive to full answers by the patient. In addition to asking open-ended questions, using a neutral tone of voice and maintaining facial

Small potato or piece of fruit: computer mouse

3 oz animal protein: deck of cards

1 oz cheese: small box of wooden matches

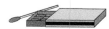

2 tbsp: golf ball

4 tbsp: four thumbs

1 cup dry measure: tightly clenched small woman's fist

Figure 12.1 Analogies for estimating portion size.

expressions that do not hint at approval or disapproval are key to appearing nonjudgmental. Combining the recall with a food frequency assessment and a focused interview will yield the best information on which to base an assessment.

Food Frequency Questionnaire

A **food frequency questionnaire** assesses intake of a variety of food groups on a daily, weekly, or longer basis. This questionnaire helps to fill in some of the missing data not captured by a 24-hour recall and helps to provide a more balanced assessment of intake. For example, in a 24-hour recall a patient may indicate no fruit intake, while during a food frequency assessment two servings of fruit and one serving of juice are reported as a daily average. When an entire category of food seems missing, the nurse can ask further questions to ascertain the reason. In this way, using both the recall and the food frequency questionnaire can uncover information that might not otherwise have surfaced in the conversation. Food intolerances, allergies, dieting, and food faddism are examples. Food frequency questionnaires can be formal instruments composed of a checklist of food groups and foods or shorter questionnaires aimed at gathering general information. All food, beverage,

and supplement groups should be included. Patients can fill out longer checklists before or after an interview but may find such tools cumbersome. Shorter questionnaires can be administered verbally and are more practical. Table 12.2 is an example of a basic food frequency questionnaire.

Food Record

Keeping a food record or diary for up to 3 days can provide supplemental information for a nutritional history. Recording two sequential weekdays and a weekend day works well. Food diaries longer than 3 days in length tend to be recorded retrospectively with a loss of accuracy. Underreporting bias should also be considered when evaluating a food diary.

Focused Nutritional History Interview

A diet recall, food frequency questionnaire, or food diary can be used alone or in combination as parameters in a quick nutritional assessment. Conducting a more focused interview along with these tools, either as part of a nursing assessment or just concerning nutrition, will give the clearest picture of nutritional status.

A nutrition-focused interview can easily occur at the same time as a diet recall. As the recall is conducted, pertinent ancillary questions can be asked. For example, a patient may report drinking cranberry juice at breakfast because of intolerance to citrus fruits. The nurse could then use that cue to ask if there are other intolerances or food allergies before getting back on track to the recall. The remainder of the needed nutrition history data can be gathered from the patient and the medical chart after the recall portion of the interview. This more extensive form of a nutritional history assesses current habits but also can assess former habits. Past chronic dieting, supplement use, and therapeutic diets are examples of important historic data to gather. Box 12.3 outlines data topics to gather during the focused interview in addition to diet recall data. Table 12.3 is an example of a nutrition assessment form combining diet recall, food frequency, and focused interview data.

Physical Assessment

The physical assessment portion of a nutritional assessment consists of two parts: **anthropometric** measurements and a head-to-toe physical assessment of a patient. Anthropometric measurements include any scientific measurement of the body. Pertinent data from the medical history and examination should be considered during this portion of a nutritional assessment. The healthcare setting and the patient's needs dictate the depth of data gathered. Height, weight, and measurements of body fat and muscle composition are anthropometric measurements. At times, estimated measurements and alternative techniques for obtaining anthropometric data may be necessary due to specific circumstances that make standard measurement difficult or impossible.

Height

Measurement of height is needed in adults to make an accurate assessment of weight status. In children, height is monitored on a continuum to assess growth and, indirectly, nutritional status. See chapter 10 for accurate height assessment methods. ∞

| TABLE 12.2 | **Food Frequency Questionnaire** | | | | |

FOOD	VARIETY	TYPE	AMOUNT PER DAY	AMOUNT PER WEEK	LESS THAN ONCE PER WEEK (LIST)
Fruit	Juice Fresh Canned/frozen	apple	12 oz		
		melon		1 cup	
		none			
Vegetables	Green Other	varied		1–2×	
		squash		1×	
Dairy	Milk Cheese Yogurt	low fat	2 cups		
					1× month
		never			
Protein	Animal Plant	poultry or fish	each night		
		soyburger or tofu		1–2×	
Fats	Saturated Unsaturated	butter	1–2 pats		
		olive oil		tbsp	
Fluids	General Caffeine Alcohol	water	4 oz 4× with meds		
		tea	each a.m.		
		wine		3×	
Sweets and Sugars		cookies	2×		
Supplements	Vitamin/mineral Herbal Other: Over-the-counter weight loss product	multivitamin	one		
		echinacea			4–5× year for cold
		cannot recall ingredients			tried once and stopped, complains of feeling dizzy

When no means of obtaining measured height is feasible, self-reported height may be used. Every effort should be made to obtain a current measured height, but this is not always possible. The accuracy of self-reported heights can be questionable. Men, women, and adolescents have been reported to overstate self-reported height by up to 2 cm (.787 in.). Adults over the age of 60 years have been reported to overstate height by approximately 2.5 cm (.984 in.). When self-reported heights are used, it should be noted in the documentation.

Weight

Current body weight and weight history are essential components of a nutritional assessment. Every effort should be made to obtain actual weight since self-reported weights are often underreported in men and women. In the individual with undetected weight loss, self-reported weight could delay proper nutritional intervention by masking the clinical change. See chapter 10 for accurate methods to determine the patient's weight. ∞

Weight history is crucial to determine the presence of any intentional or unplanned weight losses. Weight history is also followed in children and pregnant females to monitor growth and development. Weight guidelines for children and pregnant females are outlined in the Nutritional Assessment Across the Life Span section on page 203. When obtaining a weight history, the nurse should look for prior documentation of actual weight, if available. Otherwise, open-ended questions can be asked, such as "When was the last time you were weighed?" followed by "What did you weigh then?" The nurse may also ask for weights at specific points in time as a cross-check: "What did you weigh this past summer before coming to college?" The nurse should not simply ask, "Has your weight changed recently?" as the patient may not have an accurate answer or may not want to divulge any known gain or loss. The nurse can discern whether weight change has occurred by asking for specific weight information and calculating any noted differences.

Unintentional weight loss of 5% or more of body weight over a month or 10% or more over 6 months is considered clinically significant and warrants attention. Weight change is calculated using the following formula:

([prior weight − current weight]/prior weight) ×100 = % weight change

Box 12.4 on page 194 outlines an example of calculations used to determine percent weight change.

TABLE 12.3   Nutrition Assessment Form

NUTRITION EVALUATION

Name: _____   Date: _____

Home Address: _____   Referred By: _____

_____   _____

Phone: _____   _____

Age: _____   Signed Consent/Date: _____

Height (Ht) _____   Weight (Wt) _____   Recent wt change _____   Max/Min wts _____   Patient goal _____

Body fat % _____   Wt Hx _____   Exercise _____   Ex. freq/duration _____   Other activities _____

Medical Hx/Dx _____   Rx and OTC meds _____   Vits/minerals _____   Supplements _____   Herbs _____

Previous Diets _____   Food allergies/ intolerances _____   Food prep/refrig _____   Restrictive? _____   Living with _____

Binge? _____   Purge? _____   Laxatives? _____   Other? _____

Diet Hx: _____   Diet Hx: _____

M–F _____   Weekends _____

FOOD FREQUENCY

Fruit (indicate day/week/other) **Dairy** (indicate day/week/other) **Fats** (indicate day/week/other)

vit C _____   milk/yogurt _____   saturated _____

other _____   cheese _____   polyunsaturated _____

_____   other _____   monounsaturated _____

VEGETABLES   **ANIMAL PROTEIN**   **SUGARS/SWEETS**

green _____   _____   _____

other _____   _____   _____

GRAINS/STARCH   **PLANT PROTEIN**   **FLUIDS-WATER**

whole grain _____   _____   other _____

other _____   _____   caffeinated _____

_____   _____   alcohol _____

Source: Provided courtesy of Sheila Tucker, MA, RD, CSSD, LDN.

Box 12.3 Nutritional History Data

Food

- All meals and snacks—note timing to assess for large gaps or missed meals
- All liquids, including water, alcohol, and sweetened and caffeinated beverages
- Use of fortified foods
- Preparation methods, including whether food was fresh, frozen, canned, packaged, or pre-made
- Portion sizes
- Grocery habits

Beliefs and Practices

- Adherence to a therapeutic diet for medical reasons or due to food allergy or food intolerance
- Cultural or religious influences on food choices and practices
- Faddism—trendy food and nutrition beliefs
- Lifestyle diet choices—vegetarianism, vegan diet, avoidance of certain foods or food groups
- **Pica**—if craving for nonfood substances present: types of substances eaten, source, and amounts
- Meal patterns—number and frequency of meals and snacks, missed meals, location of meals

(continued)

Box 12.3 Nutritional History Data (continued)

Supplement and Medication Use

- Vitamin and mineral use—dose, frequency, and constituents
- Herbal use—dose, frequency, and constituents
- Over-the-counter weight loss or sports supplements—dose, frequency, and ingredients
- Over-the-counter and prescription medications to assess for drug-nutrient interactions or drug-herb interactions

Socioeconomic and Educational Influences

- Education and literacy level
- Knowledge and skills related to food and nutrition

- Social environment—assess for isolation and social support system
- General economic status and access to adequate food (**food security**)
- Functional capacity related to activities of daily living (ADL) and independent activities of daily living (IADL) (such as shopping, meal preparation, self-feeding)
- Activity level

Box 12.4 Calculating Weight Loss Percentage

A community health nurse is visiting the senior center for a seasonal flu shot clinic. Miss M., an 80-year-old female, complains that she needs to sew new elastic into her skirt as the old elastic is not working to keep the skirt on her waistline. The nurse wonders if she has lost some weight since the last visit and weighs her. She weighs 108 lb, down from 120 lb 6 months ago.

(120 lb prior weight − 108 lb current weight)/120 lb prior weight
= 12 lb weight loss / 120 lb prior weight = 0.10
0.10 × 100 = 10% weight loss in 6 months

TABLE 12.4   Classification of Body Mass Index (BMI) in Adults

BMI	CLASSIFICATION
<16	Severe underweight
16–16.99	Moderate underweight
17–18.49	Mild underweight
18.5–24.9	Normal
25–29.9	Overweight
30–34.9	Obese class 1
35–39.9	Obese class 2
≤40	Obese class 3

Sources: United States Department of Health and Human Services, National Heart, Lung, and Blood Institute. (n.d.). Classification of overweight and obesity by BMI, waist circumference, and associated disease risks. Retrieved from http://www.nhlbi.nih.gov/health/public/heart/obesity/lose_wt/bmi_dis .htm; World Health Organization. (2014). *BMI classification.* Retrieved from http://apps.who.int/bmi/index.jsp?introPage=intro_3.html

Body Mass Index

Body mass index (BMI) is widely used to assess appropriate weight for height using the following formula: $BMI = weight (kg)/height^2$ (meters). Parameters have been established to delineate underweight, healthy weight, and overweight standards in adults based on current scientific findings of morbidity and mortality prevalence associated with various BMI values. The National Heart, Lung, and Blood Institute (NHLBI), along with the World Health Organization (WHO), have established internationally used classifications for BMI, which are outlined in Table 12.4. Many charts, tables, and nomograms exist to make BMI calculations quick and easy for clinical application.

Exclusive use of BMI as an indicator of weight status makes the assumption that all individuals have equal body composition at each given weight. Also, it assumes that every person of the same weight has the same amount of muscle mass, body fat, and bone mineral content. This generalization has not been found to be true and, therefore, represents a clinical limitation to the use of BMI alone when assessing weight. Athletic people with little body

fat and ample muscle mass can be classified as overweight using BMI despite a visual assessment that reveals a high level of fitness. Likewise, an individual's BMI may fall within the classification of healthy, yet the person may have little muscle mass and excess body fat.

BMI classifications exist as generic standards of height–weight comparisons for the general population. Racial differences have been observed in body composition. Asian adults have been reported to have a higher proportion of body fat mass at a given BMI than Caucasians. African American adults have greater muscle mass and bone mineral density at a given BMI than Caucasians.

Additionally, ethnic differences within race categories have been observed. For example, Chinese adults have been observed to have proportionately higher body fat mass at a given BMI than Polynesians. Despite these variances, different standards for BMI do not exist for any ethnic populations. These drawbacks indicate the problem of using BMI as a sole indicator of weight status or nutritional health and are an excellent example of the need to use multiple parameters when conducting an assessment. In particular, it is recommended that BMI be used in conjunction with waist circumference when assessing the adult for health risks associated with overweight or obesity.

Height–Weight Tables

Height–weight tables have been used in the past to assess body weight in adults but are no longer a standard. Such tables outlined reference weights for given heights for both males and females or were gender specific. Table 12.5 is an example of a current height–weight table based on BMI calculations presented in an easy-to-use form.

Use of such height–weight tables has the same limitations as does use of BMI as a sole indicator of weight status. Differences in body composition go largely unaccounted for and the clinician must remember to assess each person for these individual differences.

TABLE 12.5 **Height–Weight Table with BMI Calculation**

Locate the height of interest in the leftmost column and read across the row for that height to the weight of interest. Follow the column of the weight up to the top row that lists the BMI. BMI of 19–24 is the healthy weight range, BMI of 25–29 is the overweight range, and BMI of 30 and above is in the obese range.

BMI	19	20	21	22	23	24	25	26	27	28	29	30	31	32	33	34	35
HEIGHT	WEIGHT IN POUNDS																
4'10"	91	96	100	105	110	115	119	124	129	134	138	143	148	153	158	162	167
4'11"	94	99	104	109	114	119	124	128	133	138	143	148	153	158	163	168	173
5'	97	102	107	112	118	123	128	133	138	143	148	153	158	163	158	174	179
5'1"	100	106	111	116	122	127	132	137	143	148	153	158	164	169	174	180	185
5'2"	104	109	115	120	126	131	136	142	147	153	158	164	169	175	180	186	191
5'3"	107	113	118	124	130	135	141	146	152	158	163	169	175	180	186	191	197
5'4"	110	116	122	128	134	140	145	151	157	163	169	174	180	186	192	197	204
5'5"	114	120	126	132	138	144	150	156	162	168	174	180	186	192	198	204	210
5'6"	118	124	130	136	142	148	155	161	167	173	179	186	192	198	204	210	216
5'7"	121	127	134	140	146	153	159	166	172	178	185	191	198	204	211	217	223
5'8"	125	131	138	144	151	158	164	171	177	184	190	197	203	210	216	223	230
5'9"	128	135	142	149	155	162	169	176	182	189	196	203	209	216	223	230	236
5'10"	132	139	146	153	160	167	174	181	188	195	202	209	216	222	229	236	243
5'11"	136	143	150	157	165	172	179	186	193	200	208	215	222	229	236	243	250
6'	140	147	154	162	169	177	184	191	199	206	213	221	228	235	242	250	258
6'1"	144	151	159	166	174	182	189	197	204	212	219	227	235	242	250	257	265
6'2"	148	155	163	171	179	186	194	202	210	218	225	233	241	249	256	264	272
6'3"	152	160	168	176	184	192	200	208	216	224	232	240	248	256	264	272	279
	Healthy Weight						Overweight					Obese					

Source: National Institutes of Health, National Heart, Lung, and Blood Institute (NIH/NHLBI). (n.d.). Body Mass Index Table. Retrieved from http://www.nhlbi.nih.gov/guidelines/obesity/bmi_tbl.htm

Waist Circumference

Excess, centrally located abdominal fat deposition is considered to be an independent risk factor for cardiovascular disease in adults. Measurement of waist circumference can be included in a comprehensive nutritional assessment, especially when risk factors for cardiovascular disease exist. The NHLBI considers waist circumference greater than 102 cm (40.16 in.) in males and greater than 88 cm (34.65 in.) in females indicative of risk.

Waist circumference should be measured with a spring-loaded measuring tape to ensure reliable tension is applied with each measurement. Use of the bony landmark on the lateral border of the ilium is recommended when marking a site guide for the measurement. Figure 12.2 ■ depicts the location of this landmark. Standing behind the patient and palpating the right hip can locate the lateral ilium. A line should be drawn at the uppermost lateral line of the ilium at the midaxillary point. Other references suggest measuring waist circumference just below the umbilicus, but this can be unreliable since an obese state can change the position of the umbilicus. Waist circumference should be measured at the marked midaxillary line while keeping the measuring tape parallel to the floor. Measurement should be done directly on the surface of the skin and not over clothing. It has been suggested that taking measurements with the patient in front of a mirror is helpful to ensure a true horizontal extension of the measuring tape, especially in those who are obese or have wider hips than waist. The spring-loaded measuring tape should be pulled taut but should not compress the skin. Uneven tension on the measure between sequential measurements will alter reliability of waist circumference measurements.

Waist circumference validity can be limited by obesity when increases in abdominal fat mass become pendulous due to the effects of gravity and no longer are situated along the waistline. Increases in abdominal subcutaneous fat and increases in body weight may not always be reflected by increases in waist circumference. Additionally, waist circumference is not a valid nutritional tool for use in adults with ascites, for pregnant females, or for those with other medical conditions associated with increases in fat-free abdominal girth, such as polycystic kidney disease.

Body Composition Measurement

More specific assessment of body fat and muscle mass than weight alone can be made using skinfold measurements or technologic instruments. Muscle mass is also referred to as **somatic protein** stores or skeletal muscle. This second tier of anthropometric measurements can assess body composition either in just two components, fat and fat-free mass, or in multicomponents, which can include more precise analysis of fat-free mass for muscle, bone, and fluid components. Increasing levels of technology and updating of older reference values to include multicomponent analysis will allow more valid assessment of body composition in the future.

Skinfold Measurements

Skinfold thickness measurements can estimate subcutaneous body fat stores. Measurements taken at up to eight sites on the body are believed to be predictive of overall body fat composition. Sites include the triceps, chest, subscapular, midaxillary, suprailiac, abdomen, and upper thigh.

The tricep skinfold (TSF) is the site most often used to estimate subcutaneous fat because of easy access to this measurement in most situations. Tricep measurements are done at the midpoint of the arm equidistant from the uppermost posterior edge of the acromion process of the scapula and the olecranon process of the elbow. A measuring tape should be used to determine this midpoint on the back of the upper arm, and the site should be marked for reference. It is helpful to have the patient flex the arm at a 90-degree angle while locating the bony landmarks and measuring the midpoint. However, the arm should hang freely during the skinfold measurement itself. Figure 12.3 ■ illustrates the location of the TSF measurement.

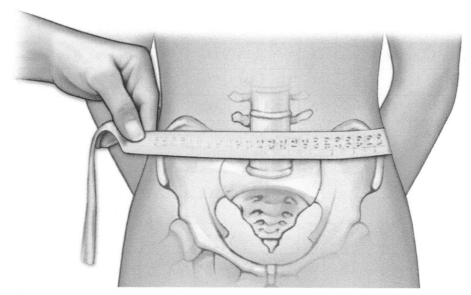

Figure 12.2 Landmarks for waist circumference.

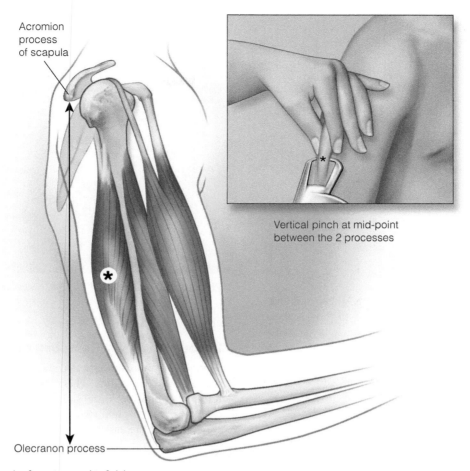

Acromion
process
of scapula

Olecranon process

Vertical pinch at mid-point
between the 2 processes

Figure 12.3 Landmarks for triceps skinfold measurement.

Skinfold measurements are made using professional grade calipers and a flexible measuring tape. Plastic calipers should not be used because they become bent or warped with use and then measurements are inaccurate. The technique for properly grasping the skinfold layers and subcutaneous fat takes practice before reliable measurements can be made. Both skinfold layers and subcutaneous fat are pinched and then held gently between the thumb and forefinger with care taken not to grasp underlying muscle. The fold is then measured between the calipers for each marked site on the body. Body composition results will not be representative if a distinct separation of subcutaneous fat and muscle cannot be accomplished when grasping the skinfold. The caliper jaws should be placed perpendicular to the fold and left in place for several seconds after tension is released to allow for even compression before the reading is taken. Three measurements should be taken at each site and then averaged. For consistency purposes, skinfold measurements should be taken on the right side of the body. Measurement values for each skinfold site can be evaluated in two ways. First, they may be used to monitor a patient over time, comparing measurements at intervals for changes in body composition. Second, they may be compared to reference values that are specific for gender, age, race, and fitness level. Reference values are simply descriptions of body composition compiled from subjects in population studies and should not be considered the same as a standard. Reference values allow the clinician to assess an individual's measurements compared to others

in a similar, well-defined population group. Standards, however, are values that are known to be desirable targets for health regardless of population norms.

Commonly used reference values to assess skinfold measurements in some populations are over 20 years old. Another problem is that these older references were not obtained from diverse population groups, which makes them difficult to apply to the wider population that exists today. Newer reference standards are constantly being published and are becoming more population specific, but no widely used single reference exists. Therefore, the nature of human diversity requires even more research to be done in this area to appreciate the variety of reference values needed for racial, ethnic, age, fitness, and gender categories. Age-related differences in body fat distribution necessitate use of the specific skinfold references established for older adults because the relationship between specific-site subcutaneous fat measurements and total body fat is different than in younger adults. Changes in skin elasticity and connective tissue also affect skinfold accuracy with age.

Midarm Muscle Circumference and Calf Circumference

Circumference measurements of limbs can be used alone or in conjunction with skinfold measurements to provide additional or confirmational body composition information. Midarm muscle circumference (MAMC) is obtained by measuring the midarm

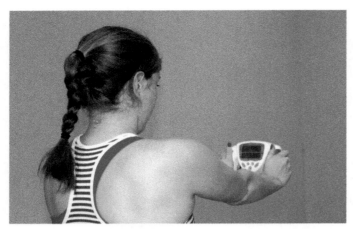

Figure 12.4 Handheld BIA device.
Source: Sheila Tucker.

circumference (MAC) at the same site as the tricep skinfold. A spring-loaded flexible measuring tape is used to provide tension without compressing the skin. Calf circumference is measured at the site of maximum calf width, which can be determined by placing the measure around the calf and sliding it along the calf until a maximum value is noted. Limb circumferences are measured in centimeters in adults.

Bioelectrical Impedance Analysis

Bioelectrical impedance analysis (BIA) is a noninvasive tool for assessing body composition employing principles of electroconduction through water, muscle, and fat. In traditional BIA, electrodes are placed on the dorsal surfaces of the right foot and hand with the patient in the supine position on a nonconductive surface. Calculations are based on the knowledge that muscle and fluids have a higher electrolyte and water content than does fat and thus conduct electric current differently. Altered hydration and altered skin temperature will cause measurement error by altering electric current flow. Patients should be well hydrated when employing BIA technology, or dehydration will slow conductivity and give a falsely high body fat measurement. Equations used to predict body fat composition with BIA need to be population specific. Standard error for BIA measurements approximates that of skinfold measurements at 3% to 4%, provided correct equations are used and the patient is hydrated. Handheld BIA devices are being manufactured for easier clinical use (see Figure 12.4 ■). This version of the device measures segmental electric impedance from arm to arm rather than the traditional whole-body method.

Near-Infrared Interactance

Near-infrared interactance devices measure body fat at specific sites by passing infrared light through tissue and measuring reflected light. Predictive equations estimate body fat composition at the site. Gender, body weight, height, frame size, and fitness level are included in the calculation to determine total body fat percentage. Generally this measurement is performed on the bicep. Small, handheld near-infrared devices are available for clinical use. Standard error for near-infrared measurement exceeds 3.5% and can be as high as 5.5%; error is greater with increased body fat.

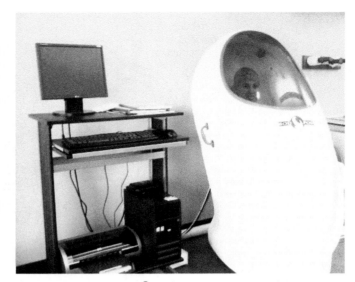

Figure 12.5 BOD POD® Body Composition Tracking System.

Laboratory Body Composition

Several other more sophisticated and expensive tools exist for measuring body composition. These are primarily used in laboratory research and not in clinical situations. Underwater weighing, dual energy x-ray absorptiometry (DEXA), and body plethysmography are examples of research tools. Underwater weighing requires the patient to be completely submersed underwater to measure water displacement by the body. Regression equations calculate body fat based on known density of fat-free and fat tissue. Underwater weighing has long been called the gold standard for body composition although it utilizes only a two-component model and does not measure bone mineral content or total body water. DEXA takes advantage of x-ray technology to measure a multicomponent model of body composition and is quickly becoming the research tool of choice. *Plethysmography* measures air volume displacement by the body using similar methodology to underwater weighing. Patients are measured in a small chamber called a BOD POD Body Composition Tracking System (see Figure 12.5 ■).

Body Fat References or Standards

Standards of body fat percentage that are associated with health or morbidity and mortality have not been established. Many sources agree that a minimum essential body fat percentage exists. A minimum of 3% body fat in men and 12% in women is considered essential. These minimums are the lowest value compatible with health, but optimal body fat is higher and should be determined on an individual basis. It is recommended that a range of body fat be given rather than a specific target due to the errors associated with predicting specific values. A range of 12% to 20% body fat in men and 20% to 30% in women has been suggested for health, but more research is necessary to develop population-specific recommendations. Research aimed at the development of future standards and references for body fat percentage is needed. Research specifically addressing the relationship between BMI and body fat percentage will allow the nurse a clearer assessment of body composition traits associated with health risks. Age-specific recommendations are also needed.

Physical Assessment

A visual head-to-toe physical assessment can yield findings that may be indicative of normal or abnormal nutritional status. Like all other components of a nutritional assessment, the physical assessment is most useful when used in conjunction with other nutritional assessment parameters. Table 12.6 outlines physical findings associated with poor nutritional health.

Data that are gathered as part of the physical assessment are also pertinent to the nutritional assessment. Existing medical diagnoses and treatment such as medication or surgical plans are important when evaluating nutritional status. Physical findings such as poor dental health; problems with chewing or swallowing; gastrointestinal complaints; functional decline in physical or mental status; and declining vision, taste, or smell all have negative effects on nutritional health.

TABLE 12.6	Clinical Findings Associated with Poor Nutritional Health		

FINDING	POTENTIAL DEFICIENT NUTRIENT	FINDING	POTENTIAL DEFICIENT NUTRIENT
Hair Dull, sparse, brittle hair Dyspigmentation (**flag sign**) Hair loss (**alopecia**) Flag sign *Source:* Centers for Disease Control and Prevention.	Protein Protein, biotin, or zinc Protein, iron, or biotin	*Face* Moon face Pallor Pallor *Source:* Dr. P. Marazzi/Science Source.	Protein Iron
Eyes Dry mucosa (**xerophthalmia**), blindness and night blindness, Bitot's spot Xerophthalmia *Source:* Centers for Disease Control and Prevention. Pale conjunctiva Yellow subdermal fat deposits around lids (**xanthelasma**) Xanthelasma *Source:* Centers for Disease Control and Prevention.	Vitamin A Iron High cholesterol	*Lips* Cracks at corners (**angular stomatitis**); inflammation (**cheilosis**) Angular stomatitis *Source:* Centers for Disease Control and Prevention.	Riboflavin

(continued)

TABLE 12.6   Clinical Findings Associated with Poor Nutritional Health (continued)

FINDING	POTENTIAL DEFICIENT NUTRIENT	FINDING	POTENTIAL DEFICIENT NUTRIENT
Tongue Smooth, beefy red or magenta (**glossitis**)	Niacin, pyridoxine (B_6), riboflavin Glossitis *Source:* E.H. Gill/Custom Medical Stock Photo.	**Teeth** Delayed eruption Caries in baby Mottled enamel	Vitamin D May indicate baby-bottle tooth decay Baby bottle caries Excess fluoride
Atrophic papillae Diminished taste (hypogeusia)	Iron Zinc Atrophic papillae *Source:* Centers for Disease Control and Prevention.	**Glands** Increased parotid size Increased thyroid (goiter)	Protein-calorie or bulimia Iodine Goiter *Source:* Wellcome Image Library/ Custom Medical Stock Photo.
Gums Spongy, bleeding (scorbutic)	Vitamin C Scorbutic gums	**Nails** Spoon-shaped (**koilonychia**) ridges	Iron Koilonychia *Source:* Dr. P. Marazzi/Science Source.

FINDING	POTENTIAL DEFICIENT NUTRIENT	FINDING	POTENTIAL DEFICIENT NUTRIENT
Skin		*Skeleton/Trunk*	
Poor wound healing/decubitus ulcer	Protein, calories, vitamin C, zinc	Stunted growth	Protein-calorie, zinc
Goosebump flesh (**follicular hyperkeratosis**)	Vitamin A	Fluid-filled abdomen (**ascites**)	Protein
Dry, scaly	Vitamin A, essential fatty acids, zinc	Beading on ribs (rachitic rosary), bowed legs (**rickets**), widened epiphysis, narrow chest (pigeon breast)	Vitamin D
Photosensitive symmetric rash (**pellagra**)	Niacin		
	Pellagra *Source:* Dr. M.A. Ansary/Science Source.	Rickets *Source:* Jessica Wilson/Science Source. Loss of fat, muscle wasting	Protein, calories
Bruising (**purpura**)	Vitamins C and K		
Pinpoint hemorrhages (**petechiae**)	Vitamin C		
Genitalia		*Limbs*	
Delayed sexual maturation (hypogonadism)	Zinc	Loss of fat, muscle wasting	Protein, calories
		Pitting edema	Protein
	Hypogonadism *Source:* Biophoto Associates/ Science Source.	Pitting edema *Source:* SPL/Science Source.	
Cardiovascular System		*Nervous System*	
Arrhythmia	Potassium, magnesium	Hyporeflexia, confabulation	Thiamine
		Dementia, confusion, ataxia, neuropathy	Vitamin B$_{12}$
		Neuropathy	Excess vitamin B$_6$
		Tetany	Calcium, magnesium

Biochemical Assessment— Laboratory Measurements

Several biochemical parameters are commonly used in a nutritional assessment. No one laboratory value is unique in its sensitivity to predict nutritional status because each has confounding reasons for abnormal values. As in the case of physical findings of malnutrition, laboratory values may not reflect current known nutrition status because half-lives and body pools of plasma components vary.

The biochemical assessment and laboratory measurements along with their significance, values, and findings are summarized in Table 12.7.

TABLE 12.7   Biochemical Assessment Laboratory Measurements

LABORATORY MEASUREMENT	SIGNIFICANCE	VALUES AND FINDINGS
Albumin	Low albumin levels can be indicative of depleted visceral protein status and malnutrition. Dehydration or overhydration will lead to false levels due to hemoconcentration or dilution. Liver disease, infection, and inflammation can alter albumin unrelated to nutrition.	Expected 3.5 to 5 g/L Half-life in days 14 to 20 Mild malnutrition 2.8 to 3.4 g/L Moderate malnutrition 2.1 to 3.4 g/L Severe malnutrition < 2.1 g/L
Prealbumin	Also called thyroxine-binding prealbumin, has a shorter half-life and is therefore felt to provide a more current picture of protein status than does albumin. Prealbumin is an acute-phase reactant protein and is affected by inflammation and infection. Hemoconcentration or dilution will cause false values.	Expected 150 to 350 mg/L Half-life in days 2 to 3 Mild malnutrition 110 to 150 mg/L Moderate malnutrition 50 to 109 mg/L Severe malnutrition < 50 mg/L
Transferrin	Responsible for iron binding and transport. Inflammation, infection, or iron deficiency can alter transferrin value.	Expected > 200 mg/dL Half-life in days 8 to 10 Mild malnutrition 180 to 200 mg/L Moderate malnutrition 160 to 180 mg/L Severe malnutrition < 160 mg/L
Total Lymphocyte Count (TLC)	Decreased value can indicate poor immunocompetence from malnutrition. Confounding medical conditions such as cancer or immunosuppressive drugs interfere with TLC usefulness in nutritional assessment.	Expected TLC is 2,000 to 3,500 cells/mm^3. Plasma level below 1,500 cells/mm^3 may indicate malnutrition and poor immunocompetence.
Delayed Skin Hypersensitivity Testing	A delayed response to intradermal injection of foreign substances such as *Streptococcus* or *Candida*.	Delayed or no response may indicate malnutrition, poor immune system, or no previous exposure.
Cholesterol	High cholesterol may indicate overnutrition or undernutrition. Low cholesterol due to drug treatment is not a risk factor for malnutrition.	≥ 200 mg/dL is associated with cardiovascular disease. ≤ 160 mg/dL may indicate malnutrition.
Nutritional Anemia Assessment	Poor nutrition may be evidenced by low stores of iron, folic acid, vitamin B$_{12}$.	*Macrocytic anemia* as evidenced by increased red blood cell volume and deficient folic acid or vitamin B$_{12}$ level. *Microcytic anemia* as evidenced by decreased red blood cell volume and iron indices. *Iron deficiency anemia* as evidenced by low plasma hemoglobin, hematocrit, ferritin, iron.

TABLE 12.7	Biochemical Assessment Laboratory Measurements (continued)	
LABORATORY MEASUREMENT	**SIGNIFICANCE**	**VALUES AND FINDINGS**
Nitrogen Balance	Measured to estimate adequacy of dietary protein intake in relation to protein losses. Nitrogen is used as the marker to measure protein losses.	*Nitrogen balance* as evidenced by nitrogen intake equals nitrogen loss. *Catabolism* occurs when there is a negative nitrogen balance because losses exceed intake. *Anabolism* occurs when the intake of protein and calories exceeds the nitrogen loss.
Plasma Proteins	Albumin, prealbumin, and transferrin are each used to assess visceral protein status.	
Immunocompetence	A depressed immune status can result from malnutrition, disease, medication, or other disease treatments.	

Cultural Considerations for the Nutritional Assessment

Religious and cultural influences on health, nutrition beliefs, and food habits vary among and within ethnic groups. It is important to ask specific questions about these influences to understand how they affect or are interpreted by the individual patient. Assumptions and generalizations based on the patient's association with a cultural or ethnic population will not provide the nurse with accurate personal information about the patient.

During the physical assessment and anthropometric portion of the assessment, careful and sensitive questioning of the patient or a translator is needed to determine whether issues exist that may interfere with the gathering of data. Removal of certain garments may be prohibited; this can interfere with obtaining accurate weight, determining body measurements, or assessing clinical signs and symptoms. Examination or touching by a member of the opposite sex may be taboo. The nurse should engage in decision making with the patient on how best to proceed when such issues are present. Box 12.5 outlines cultural nutritional considerations.

Nutritional Assessment Across the Life Span

From infancy to older adulthood, specific consideration needs to be given to each population's unique nutritional health parameters. Normal growth and development during childhood, the nutritional needs for a healthy pregnancy, and health maintenance and disease prevention in adulthood all provide additional parameters to consider when conducting a nutritional assessment.

The Pregnant Female

Nutritional health plays a primary role in a successful pregnancy. A mother's pre-conception nutritional status, appropriate weight gain, and adequate nutrition during pregnancy are important contributing factors to the health of a newborn. A comprehensive nutritional assessment of a pregnant female includes all the parameters of a general assessment with additional assessment of some pregnancy-specific data. See chapter 27, The Pregnant Female, for further details.

The Lactating Female

During lacatation, the nursing mother requires adequate nutrition to support her own nutritional needs as well as the production of sufficient breast milk for her child. In addition to assessing the general nutritional status of the mother, the nurse should assess the number and timing of all feedings; the mother's intake of all fluids, including alcohol and caffeinated beverages; the use of dietary supplements, both precribed and self-prescribed; the details of any post-pregnancy attempts at weight management; and, in the vegan mother, the daily source of vitamin B_{12} since only active intake passes to the child in breast milk.

Infants, Children, and Adolescents

Nutrition plays a crucial role in the growth, physical development, and cognitive development of infants and children. Undernutrition can lead to growth faltering and developmental delays or stunting, the effects of which can be permanent. Overnutrition can set the stage for chronic disease. Overweight and obese children, especially those with one or more overweight or obese parents, are more likely to become overweight adults. Accurate assessment of nutritional health can help ensure positive outcomes or serve as the necessary foundation for needed nutritional interventions. It is essential for a nurse to have the knowledge and skills to identify nutritionally at-risk children. In many community settings, such as schools, early intervention clinics, or well-child clinics, the nurse is often the only healthcare professional conducting an assessment that includes nutritional parameters.

Adults

Nutritional assessment of the adult focuses on evaluating the issues of both overnutrition and undernutrition. Overnutrition and undernutrition are not mutually exclusive conditions. For example, an obese individual can have nutrient deficiencies from poor quality food intake that contains excess calories. Good food habits developed early in life and maintained later may help to promote good health well into adulthood and older adulthood.

Box 12.5 Cultural Diet Influences

MODEL QUESTIONS	RATIONALES
• Do you speak or read any other languages?	• Understanding primary and secondary languages is important for both communication and education
• Is there anyone else you would like us to include in this nutrition conversation?	• In some cultures, a patient may defer to an elder or authority figure when answering questions about health
• Is there any time in the year that you change your diet for cultural reasons, including religion?	• Cultural and religious beliefs and traditions can affect food choices, beliefs, and practices in many ways, from the number of meals eaten in a day to choices of foods, preparation methods, and overall food beliefs.
• Are there any foods you avoid for cultural reasons?	• Diversity exists within cultural and religious groups. It is important to avoid applying general knowledge about cultural and religious food practices to all people within a group; instead explore individual interpretation and influences.
• What types of foods do you believe promote health or keep you well?	• Assess common dietary staples as well as foods believed to be associated with health or symbolic benefits. Some food is thought to promote health or cure conditions. Other beliefs may be related to lifespan issues, such as the proper diet during pregnancy for easy delivery or to make the "hot" condition "colder."
• Are there any foods that you would try to consume if you were sick or for certain conditions?	• Many religious groups have dietary laws that are observed differently by subgroups within the population. Consumption of kosher meats, fasting, and avoidance of certain foods such as pork, crustaceans, birds of prey, beef, or other animal products are examples.
• Do you use any health remedies or practices that are related to your culture?	• Ask about food practices and special meals for special occasions and holidays. Some religious groups fast during parts of some religious holy days.
• *For the patient with a health diagnosis or condition*: tell me what you think caused this condition.	• Discuss food preparation methods. A variety of cultures make similar types of dishes but prepare them differently—for example, using different fats like bacon drippings, lard, oils, or ghee clarified butter.
• Is there anything else that you would like me to know about your dietary practices?	• Ask about medicinal herb use because this varies among cultures and is often an important aspect of health beliefs.
• *For the patient who has immigrated*: has your diet changed in any way since you moved here? What is different? What is the same?	• Explore to what extent any acculturation has taken place and what traditional practices have changed once living in a new dominant culture. Ask whether new foods have been added along with traditional foods, whether newer or different versions of foods have been substituted, and whether any traditional foods have been omitted. In some cases, traditional diets are healthier than the diet in the new culture, and encouragement to maintain healthy traditions may be helpful.

The general components of a nutritional assessment are all pertinent when assessing an adult. The presence of a chronic disease or condition may become a significant factor affecting nutritional health. Medications can have nutritional health implications. In addition to dietary habits, lifestyle choices, socioeconomic status, education, and cultural influences can affect nutrition status. Box 12.3 outlines pertinent nutritional history data to obtain when assessing the adult.

The Older Adult

Regular nutritional assessment of the older adult is essential. Good nutritional health is an important component of ensuring autonomy into older adulthood. Undernutrition can affect quality of life, morbidity, and mortality. A BMI < 23 is associated with increased risk of mortality in the older adult despite the fact that this value is still within the normal range for all adults. Protein-energy malnutrition is considered an independent risk factor for mortality in older adults recently discharged from the hospital. Skeletal muscle loss, functional decline, altered pharmacokinetics, depressed immune status, and increased risk of institutionalization can all result from malnutrition in the older adult. Further, alterations in sensory perception negatively affect intake. Alterations in sense of smell and taste are intertwined and lead to reduced enjoyment of food. Poor vision can make food preparation difficult or unsafe for the older adult living independantly. Additionally, it can be difficult for the older adult with poor vision to discern the location and type of food on the plate when served a meal prepared by others. Reduced hearing can make social dining a challenge and cause some older adults to withdraw from group meals and eat in isolation, a risk factor for poor nutrition. Unfortunately, the prevalence of malnutrition in the elderly population is significant, affecting up to 65% of institutionalized or hospitalized older adults and up to 13% of those in the community.

Quality of life issues related to overnutrition are also important in the older population. Overweight and obesity are risk factors for degenerative joint disease and potential functional and mobility problems. Comorbid conditions associated with overweight, such as diabetes and cardiovascular disease, may require treatment intervention, therapeutic diets, and medications that impact nutritional health.

Poor nutrition occurs along a continuum. In the older adult, changes in nutrition health can go undetected if only strict cutoff values are observed to diagnose nutrition issues. Most general nutritional assessment parameters are applicable to the elderly population, but the nurse should be mindful of *any* change in nutrition status in the older adult, even when measured values and parameters remain within normal limits.

Nutritional Screening and Assessment Tools

Nutritional assessment data can be gathered and evaluated in a comprehensive fashion, or a more formal validated tool can be used to streamline the process. Numerous nutritional screening and assessment tools exist, but none is considered the gold standard for use in most populations. Until a consensus is reached defining malnutrition, a variety of nutritional screening and assessment tools will continue to be published.

Nutritional screening tools are used for quick assessment of risk factors for poor nutritional health. Screening tools are not meant for diagnostic purposes and are instead used to triage patients who may require further assessment or intervention. Screening tools give a rough estimate of nutrition risk or status. Nutritional assessment tools are generally more comprehensive than screening tools for the goal of identifying or diagnosing malnutrition. Not all assessment or screening tools are validated for use in the populations where they

are being used. The nurse should be aware that use of a screening tool that has not been validated through in-depth research may lead to frequent missed diagnoses or incorrect diagnoses of poor nutritional health. Sharp clinical judgment by the nurse is a necessary adjunct to any tool.

ChooseMyPlate

Dietary Guidelines for Americans is published jointly by the U.S. Department of Health and Human Services (USDHHS) and the U.S. Department of Agriculture (USDA). The *Guidelines* provide authoritative advice for people 2 years and older about how good dietary habits can promote health and reduce risk for major chronic diseases. The most recent guidelines provide an accompanying food guide icon called MyPlate and an interactive Web site that may be used for individual food guide planning and diet analysis (see Figure 12.6 ■). This site is located at *www.choosemyplate.gov.* The nurse can compare the diet recall or nutrition history data to the distribution of food groups recommended on MyPlate and make a general assessment of diet adequacy. The number and size of food servings included in MyPlate are generic and should be adjusted for more active or less active individuals. The comprehensive Web site has tools for calculating and tracking individual nutritional needs for calories, major nutrients, and food groups. The benefit of the new icon is that it presents an easily understood image of what an individual meal looks like that would meet current guidelines for health and therefore can be used with all levels of knowledge and literacy skills. The accompanying Web site has more in-depth information for use with a variety of learning levels.

Other Assessment Tools

In addition to dietary guideline resources such as *www.choosemyplate.gov,* there are specialized screening tools that many clinicians have found helpful.

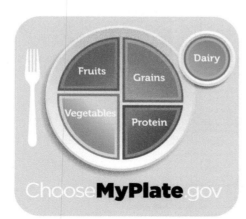

Figure 12.6 MyPlate.
Source: U.S. Department of Agriculture.

Balancing Calories
- Enjoy your food, but eat less.
- Avoid oversized portions.

Foods to Increase
- Make half your plate fruits and vegetables.
- Make at least half your grains whole grains.
- Switch to fat-free or low-fat (1%) milk.

Foods to Reduce
- Compare sodium in foods like soup, bread, and frozen meals—and choose the foods with lower numbers.
- Drink water instead of sugary drinks.

The DETERMINE Checklist

DETERMINE is an acronym standing for **D**isease, **E**ating poorly, **T**ooth loss/mouth pain, **E**conomic hardship, **R**educed social contact, **M**ultiple medicines, **I**nvoluntary weight loss/gain, **N**eeds assistance in self-care, and **E**lder years above 80 years.

The DETERMINE checklist may be used to assess the nutritional status of the older adult. The mnemonic scores the nine warning signs of poor nutrition in the older adult. The scoring of the tool provides a stratified nutritional risk score. This tool has been validated for use with community-based elderly.

The Minimum Data Set

The Minimum Data Set (MDS) is a component of the Residential Assessment Instrument mandated for all patients in Medicare-certified long-term healthcare facilities. MDS nutritional components are to be included in admission assessments for all residents as well as quarterly and annual updates. Any changes in patient status that involve a nutritional component of the MDS require a complete reassessment of nutritional status.

Mini Nutritional Assessment and Subjective Global Assessment

The Mini Nutritional Assessment (MNA) and Subjective Global Assessment (SGA) have both been validated for use in the nutritional assessment of older adults. The SGA has also been used in the assessment of other populations since its development over 20 years ago. The MNA is a newer tool with extensive data validating its use with older adults. The MNA can be included as a routine component of a physical examination or as a quick bedside tool and is available in an online version and as a mobile application.

Malnutrition Universal Screening Tool

The Malnutrition Universal Screening Tool (MUST) is a five-step tool that is validated for use with adults in all healthcare settings (see Figure 12.7 ■). BMI, unplanned weight loss, and any acute illness factor into this quick-scoring tool that helps triage the patient to further assessment, if indicated. Both online and mobile applications of this tool are available.

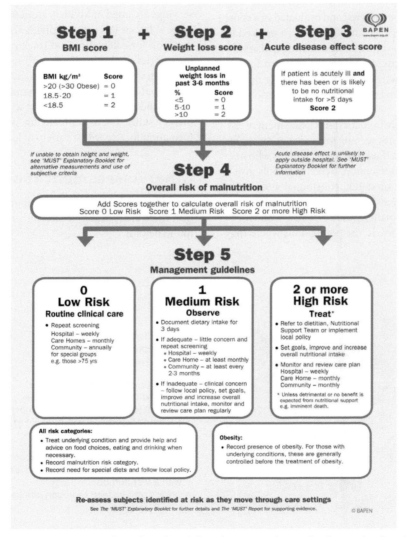

Figure 12.7 'MUST' is a five-step screening tool to identify adults who are malnourished, at risk of malnutrition (undernutrition), or obese. It also includes management guidelines that can be used to develop a care plan.
Source: © BAPEN. First published May 2003 by MAG, the Malnutrition Advisory Group, a Standing Committee of BAPEN. Reviewed and reprinted with minor changes March 2008, September 2010 and August 2011. 'MUST' is supported by the British Dietetic Association, the Royal College of Nursing, and the Registered Nursing Home Association.

Patient Education

The following are risk factors for undernutrition and overnutrition that affect health across the life span. Several factors related to nutrition are cited in *Healthy People 2020* documents. The nurse provides advice and education to promote and maintain health and reduce risks associated with the aforementioned factors that impact nutritional health across the life span.

UNDERNUTRITION

Risk Factors	Patient Education
● Insufficient gestational weight gain	▶ Provide patients with information on need for weight gain during pregnancy. Outline nutrient-dense food choices to support gain.
● Iron deficiency in pregnant female, infant, or child	▶ Teach patients or caregivers about the role of iron and important food sources. Reinforce the use of an iron supplement in pregnant females.
● Insufficient folic acid intake during pregnancy	▶ Provide patients with a list of good sources of folic acid. Emphasize the role of folic acid in avoidance of birth defects.
● Inadequate calcium and vitamin D intake	▶ Teach patients about the importance of calcium and vitamin D in bone health. Outline good sources of these nutrients.
● Inadequate dietary intake in older adults	▶ Teach patients about healthy eating and the importance of maintaining nutritional health with the aging process.

OVERNUTRITION

Risk Factors	Patient Education
● Obesity/overweight	▶ Advise patients of risks associated with excess body weight. Educate patients about healthful ways to lose weight.
● Excessive intake of cholesterol/saturated fat	▶ Discuss the relationship between diet and heart disease with patients. Educate patients on the steps to take toward lowering intake of foods that increase blood cholesterol.
● Excessive intake of dietary supplements	▶ Educate patients on dangers of oversupplementation with herbs, sports nutrition products, vitamins, and minerals. Emphasize a healthy balanced diet in place of the need for supplements.

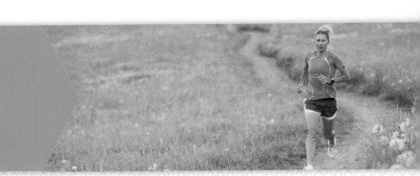

Application Through Critical Thinking

▶ Case Study

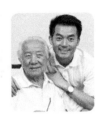

Harry Chien is an 89-year-old widower brought to the clinic by his nephew who is concerned about his diminished dietary intake. His past medical history is significant for mild hypertension, which is treated with a diuretic and a 2-g sodium therapeutic diet. Physical assessment reveals blood pressure of 110/75 and pulse of 72. Height is 5′8″, and weight is 156 lb. Weight 6 months prior was 175 lb. Significant laboratory measures: albumin 3.0 mg/dL. Urinalysis sent: sample dark and scant volume. His skin appears dry with dry axillae and petechiae on the trunk and arms. His eyes are sunken. Temporal wasting is noted as well as diminished subcutaneous fat stores on the limbs. The assessment of the oral cavity reveals poorly fitting dentures, spongy gums, and deep tongue furrows.

Upon talking to Mr. Chien, the nurse learns that food does not taste the same to him anymore. He blames this on his low-sodium diet. His nephew reports that he takes his uncle grocery shopping each week and has noticed that his pantry at home has many of the items still there from the prior week. He tells the nurse that his uncle is a retired professional chef and used to love to cook until the last few months. He has resorted to heating food in the microwave and often overcooks it. Mr. Chien states he overheats the food because the microwave is unpredictable. His nephew is reading his concerns from a list he has made and passes the list to his uncle for further comment. The nurse notices he squints at the list and then says he has nothing to add.

The nurse conducts a diet recall that reveals:

Breakfast:	Large mug black coffee
	Either cold cereal (flake type, not fortified) and whole milk or 2 pieces of toast or 1 English muffin with butter and jelly
	6 oz apple juice or cider, unfortified
Midday meal:	Sandwich on white bread—such as tuna salad, peanut butter and jelly, or sliced turkey with mayonnaise and iceberg lettuce. Used to add tomato to sandwich but "can't be bothered cutting up one."

Occasionally heats leftovers from restaurant meal with nephew; usually has enough for two or three reheated meals during week. Pasta or meat and potato- or rice-type meals. No vegetables. Overheats and discards often.

Cookie

Cup of tea with whole milk and 2 tsp sugar

Evening:	6 oz ready-to-eat pudding
	4 oz milk with comment "no liquids after 7 p.m. or I have to get up all night"

Mr. Chien takes no nutritional supplements of any kind. The nurse asks further questions about the lack of fruit and vegetables and learns that it has been almost 6 months since Mr. Chien had fruit other than applesauce or apple juice. He also has stopped eating vegetables in the same time frame. He states that he cannot be bothered preparing either type of food, but on further questioning admits that he is having difficulty chewing some foods and some vision problems that make food preparation difficult or unsafe.

▶ Complete Documentation

The following is a sample documentation from the nutrition assessment of Harry Chien.

SUBJECTIVE DATA: Brought by nephew who notes diminished intake. c/o low Na+ rx causing hypogeusia with secondary anorexia. Also c/o difficulty chewing, vision changes. Diet recall 2-meal/day pattern with no liquids after 7 p.m. Liquid intake, 32 oz/day (only 10 oz noncaffeine). No fruit/vegetable 3–6 mos.

OBJECTIVE DATA: VS: BP 110/75—Pulse 72. Height 5′8″, weight 156 lb. BMI 23.5. Weight 6 months ago 175 lb. Albumin 3.0 mg/dL, UA: sample dark and scant. Skin and axillae dry/petechiae present. Temp/limb wasting noted. Eyes sunken. Oral cavity: spongy gums, poorly fitting dentures, tongue furrows. Medications: H.Hydrochlorthiazide.

▶ Critical Thinking Questions

1. How would the data from the case study be clustered to identify the problem areas?

2. How should the nurse interpret the data related to Mr. Chien's fruit and vegetable intake?

3. What additional data would the nurse require to develop a plan of care for Mr. Chien?

4. What additional information should the nurse gather to determine why Mr. Chien is experiencing an alteration in the way food tastes to him?

5. How would the nurse address the signs and symptoms of dehydration in Mr. Chien?

▶ References

BAPEN. (2011). Malnutrition Universal Screening Tool (MUST). Retrieved from http://www.bapen.org.uk/pdfs/must/must_full.pdf

Bell, J. J., Bauer, J. D., Capra, S., & Pulle, R. C. (2014). Quick and easy is not without cost: Implications of poorly performing nutrition screening tools in hip fracture. *Journal of the American Geriatric Society, 62*, 237–243.

Centers for Disease Control and Prevention, National Center for Health Statistics. (2009). *Anthropometry procedures manual.* Retrieved from http://www.cdc.gov/nchs/data/nhanes/nhanes_09_10/BodyMeasures_09

Centers for Disease Control and Prevention (CDC). (2014). *Health, United States, 2012.* Retrieved from http://www.cdc.gov/nchs/hus.htm

Centers for Medicare and Medicaid Services (CMS). (2013). *Minimum data set manual version 3.0 for nursing homes, October 2013 update.* Retrieved from http://www.cms.gov/Medicare/Quality-Initiatives-Patient-Assessment-Instruments/NursingHomeQualityInits/MDS30RAIManual.html

Cerhan, J. R., Moore, S. C., Jacobs, E. J., Kitahara, C. M., Rosenberg, P. S., Adami, H. O., . . . Berrington de Gonzalez, A. (2014). A pooled analysis of waist circumference and mortality in 650,000 adults. *Mayo Clinic Proceedings, 89*, 335–345.

Diekmann, R., Winning, K., Uter, W., Kaiser, M. J., Sieber, C. C., Volkert, D., & Bauer, J. M. (2013). Screening for malnutrition among nursing home residents a comparative analysis of the mini nutritional assessment, the nutritional risk screening, and the malnutrition universal screening tool. *The Journal of Nutrition, Health, and Aging, 17*(4), 326–331.

Duren, D. L., Sherwood, R. J., Czerwinski, S. A., Lee, M., Choh, A. C., Siervogel, R. M., & Cameron Chumlea, W. (2008). Body composition methods: Comparisons and interpretation. *Journal of Diabetes, Science, and Technology, 2*(6), 1139–1146.

Flegal, K. M., & Graubard, B. I. (2009). Estimates of excess deaths associated with body mass index and other anthropometric indices. *American Journal of Clinical Nutrition, 89*, 1213–1219.

Forrestal, S. G. (2011). Energy misreporting among children and adolescents: A literature review. *Maternal and Child Nutrition, 7*, 112–127.

Harvard School of Public Health. (2014). *Ethnic differences in BMI and disease risk.* Retrieved from http://www.hsph.harvard.edu/obesity-prevention-source/ethnic-differences-in-bmi-and-disease-risk/

Isenring, E. A., Banks, M., Ferguson, M., & Bauer, J. D. (2012). Beyond malnutrition screening: Appropriate methods to guide nutrition care for aged care residents. *Journal of the Academy of Nutrition and Dietetics, 112*, 376–381.

Koh, K. A., Hoy, J. S., O'Connell, J. J., & Montgomery, P. (2012). The hunger-obesity paradox: Obesity in the homeless. *Journal of Urban Health, 89*, 952–964.

Mini Nutrition Assessment. (2009). *Tool and information on usage.* Retrieved from http://www.mna-elderly.com

Muurinen, S. M., Soini, H. H., Souminen, M. H., Saarela, R. K., Savikko, N. M., & Pitkala, K. H. (2014). Vision impairment and nutritional status among older assisted living residents. *Archives of Gerontology and Geriatrics, 58*, 384–387.

Ogden, C. L., Carroll, M. D., Kit, B. K., & Flegal. K. M. (2014). Prevalence of childhood and adult obesity in the United States, 2011–2012. *Journal of the American Medical Association, 311*, 806–814.

Sagna, M. L., Schopflocher, D., Raine, K., Nykiforuk, C., & Plotnikoff, R. (2013). Adjusting divergences between self-reported and measured height and weight in an adult Canadian population. *American Journal of Health Behavior, 37*, 841–850.

Sinnett, S., Bengle, R., Brown, A., Glass, A. P., Johnson, M. A., & Lee, J. S. (2010). The validity of Nutrition Screening Initiative DETERMINE Checklist reponses in older Georgians. *Journal of Nutrition for the Elderly, 29*, 393–409.

U.S. Census Bureau. (2013). *Current Population Survey Annual Social and Economic Supplement (CPS ASEC): Income, poverty, and health insurance coverage in the United States, 2012.* Retrieved from http://www.census.gov/hhes/www/poverty/data/incpovhlth/2012/index.html

United States Department of Agriculture (USDA). (n.d.a). *ChooseMyPlate.gov.* Retrieved from http://www.choosemyplate.gov/

United States Department of Agriculture (USDA). (n.d.b). *Food deserts.* Retrieved from http://apps.ams.usda.gov/fooddeserts/foodDeserts.aspx

United States Department of Health and Human Services. (2014). *Healthy people 2020.* Retrieved from http://www.healthypeople.gov/2020/topicsobjectives2020/default.aspx

United States Department of Health and Human Services. National Heart, Lung, and Blood Institute. (n.d.). *Classification of overweight and obesity by BMI, waist circumference, and associated disease risks.* Retrieved from http://www.nhlbi.nih.gov/health/public/heart/obesity/lose_wt/bmi_dis.htm

Van Bokhorst-de van der Schueren, M. A, Guaitoli, P. R., Jansma, E. P., & de Vet, H. C. (2014). Nutrition screening tools: Does one size fit all? A systematic review of screening tools for the hospital setting. *Clinical Nutrition, 33*(1), 39–58.

Winter, J. E., MacInnis, R. J., Wattanapenpaiboon, N., & Nowson, C. A. (2014). BMI and all-cause mortality in older adults: A meta-analysis. *Amercian Journal of Clinical Nutrition, 99*, 875–890.

World Health Organization. (2014). *BMI classification.* Retrieved from http://apps.who.int/bmi/index.jsp?introPage=intro_3.html

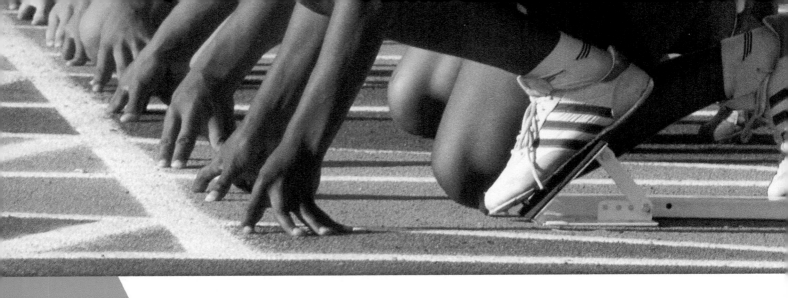

▶ Learning Outcomes

Upon completion of this chapter, you will be able to:

1. Identify the anatomy and physiology of the skin, hair, and nails.

2. Develop questions to be used when completing the focused interview.

3. Outline the techniques used for assessment of the skin, hair, and nails.

4. Explain patient preparation for assessment of the skin, hair, and nails.

5. Differentiate normal from abnormal findings in physical assessment of the skin, hair, and nails.

6. Describe developmental, psychosocial, cultural, and environmental variations in assessment techniques and findings.

7. Relate integumentary health to *Healthy People 2020* objectives.

8. Apply critical thinking to the physical assessment of the skin, hair, and nails.

Key Terms

The skin, hair, and nails are the major components of the integumentary system. The integumentary system consists of the skin and the accessory structures, the sweat and oil glands, the hair, and the nails. The largest organ of the body, the skin weighs about 20 lb (approximately 9 kg) and has a surface area of about 20 ft^2 (approximately 1.86 m^2) in adults (Colbert, Ankney, & Lee, 2011). Every square inch of the skin contains 10 to 15 ft (3 to 4.5 m) of blood vessels and nerves, hundreds of sweat and oil glands, and over 3 million cells that are constantly dying and being replaced. This complex shield protects the body against heat, ultraviolet rays, trauma, and invasion by bacteria. In addition, the skin works with other body systems to regulate body temperature, synthesize vitamin D, store blood and fats, excrete body wastes, and help humans sense the world around them.

A thorough assessment of the skin, hair, and nails provides valuable clues to a patient's general health. The skin, hair, and nails can suggest the status of a patient's nutrition, airway clearance, thermoregulation, and tissue perfusion. The skin, hair, and nails can also reveal alterations in activity, sleep and rest, level of stress, and self-care ability. A patient's ancestry, cultural practices, and physical environment, both at home and at work, can greatly influence integumentary health and are an integral part of the assessment data.

A patient's developmental stage has a tremendous influence on the appearance and functioning of these structures. Skin is very thin at birth and thickens throughout childhood. Sweat and oil glands are activated during adolescence. The function of these glands diminishes in the older adult. The appearance of the skin, hair, and nails impacts the self-concept of the individual. Skin disorders may interfere with social relationships, roles, and sexuality. Stress may also trigger or exacerbate skin disorders. The type of soap or agents used as part of the cleansing routine may contribute to dry, oily, itchy skin, or rashes. Hairstyling methods, use of hair products, chemical curling, or bleaching may be factors in damage, breakage, or loss of hair.

Anatomy and Physiology Review

The skin is composed of the epidermal, dermal, and subcutaneous layers. The cutaneous glands, which are located in the dermal layer, release secretions to lubricate the skin and to assist in temperature regulation. The hair and nails are composed of keratinized (hardened) cells and serve to protect the skin and the ends of the fingers and toes. Each of these anatomic structures is described in the following paragraphs.

Skin and Glands

The skin is composed of two distinct layers. The outer layer, called the **epidermis,** is firmly attached to an underlying layer called the **dermis.** Deep in the dermis is a layer of subcutaneous tissue that anchors the skin to the underlying body structures.

Epidermis

The epidermis is a layer of epithelial tissue that comprises the outermost portion of the skin. Where exposure to friction is greatest, such as on the fingertips, palms, and soles of the feet, the epidermis consists of five layers (or strata), as shown in Figure 13.1 ■. These five layers, from deep to superficial, are: the stratum basale, stratum spinosum, stratum granulosum, stratum lucidum, and stratum corneum.

New skin cells are formed in the stratum basale, or basal layer, which is also known as the stratum germinativum (germinating layer). These new skin cells consist mostly of a fibrous protein called **keratin,** which gives the epidermis its tough, protective qualities. About 25% of the cells in the stratum basale are *melanocytes,* which produce the skin pigment called **melanin.** All humans have the same relative number of melanocytes, but the amount of melanin they produce varies according to genetic, hormonal, and environmental factors.

Cells produced in the stratum basale gradually move through the layers of the epidermis toward the stratum corneum, where they are sloughed off. The abundance of keratin in this tough "horny layer" protects against abrasion and trauma, repels water, resists water loss, and renders the body insensitive to a variety of environmental toxins.

Dermis

The dermis is a layer of connective tissue that lies just below the epidermis. The dermis consists mainly of two types of fibers: collagen, which gives the skin its toughness and enables it to resist tearing, and the elastic fibers, which give the skin its elasticity. The dermis is richly supplied with nerves, blood vessels, and lymphatic vessels; and it is embedded with hair follicles, sweat glands, oil glands, and sensory receptors.

Subcutaneous Tissue

The subcutaneous tissue (or **hypodermis**) is a loose connective tissue that stores approximately half of the body's fat cells. Thus, it cushions the body against trauma, insulates the body from heat loss, and stores fat for energy.

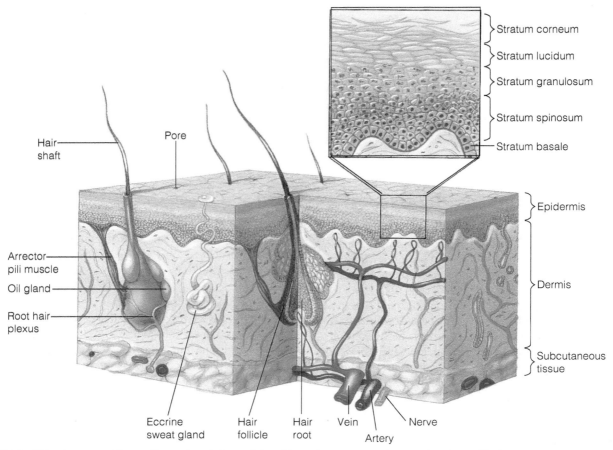

Figure 13.1 Skin structure. Three-dimensional view of the skin, subcutaneous tissue, glands, and hairs.

Cutaneous Glands

The cutaneous glands are formed in the stratum basale and push deep into the dermis. They release their secretions through ducts onto the skin surface.

There are two types of sweat (or sudoriferous) glands: eccrine and apocrine. **Eccrine glands** are more numerous and more widely distributed. They produce a clear perspiration mostly made up of water and salts, which they release into funnel-shaped pores at the skin surface. **Apocrine glands** are found primarily in the axillary and anogenital regions. They are dormant until the onset of puberty. Apocrine glands produce a secretion made up of water, salts, fatty acids, and proteins, which is released into hair follicles. When apocrine sweat mixes with bacteria on the skin surface, it assumes a musky odor.

Oil Glands

Oil glands, or **sebaceous glands,** are distributed over most of the body except the palms of the hands and soles of the feet. They produce *sebum,* an oily secretion composed of fat and keratin that is usually released into hair follicles.

The major functions of the skin are the following:

- Perceiving touch, pressure, temperature, and pain via the nerve endings.
- Protecting against mechanical, chemical, thermal, and solar damage.
- Protecting against loss of water and electrolytes.
- Regulating body temperature.
- Repairing surface wounds through cellular replacement.
- Synthesizing vitamin D.
- Allowing identification through uniqueness of facial contours, skin and hair color, and fingerprints.

The major functions of the cutaneous glands are the following:

- Excreting uric acid, urea, ammonia, sodium, potassium, and other metabolic wastes.
- Regulating temperature through evaporation of perspiration on the skin surface.
- Protecting against bacterial growth on the skin surface.
- Softening, lubricating, and waterproofing skin and hair.
- Resisting water loss from the skin surface in low-humidity environments.
- Protecting deeper skin regions from bacteria on the skin surface.

Hair

A **hair** is a thin, flexible, elongated fiber composed of dead, keratinized cells that grow out in a columnar fashion (see Figure 13.1). Each hair shaft arises from a follicle. Nerve endings in the follicle are sensitive to the slightest movement of the hair. Each hair follicle also

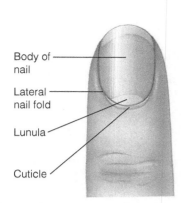
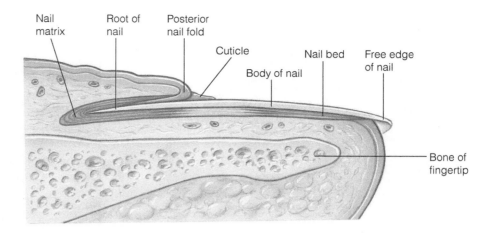

Figure 13.2 Structure of a nail.

has an arrector pili muscle that causes the hair to contract and stand upright when a person is under stress or exposed to cold.

The deep end of each follicle expands to form a hair bulb. New cells are produced at the hair bulb. Hair growth is cyclic; scalp hair typically has an active phase of about 4 years and a resting phase of a few months. Because these phases are not synchronous, only a small percentage of a person's hair follicles shed their hair at any given time.

Hair color is determined by the amount of melanin produced in the hair follicle. Black or brown hair contains the greatest amount of melanin.

The type and distribution of hair vary in different parts of the body. **Vellus hair,** a pale, fine, short strand, grows over the entire body except for the margins of the lips, the nipples, the palms of the hands, the soles of the feet, and parts of the external genitals. The **terminal hair** of the eyebrows and scalp is usually darker, coarser, and longer. At puberty, hormones signal the growth of terminal hair in the axillae, pubic region, and legs of both sexes, and on the face and chest of most males.

The major functions of the hair are to insulate against heat and cold, protect against ultraviolet and infrared rays, perceive movement or touch, protect the eyes from sweat, and protect the nasal passages from foreign particles.

Nails

Nails are thin plates of keratinized epidermal cells that shield the distal ends of the fingers and toes (see Figure 13.2 ■). Nail growth occurs at the nail matrix because new cells arise from the basal layer of the epidermis. As the nail cells grow out from the matrix, they form

a transparent layer, called the body of the nail, which extends over the nail bed. The nail body appears pink because of the blood supply in the underlying dermis. A moon-shaped crescent called a **lunula** appears on the nail body over the thickened nail matrix. A fold of epidermal skin called a **cuticle** protects the root and sides of each nail. The major functions of the nails are to protect the tips of the fingers and toes and aid in picking up small objects, grasping, and scratching.

Special Considerations

Throughout the assessment process, the nurse gathers subjective and objective data reflecting the patient's state of health. Using critical thinking and the nursing process, the nurse identifies many factors to be considered when collecting the data. Some of these factors include but are not limited to age, developmental level, race, ethnicity, work history, living conditions, social economics, and emotional well-being.

Health Promotion Considerations

Identification and reduction of environmental risk factors for skin diseases including skin cancer and occupational skin disorders are among the *Healthy People 2020* objectives related to integumentary health. See Table 13.1 for an overview of *Healthy People 2020* integumentary health objectives that are designed to promote health and wellness among individuals across the life span.

TABLE 13.1	Examples of *Healthy People 2020* Objectives Related to the Integumentary System
OBJECTIVE NUMBER	**DESCRIPTION**
C-20	Increase the proportion of persons who participate in behaviors that reduce their exposure to harmful ultraviolet (UV) irradiation and avoid sunburn
OSH-8	Reduce occupational skin diseases or disorders among full-time workers
OA-10	Reduce the rate of pressure ulcer–related hospitalizations among older adults

Source: U.S. Department of Health and Human Services (USDHHS). (2014). *Healthy People 2020.* Retrieved from http://www.healthypeople.gov/2020/default.aspx

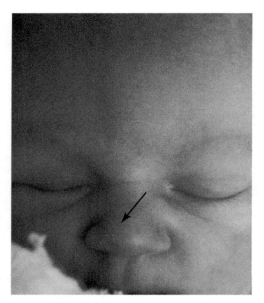

Figure 13.3 Milia.

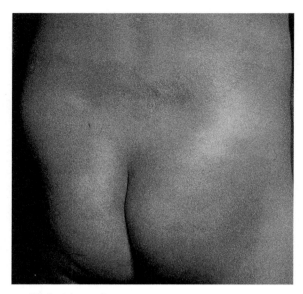

Figure 13.4 Mongolian spots.
Source: Wellcome Image Library/Custom Medical Stock Photo, Inc.

Lifespan Considerations

Growth and development are dynamic processes that describe change over time. Data collection and interpretation of these findings in relation to normative values are important. The following discussion presents specific variations for different age groups.

Infants and Children

At birth, the newborn's skin typically is covered with **vernix caseosa,** a white, cheeselike mixture of sebum and epidermal cells. The skin color of newborns is often bright red for the first 24 hours of life and then fades. Some newborns develop physiologic jaundice 3 to 4 days after birth, resulting in a yellowing of the skin, sclera, and mucous membranes. Jaundice can occur within the first 24 hours after birth or as late as 7 days postnatally. Physiologic jaundice is a temporary condition treated with fluids and phototherapy. The skin of dark-skinned newborns normally is not fully pigmented until 2 to 3 months after birth. An infant's skin is very thin, soft, and free of terminal hair.

Many harmless skin markings are common in newborns. For example, they may have areas of tiny white facial papules. These are called **milia** and are due to sebum that collects in the openings of hair follicles (see Figure 13.3 ■). Milia usually disappear spontaneously within a few weeks of birth. Vascular markings are also common. These may include stork bites, which are irregular red or pink patches found most commonly on the back of the neck. Vascular markings disappear spontaneously within a year of birth. The newborn may also have transient mottling or other transient color changes such as harlequin color change, in which a side-lying infant becomes markedly pink on the lower side and pale on the higher side. **Mongolian spots** are gray, blue, or purple spots in the sacral and buttocks areas of newborns (see Figure 13.4 ■). Mongolian spots occur in about 90% of newborns of African ancestry and in about 80% of newborns of Asian or Native American ancestry and in those with dark or olive skin tones. Mongolian spots fade early in life, usually by 3 years of age. Mongolian spots should not be interpreted as signs of abuse. Because the subcutaneous fat layer is poorly developed in infants and the eccrine sweat glands do not secrete until after the first few months of life, their temperature regulation is inefficient and absorption of topical medications is increased. The fine, downy hair of the newborn, called **lanugo,** is replaced within a few months by vellus hair. Hair growth accelerates throughout childhood.

Throughout childhood, the epidermis thickens, pigmentation increases, and more subcutaneous fat is deposited, especially in females during puberty. During adolescence, both the sweat glands and the oil glands increase their production. Increased production of sebum by the oil glands predisposes adolescents to develop acne (see Figure 13.5 ■). Increased axillary perspiration occurs as the apocrine glands mature, and body odor may develop for the first time. Pubic and axillary hair appears during adolescence, and males may develop facial and chest hair.

The Pregnant Female

Pigmentation of the skin commonly increases during pregnancy, especially in the areolae, nipples, vulva, and perianal area. Approximately 70% of pregnant women develop hyperpigmented patches on the face referred to as **chloasma,** melasma, gravidum, or "the mask of pregnancy" (see Figure 13.6 ■). This normal condition

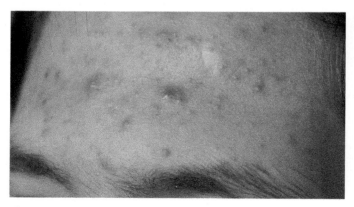

Figure 13.5 Acne.
Source: Olavs/Fotolia.

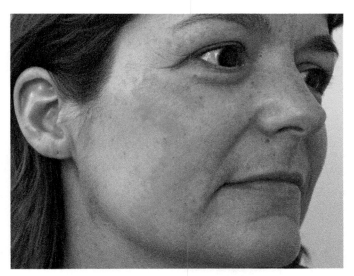

Figure 13.6 Melasma.

disappears after pregnancy in some women but may be permanent in others. Some pregnant patients may also have a dark line called a **linea nigra** running from the umbilicus to the pubic area (see Figure 13.7 ■), increased pigmentation of the areolae and nipples, and darkened moles and scars. These are all normal findings.

Many pregnant females develop striae gravidarum (stretch marks) across the abdomen. These usually fade after pregnancy but do not disappear entirely. Cutaneous tags are not uncommon, especially on the neck and upper chest.

Hormonal changes may cause the oil and sweat glands to become hyperactive during pregnancy. This increased secretion may in turn lead to a worsening of acne in the first trimester of pregnancy and an improvement in the third trimester. As more hairs enter the growth phase under hormonal influences in pregnancy, more than the usual number of hairs reach maturity and fall out in the

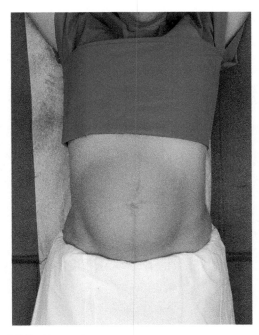

Figure 13.7 Linea nigra.

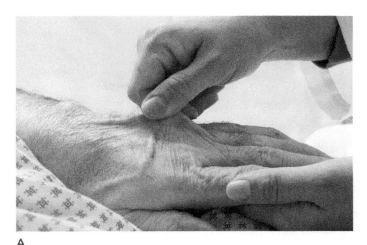

A

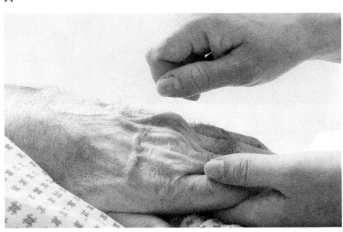

B

Figure 13.8 Tenting. A. Step one: Nurse's fingers pulling skin; B. Step two: skin released, remains pulled.

postpartum period during months 1 to 5. Usually all hair grows back by 6 to 15 months postpartum.

The Older Adult

As the skin ages, the epidermis thins and stretches out, and collagen and elastin fibers decrease, causing decreased skin elasticity and increased skin wrinkling. The skin becomes slack and may hang loosely on the frame. It may sag, especially beneath the chin and eyes, in the breasts of females, and in the scrotum of males.

The older patient's skin is also more delicate and more susceptible to injury. Decreased production of sebum leads to dryness of both the skin and the hair. The skin may appear especially thin on the dorsal surfaces of the hands and feet and over the bony prominences. Tenting of the skin is common (see Figure 13.8 ■). The sweat glands also decrease their activity, and the older adult perspires less. Decreased melanin production leads to a heightened sensitivity to sunlight, and skin cancer rates increase with age.

Some light-skinned older patients may appear pale because of decreased vascularity in the dermis, even though they may be healthy and well oxygenated. The color of a dark-skinned elderly person may appear dull, gray, or darker for the same reason.

A variety of lesions are common and some are normal changes of aging in older adults. For example, the skin of many older patients

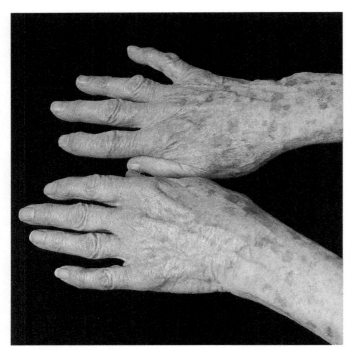

Figure 13.9 Senile lentigines.
Source: Zuber/Custom Medical Stock Photo.

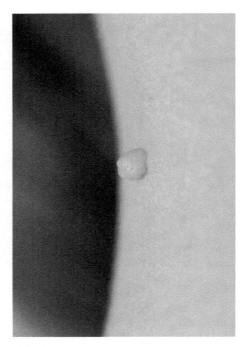

Figure 13.11 Cutaneous tag.
Source: Getty/Photolibrary/Peter Arnold, Inc.

may develop *senile lentigines* (liver spots), which look like hyperpigmented freckles, most commonly on the backs of the hands and the arms (see Figure 13.9 ■). Cherry angiomas are small, bright red spots common in older adults (see Figure 13.10 ■). They increase in number with age. Cutaneous tags may appear on the neck and upper chest (see Figure 13.11 ■), and cutaneous horns may occur on any part of the face (see Figure 13.12 ■).

The hair becomes increasingly gray as melanin production decreases. Hair thins as the number of active hair follicles decreases. Facial hair may become coarser.

The nails may show little change, or they may show the effects of decreased circulation in the body extremities, appearing thicker, harder, yellowed, oddly shaped, or opaque. They may be brittle and peeling, and may be prone to splitting and breaking.

Psychosocial Considerations

Stress may exacerbate certain skin conditions such as rashes or acne. Stress may also be a factor in compulsive behaviors such as hair twisting or plucking (**trichotillomania**) and nail biting, signaled by nails that have no visible free edge or that have short, jagged edges. A lack of cleanliness of the skin, hair, or nails also may result from emotional distress, poor self-esteem, or a disturbed body image.

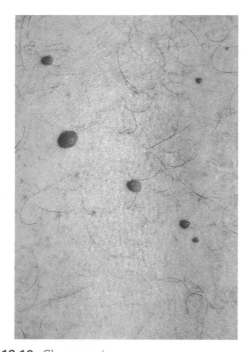

Figure 13.10 Cherry angioma.
Source: Linda Steward/Getty Images.

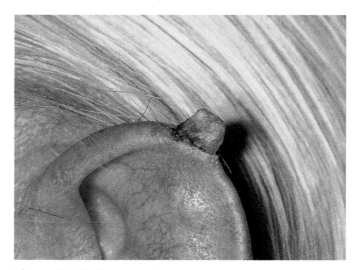

Figure 13.12 Cutaneous horn.
Source: SPL/Science Source.

If appropriate, the nurse should refer the patient to social services or a mental health professional for assistance.

However, a visible skin disorder may trigger psychosocial health problems leading to social isolation, a body image disturbance, or a self-esteem disturbance. If appropriate, the patient should be assessed further for the presence of emotional distress or anxiety related to a skin disorder.

Cultural and Environmental Considerations

A patient's culture, socioeconomic status, home environment, and means of employment may affect the health of the skin, hair, and nails. If the patient's skin, hair, and nails appear unclean, the nurse should consider the patient's job, socioeconomic status, and living situation. A patient who seems unkempt may have just come from a physically demanding job or may be ill, disabled, or depressed.

Changes in skin color may be difficult to evaluate in patients with dark skin. It is helpful to inspect areas of the body with less pigmentation, such as the lips, oral mucosa, sclerae, palms of the hands, and conjunctivae of the inner eyelids. The nurse must be careful not to mistake the normal deposition of melanin in the lips of some olive to dark-skinned people for cyanosis. Some individuals with dark skin have increased pigmentation in the creases of the palms and soles, and yellow or brown-tinged sclerae. These are normal findings (see Table 13.2 for evaluating color variations in light and dark skin).

Dry skin does not necessarily indicate dehydration and in fact may be normal for the dark-skinned patient. Additionally, since many patients use petroleum-based products to lubricate their skin, the nurse should ask about self-care before concluding that the patient has oily skin.

The skin's response to stressors such as ultraviolet radiation is similar in all races. Dark-skinned patients tan, and their skin suffers the same damaging effects from the sun, although skin damage may take longer to occur. Therefore, assessment of color, texture, moles, and other lesions should be as thorough as for light-skinned patients.

TABLE 13.2   Color Variations in Light and Dark Skin

COLOR VARIATION/ LOCALIZATION	POSSIBLE CAUSES	APPEARANCE IN LIGHT SKIN	APPEARANCE IN DARK SKIN
Pallor *Loss of color in skin due to the absence of oxygenated hemoglobin.* Widespread, but most apparent in face, mouth, conjunctivae, and nails.	May be caused by sympathetic nervous stimulation resulting in peripheral vasoconstriction due to smoking, a cold environment, or stress. May also be caused by decreased tissue perfusion due to cardiopulmonary disease, shock and hypotension, lack of oxygen, or prolonged elevation of a body part. May also be caused by anemia.	White skin loses its rosy tones. Skin with natural yellow tones appears more yellow; may be mistaken for mild jaundice.	Black skin loses its red undertones and appears ash-gray. Brown skin becomes yellow-tinged. Skin looks dull.
Absence of Color *Congenital or acquired loss of melanin pigment* Congenital loss is typically generalized, and acquired loss is typically patchy.	Generalized depigmentation may be caused by albinism. Localized depigmentation may be due to vitiligo or tinea versicolor, a common fungal infection.	Albinism appears as white skin, white or pale blond hair, and pink irises. Vitiligo is very noticeable as patchy milk-white areas. Tinea versicolor appears as patchy areas paler than the surrounding skin.	Albinism appears as white skin, white or pale blond hair, and pink irises. Vitiligo appears as patchy milk-white areas, especially around the mouth. Tinea versicolor appears as patchy areas paler than the surrounding skin.
Cyanosis *Mottled blue color in skin and its appendages due to inadequate tissue perfusion with oxygenated blood.* Most apparent in the nails, lips, oral mucosa, and tongue.	Systemic or central cyanosis is due to cardiac disease, pulmonary disease, heart malformations, and low hemoglobin levels. Localized or peripheral cyanosis is due to vasoconstriction, exposure to cold, and emotional stress.	The skin, lips, and mucous membranes look blue-tinged. The conjunctivae and nail beds are blue.	The skin may appear a shade darker. Cyanosis may be undetectable except for the lips, tongue, oral mucous membranes, nail beds, and conjunctivae, which appear pale or blue-tinged.
Reddish Blue Tone *Ruddy tone due to an increased hemoglobin and stasis of blood in capillaries.* Most apparent in the face, mouth, hands, feet, and conjunctivae.	Polycythemia vera, an overproduction of red blood cells, granulocytes, and platelets.	Reddish purple hue.	Difficult to detect. The normal skin color may appear darker in some patients. Check lips for redness.

(continued)

TABLE 13.2	Color Variations in Light and Dark Skin (continued)		
COLOR VARIATION/ LOCALIZATION	**POSSIBLE CAUSES**	**APPEARANCE IN LIGHT SKIN**	**APPEARANCE IN DARK SKIN**
Erythema *Redness of the skin due to increased visibility of normal oxyhemoglobin. Generalized, or on face and upper chest, or localized to area of inflammation or exposure.*	Hyperemia, a dilatation and congestion of blood in superficial arteries. Due to fever, warm environment, local inflammation, allergy, emotions (blushing or embarrassment), exposure to extreme cold, consumption of alcohol, or dependent position of body extremity.	Readily identifiable over entire body or in localized areas. Local inflammation and redness are accompanied by higher temperature at the site.	Generalized redness may be difficult to detect. Localized areas of inflammation appear purple or darker than surrounding skin. May be accompanied by higher temperature, hardness, swelling.
Jaundice *Yellow undertone due to increased bilirubin in the blood. Generalized, but most apparent in the conjunctivae and mucous membranes.*	Increased bilirubin may be due to liver disease, biliary obstruction, or hemolytic disease following infections, severe burns, or resulting from sickle cell anemia or pernicious anemia.	Generalized. Also visible in sclerae, oral mucosa, hard palate, fingernails, palms of hands, and soles of the feet.	Visible in the sclerae, oral mucosa, junction of hard and soft palate, palms of the hands, and soles of the feet.
Carotenemia *Yellow-orange tinge caused by increased levels of carotene in the blood and skin. Most apparent in the face, palms of the hands, and soles of the feet.*	Excess carotene due to ingestion of foods high in carotene such as carrots, egg yolks, sweet potatoes, milk, and fats. Also may be seen in patients with anorexia nervosa or endocrine disorders such as diabetes mellitus, myxedema, and hypopituitarism.	Yellow-orange tinge most visible in palms of the hands and soles of the feet. No yellowing of sclerae or mucous membranes.	Yellow-orange seen in forehead, palms, soles. No yellowing of sclerae or mucous membranes.
Uremia *Pale yellow tone due to retention of urinary chromogens in the blood. Generalized, if perceptible.*	Chronic renal disease, in which blood levels of nitrogenous wastes increase. Increased melanin may also contribute, and anemia is usually present as well.	Generalized pallor and yellow tinge, but does not affect the conjunctivae or mucous membranes. Skin may show bruising.	Very difficult to discern because the yellow tinge is very pale and does not affect the conjunctivae or mucous membranes. Rely on laboratory and other data.
Brown *An increase in the production and deposition of melanin. Generalized or localized.*	May be due to Addison's disease or a pituitary tumor. Localized increase in facial pigmentation may be caused by hormonal changes during pregnancy or the use of birth control pills. More commonly due to exposure to ultraviolet radiation from the sun or from tanning booths.	With endocrine disorders, general bronzed skin. Hyperpigmentation in nipples, palmar creases, genitals, and pressure points. Sun exposure causes red tinge in pale skin, and olive-toned skin tans with little or no reddening.	With endocrine disorders, general deepening of skin tone. Hyperpigmentation in nipples, genitals, and pressure points. Sun exposure leads to tanning in various degrees from brown to black.

Calluses (circumscribed, painless thickenings of the epidermis) tend to form on parts of the body that are regularly exposed to pressure, weight bearing, or friction. Common sites of calluses include the fingers, palms, toes, and soles of the feet.

Differences in hair color and texture are widely variable among cultural groups. Individuals of Asian origins tend to have long, straight, dark hair. Scandinavians typically have very light, blonde hair. African Americans may have straight, kinky, or long braided hair, and it can often be dry.

The patient's occupation (e.g., gardener, mechanic) may make it difficult to keep the fingers and nails unstained. Chemicals used in certain occupations and smoking tobacco may stain the nails. The patient's occupation may require frequent or prolonged immersion of the hands in water, which may lead to **paronychia.** The nail plates of dark-skinned patients may show dark pigmented streaks, which are normal findings.

Patients from many cultures use therapies that are not part of standard Western treatment. Among many Asian cultures, coining and cupping are used in treatment for a variety of illnesses. These alternative therapies include using coins, cups, or pinching on areas of the body. The use of these therapies results in lesions, including welts and bruises. These lesions can suggest abuse. Therefore, one must inquire about cultural healing practices. Box 13.1 describes these therapies. For further information about cultural concerns in health care, consult the Office of Minority Health.

Box 13.1 Coining, Cupping, Pinching

Coining	Coining refers to rubbing the skin of the back, upper chest, neck, and arms with a coin in symmetric patterns. Coining results in skin bruising.
Cupping	Cupping is sucking of the skin on the forehead, back, and upper chest. Glass cups are heated until air is removed. The heated cups are placed on the skin. Red circular lesions arise on the skin from cupping.
Pinching	When pinching, the first and second fingers pull upward on the skin of the neck, back, and chest, and between the eyebrows. The pinching produces bruises.
These treatments stimulate circulation and restore balance in children and adults with a variety of ailments.	

Gathering the Data

Assessment of the integumentary system includes gathering subjective and objective data about the skin, hair, and nails. Subjective data collection occurs during the interview, before the actual physical assessment. The nurse will use a variety of communication techniques to elicit general and specific information about the condition of the patient's skin, hair, and nails. Health records and the results of laboratory tests are important secondary sources to be reviewed and included in the data-gathering process. In physical assessment of the integumentary system, the techniques of inspection and palpation will be used. The questions in the focused interview form part of the subjective data and provide valuable information to meet the objectives related to integumentary health included in Table 13.1. See Table 13.3 for information on potential secondary sources of patient data.

Focused Interview

The focused interview for the integumentary system concerns data related to the structures and functions of that system. Subjective data related to the condition of the skin, hair, and nails are gathered during the focused interview. The nurse must be prepared to observe the patient and listen for cues related to the integumentary system. The nurse may use open-ended and closed questions to obtain information. A number of follow-up questions or requests for descriptions may be required to clarify data or gather missing information. Follow-up questions are used to identify the source of problems, determine the duration of difficulties, identify measures to alleviate problems, and provide clues about the patient's knowledge of his or her own health.

The focused interview guides the physical assessment of the integumentary system. The information is always considered in relation to norms and expectations about the function of the integument. Therefore, the nurse must consider age, gender, race, culture, environment, health practices, and past and concurrent

TABLE 13.3	**Potential Secondary Sources for Patient Data Related to the Skin, Hair, and Nails**
Laboratory Tests—Skin	
Eosinophils	Normal Value 1–4%
IgE	Normal Value <0.35 kU/L
Diagnostic Tests—Skin	
Gram stain and culture	Skin biopsy
Immunostaining	Skin scraping
Patch tests	Tzanck Test
Diagnostic Tests—Hair	
Trichogram–alopecia	
Diagnostic Tests—Nails	
Biopsy	

problems and therapies when forming questions and using techniques to elicit information. In order to address all of the factors when conducting a focused interview, categories of questions related to the status and function of each part of the integumentary system have been developed. These categories include general questions that are asked of all patients; those addressing illness and infection; questions related to symptoms, pain, and behaviors; those related to habits or practices; questions that are specific to patients according to age; those for pregnant females; and questions that address environmental concerns. One approach to questioning about symptoms would be the OLDCART & ICE method, described in detail in chapter 7. ∞

The nurse must consider the patient's ability to participate in the focused interview and physical assessment. Further, the nurse must consider that the appearance of the skin has an impact on self-image. A patient with clear, healthy skin may have a heightened self-esteem. Patients with changes in the skin due to the normal aging process or from skin disorders may be anxious about the way they appear to others. Patients with visible skin disorders are often sensitive about the condition and their appearance. The nurse must select communication techniques that demonstrate caring and preserve the dignity of the patient.

Focused Interview Questions	Rationales and Evidence

The following sections provide sample questions and bulleted follow-up questions in each of the categories for the skin. A rationale for each of the questions is provided. The list of questions is not all-inclusive but represents the types of questions required in a comprehensive focused *interview related to the skin. Questions related to the hair and nails are included but are not divided into the previously mentioned categories of questions.*

Skin

General Questions

1. **Describe your skin today.**
   - How does it compare to 2 months ago? How does it compare to 2 years ago?

   ▶ This question gives patients the opportunity to provide their own perceptions about the skin.

2. **Do you ever have trouble controlling body odor? If so, at what times?**

   ▶ Body odor becomes stronger during heavy activity because of increased excretion of uric acid. Body odor may also be related to diet. A change in body odor may indicate the presence of a systemic disorder or developmental changes (Mayo Clinic, 2014c).

3. **How much and how easily do you sweat?**

   ▶ **Diaphoresis** (profuse sweating) is a significant avenue for sodium chloride loss and may indicate the presence of a systemic disorder, including infectious disease with a fever. Increased sweating is a side effect of some medications (Wilson, Shannon, & Shields, 2013). Decreased sweating increases the risk of heat stroke (American Academy of Orthopaedic Surgeons, 2009) and may be a side effect of medications.

4. **Have you had episodes of increased sweating that occur at certain times, especially at night?**

   ▶ Such episodes can suggest the presence of an infectious process (Mayo Clinic, 2014c).

5. **Have you noticed any changes in the color of your skin?**
   - If so, did the change occur over your entire body or only in one area?

   ▶ Color changes to the skin may result from internal diseases (American Academy of Dermatology [AAD], 2013). For example, yellowing of the skin may indicate liver disease, darkening of the skin may indicate adrenal disease, and a blue tint to the skin (cyanosis) may indicate heart or respiratory diseases.

6. **Has your skin become either more oily or more dry recently?**
   - Have you noticed other changes in the way your skin feels?

   ▶ Metabolic disorders or simple age-related changes in the production of sebum may produce changes in the texture of the skin (Cleveland Clinic, 2011).

7. **Is there a history of allergies, rashes, or other skin problems in your family?**

   ▶ Some allergies and skin disorders are familial; thus, the patient may be predisposed. Follow-up is required to obtain details about specific problems, their occurrence, treatments, and outcomes.

Focused Interview Questions	Rationales and Evidence

Questions Related to Illness or Infection

1. **Have you ever had a skin problem?**
   1. When were you diagnosed with the problem?
   - What treatment was prescribed for the problem?
   - Was the treatment helpful?
   - What kinds of things did you do to help with the problem?
   - Has the problem ever recurred (acute)?
   - How are you managing the disease now (chronic)?

   ► The patient has an opportunity to provide information about specific skin problems or illnesses. If a diagnosed illness is identified, follow-up about the date of diagnosis, treatment, and outcomes is required. Data about each illness identified by the patient are essential to an accurate health assessment. Illnesses can be classified as acute or chronic, and follow-up regarding each classification will differ.

2. **Have you had any illnesses recently? If so, please describe them.**

   ► Some skin disorders are manifestations of systemic illness (AAD, 2013).

3. **An alternative to question 1 is to list possible skin problems or illnesses, such as lupus, psoriasis, lesions, burns, and trauma, and ask the patient to respond "yes" or "no" as each is stated.**

   ► This is a comprehensive and easy way to elicit information about all skin disorders. Follow-up would be carried out for each identified diagnosis as in question 1.

4. **Do you have or have you had a skin infection?**
   - When were you diagnosed with the infection?
   - What treatment was prescribed for the problem?
   - Was the treatment helpful? What kinds of things have you done in the past or are you doing now to help with the problem?
   - Has the problem ever recurred (acute)?
   - How are you managing the infection now (chronic)?

   ► If an infection is identified, follow-up about the date of infection, treatment, and outcomes is required. Data about each infection identified by the patient are essential to an accurate health assessment. Infections can be classified as acute or chronic, and follow-up regarding each classification will differ.

5. **An alternative to question 4 is to list possible skin infections, such as pruritus, warts, herpes simplex, herpes zoster, candida, and acne, and ask the patient to respond "yes" or "no" as each is stated.**

   ► This is a comprehensive and easy way to elicit information about all skin infections. Follow-up would be carried out for each identified infection as in question 1.

Questions Related to Symptoms, Pain, and Behaviors

When gathering information about symptoms, many questions are required to elicit details and descriptions that assist in the analysis of the data. Discrimination is made in relation to the significance of a symptom, in relation to specific diseases or problems, and in relation to potential follow-up examination or referral. One rationale may be provided for a group of questions in this category.

The following questions refer to specific symptoms and behaviors associated with the skin. For each symptom, questions and follow-up are required. The details to be elicited are the characteristics of the symptom; the onset, duration, and frequency of the symptom; the treatment or remedy for the symptom, including over-the-counter and home remedies; the determination if diagnosis has been sought; the effect of treatments; and family history associated with a symptom or illness.

Questions Related to Symptoms

1. **Do you have any sores or ulcers on your body that are slow in healing?**
   - Where are these?
   - Do you have frequent boils or skin infections?

   ► Delayed healing or frequent skin infections may be a sign of diabetes mellitus or inadequate nutrition (Osborn, Wraa, Watson, & Holleran, 2013).

2. **Does your skin itch? If so, where?**
   - How severe is it?
   - When does it occur?

   ► These questions may help in determining if the itching is due to an allergic reaction or eczema.

Focused Interview Questions	Rationales and Evidence

3. **Have you noticed any rashes on your body? If so, please describe.**
   - Where on your body did the rash start? Where did it spread?
   - When did you first notice it?
   - Did the rash happen at the same time as any other symptoms, such as fever or chills?
   - Have you made a recent change in any skin care products or laundry detergents that might have contributed to the rash?

▶ These factors may help in determining the cause of the rash.

4. **If you have a rash, do you notice it more after wearing certain clothes or jewelry?**
   - After using certain skin products?
   - Did it occur soon after starting a new medication?
   - Does the rash happen during or after any other activities such as gardening or washing dishes?

▶ Rashes related to clothing, jewelry, or cosmetics may be due to contact dermatitis, a type of allergy. Many medications cause allergic skin reactions. A drug reaction can occur even after the patient has taken the drug a long time. Aspirin, antibiotics, and barbiturates are a few of the drugs that fall into this category (Wilson, Shannon, & Shields, 2013).

5. **Have you noticed a change in the size, color, shape, or appearance of any moles or birthmarks?**
   - When did you first notice this?
   - Describe the change.
   - Are they painful? Do they itch? Bleed?

▶ Any changes in a mole or birthmark may signal a skin cancer (American Cancer Society, 2013).

6. **Have you noticed any other lesions, lumps, bumps, tender spots, or painful areas on your body?**
   - If so, when did you first notice them? Where?
   - Have they spread? If so, please describe how they spread and where they are now located.

▶ The time of onset and pattern of development may help determine the source of the problem. For instance, certain patterns of bruises may signal frequent falls or physical abuse (Pierce, Kaczor, Aldridge, O'Flynn, & Lorenz, 2010).

7. **Have you noticed any drainage from any skin region?**
   - If so, where does the drainage come from? What does it look like? Does it have an odor?
   - Is the drainage accompanied by any other symptoms? If so, please describe.

▶ Diagnostic cues such as pain, chills, or fever may aid in identifying the source of the problem.

8. **Please describe anything you have done to treat your skin condition.**
   - When did you begin this treatment? How has your skin responded to the treatment?

Questions Related to Pain

1. **Please describe any skin pain or discomfort.**

2. **Have you experienced any pain or discomfort in any skin folds, for example, between the toes, under the breasts, between the buttocks, or in the perianal area?**

▶ Note that the warm, dark, moist environment in skin folds may breed bacterial and fungal infections (Berman & Snyder, 2012).

3. **Where is the pain?**

▶ Questions 3 through 8 are standard questions associated with pain to determine the location, frequency, duration, and intensity of the pain.

4. **How often do you experience the pain?**

5. **How long does the pain last?**

6. **How long have you had the pain?**

7. **How would you rate the pain on a scale of 0 to 10?**

8. **Is there a trigger for the pain?**

9. **What do you do to relieve the pain?**

10. **Is this treatment effective?**

▶ Questions 9 and 10 are intended to determine if the patient has selected a treatment based on past experience, knowledge of skin disorders or use of complementary and alternative care and its effectiveness.

Focused Interview Questions	**Rationales and Evidence**

Questions Related to Behaviors

1. **Do you sunbathe, either outdoors or in a tanning bed?**

2. **Have you ever sunbathed?**

3. **Do you spend time in the sun exercising or playing sports?**

4. **Do you work outdoors?**

▶ Excessive exposure to the ultraviolet radiation of the sun thickens and damages the skin, depresses the immune system, and alters the deoxyribonucleic acid (DNA) in skin cells, predisposing an individual to cancer (Berman & Snyder, 2012).

5. **How does your skin react to sun exposure?**
   - Do you use a daily lotion with sun protection factor (SPF)?
   - What SPF lotion do you use? Do you reapply the lotion after several hours outside or after swimming?

▶ The ultraviolet radiation that accompanies sunburn is capable of disabling cells that initiate the normal immune response (World Health Organization, 2014). Individuals who burn easily or have a history of serious sunburns may have a greater risk for developing skin cancer (Mayo Clinic, 2014d). These questions determine if the patient follows recommendations by the American Cancer Society regarding skin exposure.

6. **Do you remember having a sunburn that left blisters?**

▶ A history of blistering sunburn increases the risk for skin cancer, especially if it occurred in childhood (Mayo Clinic, 2014d).

7. **How do you care for your skin?**
   - What kind of soap, cleansers, toners, or other treatments do you use?
   - How do you clean your clothes?
   - What kind of detergent do you use?
   - How often do you bathe or shower?

▶ Some skin products and laundry detergents may affect the skin of some patients. Infrequent cleansing of the skin increases the likelihood of skin infections, whereas excessive bathing decreases protective skin oils.

8. **Do you now have or have you ever had a tattoo(s)?**
   - How long have you had the tattoo(s)? Have you had any problems with that area of the skin? Further follow-up would include questions related to treatment and outcomes if skin problems accompanied tattoos.

▶ Tattoos can cause skin irritation, and the process of tattooing may increase an individual's risk for acquiring infections including hepatitis C and HIV (National Kidney Foundation, 2014).

9. **Do you now have or have you ever had piercing of any part of your body?**
   - Where are the sites of piercing?
   - How long have you had the piercing?
   - Have any piercing sites closed?
   - Have you ever had a problem at the piercing site?
   - What was the problem?
   - Did you seek treatment for the problem?
   - What was the outcome of the treatment?
   - What is the current condition of piercing site(s)?

▶ Piercing of any body part puts an individual at risk for infection and hepatitis C (National Kidney Foundation, 2014) and can result in the development of scar tissue at the site.

Questions Related to Age

The focused interview must reflect the anatomic and physiologic differences that exist along the age span. The following questions are presented as examples of those that would be specific for children, pregnant females, and older adults.

Questions Regarding Infants and Children

1. **Does the child have any birthmarks? If so, where are they?**

2. **Has the infant developed an orange hue in the skin?**

▶ Ingestion of large amounts of carotene in vegetables such as carrots, sweet potatoes, and squash can cause an orange or yellow hue (Silverberg & Lee-Wong, 2014).

Focused Interview Questions	Rationales and Evidence
3. **Does the child have a rash? If so, what seems to have caused it?** ● Have you introduced any new foods or a different kind of formula into your child's diet? ● Is it a diaper rash? If so, how often do you change the child's diaper? How do you clean the child's diaper area? Are you using anything to treat the diaper rash? ● Do you use disposable or cloth diapers? If cloth, how do you wash the child's diapers?	▶ Many children may have allergic reactions to certain foods, especially milk, chocolate, and eggs. Infrequent changing of diapers may lead to diaper rash. Harsh detergents may cause skin reactions in some children.
4. **Does the child have any burns, bruises, scrapes, or other injuries?** ● Where are the injuries? ● How did the injuries happen?	▶ A careful history can distinguish expected childhood bumps and bruises from injuries that may indicate child abuse or neglect. For example, small round burns may indicate a cigarette burn. Excessive bruising in the torso area and proximal limbs or linear whip marks may indicate physical abuse.

Questions for the Menstruating Female

1. **Female patients: Are you pregnant? If not, are you menstruating regularly? Describe your menstrual periods.**	▶ The skin may be affected by changes in hormonal balance (Osborn et al., 2013).

Questions for the Pregnant Female

1. **What changes have you noticed in your skin since you became pregnant?**	▶ The hormonal changes of pregnancy may cause various benign changes in skin pigmentation, moisture, texture, and vascularity that are entirely normal (Osborn et al., 2013).
2. **Do you use any topical medications for problems with the skin, hair, or nails?**	▶ Topical medications that can result in birth defects include Retin-A for acne, antifungal agents, and minoxidil for hair growth (Wilson, Shannon, & Shields, 2013).
3. **Do you use topical medications for other problems? If so, identify the medications.**	▶ Many medications that are absorbed through the skin may reach the baby through the bloodstream. Some of these medications may harm the developing fetus. Among the medications are antibiotics, steroids, and medications for muscle pain (Wilson, Shannon, & Shields, 2013).

Questions for the Older Adult

1. **What changes have you noticed in your skin in the past few years?**	▶ The normal changes of aging, such as increased dryness and wrinkling of the skin, may cause distress for some patients.
2. **Does your skin itch?**	▶ **Pruritus** (itching) increases in incidence with age. It is usually due to dry skin, which may in turn be caused by excessive bathing or use of harsh skin cleansers.
3. **Do you experience frequent falls?**	▶ Older adults bruise easily. Multiple bruises may result from frequent falls.

Questions Related to the Environment

Environment refers to both the internal and external environments. Questions related to the internal environment include all of the previous questions and those associated with internal or physiologic responses. Questions regarding the external environment include those related to home, work, or social environments.

Internal Environment

1. **How would you describe your level of stress? Has it changed in the past few weeks? Few months? Describe.**	▶ Emotional stress may aggravate skin disorders (Huynh, Gupta, & Koo, 2013).

Focused Interview Questions	Rationales and Evidence

2. Are you now experiencing, or have you ever experienced, intermittent or prolonged anxiety or emotional upset?
- Describe the situation.
- Can you determine precipitating factors?
- Have you sought care or treatment for the problem?
- What do you do when the problem arises?

3. Are you taking any prescription or over-the-counter medications?

▶ Patients may experience rashes or other skin eruptions in response to various drugs. Some drugs, such as antibiotics, antihistamines, antipsychotics, oral hypoglycemic agents, and oral contraceptives, can cause an adverse effect if the patient is exposed to the sun (Wilson, Shannon, & Shields, 2013).

4. Have you changed your diet recently? Have you recently tried any unfamiliar types of food? Please describe.

▶ Changes in diet or eating new foods may cause rashes and other skin reactions.

5. Has the condition of your skin affected your social relationships in any way? Has it limited you in any way? If so, how?

▶ Skin problems may affect a person's self-concept and body image, interfering with social relationships, roles, and sexuality. This is especially true for adolescents and young adults (Owoeye, Aina, Omoluabi, & Olumide, 2009). Serious skin problems may also affect a person's ability to function and maintain a job.

External Environment

The following questions deal with substances and irritants found in the physical environment of the patient. The physical environment includes the indoor and outdoor environments of the home and the workplace, those encountered for social engagements, and any encountered during travel.

1. Have you been exposed recently to extremes in temperature?
- If so, when? How long was the exposure? Where did this occur?
- Describe the temperature of your home environment. Of your work environment.

▶ Extremes in environmental temperature may exacerbate skin disorders (Osborn et al., 2013).

2. Do you work in an environment where radioisotopes or x-rays are used?
- If so, are you vigilant about following precautions and using protective gear?

▶ Excessive exposure to x-rays or radioisotopes may predispose a patient to skin cancer (Mayo Clinic, 2014d).

3. Do you wear gloves for work? If so, what types of gloves? Do you have any signs of allergy related to wearing these gloves?

▶ Certain types of gloves, especially latex, can cause mild to severe skin allergic reactions (Osborn et al., 2013).

4. How often do you travel?
- Have you traveled recently?
- If so, where?
- Have you come into contact with anyone who has a similar rash or skin problem?

▶ The nurse should suspect unfamiliar foods, water, plants, or insects as potential causes of rashes and other skin problems if the patient has traveled recently. In addition, some rashes, such as measles and impetigo, are contagious (Osborn et al., 2013).

5. Does your job or hobby require you to perform repetitive tasks?
- Does your job or hobby require you to work with any chemicals?
- Does your job or hobby require you to wear a specific type of helmet, hat, goggles, gloves, or shoes?

▶ Regular work with certain tools or regular wear of ill-fitting helmets, hats, goggles, or shoes may cause skin abrasions. Additionally, the skin absorbs certain organic solvents used in industry, such as acetone, dry-cleaning fluid, dyes, formaldehyde, and paint thinner. Excessive exposure to these and other types of irritants may contribute to rashes, skin cancers, or other skin reactions (CDC, 2013).

Focused Interview Questions	Rationales and Evidence

Hair

General Questions

1. **Describe your hair now.**
   - How does it compare to 2 months ago? How does it compare to 2 years ago?
   - Have you ever had problems with your hair? If so, please describe the problem, including any treatment and resolution.

2. **How often do you wash your hair?**
   - What kinds of shampoos do you use?
   - Do you have excessive **dandruff?**
   - Do you do anything to control it?

▶ Shampooing too frequently or using too many styling products can irritate or dry out the scalp, increasing dandruff; not shampooing frequently enough can also cause dandruff because of a buildup of dead skin cells and oil. Other skin conditions such as seborrheic dermatitis, eczema, psoriasis, and *Malassezia* infection can also contribute to dandruff (Mayo Clinic, 2014a).

3. **Have you noticed a recent increase in hair loss?**
   - If so, describe how the hair fell out.
   - What it a gradual or sudden onset?
   - It is symmetric? Are there bald or patchy areas without hair?
   - Have you been ill in the last few months?

▶ The scalp typically sheds about 50 to 90 hairs each day, and so some hair loss is normal. Progressive diffuse hair loss is natural in some men (Mayo Clinic, 2014b). Hair loss in women that follows a male pattern may be due to an imbalance of adrenal hormones such as occurs in polycystic ovarian syndrome (Setji & Brown, 2014). When patches of hair fall out, the nurse should suspect trauma to the scalp due to chemicals, infections, or blows to the head. Chemotherapeutic agents cause hair loss. Also, some people with nervous disorders pull or twist their hair, causing it to fall out (trichotillomania). If hair loss is distributed over the entire head, it may be caused by a systemic disease or fungal infection. Abnormal hair loss sometimes follows a feverish illness. Hair loss may also be the result of an autoimmune disorder called **alopecia areata** (Mayo Clinic, 2014b). Thinning or shedding of the hair on the scalp (telogen effluvium) may occur in pregnancy (Gizlenti & Ekmekci, 2013). Hair shedding may last for several months and continue for up to 15 months after delivery.

4. **Have you noticed a recent increase in hair growth?**
   - What it a gradual or sudden onset?
   - It is symmetric? Are there bald or patchy areas without hair?

▶ **Hirsutism** is shaggy or excessive hair, and is often associated with polycystic ovarian syndrome, Cushing's syndrome, congenital adrenal hyperplasia, androgen-secreting tumors, and some medications (Bode, Seehusen, & Baird, 2012).

5. **Are you taking any prescription or over-the-counter medications?**

▶ Certain medications can change the texture of the hair or lead to hair loss. For instance, oral contraceptives may change the hair texture or rate of hair growth in some women, and drugs used in the treatment of circulatory disorders and cancer may result in a temporary generalized hair loss over the entire body (Patel, Harrison, & Sinclair, 2013).

6. **How do you style your hair?**

▶ Use of styling products can dry or damage hair, as can use of hair dryers, curling irons, and heated rollers. Some methods of setting hair, and sleeping in hair rollers, may cause breakage and lead to patchy hair loss. Repeated tight braiding may damage hair and lead to patchy hair loss.

7. **Do you bleach, color, perm, or chemically straighten your hair?**
   - If so, how often? When did you last have this done?

▶ These chemical processes may damage the scalp and hair and may cause hair loss.

Focused Interview Questions	Rationales and Evidence
8. Do you pluck your eyebrows or facial hair? • Do you shave the hair on your face, on your legs, or under your arms? • Do you use chemical hair removers, wax, or electrolysis?	► Each of these hair removal methods can cause trauma to the skin. Use of unclean equipment can contaminate the skin. Plucking leaves an open portal for bacteria and may lead to infection if aseptic technique is not used (Elmann et al., 2012).
9. Do you swim regularly? How often? For how long? Where?	► Swimming regularly in salt water or chlorinated pools can dry the scalp and hair and may cause increased dandruff.

Questions Regarding Infants and Children

1. Has the child shared hair combs, brushes, or pillows with other children?	► Sharing hair care implements or pillows may expose the child to head lice.

Nails

General Questions

1. Describe your nails now. • How do they compare to 2 months ago? How do they compare to 2 years ago? • Have you ever had problems with your nails? • If so, please describe the problem, including any treatment and resolution.	► Ridged, brittle, split, or peeling fingernails may be caused by protein or vitamin B deficiencies. Changes in circulation may affect the nails. Newly acquired dark longitudinal lines may signal a nevus or melanoma in the nail root. Dark lines may be normal, especially in dark-skinned patients, or associated with some medications including antiretrovirals (Wilson, Shannon, & Shields, 2013).
2. Have you noticed any pain, swelling, or drainage around your cuticles? • If so, when did you first notice this? • What do you think might have caused it?	► Infection of the cuticles is often due to chronic trauma in a wet environment, such as occurs with nail biters or dishwashers (Tully, Trayes, & Studdiford, 2012).
3. Have you been ill recently?	► Cancer, heart disease, liver disease, anemia, and other illnesses can cause various changes in the nails such as grooves, ridges, or discoloration.
4. Have you been taking any prescription or over-the-counter medications?	► Some medication may cause nail changes in some patients. For example, patients who have been treated with the antiviral drug zidovudine (Retrovir, AZT) can develop dark, longitudinal lines on all of their fingernails (Wilson, Shannon, & Shields, 2013).
5. Do you wear nail enamel? Do you wear artificial fingernails, tips, or wraps?	► Prolonged use of nail polish may dry or discolor the nails. Additionally, some patients may have an allergic reaction to nail polish. Use of artificial nails may encourage growth of fungi or damage the nail plate (Khodavaisy, Nabili, Davari, & Vahedi, 2011).
6. Do you spend a great deal of time at work or at home with your hands in water?	► Bacterial and fungal infections of the cuticles may occur in people who submerge their hands in water for long periods (Tully et al., 2012).

Questions Regarding Infants and Children

1. Does the child have any habits such as pulling or twisting the hair, rubbing the head, or biting the nails?	► These habits may signal anxiety or emotional distress. Nail biting may also lead to impaired skin integrity.

Questions for the Pregnant Female

1. Have your nails changed? If so, what are the changes?	► Nail changes in pregnancy include brittleness, formation of grooves, or **onycholysis** (separation of the nail from the nail bed) (Osborn et al., 2013).

Focused Interview Questions	Rationales and Evidence

Questions for the Older Adult

1. **Do you find it difficult to care for your skin, hair, and nails? If so, describe any difficulties you are experiencing.**

▶ Older adults with impaired mobility may have difficulty cleansing or grooming their skin, hair, and nails. Some older adults may have trouble reaching down to their feet to groom their toenails (Osborn et al., 2013).

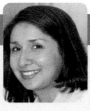

Patient-Centered Interaction

Ms. Tanish Thalia, age 32, reports to the Medi-Center with a chief complaint of pain, swelling, and redness at the nails of two fingers on her left hand. The following is an excerpt of the focused interview.

Interview

Nurse: Good morning. Ms. Thalia, I see from your information sheet that you have a problem with the fingernails of your left hand.

Ms. Thalia: Yes, I think it's my nails, but I'm not sure.

Nurse: The problem involves two fingers of the left hand.

Ms. Thalia: Yes, the thumb and index finger are the only two. The other three seem to be okay.

Nurse: Looking at your nails, I see they are highly polished.

Ms. Thalia: Yes, I have them done professionally every 7 to 10 days. They were done 5 days ago.

Nurse: Are these your natural nails?

Ms. Thalia: Yes, I have silk wraps on all my nails to help make them stronger.

Nurse: Does the manicurist push and cut your cuticles?

Ms. Thalia: Yes, she does both. Do you think this is from having the manicure?

Nurse: It could be. I'm not sure. I need more information. When did you first notice the pain and swelling?

Ms. Thalia: It started several days after I had my nails done, and now it seems to be getting worse. What is causing this?

Nurse: Is this the first time the manicurist did your nails?

Ms. Thalia: Oh no, Sally has been doing my nails for 3 years. This is the first time I have had anything like this.

Nurse: How much time are your hands and nails in water?

Ms. Thalia: Not much. I use gloves when I do the dishes.

Analysis

The nurse uses closed questions to obtain the necessary information from Ms. Thalia. The nurse seeks clarification regarding the fingers involved and also confirms the condition of the nails, the frequency of care, and the type of care regarding cutting of the cuticles. When asked, Ms. Thalia is able to provide specific information regarding date of last manicure, symptoms involved, and the relationship between these two factors. The nurse does not make a judgment and indicates that more information is needed.

Patient Education

The following are risk factors for physiologic, behavioral, and cultural considerations that affect the health of the skin, hair, and nails. Several factors are cited in *Healthy People 2020* documents. The nurse provides advice and education to reduce risks associated with these factors and to promote and maintain the health of the skin, hair, and nails across the life span.

LIFESPAN CONSIDERATIONS

Risk Factors

- Infants have permeable epidermis, increasing the risk of fluid loss through the skin, and they have active sebaceous glands, leading to milia and cradle cap.

Patient Education

▶ Teach parents and caregivers that infants require regular bathing and washing of the scalp and hair.

LIFESPAN CONSIDERATIONS

Risk Factors	Patient Education
● Infants' skin lacks the ability to contract. Therefore, they cannot shiver and do not perspire, limiting thermal regulation.	► Soap and shampoos should be mild and the skin should be thoroughly rinsed. Patting dry is recommended for sensitive young skin. Further, infants require clothing that is appropriate for the external temperature and environment since they have limited thermal regulation.
● Children's skin texture changes, but perspiration and sebaceous gland function are limited, resulting in dry skin.	► Tell parents that children's dry skin needs to be monitored and mild lotions used when dryness is excessive.
● In adolescence, skin texture continues to change. Sebaceous gland activity increases in response to hormonal changes. Eccrine glands increase function, resulting in increased perspiration, especially in response to emotional changes.	► Teach adolescents that hygiene is important in relation to increasing oil production and perspiration and that soaps and deodorants are effective in controlling body odors.
● Children and adolescents are at risk for skin trauma associated with accidents, play, and sports activity.	► Provide information about recognition and levels of skin trauma to reduce risk of infection and damage and about when to seek assistance from healthcare providers for skin trauma and problems.
● Infectious material and debris collected beneath the nails can become a source of infection.	► Teach all patients that nail care includes cleaning and drying the nails.
● Unusual nail markings or changes in the color or texture of the nails may be reflective of local or systemic health disorders.	► Advise patients to inspect their nails and to report any unusual markings or changes in nail color or texture.
● Aging results in thinning and graying of the hair and decreasing amounts of body hair. Aging skin repairs more slowly, sweat gland activity decreases, and the nails become thicker and ridged in aging.	► Tell older adults that they may require the use of lotions to maintain moisture and should limit the use of soaps to prevent increased dryness of the skin. ► Encourage older adults to "accident proof" their environments. Falls, slips, and bumps often result in tearing or injury to the increasingly fragile skin.

CULTURAL CONSIDERATIONS

Risk Factors	Patient Education
● African American males are prone to develop folliculitis.	► Teach all patients how to examine their skin (see Box 13.2).
● African Americans are more likely to have dry scalps and dry, fragile hair.	► Provide African American women with information about the risks associated with chemical treatments, excessive combing, and pulling to braid fragile hair.

Box 13.2 Self-Examination of the Skin

1. Use a room that is well lit and has a full-length mirror. Have a handheld mirror and chair available. Remove all of your clothes.

2. Examine all of your skin surface, front and back. Begin with your hands, including the spaces between your fingers. Continue with your arms, chest, abdomen, pubic area, thighs, lower legs, and toes. Next examine your face and neck. Make sure you inspect your underarms, the sides of your trunk, the back of your neck, the buttocks, and the soles of your feet.

3. Next, sit down with one leg elevated. Use the handheld mirror to examine the inside of the elevated leg, from the groin area to the foot. Repeat on the other leg.

4. Use the handheld mirror to inspect your scalp.

5. Consult your physician promptly if you see any newly pigmented area or if any existing mole has changed in color, size, shape, or elevation. Also report sores that do not heal; redness or swelling around a growth or lesion; any change in sensation such as itching, pain, tenderness, or numbness in a lesion or the skin around it; and any change in the texture or consistency of the skin.

ENVIRONMENTAL CONSIDERATIONS

Risk Factors	Patient Education
• Medication, both topical and ingested, can cause skin irritation or problems as a result of sensitivity or allergy and can exacerbate existing skin problems.	▶ Provide information about medications that may affect the skin, including side effects that may appear as skin changes. Further, information about when to seek assistance in the event of unexpected reactions to medications is essential. ▶ Instruct patients about exercise and its importance in skin maintenance across the age span and that the diet should include protein, fats, and vitamins to promote healthy skin, hair, and nails.
• Patients with diabetes, liver disease, or circulatory disease are at increased risk for problems with the skin and with healing of existing skin problems.	▶ Provide patients who have existing health problems such as diabetes with information about examination of and preventive care of the skin.
• Genetic predisposition and moles increase the risk of developing skin cancer.	▶ Teach patients to monitor moles for changes in color, size, or texture.
• Sun exposure, particularly with repeated sunburn, increases the risk of skin cancer.	▶ Tell patients that limiting sun exposure and using sunblock are important ways to decrease skin damage and reduce the risk of skin cancer. ▶ Teach all patients the steps for self-examination of the skin (see Box 13.2).
• Exposure to chemicals; allergens; and pollutants in the home, workplace, and environment can cause skin damage.	▶ Provide information about the use of protective clothing, gloves, and other equipment to reduce exposure to risks associated with chemicals, pollutants, and irritants in the home and environment.

BEHAVIORAL CONSIDERATIONS

Risk Factors	Patient Education
• Hygiene and grooming practices influence the condition of the skin, hair, and nails.	▶ Tell patients that hygiene, including regular bathing in adolescence and young adulthood, reduces risks of infection and decreases body odor.
• Proper nutrition and fluid intake influence the condition of the skin across the age span.	▶ Adequate hydration and nutrients such as Vitamin A and D are essential to skin health.
• Regular exercise and mobility are essential to promoting circulation to the skin and preventing problems of immobility.	▶ Immobility and poor circulation increase the risk for alterations in skin integrity, including skin breakdown and impaired healing.
• Tattooing and body piercing may be culturally based and are increasing among adolescents and young adults in the American culture, increasing risk for skin and systemic infection.	▶ Provide individuals, adolescents, and parents with information about the risks associated with tattooing and body piercing, including infection, scarring, and exposure to hepatitis C and HIV. ▶ Educate patients and their families about immediate and follow-up care of tattooed or pierced skin to prevent future problems.

Physical Assessment

Assessment Techniques and Findings

Physical assessment of the skin, hair, and nails requires the use of inspection and palpation. Inspection includes looking at the skin, hair, and nails to determine color, consistency, shape, and hygiene-related factors. Knowledge of norms or expected findings is essential in determining the meaning of the data as the nurse performs the physical assessment.

Skin should be clean, free from odor, and consistent in color. It should feel warm and moist and should have a smooth texture. The skin should be mobile with blood vessels visible beneath the surfaces of the abdomen and eyelids. It should be free of lesions except for findings of freckles, birthmarks, and normal age variations. The skin should be sensitive to touch and temperature.

The scalp and hair in the adult should be clean. Hair color is determined by the amount of melanin. Gray hair can occur as a result of decreased melanin, genetics, or aging. Hair texture may be coarse or thin. Hair distribution is expected to be even over the scalp. Male pattern baldness is a normal finding. Fine hair is distributed over the body with coarser, darker, longer hair in the axillae and pubic regions in adults. The nails should have a pink undertone and lie flat or form a convex curve on the nail bed.

Physical assessment of the skin, hair, and nails follows an organized pattern. It begins with a survey and inspection of the skin, followed by palpation of the skin. Inspection and palpation of the hair and nails are then carried out. When lesions are present, measurements are used to identify the size of the lesions and the location in relation to accepted landmarks.

EQUIPMENT

- examination gown and drape
- examination light
- examination gloves, clean and nonsterile
- centimeter ruler
- magnifying glass
- penlight

HELPFUL HINTS

- A warm, private environment will reduce patient anxiety.
- Provide special instructions and explain the purpose for removal of clothing, jewelry, hairpieces, nail enamel.
- Maintain the patient's dignity by using draping techniques.
- Monitor one's verbal responses to skin conditions that already threaten the patient's self-image.
- Be sensitive to cultural issues. In some cultures touching or examination by members of the opposite sex is prohibited.
- Covering the head, hair, face, or skin may be part of religious or cultural beliefs. Provide careful explanations regarding the need to expose these areas for assessment.
- Direct sunlight is best for assessment of the skin; if it is not available, lighting must be strong and direct. Tangential lighting may be helpful in assessment of dark-skinned patients.
- Use Standard Precautions throughout the assessment.

Techniques and Normal Findings	Abnormal Findings / Special Considerations

Survey

A quick survey enables the nurse to identify any immediate problem and the patient's ability to participate in the assessment. The nurse inspects the overall appearance of the patient, notes hygiene and odor, and observes for signs of anxiety.

ALERT!

The nurse must be alert for the possibility of impending shock if the patient has pallor accompanied with a drop in blood pressure, increased pulse and respirations, and marked anxiety. if these cues are present, a physician should be consulted immediately.

▶ Patients experiencing pain or discomfort may not be able to participate in the assessment. Severe pain or distress warrants evaluation by a primary care provider.

▶ Patients experiencing anxiety may demonstrate pallor and diaphoresis. Acknowledgment of the problem and discussion of the procedures often provide relief.

Techniques and Normal Findings	Abnormal Findings Special Considerations

Inspection of the Skin

1. **Position the patient.**
   - The patient should be in a sitting position with all clothing removed except the examination gown (see Figure 13.13 ▉).

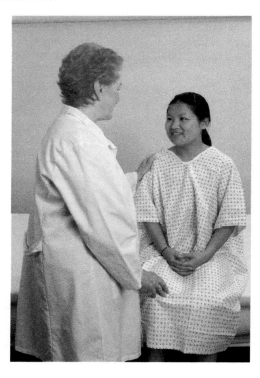

Figure 13.13 Positioning of patient.

2. **Instruct the patient.**
   - Explain that you will be looking carefully at the patient's skin.

3. **Observe for cleanliness, perspiration, or sheen on the skin and use the sense of smell to determine body odor.**
   - Some perspiration is normal and results in a sheen on the skin in healthy individuals. Body odor is produced when bacterial waste products mix with perspiration on the skin surface. During heavy physical activity, body odor increases. Amounts of urea and ammonia are excreted in perspiration.

▶ Urea and ammonia salts are found on the skin of patients with kidney disorders.

4. **Observe the patient's skin tone.**
   - Evaluate any widespread color changes such as cyanosis, pallor, erythema, or jaundice. For example, always assess patients with cyanosis for vital signs and level of consciousness. Use Table 13.2 to evaluate color variations in light and dark skin.
   - The amount of melanin and carotene pigments, the oxygen content of the blood, and the level of exposure to the sun influence skin color. Dark skin contains large amounts of melanin, while fair skin has small amounts. The skin of most Asians contains a large amount of carotene, which causes a yellow cast.

▶ Cyanosis or pallor indicates abnormally low plasma oxygen, placing the patient at risk for altered tissue perfusion. Pallor is seen in anemia.

Techniques and Normal Findings

**Abnormal Findings
Special Considerations**

5. **Inspect the skin for even pigmentation over the body.**
   - In most cases, increased or decreased pigmentation is caused by differences in the distribution of melanin throughout the body. These are normal variations. For example, the margins of the lips, areolae, nipples, and external genitalia are more darkly pigmented. Freckles (see Figure 13.14 ■) and certain *nevi* (congenital marks [see Figure 13.15 ■]) occur in people of all skin colors in varying degrees.

▶ For unknown reasons, some people develop patchy and depigmented areas over the face, neck, hands, feet, and skin folds. This condition is called **vitiligo** (see Figure 13.16 ■). Skin is otherwise normal. Vitiligo occurs in all races in all parts of the world but seems to affect dark-skinned people more severely. Patients with vitiligo may suffer a severe disturbance in body image.

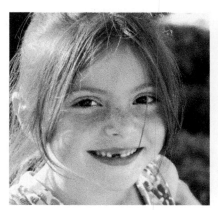

Figure 13.14 Freckles.
Source: Margot Petrowski/Shutterstock.

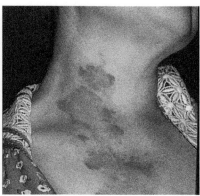

Figure 13.15 Nevus.
Source: CMSP/Custom Medical Stock Photo.

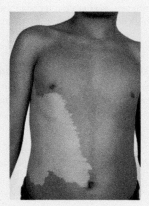

Figure 13.16 Vitiligo.
Source: Mediscan/Alamy.

6. **Inspect the skin for superficial arteries and veins.**
   - A fine network of veins or a few dilated blood vessels visible just beneath the surface of the skin are normal findings in areas of the body where skin is thin (e.g., the abdomen and eyelids).

Palpation of the Skin

1. **Instruct the patient.**
   - Explain that you will be touching the patient in various areas with different parts of your hand.

2. **Determine the patient's skin temperature.**
   - Use the dorsal surface of your fingers, which is most sensitive to temperature. Palpate the forehead or face first. Continue to palpate inferiorly, including the hands and feet, comparing the temperature on the right and left side of the body (see Figure 13.17 ■).

▶ The temperature of the skin is higher than normal in the presence of a systemic infection or metabolic disorder such as hyperthyroidism, after vigorous activity, and when the external environment is warm.

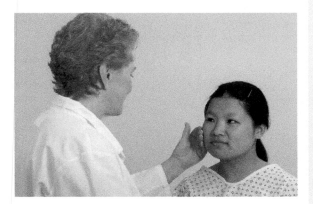

Figure 13.17 Palpating skin temperature.

Techniques and Normal Findings	Abnormal Findings Special Considerations

- Local skin temperature is controlled by the amount and rate of blood circulating through a body region. Normal temperatures range from mildly cool to slightly warm.

▶ The temperature of the skin is lower than normal in the presence of metabolic disorders such as hypothyroidism or when the external environment is cool. Localized coolness results from decreased circulation due to vasoconstriction or occlusion, which may occur from peripheral arterial insufficiency.

- The skin on both sides of the body is warm when tissue is perfused. Sometimes the hands and feet are cooler than the rest of the body, but the temperature is normally similar on both sides.

▶ A difference in temperature *bilaterally* may indicate an interruption in or lack of circulation on the cool side due to compression, immobilization, or elevation. If one side is warmer than normal, inflammation may be present on that side.

3. **Assess the amount of moisture on the skin surface.**
   - Inspect and palpate the face, skin folds, axillae, palms, and soles of the feet, where perspiration is most easily detected.

▶ Diaphoresis occurs during exertion, fever, pain, and emotional stress and in the presence of some metabolic disorders such as hyperthyroidism. It may also indicate an impending medical crisis such as a myocardial infarction.

   - A fine sheen of perspiration or oil is not an abnormal finding nor is moderately dry skin, especially in cold or dry climates.

▶ Severely dry skin typically is dark, weathered, and fissured. Pruritus frequently accompanies dry skin and may lead to abrasion and thickening if prolonged. Generalized dryness may occur in an individual who is dehydrated or has a systemic disorder such as hypothyroidism.

▶ Dry, parched lips and mucous membranes of the mouth are clear indicators of systemic dehydration. These areas should be checked if dehydration is suspected. Dry skin over the lower legs may be due to vascular insufficiency. Localized itching may indicate a skin allergy.

4. **Palpate the skin for texture.**
   - Use the palmar surface of fingers and finger pads when palpating for texture. Normal skin feels smooth, firm, and even.

▶ The skin may become excessively smooth and velvety in patients with hyperthyroidism, whereas patients with hypothyroidism may have rough, scaly skin.

5. **Palpate the skin to determine its thickness.**
   - The outer layer of the skin is thin and firm over most parts of the body except the palms, soles of the feet, elbows, and knees, where it is thicker. Normally, the skin over the eyelids and lips is thinner.

▶ Very thin, shiny skin may signal impaired circulation.

6. **Palpate the skin for elasticity.**
   - Elasticity is a combination of turgor (resiliency, or the skin's ability to return to its normal position and shape) and mobility (the skin's ability to be lifted).
     Using the forefinger and thumb, grasp a fold of skin beneath the clavicle or on the medial aspect of the wrist (see Figure 13.18 ■).

▶ When skin turgor is decreased, the skinfold "tents" (holds its pinched formation) and slowly returns to the former position (see Figure 13.8B). Decreased turgor occurs when the patient is dehydrated or has lost large amounts of weight.
  Increased skin turgor may be caused by scleroderma, literally "hard skin," a condition in which the underlying connective tissue becomes scarred and immobile.

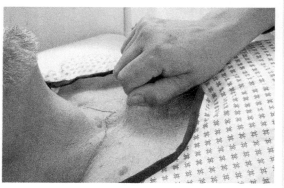

Figure 13.18 Palpating for skin elasticity.

Techniques and Normal Findings	**Abnormal Findings Special Considerations**

- Notice the reaction of the skin both as you grasp and as you release. Healthy skin is mobile and returns rapidly to its previous shape and position.
- Finally, palpate the feet, ankles, and sacrum. **Edema** is present if your palpation leaves a dent in the skin. See chapter 20 for greater detail.∞
- Grade any edema on a four-point scale: +1 indicates mild edema, and +4 indicates deep edema (see Figure 13.19 ■).
- Note that because the fluid of edema lies above the pigmented and vascular layers of the skin, skin tone in the patient with edema is obscured.

▶ *Edema* is a decrease in skin mobility caused by an accumulation of fluid in the intercellular spaces. Edema makes the skin look puffy, pitted, and tight. It may be most noticeable in the skin of the hands, feet, ankles, and sacral area (see Figure 13.20 ■).

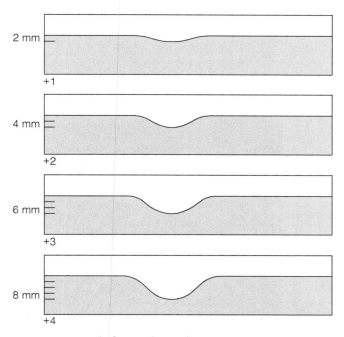

2 mm	+1
4 mm	+2
6 mm	+3
8 mm	+4

Figure 13.19 Four-point scale for grading edema.

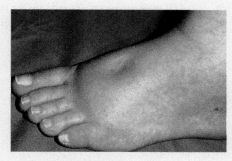

Figure 13.20 Pitting edema.
Source: Dr. P. Marazzi/Science Photo Library/Science Source.

7. **Inspect and palpate the skin for lesions.**
   - Lesions of the skin are changes in normal skin structure. **Primary lesions** develop on previously unaltered skin. Lesions that change over time or because of scratching, abrasion, or infection are called **secondary lesions** (refer to Tables 13.4 and 13.5 for more details).
   - One specific type of secondary lesion is a **pressure ulcer,** which is a localized region of damaged or necrotic tissue that is caused by the exertion of pressure over a bony prominence. Previously called decubitus ulcers, bedsores, and pressure sores, the current terminology was adopted to avoid implying that only nonambulatory, bed-bound patients are at risk for developing pressure ulcers. While reduced mobility is a significant risk factor for this condition, ambulatory patients also are at risk for developing pressure ulcers (Wake, 2010). Therefore, all patients should have their skin inspected for pressure ulcers at every assessment.
   - Pressure ulcers are staged based on their depth (see Box 13.3).

▶ The periumbilical and flank areas of the body should be observed for the presence of **ecchymosis** (bruising). Ecchymoses in the periumbilical area may signal bleeding somewhere in the abdomen (Cullen's sign). Ecchymoses in the flank area are associated with pancreatitis or bleeding in the peritoneum (Grey Turner's sign).
▶ Certain systemic disorders may produce characteristic patterns of lesions on particular body regions. Widespread lesions may indicate systemic or genetic disorders or allergic reactions. Localized lesions may indicate physical trauma, chemical irritants, or allergic dermatitis. The nurse may wish to photograph the patient's skin to document the presence, pattern, or spread of certain lesions.

ALERT!

Physical abuse should be suspected if the patient has any of the following: bruises or welts that appear in a pattern suggesting the use of a belt or stick; burns with sharply demarcated edges suggesting injury from cigarettes, irons, or immersion of a hand in boiling water; additional injuries such as fractures or dislocations; or multiple injuries in various stages of healing. A nurse must be especially sensitive if the patient is fearful of family members, is reluctant to return home, and has a history of previous injuries. When any of these diagnostic cues are evident, it is important to obtain medical assistance and follow the state's legal requirements to notify the police or local protective agency.

Techniques and Normal Findings	Abnormal Findings Special Considerations

Box 13.3 Pressure Ulcer Staging

Pressure ulcers are staged based on their depth (see Figure 13.21 ■).

- Stage I pressure ulcers demonstrate intact skin with no involvement of the underlying tissues or structures.
- Stage II pressure ulcers involve the epidermal skin layer and also may extend into the dermis.
- Stage III pressure ulcers extend into the subcutaneous tissue; however, while underlying muscle, fascia, and bone may be visible, the ulcer is not directly involved with these structures.
- Stage IV pressure ulcers involve muscle and bone (Wake, 2010).

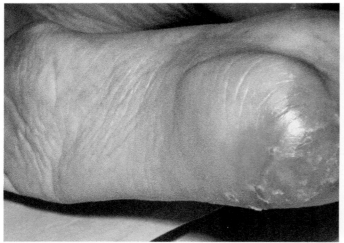

A Stage I

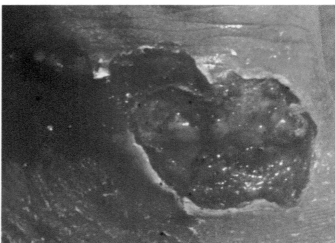

B Stage II

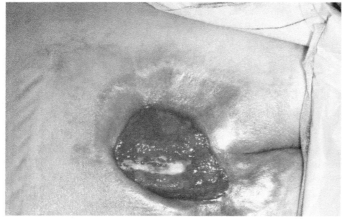

C Stage III

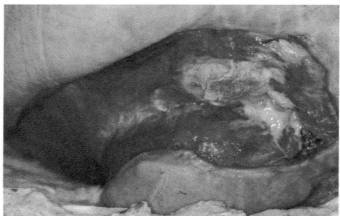

D Stage IV

Figure 13.21   The four stages of pressure ulcers.
Source: (A) SPL/Custom Medical Stock Photo; (B) David Nunuk/Science Source; (C) Tierbild Okapia/Science Source; (D) Roberto A. Penne-Casanova/Science Source.

Techniques and Normal Findings	Abnormal Findings Special Considerations

- Carefully inspect the patient's body, including skin folds and crevices, using a good source of light.
- In the obese patient this requires lifting the breasts and carefully examining the skin under folds in the abdomen, back, and perineal areas. Pressure on the bladder and bowel from the weight of the abdomen as well as reduced mobility contribute to the increased incidence of incontinence in obese patients. In addition, abdominal girth and reduced mobility contribute to difficulties with hygiene in the perineal and other areas. As a result, the obese patient is at risk for rashes and skin breakdown.
- When lesions are observed, palpate lesions between the thumb and index finger. Measure all lesion dimensions (including height, if possible) with a small, clear, flexible ruler.
- Document lesion size in centimeters. If necessary, use a magnifying glass or a penlight for closer inspection (see Figure 13.22 ■).

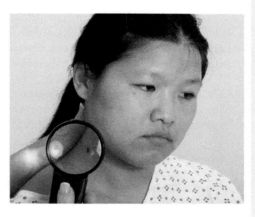

Figure 13.22 Using a magnifying glass.

- Assess any drainage for color, odor, consistency, amount, and location. If indicated, obtain a specimen of the drainage for culture and sensitivity.
- Healthy skin is typically smooth and free of lesions; however, some lesions, such as freckles, insect bites, healed scars, and certain birthmarks, are expected findings.

8. Palpate the skin for sensitivity.
- Palpate the skin in various regions of the body and ask the patient to describe the sensations.
- Give special attention to any pain or discomfort that the patient reports, especially when palpating skin lesions.
- Ask the patient to describe the sensation as closely as possible, and document the findings.
- The patient should not report any discomfort from your touch.

▶ The injection of drugs into the veins of the arms or other parts of the body results in a series of small scars called *track marks* along the course of the blood vessel. A nurse who sees track marks and suspects substance abuse should refer the patient to a mental health or substance abuse professional.

ALERT!

Localized hot, red, swollen painful areas indicate the presence of inflammation and possible infection. These areas should not be palpated, because the slightest disturbance may spread the infection deeper into skin layers.

Techniques and Normal Findings	Abnormal Findings Special Considerations

ADDITIONAL ASSESSMENT

ASSESSMENT FOR CANCEROUS LESIONS

According to the American Cancer Society (2014), more than one million cases of basal or squamous cell carcinomas go unreported each year. The number of cases of melanoma has been rising for the past thirty years. Melanoma occurs primarily in Caucasians, with rates 10 times higher than those for African Americans.

Risk factors for skin cancer include sun sensitivity, difficulty tanning, history of prolonged sun exposure, use of tanning booths, diseases in which immunosuppression occurs, a history of skin cancer, or occupational exposure to some chemicals such as coal tar and radiation. Melanoma risks include personal or family history of melanoma, the presence of moles that are atypical in growth or appearance, and the presence of more than 50 moles. Early detection of skin cancer can result in appropriate treatment and cure.

Comprehensive health assessment includes the patient interview and physical examination. Careful attention to detail during the health history interview enables the examiner to elicit information about risks for skin cancer including family history, sun exposure, and occupational hazards. Physical assessment for skin cancer includes total body skin examination, especially in those who are at high risk for development of skin cancer. Additionally, the National Cancer Institute (NCI) (2008) described the Melanoma Risk Assessment Tool as a method, when used in combination with physical examination, to calculate the risk for development of melanoma. The tool includes questions about age, gender, race, history of sunburn, geography, sun exposure, and moles. The tool is available through the NCI at www.cancer.gov/melanomarisktool/.

Screening for melanoma includes the use of the ABCDE appraisal of pigmented lesions (see Figure 13.23 ■).

The ABCDE criteria refer to size, shape, color, diameter, and change in lesions. This approach is recommended for both healthcare providers and the public to screen for melanoma. This method improves the rates of identification, diagnosis, and treatment of melanomas (Crowson, Magro, & Mihm, 2014).

> **A** = Asymmetry
> **B** = Border Irregularity
> **C** = Color Variegation
> **D** = Diameter greater than 6 mm
> **E** = Evolving Changes*
>
> *Evolving changes include changes in size, shape, symptoms (itching, tenderness), surface (bleeding), and shades of color.

Figure 13.23 ABCDE Criteria for Melanoma Assessment.

Inspection of the Scalp and Hair

1. **Instruct the patient.**
   - Explain that you will be looking at the patient's scalp and hair. Tell the patient you will be parting the hair to observe the scalp.

2. **Observe for cleanliness.**
   - Ask the patient to remove any hairpins, hair ties, barrettes, wigs, or hairpieces and to undo braids. If the patient is unwilling to do this, examine any strands of hair that are loose or undone.
   - Part and divide the hair at 1-in. intervals and observe (see Figure 13.24 ■).

▶ Lesions, including cancerous lesions, may occur on the scalp.
▶ Apply the ABCDE method (see Figure 13.23) in assessment of lesions.

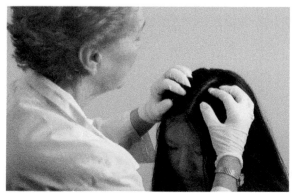

Figure 13.24 Inspecting the hair and scalp.

Techniques and Normal Findings	**Abnormal Findings Special Considerations**

- A small amount of dandruff (dead, scaly flakes of epidermal cells) may be present.

  ▶ Excessive dandruff occurs on the scalp of patients with certain skin disorders, such as psoriasis or seborrheic dermatitis, in which large amounts of the epidermis slough away. Dandruff should be distinguished from head lice.

3. **Observe the patient's hair color.**
   - Like skin color, hair color varies according to the level of melanin production. Graying is influenced by genetics and may begin as early as the late teens in some patients.

  ▶ Graying of the hair in patches may indicate a nutritional deficiency, commonly of protein or copper.

4. **Assess the texture of the hair.**
   - Roll a few strands of hair between your thumb and forefinger.
   - Hold a few strands of hair taut with one hand while you slide the thumb and forefinger of your other hand along the length of the strand.
   - Hair may be thick or fine and may appear straight, wavy, or curly.

  ▶ Hypothyroidism and other metabolic disorders, as well as nutritional deficiencies, may cause the hair to be dull, dry, brittle, and coarse.

5. **Observe the amount and distribution of the hair throughout the scalp.**
   - The amount of hair varies with age, gender, and overall health. Healthy hair is evenly distributed throughout the scalp.

  ▶ When hair loss occurs in women, it is thought to be caused by an imbalance in adrenal hormones.

   - In most men and women, atrophy of the hair follicles causes hair growth to decline by the age of 50. Male pattern baldness (see Figure 13.25 ■), a genetically determined progressive loss of hair beginning at the anterior hairline, has no clinical significance. It is the most frequent reason for hair loss in men.

  ▶ Widespread hair loss may also be caused by illness, infections, metabolic disorders, nutritional deficiencies, and chemotherapy. Patchy hair loss (*alopecia areata*) may be due to infection.

   - Remember to assess the amount, texture, and distribution of body hair. Some practitioners prefer to perform this assessment with the regions of the body.

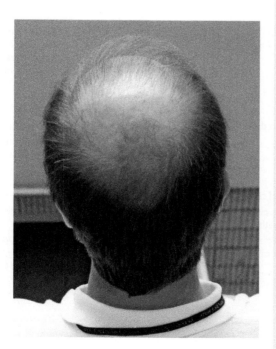

Figure 13.25 Male pattern baldness.

Techniques and Normal Findings	Abnormal Findings Special Considerations

6. Inspect the scalp for lesions.
- The healthy scalp is free from lesions.

▶ Gray, scaly patches with broken hair may indicate the presence of a fungal infection such as ringworm.

▶ Infestation by **pediculosis capitis** (head lice) is signaled by tiny, white, oval eggs (nits) that adhere to the hair shaft. Head lice usually cause intense itching. The scalp should be checked for excoriation from scratching.

Assessment of the Nails

1. Instruct the patient.
- Explain that you will be looking at and touching the patient's nails and that you will ask the patient to hold the hands and fingers in certain positions while you are inspecting the fingernails.

2. Assess for hygiene.
- Confirm that the nails are clean and well groomed.

▶ Dirty fingernails may indicate a self-care deficit but could also be related to a person's occupation.

3. Inspect the nails for an even, pink undertone.
- Small, white markings in the nail are normal findings and indicate minor trauma.

▶ The nails appear pale and colorless in patients with peripheral arteriosclerosis or anemia. The nails appear yellow in patients with jaundice, and dark red in patients with *polycythemia*, a pathologic increase in production of red blood cells. Fungal infections may cause the nails to discolor. Horizontal white bands may occur in chronic hepatic or renal disease. A darkly pigmented band in a single nail may be a sign of a melanoma in the nail matrix and should be referred to a physician for further evaluation.

4. Assess capillary refill.
- Depress the nail edge briefly to blanch, and then release. Color returns to healthy nails instantly upon release.

▶ The nail beds appear blue, and color return is sluggish in patients with cardiovascular or respiratory disorders.

5. Inspect and palpate the nails for shape and contour.
- Perform the Schamroth technique to assess clubbing. Ask the patient to bring the dorsal aspect of corresponding fingers together, creating a mirror image.
- Look at the distal phalanx and observe the diamond-shaped opening created by nails. When clubbing is present, the diamond is not formed and the distance increases at the fingertip (see Figure 13.26 ■).

▶ *Clubbing of the fingernails* occurs when there is hypoxia or impaired peripheral tissue perfusion over a long period. It may also occur with cirrhosis, colitis, thyroid disease, or long-term tobacco smoking. The ends of the fingers become enlarged, soft, and spongy, and the angle between the skin and the nail base is greater than 160 degrees. Also see Table 13.12 on page 256.

| **Techniques and Normal Findings** | **Abnormal Findings Special Considerations** |

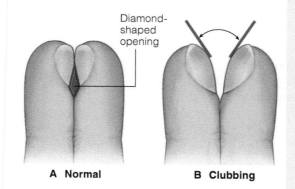

Figure 13.26 Schamroth technique. A. Healthy nail. B. Clubbing.

- The nails normally form a slight convex curve or lie flat on the nail bed. When viewed laterally, the angle between the skin and the nail base should be approximately 160 degrees (see Figure 13.27 ■).

▶ *Spoon nails* form a concave curve rather than a convex curve.

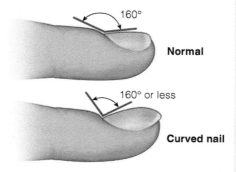

Figure 13.27 Angle of fingernail.

6. **Palpate the nails to determine their thickness, regularity, and attachment to the nail bed.**
   - Healthy nails are smooth, strong, and regular and are firmly attached to the nail bed with only a slight degree of mobility.

▶ Nails may be thickened in patients with circulatory disorders. Onycholysis occurs with trauma, infection, or skin lesions.

7. **Inspect and palpate the cuticles.**
   - The cuticles are smooth and flat in healthy nails.

▶ *Hangnails* are jagged tears in the lateral skin folds around the nail. An untreated hangnail may become inflamed and lead to a *paronychia*, an infection of the cuticle.

Abnormal Findings

Abnormal findings of the integumentary system include alterations in the skin, hair, or nails. Skin abnormalities include primary lesions (see Table 13.4), secondary lesions (see Table 13.5), and vascular lesions (see Table 13.6). Skin abnormalities also are classified based on configuration and shape (see Table 13.7). Abnormalities of the hair and nails are described at the conclusion of this chapter.

TABLE 13.4 Primary Lesions

Macule and Patch		**Papule and Plaque**	
Flat, nonpalpable change in the skin color. *Macules* are smaller than 1 cm with a circumscribed border. **Examples:** freckles, measles, petechiae.	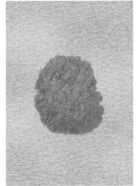 Macule.	Elevated, solid palpable masses with a circumscribed border. *Papules:* smaller than 0.5 cm. **Examples:** elevated moles, warts, lichen planus.	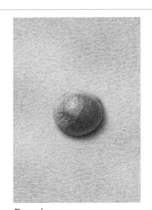 Papule.
Patches are larger than 1 cm and may have an irregular border. **Examples:** Mongolian spots, port-wine stains, vitiligo, and chloasma.	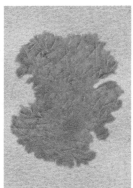 Patch.	*Plaques:* groups of papules that form lesions larger than 0.5 cm. **Examples:** psoriasis, actinic keratosis, lichen planus	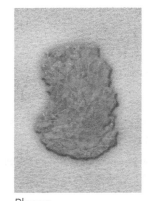 Plaque.
Nodule and Tumor		**Vesicle and Bulla**	
Elevated, solid, hard or soft palpable mass extending deeper into the dermis. *Nodules* are smaller than 2 cm and have circumscribed borders. **Examples:** small lipoma, squamous cell carcinoma, fibroma, and intradermal nevi.	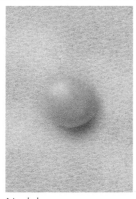 Nodule.	Elevated, fluid-filled, round or oval-shaped, palpable masses with thin, translucent walls and circumscribed borders. *Vesicles* are smaller than 0.5 cm. **Examples:** herpes simplex/zoster, early chickenpox, poison ivy, and small burn blisters.	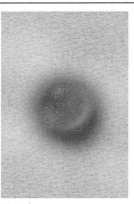 Vesicle.

TABLE 13.4	**Primary Lesions** (continued)

Tumors may have irregular borders and are larger than 2 cm.

Examples: large lipoma, carcinoma, and hemangioma.

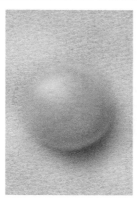

Tumor.

Bullae are larger than 0.5 cm.

Examples: contact dermatitis, friction blisters, and large burn blisters.

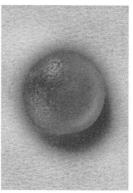

Bulla.

Pustule

An elevated, pus-filled vesicle or bulla with a circumscribed border. Size varies.

Examples: acne, impetigo, and carbuncles (large boils).

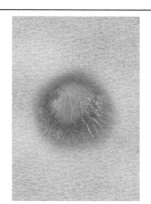

Pustule.

Wheal

An elevated, often reddish area with an irregular border caused by diffuse fluid in tissues. Size varies.

Examples: insect bites, hives (extensive wheals).

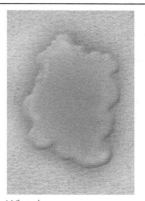

Wheal.

Cyst

Elevated, encapsulated, fluid-filled or semisolid mass originating in subcutaneous tissue or dermis, usually 1 cm or larger.

Examples: sebaceous cysts and epidermoid cysts.

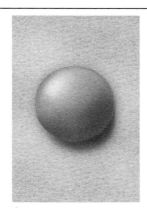

Cyst.

TABLE 13.5   **Secondary Lesions**

Atrophy

A translucent, dry, paperlike, sometimes wrinkled skin surface resulting from thinning or wasting of the skin due to loss of collagen and elastin.

Examples: striae, aged skin.

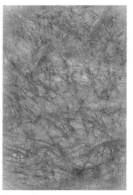

Atrophy.

Crust

Dry blood, serum, or pus on the skin surface from burst vesicles or pustules. It can be red-brown, orange, or yellow. Large crusts are called scabs.

Examples: eczema, impetigo, herpes, or scabs following abrasion.

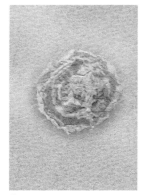

Crust.

Erosion

Wearing away of the superficial epidermis causing a moist, shallow depression. Usually heal without scarring.

Examples: scratch marks, ruptured vesicles

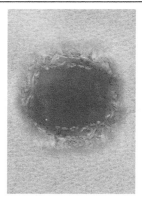

Erosion.

Fissure

A linear crack with sharp edges extending into the dermis.

Examples: cracks at the corners of the mouth or in the hands, athlete's foot.

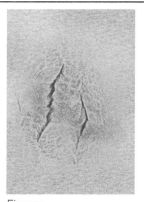

Fissure.

Keloid

An elevated, irregular, darkened area of excess scar tissue caused by excessive collagen formation during healing that extends beyond the site of the original injury.

Example: keloid from ear piercing or surgery

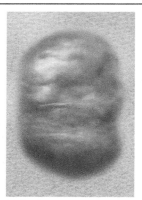

Keloid.

Lichenification

A rough, thickened, hardened area of epidermis resulting from chronic irritation such as scratching or rubbing.

Example: chronic dermatitis

Lichenification.

Scales

Shedding flakes of greasy, keratinized skin tissue. Color may be white, gray, or silver. Texture may vary from fine to thick.

Examples: dry skin, dandruff, psoriasis, and eczema.

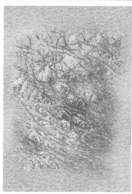

Scales.

Scar

A flat, irregular area of connective tissue left after a lesion or wound has healed. New scars may be red or purple; older scars may be silvery or white.

Examples: healed surgical wound or injury, healed acne.

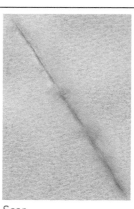

Scar.

TABLE 13.5	**Secondary Lesions** (continued)

Ulcer

A deep, irregularly shaped area of skin loss extending into the dermis or subcutaneous tissue. May be caused by venous hypertension, arterial insufficiency, **neuropathy,** or **lymphedema.** Ulcerated skin may bleed or leave a scar.

Examples: stasis ulcers, chancres.

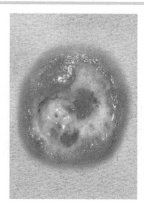

Ulcer.

TABLE 13.6	**Vascular Lesions**

NAME/DESCRIPTION	CAUSES	LOCALIZATION/DISTRIBUTION
Ecchymosis Flat, irregularly shaped lesion of varying size with no pulsation; does not blanch with pressure. • In light skin, it begins as a bluish purple mark that changes to greenish yellow. • In brown skin, it varies from blue to deep purple. • In black skin, it appears as a darkened area.	Release of blood from superficial vessels into surrounding tissue due to trauma, hemophilia, liver disease, or deficiency of vitamins C or K.	May occur anywhere on the body at the site of trauma or pressure. Ecchymosis. *Source:* P. Marazzi/Science Source.

(continued)

TABLE 13.6   Vascular Lesions (continued)

NAME/DESCRIPTION	CAUSES	LOCALIZATION/DISTRIBUTION
Hemangioma A bright red, raised lesion about 2–10 cm in diameter that does not blanch with pressure and is usually present at birth or within a few months of birth. Typically, it disappears by age 10.	A cluster of immature capillaries. Cause is unknown; may be hereditary.	May appear on any part of the body. Hemangioma. *Source:* H.C. Robinson/Science Source.
Hematoma A raised, irregularly shaped lesion similar to an ecchymosis except that it elevates the skin and looks like a swelling.	A leakage of blood into the skin and subcutaneous tissue as a result of trauma or surgical incision.	May occur anywhere on the body at the site of trauma, pressure, or surgical incision. Hematoma. *Source:* P. Barber/Getty Images.
Petechiae Flat, red or purple rounded "freckles" approximately 1 to 3 mm in diameter. They are difficult to detect in dark skin and do not blanch.	Minute hemorrhages resulting from fragile capillaries that are caused by septicemias, liver disease, vitamins C or K deficiency, or anticoagulant therapy.	Most commonly appear on body's dependent surfaces (back, buttocks) but may occur in oral mucosa and conjunctivae. Petechiae on palate. *Source:* Heinz F. Eichenwald/Centers for Disease Control and Prevention (CDC).

TABLE 13.6   Vascular Lesions (continued)

NAME/DESCRIPTION	CAUSES	LOCALIZATION/DISTRIBUTION
Port-Wine Stain A flat, irregularly shaped lesion ranging from pale red to deep purple-red. Color deepens with exertion, emotional response, or exposure to extremes of temperature. Present at birth and typically does not fade.	A large, flat mass of blood vessels on the skin surface that is likely caused by a genetic mutation (Shirley, Tang, Gallione, Baugher, Frelin, Cohen & Pevsner, 2013).	Most commonly appears on the face and head but may occur in other sites. Port-wine stain (nevus flammeus). *Source:* Custom Medical Stock Photo.
Purpura Flat, reddish-blue, irregularly shaped extensive patches of varying size.	Bleeding disorders, scurvy, and capillary fragility in the older adult (senile purpura).	May appear anywhere on the body but are most noticeable on the legs, arms, and backs of hands. Purpura. *Source:* Biophoto Associates/Photo Researchers/Getty Images.
Spider Angioma A flat, bright red dot with tiny radiating blood vessels ranging in size from a pinpoint to 2 cm. It blanches with pressure.	A type of telangiectasis (vascular dilatation) caused by elevated estrogen levels, pregnancy, estrogen therapy, vitamin B deficiency, or liver disease, or it may not be pathologic.	Most commonly appears on the upper half of the body. Spider (star) angioma. *Source:* Southern Illinois University/Photo Researchers/Getty Images.

(continued)

TABLE 13.6   Vascular Lesions (continued)

NAME/DESCRIPTION	CAUSES	LOCALIZATION/DISTRIBUTION
Venous Lake A soft, compressible, slightly elevated vascular lesion. Color typically ranges from dark blue to purple.	Venule dilation; most commonly occurs in individuals who are over age 50 and have a history of sun exposure.	Most commonly found on sun-exposed areas, including the lips, ears, neck, face, and posterior hand. Venous lake. *Source:* Science Photo Library/Science Source.

TABLE 13.7   Configurations and Shapes of Lesions

NAME	EXAMPLE	NAME	EXAMPLE
Annular Lesions with a circular shape ***Examples:*** Tinea corporis, pityriasis rosea.	 Annular lesions. *Source:* Dr. Lucille K. Georg/Centers for Disease Control and Prevention (CDC).	**Confluent** Lesions that run together. ***Example:*** Urticaria.	 Confluent lesions. *Source:* Konmesa/Shutterstock.

TABLE 13.7	**Configurations and Shapes of Lesions** (continued)		
NAME	**EXAMPLE**	**NAME**	**EXAMPLE**
Discrete Lesions that are separate and discrete. ***Example:*** Molluscum.	 Discrete lesions. *Source:* Jodi Jacobson/Getty Images.	**Grouped** Lesions that appear in clusters. ***Example:*** Purpural lesion.	 Grouped lesions. *Source:* P. Barber/RBP/Custom Medical Stock Photo.
Target Lesions with concentric circles of color. ***Example:*** Erythema multiforme.	 Target lesions. *Source:* Arthur E. Kaye/Centers for Disease Control and Prevention (CDC).	**Linear** Lesions that appear as a line. ***Example:*** Scratches.	 Linear lesions. *Source:* CMSP/Custom Medical Stock Photo.

(continued)

TABLE 13.7	Configurations and Shapes of Lesions (continued)		
NAME	**EXAMPLE**	**NAME**	**EXAMPLE**
Polycyclic Polycyclic lesions are lesions that are circular but united. *Example:* Psoriasis.	Polycyclic lesions. *Source:* CMSP/Custom Medical Stock Photo.	**Zoosteriform** Lesions arranged in a linear manner along a nerve route. *Example:* Herpes zoster (shingles).	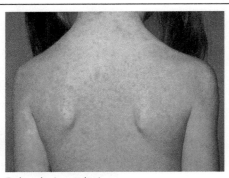Zosteriform lesions. *Source:* John Noble, Jr., MD/Centers for Disease Control and Prevention (CDC).

Overview of Skin Lesions

Skin lesions may have a variety of causes, or etiologies. For example, the etiology of a skin lesion may be an infectious disease, an allergic or inflammatory disorder, or a cancerous condition (malignancy). The following sections provide an overview of these categories of skin lesions.

INFECTIOUS SKIN LESIONS

Skin lesions may be caused by infectious organisms, such as viruses, bacteria, and fungi. In some cases, the lesions may be caused by a combination of organisms. Examples of infectious skin lesions include tinea, measles (rubeola), German measles (rubella), chickenpox (varicella), herpes simplex, and herpes zoster (shingles) (see Table 13.8).

TABLE 13.8	Common Infectious Skin Lesions
TINEA	**RUBEOLA (MEASLES)**
Fungal infection affecting the body (tinea corporis); scalp (tinea capitis); or feet (tinea pedis, athlete's foot). Secondary bacterial infection may also be present. Appearance of tinea lesions varies. 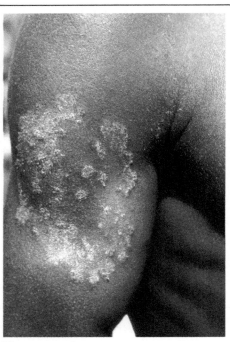Tinea corporis. *Source:* K. Mae Lennon/Centers for Disease Control and Prevention (CDC).	A highly contagious viral disease that causes a rash of red to purple macules or papules that begins on the face, and then progresses over the neck, trunk, arms, and legs. Lesions do not blanch. Oral mucosa may demonstrate tiny, white spots that look like grains of salt (Koplik's spots). Rubeola (measles). *Source:* Wellcome Image Library Custom Medical Stock Photo.

TABLE 13.8   Common Infectious Skin Lesions (continued)

RUBELLA (GERMAN MEASLES)

A highly contagious disease caused by the rubella virus. Typically it begins as a pink, papular rash that is similar to measles but paler. Skin lesions begin on the face and then spread over the body.

Unlike measles, German measles may be accompanied by swollen glands, but not by Koplik's spots. Most common in children.

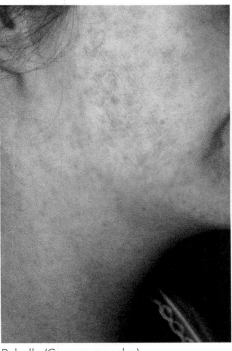

Rubella (German measles).
Source: Wellcome Image Library/Custom Medical Stock Photo.

VARICELLA (CHICKENPOX)

A mild infectious disease caused by a primary infection with the varicella zoster virus that begins as groups of small, red, fluid-filled vesicles usually on the trunk from which the rash progresses to the face, arms, and legs. Vesicles erupt over several days, forming pustules, then crusts; may cause intense itching. Most common in children.

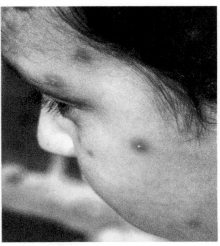

Varicella (chickenpox).

HERPES SIMPLEX

A chronic viral infection. Lesions progress from vesicles to pustules and then crusts. There are two different types of herpes simplex: oral (HSV-1) and genital (HSV-2). HSV-1 causes lesions on the lips and oral mucosa. HSV-2 causes lesions on the penis, vagina, buttocks, or anus. Although lesions are often confined to the oral mucosa or genitals, lesions from both types of herpes can appear anywhere on the body.

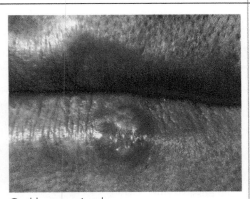

Oral herpes simplex.
Source: National Archives and Records Administration.

HERPES ZOSTER (SHINGLES)

A reactivation of the dormant varicella zoster virus, which typically has invaded the body during an attack of chickenpox. Clusters of small vesicles form on the skin along the route of sensory nerves. Vesicles progress to pustules and then crusts and cause intense pain and itching. More common and more severe among older adults.

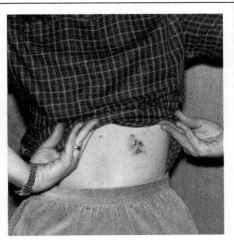

Herpes zoster (shingles).
Source: E. H. Gill/Custom Medical Stock Photo.

(continued)

TABLE 13.8	**Common Infectious Skin Lesions** (continued)

IMPETIGO

A contagious bacterial skin infection that usually appears on the skin around the nose and mouth. Lesions may begin as a barely perceptible patch of blisters that breaks, exposing red, weeping area beneath. Tan crust soon forms over this area, and the infection may spread out of the edges. Common in children.

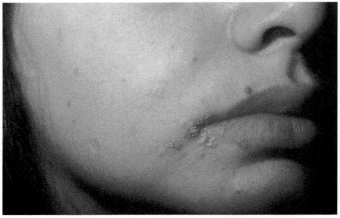

Impetigo
Source: Lester V. Bergman/Corbis.

ALLERGIC OR INFLAMMATORY SKIN LESIONS

Allergies and inflammatory responses also may cause skin lesions to develop. For example, contact dermatitis is caused by an allergic reaction, while eczema and psoriasis are caused by inflammatory responses (see Table 13.9).

TABLE 13.9	**Common Allergic or Inflammatory Skin Lesions**

CONTACT DERMATITIS	ECZEMA
Inflammation of the skin due to an allergy to a substance that comes into contact with the skin, such as clothing, jewelry, plants, chemicals, or cosmetics. Lesion location may help identify the allergen. May progress from redness to hives, vesicles, or scales; usually accompanied by intense itching. 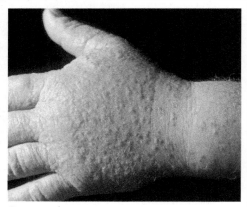 Contact dermatitis. *Source: Getty/Photolibrary/Peter Arnold, Inc.*	Internally provoked inflammation of the skin causing reddened papules and vesicles that ooze and weep and possible crust formation. Lesions usually located on the scalp, face, elbows, knees, forearms, torso, and wrists; usually accompanied by intense itching. 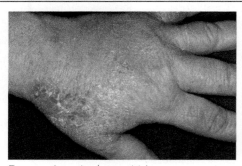 Eczema (atopic dermatitis). *Source: Scott Camazine/Visuals Unlimited/Corbis.*

TABLE 13.9   **Common Allergic or Inflammatory Skin Lesions** (continued)

PSORIASIS

Thickening of the skin in dry, silvery, scaly patches that occurs with overproduction of skin cells, resulting in buildup of cells faster than they can be shed. May be triggered by emotional stress or generally poor health. Lesions may form on the scalp, elbows and knees, lower back, and perianal area.

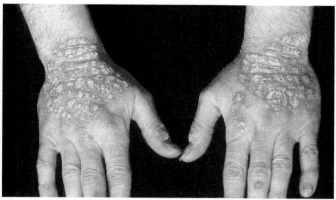

Psoriasis.
Source: Custom Medical Stock Photo, Inc.

MALIGNANT SKIN LESIONS

Certain forms of skin lesions are malignant, or cancerous. Examples of malignant skin lesions include basal cell carcinoma, squamous cell carcinoma, malignant melanoma, and Kaposi's sarcoma (see Table 13.10).

TABLE 13.10   **Malignant Skin Lesions**

BASAL CELL CARCINOMA

The most common but least malignant type of skin cancer. A proliferation of the cells of the stratum basale into the dermis and subcutaneous tissue.

Lesions begin as shiny papules that develop central ulcers with rounded, pearly edges and occur most often on regions regularly exposed to the sun.

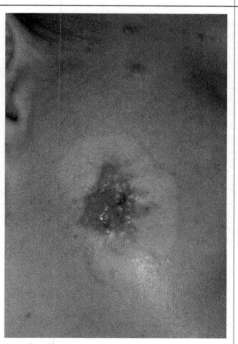

Basal cell carcinoma.
Source: Dr. Kenneth Greer/Getty Images.

SQUAMOUS CELL CARCINOMA

Arises from the cells of the stratum spinosum, and begins as a reddened, scaly papule that then forms a shallow ulcer with a clearly delineated, elevated border. Commonly appears on the scalp, ears, backs of the hands, and lower lip. Believed to be caused by sun exposure; grows rapidly.

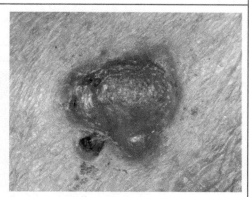

Squamous cell carcinoma.
Source: P. Marazzi/Science Source.

(continued)

TABLE 13.10	**Malignant Skin Lesions** (continued)

MALIGNANT MELANOMA	KAPOSI'S SARCOMA
The least common but most serious type of skin cancer, because it spreads rapidly to lymph and blood vessels. Lesion contains areas of varied pigmentation and may be black, brown, blue, or red, often with irregular edges with notched borders; diameter is greater than 6 mm. 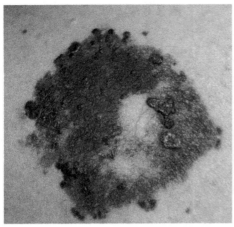 Malignant melanoma. *Source:* Kenneth Greer/Getty Images.	Malignant tumor of the epidermis and internal epithelial tissues. Painless lesions are typically soft, blue to purple; other characteristics are variable. Lesions may be macular or papular and may resemble keloids or bruises. Most commonly occurs in people who are HIV positive. 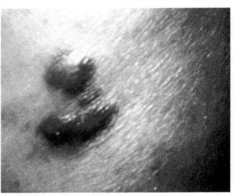 Kaposi's sarcoma. *Source:* Steve Kraus/Centers for Disease Control and Prevention (CDC).

Overview of Hair and Scalp Abnormalities

Certain disorders of the integumentary system tend to affect the hair, the scalp, or a combination of these two regions (see Table 13.11).

TABLE 13.11	**Hair and Scalp Abnormalities**

SEBORRHEIC DERMATITIS	TINEA CAPITIS
Yellow-white greasy scales on the scalp and forehead, similar to eczema, but without the significant itching or discomfort characteristic of eczema (Mayo Clinic, 2012). Common in infants. Also called cradle cap. 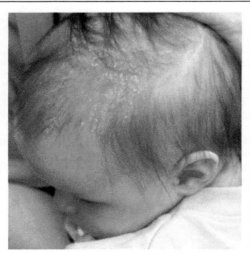 Seborrheic dermatitis (cradle cap).	Highly contagious fungal disease (Mayo Clinic, 2014e) that causes patchy hair loss on the head with skin pustules. Transmitted from the soil, from animals, or from person to person. Most common among toddlers and school-age children. Also called scalp ringworm. 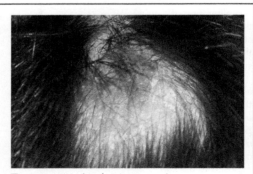 Tinea capitis (scalp ringworm). *Source:* SPL/Science Source.

| TABLE 13.11 | **Hair and Scalp Abnormalities** (continued) |

ALOPECIA AREATA

There is no known cause for this condition, which produces a sudden loss of hair in a round balding patch on the scalp.

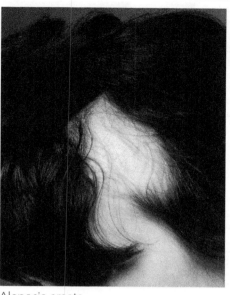

Alopecia areata.
Source: Wellcome Image Library/Custom Medical Stock Photo.

FOLLICULITIS

Infections of hair follicles, appears as pustules with underlying erythema.

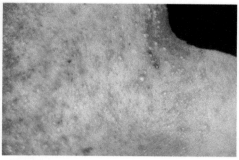

Folliculitis.
Source: BioPhoto Associates/Photo Researchers/Getty Images.

HIRSUTISM

Excess body hair in females on the face, chest, abdomen, arms, and legs, following the male pattern that is typically due to endocrine or metabolic dysfunction. Also may be idiopathic, or of unknown origin.

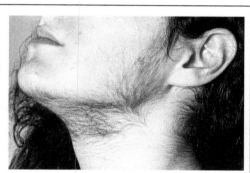

Hirsutism.
Source: John Radcliffe/Science Source.

FURUNCLE/ABSCESS

Infected hair follicles give rise to *furuncles*, hard, erythematous, pus-filled lesions. *Abscesses* are caused by bacteria entering the skin. These are larger lesions than furuncles.

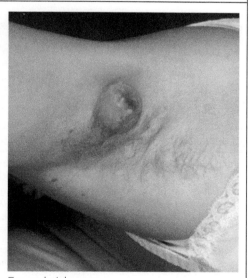

Furuncle/abscess.
Source: Wellcome Image Library/Custom Medical Stock Photo.

Overview of Nail Abnormalities

Abnormalities of the nails can stem from numerous etiologies, including genetic factors, infectious disease processes, and traumatic injuries. Nail abnormalities also can provide clues to the presence of underlying disease processes involving other body systems. Examples of nail abnormalities include spoon nails, paronychia, Beau's line, splinter hemorrhage, clubbing, and onycholysis (see Table 13.12).

TABLE 13.12 **Nail Abnormalities**

KOILONYCHIA

Concavity and thinning of the nails, koilonychia, or spoon nails, are commonly a congenital condition or result from an iron deficiency.

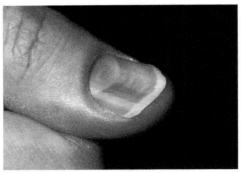

Koilonychia (spoon nails).
Source: Dr. P. Marazzi/Science Source.

PARONYCHIA

An infection of the skin adjacent to the nail, usually caused by bacteria or fungi. Affected area becomes red, swollen, and painful; pus may ooze from affected area.

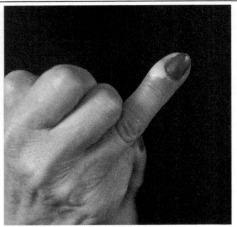

Paronychia.
Source: Marcel Jancovic/Shutterstock.

BEAU'S LINES

Occur due to trauma or illness affecting nail formation. A linear depression develops at the base and moves distally as the nail grows.

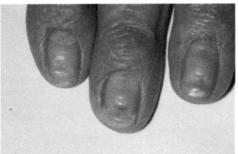

Beau's Line.
Source: Dr. P. Marazzi/Science Source.

SPLINTER HEMORRHAGE

Can occur as a result of trauma or in endocarditis. These appear as reddish-brown spots in the nail.

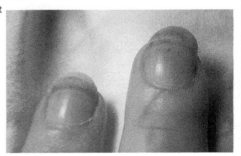

Splinter hemorrhages.
Source: CDC/Dr. Thomas F. Sellers/Emory University.

CLUBBING

The nail appears more convex and wide; the nail angle is greater than 160 degrees. Occurs in chronic respiratory and cardiac conditions in which oxygenation is compromised (lung disease, lung cancer, bronchiectasis, cystic fibrosis) (Mason et al., 2010). Additional causes may include liver disease, congenital heart disease, hypertrophic osteoarthropathy, and HIV (Mason et al., 2010).

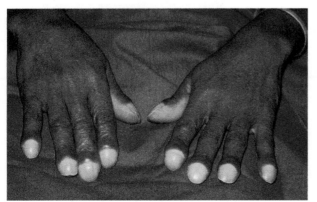

Clubbing of fingernails.
Source: BioPhoto Associates/Getty Images.

ONYCHOLYSIS

Fungal nail infection that causes the nails to thicken and lift off the nail bed and appear white, yellow, or opaque. Most commonly occurs on toenails; more common in adults. Also called tinea unguium.

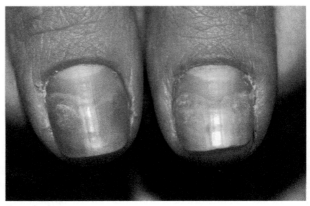

Onycholysis.
Source: Dr. Harout Tanielian/Science Source.

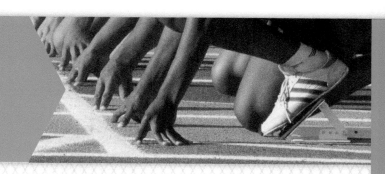

Application Through Critical Thinking

▶ **Case Study**

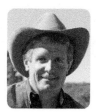

Mr. Shelley is a 54-year-old groundskeeper for a large corporation in the Southwest. Today, he visits the company's health and wellness office saying, "My wife told me to have someone check my leathery skin."

Julieta Caredenas, RN, asks Mr. Shelley how much time he spends outdoors. He reveals that he is outside from about 8:00 a.m. until 4:00 p.m. each day, except for his lunch break, which he usually takes in the cafeteria. He reports that he does not use sunscreen. In the summertime, he works in a short-sleeved shirt, shorts, and a hat. He doesn't recall ever having had a bad sunburn. He states that he has a mole on his left thigh that has been present since birth, but to his knowledge it has not changed. He is not aware of any other birthmarks or skin lesions. He has never performed a skin self-assessment. He reports no family history of skin cancer. He states that he never sunbathes or swims, and that he plays outdoor baseball only at the annual family picnic. He showers each day before going home and uses deodorant soap. He admits that his skin is often quite dry but said he feels that sunscreens and lotions "are for women."

The nursing assessment of Mr. Shelley's skin reveals the following data: His skin is clean. It is a ruddy brown color where frequently exposed to the sun and a pinkish tan elsewhere. His temperature is warm bilaterally, and he has a mild sheen of perspiration on his face, neck, and upper trunk. Where exposed to the sun, his skin is thick with decreased elasticity. There are no unexpected visible blood vessels or vascular lesions. There is a mole approximately 2 cm by 2 cm on the anterior surface of his left thigh. No drainage is noted. Mr. Shelley's scalp and hair appear dry but clean and free of lesions. Soil is embedded beneath the free edge of his nails. He states that he had been transplanting cuttings.

▶ Complete Documentation

The following information is summarized from the case study.

SUBJECTIVE DATA: Seeks checkup for "leathery skin." Works as groundskeeper. Outdoors 7 hours a day. No sunscreen, protective clothing. No recall of sunburn. Mole left thigh since birth, reports unchanged. No other lesions. No self-skin assessment. No family history of skin cancer. Denies sunbathing or swimming. Occasional outdoor baseball. Showers daily with deodorant soap. Feels skin is "dry." "Sunscreens and lotions are for women."

OBJECTIVE DATA: Skin clean, ruddy brown where exposed, pinkish tan in unexposed areas. Temperature warm, bilaterally, mild perspiration face, neck, upper trunk. Exposed skin thick, decreased elasticity. No unexpected vessels, vascular lesions. Mole 2 cm × 2 cm anterior (L) thigh, no drainage. Scalp and hair, no lesions. Nails, soil embedded beneath free edge.

A sample assessment form appears on the next page.

▶ Critical Thinking Questions

1. Describe the findings from the case study.

2. Identify the findings as normal or abnormal.

3. Determine the categories that emerge from clustering of the data.

4. Analyze the categories to identify the physical and psychosocial nursing care priorities for Mr. Shelley.

5. What might the nurse do help Mr. Shelley understand the risks of not using sunscreen?

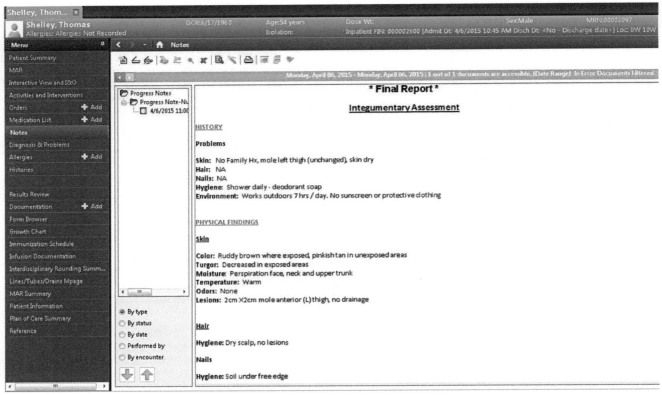

Source: From Cerner Electronic Health Record. Copyright © by Cerner Corporation. Used by permission of Cerner Corporation.

▸ Prepare Teaching Plan

LEARNING NEED: The data from the case study reveal that Mr. Shelley is concerned about his "leathery skin." His skin condition is associated with unprotected skin exposure to the sun for long periods of the daytime. Mr. Shelley is at risk for skin cancer.

The case study provides data that are representative of risks, symptoms, and behaviors of many individuals. Therefore, the following teaching plan is based on the need to provide information to members of any community about skin cancer.

GOAL: The participants in this learning program will have increased awareness of risk factors and strategies to prevent skin cancer.

OBJECTIVES: At the completion of this learning session, the learner will be able to:

1. Identify risk factors associated with skin cancer.
2. List the symptoms of skin cancer.
3. Describe the types of skin cancer.
4. Discuss strategies to prevent skin cancer.

Following is an example of the teaching plan for Objective 1.

APPLICATION OF OBJECTIVE 1: Identify risk factors associated with skin cancer

Content	Teaching Strategy	Evaluation
• *Moles.* Usually harmless pigmented growth. Multiple moles or large moles indicate risk. • *Fair complexion.* Skin cancer risk is higher in those with fair skin, freckles, blue eyes, and blond hair. • Family history of skin cancer. • Too much time in the sun or tanning booth. Severe sunburn as child or teen. • Age. Half of skin cancer occurs after age 50.	• Lecture • Discussion • Audiovisual materials • Printed materials Lecture is appropriate when disseminating information to large groups. Discussion allows participants to bring up concerns and to raise questions. Audiovisual materials such as illustrations of the moles reinforce verbal presentation. Printed material, especially to be taken away with learners, allows review, reinforcement, and reading at the learner's pace.	• Written examination. May use short answer, fill-in, or multiple-choice items, or a combination of items. If these are short and easy to evaluate, the learner receives immediate feedback.

▶ References

American Academy of Dermatology. (2013). *Skin can show first sign of some internal diseases*. Retrieved from http://www.aad.org/stories-and-news/news-releases/skin-can-show-first-signs-of-some-internal-diseases—

American Academy of Dermatology. (n.d.). *Herpes simplex: Signs and symptoms*. Retrieved from http://www.aad.org/dermatology-a-to-z/diseases-and-treatments/e—h/herpes-simplex/signs-symptoms

American Academy of Orthopaedic Surgeons. (2009). *Heat injury and heat exhaustion*. Retrieved from http://orthoinfo.aaos.org/topic.cfm?topic=a00319

American Cancer Society. (2013). *Signs and symptoms of melanoma skin cancer*. Retrieved from http://www.cancer.org/cancer/skincancer-melanoma/detailedguide/melanoma-skin-cancer-signs-and-symptoms

American Cancer Society. (2014). *Cancer facts and statistics*. Retrieved from http://www.cancer.org/research/cancerfactsstatistics/index

Andrews, M. M., & Boyle, J. S. (2011). *Transcultural concepts in nursing care* (6th ed.). Philadelphia, PA: Lippincott Williams & Wilkins

Berman, A., & Snyder, S. J. (2012). *Kozier and Erb's fundamentals of nursing: Concepts, process, and practice* (9th ed.). Upper Saddle River, NJ: Prentice Hall.

Bickley, L. S. (2012). *Bates' guide to physical examination and history taking* (11th ed.). Philadelphia: Lippincott.

Bode, D., Seehusen, D. A., & Baird, D. (2012). Hirsutism in women. *American Family Physician, 85*(4), 373–380.

Centers for Disease Control and Prevention (CDC). (2013). *Workplace safety and health topics: Skin exposures & effects*. Retrieved from http://www.cdc.gov/niosh/topics/skin/

Cleveland Clinic. (2011). *Diseases and conditions: Metabolic syndrome*. Retrieved from http://my.clevelandclinic.org/disorders/metabolic_syndrome/hic_metabolic_syndrome.aspx

Colbert, B. J., Ankney, J., Lee, K. T. (2011). *Anatomy & physiology for health professions: An interactive journey*. (2nd ed.) Upper Saddle River, NJ: Pearson.

Crowson, A. N., Magro, C. M., & Mihm, M. C. (2014). *The melanocytic proliferations: A comprehensive textbook of pigmented lesions*. Hoboken, NJ: John Wiley & Sons.

Elmann, S., Pointdujour, R., Blaydon, S., Nakra, T., Connor, M., Mukhopadhyay, C., . . . Shinder, R. (2012). Periocular abscesses following brow epilation. *Ophthalmic Plastic & Reconstructive Surgery, 28*(6), 434–437.

Gizlenti, S., & Ekmekci, T. R. (2013). The changes in the hair cycle during gestation and the post-partum period. *Journal of the European Academy of Dermatology and Venereology*. Advance online publication. doi: 10.1111/jdv.12188

Huynh, M., Gupta, R., & Koo, J. Y. (2013). Emotional stress as a trigger for inflammatory skin Disorders. *Seminars in Cutaneous Medicine and Surgery, 32*, 68–72.

Khodavaisy, S., Nabili, M., Davari, B., & Vahedi, M. (2011). Evaluation of bacterial and fungal contamination in the health care workers' hands and rings in the intensive care unit. *Journal of Preventive Medicine and Hygiene, 52*(4), 215–218.

Marieb, E. (2009). *Essentials of human anatomy and physiology* (9th ed.). Redwood City, CA: Benjamin/Cummings/Pearson Education.

Mason, R. J., Broaddus, V. C., Martin, T. R., King, T. E. Jr., Schraufnagel, D. E., Murray, J. F., & Nadel, J. A. (2010). *Murray and Nadel's textbook of respiratory medicine* (5th ed.). Philadelphia, PA: Elsevier.

Mayo Clinic. (2012). *Diseases and conditions: Cradle cap*. Retrieved from http://www.mayoclinic.org/diseases-conditions/cradle-cap/basics/definition/con-20032328

Mayo Clinic. (2014a). *Diseases and conditions: Dandruff*. Retrieved from http://www.mayoclinic.org/diseases-conditions/dandruff/basics/definition/con-20023690

Mayo Clinic. (2014b). *Diseases and conditions: Hair loss*. Retrieved from http://www.mayoclinic.org/diseases-conditions/hair-loss/basics/definition/con-20027666

Mayo Clinic. (2014c). *Diseases and conditions: Sweating and body odor*. Retrieved from http://www.mayoclinic.org/diseases-conditions/sweating-and-body-odor/basics/definition/con-20014438

Mayo Clinic. (2014d). *Diseases and conditions: Skin cancer:Risk factors*. Retrieved from http://www.mayoclinic.org/diseases-conditions/skin-cancer/basics/risk-factors/con-20031606

Mayo Clinic. (2014e). *Diseases and conditions: Ringworm (scalp)*. Retrieved from http://www.mayoclinic.org/diseases-conditions/ringworm/basics/definition/con-20029923

Mayo Foundation for Medical Education and Research. (2014). Rochester test catalog: 2014 online test catalog. Available at http://www.mayomedicallaboratories.com/test-catalog/

National Cancer Institute (NCI). (2008). *Melanoma risk assessment tool*. Retrieved from http://www.cancer.gov/melanomarisktool/

National Kidney Foundation. (2014). *What you should know about infectious diseases: A guide for hemodialysis patients and their families*. Retrieved from http://www.kidney.org/atoz/content/what_infectdiseases.cfm

Osborn K. S., Wraa, C. E., Watson, A., & Holleran, R. S. (2013). *Medical-surgical nursing: Preparation for practice* (2nd ed.). Upper Saddle River, NJ: Pearson.

Owoeye, O. A., Aina, O. F., Omoluabi, P. F., & Olumide, Y. M. (2009). Self-esteem and suicidal risk among subjects with dermatological disorders in a West African teaching hospital. *Journal of the Islamic Medical Association of North America, 41*(2).

Patel, M., Harrison, S., & Sinclair, R. (2013). Drugs and hair loss. *Dermatologic Clinics, 31*(1), 67–73.

Pierce, M. C., Kaczor, K., Aldridge, S., O'Flynn, J., & Lorenz, D. J. (2010). Bruising characteristics discriminating physical child abuse from accidental trauma. *Pediatrics, 125*(1), 67–74.

Setji, T. L., & Brown, A. J. (2014). Polycystic ovarian syndrome: Update on diagnosis and treatment. *American Journal of Medicine*. Advance online publication. doi: 10.1016/j.amjmed.2014.04.017

Shirley, M. D., Tang, H., Gallione, C. J., Baugher, J. D., Frelin, L. P., Cohen, B., . . . & Pevsner, J. (2013). Sturge-Weber syndrome and port-wine stains caused by somatic mutation in GNAQ. *New England Journal of Medicine, 368*(21), 1971–1979.

Silverberg, N. B., & Lee-Wong, M. (2014). Generalized yellow discoloration of the skin. *Cutis, 93*(5), E11–E12.

Tortora, G. J., & Derrickson, B. H. (2009). *Principles of anatomy and physiology* (12th ed.). New York: John Wiley & Sons.

Tully, A. S., Trayes, K. P., & Studdiford, J. S. (2012). Evaluation of nail abnormalities. *American Family Physician, 85*(8), 779–787.

U.S. Department of Health and Human Services (USDHHS). (2010). *Healthy People 2020*. Retrieved from http://www.healthypeople.gov/2020/default.aspx

Wake, T. W. (2010). Pressure ulcers: What clinicians need to know. *The Permanente Journal, 14*(2), 56–60.

Wilson, B. A., Shannon, M. T., & Shields, K. M. (2013). *Pearson nurse's drug guide*. Upper Saddle River, NJ: Pearson.

World Health Organization (WHO). (2014). *Health effects of UV radiation: UV health effects on the immune system*. Retrieved from http://www.who.int/uv/health/uv_health2/en/index3.html

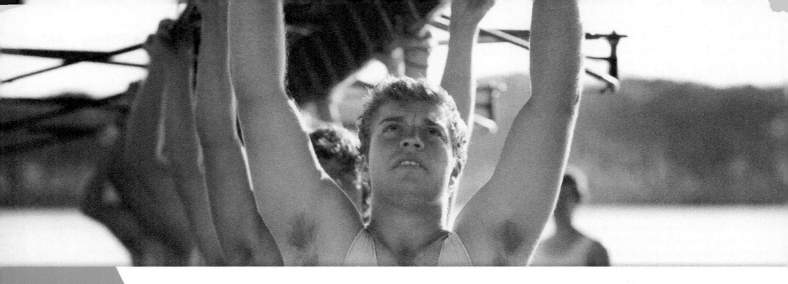

CHAPTER

14 Head, Neck, and Related Lymphatics

▶ Learning Outcomes

Upon completion of this chapter, you will be able to:

1. Describe the anatomy and physiology of the structures of the head, neck, and related lymphatics.

2. Develop questions to be used when completing the focused interview.

3. Outline the techniques used for assessment of the head, neck, and related lymphatics.

4. Explain patient preparation for assessment of the head, neck, and related lymphatics.

5. Differentiate normal from abnormal findings in the physical assessment of the head, neck, and related lymphatics.

6. Describe developmental, psychosocial, cultural, and environmental variations in assessment techniques and findings.

7. Relate overall health of the head, neck, and related lymphatics to *Healthy People 2020* objectives.

8. Apply critical thinking to the physical assessment of the head, neck, and related lymphatics.

Key Terms

acromegaly, 282
anterior triangle, 262
atlas, 262
axis, 262
Bell's palsy, 282
cerebrovascular accident, 282
craniosynostosis, 282
crepitation, 276
Cushing's syndrome, 283
Down syndrome, 283
fetal alcohol syndrome, 283
goiter, 267
hydrocephalus, 283
hyoid, 262
hyperthyroidism, 278
hypothyroidism, 278
lymphadenopathy, 279
Parkinson's disease, 284
posterior triangle, 262
sutures, 261
thyroid gland, 262
torticollis, 284

260

Because it houses the brain and several endocrine glands that control body functions, the head and neck region is vital to survival. Several systems are integrated in the head and neck. For example, the musculoskeletal system permits movement of the neck and face, while the bones protect the brain, spinal cord, and eyes.

Several body systems interconnect in the head and neck region. The nurse will be assessing several systems at the same time. For instance, the integumentary system provides covering and protection. Food is taken in (ingested) through the mouth, which is the beginning of the gastrointestinal system. Air enters the lungs through the nose, mouth, and trachea, which make up the upper respiratory system. The cardiovascular system carries oxygen and other nutrients to the region and transports wastes. The nurse must consider this close interrelationship of systems when assessing the patient's head and neck, where clues to the patient's nutritional status, airway clearance, tissue perfusion, metabolism, level of activity, sleep and rest, level of stress, and self-care ability may be apparent.

When performing an assessment of the head and neck, one must be aware of psychosocial factors such as stress and anxiety that can influence the health of this body area. It is also important for the nurse to consider the patient's self-care practices. Many patients spend a great deal of time caring for this area of the body, and alterations in health may affect their ability to provide this care. A patient's ancestry, cultural practices, socioeconomic status, and physical environment both at home and at work can greatly influence the health of the head and neck and are an integral part of the assessment data. Additionally, a patient's developmental stage has a tremendous influence on the appearance and functioning of the region.

Healthy People 2020 identifies the prevention of injury and violence as national objectives. The goal is to reduce the number of injuries, disabilities, and deaths from a multitude of causes, including head injuries, as described later in this chapter.

Anatomy and Physiology Review

The structures of the head include the skull and facial bones. The vertebrae, hyoid bone, cartilage, muscles, thyroid gland, and major blood vessels are found within the neck. A large supply of lymph nodes is located in the head and neck region. Each of these structures is described in the following paragraphs.

Head

The skull is a protective shell made up of the bones of the cranium (see Figure 14.1 ■) and face. The major bones of the cranium are the frontal, parietal, temporal, and occipital bones. These bones are connected to each other by means of **sutures**, or nonmovable joints. The solidification process of the sutures is completed by the second year of life. The primary function of the skull is to protect the brain. The bones of the skull are covered by muscles and skin, which is commonly called the scalp. The bones provide landmarks for assessment. Fourteen bones form the anterior region of the skull, commonly called the face. These bones are the frontal, maxillae, zygomatic, nasal, ethmoid, lacrimal, sphenoid, and mandible. The intricate fusion of these bones provides structure for the face and cavities for the eyes, nose, and mouth. It also allows movement of the mandible at the temporomandibular joint (TMJ). The TMJ is located anterior to the tragus of the ear and allows a person to open and close the mouth, protract and retract the chin, and slide the lower jaw from side to side. These actions are used for chewing and speaking.

The skin, muscles, and bones of the face provide landmarks for assessment, as do the bones of the skull. The eyebrows, appendages of the skin, are over the supraorbital margins of the skull. The lateral canthus of the eye forms a straight line with the pinna, and the nasolabial folds are equal (see Figure 14.2 ■).

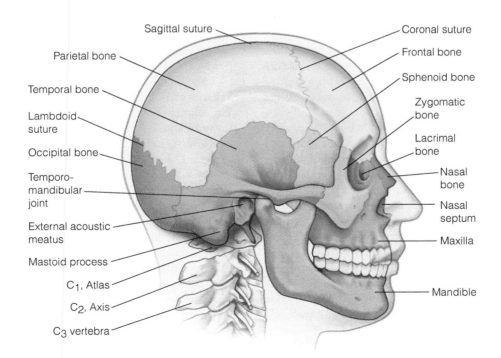

Figure 14.1 Bones of the head.

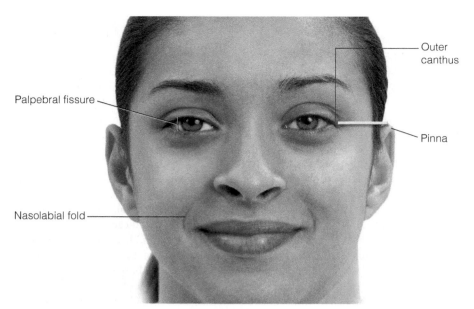

Figure 14.2 Facial landmarks.

Figure 14.3 ■ identifies the main muscles of the scalp, face, and neck. These muscles play a major role in expressing emotions through facial expressions. They also contribute to movement of the head and neck. Details regarding movement of the structures of the head and neck are discussed in chapter 25 of this text. ∞ Cranial nerve innervation of muscles, senses, and balance are discussed in detail in chapter 26 of this text. ∞

Neck

The neck is formed by the seven cervical vertebrae, ligaments, and muscles, which support the cranium. The first cervical vertebra (C1), commonly called the **atlas**, carries the skull. The second cervical vertebra (C2), commonly called the **axis**, allows for movement of the head (see Figure 14.1). The greatest mobility is at the level of C4, C5, and C6. The seventh cervical vertebra (vertebra prominens) has the largest spinous process. This vertebral process is visible and easily palpated, making it a definite landmark during patient assessment.

The sternocleidomastoid and trapezius muscles are the primary muscles of the neck. The sternocleidomastoid muscles, innervated by cranial nerve XI (Accessory), originate at the manubrium of the sternum and the medial portion of the clavicles. The insertion of this muscle is at the mastoid process of the temporal bones.

Each trapezius muscle, also innervated by cranial nerve XI (Accessory), originates on the occipital bone of the skull and spine of several vertebrae. The insertion of these muscles is on the scapulae and lateral third of the clavicles.

These two muscle groups form the anterior and posterior triangles of the neck. The mandible, the midline of the neck, and the anterior aspect of the sternocleidomastoid muscles border the **anterior triangle**. The trapezius muscle, the sternocleidomastoid muscle, and the clavicle form the **posterior triangle** (see Figure 14.4 ■).

The **hyoid** bone is suspended in the neck (see Figure 14.5 ■) approximately 2 cm (1 in.) above the larynx. The hyoid is the only

bone in the body that does not articulate directly with another bone. The base of the tongue rests on the curved body of this bone. The curved shape of the bone produces a horn at each end that is palpable just inferior to the angle of the jaw. This serves as a landmark for assessing structures of the neck, especially the trachea and thyroid gland.

The thyroid cartilage is the largest cartilage of the larynx and is formed by the joining of two pieces of cartilage. This fusion forms a ridge called the Adam's apple. This ridge is significantly larger in males (see Figure 14.5). The cricoid cartilage, a C-shaped ring, is the first cartilage ring anchored to the trachea. The trachea, commonly called the windpipe, descends from the larynx to the bronchi of the respiratory system. The trachea has slight mobility and flexibility. The C-shaped rings help maintain the shape of the trachea and are palpable superior to the sternum at the midline of the neck (see Figure 14.5).

The **thyroid gland,** which is part of the endocrine system, is butterfly shaped. It is located in the anterior portion of the neck. The isthmus of the thyroid connects the right and left lobes of the thyroid gland. The isthmus is located beneath the cricoid cartilage (or the first tracheal ring). The isthmus is inferior to the thyroid cartilage (Adam's apple). The thyroid gland lies over the trachea, and the sternocleidomastoid muscles cover the lateral aspects of the lobes (see Figure 14.5).

The carotid arteries and the jugular veins are located in the neck. The carotid artery is palpated in the groove between the trachea and the sternocleidomastoid muscle below the angle of the jaw. The external and internal jugular veins are also in the neck, in proximity to the common carotid artery. The external jugular veins are more superficial and lateral to the sternocleidomastoid muscle. The internal jugular veins are larger and not visible; however, a reflection of the undulation is seen at the sternal notch (see Figure 14.6 ■). These vessels are deep and medial to the muscle. The carotid arteries and jugular veins are discussed in detail in chapter 19 of this text. ∞

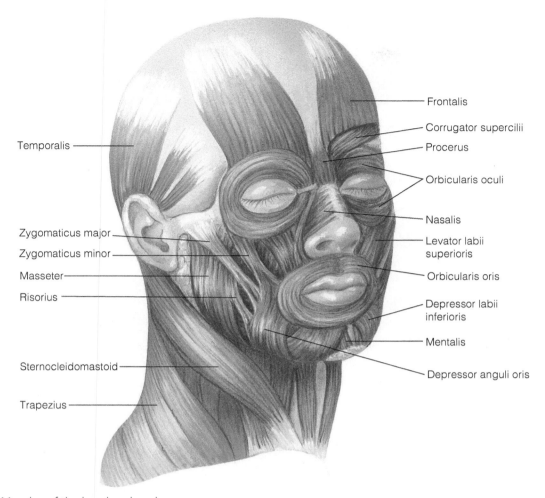

Figure 14.3 Muscles of the head and neck.

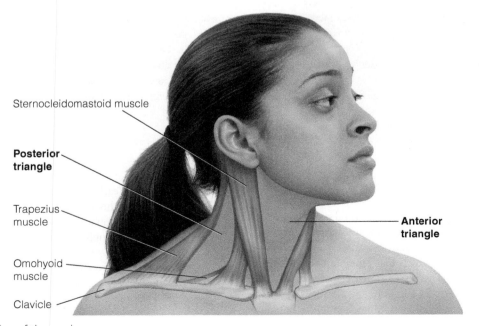

Figure 14.4 Triangles of the neck.

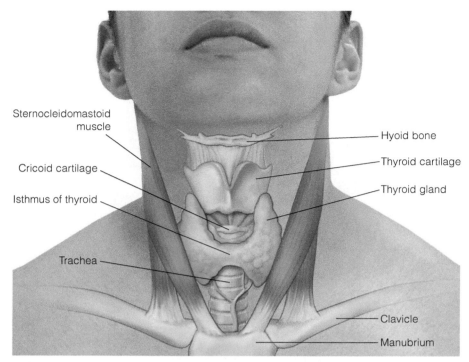

Figure 14.5 Structures of the neck.

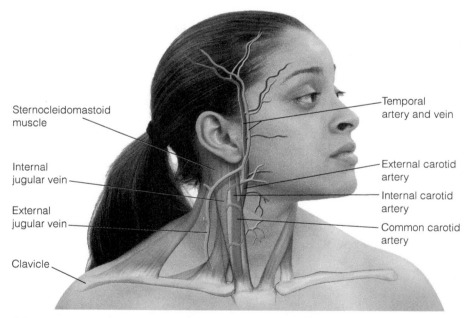

Figure 14.6 Vessels of the neck.

Lymphatics

Numerous lymph nodes are located in the head and neck region of the body. These nodes provide defense against invasion of foreign substances by producing lymphocytes and antibodies. The lymph nodes are clustered along lymphatic vessels that infiltrate tissue capillaries and pick up excess fluid called *lymph*. The nurse palpates various areas of the head and neck, looking for lymph nodes. Normally, the nodes are nonpalpable. Occasionally, an isolated node is found on palpation. This is usually not considered an abnormal finding. Nodes are palpable when infected or enlarged. This finding may be significant in

recognizing signs of early infection. The names of the nodes may vary depending on the author or practitioner; however, they usually correspond to adjacent anatomic structures or locations (see Figure 14.7 ■). The nodes most commonly assessed are the following:

- *Preauricular*—in front of the ear
- *Occipital*—at the base of the skull
- *Postauricular*—behind the ear, over the outer surface of the mastoid bone
- *Submental*—behind the tip of the mandible at the midline

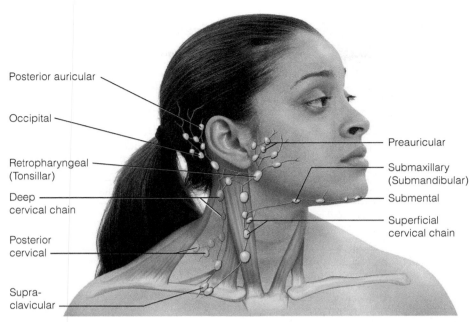

Posterior auricular

Occipital

Retropharyngeal
(Tonsillar)

Deep
cervical chain

Posterior
cervical

Supra-
clavicular

Preauricular

Submaxillary
(Submandibular)

Submental

Superficial
cervical chain

Figure 14.7   Lymph nodes of the head and neck.

- *Submandibular*—on the medial border of the mandible
- *Retropharyngeal (tonsillar)*—at the junction of the posterior and lateral walls of the pharynx at the angle of the jaw
- *Anterior/Superficial cervical*—anterior to the sternocleidomastoid muscle
- *Deep and posterior cervical*—posterior to the sternocleidomastoid muscle
- *Supraclavicular*—above the clavicle

A detailed description of the lymphatic system is provided in chapter 20 of this text. ∞

Special Considerations

Throughout the assessment process, the nurse gathers subjective and objective data reflecting the patient's state of health. Using critical thinking and the nursing process, the nurse identifies many factors to be considered when collecting the data. Some of these factors include but are not limited to age, developmental level, race, ethnicity, work history, living conditions, social economics, and emotional well-being.

Health Promotion Considerations

Goals of *Healthy People 2020* include preventing injuries and fatalities, including those attributed to violence, motor vehicle crashes, falls, and accidents related to sports and recreation. In particular, traumatic head injuries are a primary source of disability and death. Along with promoting increased use of seat belts and other vehicular restraint systems, *Healthy People 2020* seeks to encourage the appropriate use of helmets and other protective gear during sports and recreational activities.

Healthy People 2020 also aims to decrease the incidence of fetal alcohol syndrome (FAS), which comprises manifestations that are caused by maternal alcohol consumption during the prenatal period. FAS is associated with neurologic dysfunction, developmental delays, and cardiac defects. On observation, assessment findings of the infant with FAS may include characteristic deformities of the head and facial structures.

Among the many *Healthy People 2020* goals related to cancer, key concerns include detecting and preventing cancer, as well as promoting survival among individuals who undergo cancer treatment. Almost every form of cancer, including breast cancer, lung cancer, and prostate cancer, can spread to the lymph nodes through metastasis, which may then cause the lymph nodes to become firm and inflamed. Routine screenings that include assessment and palpation of the lymph nodes located in the neck may help with identification and early treatment of cancer (American Cancer Society [ACS], 2013). In turn, early detection and early treatment of cancer may improve survival rates among individuals who experience cancer.

See Table 14.1 for examples of *Healthy People 2020* objectives that are designed to promote health and wellness among individuals across the life span.

Lifespan Considerations

Growth and development are dynamic processes that describe change over time. It is important to understand data collection and interpretation of findings regarding growth and development in relation to normative values. The following discussion presents specific variations in the head and neck for different age groups.

Infants and Children

An infant's head should be measured at each visit until 2 years of age. The newborn's head is about 34 cm (13 to 14 in.), and this is generally equal to the chest circumference. The shape of the head may indicate *molding*, the shaping of the head by pressure on the bony structures as the head moves through the vaginal canal during delivery.

TABLE 14.1	Examples of *Healthy People 2020* Objectives Related to the Head, Neck, and Related Lymphatics
OBJECTIVE NUMBER	**DESCRIPTION**
IVP-2	Reduce fatal and nonfatal traumatic brain injuries
IVP-15	Increase use of safety belts
IVP-16	Increase age-appropriate vehicle restraint system use in children between 0 and 12 years of age
IVP-20	Reduce pedalcyclist deaths on public roads
IVP-22	Increase the proportion of motorcycle operators and passengers using helmets
IVP-23	Prevent an increase in fall-related deaths
IVP-26	Reduce sports and recreation injuries
IVP-27	Increase the proportion of public and private schools that require students to wear appropriate protective gear when engaged in school-sponsored physical activities
MICH-25	Reduce the incidence of fetal alcohol syndrome (FAS)
C-1	Reduce the overall cancer death rate.

Source: U.S. Department of Health and Human Services (USDHHS). (2014). *Healthy People 2020.* Retrieved from http://www.healthypeople.gov/2020/default.aspx

The degree of molding will be influenced by the presenting part of the head and type of delivery. Usually, it takes several days for the head to take on the more normal round shape. Suture lines should be open as are the fontanels. The anterior fontanel is diamond shaped, and the posterior fontanel is triangular in shape (see Figure 14.8 ■). The fontanels should be firm and even with the skull. Slight pulsations are normal. The posterior fontanel closes at approximately 2 months of age; the anterior fontanel closes between 12 and 18 months of age. The neck of the newborn is short with many skin folds and begins to lengthen over time. By about 4 months of age the infant begins to demonstrate control of the head. In toddlers, the head is relatively large and the muscles of the neck are underdeveloped compared to adults. The proportions change throughout the preschool years, and by school age the proportions are similar to those of adults.

The thyroid gland, located in the neck, plays an important role in growth and development. Infants have shorter necks than older children and adults. The thyroid is difficult to palpate on an infant, but it can be accomplished on a child using two or three fingers. Abnormalities in thyroid function are generally detected by assessment of growth and development and through laboratory testing. All U.S. states require newborn screening for congenital hypothyroidism, or reduced thyroid function. This screening is conducted through blood testing for thyroid-stimulating hormone

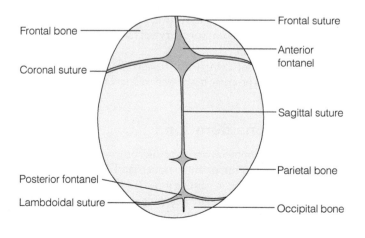

A Superior view

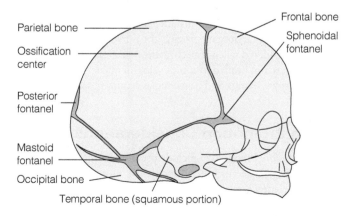

B Lateral view

Figure 14.8 The newborn's skull.

levels (MedlinePlus, 2013a). Blood samples for this test should ideally be taken when the newborn is 2 to 4 days old.

The lymph nodes are present at birth, but differentiation and growth of lymphatic tissue occurs primarily between ages 4 and 8 years. As such, preschoolers and school-age children often have "shotty" lymph nodes and slightly enlarged tonsils. Shotty nodes are noninfected, nontender, slightly enlarged lymph nodes that move when palpated and feel firmer than normal. Most children under 6 to 7 years have palpable, shotty femoral or cervical lymph nodes. Newborns and infants with a history of internal fetal monitoring during labor often have palpable occipital lymph nodes.

The Pregnant Female

The pregnant female may develop blotchy pigmented spots (melasma) on her face (see Figure 13.6 on page 215), facial edema, and enlargement of the thyroid. ∞ All of these symptoms are considered normal and subside after childbirth. The pregnant female may also complain of headaches during the first trimester, which may be related to rapidly increasing estrogen levels; however, most women find relief from headaches, especially migraines, during pregnancy as hormone levels stabilize. Severe persistent headaches should be evaluated, because headaches may be an indication of preeclampsia (see chapter 27). ∞

The Older Adult

The older adult loses subcutaneous fat in the face. This increases the wrinkles in the skin, yielding an older appearance. A decrease in reproductive hormones results in the development of coarse, long eyebrows and nasal hair in males and coarse hair, usually on the chin, in females. Loss of teeth and improperly fitting dentures provide a change to facial expressions and symmetry. Rigidity of the cervical vertebrae is common, causing limited range of motion of the neck. The thyroid gland produces fewer hormones with age. In addition to female gender, one of the highest risk factors for developing hypothyroidism is being over the age of 50 (University of Maryland Medical Center, 2013).

Among older adults, complaints of feeling tired, weak, or unwell may be related to thyroid dysfunction. Some symptoms that many people expect with aging, such as weight changes, decreased cognitive function, slowed physical movement, and feeling unwell, may be signs of thyroid disorders, as well.

Psychosocial Considerations

A patient who is under a great deal of stress may be prone to headaches, including tension headaches, neck pain, and mouth ulcers. Pain in the TMJ may be due to unconscious clenching of the jaw during stressful situations, such as driving in heavy traffic or taking an exam. It may also be caused by nighttime teeth grinding. Chronic TMJ syndrome may eventually result in a wearing down of the teeth, and the patient may need to consult a dentist or orthodontist.

Other indications of psychosocial disturbances include tics (involuntary muscle spasms), hair twisting or pulling, lip biting, and excessive blinking. Relaxation techniques such as meditation and guided imagery may help relieve head and neck symptoms related to stress. If appropriate, the nurse should refer the patient to a mental health professional for assistance.

The nurse should also be aware of psychosocial implications of face, head, and neck disorders that alter the appearance of the patient. The nurse may need to discuss self-esteem issues with the patient or refer the patient to a psychologist for counseling. Depending on the disorder, the nurse may also refer patients to orthodontists, otolaryngologists, cosmetic surgeons, or other specialists.

Psychosocial factors can also contribute to changes in the efficiency of the lymphatic system. Because lymph is moved through the lymphatic system by muscle contraction, lack of movement may cause pooling lymph. Blocked or pooled lymph may lead to edema, frequent infection, fatigue, gastrointestinal issues, and cellulite buildup. These conditions may decrease productiveness at work or at home, leading to job difficulties or strained relationships.

Cultural and Environmental Considerations

Within some cultures, eye contact and smiling are considered rude or aggressive. Furthermore, sharing of personal information with strangers is not permitted. This makes obtaining a detailed health history or conducting a focused interview most difficult. Some cultures and religions, such as Muslims and Sikhs, require the individual to cover the head or face. Touching the head is prohibited in cultures in which the soul or spirit is believed to reside in the head. These cultural groups include, but are not limited to, individuals who are of Hmong and Cambodian heritage (Owens, 2007; Mony, 2008).

Facial malformations are a frequent occurrence in children with FAS. Some infants have a flat occipital prominence (plagiocephaly), which may result from putting them to sleep on their backs. Placing infants on their backs for sleep has become a common practice to reduce the incidence of sudden infant death syndrome (SIDS). Flattening of the head may also occur when infant boards are used, for example, as in Central American cultures. Over time, the flattening of the head can reverse itself.

Thyroid disease is common in areas where iodine is limited. Iodine deficiency disorders, including **goiter** (enlarged thyroid) and hypothyroidism, are significant health problems in India and China. Iodine deficiencies occur in areas where the soil is poor in iodine. These areas include eastern Europe, parts of South America, Australia, and the western United States. Use of iodized salt has generally obliterated iodine deficiencies in the United States. The World Health Organization (WHO) is overseeing global programs to increase the use of iodized salt to prevent these deficiencies.

Gathering the Data

Health assessment of the head and neck includes gathering subjective and objective data. Recall that subjective data collection occurs during the patient interview, before the physical assessment, with the collection of the objective data. During the interview, the nurse uses a variety of communication techniques to elicit general and specific information about the structures of the patient's head and neck. Health records, the results of laboratory tests, and radiologic and imaging reports are important secondary sources to be reviewed and included in the data-gathering process. During physical assessment of the head and neck, the techniques of inspection, palpation, and auscultation will be used to gather the objective data.

See Table 14.2 for information on potential secondary sources of patient data.

Focused Interview

The focused interview for the head and neck concerns data related to the head, the face, and the structures of the neck including the thyroid, trachea, and lymph nodes. Subjective data are gathered during the focused interview. The nurse must be prepared to observe the patient and listen for cues related to the functions of structures within the head and neck. The nurse may use open-ended and closed

TABLE 14.2	Potential Secondary Sources for Patient Data Related to the Head, Neck, and Related Lymphatics	
LABORATORY TESTS	**NORMAL VALUES**	
Thyroid		
TSH	0.3–5.0 mIU/L	
T_3	80–190 ng/dL	
T_4	5.0–12.5 mcg/dL	
Calcitonin	Male: <16 pg/mL	
	Female: <8 pg/mL	
Lymph Nodes		
Complete Blood Count with Differential	Red Blood Cells (RBC)	
	Male: 4.32–5.72 million/microliter (mcL)	
	Female: 3.90–5.03 million/microliter (mcL)	
	Hemoglobin (Hgb)	
	Male: 13.5–17.5 g/dL	
	Female: 12.0–15.5 g/dL	
	Hematocrit (Hct)	
	Male: 38%–50%	
	Female: 34%–44.5%	
	White Blood Cells	
	Leukocytes 4,500–10,000/mcl	
	Bands 0%–3%	
	Basophils 0.5%–1%	
	Eosinophils 1%–4%	
	Lymphocytes 20%–40%	
	B-Lymphocytes 4%–25%	
	T-Lymphocytes 60%–95%	
	Monocytes 2%–8%	
	Neutrophils 40%–60%	
	Platelets 150–450 billion/L	
	Erythrocyte Sedimentation Rate (ESR)	
	Males: <23 mm/hr	
	Females: <29 mm/hr	
Diagnostic Tests		
Biopsy		
Chest X-ray		
Liver/Spleen Scan		
Lymph Nodes		
Biopsy		
Thyroid		
Thyroid Scan		
Ultrasonography		

questions to obtain information. Follow-up questions or requests for descriptions are required to clarify data or gather missing information. Follow-up questions are intended to identify the source of problems, explain the duration of problems, discuss ways to alleviate problems, and provide clues about the patient's knowledge about his or her own health. Remember, the subjective data collected and the questions asked during the health history and focused interview will provide information to help meet the goal of safety with reduced injuries and disabilities as described in *Healthy People 2020*.

The focused interview guides the physical assessment of the head and neck. The information is always considered in relation to normative values and expectations regarding function of the specific structure. Therefore, the nurse must consider age, gender, race, culture, environment, health practices, past and concurrent problems, and therapies when framing questions and using techniques

to elicit information. In order to address all of the factors when conducting a focused interview, categories of questions related to status and function of the head and neck have been developed. These categories include general questions that are asked of all patients; those addressing acute and chronic illness and infections; questions related to symptoms, pain, and behaviors; those related to habits or practices; questions that are specific to patients according to age; those for pregnant females; and questions that address environmental concerns. One approach to elicit data about symptoms is the OLDCART & ICE method as described in chapter 7. See Figure 7.3 on page 120. ∞

The nurse must consider the patient's ability to participate in the focused interview and physical assessment of the head and neck. If a patient is experiencing pain, stiffness, or anxiety that accompanies any of these problems, attention must focus on relief of symptoms.

Focused Interview Questions	Rationales and Evidence

The following section provides sample questions and follow-up questions in each of the previously mentioned categories. A rationale for each of the questions is provided. The list of questions is not inclusive, but rather represents the types of questions required in a comprehensive focused interview related to the head and neck. The follow-up bulleted

questions are asked to seek clarification with additional information from the patient to enhance the subjective database. The subjective data collected and the questions asked during the health history and the focused interview will provide data to help meet the goal of preventing head injuries and resulting disabilities.

General Questions

1. **Describe the condition of your scalp today.**
   - Is it different from 2 months ago? From 2 years ago?

   ▶ This question gives patients the opportunity to provide their own perceptions about the condition of the scalp.

2. **Do you have any problems that affect your scalp?**

   ▶ This question elicits information about problems or illnesses, which may be localized or systemic, that impact the scalp. If the patient identifies any problems, follow-up is required to obtain descriptions and details about what, when, and how problems occur, and the duration of each problem.

3. **Is there anyone in your family who has had a problem with his or her scalp or a problem that indirectly affected his or her scalp?**

   ▶ This question may elicit information about illnesses with a familial or genetic predisposition. Follow-up is required to obtain details about specific problems related to occurrence, treatment, and outcomes.

4. **Questions 1, 2, and 3 would be repeated for the skull, face, trachea, thyroid, and lymph nodes.**

Questions Related to Illness, Infection, or Injury

1. **Have you ever been diagnosed with an illness affecting your head, face, or neck?**
   - When were you diagnosed with the problem?
   - What treatment was prescribed for the problem?
   - Do you use or have you used any strategies to minimize discomfort or otherwise cope with this problem? Was the strategy successful?
   - Has the problem ever recurred (acute)?
   - How are you managing the disease now (chronic)?

   ▶ The patient has an opportunity to provide information about specific illnesses. If a specific disease or illness is identified, follow-up about the date of diagnosis, treatment, and outcomes is required. Data about each illness identified by the patient are essential to an accurate health assessment. Illnesses are classified as acute or chronic, and follow-up regarding each classification will differ.

Focused Interview Questions	Rationales and Evidence
2. Do you now have or have you ever had an infection affecting your head, face, or neck?	▶ The patient has an opportunity to provide information about infectious processes. Follow-up would be carried out as in question 1.
3. Have you ever had any problem with your thyroid gland? Have you had thyroid surgery? Are you currently taking thyroid medication? What symptoms do you associate with your thyroid problem?	▶ Over- or undersecretion by the thyroid gland may cause rapid weight gain or loss, heat or cold intolerance, fatigue, mood swings, tremor, anxiety, tachycardia and palpitations, muscle weakness, changes in skin and hair, and other alterations in health (Sharma, Aronow, Patel, Gandhi, & Desai, 2011; Gaitonde, Rowley, & Sweeney, 2012).
4. Describe any recent or past injury to your head. • Did you lose consciousness? • How long were you unconscious? • How did it occur? • Have problems recurred (acute)? • How are you managing the problem now (chronic)?	▶ Head injury can result in acute or chronic neurologic problems.

Questions Related to Symptoms, Pain, and Behaviors

When gathering information about symptoms, many questions are required to elicit details and descriptions. Questions are asked in relation to the significance of a symptom, specific diseases or problems, and potential follow-up examination or referral. One rationale may be provided for a group of questions in this category.

Questions Related to Symptoms

The following questions refer to specific symptoms associated with the head and neck. For each symptom, questions and follow-up are required. The details to be elicited are: the characteristics of the symptom; the onset, duration, and frequency of the symptom; the treatment or remedy for the symptom, including over-the-counter and home remedies; the determination if diagnosis has been sought; the effect of treatments; and family history associated with a symptom or illness.

1. Have you had any dizziness, loss of consciousness, seizures, or blurred vision? When did each symptom occur? How long did the symptom last? What did you do to relieve the symptom? Does the treatment help?	▶ These symptoms may indicate problems with carotid arteries, cerebral clots or bleeding, recent head injury, or neurologic disease (Osborn, Wraa, Watson, & Holleran, 2013).
2. Have you noticed any swelling, lumps, bumps, or skin sores on your head that did not heal?	▶ Swellings, masses, and lesions that do not heal may indicate cancer (CDC, 2013a).
3. Have you noticed any lumps or swellings on your neck?	▶ Lateral neck masses are usually due to enlargement of the cervical lymph nodes, indicative of infection or malignancy. Swelling in the medial aspect of the neck may be indicative of thyroid pathology (Berman & Snyder, 2012).

Focused Interview Questions	Rationales and Evidence

Questions Related to Pain

1. **Do you have headaches? If so, please tell me about them.**
   - *Frequency:* How often?
   - *Onset:* How long have you been bothered with this type of headache? When does the headache begin?
   - *Duration:* How long does a typical headache last?
   - *Location:* Where is the pain? On one side of the head? Behind the eyes? In the sinus area?
   - *Character:* Is the pain throbbing, steady, dull, or sharp? On a scale of 0 to 10, with 10 being the strongest, how severe is the pain?
   - *Associated symptoms:* Do you experience any nausea, vomiting, sensitivity to light or noise, muscle pain, or other symptoms along with the headache?
   - *Precipitating factors:* Do you feel that the headaches usually are triggered by stress, alcohol intake, anxiety, menstrual cycle, allergies, or any other factors? Please describe.
   - *Treatment:* What seems to relieve the symptoms? Resting? Medication? Exercise?

   ▶ Questions 1, 2, and 3 encourage the patient to provide a detailed description of the headache necessary to help determine the cause and possible treatments.

2. **Do you experience any problems that precede the headache, such as visual problems?**

   ▶ Bright or rapidly changing lights, such as strobe lights, can trigger migraines. Migraines are often accompanied by visual symptoms such as blurry vision, photophobia, and eyelid ptosis (Kurlander, Punjabi, Liu, Sattar, & Guyuron, 2014).

3. **Do your headaches occur in episodes? If so, describe the episodes.**
   - Do your headaches increase in severity with each episode?

4. **Have you recently had an infection or cold?**

   ▶ These conditions may be accompanied by headaches.

5. **Has your neck been weak, sore, or stiff?**

   ▶ Neck symptoms may indicate problems with the muscles of the neck or the cervical spinal cord or an infectious problem such as meningitis (CDC, 2014).

Questions Related to Behaviors

1. **Do you now use or have you ever used alcohol, recreational drugs, tobacco products, or caffeine?**
   - How much of the product do you use?
   - When did you start using the product?
   - How long have you used the product?
   - Have you had problems associated with the product?
   - What have you done to deal with the problem?

   ▶ Use of alcohol, tobacco, and street drugs, as well as caffeine withdrawal, can affect neurologic and neurovascular function and increase headaches (Welch, 2011).

Questions Related to Age

The focused interview must reflect the anatomic and physiologic differences that exist along the age span. The following questions are examples of those that would be specific for infants and children, the pregnant female, and the older adult.

Questions Regarding Infants and Children

1. **Did you use alcohol or recreational drugs during your pregnancy?**

   ▶ FAS causes neurologic disorders, developmental delays, and characteristic head and facial deformities. Use of cocaine during pregnancy can result in neurologic and cardiovascular problems in the infant (Meyer & Zhang, 2009).

2. **Have you noticed any depression or bulging over the infant's "soft spots" (fontanels)?**

   ▶ A depressed fontanel can indicate dehydration, and a bulging fontanel can indicate an infection (Goldberg, 2013).

Focused Interview Questions	Rationales and Evidence

Questions for the Pregnant Female

1. **Do you have frequent headaches?**

   ▶ Headaches are common during the first trimester, but it is important to rule out other possible complications of pregnancy such as preeclampsia.

2. **Have you noticed changes in the skin on your face? If yes, what changes have occurred?**

   ▶ Increasing hormonal changes can result in melasma or chloasma, which are pigmented areas on the face. In addition, the hormonal changes cause increased secretions of oils from the skin's sebaceous glands, which may result in acne.

3. **Do you have a history of thyroid disease? If yes, what is the disease and treatment?**

   ▶ Thyroid diseases can result in problems with the developing fetus (Stagnaro-Green et al., 2011). Existing thyroid problems require careful monitoring of medications.

Questions for the Older Adult

1. **Do you carry out safety precautions in your home? When driving or away from home?**
   - Do you have safety rails installed in the bathroom?
   - Do you keep your floors clear of clutter and rugs that can slip?
   - Is your home well-lit?
   - Do you wear your seatbelt while driving?
   - Do you use an assistive device while walking when away from home?

   ▶ Safety precautions can reduce the risk for falls and injuries to the head and neck. Older adults are at increased risk for falls.

Questions Related to the Environment

Environment refers to both the internal and external environments. Questions related to the internal environment include all of the previous questions and those associated with internal or physiologic responses. Questions regarding the external environment include those related to home, work, or social environments.

Internal Environment

1. **Are you now experiencing or have you ever had an experience of intermittent or prolonged anxiety or emotional upset?**

   ▶ Anxiety and situations of emotional upset impact the sympathetic nervous system, producing hormonal responses that affect vascular function. The resultant vasoconstriction can contribute to headache, hypertension, and risk for cardiovascular problems. Stress and tension may precipitate and increase neck pain or stiffness.

2. **Do you now use or have you used prescribed or over-the-counter (OTC) medications, home remedies, cultural treatments, or therapies for problems with your head and neck or for any other purpose?**

   ▶ Medications can have side effects and interactions that exacerbate or enhance symptoms. Knowledge of medication usage provides information that assists in the analysis of patient situations and determination of the significance of findings in a comprehensive assessment.

External Environment

The following questions deal with substances and irritants found in the physical environment of the patient. These include the indoor and outdoor environments of the home and the workplace and those encountered during travel.

1. **Have you ever had irradiation of the head or neck?**

   ▶ Radiation exposure increases the risk for thyroid tumors (Ron et al., 2012).

2. **Are you exposed to chemicals or toxins in your home or work environment (e.g., radiation, acids, bases, detergents, pesticides, fertilizers, solvents, metals, etc.)?**

   ▶ Environmental chemicals and toxins can be precipitating factors for headache and neurologic problems (CDC, 2013b).

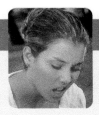

Patient-Centered Interaction

Ms. Dowd, a 20-year-old college sophomore, reports to the university health office with a "very bad headache." Following is part of the focused interview taken by the nurse.

Interview

Nurse: Ms. Dorothy Dowd, you have already told me you have a headache, and I would like to know more about it. On a scale of 0 to 10, with 10 being the worst pain, please rate your headache.

Ms. Dowd: **Right now my headache is an 8.**

Nurse: During the interview, should you need to stop, close your eyes, and relax for a few minutes, let me know.

Ms. Dowd: **Okay, but I should be all right.**

Nurse: Tell me about your headaches.

Ms. Dowd: **I have had this for 2 to 3 weeks, on and off. Now it feels like it is all the time, but it is not always 8. Sometimes it is 5.**

Nurse: Using one or two words, can you describe the pain?

Ms. Dowd: **It is usually a dull, constant ache.**

Nurse: Describe the location of this dull ache in your head.

Ms. Dowd: **It always seems to start at the top of my neck. As it gets worse, it moves up to the top of my head.**

Nurse: Are you talking about the right or left side?

Ms. Dowd: **Right now it is both sides. That's why I'm here. I can't stand it anymore. Sometimes it's only one side. Sometimes it stays low (pointing to the occipital region) and doesn't come high.**

Nurse: Have you always had headaches?

Ms. Dowd: **I would have an occasional headache. Sometimes a day or two before my period and then it would go away. Nothing like this, though.**

Nurse: What do you think is causing your headaches?

Ms. Dowd: **I don't know. I have not been sleeping very well lately. I'm worried about this one course. I can't seem to "get it" and I'm afraid it will kill my GPA. If that happens I will lose my scholarship. I'm working so hard in this course that some of my other work is beginning to slide.**

Analysis

The nurse begins the interview with confirmation of the reason for seeking help and then asks the patient to confirm the severity of the pain. The nurse acknowledges Ms. Dowd's pain before seeking more specific subjective data from the patient. Using an open-ended approach encourages Ms. Dowd to communicate more openly.

Patient Education

The following are physiologic, behavioral, and cultural factors that affect the head and neck across the age span. Several of these factors reflect trends cited in *Healthy People 2020* documents. The nurse provides advice and education to reduce risks associated with these factors and to promote and maintain health and function of the structures of the head and neck.

LIFESPAN CONSIDERATIONS

Risk Factors	Patient Education
• Alcohol use during pregnancy can result in facial deformities in the newborn.	▶ Encourage prenatal care to pregnant females and stress cessation of alcohol consumption during pregnancy.
• Congenital hypothyroidism can result in physical and mental retardation.	▶ Teach parents the signs of hypothyroidism in newborns, and teach them the importance of newborn metabolic screening for low TSH levels.
• Thyroid disease occurs with greater frequency in females than in males.	▶ Advise females of all ages to have thyroid screening performed if there is a family history of thyroid disease.

LIFESPAN CONSIDERATIONS

Risk Factors

- The development of thyroid dysfunction occurs more frequently in males and females after age 60.

- Production of thyroid hormone decreases with age.

Patient Education

▶ Depression in old age may be associated with hypothyroidism. Advise patients and families to consult with healthcare providers if the symptom arises.

▶ Advise older adults to have thyroid screening and annual monitoring of thyroid hormone levels.

CULTURAL CONSIDERATIONS

Risk Factor

- Iodine deficiency leads to thyroid dysfunction and may occur in immigrant populations.

Patient Education

▶ Advise immigrants to include iodized salt in their diet if they are at risk for thyroid dysfunction.

ENVIRONMENTAL CONSIDERATIONS

Risk Factors

- Medications with iodine can cause hyperthyroidism.

- Thyroid diseases such as Hashimoto's (an autoimmune disorder causing hypothyroidism) are genetic disorders.

Patient Education

▶ Provide information about potential side effects of medications, especially those with iodine (e.g., iodine supplements, amiodarone).

▶ Teach at-risk patients (those with a family history of Hashimoto's) about the signs and symptoms of the disorder.

Physical Assessment

Assessment Techniques and Findings

Physical assessment of the head and neck requires the use of inspection, palpation, and auscultation. During each of the procedures, the nurse is gathering objective data related to the structures of the head and neck and the functions of the structures within them. Inspection includes looking at skin color, the scalp, the skull, and the face for symmetry of bones and structure. The trachea is palpated for position. The thyroid is palpated for movement, texture, and identification of size or abnormalities. The lymph nodes of the head and neck are palpated to evaluate enlargement, tenderness, and mobility. The temporal artery is auscultated. Knowledge of normal parameters and expected findings is essential to interpreting data as the nurse performs the assessment.

In adults and children over 12–18 months of age, the skull should be normocephalic, that is, a rounded and symmetric shape. In children under 12–18 months of age, the cranial bones are not yet fused and the head shape may be misshapen, especially in newborns who underwent a vaginal birth. In all individuals, the frontal parietal and occipital prominences are present and symmetric. The scalp is clear and free of lesions; the hair is evenly distributed. The face is symmetric in shape; the eyes, ears, nose, and mouth are symmetrically placed. The facial movements are smooth and coordinated, and demonstrate a variety of expressions. In adults, the temporal artery feels smooth and firm with no tenderness to palpation and without bruits on auscultation; children may occasionally have innocuous

EQUIPMENT

- examination gown
- clean, nonsterile examination gloves
- glass of water
- stethoscope

HELPFUL HINTS

- Explain what is expected of the patient for each step of the assessment.
- Tell the patient the purpose of each procedure and when and if discomfort will accompany any examination.
- Identify and remedy language or cultural barriers at the outset of the patient interaction.
- Explain to the patient the need to remove any items that would interfere with the assessment, including jewelry, hats, scarves, veils, hairpieces, and wigs.
- Use Standard Precautions.

bruits upon auscultation. The TMJ has nonpainful, full, and smooth range of motion. The head is held erect without tremors. The neck is symmetric without swelling and has full range of motion. Carotid artery pulsation is usually visible bilaterally when the patient is lying down. The trachea is midline, and the hyoid bone and tracheal cartilage move with swallowing. The thyroid is not enlarged and is without palpable nodules. The lymph nodes of the head and neck are nonpalpable in adults, infants, and adolescents. Cervical lymph nodes are usually small and palpable in children between the ages of 1 and 11 years old.

Techniques and Normal Findings	Abnormal Findings Special Considerations

The Head

1. **Position the patient.**
   - Ask the patient to sit comfortably on the examination table (see Figure 14.9 ■).

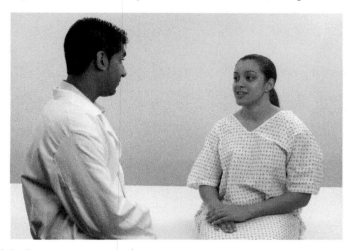

Figure 14.9   Patient is positioned.

2. **Instruct the patient.**
   - Explain that you will be looking at the patient and touching the head, hair, and face. Explain that no discomfort should occur, but if the patient experiences pain or discomfort you will stop that part of the examination.

3. **Inspect the head and scalp.**
   - Note the size, shape, symmetry, and integrity of the head and scalp. Identify the prominences—frontal, parietal, and occipital—that determine the shape and symmetry of the head.
   - Part the hair and look for scaliness of the scalp, lesions, or foreign bodies. (Refer to Figure 13.24 on page 238. ∞)
   - Check hair distribution and hygiene.

4. **Inspect the face.**
   - Note the facial expression and symmetry of structures. The eyes, ears, nose, and mouth should be symmetrically placed. Inspect the symmetry of the lips at rest and when speaking. The nasolabial folds should be equal. The palpebral fissures should be equal. The top of the pinnae of the ear should be at the level of the outer canthi of the eyes (see Figure 14.2 on page 262).

5. **Observe movements of the head, face, and eyes.**
   - All movements should be smooth and with purpose. Cranial nerves III (Oculomotor), IV (Trochlear), and VI (Abducens) control movement of the eye. Cranial nerve V (Trigeminal) stimulates movement for mastication. Cranial nerve VII (Facial) controls movement of the face. A detailed discussion of the cranial nerves is found in chapter 26. ∞

▶ Jerky movements or tics may be the result of neurologic or psychologic disorders.

Techniques and Normal Findings	Abnormal Findings / Special Considerations

6. **Palpate the head and scalp.**
   - Note the texture of the scalp and the contour and size of the head. Ask the patient to report any tenderness as you palpate. Normally there is no tenderness with palpation.

▶ Note any tenderness, swelling, edema, or masses, which require further evaluation. Ask permission prior to palpation, because touching of the head is prohibited in some cultures.

7. **Confirm skin and tissue integrity.**
   - The skin should be intact.

▶ Note any alteration in skin or tissue integrity related to ulcerations, rashes, discolorations, or swellings.

8. **Palpate the temporal artery.**
   - Palpate between the eye and the top of the ear (see Figure 14.10 ■). The artery should feel smooth.

▶ Any thickening or tenderness could indicate inflammation of the artery.

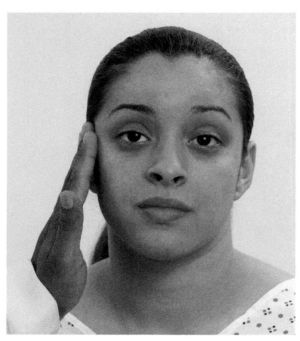

Figure 14.10 Palpating the temporal artery.

9. **Auscultate the temporal artery.**
   - Use the bell of the stethoscope to auscultate for a bruit (a soft blowing sound). Bruits are not normally present.

▶ A bruit is indicative of stenosis (narrowing) of the vessel.

10. **Test the range of motion of the TMJ.**
    - Place your fingers in front of each ear and ask the patient to open and close the mouth slowly. There should be no limitation of movement or tenderness. You should feel a slight indentation of the joint. (For more detail on assessment of the TMJ, see chapter 25.) ∞
    - Soft clicking noises on movement are sometimes heard and are considered normal.

▶ Any limitation of movement or tenderness on movement requires further evaluation.
   Crepitation, a crackling sound on movement, may indicate joint problems.

The Neck

1. **Instruct the patient.**
   - Explain that you will be looking at and touching the front and sides of the patient's neck. Tell the patient that you will provide specific instructions for special tests. Advise the patient to inform you of any discomfort.

▶ In the obese patient with a short neck, any assessments of structures in the neck can be difficult. Alternate methods may be required, for example, a Doppler stethoscope to assess pulses.

Techniques and Normal Findings	Abnormal Findings Special Considerations

2. **Inspect the neck for skin color, integrity, shape, and symmetry.**
   - Observe for any swelling of the lymph nodes below the angle of the jaw and along the sternocleidomastoid muscle.
   - The head should be held erect with no tremors.

▶ Excessive rigidity of the neck may indicate arthritis. Inability to hold the neck erect may be due to muscle spasms. Swelling of the lymph nodes may indicate infection and requires further assessment.

3. **Test the range of motion of the neck.**
   - Ask the patient to slowly move the chin to the chest, turn the head right and left, then touch the left ear to left shoulder and the right ear to right shoulder (without raising the shoulders). Then ask the patient to extend the head back.
     There should be no pain and no limitation of movement (for further discussion, see chapters 25 and 26.) ∞

▶ Any pain or limitation of movement could indicate arthritis, muscle spasm, or inflammation. Rapid movement and compression of the cerebral vertebrae may cause dizziness.

4. **Observe the carotid arteries and jugular veins.**
   - The carotid artery runs just below the angle of the jaw, and its pulsations can frequently be seen. Assessment of the carotid arteries and jugular veins is discussed fully in chapter 19. ∞

▶ Any distention or prominence may indicate a vascular disorder.

5. **Palpate the trachea.**
   - Palpate the sternal notch. Move the finger pad of the palpating finger off the notch to the midline of the neck. Lightly palpate the area. You will feel the C rings (cricoid cartilage) of the trachea.
     Move the finger laterally, first to the right and then to the left. You have now identified the lateral borders of the trachea (see Figure 14.11 ■).
   - The trachea should be midline, and the distance to the sternocleidomastoid muscles on each side should be equal. Place the thumb and index finger on each side of the trachea and slide them upward. As the trachea begins to widen, you have now identified the thyroid cartilage. Continue to slide your thumb and index finger high into the neck. Palpate the hyoid bone. The greater horns of the hyoid bone are most prominent. Confirm that the hyoid bone and tracheal cartilages move when the patient swallows.

▶ Tracheal displacement is the result of masses in the neck or mediastinum, pneumothorax, or pulmonary fibrosis.

▶ Palpating the trachea may be difficult in children under 3 years of age because their necks are short and thick (Chiocca, 2011).

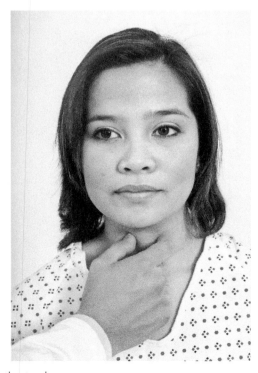

Figure 14.11 Palpating the trachea.

Techniques and Normal Findings	Abnormal Findings / Special Considerations

6. Inspect the thyroid gland.

- The thyroid is not observable normally until the patient swallows. Give the patient a cup of water.
- Distinguish the thyroid from other structures in the neck by asking the patient to drink a sip of water.
- The thyroid tissue is attached to the trachea, and, as the patient swallows, it moves superiorly. You may want to adjust the lighting in the room if possible so that shadows are not cast on the patient's neck. This may help you to visualize the thyroid.

▶ If the patient has any enlargement of the thyroid or masses near the thyroid, they appear as bulges when the patient swallows.

7. Palpate the thyroid gland from behind the patient.

- Palpation of the thyroid gland is difficult and requires practice. While not all nurses will be required to perform this assessment skill, the nurse should be familiar with the basic steps involved, as well as its purpose.
- Stand behind the patient.
- Ask the patient to sit up straight, lower the chin, and turn the head slightly to the right.
- This position causes the patient's neck muscles to relax.
- Using the fingers of your left hand, push the trachea to the right. Use light pressure during palpation to avoid obliterating findings.
- With the fingers of the right hand, palpate the area between the trachea and the sternocleidomastoid muscle. Slowly and gently retract the sternocleidomastoid muscle and then ask the patient to drink a sip of water. Palpate as the thyroid gland moves up during swallowing (see Figure 14.12 ■). Normally, you will not feel the thyroid gland, although in some patients with long, thin necks, you may be able to feel the isthmus. You may be able to feel the fullness of the thyroid as it moves up upon swallowing.
- Reverse the procedure for the left side.

▶ An enlarged thyroid gland may be due to a metabolic disorder such as **hyperthyroidism** or **hypothyroidism**. Palpable masses of 5 mm or larger are alterations in health. Their location, size, and shape should be documented, and the patient should be evaluated further. In pregnancy, a slightly enlarged thyroid can be a normal finding. Most pathologic hyperthyroidism in pregnancy is caused by Graves' disease, an autoimmune disorder that causes increased production of thyroid hormones.

▶ The thyroid usually cannot be palpated in newborns and is difficult to palpate in infants and young children unless the thyroid is enlarged (Chiocca, 2011)

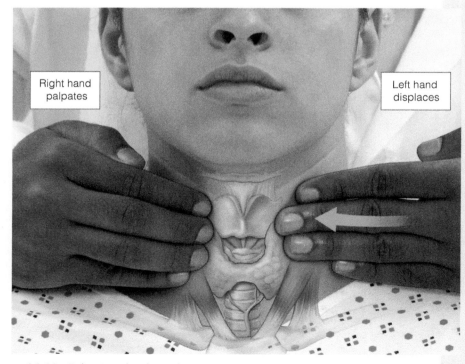

Right hand palpates

Left hand displaces

Figure 14.12 Palpating the thyroid using a posterior approach.

Techniques and Normal Findings	Abnormal Findings Special Considerations

8. Palpate the thyroid gland from in front of the patient.

- This is an alternative approach. Stand in front of the patient. Ask the patient to lower the head and turn slightly to the right. Using the thumb of your right hand, push the trachea to the right (see Figure 14.13 ■).
- Place your left thumb and fingers over the sternocleidomastoid muscle and feel for any enlargement of the right lobe as the patient swallows. Have water available to make swallowing easier. Reverse the procedure for the left side.

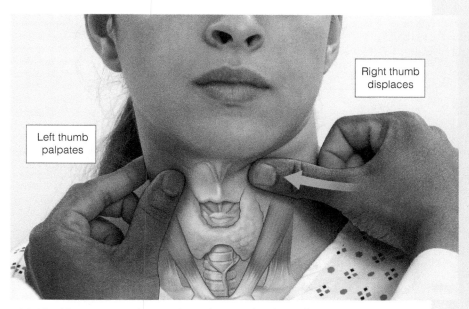

Right thumb displaces

Left thumb palpates

Figure 14.13 Alternative technique for palpating the thyroid.

9. Auscultate the thyroid.

- If the thyroid is enlarged, the area over the thyroid is auscultated to detect any bruits. In an enlarged thyroid, blood flows through the arteries at an accelerated rate, producing a soft, rushing sound. This sound can best be detected with the bell of the stethoscope.

▶ The presence of a bruit is abnormal and is an indication of increased blood flow.

10. Palpate the lymph nodes of the head and neck.

- Palpate the lymph nodes by exerting gentle circular pressure with the finger pads of two or three fingers of both hands. It is important to avoid strong pressure, which can push the nodes into the muscle and underlying structures, making them difficult to find. It is also important to establish a routine for assessment; otherwise, it is possible to omit one or more of the groups of nodes.

▶ Enlargement of lymph nodes is called **lymphadenopathy** and can be due to infection, allergies, or a tumor.

Techniques and Normal Findings

- The following is one suggested order of assessment (see Figure 14.14A ■).
  1. Preauricular
  2. Postauricular
  3. Occipital
  4. Retropharyngeal (tonsillar)
  5. Submandibular
  6. Submental (with one hand)
  7. Anterior/superficial cervical chain
  8. Posterior and deep cervical chain
  9. Supraclavicular

Abnormal Findings Special Considerations

▶ Lymph nodes are normally nonpalpable in adults, infants, and adolescents. They may be palpable in children between the ages of 1 and 11 years old (see Figure 14.14B ■).

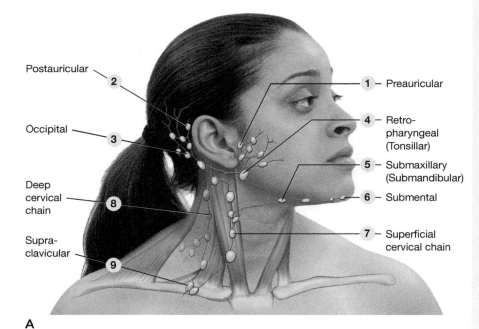

Postauricular   2

Occipital   3

Deep cervical chain   8

Supra-clavicular   9

1 – Preauricular

4 – Retro-pharyngeal (Tonsillar)

5 – Submaxillary (Submandibular)

6 – Submental

7 – Superficial cervical chain

A

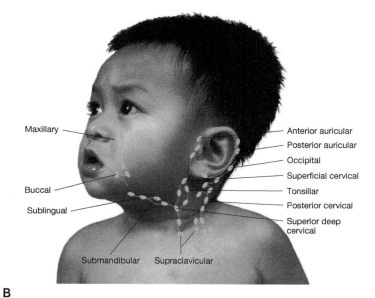

Maxillary

Buccal

Sublingual

Anterior auricular
Posterior auricular
Occipital
Superficial cervical
Tonsillar
Posterior cervical
Superior deep cervical

Submandibular   Supraclavicular

B

Figure 14.14 A. Suggested sequence for palpating lymph nodes. B. Location of the head and neck lymph nodes in children.

- Ask the patient to relax the muscles of the neck to make the nodes easier to palpate. It is helpful to have the patient shrug the shoulders when palpating the supraclavicular nodes. If any lymph nodes are palpable, make a note of their location, size, shape, fixation or mobility, and tenderness (see Figure 14.15 ■).

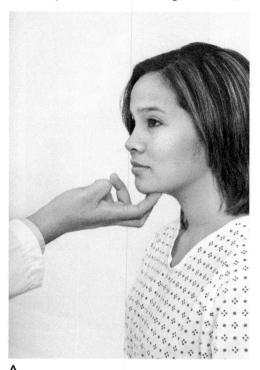

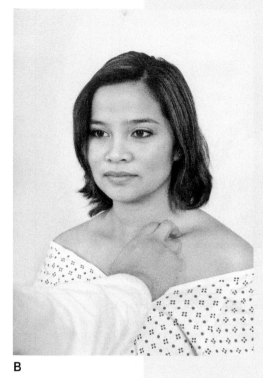

A   B

Figure 14.15 Palpating lymph nodes. A. Submental. B. Supraclavicular.

Abnormal Findings

Abnormal findings in the head and neck include headaches, abnormalities in the size and contour of the skull, malformations or abnormalities of the face and neck, and thyroid disorders. Table 14.3 provides an overview of skull and face abnormalities that are associated with common disorders. Headaches and thyroid disorders are discussed in the following sections.

Headaches

Headaches vary in terms of type and duration. Likewise, the cause of a headache, or its trigger, may vary among individuals. Especially with regard to migraine headaches, tyramine-rich foods are believed to be headache triggers (see Box 14.1). Certain food additives, including food coloring and nitrates, are believed to be potential headache triggers, as well.

TABLE 14.3   Abnormalities of the Head and Neck

Acromegaly

Enlargement of the bones, facial features, hands, and feet due to the increased production of growth hormone by the pituitary gland.

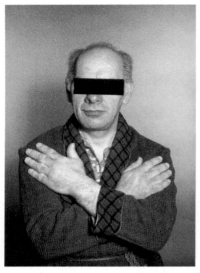

Figure 14.16   Acromegaly.
Source: John Radcliffe Hospital/Science Source.

Bell's Palsy

A sudden, temporary disorder affecting cranial nerve VII (Facial) that produces unilateral facial paralysis. It may be caused by a virus.

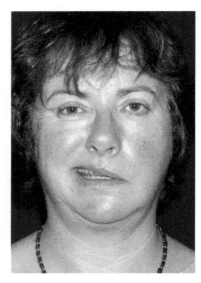

Figure 14.17   Bell's palsy.
Source: Dr. P. Marazzi/Science Source.

Cerebrovascular Accident (CVA, stroke, brain attack)

As with Bell's palsy, neurologic deficits associated with CVA can include facial paralysis. However, unlike Bell's palsy, neurologic effects of a CVA extend to other body regions, as well.

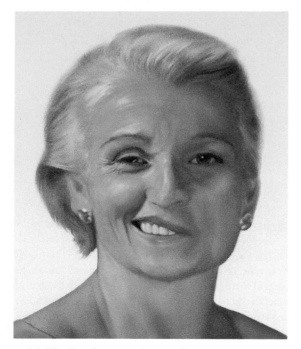

Figure 14.18   Cerebrovascular accident.

Craniosynostosis

Early closure of sagittal sutures causes the head to elongate; early closure of coronal sutures alters the head, face, and orbits.

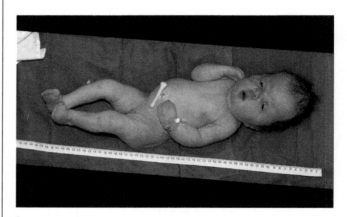

Figure 14.19   Craniosynostosis.
Source: Wellcome Image Library/Custom Medical Stock Photo.

TABLE 14.3	**Abnormalities of the Head and Neck** (continued)

Cushing's Syndrome

Increased cortisol production by the adrenal gland leads to a rounded "moon" face, ruddy cheeks, prominent jowls, and excess facial hair.

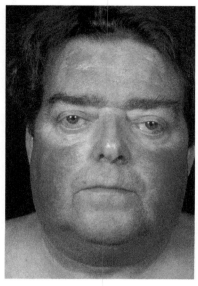

Figure 14.20 Cushing's syndrome.
Source: BioPhoto Associates/Getty Images.

Down Syndrome

A chromosomal defect causing varying degrees of intellectual disability and characteristic facial features such as slanted eyes; a flat nasal bridge; a flat nose; a protruding tongue; and a short, broad neck.

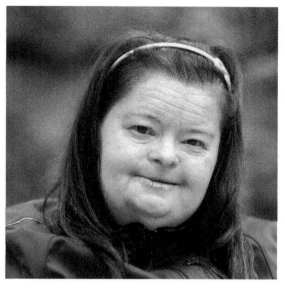

Figure 14.21 Down syndrome.
Source: Marcel Jancovic/Shutterstock.

Fetal Alcohol Syndrome (FAS)

A disorder characterized by epicanthal folds, narrow palpebral fissures, a deformed upper lip below the septum of the nose, and some degree of intellectual disability; caused by fetal exposure to high levels of alcohol.

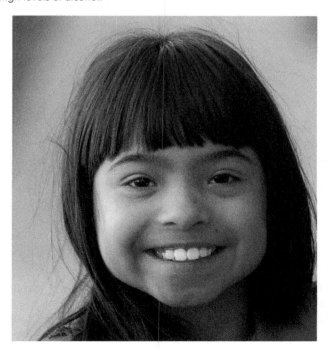

Figure 14.22 Fetal alcohol syndrome.
Source: Lyn Alweis/The Denver Post/Getty Images.

Hydrocephalus

Enlargement of the head caused by inadequate drainage of cerebrospinal fluid, resulting in abnormal growth of the skull.

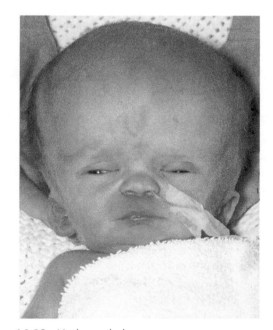

Figure 14.23 Hydrocephalus.
Source: M.A. Ansary/Custom Medical Stock Photo.

(continued)

| TABLE 14.3 | Abnormalities of the Head and Neck (continued) |

Parkinson's Disease

A masklike expression occurs in Parkinson's disease. The disease is the result of a decrease in the production of the neurotransmitter dopamine.

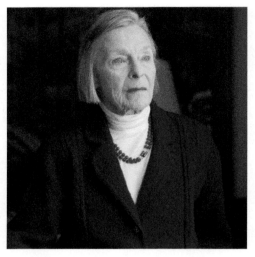

Figure 14.24 Parkinson's disease.
Source: Scott Houston/Corbis.

Torticollis

A spasm of the muscles supplied by the spinal accessory nerve, causing lateral flexion contracture of the cervical spine musculature. Caused by cervical problems such as trauma, tumors, or scars.

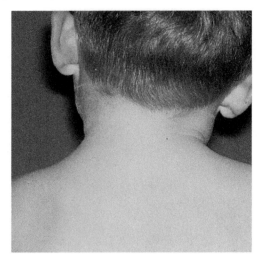

Figure 14.25 Torticollis.
Source: Wellcome Image Library/Custom Medical Stock Photo.

CLASSIC MIGRAINE

A classic migraine is usually preceded by an aura during which the patient may feel depressed, restless, or irritable; see spots or flashes of light; feel nauseated; or experience numbing or tingling in the face or extremities. The pain of the migraine itself may be mild or debilitating, requiring the patient to lie down in the darkness in silence. It is usually a pulsating pain that is localized to the side, front, or back of the head and may be accompanied by nausea, vertigo, tremors, and other symptoms. The acute phase of a classic migraine typically lasts from 4 to 6 hours.

CLUSTER HEADACHE

A cluster headache is so named because numerous episodes occur over a period of days or even months and then are followed by a period of remission during which no headaches occur. Cluster headaches have no aura. Their onset is sudden and may be associated with alcohol consumption, stress, or emotional distress. They often begin suddenly at night with an excruciating pain on one side of the face spreading upward behind one eye. The nose and affected eye water, and nasal congestion is common. Cluster headaches may last for only a few minutes or up to a few hours.

TENSION HEADACHE

A tension headache, also known as a muscle contraction headache, is due to sustained contraction of the muscles in the head, neck, or upper back. The onset is gradual, not sudden, and the pain is usually

| Box 14.1 | Tyramine-Rich Foods |

- Aged cheese, including Swiss, mozzarella, cheddar, and blue cheese
- Avocados
- Beer on tap
- Canned soup
- Cured meats
- Homemade yeast breads
- Nuts
- Olives
- Onions
- Raisins
- Red wine
- Sauerkraut
- Soy sauce

Sources: Mayo Clinic. (2013). *I just started taking MAOIs for depression. Do I really need to follow a low-tyramine diet?* Retrieved from http://www.mayoclinic.org/diseases-conditions/depression/expert-answers/maois/faq-20058035; Northwestern Memorial Hospital. (2008). *Low tyramine diet.* Retrieved from http://www.nmh.org/ccurl/504/151/Low-tyramine-diet-08.pdf; WebMD. (2012a). *Tyramine and migraines.* Retrieved from http://www.webmd.com/migraines-headaches/guide/tyramine-and-migraines; WebMD (2012b). *Frequently asked questions about food triggers, migraines, and headaches.* Retrieved from http://www.webmd.com/migraines-headaches/guide/triggers-specific-foods

steady, not throbbing. The pain may be unilateral or bilateral and typically ranges from the cervical region to the top of the head. Tension headaches may be associated with stress, overwork, position, dental problems, premenstrual syndrome, sinus inflammation, and other health problems.

Thyroid Abnormalities

Thyroid disorders may stem from various causes. The primary manifestations of a thyroid disorder depend on whether the thyroid is producing too much or too little thyroid hormones.

HYPERTHYROIDISM

Hyperthyroidism is excessive production of thyroid hormones.

Subjective findings:

- Irritability/nervousness.
- Muscle weakness and fatigue.
- Amenorrhea.
- Insomnia.
- Heat intolerance.

Objective findings:

- Thyroid gland enlargement.
- Exophthalmos (bulging eyes).
- Cardiac changes, including tachycardia (heart rate > 100 bpm) and cardiac dysrhythmias (abnormal heart rhythms).
- Integumentary changes, including skin thinning and fine, brittle hair.
- Weight loss.
- Increased diaphoresis (sweating).

HYPOTHYROIDISM

Hypothyroidism occurs when there is a decrease in production of thyroid hormones. The decrease in thyroid hormones results in lowered basal metabolism. The most common occurrence in hypothyroidism is loss of thyroid tissue as a result of iodine deficiency or an autoimmune response. It may be a result of decreased pituitary stimulation of the thyroid gland or lack of hypothalamic thyroid-releasing factor. Hypothyroidism occurs most frequently in females between the ages of 30 and 50.

Subjective findings:

- Weakness/feeling tired.
- Depression.
- Heavy menstrual periods.
- Difficulty concentrating.
- Cold intolerance.

Objective findings:

- Constipation.
- Integumentary changes, including dry skin and weak nails.
- Weight gain.
- Cool skin.

THYROID-RELATED DISORDERS

Manifestations of thyroid disorders vary depending on whether the disorder involves hypothyroidism or hyperthyroidism. Goiter, which is an enlargement of the thyroid gland, may be caused by increased (hyper) or decreased (hypo) thyroid function. An overview of other selected thyroid disorders is provided in Table 14.4.

TABLE 14.4 Overview of Selected Thyroid Disorders

CONDITION	DESCRIPTION
Graves' Disease	• Most common type of hyperthyroidism • No known cause; may be an autoimmune response or related to hereditary factors
Thyroid adenoma	• Benign thyroid nodules that occur most frequently in older adults • No known cause
Thyroid carcinoma	• Involves presence of malignant tumors in hormone-producing cells or supporting cells • Excess thyroid hormone is produced in the tumors • May occur following radiation of the thyroid, chronic goiter, or as a result of hereditary factors
Medication-induced hyperthyroidism	• Excessive iodine in some medications may cause oversecretion of thyroid hormones
Congenital hypothyroidism	• Thyroid is nonfunctioning at birth • Left untreated, results in retardation of physical and mental growth
Myxedema	• Severe form of hypothyroidism • Causes nonpitting edema throughout the body and thickening of facial features • Complications may adversely affect major organ systems • Myxedema coma results in cardiovascular collapse, electrolyte disturbances, respiratory depression, and cerebral hypoxia

(continued)

TABLE 14.4	**Overview of Selected Thyroid Disorders** (continued)
CONDITION	**DESCRIPTION**
Thyroiditis	• Inflammation of the thyroid gland • Inflammation may cause release of stored hormones, resulting in temporary hyperthyroidism that may last weeks or months • May manifest as hypothyroidism (American Thyroid Association, 2014)
Postpartum thyroiditis	• Temporary condition occurring in 5% to 9% of females postpartum • May manifest as temporary thyrotoxicosis (hyperthyroidism) followed by temporary hypothyroidism (American Thyroid Association, 2014)
Hashimoto's thyroiditis	• Autoimmune disease that results in primary hypothyroidism • Occurs most frequently in females • Tends to be familial

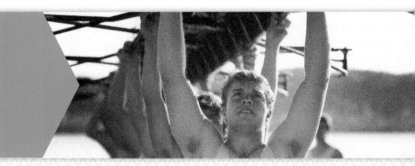

Application Through Critical Thinking

▶ Case Study

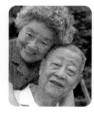

A married couple has come to the clinic for renewal of prescriptions and annual flu shots. During the encounter, the husband mentions to the nurse that he is concerned about his 69-year-old wife. He tells the nurse that she has become very forgetful. She eats very little but has seemed to gain weight. She seems "down" all the time. When questioned, the wife states she "just hasn't been herself." She admits she doesn't have much of an appetite. She explains that she has not been as active as she used to be and as a result her bowels are not as regular. She thinks those are the reasons she feels "out of sorts." She chides her husband that his memory "isn't so hot either." He insists that she is forgetting simple things while he has always forgotten to write down phone messages and birthdays and such.

The nurse is concerned about this patient and carries out a further interview, which reveals the following findings: The patient is generally cold, feels tired all of the time, and really doesn't have the energy to do much around the house. She finds the thought of going out exhausting. She tells the nurse that her tongue feels thick and she thinks her voice has changed.

The patient agrees to a physical examination. The findings include a weight gain of 10 lb from her last clinic visit, 6 months ago. Her thyroid is enlarged and palpable. Her skin is dry, she has edema of the lower extremities, and her speech is slow. Her abdomen is distended with bowel sounds in all quadrants.

The nurse recommends that this woman have laboratory testing for thyroid dysfunction and arranges for consultation with a physician. The nurse schedules a follow-up appointment and makes some recommendations for this patient that include increasing fluid intake and fiber to improve bowel function. The patient is advised to wear warm clothing and to rest frequently. The nurse explains the functions of the thyroid and that medication can improve all aspects of her current condition when taken regularly.

▶ Complete Documentation

The following information is summarized from the case study.

SUBJECTIVE DATA: "Just haven't been myself." Loss of appetite, decreased activity, irregular bowel function. Generally cold, tired, lack of energy, thick tongue, and change in voice. Husband states that wife is forgetful, eats very little, has gained weight, and seems "down."

OBJECTIVE DATA: BP 120/76—P 64—T 98.4. Alert and oriented. Unable to repeat list of five words after 5 minutes. Weight gain 10 lb over 6 months. Thyroid enlarged and palpable. Skin cool, dry, edema lower extremities. Slow speech. Abdomen distended. Bowel sounds present all quadrants.

A sample assessment form appears below.

▶ Critical Thinking Questions

1. What may be responsible for the findings about this 69-year-old female?

2. What further data should the nurse collect?

3. What aspects of physical assessment and what tests are important in arriving at a diagnosis for this patient?

4. How could you determine if depression was causing the symptoms of "feeling down" and lack of energy?

5. How would you approach the situation if the patient and her husband are Muslims and she is required to keep her head covered?

▶ Prepare Teaching Plan

LEARNING NEED: The case study includes subjective and objective data indicative of a thyroid dysfunction. The nurse provides for diagnostic studies, follows up with a physician, and provides information about the thyroid gland and medication as treatment for the problem. The nurse's actions are based on the determination that the patient needs suggestions to ease her current symptoms and that information will reassure her and assist her in decision making about the diagnosis and treatment of her problem.

The patient is representative of a population at risk for hypothyroidism; that is, female and over 50 years of age. Aging individuals could benefit from education about hypothyroidism. The following teaching plan is intended to provide information about hypothyroidism for a group of learners.

GOAL: The participants will acquire information of value in promotion of thyroid health.

OBJECTIVES: Upon completion of the learning session, the participants will be able to:

1. Discuss thyroid function.

2. Describe hypothyroidism.

3. List symptoms of hypothyroidism.

4. Identify diagnostic tests for hypothyroidism.

5. Discuss treatment for hypothyroidism.

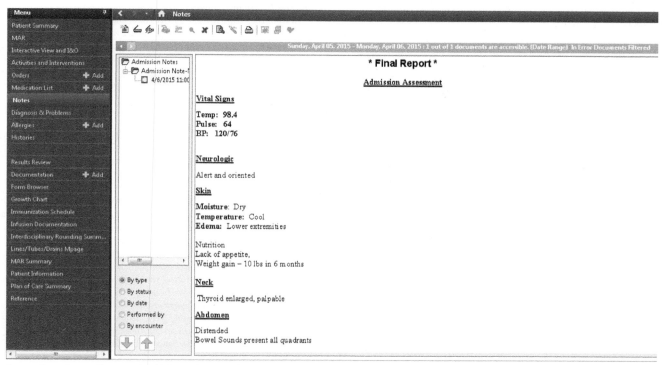

Source: From Cerner Electronic Health Record. Copyright © by Cerner Corporation. Used by permission of Cerner Corporation.

Following is an example of the teaching plan for Objective 2.

APPLICATION OF OBJECTIVE 2: Describe hypothyroidism

Content	Teaching Strategy	Evaluation
• Hypothyroidism occurs when the thyroid does not produce enough of the thyroid hormones.	• Lecture	• Written examination.
• Hypothyroidism can occur as a result of inflammation of the thyroid leading to failure of parts of the gland.	• Discussion	May use short answer, fill-in, or multiple-choice items or a combination of items.
• Hashimoto's disease is an autoimmune disease that leads to thyroid failure. The immune system attacks the thyroid.	• Printed materials	If these are short and easy to evaluate, the learner receives immediate feedback.
• Other causes include surgical removal of part of the gland, irradiation of the gland, or other inflammatory processes.	Lecture is appropriate when disseminating information to large groups.	
• Hypothyroidism occurs more frequently in females and after 50 years of age.	Discussion allows participants to bring up concerns and to raise questions.	
• Risk factors include obesity, x-ray exposure in the neck area, or radiation treatment of the thyroid.	Printed material, especially to be taken away with learners, allows review, reinforcement, and reading at the learner's pace.	

▶ References

American Cancer Society (ACS). (2013). *Cancer—unknown primary.* Retrieved from http://www.cancer.org/cancer/cancerofunknownprimary/detailedguide/cancer-unknown-primary-diagnosed

American Thyroid Association. (2014). *What is thyroiditis?* Retrieved from http://www.thyroid.org/what-is-thyroiditis/

Berman, A., & Snyder, S. J. (2012). *Kozier and Erb's fundamentals of nursing: Concepts, process, and practice* (9th ed.). Upper Saddle River, NJ: Prentice Hall.

Bikley, L. S. (2012). *Bates' guide to physical examination and history taking* (11th ed.). Philadelphia: Lippincott.

Centers for Disease Control and Prevention (CDC). (2013a). *Skin cancer—what are the symptoms?* Retrieved from http://www.cdc.gov/cancer/skin/basic_info/symptoms.htm

Centers for Disease Control and Prevention (CDC). (2013b). *Workplace safety & health topics: Indoor environmental quality.* Retrieved from http://www.cdc.gov/niosh/topics/indoorenv/chemicalsodors.html

Centers for Disease Control and Prevention (CDC). (2014). *Meningitis: Viral meningitis.* Retrieved from http://www.cdc.gov/meningitis/viral.html

Chiocca, E. M. (2011). *Advanced pediatric assessment.* Philadelphia, PA: Lippincott Williams & Wilkins.

Gaitonde, D. Y., Rowley, K. D., & Sweeney, L. B. (2012). Hypothyroidism: An update. *American Family Physician, 86*(3), 244–251.

Goldberg, E. M. (2013). Fever and bulging fontanelle mimicking meningitis in an infant diagnosed with benign intracranial hypertension. *Pediatric Emergency Care, 29*(4), 513–514.

Kurlander, D. E., Punjabi, A., Liu, M. T., Sattar, A., & Guyuron, B. (2014). In-depth review of symptoms, triggers, and treatment of temporal migraine headaches (Site II). *Plastic and Reconstructive Surgery, 133*(4), 897–903.

Marieb, E. (2009). *Essentials of human anatomy and physiology* (9th ed.). San Francisco: Benjamin/Cummings.

Mayo Clinic. (2013). *I just started taking MAOIs for depression. Do I really need to follow a low-tyramine diet?* Retrieved from http://www.mayoclinic.org/diseases-conditions/depression/expert-answers/maois/faq-20058035

Mayo Clinic. (2013). *Tests and procedures: Sed rate (erythrocyte sedimentation rate).* Retrieved from http://www.mayoclinic.org/tests-procedures/sed-rate/basics/results/prc-20013502

Mayo Foundation for Medical Education and Research. (2014). *Rochester test catalog: 2014 online test catalog.* Available at http://www.mayomedicallaboratories.com/tests-catalog

MedlinePlus. (2013a). *Newborn screening tests.* Retrieved from http://www.nlm.nih.gov/medlineplus/ency/article/007257.htm

MedlinePlus. (2013b). *Blood differential.* Retrieved from http://www.nlm.nih.gov

Meyer, K. D., & Zhang, L. (2009). Short- and long-term adverse effects of cocaine abuse during pregnancy on the heart development. *Therapeutic Advances in Cardiovascular Disease, 3*(1), 7–16.

Mony, K. (2008). *General etiquette in Cambodian society.* Retrieved from http://ethnomed.org/culture/cambodian/general-etiquette-in-cambodian-society/?searchterm=touching%20the%20head

Northwestern Memorial Hospital. (2008). *Low tyramine diet.* Retrieved from http://www.nmh.org/ccurl/504/151/Low-tyramine-diet-08.pdf

Osborn K. S., Wraa, C. E., Watson, A., & Holleran, R. S. (2013). *Medical-surgical nursing: Preparation for practice* (2nd ed.). Upper Saddle River, NJ: Pearson.

Owens, C. W. (2007). *Hmong cultural profile.* Retrieved from http://ethnomed.org/culture/hmong/hmong-cultural-profile

Pagana, K.D. (2013). *Mosby's manual of diagnostic and laboratory tests.* (5th ed.). St. Louis, MO: Elsevier.

Ricci, S. S., Kyle, T., & Carman, S. (2012). *Maternal and pediatric nursing* (2nd ed.). Philadelphia, PA: Lippincott Williams & Wilkins.

Ron, E., Lubin, J. H., Shore, R. E., Mabuchi, K., Modan, B., Pottern, L. M., . . . Boice, Jr., J. D. (2012). Thyroid cancer after exposure to external radiation: A pooled analysis of seven studies. *Radiation Research, 178*(2), AV43–AV60.

Sharma, M., Aronow, W. S., Patel, L., Gandhi, K., & Desai, H. (2011). Hyperthyroidism. *Medical Science Monitor, 17*(4), RA85–RA91.

Stagnaro-Green, A., Abalovich, M., Alexander, E., Azizi, F., Mestman, J., Negro, R., . . . Wiersinga, W. (2011). Guidelines of the American Thyroid Association for the diagnosis and management of thyroid disease during pregnancy and postpartum. *Thyroid, 21*(10), 1081–1125.

University of Maryland Medical Center. (2013). *Hypothyroidism.* Retrieved from http://umm.edu/health/medical/reports/articles/hypothyroidism

U.S. Department of Health and Human Services (USDHHS). (2014). *Healthy people 2020.* Retrieved from http://www.healthypeople.gov/2020/default.aspx

WebMD. (2012a). *Tyramine and migraines.* Retrieved from http://www.webmd.com/migraines-headaches/guide/tyramine-and-migraines

WebMD. (2012b). *Frequently asked questions about food triggers, migraines, and headaches.* Retrieved from http://www.webmd.com/migraines-headaches/guide/triggers-specific-foods

Welch, K. A. (2011). Neurological complications of alcohol and misuse of drugs. *Practical Neurology, 11,* 206–219.

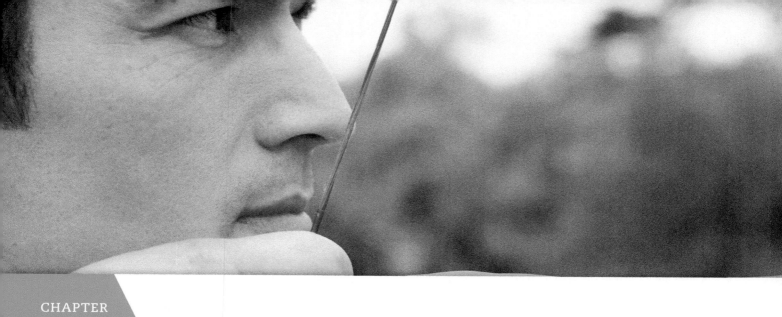

15 ❯ Eye

❯ Learning Outcomes

Upon completion of this chapter, you will be able to:

1. Describe the anatomy and physiology of the eye.

2. Develop questions to be used when completing the focused interview.

3. Outline the techniques used for assessment of the eye.

4. Explain patient preparation for assessment of the eye.

5. Explain the use of the ophthalmoscope.

6. Differentiate normal from abnormal findings in physical assessment of the eye.

7. Describe developmental, psychosocial, cultural, and environmental variations in assessment techniques and findings of the eye.

8. Discuss the objectives related to overall health of the eyes and vision as presented in *Healthy People 2020*.

9. Apply critical thinking to the physical assessment of the eye.

Key Terms

accommodation, 312
aqueous humor, 291
arcus senilis, 295
astigmatism, 323
blepharitis, 316
cataract, 295
choroid, 290
consensual constriction, 311
convergence, 312
cornea, 290
ectropion, 317
emmetropia, 291
entropion, 317
esophoria, 324
exophoria, 325
fundus, 312
hyperopia, 291
iris, 290
iritis, 318
lens, 291
macula, 291
miosis, 290
mydriasis, 290

The eyes are located in the orbital cavities of the skull. Only the anterior aspect of the eye is exposed. The eyes are the sensory organs responsible for vision. Vision affects how an individual interacts and communicates with the world, including while learning, working, and playing (U.S. Department of Health and Human Services [USDHHS], 2013). Therefore, *Healthy People 2020* objectives have been created to improve visual health through prevention, early diagnosis, prompt treatment, and rehabilitation as described later in this chapter.

Anatomy and Physiology Review

The eye is the structure through which light is gathered to produce vision. Layers and membranes serve several purposes. The accessory structures of the eye provide protection and are responsible for movement of the eye. Each anatomic structure is described in the following section.

Eye

The eye, commonly called the eyeball, is a fluid-filled sphere having a diameter of approximately 2.5 cm (1 in.). The eye receives light waves and transmits these waves to the brain for interpretation as visual images. Only a small portion of the eye is seen. Most of the eye is set into and protected by the bony orbit of the skull (see Figure 15.1 ■).

The eye is composed of three layers: the sclera, the choroids, and the retina. The **sclera**, the outermost layer, is an extremely dense, hard, fibrous membrane that helps to maintain the shape of the eye. It is the white fibrous part of the eye that is seen anteriorly. Its primary function is to support and protect the structures of the eye (see Figure 15.2 ■).

The **cornea** is the clear, transparent part of the sclera and forms the anterior one sixth of the eye. It is considered to be the window of the eye, allowing light to enter. The extensive nerve endings in the cornea are responsible for the blink reflex, an increase in the secretion of tears for protection, and are most sensitive to pain.

The **choroid**, the middle layer, is the vascular-pigmented layer of the eye. The **iris** is the circular, colored, muscular aspect of this layer of the eye and is located in the anterior portion of the eye. In the center of the iris is an opening called the **pupil**, which allows light to travel inside the eye. The iris responds to light by making the pupil larger or smaller, thereby controlling the amount of light that enters the eye. A dim light will cause the iris to respond, enlarging the pupil size (**mydriasis**). This increases the amount of light entering the eye, enhancing distant vision. A bright light causes the iris to respond by decreasing pupil size (**miosis**), thus decreasing the amount of light entering the eye, accommodating near vision. The third cranial nerve controls pupillary constriction and dilation. The parasympathetic branch of this nerve stimulates pupillary constriction while the sympathetic branch stimulates dilation of the pupil.

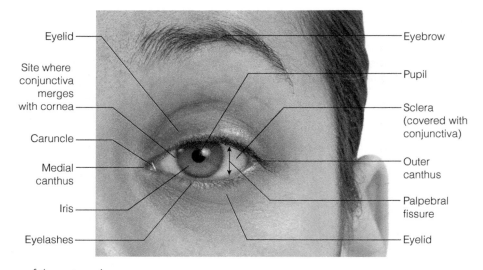

Figure 15.1 Structures of the external eye.

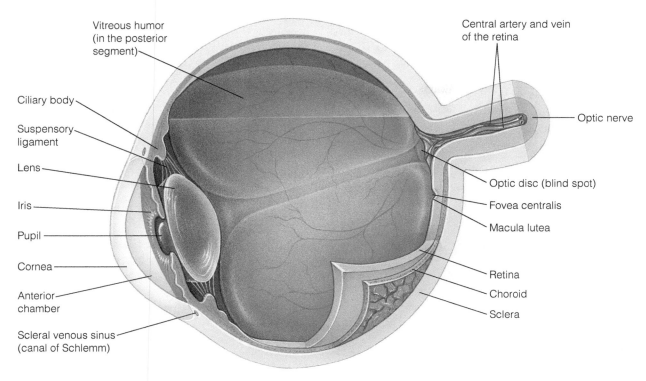

Vitreous humor
(in the posterior
segment)

Central artery and vein
of the retina

Ciliary body

Suspensory
ligament

Lens

Iris

Pupil

Cornea

Anterior
chamber

Scleral venous sinus
(canal of Schlemm)

Optic nerve

Optic disc (blind spot)

Fovea centralis

Macula lutea

Retina

Choroid

Sclera

Figure 15.2 Interior of the eye.

The third and innermost membrane, the **retina,** is the sensory portion of the eye. The retina, a direct extension of the optic nerve, helps to change light waves to neuroimpulses for interpretation as visual impulses by the brain. The retina contains many rods and cones. The rods function in dim light and are also considered to be peripheral vision receptors. The cones function in bright light, are central vision receptors, and provide color to sight.

The **optic disc,** on the nasal aspect of the retina, is round with clear margins. It is usually creamy yellow and is the point at which the optic nerve and retina meet. The color of the disc and the retinal background differ according to skin color. The color is lighter in persons with light skin and darker in individuals with darker skin color. The center of this disc, the physiologic cup, is the point at which the vascular network enters the eye.

The **macula** is responsible for central vision. The macula, with its yellow, pitlike center called the *fovea centralis,* appears as a hyperpigmented spot on the temporal aspect of the retina.

Refraction of the Eye

Light rays travel in a straight line. For vision to occur, light rays must be reflected off an object, and then transmitted through the cornea. The cornea refracts (bends) the light rays, directing them to pass through the pupil and into the eye. As light travels through the eye, each structure in its pathway has a different density. Several structures of the eye help with the deflection or refraction of the light rays. The structures responsible for refraction include the cornea, aqueous humor, crystalline lens, and vitreous humor.

Refraction allows the light rays to enter the eye and be aimed (reflected) to the correct part of the retina for most accurate vision. **Emmetropia** is the normal refractive condition of the eye. **Myopia**

(nearsightedness) is a condition in which the light rays focus in front of the retina. In **hyperopia** (farsightedness) the light rays focus behind the retina.

The **aqueous humor** is a clear, fluidlike substance found in the anterior segment of the eye that helps maintain ocular pressure. The aqueous humor is a refractory medium of the eye that is constantly being formed and is always flowing through the pupil and draining into the venous system. The **vitreous humor,** another refractory medium, is a clear gel located in the posterior segment of the eye. This gel helps maintain the intraocular pressure and the shape of the eye, and transmits light rays through the eye.

The **lens,** situated directly behind the pupil, is a biconvex (convex on both surfaces), transparent, and flexible structure. It separates the anterior and posterior segments of the eye. The ability of the lens to accommodate or change its shape permits light to focus properly on the retina and enhances fine focusing of images.

Visual Pathways

An object external to the body is perceived by the eye to create an image. Via light waves, this image is transported to the brain for interpretation as vision. Light waves must bend to focus correctly on the retina. The refractory structures—the cornea, aqueous humor, anterior and posterior chambers, lens, and vitreous humor—help bend the light waves onto the retina. This retinal image, via the nerve fibers, is conducted to the optic nerve (cranial nerve II). At the optic chiasm, the optic fibers of the nerves cross over and join the temporal fibers from the opposite eye. Optic tracts encircle the brain and the impulse is transmitted to the occipital lobe of the brain for interpretation (see Figure 15.3 ■).

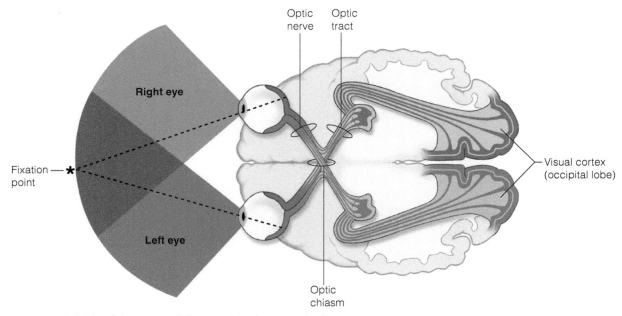

Figure 15.3 Visual fields of the eye and the visual pathway to the brain.

Accessory Structures of the Eye

The eye has several external accessory structures. The eyebrows are the coarse short hairs that are located on the lower portion of the forehead at the orbital margins. The primary function of the eyebrow is to protect the eye (see Figure 15.1).

The eyelids, or **palpebrae**, are the movable folds of skin that cover and protect the eyes. The opening between the upper and lower eyelids is called the **palpebral fissure**. The eyelids meet medially and laterally to form the medial canthus and the outer canthus. The meibomian glands, embedded in the eyelids, are modified sebaceous glands that produce an oily substance to help lubricate the eyes and eyelids. The eyelashes are hairs that project from

the eyelids and curl outward. The high supply of nerve fibers helps support the blink reflex, thereby protecting the eye.

The conjunctiva, a thin mucous membrane, lines the interior of the eyelids and continues over the anterior portion of the eye, meeting the cornea but not covering it. The conjunctiva protects the eye by preventing foreign objects from entering the eye. The conjunctiva also produces a lubricating fluid that prevents the eyes from drying.

The lacrimal apparatus consists of the lacrimal glands and ducts. Lacrimal secretions, commonly called tears, are secreted and spread over the conjunctiva when blinking. The tears enter the lacrimal puncta and drain via the many ducts into the posterior nasal passage (see Figure 15.4 ■).

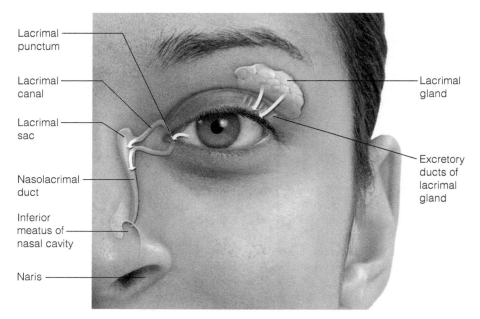

Figure 15.4 Lacrimal glands of the eye.

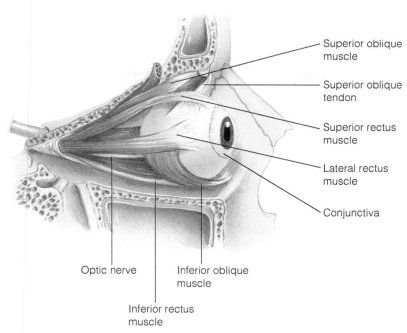

Figure 15.5 Extraocular muscles.

Each eye has six extrinsic or extraocular muscles. They help hold the eye in place within the bony orbit. These muscles are the lateral rectus, medial rectus, superior rectus, inferior rectus, inferior oblique, and superior oblique (see Figure 15.5 ■). With the coordination of these muscles, the individual experiences one image sight. These muscles are innervated by cranial nerves III, IV, and VI. Figure 15.6 ■ on page 294 depicts the correlation of eye movement with eye muscles and cranial nerves.

Special Considerations

Throughout the assessment process, the nurse gathers subjective and objective data reflecting the patient's state of health. Using critical thinking and the nursing process, the nurse identifies many factors to be considered when collecting the data. Vision and eye health are influenced by a number of factors, including age, developmental level, race, ethnicity, occupation, socioeconomics, and emotional well-being. The nurse must consider these factors when gathering subjective and objective data during a comprehensive health assessment.

Health Promotion Considerations

While vision is essential to overall health, the eyes often are overlooked during health assessment (USDHHS, 2013). Goals of *Healthy People 2020* related to vision and eye health include prevention of eye diseases, disorders, and injuries. For individuals who experience eye disorders and vision impairment, *Healthy People 2020* goals include early detection, prompt treatment, and rehabilitation (USDHHS, 2013). See Table 15.1 for examples of *Healthy People 2020* objectives that are designed to promote eye health and preservation of vision among individuals across the life span.

TABLE 15.1	Examples of *Healthy People 2020* Objectives Related to Eye Health
OBJECTIVE NUMBER	**DESCRIPTION**
V-1	Increase the proportion of preschool children aged 5 years and under who receive vision screening
V-2	Reduce blindness and visual impairment in children and adolescents aged 17 years and under
V-3	Reduce occupational eye injuries
V-4	Increase the proportion of adults who have a comprehensive eye examination, including dilation, within the past 2 years
V-5	Reduce visual impairment
V-6	Increase the use of personal protective eyewear in recreational activities and hazardous situations around the home
V-7	Increase vision rehabilitation
V-8	(Developmental) Increase the proportion of Federally Qualified Health Centers (FQHCs) that provide comprehensive vision health services

Source: U.S. Department of Health and Human Services (USDHHS). (2014). *Healthy People 2020.* Retrieved from http://www.healthypeople.gov/2020/default.aspx

Right Eye	Eye Movements	Left Eye

Inferior oblique muscle Cranial nerve III	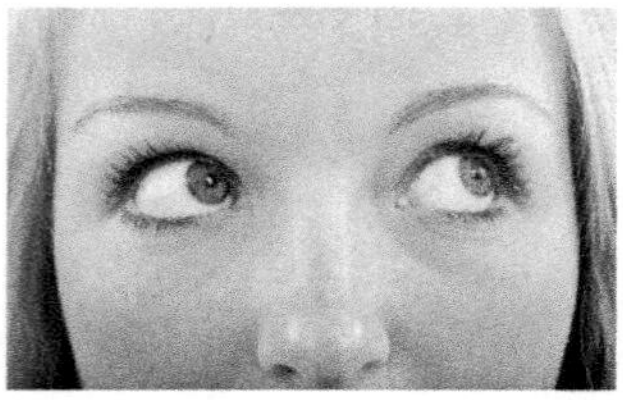	Superior rectus muscle Cranial nerve III
Medial rectus muscle Cranial nerve III	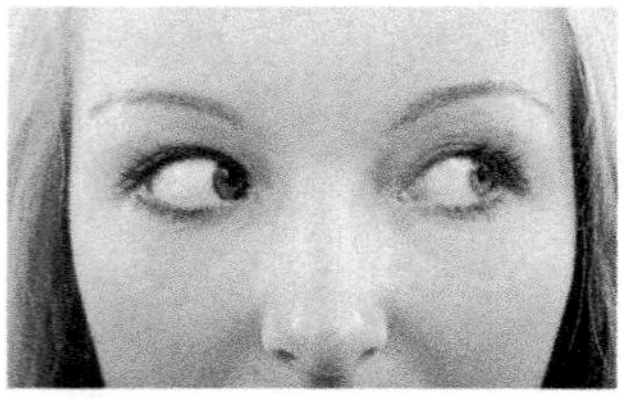	Lateral rectus muscle Cranial nerve VI
Superior oblique muscle Cranial nerve IV	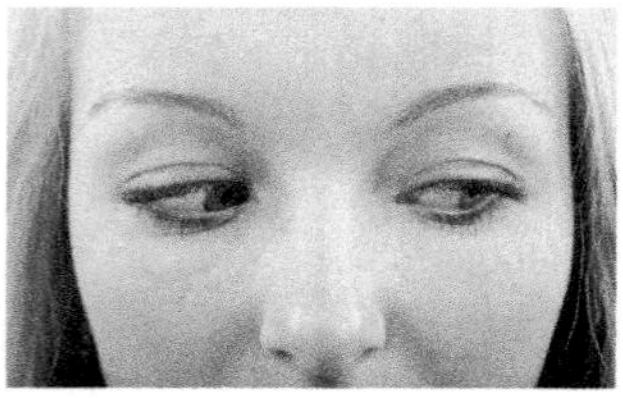	Inferior rectus muscle Cranial nerve III
Superior rectus muscle Cranial nerve III	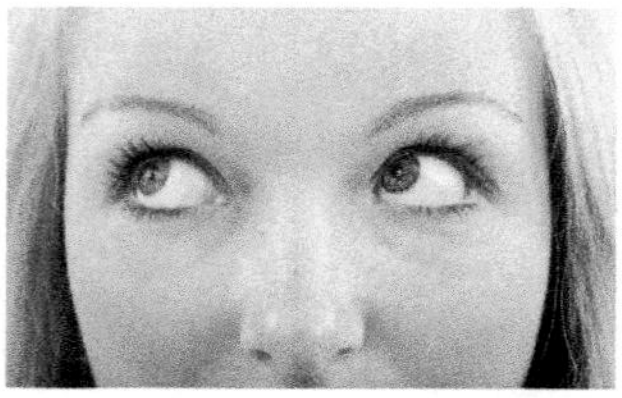	Inferior oblique muscle Cranial nerve III
Lateral rectus muscle Cranial nerve III	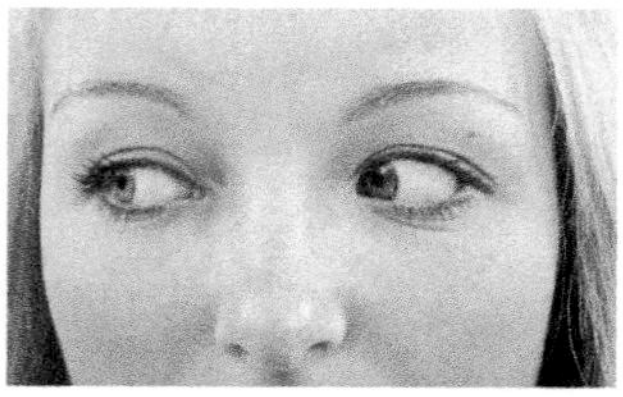	Medial rectus muscle Cranial nerve III
Inferior rectus muscle Cranial nerve III	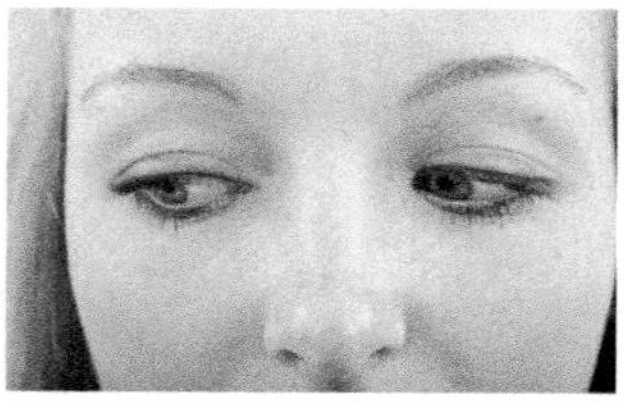	Superior oblique muscle Cranial nerve IV

Figure 15.6 Eye movements with muscle and nerve coordination.

Lifespan Considerations

Comprehensive health assessment includes interpretation of findings in relation to normative values. The following sections describe normal variations in structures and functions of the eye for different age groups.

Infants and Children

Babies can see at birth, but the visual acuity of newborns is not as sharp as adults. Children typically have 20/20 vision by the age of 7 years. At birth, the eyes of the neonate should be symmetric. The pupils are equal and respond to light. The iris is generally brown in dark-skinned neonates, and slate gray-blue in light-skinned neonates. By about the third month of age, the color of the eyes begins to change to a more permanent shade. Many times the eyelids are edematous at birth. Little to no tears are present at birth but begin to appear by the fourth week. Binocular vision (vision in both eyes) begins to develop by 6 weeks of age. Before this time, neonates will fixate on a bright or moving object. An infant who cannot focus on objects at birth needs further evaluation.

The eyes reach adult size by 8 years of age. The *red reflex,* a glowing red color that fills the pupil as light from the ophthalmoscope reflects off the retina, should be elicited from birth. A whitened red reflex occurs with congenital cataracts. Infants and preschool children with the cancer retinoblastoma often present a history of a diminished red reflex or a "white glow" in the pupil.

Peripheral vision may be assessed by confrontation in children older than 3 years of age. It is important to assess extraocular muscle function as early as possible in young children because delay can lead to permanent visual damage. The corneal light reflex, Hirschberg's test, can be used to determine symmetry of muscle function. Lateral deviations of the eye (disconjugate gaze) are normal findings until 2 months of age (Medscape, 2012a).

The Pregnant Female

The pregnant female may complain of dry eyes and may discontinue wearing contact lenses during her pregnancy. The pregnant patient may also describe visual changes due to shifting fluid in the cornea. These symptoms are usually not significant and disappear after childbirth. Changes in eyesight, such as refraction changes requiring a new prescription for glasses or contact lenses, blurriness, or distorted vision, can occur because of temporary changes in the shape of the eye during the last trimester of pregnancy and the first 6 weeks postpartum.

The Older Adult

Several alterations are associated with normal aging and are not related to vision or eye problems. **Xanthelasma** are soft, yellow plaques on the lids at the inner canthus. These plaques are sometimes associated with cholesterolemia but usually have no pathologic significance because they appear on persons with normal cholesterol counts. **Pingueculae** are yellowish nodules that are thickened areas of the bulbar conjunctiva caused by prolonged exposure to sun, wind, and dust. They may be on either side of the pupil and cause no problems. However, they must be differentiated from **pterygium**, opacity of the bulbar conjunctiva that can grow over the cornea and block vision.

By age 45, the lens of the eye loses elasticity, and the ciliary muscles become weaker, resulting in a decreased ability of the lens to change shape to accommodate for near vision. This condition is called **presbyopia**. The loss of fat from the orbit of the eye produces a drooping appearance. The lacrimal glands decrease tear production, and the patient may complain of a burning sensation in the eyes. The cornea of the eye may appear cloudy, and the nurse may detect a light gray or white ring surrounding the iris at the corneal margin due to the deposition of lipids. This common finding, known as **arcus senilis**, does not affect vision. The pupillary light reflex is slower with age, and the pupils may be smaller in size.

Within the eye, the blood vessels are paler in color, and the nurse may detect small, round, yellow dots scattered on the retina. These yellow dots do not interfere with vision. As the patient ages, the lens continues to thicken and yellow, forming a dense area that reduces lens clarity. This condition is the beginning of a **cataract** formation. Macular degeneration can occur in the older patient, resulting in a loss of central vision. The ophthalmoscopic examination may reveal narrowed blood vessels with a granular pigment in the macula.

Psychosocial Considerations

Decreased visual acuity and visual impairment can impact individuals across the age span. Visually impaired children may have developmental delays and may require special assistive social and educational services into adulthood. Adults with visual impairments may lose some personal independence, may experience decreased quality of life, and may find it difficult to obtain or maintain employment. Visual impairment results in stress for individuals and families as they adapt to alterations in activities of daily living (ADLs) and as they navigate the healthcare and social service systems for diagnosis, treatment, and assistance.

Eye contact with other people varies, especially during the communication process. Age, gender, and culture influence the type and amount of eye contact people make with others.

Cultural and Environmental Considerations

Cultural factors affect physical appearance of the eyes and their structures. For example, Asian patients have prominent epicanthic folds (a vertical fold of skin) covering the inner canthus of the eye. Dark-skinned individuals may have dark pigmented spots on the sclera, and their retinae may appear darker. People with light-colored eyes typically have lighter retinae and better night vision but are more sensitive to bright sunlight and artificial light.

Cultural factors also influence the incidence and prevalence of eye-related disorders. For example, among older adults, age-related macular degeneration occurs more frequently among Caucasians than in other groups (Lim, Mitchell, Seddon, Holz, & Wong, 2012). Among African Americans, cataracts are the leading cause of blindness, followed by glaucoma (Glaucoma Research Foundation, 2013). Glaucoma is approximately five times more common among African Americans than in individuals of other cultural backgrounds (Glaucoma Research Foundation, 2013). Excessive sun exposure without the use of sunglasses may promote cataract formation (World Health Organization [WHO], n.d.). A deficiency of vitamin A in the diet may cause night blindness (Gilbert, 2013). Some medications have side effects that may cause excessive corneal dryness, vision changes, or increased intraocular pressure (Wilson, Shannon, & Shields, 2013). When assessing a patient who wears contact lenses, it is important to determine what type of contact lens is worn (hard versus soft, extended wear versus daily change) and evaluate the patient's cleansing routine (WebMD, 2012a). Makeup and applicators should be discarded after 3 months and, to reduce the risk of infection, makeup should not be shared (University of Iowa, 2014). Trauma or damage to the eye can occur in work, recreational, and social environments. Safety glasses or protective goggles are recommended when the eye is at risk. For example, protective eyewear is used in carpentry, welding, chemical laboratories, and in many healthcare fields to prevent debris or splashes from entering the eye.

Gathering the Data

Health assessment of the eye includes the gathering of subjective and objective data. The subjective data are collected during the interview in which the professional nurse uses a variety of communication techniques to elicit general and specific information about the health of the eye. Health records combine subjective and objective data. The results of laboratory tests and radiologic studies are important secondary sources of objective data. Physical assessment of the eye, during which objective data are collected, includes the technique of inspection, the application of specific tests of vision and structures of the eye, and the use of the ophthalmoscope to assess the inner eye. See Table 15.2 for information on potential secondary sources of patient data.

Focused Interview

The focused interview for assessment of the eye concerns data related to the structures of the internal and external eye and those data concerned with vision. The nurse will observe the patient and listen for cues that relate to the status and function of the eye. The nurse may use open-ended and closed questions to obtain information. Follow-up questions or requests for descriptions are required to clarify data or to supply missing information. Follow-up questions are used to identify the source of problems, duration of difficulties, measures to alleviate problems, and cues about the patient's knowledge of his or her own health and health practices.

The focused interview guides the physical assessment of the eye. The information obtained is considered in relation to norms and expectations about the function of the eye and structures of the eye. Therefore, the nurse must consider age, gender, race, culture, environment, health practices, past and current problems, and therapies when framing questions and using techniques to elicit information. Remember, the subjective data collected and the questions asked during the health history and focused interview will provide data to

TABLE 15.2	Potential Secondary Sources for Patient Data Related to the Eye

Diagnostic Testing

Automated Perimetry Examination

Electroretinography

Fluorescein Angiography

Fluorescein Eye Stain

Refraction Test

Retinal Imaging

Tonometry (Intraocular Pressure [IOP] Measurement)—Normal Range 12 to 22 mmHg

Ultrasonography of the Eye and Orbit

help meet the objectives related to promoting visual acuity as stated in *Healthy People 2020*. In order to address all of the factors, categories of questions related to status and functions of the eye have been developed. These categories include general questions that are asked of all patients; those addressing illness and infection; questions related to symptoms, pain, and behaviors; those related to habits or practices; questions that are specific to patients according to age and for the pregnant female; and questions to address environmental concerns. One method to elicit information about symptoms is the OLDCART & ICE method, described in chapter 7.

The nurse must consider the patient's ability to participate in the focused interview and physical assessment of the eye. The ability to communicate is essential to the focused interview. If language barriers exist, a translator must be used. If the patient is experiencing discomfort or anxiety, efforts to address those problems have priority over other aspects of health assessment.

Focused Interview Questions	Rationales and Evidence

The following section provides sample questions and bulleted follow-up questions in each of the previously mentioned categories. A rationale for each of the questions is provided. The list of questions is not all-inclusive

but rather represents the types of questions required in a comprehensive focused interview related to the eye.

General Questions

1. **Describe your vision today.**

▶ Open-ended discussion provides an opportunity for patients to describe their own perceptions about vision.

Focused Interview Questions	Rationales and Evidence

2. **What was the date of your last eye examination? What were the results of that examination? Have you had any vision changes or problems in the past few months? If so, please describe your vision problems.**
   - What medications were prescribed or measures taken to relieve the problem?
   - Have the medications or measures been effective in relieving the problem?
   - Has the problem affected your activities of daily living?

▶ These questions provide specific information about healthcare practices and identify any known visual problems.

Follow-up questions would be required when a problem with vision or with the structures of the eye has been identified as a result of an eye examination.

3. **Do you wear glasses or contact lenses?**
   - How long have you used glasses or contact lenses?
   - Describe your vision with and without the use of glasses or contact lenses.

▶ These questions elicit information about vision correction and the effectiveness of the correction.

4. **Have you or any member of your family been diagnosed with hypertension, diabetes, or glaucoma?**

▶ This question may reveal information about diseases associated with genetic or familial predisposition. Each of the diseases mentioned can lead to vision problems. Hypertension can cause arteriosclerosis of the retina. Diabetes can cause bleeding in the capillaries of the retina (Grosso, Cheung, Veglio, & Wong, 2011).

Questions Related to Illness or Infection

1. **Have you ever been diagnosed with a disease of the eye?**
   - When were you diagnosed with the problem?
   - What treatment was prescribed for the problem?
   - Was the treatment helpful?
   - Describe things you have done or currently do to cope with this problem.
   - Has the problem ever recurred (acute)?
   - How are you managing the disease now (chronic)?

▶ The patient has an opportunity to provide information about a specific eye disease or problem. If a diagnosed illness is identified, follow-up is required about the date of diagnosis, treatment, and outcomes. Data about each illness identified by the patient are essential to an accurate health assessment. Illnesses can be classified as acute or chronic, and follow-up about each classification will differ.

2. **An alternative to question 1 is to list possible eye diseases, such as glaucoma, cataracts, corneal injury, Horner's syndrome, and exophthalmos, and ask the patient to respond "yes" or "no" as each is stated.**

▶ This is a comprehensive and efficient way to elicit information about all eye-related diseases. Follow-up would be carried out for each identified diagnosis as in question 1.

3. **Do you now have or have you had an infection of the eye?**

▶ If an infection is identified, follow-up about the date of the infection, treatment, and outcomes is required. Data about each infection identified by the patient are essential to an accurate health assessment. Infections can be classified as acute or chronic, and follow-up about each classification will differ.

4. **An alternative to question 3 is to list possible eye infections, such as conjunctivitis, iritis, uveitis, blepharitis, dacryocystitis, stye (hordeolum), and episcleritis, and ask the patient to respond "yes" or "no" as each is stated.**

▶ This is a comprehensive and efficient way to elicit information about all eye infections. Follow-up would be carried out for each identified infection as in question 3.

5. **Have you had an injury to the eye?**

6. **Have you had eye surgery?**

▶ Questions 5 and 6 require follow-up regarding the type of injury or surgery, the causes and treatments, and the adaptations the individual has made to overcome visual or other deficits as a result of the injury or surgery.

Focused Interview Questions	Rationales and Evidence

Questions Related to Symptoms, Pain, and Behaviors

When gathering information about symptoms, many questions are required to elicit details and descriptions that assist in analysis of the data. Discrimination is made in relation to the significance of the symptom associated with a specific disease or problem, or in association with the need for referrals and follow-up. One rationale may be provided for a group of questions about symptoms.

The following questions refer to specific symptoms and behaviors associated with the eyes and vision. For each symptom, questions and follow-up are required. The details to be elicited are the characteristics of the symptom; the onset, duration, and frequency of the symptom; the treatment or remedy for the symptom, including over-the-counter and home remedies; the determination if diagnosis has been sought; the effect of treatments; and family history associated with a symptom or illness.

Questions 1 through 14 refer to blurred vision as a symptom. The rationales and follow-up questions provide examples of the number and types of questions required in a focused interview when symptoms exist. The remaining questions refer to other symptoms associated with problems with the eyes or vision. Follow-up is included only when required for clarification.

Questions Related to Symptoms

1. **Have you ever experienced blurred vision?**

2. **How long have you had blurred vision?**

   ▶ Determining the duration of symptoms is helpful in determining the significance of symptoms in relation to specific diseases and problems. Blurred vision can be an indication of a neurologic, cardiovascular, or endocrine problem; a need for corrective lenses; or cataracts (Osborn, Wraa, Watson, & Holleran, 2013; Berman & Snyder, 2012).

3. **Is your vision blurred all of the time?**

   ▶ It is important to determine if a symptom is constant or intermittent.

4. **Do you know what causes the blurred vision?**

   ▶ This question permits patients to identify whether an actual diagnosis has been made in regard to the symptom or to express their beliefs or perceptions about the cause of the symptom.

5. **Describe your blurred vision.**

   ▶ Descriptions provide information about symptoms in the patient's own words. The descriptions often provide cues for further follow-up questions.

6. **Have you sought treatment for the blurred vision?**

   ▶ Questions 6 through 10 provide information about the need for diagnosis, referral, or continued evaluation of the symptom as well as information about the patient's knowledge of a current diagnosis and the response to intervention.

7. **When was that treatment sought?**

8. **What occurred when you sought treatment?**

9. **Was something recommended or prescribed to help with the blurred vision?**

10. **What was the effect of the treatment?**

11. **Do you use any over-the-counter or home remedies for the blurred vision?**

    ▶ Questions 11 through 14 provide information about drugs and/or remedies that may relieve symptoms or provide comfort. Conversely, some remedies may interfere with the effect of prescribed treatments or medications and may harm the patient.

12. **What are the remedies that you use?**

13. **How often do you use them?**

14. **How much of them do you use?**

Focused Interview Questions	Rationales and Evidence
15. Have you ever experienced double vision?	▶ Double vision can be caused by muscle or nerve complications and some medications (Osborn et al., 2013; Wilson et al., 2013).
16. Are you now or have you ever been sensitive to light?	▶ Sensitivity to light (photophobia) may indicate an eye disorder. However, other disorders and certain medications may also cause photophobia.
17. Do you experience burning or itching of the eyes?	▶ Burning and itching of the eyes are often associated with altered tear production and allergies (Greiner, Hellings, Rotiroti, & Scadding, 2012).
18. Do you ever see small black dots that seem to move when you are looking at something?	▶ Black dots or spots are known as floaters. Floaters are considered normal unless they obstruct vision (WebMD, 2012b).
19. Do you see halos around lights?	▶ Halos around lights are associated with glaucoma, a disease marked by increased intraocular pressure (Mayo Clinic, 2012).
20. Do you have trouble seeing at night? 21. Do you have trouble driving at night?	▶ If the patient responds affirmatively to any of these questions, follow-up is required. Follow-up would include determination of onset, duration, and frequency of the symptom; identification of treatment and the effectiveness of the treatment; and determination of a diagnosis for the problem.

Questions Related to Pain

1. Have you had any eye pain?	▶ Eye pain can be superficial, affecting the outer eye only, or deep and throbbing, possibly associated with glaucoma. Any sudden onset of eye pain should be referred immediately to a physician.
2. Where is the pain?	▶ Questions 2 through 11 are standard questions associated with pain to determine the duration, location, frequency, and intensity of the pain.
3. How often do you experience the pain?	
4. How long does the pain last?	
5. How long have you had the pain?	
6. How would you rate the pain on a scale of 0 to 10?	
7. Is there a trigger for the pain?	
8. Can you describe the pain?	
9. Does the pain radiate to any other areas?	
10. What do you do to relieve the pain?	
11. Is this treatment effective?	

Focused Interview Questions	Rationales and Evidence

Questions Related to Behaviors

1. How do you clean and care for your eyes?

2. If you use eye makeup, how do you apply it and remove it? How often do you replace the makeup and applicators?

3. How do you clean and care for your contact lenses, if used?

4. Do you wear sunglasses when outside?

5. Do you use a tanning salon?

▶ Some eye care products, facial cleansers, and skin care products can be irritating to the eyes. Products used in applying makeup to the eyes and improper care of contact lenses can irritate the eye or cause infection if they are not cleaned or changed frequently (WebMD, 2012a).

▶ Ultraviolet (UV) radiation can cause temporary loss of vision, often referred to as "snow blindness," and pterygium (WHO, n.d.). UVA radiation can cause browning of the lens or loss of elasticity.
 Overexposure to UVB radiation can cause cataracts (WHO, n.d.). Tanning indoors, through tanning salons and sunlamps, can result in eye injuries because of exposure to UV and visible light from sunlamp products.

Questions Related to Age

The focused interview must reflect the anatomic and physiologic differences that exist along the age span. The following questions are presented as examples of those that would be specific for children, the pregnant female, and the older adult.

Questions Regarding Infants and Children

1. Did the mother have any vaginal infections at the time of delivery?

▶ Vaginal infections in the mother can cause eye infections in the newborn (Zuppa, D'Andrea, Catenazzi, Scorrano, & Romagnoli, 2011).

2. Did the baby get eye ointment after birth?

3. Was the infant preterm or full term?

▶ If the infant was born preterm, resuscitation and oxygen may have been required, which can damage the eyes (Chen, Guo, Smith, Dammann, & Dammann, 2010).

4. Does the infant look directly at you? Does your infant follow objects with the eyes?

▶ The infant may have crossed eyes or eyes that move in different directions normally until 2 months of age; then the findings may be associated with weakness of the eye muscles (Medscape, 2012a).

5. Do you have concerns about the child's ability to see? Does the school-age child like to sit at the front of the classroom?

▶ Poor eyesight may necessitate sitting at the front of the room.

6. Has the child had a vision examination? When was the last eye examination?
   - How often has the child's vision been checked?
   - By whom?
   - What were the results?

7. Does the child rub his or her eyes frequently?

▶ Rubbing of the eyes can be associated with infection, allergy, or visual problems (WebMD, 2012c). Some children rub their eyes when fatigued.

Focused Interview Questions	Rationales and Evidence

Questions for the Pregnant Female

1. Have you had any changes in your eyesight during your pregnancy?

▶ Changes in vision should be referred to an ophthalmologist.

Questions for the Older Adult

1. Do you experience dryness or burning in your eyes?

▶ Dryness is usually due to decreased tear production, which occurs with aging (Osborn et al., 2013).

2. Do you have problems seeing at night?

▶ Night blindness is associated with cataracts and some retinal diseases (Osborn et al., 2013).

3. Do bright lights bother you?

▶ The lens of the eye thickens with aging; therefore, accommodation to light is not as rapid (Osborn et al., 2013).

4. Are you routinely tested for glaucoma?

5. What was the date of your last eye examination?

Questions Related to the Environment

Environment refers to both the internal and external environments. Questions related to the internal environment include all of the previous questions and those associated with internal or physiologic responses. Questions regarding the external environment include those related to home, work, or social environments.

Internal Environment

1. What medications are you taking?

▶ Some medications have side effects that impact the eye (Wilson et al., 2013).

2. Are you taking any medications specifically for the eyes?

3. Have you or any family member had diabetes, hypertension, or glaucoma?

▶ All of these diseases can be hereditary and can cause visual difficulties. Hypertension can cause arteriosclerosis of the retina. Diabetes can cause bleeding of the capillaries of the retina, eventually affecting vision (Grosso et al., 2011).

External Environment

The following questions deal with substances, irritants, and other factors found in the physical environment of the patient that could impact the eyes or vision. The physical environment includes the indoor and outdoor environments of the home and the workplace, those encountered for social engagements, and any encountered during travel.

1. Have you been exposed to inhalants such as dust, pollen, chemical fumes, or flying debris that caused eye irritation?

▶ Substances such as dust and pollen can cause eye irritation. Debris can cause a variety of eye injuries, including corneal abrasion. Exposure to chemical fumes can cause corneal burns and other eye injuries.

Focused Interview Questions	Rationales and Evidence

2. **What were those irritants?**

3. **What was the effect on your eyes?**

4. **What have you done to remedy the eye problem?**

5. **What have you done to decrease the exposure to the irritant?**

6. **What kind of activities do you perform at work?**

7. **Do you need or wear safety glasses at work?**

8. **How many hours in the workday are you using a coamputer?**

9. **What sports or hobbies do you participate in?**

10. **Do you routinely wear sunglasses when outside in bright light?**
    - Follow-up questions would include all of the questions previously mentioned that address symptoms and problems.

▶ Use of equipment at work or at home may require the use of safety glasses to prevent eye injury from debris. Prolonged work under bright lights or at a computer screen can cause eyestrain. Some athletic activities put the patient at risk for eye injury, and shields or masks are recommended to prevent or reduce the risk for injury.

Patient-Centered Interaction

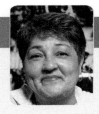

Sophia Rodriguez, a 62-year-old Mexican immigrant, is employed as a sewing machine operator at the local shirt factory. The operators are paid based on work production. Sophia has always received a monthly bonus for her production. Lately, her productivity has decreased and her supervisor tries to help determine the reason. Sophia tells the supervisor she needs a better, stronger light on the sewing machine since it is very hard to see the stitches and thread. Sophia is directed to the local eye clinic. Following is an excerpt of the focused interview.

Interview

Nurse: Mrs. Rodriguez, tell me your reason for coming to the eye clinic today.

Mrs. Rodriguez: **I can't see the thread or the stitches like I used to. I don't sew as many sleeves like I used to. I make mistakes now, and that slows me down.**

Nurse: Have you ever had your eyes examined?

Mrs. Rodriguez: **Yes, several years ago. They told me everything was okay. No glasses.**

Nurse: Describe your vision.

Mrs. Rodriguez: **I don't know what you want me to say. I just can't see like I used to.**

Nurse: Can you see to read the newspaper?

Mrs. Rodriguez: **Yes.**

Nurse: Do you need to hold the newspaper closer to your eyes or farther away when reading?

Mrs. Rodriguez: **A little farther away. But I can't read it at night unless I'm next to the light in the room.**

Nurse: Can you see the street signs when you are driving?

Mrs. Rodriguez: **Yes, that is not a problem.**

Nurse: Is your vision blurred?

Mrs. Rodriguez: **Sometimes, especially if I'm tired.**

Nurse: Do you ever see black spots floating in your eyes?

Mrs. Rodriguez: **No.**

Nurse: Are your eyes sensitive to light?

Mrs. Rodriguez: **No.**

Nurse: Do you see halos or rings around lights?

Mrs. Rodriguez: **No.**

Nurse: Do you have any pain or burning in your eyes?

Mrs. Rodriguez: **No.**

Analysis

The nurse knows presbyopia is a common change of the eye associated with aging. The nurse begins the interview using open-ended statements to gather data associated with presbyopia and other medical diagnoses. Using open-ended statements, the nurse obtains clear baseline data. When the patient indicates she is not clear how to respond, the nurse proceeds using closed-ended statements. This allows the patient to respond "yes" or "no." The nurse must be sure to present the many questions in a non-threatening manner.

Patient Education

The following are physiologic, behavioral, and cultural factors that affect the health of the eye across the life span. Several factors related to the eye are cited in *Healthy People* documents. The nurse provides advice and education to promote and maintain health and reduce risks associated with the aforementioned factors that impact the eye across the life span.

LIFESPAN CONSIDERATIONS

Risk Factors

- Children with fetal alcohol syndrome (FAS) experience changes in the structure of the eye, ptosis, and visual disturbances including reduced visual acuity, nystagmus, cataracts, and strabismus.

- Visual disturbances in children are often discovered as a result of learning or behavioral problems.

- Presbyopia, the gradual decrease in near vision, occurs in all individuals, with an onset at around age 45.
- Senile ptosis and ectropion or entropion accompany loss of muscle tone in older adults.

- Older adults experience a decrease in lacrimal secretions, resulting in a dryness of the eyes.

Patient Education

▶ Discuss risks of alcohol abuse with females of childbearing age.
▶ Provide information about support services and agencies to assist those with alcohol addiction.

▶ Provide information to parents about the development of vision from infancy to adolescence.
▶ Guide patients to recognize symptoms of problems with the structures of the eye or neuromuscular functions.

▶ Provide information about recommendations for eye examinations across the life span.

▶ Provide information about lubricating agents for older adults with drying of the eyes.

CULTURAL CONSIDERATIONS

Risk Factors

- African Americans and Hispanic Americans are at higher risk for glaucoma than other racial groups.

- Diabetic retinopathy is the leading cause of blindness in the United States. Retinal changes occur in diabetes types 1 and 2.

- Type 2 diabetes occurs more frequently in African Americans, Asian Americans, Hispanic Americans, and Native Americans than in Caucasians.

Patient Education

▶ Instruct susceptible populations to have a glaucoma check every 1–2 years after the age of 35, especially if they also have high blood pressure.

▶ Instruct patients with diabetes or those with a family history of diabetes to have a vision and retinal examination annually.

▶ Patients in these populations, especially obese patients, should have fasting blood test performed with each annual checkup.

ENVIRONMENTAL CONSIDERATIONS

Risk Factors

- Environmental factors including pollutants and ultraviolet light can affect the health of the eye and vision.

- Medications can affect the integrity and function of the eye.

Patient Education

▶ Advise patients to use sunglasses to avoid environmental hazards.

▶ Instruct the patient regarding prescription and over-the-counter (OTC) medications in terms of proper instillation of eye medications as well as side effects and potential interactions between and among medications.

BEHAVIORAL CONSIDERATIONS

Risk Factor	Patient Education
• Trauma to the eye can occur during recreational activities, in the workplace, and in the home.	► Provide information about eye safety in the home, in the workplace, and during recreational activity, including the use of protective eyewear.
	► Instruct the patient in emergency eye care for substances in the eye, chemical splash, cuts in or near the eye, and blunt injury to the eye.

Physical Assessment

Assessment Techniques and Findings

Physical assessment of the eyes requires the use of inspection, palpation, and tests of the function of the eyes. The ophthalmoscope is used to assess the internal eye. During each of the assessments, the nurse is gathering data related to the patient's vision and the internal and external structures and functions of the eye. Inspection includes looking at the size, shape, and symmetry of the eye, eyelids, eyebrows, and eye movements. Knowledge of the norms and expectations related to the eyes and vision according to age and development is essential in determining the meaning of the data.

Presbyopia, the inability to accommodate for near vision, is common in patients over the age of 45. The size, shape, and position of the eyes should be symmetric. The sclerae are white, the cornea is clear, and the pupils are round and symmetric in size and respond briskly to light. The eyebrows are located equally above the eyes; the eyelashes are full and everted. The eyes are moist, indicating tear production. The movements of the eye are smooth and symmetric. Upon ophthalmoscopic examination, the red reflex is visible in each eye and the retinae are a uniform yellowish pink with a sharply defined disc and visible vessels.

Physical assessment of the eyes follows an organized pattern. It begins with assessment of visual acuity and is followed by assessments of visual fields, muscle function, and external eye structures. The assessment of the eye concludes with the ophthalmoscopic examination. Additional information about the eye, vision screening and assessment can be obtained through the National Eye Institute at www.nei.nih.gov.

EQUIPMENT

- visual acuity charts (Snellen or E for distant vision, Rosenbaum for near vision). For patients who cannot read, including children, charts with pictures or numbers are used (MedlinePlus, 2013).
- opaque card or eye cover
- penlight
- cotton-tipped applicator
- ophthalmoscope

HELPFUL HINTS

- Provide specific instructions about what is expected of the patient. This would include telling the patient clearly which eye to cover when conducting an assessment of visual acuity.
- The ability to read letters will determine the type of acuity chart to be used. Children and non–English-speaking patients can use the E chart or a chart with figures and images for visual acuity.
- An opaque card or eye cover is used for covering the eye in several assessments. The patient must be instructed not to close or apply pressure to the covered eye.
- Several types of lighting are required. Visual acuity requires bright lighting, while the room is darkened to assess pupillary responses and the internal eye.
- The room must provide 20 feet from the Snellen chart.
- The assessment may be conducted with the patient seated or standing. The nurse stands or sits at eye level with the patient.
- Use Standard Precautions.

Techniques and Normal Findings	Abnormal Findings Special Considerations

Vision

Testing Distant Vision

1. **Position the patient.**
   - Position the patient exactly 20 ft, or 6.1 meters (m), from the Snellen chart. The patient may be standing or seated. The chart should be at the patient's eye level.

2. **Instruct the patient.**
   - Explain that you are testing distant vision. Explain that the patient will read the letters from the top of the chart down to the smallest line of letters that the patient can see, reading each line left to right. Explain that each line of the chart has a number that indicates what the patient's vision is in relation to that of a person with normal vision.

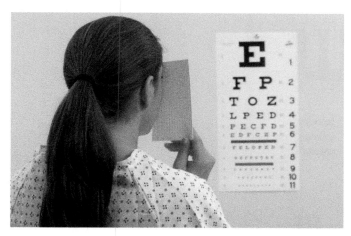

Figure 15.7 Testing distant vision.

3. Ask the patient to cover one eye with the opaque card or eye cover (see Figure 15.7 ■). Tell the patient to read, left to right, from the top of the chart down to the smallest line of letters that the patient can see.

4. Ask the patient to cover the other eye and to read from the top of the chart down to the smallest line of letters that the patient can see.

5. Ask the patient to read from the top of the chart down to the smallest line of letters that the patient can see with both eyes uncovered.

6. If a patient uses corrective lenses for distance vision, test first with eyeglasses or contact lenses. Then test without glasses or contact lenses.
   - The results are recorded as a fraction. The numerator indicates the distance from the chart (20 ft). The denominator indicates the distance at which a person with normal vision can read the last line.
   - Normal vision is 20/20; therefore, at 20 ft the patient can read the line numbered 20. If a patient's vision is 20/30, the patient reads at 20 ft what a person with normal vision reads at 30 ft. Observe while the patient is reading the chart.
   - If the patient is unable to read more than one half of the letters on a line, record the number of the line above.

▶ Frowning, leaning forward, and squinting indicate visual or reading difficulties.

Techniques and Normal Findings	Abnormal Findings Special Considerations

The Snellen E Chart

The Snellen E chart has *E*'s pointing in different directions (see Figure 15.8 ■). For patients who cannot read, including children, charts that feature numbers or pictures are used (MedlinePlus, 2013).

- The letter *E* becomes smaller as one proceeds from the top to the bottom of the chart. Numbers on each line correspond to the patient's vision in relation to that of a person with normal vision that would be seen testing distant vision with the E chart.
- Repeat steps 1 to 6 as previously noted but ask the patient to start at the top of the chart and to point in the direction the letter faces on each line until the patient can no longer see the Es.
- Observe while the patient is reading the chart.

▶ Inability to see objects at a distance is myopia. The smaller the fraction, the worse the vision. Vision of 20/200 is considered legal blindness. Changes in vision may be related to dysfunction of cranial nerve II.

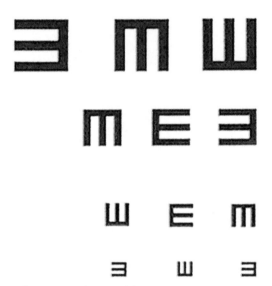

Figure 15.8 E chart for testing distant vision.

Testing Near Vision

1. **Position the patient.**
   - The patient is sitting with a Jaeger or Rosenbaum chart held at a distance of 12 to 14 in. (30.5 to 35.5 cm) from the eyes.

2. **Instruct the patient.**
   - Explain that you are testing near vision, and the patient will read the letters from the top of the card down to the smallest line the patient can see. Tell the patient to hold the card at the same distance throughout the test. Explain that each line on the card has a number that indicates what the patient's vision is in relation to that of a person with normal vision (see Figure 15.9 ■).

3. **Ask the patient to cover one eye with the opaque card or eye cover.**

4. **Repeat the test with the other eye and then with both eyes uncovered. The results are recorded as a fraction. A normal result is 14/14 in each eye.**

5. **If a patient uses corrective lenses for reading, test with the corrective lenses.**

▶ Inability to see objects at close range is called hyperopia. Presbyopia, the inability to accommodate for near vision, is common in persons over 45 years of age; however, this condition may occur among individuals of other ages, as well.

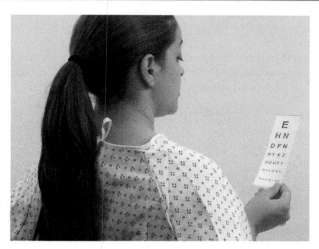

Figure 15.9 Testing near vision.

Testing Peripheral Vision

1. **Position the patient.**
   - For direct confrontation visual field testing, the patient and examiner sit facing one another. To test peripheral vision, the patient should be sitting 2 to 3 ft (0.6 to 0.9 m) from you and at eye level.

2. **Instruct the patient.**
   - Explain that you are testing peripheral vision. In this test, the patient's peripheral visual fields are compared to that of the examiner. The patient will alternately cover an eye and must look directly into your open eye. A pen or penlight will be moved into the patient's field of vision, sequentially from four directions. The patient is to indicate by saying "now" or "yes" when the object is first seen.

3. **Ask the patient to cover one eye with a card while you cover your opposite eye with a card.**

4. **Holding a penlight in one hand, extend your arm upward, and advance it in from the periphery to the midline point (see Figure 15.10 ■).**

► If the patient is not able to see the object at the same time that the examiner does, there may be some peripheral vision loss. The patient should be evaluated further.

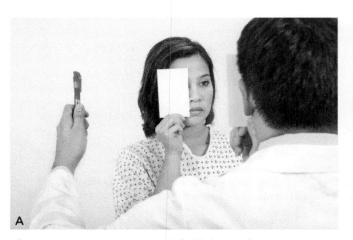
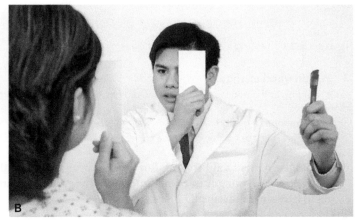

Figure 15.10 A. Testing visual fields by confrontation, nurse's view. B. Testing visual fields by confrontation, patient's view.

Techniques and Normal Findings	Abnormal Findings Special Considerations

5. Be sure to keep the penlight equidistant between the patient and yourself.

6. Ask the patient to report when the object is first seen. Repeat the procedure upward, toward the nose, and downward. Then repeat the entire procedure with the other eye covered. This test assumes the examiner has normal peripheral vision.

Extraocular Movements (EOM)

Testing the Six Fields of Cardinal Gaze

1. **Position the patient.**
   - The patient is sitting in a comfortable position. You are at eye level with the patient.

2. **Instruct the patient.**
   - Explain that you will be testing eye movements and the muscles of the eye. Explain that the patient must keep the head still while following a pen or penlight that you will move in several directions in front of the patient's eyes.

3. **Stand about 2 ft (0.6 m) in front of the patient.**

4. **Letter "H" method.**
   - Starting at midline, move the penlight to the left, then straight up, then straight down.
   - Drop your hand. Position the penlight against the midline.
   - Now move the penlight to the right, then straight up, then straight down (see Figure 15.11 ■).

▶ This method does not allow the nurse to scatter the movement of the penlight.

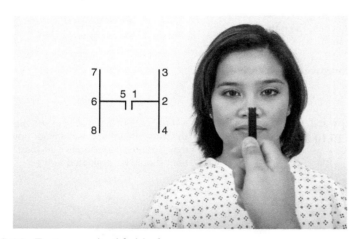

Figure 15.11   Testing cardinal field of gaze.

5. **Wagon wheel method.**
   - Starting at the midline, move the pen or light in the direction to form a star or wagon wheel.
   - Use random direction pattern to create the movement.
   - Always return the light or pen to the center before changing direction (see Figure 15.12 ■).

6. **Assess the patient's ability to follow your movements with the eyes (see Figure 15.11). Nystagmus, rapid fluttering of the eyeball, occurs at completion of rapid lateral eye movement.**

▶ If **nystagmus** occurs during testing, there could be a weakness in the extraocular muscles or cranial nerve III.

Techniques and Normal Findings	Abnormal Findings Special Considerations

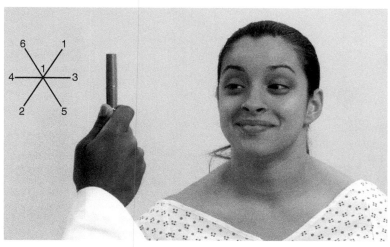

Figure 15.12 Alternative method of testing cardinal field of gaze.

Assessing Corneal Light Reflex

1. **Position the patient.**
   - You will sit at eye level with the patient.

2. **Instruct the patient.**
   - Explain that you are examining the cornea of the eyes. Instruct the patient to stare straight ahead while you hold a penlight 12 in. (30.5 cm) from both eyes.

3. **Shine the light into the eyes from a distance of 12 inches (see Figure 15.13 ■).**
   - The reflection of light should appear in the same spot on both pupils. This appears as a "twinkle" in the eye.

▶ If the reflection of light is not symmetric, there could be a weakness in the extraocular muscles.

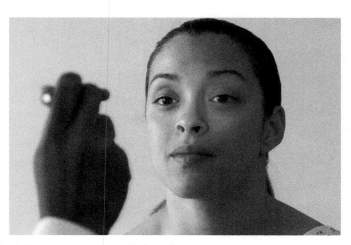

Figure 15.13 Testing the corneal light reflex.

| Techniques and Normal Findings | Abnormal Findings Special Considerations |

Performing the Cover/Uncover Test

1. **Position the patient.**
    - You should be sitting at eye level with the patient.

2. **Instruct the patient.**
    - Explain that this test determines the balance mechanism (fusion reflex) that keeps the eyes parallel. Explain that the patient will look at a fixed point while covering each eye. You will observe the eyes.

3. **Cover one eye with a card and observe the uncovered eye, which should remain focused on the designated point (see Figure 15.14 ■).**

4. **Quickly remove the card from the covered eye and observe the newly uncovered eye for movement. it should focus straight ahead.**

▶ If there is a weakness in one of the eye muscles, the fusion reflex is blocked when one eye is covered and the weakness of the eye can be observed.

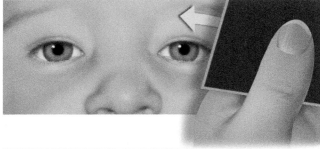

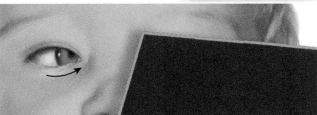

A Right, or uncovered eye, is weaker.

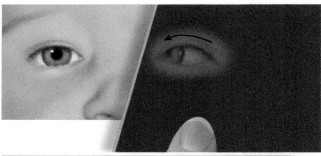

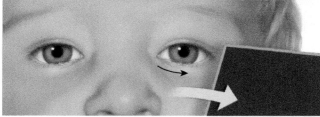

Figure 15.14
Cover/Uncover test.   **B** Left, or covered eye, is weaker.

5. **Repeat the procedure with the other eye.**

Techniques and Normal Findings	Abnormal Findings Special Considerations

Inspection of the Eyes

Assessing the Eye

1. **Instruct the patient.**
   - Explain that you will be examining the patient's eye. You will be looking at the patient's eyes and touching them to see inside the lids. Explain that you will provide specific instructions before each test.

2. **Stand directly in front of the patient and focus on the external structures of the eye.**
   - The eyebrows should be symmetric in shape and the eyelashes similar in quantity and distribution. The eyebrows and eyelashes should be free of flakes and drainage.

► Absence of the lateral third of the eyebrow is associated with hypothyroidism. Absent eyelashes may indicate pulling or plucking associated with obsessive-compulsive behavior.

3. **Ask the patient to open the eyes.**
   - The distances between the palpebral fissures should be equal.
   - The upper eyelid covers a small arc of the iris.

4. **Ask the patient to close the eyes.**
   - The eyelids should symmetrically cover the eyeballs when closed.
   - The eyeball should be neither protruding nor sunken.

5. **Gently separate the eyelids and ask the patient to look up, down, and to each side.**
   - The conjunctiva should be moist and clear, with no redness or drainage, and with small blood vessels visible beneath the conjunctival surface.
   - The lens should be clear, and the sclera white.
   - The irises should be round and both of the same color, although irises of different colors can be a normal finding.

► One eyelid drooping (**ptosis**) can be caused by a dysfunction of cranial nerve III (oculomotor). Eyes that protrude beyond the supraorbital ridge can indicate a thyroid disorder; however, this trait may be normal for the patient. Edema of the eyelids can be caused by allergies, heart disease, or kidney disease. Inability to move the eyelids can indicate dysfunction of the nervous system, including facial nerve paralysis.

6. **Inspect the cornea by shining a penlight from the side across the cornea.**
   - The cornea should be clear with no irregularities.
   - The pupils should be round and equal in size (see Figure 15.15 ■).

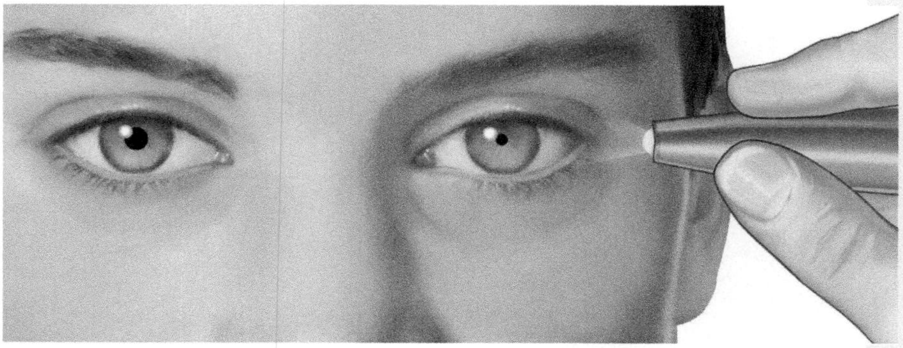

Figure 15.15 Inspecting the cornea.

7. **Observe the constriction in the illuminated pupil.**
   - Also observe the simultaneous reaction (**consensual constriction**) of the other pupil. The direct reaction should be faster and greater than the consensual reaction.

► If the illuminated pupil fails to constrict, there is a defect in the direct pupillary response. If the unilluminated pupil fails to constrict, there is a defect in the consensual response, controlled by cranial nerve III (oculomotor).

Techniques and Normal Findings	Abnormal Findings Special Considerations

Testing Near Vision

1. **Instruct the patient.**
   - Explain that you are testing muscles of the eye. Explain that the patient will shift the gaze from the far wall to an object held 4 to 5 in. (10 to 12 cm) from the patient's nose.

2. **Ask the patient to stare straight ahead at a distant point.**

3. **Hold a penlight about 4 to 5 in. (10 to 12 cm) from the patient's nose; then ask the patient to shift the gaze from the distant point to the penlight.**
   - The eyes should converge (turn inward) and the pupils should constrict as the eyes focus on the penlight. This pupillary change is **accommodation,** a change in size to adjust vision from far to near.
   - A normal response to pupillary testing is recorded as PERRLA (pupils equal, round, react to light, and accommodation).

▶ Lack of **convergence** (turning inward of the eye) and failure of the pupils to constrict indicates dysfunction of cranial nerves III, IV, and VI.

ADVANCED SKILL

Inspecting Fundus With Ophthalmoscope

1. **Instruct the patient.**
   - Explain that you will be using the ophthalmoscope to look into the inner deep part of the eye (**fundus**) and that the lights in the room will be dimmed. Explain that the patient must stare ahead at a fixed point while you move in front with the ophthalmoscope. Tell the patient to maintain a fixed gaze, as if looking through you. Explain that you will place your hand on the patient's head so you both remain stable.

2. **To examine the right eye, hold the ophthalmoscope in your right hand with the index finger on the lens wheel.**

3. **Begin with the lens on the 0 diopter. With the light on, place the ophthalmoscope over your right eye (see Figure 15.16 ■).**

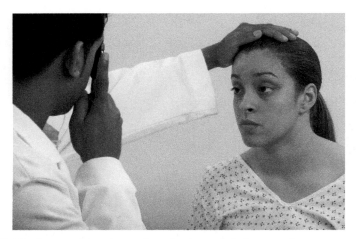

Figure 15.16 Approaching the patient for the ophthalmoscopic exam.

4. **Stand at a slight angle lateral to the patient's line of vision.**

5. **Approach the patient at about a 15-degree angle toward the patient's nose.**

6. **Place your left hand on the patient's shoulder or head.**

7. Hold the ophthalmoscope against your head, directing the light into the patient's pupil. Keep your other eye open.

8. Advance toward the patient.

9. As you look into the patient's pupil, you will see the *red reflex*, which is the reflection of the light off the retina. Remember to examine the patient's right eye with your right eye, and the patient's left eye with your left eye. At this point you may need to adjust the lens wheel to bring the ocular structures into focus. Normally, you will see no shadows or dots interrupting the red reflex. If the light strays from the pupil, you will lose the red reflex. Adjust your angle until you see the red reflex again.

▶ Persistent absence of the red reflex may indicate a cataract, an opacity of the lens.

10. Keep advancing toward the patient until the ophthalmoscope is almost touching the patient's eyelashes (see Figure 15.17 ■).

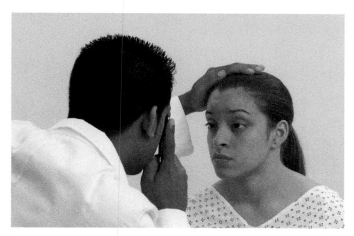

Figure 15.17 Examining the eye using the ophthalmoscope.

11. Rotate the diopter wheel if necessary to bring the ocular fundus into focus.

12. If the patient's vision is myopic, you will need to rotate the wheel into the minus numbers (see Figure 15.18 ■).

13. If the patient's vision is hyperopic, rotate the wheel into the plus numbers.

14. **Begin to look for the optic disc by following the path of the blood vessels.** As they grow larger, they lead to the optic disc on the nasal side of the retina (see Figure 15.19 ■).

    The optic disc normally looks like a round or oval yellow-orange depression with a distinct margin. It is the site where the optic nerve and blood vessels exit the eye.

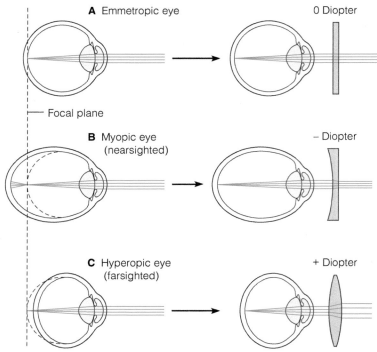

A Emmetropic eye   0 Diopter

Focal plane

B Myopic eye
(nearsighted)   – Diopter

C Hyperopic eye
(farsighted)   + Diopter

Figure 15.18 Use of diopter to adjust for problems of refraction. A. In the emmetropic (normal) eye, light is focused properly on the retina, and the 0 diopter is used. B. In the myopic eye, light from a distant source converges to a focal point before reaching the retina. Negative diopter numbers are used. C. In the hyperopic eye, light from a near source converges to a focal point past the retina. Positive diopter numbers are used.

15. **Follow the vessels laterally to a darker circle. This is the *macula*, or area of central vision.**

The *fovea centralis*, a small white spot located in the center of the macula, is the area of sharpest vision.

▶ Degeneration of the macula is common in older adults and results in impaired central vision. It may be due to hemorrhages, cysts, or other alterations.

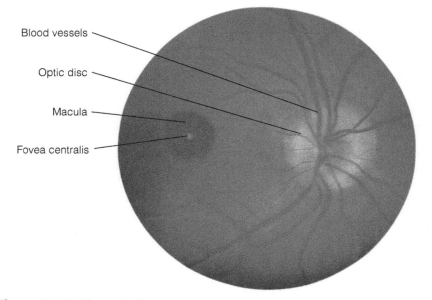

Blood vessels

Optic disc

Macula

Fovea centralis

Figure 15.19 The optic disc.
Source: Don Wong/Science Source

Techniques and Normal Findings	Abnormal Findings Special Considerations

16. **Systematically inspect these structures. A crescent shape around the margin of the optic disc is a normal finding. A *scleral crescent* is an absence of pigment in the choroid and is a dull white color. A *pigment crescent*, which is black, is an accumulation of pigment in the choroid.**

▶ Abnormalities of the retinal structures present as dark or opaque spots on the retina, an irregularly shaped optic disc, and lesions or hemorrhages on the fundus.

17. **Use the optic disc as a clock face for documenting the position of a finding and the diameter of the disc (DD) for noting its distance from the optic disc. For instance, "at 2:00, 2 DD from the disc" describes the finding in Figure 15.20 ■.**

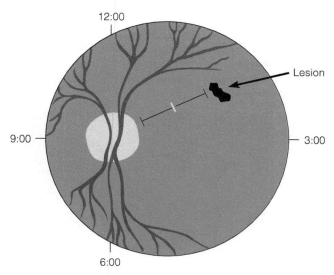

Figure 15.20 Documenting a finding from the ophthalmoscopic examination.

18. **Trace the path of a paired artery and vein from the optic disc to the periphery in the four quadrants of the eyeball.**

▶ An absence of major vessels in any of the four quadrants is an abnormal finding. Constricted arteries look smaller than two-thirds the diameter of accompanying veins. Crossing of the vessels more than 2 DD away from the optic disc requires further evaluation.

19. **Note the number of major vessels, color, width, and any crossing of the vessels.**

Palpation of the Eye

1. **Ask the patient to close both eyes.**

2. **Using the first two or three fingers, gently palpate the lacrimal sacs, the eyelids, and erythematous areas for warmth or tenderness.**

▶ Erythema may be a symptom of injury or infection, cardiovascular problems, or renal problems.

3. **Confirm that there is no swelling or tenderness and that the eyeballs feel firm.**

Abnormal Findings

Abnormalities of the eye arise for a variety of reasons and can be associated with vision, eye movement, and the internal and external structures of the eye. The following sections address abnormal findings associated with the eyelids (see Table 15.3), the eye (see Table 15.4), and the fundus (see Table 15.5). In addition, an overview of conditions that may be associated with an impaired pupillary response is provided (see Table 15.6).

TABLE 15.3   Abnormalities of the Eyelids

Blepharitis

Blepharitis is inflammation of the eyelids. Staphylococcal infection leads to red, scaly, and crusted lids. The eye burns, itches, and tears.

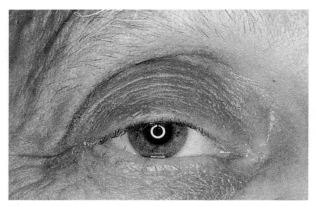

Figure 15.21 Blepharitis.
Source: BSIP SA/Alamy.

Basal Cell Carcinoma

Usually seen on the lower lid and medial canthus. It has a papular appearance.

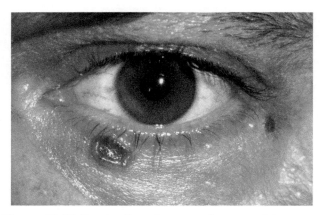

Figure 15.22 Basal cell carcinoma on lower eyelid.
Source: BSIP SA/Alamy.

Chalazion

A firm, nontender nodule on the eyelid, arising from infection of the meibomian gland. Not painful unless inflamed.

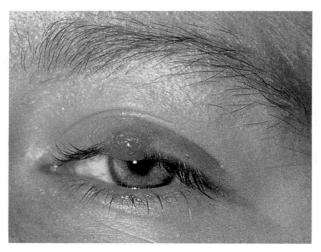

Figure 15.23 Chalazion.
Source: SLP/Custom Medical Stock Photo.

Hordeolum

The result of a staphylococcal infection of hair follicles on the margin of the lids. Affected eye is swollen, red, and painful. Also called a stye.

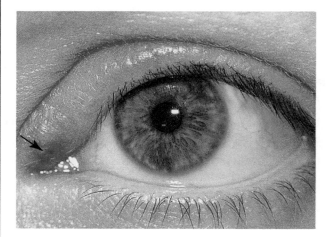

Figure 15.24 Hordeolum (stye).
Source: Science Photo Library/Science Source.

TABLE 15.3   Abnormalities of the Eyelids (continued)

Entropion

Entropion is an inversion of the lid and lashes caused by muscle spasm of the eyelid. Friction from lashes can cause corneal irritation.

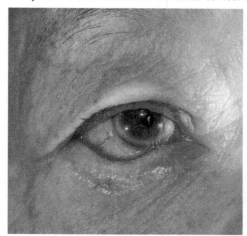

Figure 15.25 Entropion.
Source: Arztsamui/Shutterstock.

Ectropion

Ectropion is eversion of the lower eyelid caused by muscle weakness, exposing the palpebral conjunctiva.

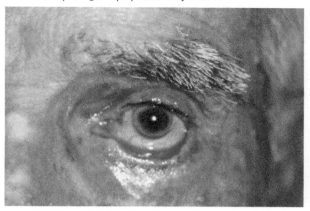

Figure 15.26 Ectropion.
Source: JPD/Custom Medical Stock Photo.

Ptosis

Drooping of the eyelid; occurs with cranial nerve damage or systemic neuromuscular weakness.

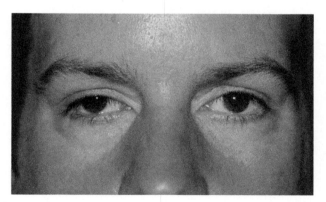

Figure 15.27 Ptosis.
Source: Dr. P. Marazzi/Science Source.

Periorbital Edema

Periorbital edema refers to swollen, puffy lids; occurs with crying, infection, trauma, and systemic problems including kidney failure, heart failure, and allergy.

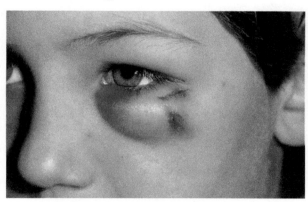

Figure 15.28 Periorbital edema.
Source: SPL/Custom Medical Stock Photo.

Exophthalmos

Abormal protrusion of one or both eyeballs; usually occurs secondary to Graves' disease; causes also may include infectious disease, certain forms of cancer, and other disorders.

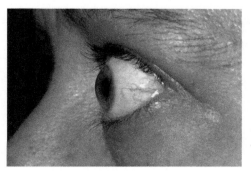

Figure 15.29 Exophthalmos.
Source: Dr. P. Marazzi/Science Source.

TABLE 15.4	**Abnormalities of the Eye**

Conjunctivitis

Infection of the conjunctiva usually due to bacteria or virus but which may result from chemical exposure. It is commonly called pink eye.

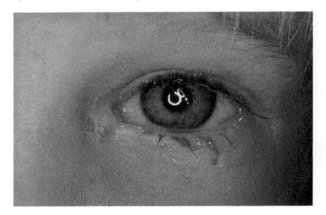

Figure 15.30 Conjunctivitis.
Source: Steve Gorton/Dorling Kindersley Ltd.

Iritis

Iritis is a serious disorder characterized by redness around the iris and cornea, decreased vision, and deep, aching pain; pupil is often irregular.

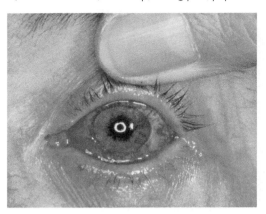

Figure 15.31 Iritis.
Source: Custom Medical Stock Photo, Inc.

Subconjunctival Hemorrhage

Results from ruptured blood vessel that leads to blood accumulation in the subconjunctival space. Causes include trauma, anticoagulant therapy, hypertension, and elevated venous pressure (Tarlan & Kiratli, 2013).

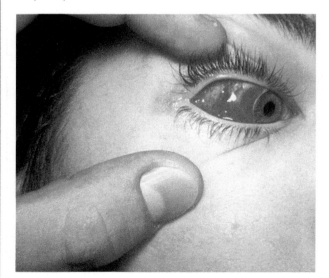

Figure 15.32 Subconjunctival hemorrhage.
Source: Dr. Thomas F. Sellers/Emory University/Centers for Disease Control and Prevention (CDC).

Pterygium

Non-cancerous growth that develops from the conjunctiva and extends onto the sclera; may also extend to the cornea (MedlinePlus, 2012).

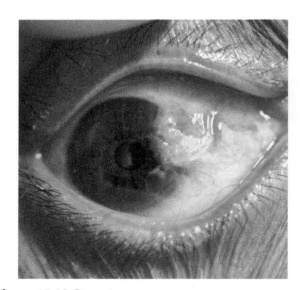

Figure 15.33 Pterygium.
Source: Arztsamui/Shutterstock.

TABLE 15.4 **Abnormalities of the Eye** (continued)

Hyphema

Collection of blood in the anterior chamber of the eye that is most often caused by blunt trauma to the eye. Additional causes include eye surgery, blood vessel abnormalities, and medical problems (cancer).

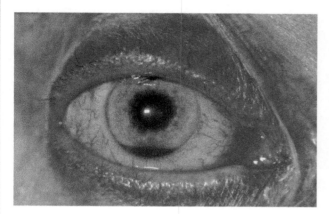

Figure 15.34 Hyphema.
Source: SPL/Science Source.

Acute Glaucoma

The result of sudden increase in intraocular pressure resulting from blocked flow of fluid from the anterior chamber. Pupil is oval-shaped and dilated; cornea appears cloudy with circumcorneal redness. Pain onset is sudden and accompanied by decrease in vision and halos around lights. Acute glaucoma requires immediate intervention.

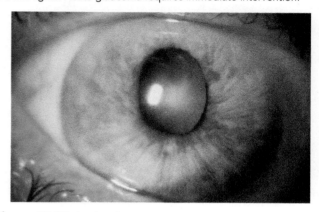

Figure 15.35 Acute glaucoma.
Source: Wellcome Image Library/Custom Medical Stock Photo.

Cataract

An opacity in the lens; usually occurs in aging.

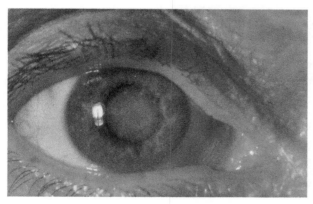

Figure 15.36 Cataract.
Source: Biophoto Associates/Getty Images.

Pinguecula

Yellowish nodules that are thickened areas of the bulbar conjunctiva. Caused by prolonged exposure to sun, wind, and dust.

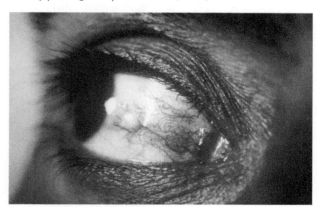

Figure 15.37 Pinguecula.
Source: Centers for Disease Control (CDC).

TABLE 15.5 Abnormalities of the Fundus

Diabetic Retinopathy

Refers to the changes that occur in the retina and its vasculature, including microaneurysms, hemorrhages, macular edema, and retinal exudates.

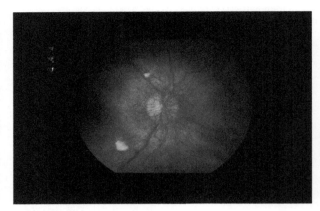

Figure 15.38 Diabetic retinopathy.
Source: Mediscan/Alamy.

Hypertensive Retinopathy

Refers to changes in the retina and its vasculature in response to high blood pressure. Include flame hemorrhages, nicking of vessels, and "cotton wool" spots that arise from nerve fiber infarction.

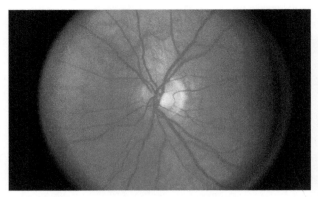

Figure 15.39 Hypertensive retinopathy.
Source: Science Source.

Age-Related Macular Degeneration (ARMD)

A degenerative condition of the macula, the central retina, causing the gradual loss of central vision while peripheral vision remains intact. The eyes are affected at different rates. Risk factors for macular degeneration include hypertension and cigarette smoking (Lim et al., 2012).

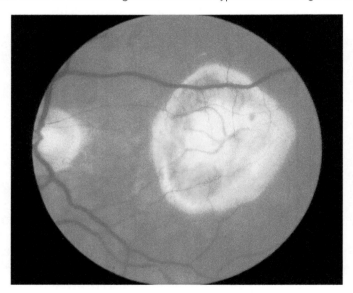

Figure 15.40 Macular degeneration.
Source: Paul Parker/Science Source.

TABLE 15.6 **Conditions Associated with Impaired Pupillary Response**

Adie's Pupil

Also known as tonic pupil, Adie's pupil is sluggish pupillary response. Usually unilateral, but can be bilateral. Occurs due to damage to parasympathetic nerves that innervate the eye.

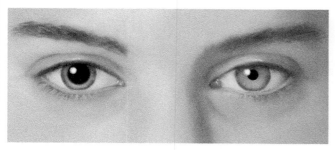

Figure 15.41 Adie's pupil.

Argyll Robertson Pupils

Small, irregular, pupils that exist bilaterally and are nonreactive to light. Occur with CNS disorders including tumor, syphilis, and narcotic use.

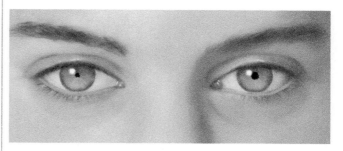

Figure 15.42 Argyll Robertson pupils.

Anisocoria

Unequal pupillary size, which may be a normal finding or may indicate CNS disease.

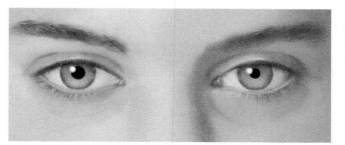

Figure 15.43 Anisocoria.

Cranial Nerve III Damage

Results in a unilaterally dilated pupil. There is no reaction to light. Ptosis may be seen.

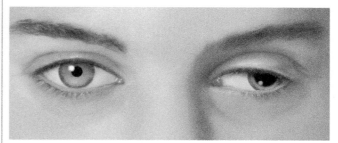

Figure 15.44 Cranial nerve III damage.

Horner's Syndrome

A result of blockage of sympathetic nerve stimulation. Findings include a unilateral, small regular pupil that is nonreactive to light. Ptosis and anhidrosis of the same side accompany the pupillary signs.

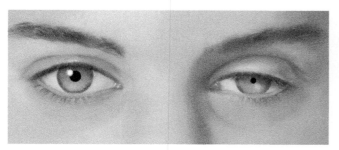

Figure 15.45 Horner's syndrome.

Mydriasis

Refers to fixed and dilated pupils; may occur with sympathetic nerve stimulation, glaucoma, CNS damage, or deep anesthesia.

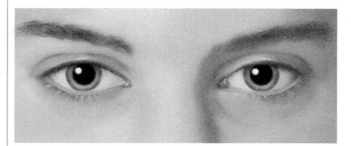

Figure 15.46 Mydriasis.

(continued)

TABLE 15.6	Conditions Associated with Impaired Pupillary Response (continued)

Miosis

Miosis refers to fixed and constricted pupils; may occur with the use of narcotics, with damage to the pons, or as a result of treatment for glaucoma.

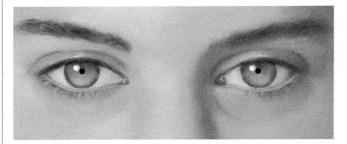

Figure 15.47 Miosis.

Monocular Blindness

Results in direct and consensual response to light directed in the normal eye and absence of response in either eye when light is directed in the blind eye.

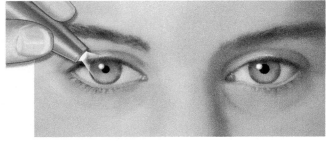

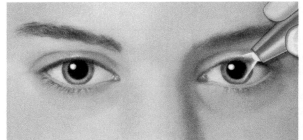

Figure 15.48 Monocular blindness.

Disorders of Visual Acuity

Visual acuity is dependent on the ability of the eye to refract light rays and focus them on the retina. The shape of the eye is one determinant in the refractive and focusing processes of vision.

Emmetropia is the normal refractive condition of the eye in which light rays are brought into sharp focus on the retina (see Figure 15.49 ■).

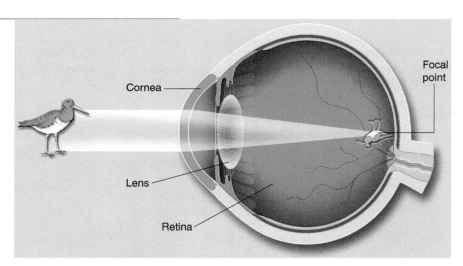

Figure 15.49 Emmetropia.

MYOPIA

Myopia (nearsightedness) is generally inherited and occurs when the eye is longer than normal. As a result, light rays focus in front of the retina (see Figure 15.50 ■).

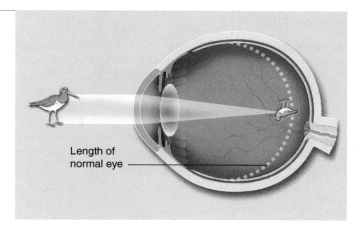

Figure 15.50 Myopia.

HYPEROPIA

Hyperopia (farsightedness) is also an inherited condition in which the eye is shorter than normal. In hyperopia the light rays focus behind the retina (see Figure 15.51 ■).

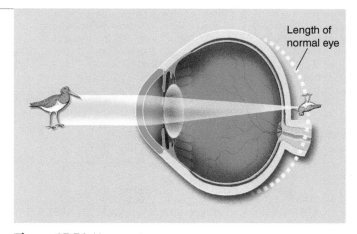

Figure 15.51 Hyperopia.

ASTIGMATISM

Astigmatism is often a familial condition in which the refraction of light is spread over a wide area rather than on a distinct point on the retina. In the normal eye, the cornea is round in shape, whereas in astigmatism the cornea curves more in one direction than another. As a result, light is refracted and focused on two focal points on or near the retina. Vision in astigmatism may be blurred or doubled (see Figure 15.52 ■).

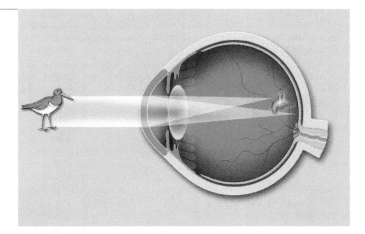

Figure 15.52 Astigmatism.

PRESBYOPIA

Presbyopia is an age-related condition in which the lens of the eye loses the ability to accommodate. As a result, light is focused behind the retina, and focus on near objects becomes difficult.

VISUAL FIELDS

The **visual field** refers to the total area in which objects can be seen in the periphery while the eye remains focused on a central point. Testing visual fields enables the examiner to detect and map losses in peripheral vision. The mapping aids in determination of the problem. Changes in visual fields accompany damage to the retina, lesions in the optic nerve or chiasm, increased intraocular pressure, and retinal vascular damage. The normal visual pathways and loss of visual fields in relation to the previously mentioned conditions are depicted in Figures 15.53 and 15.54 ■, respectively.

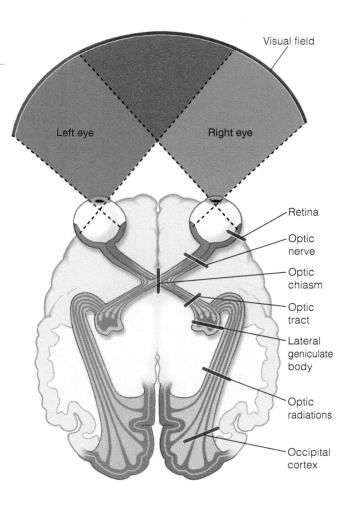

Figure 15.53 Normal visual pathways.

LEFT EYE   RIGHT EYE

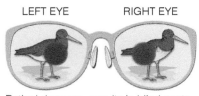

Retinal damage—results in blind spots in localized damaged areas.

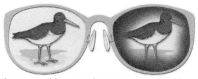

Increased intraocular pressure resulting in decreased peripheral vision.

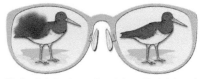

Retinal detachment—vision diminishes in affected area.

Right optic tract or optic radiation lesion resulting in loss of right nasal and left temporal fields. Homonymous hemianopsia.

LEFT EYE   RIGHT EYE

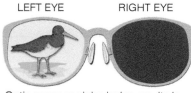

Optic nerve or globe lesion results in unilateral blindness.

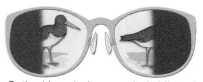

Optic chiasm lesion—results in bilateral heteronymous hemianopsia (loss of temporal visual fields).

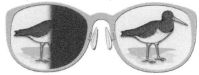

Lesion occurs in uncrossed fibers of optic chiasm resulting in left hemianopsia (nasal).

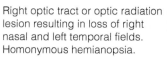

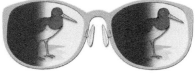

Figure 15.54 Patient's view with visual field loss.

CARDINAL FIELDS OF GAZE

Eye movement is controlled by six extraocular muscles and by cranial nerves III, IV, and VI. Muscle weakness or dysfunction of a cranial nerve can be identified by assessing the fields of gaze, assessing corneal light reflex, and performing the cover test.

Strabismus is a condition in which the axes of the eyes cannot be directed at the same object. Strabismus can be classified as convergent (esotropia) in which the eye deviates inward, and divergent (exotropia) in which the deviation is outward. In strabismus, light can be seen to reflect in different axes (see Figure 15.55 ■).

Esophoria (inward turning of the eye) and **exophoria** (outward turning of the eye) are detected in the cover test. Esotropic findings are depicted in Figure 15.14. Unlike esotropia and exotropia, which are associated with strabismus, the eye misalignment that is associated with esophoria and exophoria is not always apparent. Instead, with esophoria and exophoria, the eye deviation is a tendency, and the eyes tend to function normally. However, if the misalignment is significant, it may cause eye strain and headache.

Nonparallel eye movements and failure of the eyes to follow in a certain direction are indicative of problems with extraocular muscles or cranial nerves. Figure 15.56 ■ provides details about the specific muscles and nerves associated with abnormal eye movement.

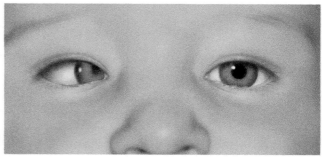

Esotropia

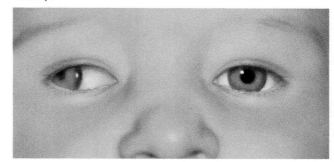

Exotropia

Figure 15.55 Strabismus.

Disruption of Function		
Muscle	**Cranial Nerve**	**Results**
Superior rectus	Oculomotor	Inability to move eye upward or temporally
Superior oblique	Trochlear	Inability to move eye down or nasally
Lateral rectus	Abducens	Inability to move eye temporally
Inferior oblique	Oculomotor	Inability to move eye upward or temporally
Inferior rectus	Oculomotor	Inability to move eye downward or temporally
Medial rectus	Oculomotor	Inability to move eye nasally

Figure 15.56 Extraocular muscle abnormalities.

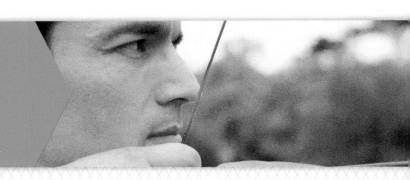

Application Through Critical Thinking

▌ Case Study

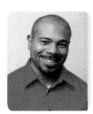

John Jerome is a 45-year-old African American male who made an appointment for an annual employment physical assessment. Mr. Jerome completed a written questionnaire in preparation for his meeting with a healthcare professional. He checked "none" for all categories of family history of disease except diabetes. He indicated that he knew of no changes in his health since his last assessment.

The following observations are made during the initial encounter with Mr. Jerome.

A tall, African American male wearing eyeglasses entered the room. He turned his head to the left and right and looked about the room before sitting across from the examiner. The patient had some redness in the sclera of both eyes. During the interview, the patient reveals that his last eye examination occurred 6 months ago, and he received a prescription for new glasses. He states that he is still having a problem with the new glasses and needs to have them checked. When asked to describe the problem, Mr. Jerome replies, "I just don't feel right with these glasses, and these are the second pair in a little over a year." He further states, "I just think I am overworking my eyes lately. I need to rest them more than ever and I have had some headaches. I thought the glasses would help, but it hasn't gotten better." The patient denies any other problems. In response to inquiries about family history, he reports that his mother had diabetes but had no problems with her eyes. He doesn't know of any other eye problems in his family, except his mother had told him that an aunt of hers had been blind for some time. He reiterates that his only problem of late had been "this thing with my glasses, otherwise I feel fine."

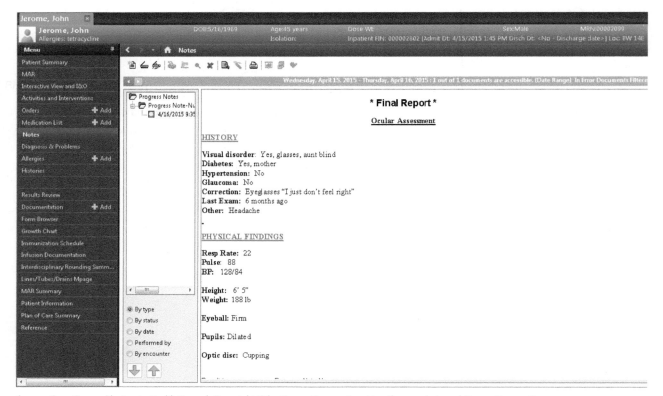

The physical assessment reveals the following:

- Vital signs: BP 128/84—P 88—RR 22

- Height 6′ 3″, weight 188 lb

- Eyeballs firm to palpation

- Moderately dilated pupils

- Cupping of the optic discs

▶ Complete Documentation

The following information is summarized from the case study.

SUBJECTIVE DATA: Visit for annual employment physical assessment. Negative family history except diabetes. No changes in health since last assessment. Last eye assessment 6 months ago—result prescription for new glasses. Stated he was having a problem with the new glasses. "I don't feel right with them." Stated, "I think I'm overworking my eyes lately. I thought the new glasses would help, but it hasn't gotten better." History of aunt with blindness.

OBJECTIVE DATA: Turns head to left and right and looked around room before sitting across from examiner. Scleral redness bilaterally. Eyeballs firm to palpation. Pupils moderate dilation. Cupping of optic discs. Height 6′3″, weight 188 lb. VS: BP 128/84—P 88—RR 22.

▶ Critical Thinking Questions

1. What conclusions would the nurse reach based on the data?

2. How was this conclusion formulated?

3. What information is missing?

4. What is the priority for this patient and what options would apply?

5. As Mr. Jerome ages, for what age-related vision changes will he be at risk?

▶ Prepare Teaching Plan

LEARNING NEED: The data in the case study revealed that Mr. Jerome was experiencing eye problems and had a family history of diabetes and blindness. Because of his history, he would be tested for diabetes and screened for diabetic retinopathy. His eye examination revealed cupping of the optic disc and slightly dilated pupils, both of which are associated with glaucoma. Blindness can occur with glaucoma and may have caused his aunt's blindness. Mr. Jerome will be referred for further evaluation of two suggested problems.

The case study provides data that are representative of risks, symptoms, and behaviors of many individuals. Therefore, the following teaching plan is based on the need to provide information to members of any community about glaucoma.

GOAL: The participants in this learning program will have increased awareness about glaucoma and follow recommendations for eye care.

OBJECTIVES: At the completion of this learning session, the participants will be able to:

1. Discuss glaucoma.

2. Identify risk factors associated with glaucoma.

3. List the diagnostic tests for glaucoma.

4. Describe recommendations for eye care.

APPLICATION OF OBJECTIVE 2: Identify risk factors associated with glaucoma

Content	Teaching Strategy	Evaluation
African Americans. Glaucoma is six to eight times more common in African Americans.	Lecture	Written examination.
Age. Individuals over the age of 60 are six times more likely to get glaucoma than younger people.	Discussion Audiovisual materials Printed materials	May use short answer, fill-in, or multiple choice items or a combination of items. If these are short and easy to evaluate, the learner receives immediate feedback.
Heredity. Individuals with a family history, especially immediate family, of glaucoma are at greater risk. Family history increases risk four to nine times.	Lecture is appropriate when disseminating information to large groups.	
Steroid use. Some evidence links glaucoma with steroid use. It is associated with high doses of steroids, for example, that would be used for severe asthma.	Discussion allows participants to bring up concerns and to raise questions. Audiovisual materials such as illustrations of the structures of the eye reinforce verbal presentation.	
Eye injury. Blunt trauma such as occurs with a blow to the head or blunt trauma to the eye in baseball or boxing can cause glaucoma immediately or years later.	Printed material, especially to be taken away with learners, allows review, reinforcement, and reading at the learner's pace.	

References

American Association for Pediatric Ophthalmology and Strabismus (AAPOS). (2012). *Hyphema*. Retrieved from http://www.aapos.org/terms/conditions/58

Berman, A., & Snyder, S. J. (2012). *Kozier and Erb's fundamentals of nursing: Concepts, process, and practice* (9th ed.). Upper Saddle River, NJ: Prentice Hall.

Bikley, L. S. (2008). *Bates' guide to physical examination and history taking* (10th ed.). Philadelphia: Lippincott.

Chen, M. L., Guo, L., Smith, L. E., Dammann, C. E., & Dammann, O. (2010). High or low oxygen saturation and severe retinopathy of prematurity: A meta-analysis. *Pediatrics, 125*(6), e1483–e1492.

Gilbert, C. (2013). The eye signs of vitamin A deficiency. *Community Eye Health Journal, 26*(84), 66–67.

Glaucoma Research Foundation. (2013). *African Americans and glaucoma*. Retrieved from http://www.glaucoma.org/glaucoma/african-americans-and-glaucoma.php

Glaucoma Research Foundation. (2012). *What is considered normal eye pressure?* Retrieved from http://www.glaucoma.org/q-a/what-is-considered-normal-pressure.php

Greiner, A. N., Hellings, P. W., Rotiroti, G., & Scadding, G. K. (2012). Allergic rhinitis. *Lancet, 378*(9809), 2112–2122.

Grosso, A., Cheung, N., Veglio, F., & Wong, T. Y. (2011). Similarities and differences in early retinal phenotypes in hypertension and diabetes. *Journal of Hypertension, 29*(9), 1667–1675.

Lim, L. S., Mitchell, P., Seddon, J. M., Holz, F. G., & Wong, T. Y. (2012). Age-related macular degeneration. *Lancet, 379*(9827): 1728–1738.

Marieb, E. (2009). *Essentials of human anatomy and physiology* (9th ed.). Redwood City, CA: Benjamin Cummings/Pearson Education.

Mayo Clinic. (2012). *Glaucoma: Symptoms*. Retrieved from http://www.mayoclinic.org/diseases-conditions/glaucoma/basics/symptoms/con-20024042

Mayo Foundation for Medical Education and Research. (2014). *Rochester test catalog: 2014 online test catalog*. Available at http://www.mayomedicallaboratories.com/tests-catalog

MedlinePlus. (2012). *Pterygium*. Retrieved from http://www.nlm.nih.gov/medlineplus/ency/article/001011.htm

MedlinePlus. (2013). *Visual acuity test*. Retrieved from http://www.nlm.nih.gov/medlineplus/ency/article/003396.htm

Medscape. (2012a). *Strabismus in infants: Screening in primary care*. Retrieved from http://www.medscape.com/viewarticle/759741

Medscape. (2012b). *Exophthalmos clinical presentation*. Retrieved from http://emedicine.medscape.com/article/1218575-overview

Murray, R. B., & Zentner, J. P. (2008). *Health promotion strategies, through the life span* (8th ed.). Upper Saddle River, NJ: Prentice Hall.

Osborn K. S., Wraa, C. E., Watson, A., & Holleran, R. S. (2013). *Medical-surgical nursing: Preparation for practice* (2nd ed.). Upper Saddle River, NJ: Pearson.

Pender, N. J., Murdaugh, C. L., & Parsons, M. A. (2011). *Health promotion in nursing practice* (6th ed.). Upper Saddle River, NJ: Prentice Hall.

Tarlan, B., & Kiratli, H. (2013). Subconjunctival hemorrhage: Risk factors and potential indicators. *Clinical Ophthalmology, 7*, 1163.

Tortora, G. J., & Derrickson, B. H. (2009). *Principles of anatomy and physiology* (12th ed.). New York: John Wiley & Sons.

United States Department of Health and Human Services (USDHHS). (2014). *Healthy people 2020*. Retrieved from http://www.healthypeople.gov/2020/default.aspx

University of Iowa. (2014). *Instructions for handling contact lenses*. Retrieved from https://www.uihealthcare.org/2column.aspx?id=225660

WebMD. (2012a). *Caring for your contact lenses and your eyes*. Retrieved from http://www.webmd.com/eye-health/caring-contact-lens

WebMD. (2012b). *Eye floaters: Benign*. Retrieved from http://www.webmd.com/eye-health/benign-eye-floaters

WebMD. (2012c). *Signs of vision problems in young kids*. Retrieved from http://www.webmd.com/eye-health/features/child-eye-and-vision-problems

Wilson, B. A., Shannon, M. T., & Shields, K. M. (2013). *Pearson nurse's drug guide*. Upper Saddle River, NJ: Pearson.

World Health Organization (WHO). (n.d.). *Ultraviolet radiation and the INTERSUN programme: Health effects of UV radiation*. Retrieved from http://www.who.int/uv/health/en/

Zuppa, A. A., D'Andrea, V., Catenazzi, P., Scorrano, A., & Romagnoli, C. (2011). Ophthalmia neonatorum: What kind of prophylaxis? *Journal of Maternal-Fetal and Neonatal Medicine, 24*(6), 769–773.

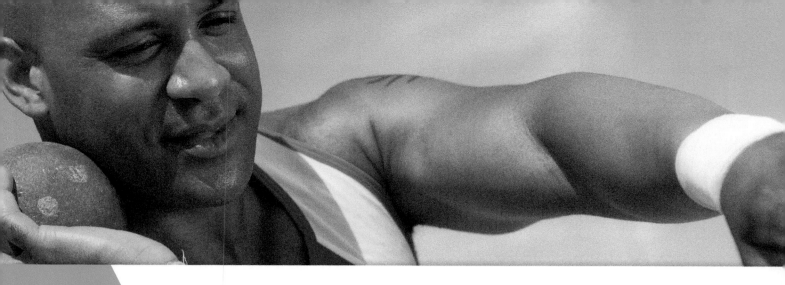

▌ Learning Outcomes

Upon completion of this chapter, you will be able to:

1. Describe the anatomy and physiology of the ear, nose, mouth, and throat.

2. Develop questions to be used when completing the focused interview.

3. Outline the techniques used for assessment of the structures of the ear, nose, mouth, and throat.

4. Demonstrate correct use of the otoscope.

5. Differentiate normal from abnormal findings in the physical assessment of the ear, nose, mouth, and throat.

6. Describe the developmental, psychosocial, cultural, and environmental variations in assessment techniques and findings.

7. Relate ear, nose, and throat health to *Healthy People 2020* objectives.

8. Apply critical thinking to the physical assessment of the structures of the ear, nose, mouth, and throat.

▌ Key Terms

air conduction, 352
auricle, 330
bone conduction, 352
cerumen, 330
cheilitis, 338
cochlea, 330
cold sores, 358
eustachian tube, 330
fever blisters, 358
helix, 330
lobule, 330
mastoiditis, 349
nasal polyps, 355
ossicles, 330
otitis externa, 341
otitis media, 337
palate, 333
paranasal sinuses, 331
pinna, 330
presbycusis, 338
tragus, 330
tympanic membrane, 330
uvula, 332

The structures of the ear, nose, mouth, and throat are responsible for the senses of hearing, smell, and taste. Each of these body systems is discussed in this chapter and again when describing the neurologic assessment in chapter 26. ∞

The interrelationships of the senses, and their structures, provide data for several body systems. For example, the sense of smell in the nose also impacts the respiratory and digestive systems. Hearing and oral health are discussed in *Healthy People 2020*. Objectives related to these areas include improvement in hearing and the prevention and control of oral diseases and conditions, as discussed later in this chapter.

Anatomy and Physiology Review

The anatomic structures of the ear, nose, mouth, and throat include the internal and external ear, the nose and sinuses, the oral cavity, and the pharynx (throat). Each of the structures is described in the following sections.

Ear

The ear is the sensory organ that functions in hearing and equilibrium. It is divided into the external, middle, and inner ear. The external portion, or what most people think of as the ear, is called the **auricle** or **pinna.** It has a shell of cartilage covered with skin that funnels sound into the meatus (opening) of the external auditory canal.

External Ear

Figure 16.1 ■ depicts the surface anatomy of the external ear. The external large rim of the auricle is called the **helix.** The **tragus** is a stiff projection that protects the anterior meatus of the auditory canal. The **lobule** of the ear is a small flap of flesh at the inferior end of the auricle. The external auditory canal is about 1 in. (2.54 cm) in length, is S-shaped, and leads to the middle ear. It is lined with glands that secrete a yellow-brown wax called **cerumen.** These secretions lubricate and protect the ear. The functions of chewing and talking help move the cerumen in the canal. The mastoid process, part of the temporal bone of the skull, is adjacent to the cavity of the middle ear. It contains many air cells and is assessed with the ear. This process has no role in hearing or balance. The mastoid process may become infected following ear infections in the adult.

Middle Ear

The external ear and middle ear are separated by the **tympanic membrane** or eardrum (see Figure 16.2 ■). This thin, translucent membrane is pearly gray in color and lies obliquely in the canal. Sound waves entering the auditory canal strike the membrane, causing it to vibrate. The vibrations are transferred to the **ossicles,** or bones of the middle ear: the malleus, the incus, and the stapes. The ossicles, in turn, transfer the vibration to the oval window of the inner ear. Note that the malleus projects inferiorly and laterally and can be seen through the translucent tympanic membrane when viewed with the otoscope. The **eustachian tube** or auditory tube connects the middle ear with the nasopharynx. These tubes help to equalize air pressure on both sides of the tympanic membrane. The middle ear functions to conduct sound vibrations from the external

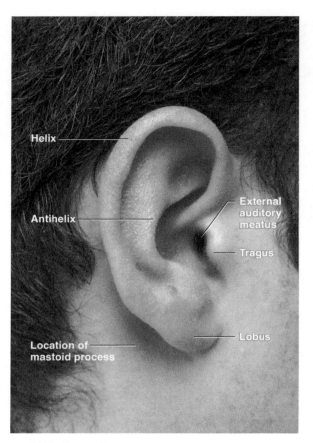

Figure 16.1 External ear.

ear to the inner ear. It also protects the inner ear by reducing loud sound vibrations.

Inner Ear

The inner ear contains the bony labyrinth, which consists of a central cavity called the vestibule; three semicircular canals responsible for the sense of equilibrium; and the **cochlea,** a spiraling chamber that contains the receptors for hearing. Impulses from the equilibrium receptors of the inner ear are sent via the eighth cranial nerve to the brain. Responses are then initiated to activate the eyes and muscles of the body to maintain balance. The cochlea transmits sound vibrations to the auditory nerve (cranial nerve VIII), which in turn carries the impulse to the auditory cortex in the temporal lobe of the brain for interpretation as hearing.

The major functions of the ears are collecting and transporting sound vibrations to the brain and maintaining the sense of equilibrium.

Nose and Sinuses

The nose is a triangular projection of bone and cartilage situated midline on the face (see Figure 16.3 ■). It is the only externally visible organ of the respiratory system. During inspiration, air enters the nasal cavity where it is filtered, warmed, and moistened before it moves toward the trachea and lungs.

The nose consists of external and internal structures. Externally, the bridge of the nose is on the superior aspect of the nose, medial to each orbit of the eyes. Inferior to the bridge and free of attachment

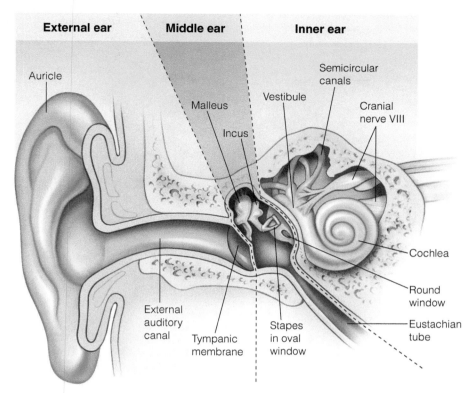

Figure 16.2 The three parts of the ear.

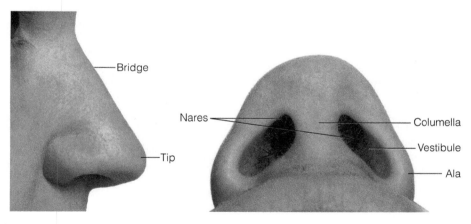

Figure 16.3 The nose.

to the face is the tip of the nose. The nares, two oval external openings at the base of the nose, are surrounded by the columella and ala structures of cartilage. Each nare widens into the internal vestibule and nasal cavity. The nasal septum is a continuation of the columella, dividing the nose into a right and left side.

The nasal mucosa with its rich blood supply helps filter inspired air and has a redder appearance than the oral mucosa. Three turbinates (superior, middle, and inferior) project from the medial wall into each side of the nasal cavity. These bony projections, covered with nasal mucosa, add surface area for cleaning, moistening, and warming air entering the respiratory tract. Each side of the posterior nasal cavity opens into the nasopharynx (see Figure 16.4 ■).

The olfactory cells, located in the roof of the nasal cavity, form filaments that connect to the olfactory nerve (cranial nerve I) and are responsible for the sense of smell.

The **paranasal sinuses** are mucus-lined, air-filled cavities that surround the nasal cavity and perform the same air-processing functions of filtration, moistening, and warming. They are named for the bones of the skull in which they are contained: sphenoid, frontal, ethmoid, and maxillary. The frontal and maxillary sinuses are accessible to examination and are discussed later in this chapter (see Figure 16.5 ■).

The major functions of the nose and sinuses are the following:

- Providing an airway for respiration.
- Filtering, warming, and humidifying air flowing into the respiratory tract.
- Providing resonance for the voice.
- Housing the receptors for olfaction.

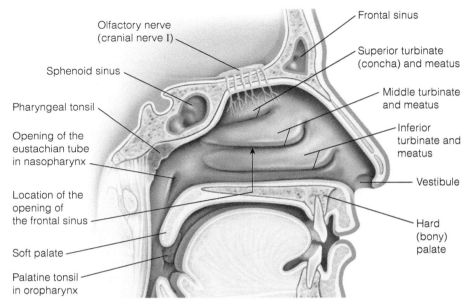

Figure 16.4 Internal structure of the nose—lateral view.

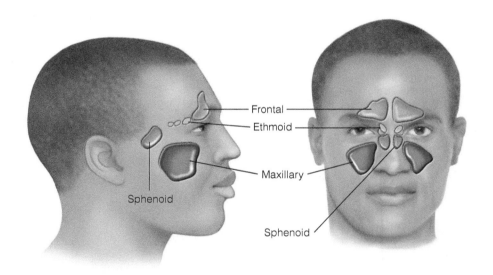

Figure 16.5 Nasal sinuses.

Mouth

The oral cavity, an oval-shaped cavity, is the beginning of the alimentary canal and digestive system (see Figure 16.6 ■). The oral cavity is divided into two parts by the teeth: the vestibule and the mouth. The vestibule, the anterior and smaller of the two regions, is composed of the lips, the buccal mucosa, the outer surface of the gums and teeth, and the cheeks. At the posterior aspect of the teeth, the mouth is formed and includes the tongue, the hard and soft palate, the **uvula,** and the mandibular arch and maxillary arch.

The lips are folds of skin that cover the underlying muscle. They help keep food in place when chewing, and they play a role in speech. The cheeks form the side of the face and are continuous with the lips. Like the lips, the skin covers the underlying

muscle. Both the lips and cheeks are lined internally with mucous membranes.

The gingivae or gums are bands of fibrous tissue that surround each tooth. The gums cover the mandibular and maxillary arches.

Thirty-two permanent teeth in the adult and 20 deciduous teeth (also called baby teeth or primary teeth) in the child sit in the alveoli sockets of the mandible and maxilla (see Figure 16.7 ■). The enamel-covered crown is the visible portion of the tooth. The root, embedded in the jawbone, helps hold the tooth in place. Teeth are used for biting and chewing of food.

The tongue, the organ for taste, sits on the floor of the mouth. Its base sits on the hyoid bone. The anterior portion of the tongue is attached to the floor of the mouth by the frenulum. The ventral

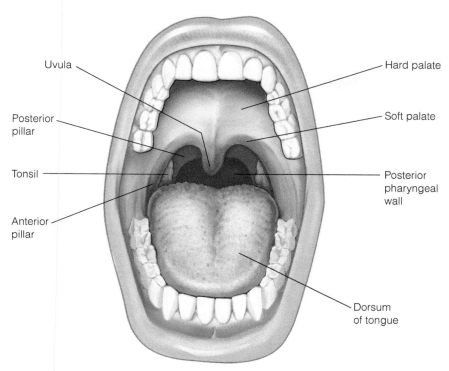

Uvula

Posterior
pillar

Tonsil

Anterior
pillar

Hard palate

Soft palate

Posterior
pharyngeal
wall

Dorsum
of tongue

Figure 16.6 Oral cavity.

surface (undersurface) of the tongue is smooth with visible vessels. The dorsal (top) surface of the tongue is rough and supports the papillae. Papillae contain the taste buds and assist with moving food in the mouth. Taste buds are distributed throughout the tongue and are innervated by the facial and glossopharyngeal nerves (see Figure 16.8 ■). The tongue also assists with speech and swallowing. These actions are stimulated by the hypoglossal nerve (cranial nerve XII).

Hard and soft palates form the roof of the mouth. The hard **palate,** formed by bones, is the anterior portion of the roof of the mouth. The soft palate, formed by muscle, does not have a bony structure and is the posterior and somewhat mobile aspect of the roof of the mouth. The uvula hangs from the free edge of the soft palate. The uvula and soft palate move with swallowing, breathing, and phonation and are innervated by cranial nerves IX and X.

Parotid, submandibular, and sublingual salivary glands are responsible for the production of saliva (see Figure 16.9 ■). The parotid glands are situated anterior to the ear within the cheek. Saliva enters the mouth via Stensen's duct located in the buccal mucosa opposite the second upper molar. The submandibular glands sit beneath the mandible at the angle of the jaw. Saliva from these glands enters the mouth via Wharton's duct. The orifice of these ducts is on either side of the frenulum on the floor of the mouth. The sublingual salivary glands, the smallest of the glands, are situated in the floor of the mouth and have many ducts that empty into the floor of the mouth.

Throat

The throat, known as the pharynx, connects the nose, mouth, larynx, and esophagus. The three sections of the throat are the nasopharynx (behind the nose), the oropharynx (behind the mouth),

and the laryngopharynx (behind the larynx). The nasopharynx is behind the nose and above the soft palate. The adenoids and openings of the eustachian tubes are located in the nasopharynx.

The oropharynx is behind the mouth and below the nasopharynx. It extends to the epiglottis and serves as a passageway for air and food. The tonsils are located behind the pillars (palatopharyngeal folds) on either side.

Special Considerations

The nurse must be aware that variations in findings from health assessment occur in relation to age, developmental level, race, ethnicity, work history, living conditions, socioeconomics, and emotional well-being. The following sections describe some factors to consider when collecting subjective and objective data.

Health Promotion Considerations

As part of preventing hearing loss, screening for hearing deficits is included among the *Healthy People 2020* objectives related to promoting health of the ears, nose, and throat. Goals of this national initiative also include encouraging individuals to seek assessment and treatment of sensory-related disorders. In addition, *Healthy People 2020* aims to increase healthcare-related use of the Internet among individuals who are experiencing sensory loss, including hearing deficits.

With regard to promotion of oral health, *Healthy People 2020* objectives center on prevention of tooth decay and increasing access to care for individuals who develop tooth decay. In addition, increasing access to preventative dental care is emphasized.

Upper deciduous teeth

Age tooth comes in

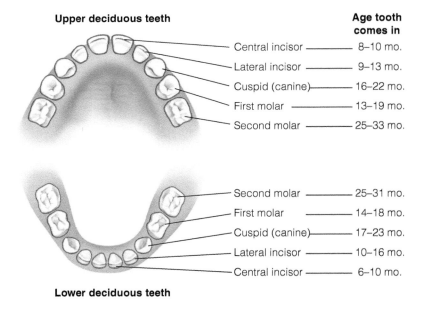

Central incisor	8–10 mo.
Lateral incisor	9–13 mo.
Cuspid (canine)	16–22 mo.
First molar	13–19 mo.
Second molar	25–33 mo.
Second molar	25–31 mo.
First molar	14–18 mo.
Cuspid (canine)	17–23 mo.
Lateral incisor	10–16 mo.
Central incisor	6–10 mo.

Lower deciduous teeth

Age tooth comes in

Upper permanent teeth

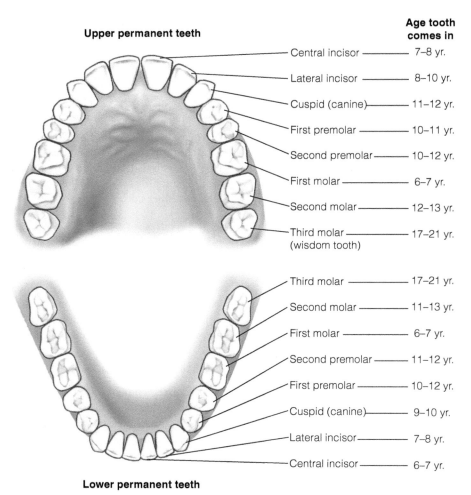

Central incisor	7–8 yr.
Lateral incisor	8–10 yr.
Cuspid (canine)	11–12 yr.
First premolar	10–11 yr.
Second premolar	10–12 yr.
First molar	6–7 yr.
Second molar	12–13 yr.
Third molar (wisdom tooth)	17–21 yr.
Third molar	17–21 yr.
Second molar	11–13 yr.
First molar	6–7 yr.
Second premolar	11–12 yr.
First premolar	10–12 yr.
Cuspid (canine)	9–10 yr.
Lateral incisor	7–8 yr.
Central incisor	6–7 yr.

Lower permanent teeth

Figure 16.7 Deciduous and permanent teeth.

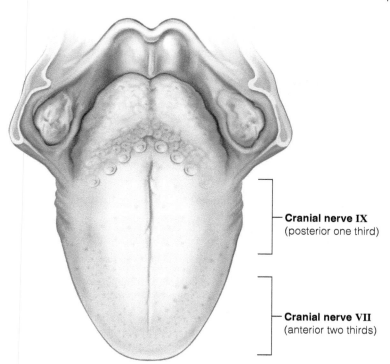

Figure 16.8 Innervation of the tongue.

Cranial nerve IX
(posterior one third)

Cranial nerve VII
(anterior two thirds)

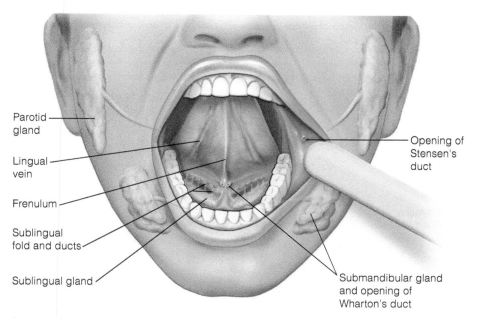

Parotid
gland

Lingual
vein

Frenulum

Sublingual
fold and ducts

Sublingual gland

Opening of
Stensen's
duct

Submandibular gland
and opening of
Wharton's duct

Figure 16.9 Salivary glands.

See Table 16.1 for selected examples of *Healthy People 2020* objectives that are designed to promote health and wellness among individuals across the life span.

Lifespan Considerations

Changes in anatomy and physiology occur during growth and development. The ability to interpret data in relation to the normative values at various ages is important in the assessment process.

Specific variations for different age groups are presented in the following sections.

Infants and Children

The infant's auditory canal is shorter than the adult's and has an upward curve, which persists until about 3 years of age. The nurse should pull the earlobe down and back when examining the tympanic membrane with the otoscope of children age 3 years and younger, as illustrated in Figure 16.10 ■.

TABLE 16.1	Examples of *Healthy People 2020* Objectives Related to Ear, Nose, and Throat Health
OBJECTIVE NUMBER	**DESCRIPTION**
ENT-VSL-1	Increase the proportion of newborns who are screened for hearing loss by no later than age 1 month, have audiologic evaluation by age 3 months, and are enrolled in appropriate intervention services no later than age 6 months
ENT-VSL-2	Reduce otitis media in children and adolescents
ENT-VSL-3	Increase the proportion of persons with hearing impairments who have ever used a hearing aid or assistive listening devices or who have cochlear implants
ENT-VSL-4	Increase the proportion of persons who have had a hearing examination on schedule
ENT-VSL-5/6	Increase the number of persons who are referred by their primary care physician or other healthcare provider for hearing evaluation and treatment. Increase the use of hearing protection devices
ENT-VSL-9	Increase the proportion of adults bothered by tinnitus who have seen a doctor or other healthcare professionals
ENT-VSL-16	(Developmental) Increase the proportion of adults with chemosensory (smell or taste) disorders who have seen a healthcare provider about their disorder in the past 12 months
ENT-VSL-23	(Developmental) Increase the proportion of persons with hearing loss and other sensory or communication disorders who have used Internet resources for healthcare information, guidance, or advice in the past 12 months
OH-1	Reduce the proportion of children and adolescents who have dental caries experience in their primary or permanent teeth
OH-2	Reduce the proportion of children and adolescents with untreated dental decay
OH-3	Reduce the proportion of adults with untreated dental decay
OH-9	Increase the proportion of school-based health centers with an oral health component
OH-14	(Developmental) Increase the proportion of adults who receive preventive interventions in dental offices

Source: U.S. Department of Health and Human Services (USDHHS). (2014). *Healthy People 2020.* Retrieved from http://www.healthypeople.gov/2020/default.aspx

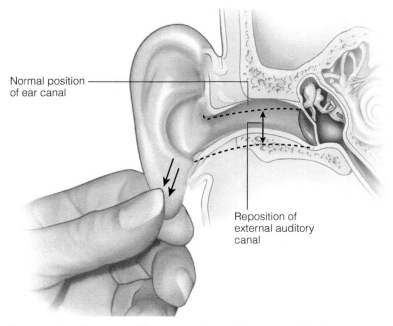

Normal position of ear canal

Reposition of external auditory canal

Figure 16.10 Positioning of external auditory canal for tympanic membrane visualization.

The eustachian tubes of infants, toddlers, and preschoolers are shorter, straighter, and more level than those in older children and adults. This normal variant, in combination with increased frequency of colds and respiratory infections, results in an increased incidence of **otitis media,** or middle ear infections, in children under the age of 4. The occurrence of otitis media peaks between 6 and 18 months of age. Children with middle ear infections typically present with fever, decreased appetite, irritability, and the inability to sleep lying down. The tympanic membrane is a vascular tissue that appears red with infection, fever, or any condition that results in skin flushing. Children with red tympanic membranes and no purulent discharge in the middle ear space do not have bacterial otitis media.

The nose of a child is too small to examine with a speculum. The maxillary and ethmoid sinuses are present at birth, but they are proportionately smaller than in adults. The sphenoid sinuses develop before age 5 and the frontal sinuses by age 10. Children rarely have infections of the ethmoid sinuses. The frontal sinuses cause infection only in older school-age and adolescent children. Children under the age of 5 years often have yellow-green nasal discharge during upper respiratory infections because they cannot efficiently clear their nasal passages.

Both sets of teeth develop before birth. Deciduous (baby) teeth begin to erupt between 6 months and 2 years of age. Eruption of permanent teeth begins at around age 6 and continues through adolescence. Salivation begins at 3 months of age. Drooling of saliva occurs for several months until swallowing saliva is learned. Figure 16.11 ■ shows a typical sequence of tooth eruption for both deciduous and permanent teeth.

Because differentiation and growth of lymphatic tissue occur primarily between ages 4 and 8 years, preschoolers and school-age children often have slightly enlarged tonsils. Enlarged, noninfected tonsils are common in children ages 4 to 8.

The Pregnant Female

Changes in estrogen levels cause increased vascularity throughout the body in pregnancy. Vessel changes of the middle ear may cause a feeling of fullness or earaches. Increased blood flow (hyperemia) to the sinuses can cause rhinitis (inflammation of the nasal cavity) and epistaxis (nosebleed). The sense of smell is heightened in pregnancy. Edema of the vocal cords may cause hoarseness or deepening of the voice. Hyperemia of the throat can lead to an increase in snoring. Small blood vessels and connective tissue increase in the mouth. As a result, gingivitis or inflammation of the gums occurs in many females, which leads to bleeding and discomfort with brushing of the teeth and eating. Occasionally, a hyperplastic overgrowth forms a mass on the gums called *epulis,* which bleeds easily and recedes after birth.

The Older Adult

The older adult may have coarse hairs at the opening of the auditory meatus. The ears may appear more prominent, because cartilage formation continues throughout life. The tympanic membrane becomes paler in color and thicker in appearance with aging. Assessment of hearing may reveal a loss of high-frequency tones, which is consistent with aging. Over time, this loss often progresses to

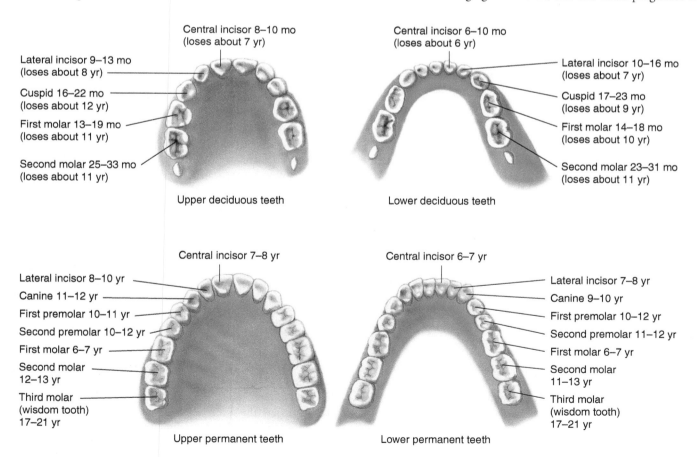

Figure 16.11 Typical sequence of tooth eruption for both deciduous and permanent teeth.

lower-frequency sounds as well. Gradual hearing loss with age is called **presbycusis.** Older patient may complain that they do not hear consonants well when listening to normal conversation. This is due to the loss of hair cells in the organ of Corti in the inner ear. However, conductive sound loss can often occur due to an accumulation of earwax that is drier and becomes more impacted than in a younger person. Any older persons complaining of difficulty in hearing should be checked for outer ear canal blockage and have their ears cleaned before any further testing is performed.

The senses of smell and taste diminish with age because of a decrease in olfactory fibers, taste buds, and saliva production. In some older persons, however, saliva increases, causing **cheilitis** (angular stomatitis), which manifests as tissue inflammation at the corners of the mouth. The lips and buccal mucosa become thinner and less vascular with age. Gums are paler in color. The tongue develops more fissures, and motor function may become impaired, resulting in problems with swallowing. Senile tremors may cause slight protrusion of the tongue. A decreased sense of taste and smell may contribute to a decreased appetite and poor nutrition. There may also be a decreased production of saliva. This may be due to atrophy of the salivary glands or a side effect of a medication.

Older adults typically demonstrate gum recession. Tooth loss may occur due to osteoporosis. Partial or complete loss of teeth may also be found, especially in the oldest adults who lived half of their lives before the use of prophylactic fluoride and other modern dental care. Poor dental health is decreasing, dental care is improving for people of all ages, and the current generation of older adults has lived most of their lives drinking fluoridated water and observing modern dental hygiene. Lost teeth may cause the remaining teeth to drift. Ill-fitting dentures can produce oral lesions. Edentulism can give the mouth a pursed or sunken look. Individuals with and without teeth should be examined for gingivitis and signs of periodontal disease. This pathology must be differentiated from normal gums that may recede to an extent, making teeth appear longer.

Psychosocial Considerations

A patient who is under a great deal of stress may be prone to mouth ulcers and lip biting. Tics (involuntary muscle spasms) and unconscious clenching of the jaw may indicate psychosocial disturbances. Relaxation techniques such as meditation and guided imagery may help relieve these stress-related behaviors.

Cultural and Environmental Considerations

Dark-skinned patients may have darker cerumen in the ear, and their oral mucosa may be darker. People of European ancestry tend to have more tooth decay and tooth loss than people of African ancestry. The size of the teeth varies with cultural ancestry. People of European descent have the smallest teeth; Asians, Alaska Natives, and Australian Aborigines have the largest.

A patient's occupation may increase the risk for hearing loss if the nature of the work or work environment exposes the patient to high noise levels. For example, construction workers, welders, groundskeepers, and musicians should be evaluated for hearing acuity and also should be advised to use earplugs. Noise levels in the home may also need to be evaluated.

Cerumen appearance may vary based on cultural background. For example, individuals who are of East Asian descent tend to produce dry, colorless cerumen, while individuals who are of African descent commonly produce moist cerumen that is yellowish-brown in color. Among White individuals, cerumen tends to be sticky and yellow (Prokop-Prigge, Thaler, Wysocki, & Preti, 2014).

Among pediatric patients, socioeconomic status is one of the most significant predictors of the development of otitis media. Children of lower socioeconomic status are at increased risk for development of this form of ear infection (Smith & Boss, 2010).

A patient's socioeconomic status may affect the appearance and function of the structures of the mouth. For example, many patients do not have dental insurance and cannot afford regular dental care. Referral to a low-cost dental clinic or a dental school offering free care may be appropriate. The incidence of cleft lip and cleft palate is highest among individuals who are of Asian descent (USDHHS Office of Minority Health, 2009).

A patient's enthic background may contribute to cleft uvula, also called bifid uvula or split uvula. Native Americans have a high rate of cleft uvula, with 8%–11% of infants being born with cleft uvula. In contrast, African Americans have a low rate of cleft uvula, with less than 1% of infants being born with cleft uvula. Cleft uvula is usually a sign of submucosal cleft palate or Loeys-Dietz syndrome (McMillan, Feigin, DeAngelis, & Jones, 2006).

Gathering the Data

Health assessment of the ears, nose, mouth, and throat includes gathering subjective and objective data. Recall that subjective data collection occurs during the patient interview, before the actual physical assessment. During the interview the nurse uses a variety of communication techniques to elicit general and specific information about the state of health or illness of the patient's ears, nose, mouth, and throat. Health records, the results of laboratory tests, and x-rays are important secondary sources to be reviewed and included in the data-gathering process. The techniques of inspection, palpation, and percussion will be used in the physical assessment of the ears, nose, mouth, and throat. Before proceeding, it may be helpful to review the information about each of the data-gathering processes and practice the techniques of health assessment. Some special equipment and assessments are included—for example, the use of the otoscope. See Table 16.2 for information on potential secondary sources of patient data.

TABLE 16.2 **Potential Secondary Sources for Patient Data Related to the Ears, Nose, Mouth, and Throat**

Laboratory Tests for the Ear, Nose, Mouth, and Throat
Cultures and Sensitivity
Diagnostic Tests
Ear
>   Audiometric Screening
>   Auditory Screening
>   Electronystagmography
>   X-ray

Nose and Sinuses
>   Computed Tomography (CT)
>   X-ray

Teeth
>   X-ray

Throat
>   Laryngoscopy

The nurse must be prepared to observe the patient and listen for cues related to the functions of these structures. The nurse may use open-ended and closed questions to obtain information. Follow-up questions or requests for descriptions are required to clarify data or gather missing information. Follow-up questions identify the source of problems, duration of difficulties, and measures to alleviate problems. They also provide clues about the patient's knowledge about his or her own health.

The focused interview guides the physical assessment of the ears, nose, mouth, and throat. The information is always considered in relation to normative parameters and expectations about function. Therefore, the nurse must consider age, gender, race, culture, environment, health practices, past and concurrent problems, and therapies when framing questions and using techniques to elicit information. In order to address all of the factors when conducting a focused interview, categories of questions have been developed. These categories include general questions that are asked of all patients; those addressing illness, infection; questions related to symptoms, pain, behaviors; those related to habits or practices; questions that are specific to patients according to age; those for the pregnant female; and questions that address environmental concerns. One method to elicit information about symptoms is the OLDCART & ICE method, described in chapter 7. ∞

The nurse must consider the patient's ability to participate in the focused interview and physical assessment of the ears, nose, mouth, and throat. If a patient is experiencing pain, discomfort, or anxiety, attention must focus on relief of symptoms.

Focused Interview

The focused interview concerns data related to the structures and functions of the ears, nose, mouth, and throat. Subjective data related to these structures are gathered during the focused interview.

Focused Interview Questions	Rationales and Evidence
The following section provides sample questions and bulleted follow-up questions in each of the previously identified categories. For assessment of the ears, a rationale for each of the questions is provided. The list of questions is not all inclusive but represents the types of questions required in a comprehensive focused interview related to the ears. Questions for the nose, mouth, and throat are included. These questions would follow the same format and be categorized as those for the ear. The bulleted	*follow-up questions are asked to seek clarification. This additional information from the patient expands the subjective database. Remember that the subjective data collected and the questions asked during the health history and the focused interview will provide information to help meet the goals of improving hearing and preventing and controlling oral diseases as described in* Healthy People 2020.

General Questions

1. **Describe your hearing. Have you noticed any change in your hearing? If so, tell me about:**
   - *Onset:* Gradual or sudden?
   - *Character:* Just certain sounds or tones, or all hearing?
   - *Situations:* When using a telephone? Watching television? During conversations?

   ▶ The patient's failure to respond to questions, or asking the nurse to repeat questions, may indicate a hearing loss. Hearing acuity decreases gradually with age. Any sudden loss of hearing should be investigated.

2. **When was your last hearing test?**
   - What were the results?
   - Does your hearing seem better in one ear than the other?
   - Which ear?

   ▶ Infants should have a full hearing test before 3 months of age. In children, hearing tests should be conducted prior to beginning school and whenever hearing problems are suspected (CDC, 2012a). Individuals who live or work in noisy environments should have annual hearing tests (CDC, 2011). Hearing loss in one ear could indicate an obstruction with cerumen or a ruptured tympanic membrane (American Speech-Language-Hearing Association [ASHA], n.d.).

3. **Has any member of your family had ear problems or hearing loss?**

   ▶ Hearing loss can be hereditary (ASHA, n.d.).

Focused Interview Questions	Rationales and Evidence

Questions Related to Illness or Infection

1. **Have you ever been diagnosed with a disease affecting the ears?**
   - When were you diagnosed with the problem?
   - What treatment was prescribed for the problem?
   - What kinds of things do you do to help with the problem?
   - Has the problem ever recurred (acute)?
   - How are you managing the disease now (chronic)?

▶ The patient has an opportunity to provide information about specific illnesses affecting the ears. If a diagnosed illness is identified, follow-up about the diagnosis, treatment, and outcomes is required. Data about each illness identified by the patient are essential to an accurate health assessment. Illnesses are classified as acute or chronic, and follow-up regarding each classification will differ.

2. **An alternative to question 1 is to list possible illnesses of the ears, such as Ménière's disease, vertigo, and acoustic neuroma, and ask the patient to respond "yes" or "no" as each is stated.**

▶ This is a comprehensive and easy way to elicit information about all diagnoses related to the ear. Follow-up would be carried out for each identified diagnosis as in question 1.

3. **Do you now have or have you had an ear infection?**
   - When were you diagnosed with the infection?
   - What treatment was prescribed for the problem?
   - Was the treatment helpful?
   - What kinds of things do you do to help with the problem?
   - Has the problem ever recurred (acute)?
   - How are you managing the infection now (chronic)?

▶ If an infection is identified, follow-up about the date of infection, treatment, and outcomes is required. Data about each infection identified by the patient are essential to an accurate health assessment. Infections can be classified as acute or chronic, and follow-up regarding each classification will differ.

4. **An alternative to question 3 is to list possible ear infections, such as external otitis, otitis media, labyrinthitis, and mastoiditis, and ask the patient to respond "yes" or "no" as each is stated.**

▶ This is a comprehensive and easy way to elicit information about all ear infections. Follow-up would be carried out for each identified infection as in question 3.

Questions Related to Symptoms, Pain, and Behaviors

When gathering information about symptoms, many questions are required to elicit details and descriptions that assist in the analysis of the data. Discrimination is made in relation to the significance of a symptom, in relation to specific diseases or problems, and in relation to potential follow-up examination or referral. One rationale may be provided for a group of questions in this category.

The following questions refer to specific symptoms and behaviors associated with the ear. For each symptom, questions and follow-up are required. The details to be elicited are the characteristics of the symptom; the onset, duration, and frequency of the symptom; the treatment or remedy for the symptom including over-the-counter and home remedies; the determination if diagnosis has been sought; the effect of treatments; and family history associated with a symptom or illness.

Questions Related to Symptoms

1. **Have you had any ear drainage? If so, describe it.**

▶ Ear drainage may indicate an infection. Bloody or purulent drainage could indicate otitis media, or infection of the middle ear. Serous drainage could indicate allergic reaction. Clear drainage could be cerebrospinal fluid following trauma (Osborn, Wraa, Watson, & Holleran, 2013).

2. **Have you had dizziness, nausea, vomiting, or ringing in your ears?**

▶ These symptoms could indicate a problem with the inner ear, could be related to a neurologic problem, or could be drug related (ASHA, n.d.).

Questions Related to Pain

1. **Do you have any pain in your ears?**
   - If so, describe it. If yes, have you recently had a cold or sore throat?
   - Have you had any problems lately with your sinuses or your teeth?
   - Have you had any ear trauma or ear surgery?

▶ Pain in one or both ears may be caused by acute otitis media, otitis externa, foreign bodies or trauma, temporomandibular joint syndrome, dental problems, pharyngitis, tonsillitis, and other diseases (Ely, Hansen, & Clark, 2008).

Focused Interview Questions	Rationales and Evidence

Questions Related to Behaviors

1. **How do you clean your ears?**

▶ Many people use cotton-tipped applicators to remove cerumen. This practice can cause trauma to the eardrum and cause cerumen to become impacted. Ear canals should never be cleaned. Cerumen moves to the outside naturally. Commercial cerumen removal products are available but should be used with the guidance of a healthcare provider (Mason, 2013).

2. **Do you either own or use a hearing aid?**

▶ Some patients have hearing aids but will not use them because of increased background noise, embarrassment, or inability to pay for the necessary batteries.

Questions Related to the Environment

Environment refers to both the internal and external environments. Questions related to the internal environment include all of the previous questions and those associated with internal or physiologic responses. Questions regarding the external environment include those related to home, work, or social environments.

Internal Environment

1. **Are you taking any medications?**
   - What are they?
   - How often do you take them?

▶ Certain medicines affect the ears. Aspirin can cause ringing in the ears (tinnitus). Some antibiotics can cause hearing loss and dizziness (Wilson, Shannon, & Shields, 2013).

External Environment

The following questions deal with substances and irritants found in the physical environment of the patient. The physical environment includes the indoor and outdoor environments of the home and workplace, those encountered for social engagements, and any encountered during travel.

1. **Are you frequently exposed to loud noise?**
   - When?
   - How often?
   - Are protective devices available and do you use them?

▶ Long-term exposure to loud noise can result in hearing loss. Patients at risk are those with jobs in noisy factories; jobs at airports; jobs requiring the use of explosives, firearms, jackhammers, or other loud equipment; and jobs in nightclubs. Frequent exposure to loud music, either live or from stereos or headphones, can also contribute to hearing loss (ASHA, n.d.).

2. **Do you experience ear infections or irritations after swimming or being exposed to dust or smoke? If so, describe them.**

▶ Contaminated water left in the ear may cause **otitis externa,** or swimmer's ear. Irritation of the ear after exposure to certain substances may indicate an allergy to such substances (Osborn et al., 2013).

Questions Related to Age

The focused interview must reflect the anatomic and physiologic differences that exist along the age span. The following questions are presented as examples of those that would be specific for infants and children, pregnant females, and older adults.

Questions Regarding Infants and Children

1. **Does the child have recurrent ear infections?**
   - How many ear infections has the child had in the last 6 months?
   - How were they treated?
   - Has the child had any ear surgery such as insertion of ear tubes?
   - When?
   - What were the results?
   - Does the child attend day care?

▶ Recurrent or chronic ear infections may lead to more serious conditions, including perforation of the tympanic membrane (eardrum). Especially in infants and toddlers, significant periods of hearing impairment can lead to delayed speech development. In rare cases, untreated recurrent ear infections may spread to structures in the skull, including the brain (Mayo Clinic, 2013).

Focused Interview Questions	Rationales and Evidence
2. Does the child tug at his or her ears?	▶ Tugging at the ears can be an early sign of infection (Shaikh et al., 2009).
3. Does the child respond to loud noises?	▶ A lack of response could indicate hearing loss (CDC, 2012a).
4. If the child is over 6 months of age, does the child babble?	▶ A child who does not babble may have a hearing impairment (CDC, 2012a).
5. Have you ever had the child's hearing tested? ● What were the results?	
6. Has the child had measles, mumps, or any disease with a high fever? ● Has the child been treated recently with any antibiotics such as streptomycin or neomycin?	▶ High fevers and certain drugs can cause hearing loss (Osborn et al., 2013).
7. How do you clean the child's ears?	▶ The nurse should ascertain whether the procedure the caregiver uses is harmful, such as cleaning ears with cotton swabs, which may cause impacted cerumen (ASHA, n.d.).

Questions for the Pregnant Female

1. Have you ever experienced a ringing in your ears?	▶ Ringing in the ears during pregnancy may occur with hypertension associated with preeclampsia (a serious condition that can threaten maternal and fetal health) (Smith & Hoare, 2012).
2. Have you experienced an earache or a feeling of fullness in your ears?	▶ Changes in estrogen produce increased vascularity throughout the systems of the body during pregnancy. The vascularity may cause a feeling of fullness or an aching in the ears (Kumar, Hayhurst, & Robson, 2011).

Questions for the Older Adult

1. Do you wear a hearing aid?
  ● If so, is it effective?
  ● How often do you wear your hearing aid?
	▶ Many older adults have a hearing loss but cannot adjust to using a hearing aid or cannot afford batteries for the hearing aid.

2. Do you have any difficulty operating the hearing aid? ● How do you clean the hearing aid?	▶ Some patients forget to clean the tubes of the hearing aid periodically.

Nose and Sinuses

1. Are you having any problems with your nose or sinuses? If so, describe them. Are you able to breathe through your nose?
  ● Can you breathe through both nostrils?
  ● Is one side obstructed?
  ● Describe any problems you have had breathing in the last few days. In the last few weeks.
	▶ A history of frequent respiratory problems may indicate an underlying respiratory problem such as allergies or recurring infections (Sly & Holt, 2011).

2. Do you have nasal discharge?
  ● If so, is it continuous or occasional?
  ● Describe the discharge.
	▶ A thin, watery discharge is the result of acute rhinitis from either a viral infection, such as the common cold, or an allergic reaction. Allergies that cause nasal discharge can also produce itchy eyes, postnasal drip, sore throats, ear infections, or headaches. Some allergies are seasonal; others are constant (Marrs, Anagnostou, Fitzsimons, & Fox, 2013).

3. Do you have nosebleeds?
  ● How often?
  ● What is your usual blood pressure?
  ● Do you use nasal sprays?
  ● How do you treat your nosebleeds?
	▶ Nosebleeds can occur as a result of high blood pressure, overuse of nasal sprays, and certain blood disorders (Mayo Clinic, 2012).

Focused Interview Questions	Rationales and Evidence

4. **Have you ever had any nose injury or nose surgery?**
   - If so, describe it.
   - How was the injury treated?
   - Do you have any residual problems from the injury or surgery?

5. **Describe your sense of smell.**
   - Are there any circumstances, objects, places, or activities that affect your sense of smell? If so, describe them.

   ▶ Anosmia, the inability to smell, may be neurologic, hereditary, or due to a deficiency of zinc in the diet (CDC, 2014).

6. **What prescribed or over-the-counter drugs do you take to relieve your nasal symptoms?**
   - Do you use a nasal inhalant, oxygen, or a humidifier to help you breathe?
   - What other medications do you take regularly?

   ▶ Certain medications can produce unpleasant side effects in the nose such as nasal stuffiness or nosebleeds. Many drugs administered by nasal inhalers may irritate the nasal mucosa and cause nosebleeds. Steroid inhalers can cause growth of *Candida* in the nose, mouth, or throat (Wilson et al., 2013).

7. **Do you use recreational drugs?**
   - If so, what drugs? How often?

   ▶ Some inhaled drugs, such as cocaine, gradually break down the nasal lining by vasoconstriction. Regular nasal inhalation of cocaine may cause nasal perforation (Guyuron & Afrooz, 2008).

Questions Regarding Infants and Children

1. **Does the child put objects into his or her nose?**

   ▶ Foreign objects can cause trauma to nasal tissues.

2. **Does the child frequently have drainage from the nose?**

   ▶ Frequent drainage can indicate an infection or allergies.

Questions for the Pregnant Female

1. **Have you had nosebleeds during your pregnancy? If so, how often?**

   ▶ During pregnancy, increased circulatory blood flow leads to swelling of mucous membranes, including those in the nasal passages. Swollen mucous membranes are more susceptible to bleeding (Mayo Clinic, 2014).

Mouth and Throat

1. **How would you describe the condition of your mouth and teeth?**
   - Have you noticed any changes in the last few months?

2. **Do you have any problems swallowing?**

   ▶ Dysphagia, or difficulty in swallowing, is frequently related to age-related changes in swallowing physiology; stroke; dementia and other neurological diseases; cancers of the head, neck, or esophagus; and other disorders (Sura, Madhavan, Carnaby, & Crary, 2012). Achalasia is a motility disorder associated with loss of esophageal peristalsis and failure of the lower esophageal sphyincter to relax upon swallowing; the cause of achalasia is unknown (O'Neill, Johnston, & Coleman, 2013).

3. **Do you have any sores or lesions in your mouth or on your tongue?**
   - If so, describe them.
   - Are they present constantly or do they come and go periodically?

   ▶ Lesions of the mouth or tongue may be cold sores, mouth ulcers, or cysts. They may accompany gum infections, viral infections such as HIV or HPV, trauma, or inflammatory reactions. Lesions are frequently found in chronic tobacco users. Lesions may be benign or malignant, so any lesion of the mouth that does not heal should be evaluated for oral cancer (Gonsalves, Chi, & Neville, 2007a; Gonsalves, Chi, & Neville, 2007b).

Focused Interview Questions	Rationales and Evidence
4. Do your gums bleed frequently?	▶ Gum diseases such as gingivitis and periodontitis may cause gums to bleed easily. Gums may also bleed easily with ill-fitting braces or dentures (Osborn et al., 2013).
5. Have you noticed a change in your sense of taste recently?	▶ Loss of the sense of taste commonly accompanies colds. A foul taste in the mouth may signal a gum infection or inadequate care of teeth or dentures.
6. What dental problems, surgeries, or procedures have you had in the past? • Describe them.	
7. Do you wear dentures, partial plates, retainers, or any other removable or permanent dental appliance? • Does it fit well? Is it comfortable? • Why are you wearing the appliance? • Does it help resolve the problem? • Are any of your teeth capped? Which ones?	
8. How often do you brush your teeth or dentures? • Do you use floss regularly?	▶ Regular mouth care is important in maintaining healthy teeth and gums and preventing gum diseases such as gingivitis and periodontitis.
9. When was your last dental examination? • Are you unable to eat some foods because of problems with your teeth? • Do you have any pain in one or more teeth?	
10. Do you have frequent sore throats?	▶ A sore throat may be the result of irritation from sinus drainage, viral or bacterial infection, or the first sign of throat cancer (National Cancer Institute [NCI], n.d.).
11. Have you noticed any hoarseness or loss of your voice?	▶ Hoarseness is a common finding in disorders of the throat. Recurrent or persistent hoarseness may indicate cancer of the larynx (NCI, n.d.). Hoarseness may also be due to anxiety, overuse of the voice, or a cold. Smoking and drinking alcohol can lead to inflammation of the vocal cords and result in hoarseness.
12. Do you now or did you ever smoke a pipe, cigarettes, or cigars? • Chew tobacco or dip snuff? • How much? How often?	▶ Smoking, dipping snuff, or chewing tobacco may result in cancer of the lips, mouth, and throat (NCI, n.d.).

Questions Regarding Infants and Children

1. Does the child suck his or her thumb or a pacifier?	▶ These behaviors can interfere with alignment of secondary teeth.
2. When did the child's teeth begin to erupt?	▶ Late eruption of teeth could indicate delayed development.
3. Does the child go to bed with a bottle at night? • What is in the bottle?	▶ Frequent use of a bottle with milk or juice at night can cause decay of teeth.

Focused Interview Questions	**Rationales and Evidence**

4. Does the child know how to brush teeth?
- Does the child brush daily?

5. How often does the child go to the dentist?

▶ Children should begin annual visits to the dentist no later than or by 1 year of age, with follow-up visits recommended every 6 months (American Academy of Pediatric Dentists [AAPD], n.d.).

6. Is the child's drinking water fluoridated?

▶ Fluoride in the water supply helps prevent tooth decay (Parnell, Whelton, & O'Mullane, 2009).

Questions for the Older Adult

1. Are you able to chew all types of food?

▶ If teeth are missing or dentures fit improperly, the patient may not be able to chew meat or certain vegetables, resulting in undernutrition.

2. Do you experience dryness in your mouth?

▶ Certain medications may cause dryness, which may interfere with the patient's appetite or digestion (Wilson et al., 2013).

3. Do you wear dentures?
- If so, do they fit properly?

▶ Ill-fitting dentures can interfere with proper nutrition because of food avoidance and other digestive problems (Altenhoevel, Norman, Smoliner, & Peroz, 2012).

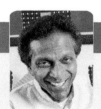

Patient-Centered Interaction

Mr. Sanji, age 65, comes to the Medi-Center with a chief complaint of "having trouble hearing." The intake sheet that Mr. Sanji completed reveals a slow progressive loss of hearing with no pain in the ears or head. Following is an excerpt of the focused interview.

Interview

Nurse: Good morning, Mr. Sanji. Please have a seat and tell me about your deafness.

The nurse and Mr. Sanji sit down across the desk from each other. During the interview, the nurse's head is down. The nurse maintains some eye contact by looking over the rim of the eye glasses.

Mr. Sanji: I'm not deaf. I just can't hear like before.

Nurse: How long have you noticed this progressive loss of hearing?

Mr. Sanji: I'm not sure, a while, but I'm not deaf!

Nurse: Have you had any purulent drainage from your ears?

Mr. Sanji: Hum!

Nurse: Do you have a history of having otitis media or a tympanoplasty?

Mr. Sanji does not answer the question.

Nurse: Would you like me to repeat the question?

Mr. Sanji: Yeah, louder and in simple language!

Analysis

In this situation the nurse has utilized several strategies that act as a hindrance to effective communication. The first problem is the nurse's body position and lack of eye contact. Keeping the head down muffles the sound for any person, especially one with a hearing deficit. The nurse should look up, speak directly to the patient, and maintain eye contact. Twice the patient says he is not deaf and the nurse does not seek clarification. Using language and terminology the individual does not understand is another obstacle. Mr. Sanji tells the nurse to speak louder and in simple terms.

Patient Education

The following are physiologic, behavioral, and cultural factors that affect the health of the ears, nose, mouth, and throat across the age span. Several factors reflect trends cited in *Healthy People 2020* documents. The nurse provides advice and education to reduce risks associated with the previously mentioned factors and to promote and maintain health of the ears, nose, mouth, and throat.

LIFESPAN CONSIDERATIONS

Risk Factors	Patient Education
• Bottles at bedtime or propped in the crib with infants increase the risk for dental disease and ear infection.	▶ Provide information about bottles at bedtime in relation to dental health and prevention of ear problems.
• Children are likely to insert foreign objects into the nose and ears.	▶ Teach parents about safety in relation to toys and objects that may have small parts or easily loosened small parts. Advise them to seek assistance from healthcare providers to remove foreign bodies from the ears or nose.
• Hearing acuity diminishes with aging.	▶ Advise adults to have annual hearing tests after age 55, and provide information about use of hearing aids for older adults.
• The sense of smell diminishes with aging.	▶ Advise patients with decreased sense of smell about the use of smoke alarms in the home and to establish the practice of monitoring pilot lights or dials of gas appliances.

ENVIRONMENTAL CONSIDERATIONS

Risk Factors	Patient Education
• Loud noise from machinery and music in the workplace or home can result in diminished hearing.	▶ Educate patients across the age span that noise in the work, home, and social environments can increase the risk of hearing loss. Provide advice about safety.
• Respiratory infections are easily transmissible through diffusion of droplets and spraying of nasal and oral secretions.	▶ Instruct all patients about use of tissues and hand hygiene to reduce the risk of spread of respiratory infections. Hand hygiene may include washing hands with non-antimicrobial soap and water, or using antiseptic hand cleanser or an alcohol-based hand rub (CDC, 2012b). ▶ Teach patients and family members principles of cough etiquette, including covering the mouth and nose with a tissue when sneezing or coughing; promptly disposing of used tissues in the nearest waste receptable; and performing hand hygiene immediately after being in contact with respiratory secretions or potentially contaminated materials (CDC, 2012b).
• Some medications, including Dilantin and steroids in infants, may promote problems with the gums or oral mucosa.	▶ Inform patients about medications. Teach self-assessment regarding side effects that affect the gums and mouth, including gingivitis and fungal infections.

BEHAVIORAL CONSIDERATIONS

Risk Factors

- Smoking and the use of oral tobacco products increase the risk for oral cancer.

Patient Education

▶ Advise patients about smoking cessation. Inform individuals and parents about recommendations for dental examination and hygiene measures.

Physical Assessment

Assessment Techniques and Findings

Physical assessment of the ears, nose, mouth, and throat requires the use of inspection, palpation, percussion, and transillumination of the sinuses. In addition, special examination techniques include the use of the otoscope, tuning fork, and nasal speculum. These techniques are used to gather objective data. Knowledge of normal or expected findings is essential in determining the meaning of data as the nurse proceeds.

Adults and children normally have binaural hearing, meaning that the brain is capable of simultaneously integrating information that is received from both ears. The ears are symmetric in size, shape, color, and configuration. The external auditory canal is patent and free of drainage. The external ear and mastoid process are free of lesions, and the tragus is movable. Under otoscopic examination the external ear canal is open; is nontender; and is free of lesions, inflammation, or foreign substances. Cerumen, if present, is soft and in small amounts. The tympanic membrane is flat, gray, and translucent without lesions. The malleolar process and reflected light are visible on the tympanic membrane. The tympanic membrane flutters with the Valsalva maneuver. During hearing tests, air conduction is longer than bone conduction. Adults and healthy children other than infants are able to maintain balance.

The external nose is free of lesions, the nares are patent, and the mucosa of the nasal cavity is dark pink and smooth. The nasal septum is midline, straight, and intact. The sinuses are nontender and transilluminate.

The lips are smooth, symmetric, and lesion-free. Typically, children begin losing their deciduous teeth by 6 years of age. On average, most children lose their last deciduous tooth at approximately 12 to 13 years of age (Mayo Clinic, 2011). Healthy adults and children who are 13 years and older have 32 permanent teeth, including four wisdom teeth, all of which are white with smooth edges. The tongue is mobile, is pink, and has papillae on the dorsum. The oral mucosa is pink, moist, and smooth. Salivary ducts are visible and not inflamed. The membranes and structures of the throat are pink and moist. The uvula is midline and, like the soft palate, rises when the patient says "aah." This movement is related to the proper functioning of cranial nerves IX and X.

Physical assessment of the ears, nose, mouth, and throat follows an organized pattern. It begins with instruction of the patient and proceeds through inspection, palpation, and otoscopic examination of the ears, followed by hearing assessment and the Romberg test. The nose is inspected and the internal aspect visualized while using a speculum. The sinuses are palpated, percussed, and transilluminated. The assessment concludes with inspection of the external mouth, the internal structures of the mouth, and assessment of the throat.

EQUIPMENT

- examination gown
- clean, nonsterile exam gloves
- otoscope with specula of various sizes
- tuning fork, 512 or 1024 Hz
- nasal speculum
- penlight
- gauze pads
- tongue blade

HELPFUL HINTS

- Provide specific instructions about what is expected of the patient. The nurse would state whether the head must be turned or the mouth opened.
- Consider the age of the patient. Response to directions varies across the life span.
- Pay attention to nonverbal cues throughout the assessment.
- Hearing difficulties may affect the data gathering process. Clarify problems and possible remedies before beginning the assessment. The patient may use sign language, hearing aids, lip reading, or written communication.
- Explain the use of each piece of equipment throughout the assessment.
- Use Standard Precautions.

Techniques and Normal Findings	Abnormal Findings Special Considerations

Ear

1. Position the patient.
- The patient should be in a sitting position. Lighting must be adequate to detect skin color changes, discharge, and lesions.

2. Instruct the patient.
- Explain that you will be carrying out a variety of assessments of the ear. Tell the patient you will be touching the ear areas, that it should cause no discomfort, and that any pain or discomfort should be reported.

3. Note that you will have begun to evaluate the patient's hearing while taking the health history.
- Did the patient hear the questions you asked?
- Did the patient answer appropriately?
- Generally, the formal evaluation of hearing is performed after otoscopic examination so that physical barriers to hearing, such as large amounts of cerumen, can be identified.

4. Inspect the external ear for symmetry, proportion, color, and integrity.
- Confirm that the external auditory meatus is patent with no drainage. The color of the ear should match that of the surrounding area and the face, with no redness, nodules, swelling, or lesions.

▶ Any discharge, redness, or swelling may indicate an infection or allergy.

5. Palpate the auricle and push on the tragus (Figure 16.12 ■).
- Confirm that there are no hard nodules, lesions, or swelling. The tragus should be movable.
- This technique should not cause pain.

▶ Lesions accompanied by a history of long-term exposure to the sun may be cancerous.
Pain could be the result of an infection of the external ear (otitis externa). Pain could also indicate temporomandibular joint dysfunction with pressure on the tragus. Hard nodules (tophi) are uric acid crystal deposits, which are a sign of gout.

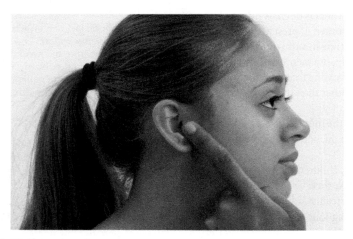

Figure 16.12 Palpating the tragus.

Techniques and Normal Findings	Abnormal Findings Special Considerations

6. **Palpate the mastoid process lying directly behind the ear (see Figure 16.13 ▪).**
   - Confirm that there are no lesions, pain, or swelling.

▶ **Mastoiditis** refers to inflammation or infection of the mastoid bone. It is a complication of either a middle ear infection or a throat infection. Mastoiditis is very difficult to treat. It spreads easily to the brain since the mastoid area is separated from the brain by only a thin, bony plate.

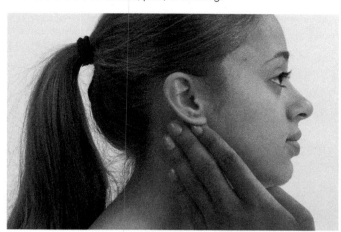

Figure 16.13 Palpating the mastoid process.

7. **Inspect the auditory canal using the otoscope.**
   - For the best visualization, use the largest speculum that will fit into the auditory canal.
   - Ask the patient to tilt the head away from you toward the opposite shoulder.
   - Hold the otoscope between the palm and first two fingers of the dominant hand. The handle may be positioned upward or downward (see Figure 16.15 on page 350).
   - Use your other hand to straighten the canal.
   - In the adult patient, pull the pinna up, back, and out to straighten the canal (see Figure 16.14 ▪).

▶ In infants the pinna is pulled down and back due to the shorter, straight external ear canal (see Figure 16.10).

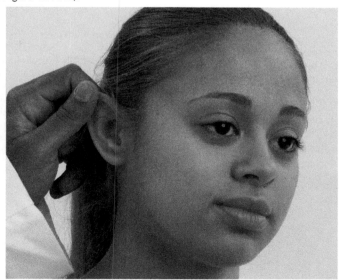

Figure 16.14 Pulling the pinna to straighten the canal.
   - Be sure to maintain this position until the speculum is removed.
   - Instruct the patient to tell you if any discomfort is experienced but not to move the head or suddenly pull away.

ALERT!

One must use care when inserting the speculum of the otoscope into the ear. The inner two thirds of the ear are very sensitive, and pressing the speculum against either side of the auditory canal will cause pain.

Techniques and Normal Findings	**Abnormal Findings Special Considerations**

- With the light on, use the upward or downward position of the handle to insert the speculum into the ear (see Figure 16.15A and B ■). Brace the otoscope with the dorsal surface of the fingers or hand. The external canal should be open and without tenderness, inflammation, lesions, growths, discharge, or foreign substances.
- Note the amount, color, and texture of the cerumen that is present.

▶ If the ear canal is occluded with cerumen, the cerumen must be removed. Most cerumen can be removed with a cerumen spoon. If the cerumen is dry, the external canal should be irrigated using a bulb syringe and a warmed solution of mineral oil and hydrogen peroxide, followed by warm water.

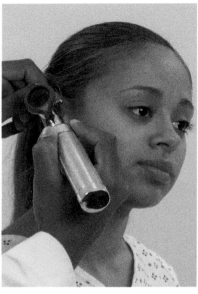 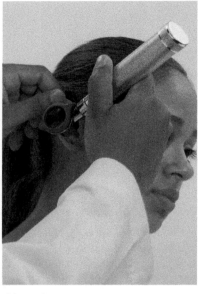

A   B

Figure 16.15 Two techniques for holding and inserting an otoscope.
A. Otoscopic examination with otoscope handle in downward position.
B. Otoscopic examination with otoscope handle in upward position.

8. **Examine the tympanic membrane using the otoscope.**
- The membrane should be flat, gray, and translucent with no scars (see Figure 16.16 ■). A cone-shaped reflection of the otoscope light should be visible at the 5 o'clock position in the right ear and the 7 o'clock position in the left ear. The short process of the malleus should be seen as a shadow behind the tympanic membrane. The membrane should be intact.
- If you cannot visualize the tympanic membrane, remove the otoscope, reposition the auricle, and reinsert the otoscope. Do not reposition the auricle with the otoscope in place.

▶ White patches on the tympanic membrane indicate scars from prior infections. If the membrane is yellow or reddish, it could indicate an infection of the middle ear. A bulging membrane may indicate increased pressure in the middle ear, whereas a retracted membrane may indicate a vacuum in the middle ear due to a blocked eustachian tube. Failure to visualize the tympanic membrane may result from cerumen impaction. If needed, clean out the cerumen before attempting to visualize the tympanic membrane again.

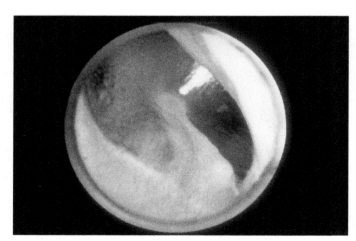

Figure 16.16 Normal tympanic membrane with cone of light and process of malleus.
Source: Lester V. Bergman/Corbis.

Techniques and Normal Findings	**Abnormal Findings** **Special Considerations**

9. **Perform the whisper test.**
   - This test evaluates hearing acuity of high-frequency sounds.
   - Ask the patient to occlude the left ear or the ear may be occluded by the nurse.
   - Cover your mouth so that the patient cannot see your lips.
   - Standing at the patient's side at a distance of 1 to 2 ft, (approximately 0.3 to 0.6 m), whisper a simple phrase such as, "The weather is hot today." Ask the patient to repeat the phrase. Then do the same procedure to test the right ear using a different phrase. The patient should be able to repeat the phrases correctly (Figure 16.17 ■).

▶ Inability to repeat the phrases may indicate a loss of the ability to hear high-frequency sounds.

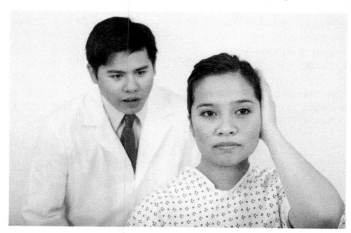

Figure 16.17 Performing the whisper test.

   - Tuning forks are also used to evaluate auditory acuity. The tines of the fork, when activated, produce sound waves. The frequency, or cycles per second (cps), is the expression used to describe the action of the instrument. A fork with 512 cps vibrates 512 times per second and is the size of choice for auditory evaluations. The tines are set into motion by squeezing, stroking, or lightly tapping against your hand. The fork must be held at the handle to prevent interference with the vibration of the tines (see Figure 16.18 ■).

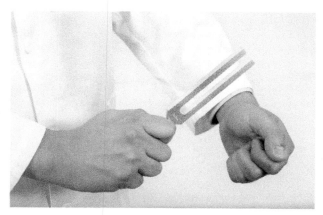

Figure 16.18 Activating the tuning fork.

| Techniques and Normal Findings | Abnormal Findings Special Considerations |

- The following tests use a tuning fork primarily to evaluate conductive versus perceptive hearing loss. **Air conduction** (AC) is the transmission of sound through the tympanic membrane to the cochlea and auditory nerve. **Bone conduction** (BC) is the transmission of sound through the bones of the skull to the cochlea and auditory nerve.

10. **Perform the Rinne test.**
    - The Rinne test compares air and bone conduction. This is an advanced assessment technique. Hold the tuning fork by the handle and gently strike the fork on the palm of your hand to set it vibrating.
    - Place the base of the fork on the patient's mastoid process (see Figure 16.19A ■).
    - Ask the patient to tell you when the sound is no longer heard.
    - Note the number of seconds. Then immediately move the tines of the still-vibrating fork in front of the external auditory meatus (see Figure 16.19B ■). It should be 1 to 2 cm (about 1/2 in.) from the meatus.
    - Ask the patient to tell you again when the sound is no longer heard. Again note the number of seconds. Normally, the sound is heard twice as long by air conduction than by bone conduction after bone conduction stops. For example, a normal finding is AC 30 seconds, BC 15 seconds.

▶ If the patient hears the bone-conducted sound as long as or longer than the air-conducted sound, the patient may have some degree of conductive hearing loss.

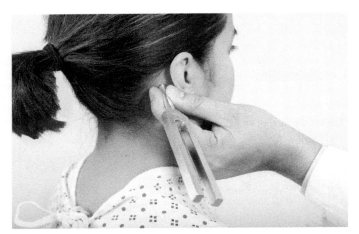

Figure 16.19A Rinne test. Bone conduction.

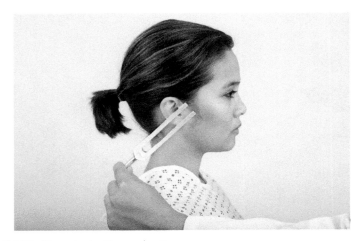

Figure 16.19B Rinne test. Air conduction.

Techniques and Normal Findings	Abnormal Findings Special Considerations

11. Perform the Weber test.

- The Weber test uses bone conduction to evaluate hearing in a person who hears better in one ear than in the other. Hold the tuning fork by the handle and strike the fork on the palm of the hand. Place the base of the vibrating fork against the patient's skull. The midline of the anterior portion of the frontal bone is used (Figure 16.20 ■). The midline of the forehead is an alternative choice.

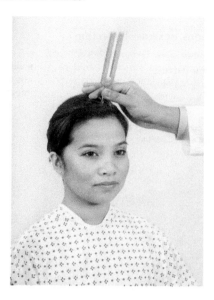

Figure 16.20 Weber test.

- Ask the patient if the sound is heard equally on both sides, or better in one ear than the other. The normal response is bilaterally equal sound, which is recorded as "no lateralization." If the sound is lateralized, ask the patient to tell you which ear hears the sound better.

12. Perform the Romberg test.

- The Romberg test assesses equilibrium. Ask the patient to stand with feet together and arms at sides, first with eyes opened and then with eyes closed (Figure 16.21 ■).

▶ If the patient hears the sound in one ear better than the other ear, the hearing loss may be due to either poor conduction or nerve damage. If the patient has poor conduction in one ear, the sound is heard better in the impaired ear because the sound is being conducted directly through the bone to the ear, and the extraneous sounds in the environment are not being picked up. Conductive loss in one ear may be due to impacted cerumen, infection, or a perforated eardrum. If the patient has a hearing loss due to nerve damage, the sound is referred to the better ear, in which the cochlea or auditory nerve is functioning better.

▶ The abnormal findings are recorded as "sound lateralizes to (right or left) ear."

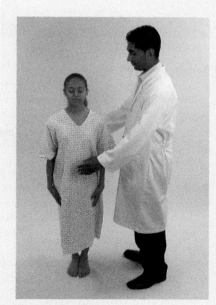

Figure 16.21 Romberg test.

- Wait about 20 seconds. The person should be able to maintain this position, although some mild swaying may occur. Mild swaying is documented as a negative Romberg. it is important to stand nearby and prepare to support the patient if there is a loss of balance. Hearing and balance are functions of cranial nerve VIII and are discussed in chapter 26. ∞

▶ If the patient is unable to maintain balance or needs to have the feet farther apart, there may be a problem with functioning of the vestibular apparatus.

Techniques and Normal Findings	Abnormal Findings Special Considerations

Nose and Sinuses

Note: The sense of smell and function of cranial nerve I are evaluated with the neurologic assessment presented in chapter 26. ∞

1. **Instruct the patient.**
   - Explain that you will be looking at and touching the patient's nose. Tell the patient to inform you of discomfort.

2. **Inspect the nose for size, symmetry, shape, skin lesions, or signs of infection in frontal and lateral views.**
   - Confirm that the nose is straight, in proportion to the other facial structures, midline, without deformities, the nares are equal in size, the skin is intact, and no drainage or inflammation is present (see Figure 16.22 ■).

▶ If breathing is noisy or a discharge is present, the patient may have an obstruction or an infection.

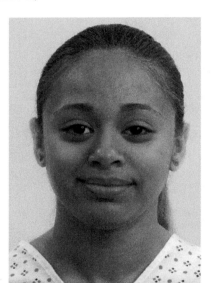

Figure 16.22 Inspection of the nose.

3. **Test for patency.**
   - Press your finger on the patient's nostril to occlude one naris, and ask the patient to breathe through the opposite side with the mouth closed.
   - Repeat with the other nostril.
   - The patient should be able to breathe through each naris.

▶ If the patient cannot breathe through each naris, severe inflammation or an obstruction may be present.

▶ Ineffective breathing patterns or mouth breathing may be related to nasal swelling or trauma.

4. **Palpate the external nose for tenderness, swelling, and stability.**
   - Using two fingers, palpate the nose from the bridge to the tip and along the entire lateral surfaces, around the nares and along the columella.
   - Note the smoothness and stability of the underlying soft tissue and cartilage.

5. **Inspect the nasal cavity using an otoscope.**
   - Apply a disposable cover to the tip of the otoscope. With your nondominant hand, stabilize the patient's head. With the otoscope in your dominant hand, gently insert the speculum horizontally into the naris (see Figure 16.23 ■). The speculum should be in the dominant hand for better control at the time of insertion to avoid hitting the sensitive septum.

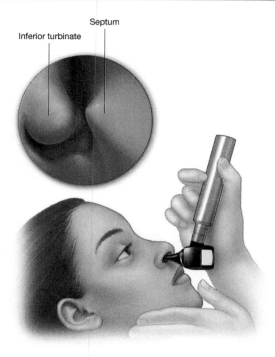

Inferior turbinate · Septum

Figure 16.23 Using the otoscope for nasal inspection.

- With the patient's head erect, inspect the vestibule and then the inferior turbinates (see Figure 16.23).
- With the patient's head tilted back, inspect the middle meatus and middle turbinates. Mucosa should be dark pink and smooth without swelling, discharge, bleeding, or foreign bodies. The septum should be midline, straight, and intact.
- When finished with inspection, gently remove the speculum. Again, do not hit the sensitive septum.
- Repeat on other side.

6. **Palpate the sinuses.**
   - Begin by pressing your thumbs over the frontal sinuses below the superior orbital ridge. Palpate the maxillary sinuses below the zygomatic arches of the cheekbones (see Figures 16.24A and B ■).
   - Observe the patient for signs of discomfort. Ask the patient to inform you of pain.

▶ If the mucosa is swollen and red, the patient may have an upper respiratory infection. If the mucosa is pale and boggy or swollen, the patient may have chronic allergies. A *deviated septum* appears as an irregular lump in one nasal cavity. Slight deviations do not present problems for most patients. **Nasal polyps** are smooth, pale, benign growths found in many patients with chronic allergies.

▶ Tenderness upon palpation may indicate chronic allergies or sinusitis.

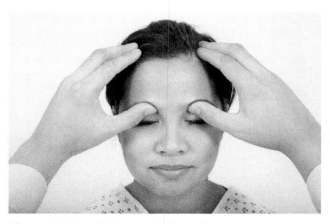

Figure 16.24A Palpating the frontal sinuses.

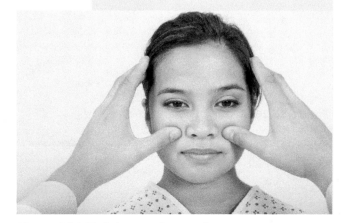

Figure 16.24B Palpating the maxillary sinuses.

Techniques and Normal Findings	Abnormal Findings Special Considerations

7. Percuss the sinuses.

- To determine if there is pain in the sinuses, directly percuss over the maxillary and frontal sinuses by lightly tapping with one finger (see Figures 16.25A and B ■).

▶ Pain may indicate sinus fullness, allergies, or infection.

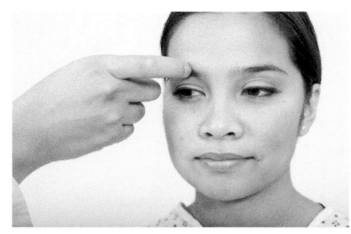

Figure 16.25A Percussion of frontal sinuses.

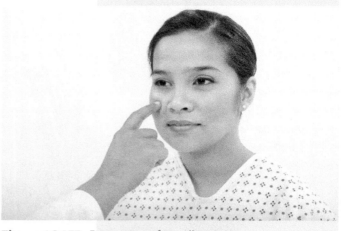

Figure 16.25B Percussion of maxillary sinuses.

8. Transilluminate the sinuses.

- If you suspect a sinus infection, the maxillary and frontal sinuses may be transilluminated.
- To transilluminate the frontal sinus, darken the room and hold a penlight under the superior orbit ridge against the frontal sinus area (see Figure 16.26A ■).

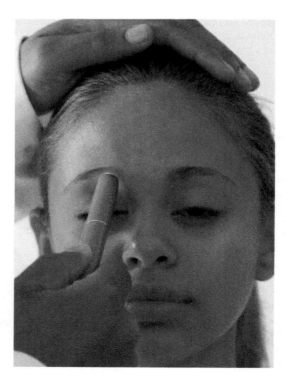

Figure 16.26A Transillumination of the frontal sinuses.

Techniques and Normal Findings	Abnormal Findings Special Considerations

- Cover the frontal sinus with your hand. There should be a red glow over the frontal sinus area (see Figure 16.26B ■).

▶ If the sinus is filled with fluid, it will not transilluminate.

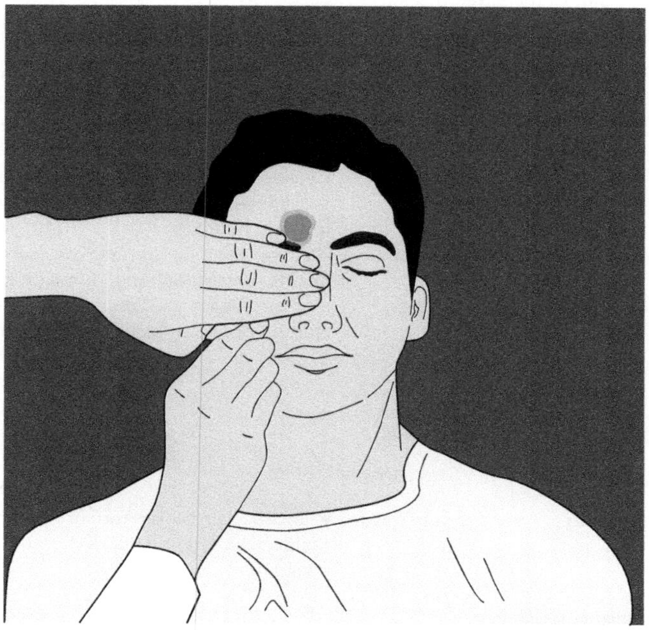

Figure 16.26B Observing transillumination of the frontal sinuses.

- To test the maxillary sinus, place a clean penlight in the patient's mouth and shine the light on one side of the hard palate, then the other. Gently cover the patient's mouth with one hand.
- There should be a red glow over the cheeks (see Figure 16.27A ■). Make sure the penlight is cleaned before using it again.
- An alternate technique is to place the penlight directly on the cheek and observe the glow of light on the hard palate (see Figure 16.27B ■).

▶ If there is no red glow under the eyes, the sinuses may be inflamed.

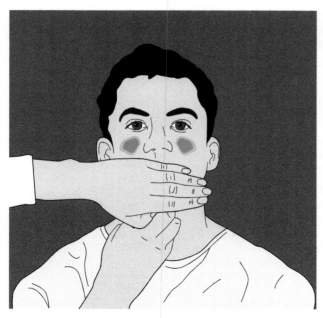

Figure 16.27A Transillumination of the maxillary sinuses.

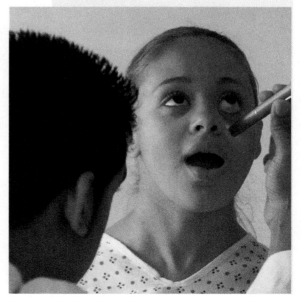

Figure 16.27B Transillumination of the maxillary sinuses using alternate technique.

Techniques and Normal Findings	Abnormal Findings Special Considerations

Mouth and Throat

Note: Be sure to wear clean, nonsterile examination gloves for this part of the assessment.

1. **Inspect and palpate the lips.**
   - Confirm that the lips are symmetric, smooth, pink, moist, and without lesions. Makeup or lipstick should be removed.

   - Note the presence, shape, and color of the vermilion border, which is the darker line that forms a boundary between the lips and the skin.

▶ Lesions or blisters on the lips may be caused by the herpes simplex virus. These lesions are also known as **fever blisters** or **cold sores.** However, lesions must be evaluated for cancer, because cancer of the lip is the most common oral cancer. Pallor or cyanosis of the lips may indicate hypoxia.

▶ A thin vermilion border may be a sign of fetal alcohol syndrome. The vermilion border may also be absent after reconstructive surgery for cleft lip or hemangioma resection.

2. **Inspect the teeth.**
   - Observe the patient's dental hygiene. Ask the patient to clench the teeth and smile while you observe occlusion (see Figure 16.28 ■).
   - Note dentures and caps at this time.
   - The teeth should be white, with smooth edges, and free of debris. Adults should have 32 permanent teeth, if wisdom teeth are intact.

▶ Loose, painful, broken, or misaligned teeth; malocclusion; and inflamed gums need further evaluation.

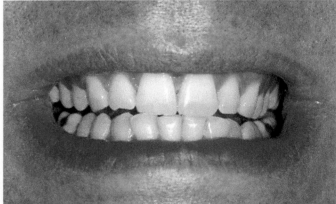

Figure 16.28 Inspecting the teeth.

3. **Inspect and palpate the buccal mucosa, gums, and tongue.**
   - Look into the patient's mouth under a strong light.
   - Confirm that the tongue is pink and moist with papillae on the dorsal surface.

- Ask the patient to touch the roof of the mouth with the tip of the tongue. The ventral surface should be smooth and pink. Palpate the area under the tongue.
- Check for lesions or nodules. Using a gauze pad, grasp the patient's tongue and inspect for any lumps or nodules (see Figure 16.29 ■). The tissue should be smooth.

▶ A smooth, coated, or hairy tongue is usually related to dehydration or disease. A small tongue may indicate undernutrition. Tremor of the tongue may indicate a dysfunction of the hypoglossal nerve (cranial nerve XII).

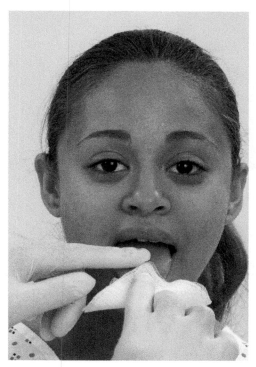

Figure 16.29 Palpating the tongue.

- Use a tongue blade to hold the tongue aside while you inspect the mucous lining of the mouth and the gums.
- Confirm that these areas are pink, moist, smooth, and free of lesions.
- Confirm the integrity of both the soft and the hard palate.
- Inspect the frenula of the tongue, upper lip, and lower lip. The frenulum is the small flap of tissue connecting the protruding portion of the lip or tongue to the rest of the mouth.
- The sense of taste (cranial nerves VII and IX) and movement of the tongue (cranial nerve XII) are discussed in detail in chapter 26. ∞

▶ Persistent lesions on the tongue must be evaluated further. Cancerous lesions occur most commonly on the sides or at the base of the tongue. The gums are diseased if there is bleeding, retraction, or overgrowth onto the teeth.
▶ The frenula are delicate flaps of skin and are easily damaged by a direct blow to the mouth during abuse or other trauma.

4. **Inspect the salivary glands.**
   - The salivary glands open into the mouth. Wharton's ducts (submandibular) open close to the lingual frenulum. Stensen's ducts (parotid) open opposite the second upper molars. Both ducts are visible, whereas the ducts of the sublingual glands are not visible.
   - Confirm that Wharton's and Stenson's salivary ducts are visible, with no pain, tenderness, swelling, or redness.
   - Touch the area close to the ducts with a sterile applicator, and confirm the flow of saliva.

▶ Pain or the lack of saliva can indicate infection or an obstruction.

Techniques and Normal Findings	Abnormal Findings Special Considerations

5. **Inspect the throat.**

- Use a tongue blade and penlight to inspect the throat (see Figure 16.30 ■).

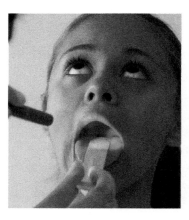

Figure 16.30 Inspecting the throat.

- Ask the patient to open the mouth wide, tilt the head back, and say "aah." The uvula should rise in the midline.
- Use the tongue blade to depress the middle of the arched tongue enough so that you can clearly visualize the throat but not so much that the patient gags. Ask the patient to say "aah" again.
- Confirm the rising of the soft palate, which is a test for cranial nerve X.
- Confirm that the tonsils, uvula, and posterior pharynx are pink and are without inflammation, swelling, or lesions. Observe the tonsils behind the anterior tonsillar pillar. The color should be pink with slight vascularity present. Tonsils may be partially or totally absent.
- Visualization of tonsils may be described based on size (Figure 16.31 ■) as follows:
  - Grade 0: Absent
  - Grade 1 (normal): Tonsils are hidden behind the tonsillar pillars
  - Grade 2: Tonsils extend to the edges of the tonsillar pillars
  - Grade 3: Tonsils extend beyond the edges of the tonsillar pillars but not to the midline
  - Grade 4: Tonsils extend to the midline
- As you inspect the throat, note any mouth odors.
- Discard the tongue blade.

▶ Viral pharyngitis may accompany a cold. Tonsils may be bright red and swollen and may have white spots on them.

▶ Patients with diabetic acidosis have a sweet, fruity breath. The breath of patients with kidney disease smells of ammonia.

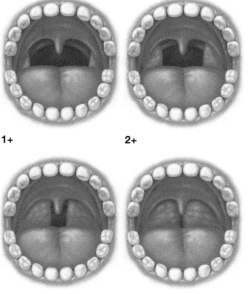

1+　　　　2+

3+　　　　4+

Figure 16.31 Tonsil size grading.

Abnormal Findings

Abnormal findings in the ears, nose, mouth, and throat include lesions, deformities, infectious processes, and dental problems. See Table 16.3 and Table 16.4 for an overview of ear-related disorders. Table 16.5 provides examples of disorders of the nose and sinuses. An overview of disorders of the mouth and throat is presented in Table 16.6.

TABLE 16.3	Overview of Disorders of the External Ear

Keloid

Scar tissue that forms following tissue injury. Ear piercing may cause keloid formation. Keloid tissue may be pink, red, or flesh-colored.

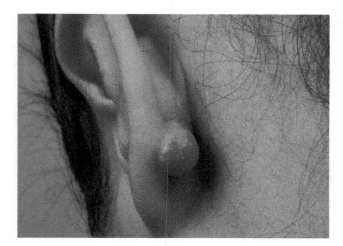

Figure 16.32 Keloid.
Source: BSIP/Getty Images.

Otitis Externa

Infection of the outer ear that causes redness and swelling of the auricle and ear canal and scanty drainage; may be accompanied by itching, fever, and enlarged lymph nodes. Also called swimmer's ear.

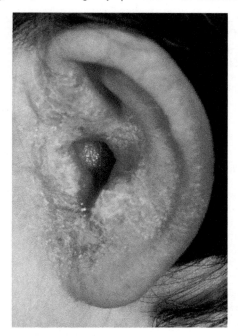

Figure 16.33 Otitis externa (swimmer's ear).
Source: BioPhoto Associates/Photo Researchers/Getty Images.

Tophi

Small white nodules on the helix or antihelix of the ear that contain uric acid crystals and are a sign of gout, which is a type of arthritis that is caused by a build-up of uric acid in the joints. Tophi may also occur in the olecranon process (elbow), knee joint, palm, and Achilles tendon.

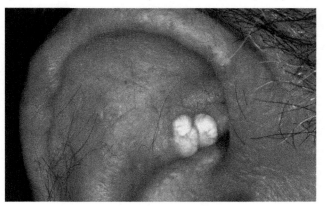

Figure 16.34 Tophi.
Source: Science Photo Library/Science Source.

TABLE 16.4   **Overview of Disorders of the Middle and Internal Ear**

Otitis Media

Infection of the middle ear producing a red, bulging eardrum; fever; and hearing loss. Otoscopic examination reveals absent light reflex.

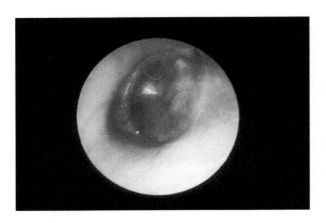

Figure 16.35 Otitis media.
Source: Southern Illinois University/Getty Images.

Perforation of the Tympanic Membrane

A rupturing of the eardrum due to trauma or infection. During otoscopic inspection, the perforation may be seen as a dark spot on the eardrum.

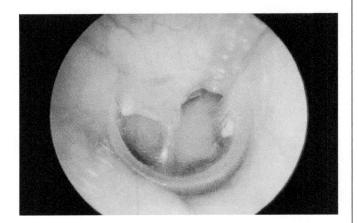

Figure 16.36 Perforation of tympanic membrane.
Source: Professor Tony Wright, Institute of Laryngology & Otology/Science Source.

Scarred Tympanic Membrane

A condition in which the eardrum has white patches of scar tissue due to repeated ear infections. Chronic irritation of the tympanic membrane without infection also can cause scarring. In most cases, this condition does not cause hearing loss.

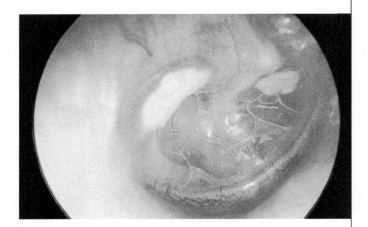

Figure 16.37 Scarred tympanic membrane.
Source: Professor Tony Wright/Science Source.

TABLE 16.5   ## Overview of Disorders of the Nose and Sinuses

Deviated Septum

A displacement of the lower nasal septum. When viewed with a nasal speculum, one nasal cavity appears to have an outgrowth or shelf.

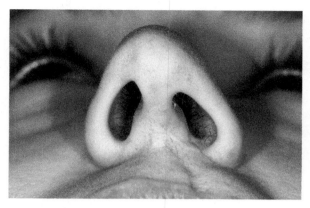

Figure 16.38 Deviated septum.
Source: Dr. P. Marazzi/Science Source.

Epistaxis

A nosebleed may follow trauma, such as a blow to the nose, or it may accompany another alteration in health, such as rhinitis, hypertension, or a blood coagulation disorder.

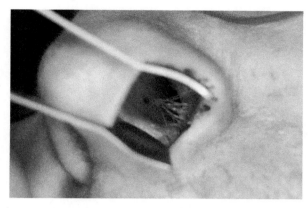

Figure 16.39 Epistaxis (nosebleed).
Source: Dr. P. Marazzi/Science Source.

Nasal Polyp

Pale, round, firm, nonpainful overgrowth of nasal mucosa usually caused by chronic allergic rhinitis.

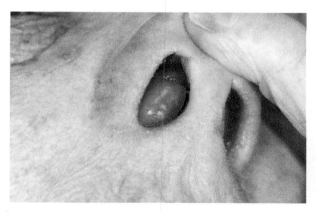

Figure 16.40 Nasal polyp.
Source: Science Photo Library/Science Source.

Perforated Septum

A hole in the septum caused by chronic infection, trauma, or sniffing cocaine. It can be detected by shining a penlight through the naris on the other side.

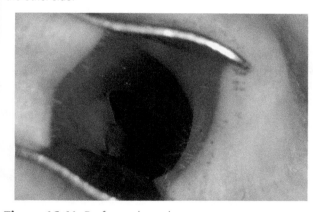

Figure 16.41 Perforated nasal septum.
Source: Dr. P. Marazzi/Science Source.

(continued)

| TABLE 16.5 | **Overview of Disorders of the Nose and Sinuses (continued)** |

Rhinitis

Nasal inflammation usually due to a viral infection or allergy, accompanied by watery and often copious discharge, sneezing, and congestion. *Acute rhinitis* is caused by a virus, whereas *allergic rhinitis* results from contact with allergens such as pollen and dust.

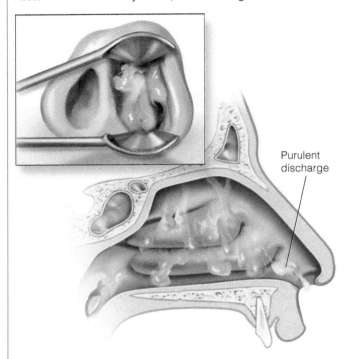

Figure 16.42 Acute rhinitis.

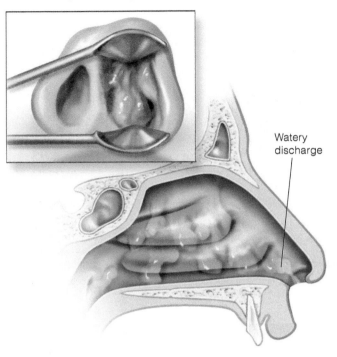

Figure 16.43 Allergic rhinitis.

Sinusitis

Inflammation of the sinuses usually following an upper respiratory infection. The inflammation causes facial pain and discharge. Fever; chills; frontal headache; or a dull, pulsating pain in the cheeks or teeth may accompany sinusitis.

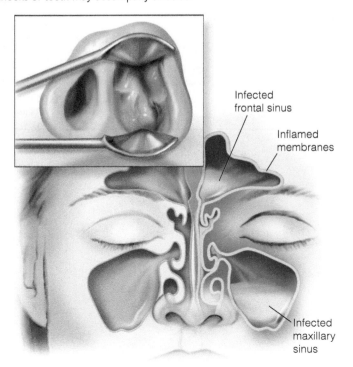

Figure 16.44 Sinusitis.

TABLE 16.6 **Overview of Disorders of the Mouth and Throat**

Ankyloglossia

Fixation of the tip of the tongue to the floor of the mouth due to a shortened lingual frenulum. The condition is usually congenital and may be corrected surgically.

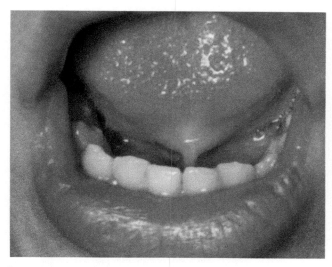

Figure 16.45 Ankyloglossia.
Source: Dr. P. Marazzi/Science Source.

Aphthous Ulcers

Small, round, white, painful lesions occurring singularly or in clusters on the oral mucosa. Commonly result from oral trauma; also associated with stress, exhaustion, and food allergies. Also called canker sores.

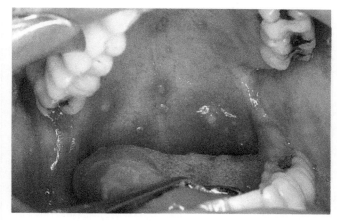

Figure 16.46 Aphthous ulcers.
Source: Sol Silverman, Jr., DDS/Centers for Disease Control and Prevention (CDC).

Black Hairy Tongue

A temporary condition caused by the inhibition of normal bacteria and the overgrowth of fungus on the papillae of the tongue. It is usually associated with the use of antibiotics.

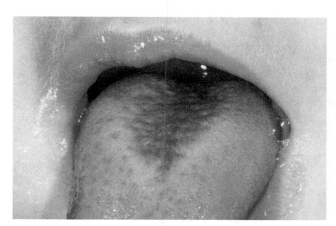

Figure 16.47 Black hairy tongue.
Source: Dr. P. Marazzi/Science Source.

Oral Carcinoma

Most commonly found on the lower lip or the base of the tongue. Cancer is suspected if a sore or lesion does not heal within a few weeks. Heavy smoking, chewing tobacco, and chronic heavy alcohol use increase the risk.

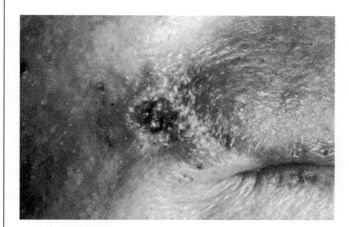

Figure 16.48 Carcinoma on left cheek and lips.
Source: O.J.Staats MD/Custom Medical Stock Photo.

(continued)

TABLE 16.6 **Overview of Disorders of the Mouth and Throat** (continued)

Cleft Lip

A separation or splitting of the two sides of the upper lip; appears as a gap or narrow opening in the skin of the upper lip. May occur alone or along with cleft palate.

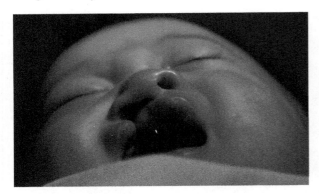

Figure 16.49 Cleft lip.
Source: Melyn R. Acosta/epa/Corbis.

Cleft Palate

An opening or separation in the roof of the mouth; may involve the hard palate, the soft palate, or both of these structures. May or may not occur along with cleft lip.

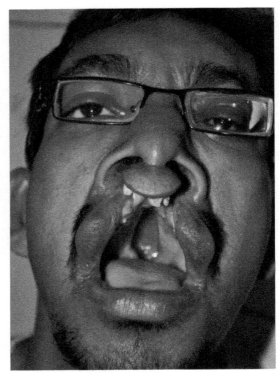

Figure 16.50 Cleft palate.
Source: Yameen Qureshi/Demotix/Corbis.

Gingival Hyperplasia

An enlargement of the gums; frequently seen in pregnancy, leukemia, or after prolonged use of phenytoin (Dilantin).

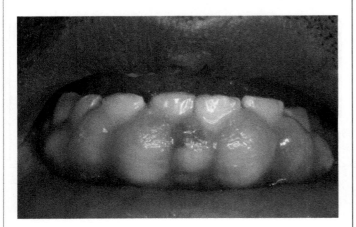

Figure 16.51 Gingival hyperplasia.
Source: Wellcome Image Library/Custom Medical Stock Photo.

Gingivitis

Gum inflammation that may be caused by poor dental hygiene or vitamin C deficiency. Untreated, it may progress to periodontal disease and tooth loss.

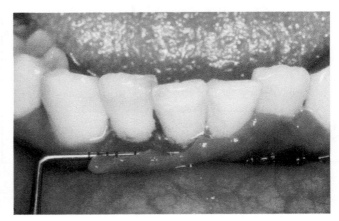

Figure 16.52 Gingivitis.
Source: Custom Medical Stock Photo, Inc.

TABLE 16.6   **Overview of Disorders of the Mouth and Throat (continued)**

Herpes Simplex

A virus that is often accompanied by clear vesicles (*cold sores, fever blisters*) usually at the junction of the skin and the lip that erupt, crust over, and heal within 2 weeks. Usually recur, especially after heavy exposure to bright sunlight.

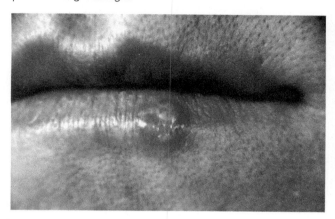

Figure 16.53 Herpes simplex.
Source: Dr. Herrmann/Centers for Disease Control and Prevention (CDC).

Leukoplakia

A whitish thickening of the mucous membrane in the mouth or tongue that cannot be scraped off. Most often associated with heavy smoking or drinking, it can be a precancerous condition.

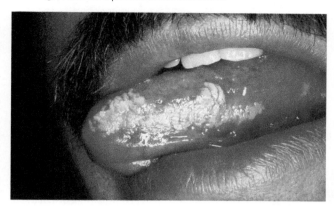

Figure 16.54 Leukoplakia.
Source: J.S. Greenspan, B.D.S., University of California, San Francisco; Sol Silverman, Jr., D.D.S Centers for Disease Control and Prevention (CDC).

Atrophic glossitis

The surface of the tongue is smooth and red with a shiny appearance; occurs as a result of vitamin B and iron deficiency.

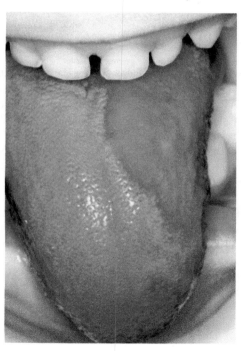

Figure 16.55 Atrophic glossitis (smooth, glossy tongue).
Source: Custom Medical Stock Photo, Inc.

Tonsillitis

Inflammation of the tonsils. The throat is red and the tonsils are swollen and covered by white or yellow patches (exudate); may include high fever and enlarged cervical chain lymph nodes.

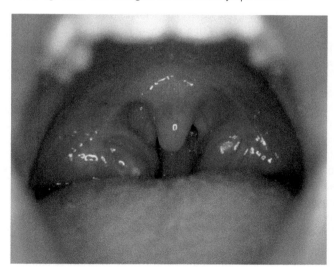

Figure 16.56 Tonsillitis.
Source: Dr. P. Marazzi/Science Source.

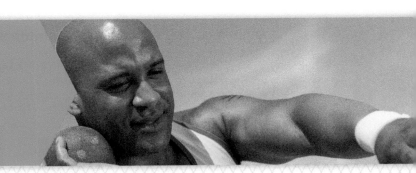

Application Through Critical Thinking

▌ Case Study

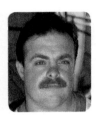

Harold Chandler is a 35-year-old executive in a computer firm who comes to the employees' wellness center complaining of a marked loss of hearing in his left ear. He says that he woke up yesterday with a "feeling of fullness" in his left ear but no pain. He further relates that his 3-year-old daughter has a "bad cold and an earache," and he wonders if he has "the same thing." He denies any other symptoms of infection, has had no discharge from either ear, and is not taking any medicine at this time. He has not had an audiometric assessment since his last physical 3 years ago. He further volunteers that he has just returned from a business trip to Europe and wonders whether the pressurized atmosphere of the airplane "created a problem with his hearing." He also tells you he spent summers working construction jobs when he was in college.

Nurse Michael Navarro's assessment of Mr. Chandler reveals normal vital signs. His left ear's external canal is of a uniform pink color with no redness, swelling, lesions, or discharge. The Weber test reveals lateralization to the left ear. The otoscopic assessment reveals a left ear impacted with brown-gray cerumen, and the tympanic membrane cannot be visualized. Assessment of the right ear shows the external canal is of a uniform pink color with no redness, swelling, lesions, or discharge. During the otoscopic assessment, the tympanic membrane is easily visualized. It is translucent and pearl-gray with the cone of light at the 5 o'clock position. No perforations are noted.

To visualize the tympanic membrane of the left ear, Mr. Navarro prepares a solution of mineral oil and hydrogen peroxide and instills the solution into the left ear canal to soften the cerumen. Then he irrigates the canal with warm water using a bulb syringe. After Mr. Navarro completes the irrigation, Mr. Chandler is surprised to discover that his hearing has returned in his left ear. Now Mr. Navarro completes the otoscopic assessment. He is able to visualize the tympanic membrane, which is translucent and pearl-gray with the cone of light at the 7 o'clock position. No perforations are noted.

To be sure that Mr. Chandler's hearing has been restored, Mr. Navarro performs a screening evaluation of his auditory function. He is able to hear a low whisper at 2 ft. His Rinne test is positive, and his Weber test indicates equal lateralization.

▌ Complete Documentation

The following is sample documentation for Harold Chandler.

SUBJECTIVE DATA: 35-year-old c/o hearing loss (Left) ear. Woke up yesterday with fullness, no pain (Left) ear. His 3-year-old daughter has "bad cold and earache," wonders if he has the same. Denies signs of infection, no discharge, and no medication. Audiometric assessment 3 years ago. Recent air travel, wonders if pressurized atmosphere created hearing problem.

OBJECTIVE DATA: Ears, equal in size, shape. Tragus mobile, nontender bilaterally. Left ear canal pink, no redness, edema, lesions, discharge. Weber—lateralization to left. Otoscopic assessment: Left ear impacted—brown-gray cerumen, no visualization tympanic membrane. Right ear—canal pink, clear, no edema, tympanic membrane gray with no lesions.

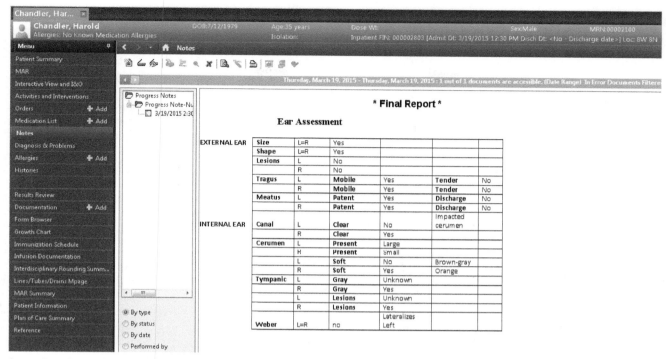

Source: From Cerner Electronic Health Record. Copyright © by Cerner Corporation. Used by permission of Cerner Corporation.

▶ Critical Thinking Questions

1. Describe the application of critical thinking to the situation.
2. How was information clustered to guide decision making?
3. What recommendations should the nurse provide for this patient?
4. What special considerations should the nurse take into account in this situation?
5. Why is it important to understand whether the hearing loss was acute or gradual?

▶ Prepare Teaching Plan

LEARNING NEED: Mr. Chandler experienced a hearing problem and sought treatment because he was unsure of the cause. The data revealed his concern that the hearing loss and ear discomfort he experienced were from "a cold, like my daughter" or "pressure changes due to air travel." After the assessment, it was determined that the cause of Mr. Chandler's problem was impacted cerumen.

The case study provides data that are representative of symptoms and behaviors of a variety of hearing and ear problems. Individuals and groups could benefit from education about the ear, hearing loss, and care of the ear. The following teaching plan is intended for a group of learners and focuses on ear care.

GOAL: The participants will practice safe care of the ear.

OBJECTIVES: Upon completion of this educational session, the participants will be able to:

1. Identify the structures of the ear.
2. Discuss common problems with the ear.
3. Describe measures for care of the ear.

APPLICATION OF OBJECTIVE 3: Describe measures for care of the ear

Content	Teaching Strategy and Rationale	Evaluation
An old adage: Never put anything smaller than your elbow in your ear. Ear canals should never have to be cleaned. The cerumen moves to the outside naturally. Sometimes, the cerumen is excreted in large amounts or it is not effectively cleared. Do's and Don'ts Do consult your physician when you have ear symptoms. Do follow the instructions for use of commercial ear wax removal products. Don't use cotton swabs, hairpins, or paper clips to attempt to remove cerumen. You may perforate the eardrum or merely push the cerumen farther into the canal.	Lecture Discussion Audiovisual materials Printed materials Lecture is appropriate when disseminating information to large groups. Discussion allows participants to bring up concerns and to raise questions. Audiovisual materials, such as illustrations of the structures of the ear, reinforce verbal presentation. Printed material, especially to be taken away with learners, allows review, reinforcement, and reading at the learner's own pace.	Written examination. May use short answer, fill-in, or multiple-choice items or a combination of items. If these are short and easy to evaluate, the learner receives immediate feedback.

▶ References

Altenhoevel, A., Norman, K., Smoliner, C., & Peroz, I. (2012). The impact of self-perceived masticatory function on nutritional and gastrointestinal complaints in the elderly. *Journal of Nutrition, Health, and Aging, 16*(2), 175–178.

American Academy of Pediatric Dentistry (AAPD). (n.d.). *Frequently asked questions.* Retrieved from http://www.aapd.org/resources/frequently_asked_questions/

American Speech-Language-Hearing Association (ASHA). (n.d.) Causes of hearing loss in adults. Retrieved from http://www.asha.org/public/hearing/Causes-of-Hearing-Loss-in-Adults/

Berman, A., & Snyder, S. J. (2012). *Kozier and Erb's fundamentals of nursing: Concepts, process, and practice* (9th ed.). Upper Saddle River, NJ: Prentice Hall.

Centers for Disease Control and Prevention (CDC). (2011). *Workplace safety & health topics: Noise and hearing loss prevention.* Retrieved from http://www.cdc.gov/niosh/topics/noise/faq.html

Centers for Disease Control and Prevention (CDC). (2012a). *Hearing loss in children: Facts.* Retrieved from http://www.cdc.gov/ncbddd/hearingloss/facts.html

Centers for Disease Control and Prevention (CDC). (2012b). *Respiratory hygiene/cough etiquette in healthcare settings.* Retrieved from http://www.cdc.gov/flu/professionals/infectioncontrol/resphygiene.htm

Centers for Disease Control and Prevention (CDC). (2014). *Loss of smell (anosmia)—causes.* Retrieved from http://www.mayoclinic.org/symptoms/loss-of-smell/basics/causes/sym-20050804

Ely, J. W., Hansen, M. R., & Clark, E. C. (2008). Diagnosis of ear pain. *American Family Physician, 77*(5), 621–626.

Gonsalves, W. C., Chi, A. C., & Neville, B. W. (2007a). Common oral lesions: Part I. Superficial musocal lesions. *American Family Physician, 75*(4), 501–506.

Gonsalves, W. C., Chi, A. C., & Neville, B. W. (2007b). Common oral lesions: Part II. Masses and neoplasia. *American Family Physician, 75*(4), 509–512.

Guyuron, B., & Afrooz, P. N. (2008). Correction of cocaine-related nasal defects. *Plastic and Reconstructive Surgery, 121*(3), 1015–1023.

Kumar, R., Hayhurst, K. L., & Robson, A. K. (2011). Ear, nose, and throat manifestations during pregnancy. *Otolaryngology—Head and Neck Surgery, 145*(2), 188–198.

Marieb, E. (2009). *Essentials of human anatomy and physiology* (9th ed.). Redwood City, CA: Benjamin Cummings/Pearson Education.

Marrs, T., Anagnostou, K., Fitzsimons, R., & Fox, A. T. (2013). Optimising treatment of allergic rhinitis in children. *Practitioner, 257*(1762), 13–18.

Mason, P. (2013). Nothing smaller than your elbows, please [Web log post]. Retrieved from http://blog.asha.org/2013/01/08/nothing-smaller-than-your-elbow-please/

Mayo Clinic. (2011). *At what age do children start losing their baby teeth?* Retrieved from http://www.mayoclinic.org/healthy-living/childrens-health/expert-answers/baby-teeth/faq-20058532

Mayo Clinic. (2012). *Nosebleeds: Causes.* Retrieved from http://www.mayoclinic.org/symptoms/nosebleeds/basics/causes/sym-20050914

Mayo Clinic. (2013). *Ear infection (middle ear): Complications.* Retrieved from http://www.mayoclinic.org/diseases-conditions/ear-infections/basics/complications/con-20014260

Mayo Clinic (2014). *Second trimester pregnancy: What to expect.* Retrieved from http://www.mayoclinic.org/diseases-conditions/ear-infections/basics/complications/con-20014260

McMillan, J. A., Feigin, R. D., DeAngelis, C. D., & Jones, M. D., Jr. (2006). *Oski's pediatrics: Principles and practice* (4th ed.). Philadelphia, PA: Lippincott.

National Cancer Institute (NCI). (n.d.). *Head and neck cancer.* Retrieved from http://www.cancer.gov/cancertopics/factsheet/Sites-Types/head-and-neck

O'Neill, O. M., Johnston, B. T., & Coleman, H. G. (2013). Achalasia: A review of clinical diagnosis, epidemiology, treatment and outcomes. *World Journal of Gastroenterology, 19*(35), 5808–5812.

Osborn, K. S., Wraa, C. E., Watson, A., & Holleran, R. S. (2013). *Medical-surgical nursing: Preparation for practice* (2nd ed.). Upper Saddle River, NJ: Pearson.

Parnell, C., Whelton, H., & O'Mullane, D. (2009). Water fluoridation. *European Archives of Paediatric Dentistry, 10*(3), 141–148.

Prokop-Prigge, K. A., Thaler, E., Wysocki, C. J., & Preti, G. (2014). Identification of volatile organic compounds in human cerumen. *Journal of Chromatography B, 953*, 48–52.

Shaikh, N., Hoberman, A., Paradise, J. L., Wald, E. R., Switze, G. E., Kurs-Lasky, M., ... Zoffel, L. M. (2009). Development and preliminary evaluation of a parent-reported outcome instrument for clinical trials in acute otitis media. *Pediatric Infectious Disease Journal, 28*(1), 5–8.

Sly, P. D., & Holt, P. G. (2011). Role of innate immunity in the development of allergy and asthma. *Current opinion in allergy and clinical immunology, 11*(2), 127–131.

Smith, D. F., & Boss, E. F. (2010). Racial/ethnic and socioeconomic disparities in the prevalence and treatment of otitis media in children in the United States. *The Laryngoscope, 120*(11), 2306–2312.

Smith, S., & Hoare, D. (2012). Ringing in my ears: Tinnitus in pregnancy. *Practising Midwife, 15*(8), 20–23.

Sura, L., Madhavan, A., Carnaby, G., & Crary, M. A. (2012). Dysphagia in the elderly: Management and nutritional considerations. *Clinical Interventions in Aging, 7*, 287–298.

U.S. Department of Health and Human Services (USDHHS). (2014). *Healthy people 2020.* Retrieved from http://www.healthypeople.gov/2020/default.aspx

U.S. Department of Health and Human Services (USDHHS) Office of Minority Health. (2009). *Cleft lip/palate more prevalent in Asians.* Retrieved from http://minorityhealth.hhs.gov/templates/content.aspx?ID=7590&lvl=3&lvlID=287

Wilson, B. A., Shannon, M. T., & Shields, K. M. (2013). *Pearson nurse's drug guide.* Upper Saddle River, NJ: Pearson.

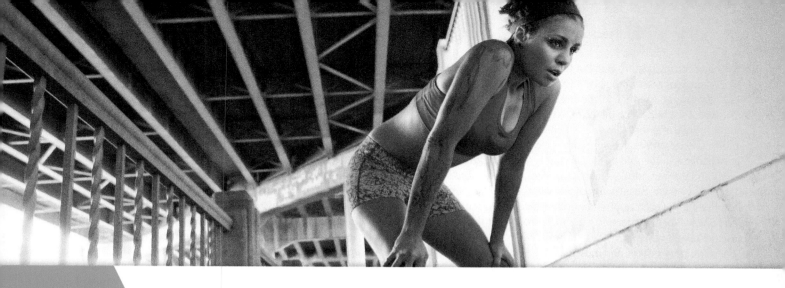

▶ Learning Outcomes

Upon completion of this chapter, you will be able to:

1. Describe the anatomy and physiology of the respiratory system.

2. Identify landmarks that guide assessment of the respiratory system.

3. Develop questions to be used when completing the focused interview.

4. Explain patient preparation for assessment of the respiratory system.

5. Describe the techniques required for assessment of the respiratory system.

6. Differentiate normal from abnormal findings in physical assessment of the respiratory system.

7. Describe developmental, psychosocial, cultural, and environmental variations in assessment techniques and findings related to the respiratory system.

8. Discuss the objectives related to the overall health of the respiratory system as presented in *Healthy People 2020*.

9. Apply critical thinking to the physical assessment of the respiratory system.

Key Terms

adventitious sounds, 404
angle of Louis, 376
bronchial sounds, 402
bronchophony, 404
bronchovesicular sounds, 402
choanal atresia, 382
dullness, 400
dyspnea, 375
egophony, 404
eupnea, 375
fremitus, 398
landmarks, 375
laryngomalacia, 382
manubrium, 376
mediastinum, 372
orthopnea, 386
rales, 404
resonance, 399
respiratory cycle, 373
rhonchi, 404
tracheal sounds, 402
tracheomalacia, 382
vesicular sounds, 402
wheezes, 404
whispered pectoriloquy, 404

The primary responsibility of the respiratory system is the exchange of gases in the body. Exchange of oxygen and carbon dioxide is essential to the homeostatic and hemodynamic processes of the body. The intake of oxygen needed for metabolism and the release of carbon dioxide, which is the waste product of metabolism, occur with each respiratory cycle. This delicate balance of gas exchange is influenced by the nervous system, the cardiovascular system, and the musculoskeletal system. The central nervous system, influenced by the concentration of gases in the blood, regulates the rate and depth of each respiratory cycle. The cardiovascular system is responsible for transporting the gases throughout the body. The musculoskeletal system provides the bones to protect the structures of the respiratory system, and muscular activity allows for the rhythmic movement of the thoracic cavity. This coordinated movement, together with pressure changes in the thoracic cavity, lead to the exchange of the oxygen and carbon dioxide.

The respiratory system has a major role in helping the body to maintain acid–base balance. The concentration of carbon dioxide in the blood directly influences the blood concentration of carbonic acid and hydrogen ions. The respiratory system responds to the needs of the body to either retain or excrete carbon dioxide. This action will help maintain the delicate balance of carbonic acid and bicarbonate ions at the 1:20 ratio, keeping the plasma pH between 7.35 and 7.45, which is the normal range.

The respiratory system is also influential in the production of vocal sounds. The sounds commonly referred to as speech are produced as air moves out of the lungs and passes over the vocal cords. The pitch and volume of one's speech are influenced by the length and tension of the vocal cords, the movement of the glottis, and the force of the air across the vocal cords. The quality of the voice is further influenced by other structures including the pharynx, tongue, palate, mouth, and lips.

Assessment of respiratory function is an integral aspect of the total patient assessment performed by the professional nurse. Developmental factors are considered during assessment of the respiratory system. For example, newborns have a high respiratory rate. In the pediatric patient, respirations are abdominal in nature. In pregnant patients, as the uterus enlarges, increasing pressure in the abdominal cavity limits diaphragmatic excursion and can result in more rapid and shallow respirations.

Environmental factors also contribute to respiratory difficulty and pathology, which ultimately can affect respiratory function. Assessment must identify exposure to irritants such as dust, tobacco, smoke, pollen, smog, asbestos, and vapors from household cleaners. Tobacco use is one of the topics discussed in *Healthy People 2020*, which also includes objectives to promote respiratory health through prevention, detection, treatment, and education (see Table 17.1 on page 383). The nurse must be cognizant of factors that influence respiratory health as questions for the focused interview are formulated and physical assessment is performed.

Anatomy and Physiology Review

The thorax, commonly called the chest, is a closed cavity of the body, containing structures needed for respiration. The thorax, or thoracic cavity, is surrounded by ribs and muscles and extends from the base of the neck to the diaphragm. It has three sections: the mediastinum and the right and left pleural cavities. The **mediastinum** contains the heart, trachea, esophagus, and major blood vessels of the body. Each pleural cavity contains a lung (see Figure 17.1 ■).

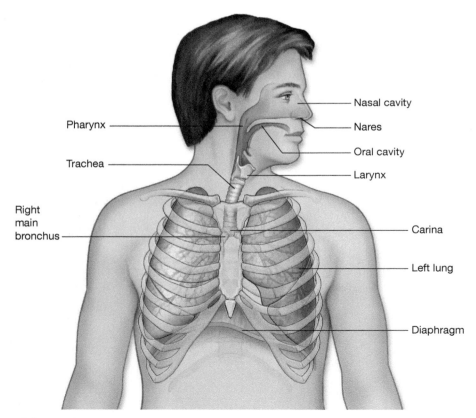

Figure 17.1 Anatomy of the respiratory system.

The major structures of the respiratory system are situated in the thoracic cavity. The main function of the respiratory system is to supply the body with oxygen and expel carbon dioxide. Air moves in and out of the lungs with each **respiratory cycle.** A complete respiratory cycle consists of an inspiratory phase and an expiratory phase of breathing. The exchange of oxygen and carbon dioxide at the alveoli level of the lung is *external respiration.* Gases are transported from the lungs via the blood to the cells of the body. As the gases move across the systemic capillaries, exchange of oxygen and carbon dioxide occurs at the cellular level and *internal respiration* occurs.

The respiratory system consists of the upper and lower respiratory tracts. The structures of the upper respiratory tract include the nose, the mouth, the sinuses, the pharynx, the larynx, and the proximal portion of the trachea. The lower respiratory tract includes the distal portion of the trachea, as well as the bronchi and lungs. Pleural membranes, the muscles of respiration, and the mediastinum complete the lower respiratory tract.

The anatomy and physiology review and assessment of the structures of the upper respiratory tract are discussed in chapter 14 ∞ on pages 262–264. Before proceeding, it may be helpful to review that information.

Lower Respiratory Tract

The lower respiratory tract includes the trachea, bronchi, and lungs. Additional structures of the pleural membranes, the mediastinum, and the muscles of respiration are also discussed at this time. Consideration must be given to all structures during the assessment process.

Trachea

The trachea, located in the mediastinum, descends from the larynx in the neck to the main bronchi at the distal point. In adults, the trachea is approximately 10 to 12 cm (4 in.) long and 2.5 cm (1 in.) in diameter. The trachea is a very flexible and mobile structure, bifurcating anteriorly at about the sternal angle and posteriorly at about the vertebrae T3 to T5. The trachea contains 16 to 20 rings of hyaline cartilage. These C-shaped rings help maintain the shape of the trachea and prevent its collapse during inspiration and expiration. Just above the point of bifurcation, the last tracheal cartilage, known as the carina, is expanded. The carina separates the openings of the two main bronchi. The trachea, like other structures of the respiratory tract, is lined with a mucus-producing membrane that traps dust, bacteria, and other foreign bodies. This membrane at the level of the carina is most sensitive to foreign substances. Coughing and cilia, which are hairlike projections of the membrane, help sweep debris toward the mouth for removal.

Bronchi

Anteriorly, the trachea bifurcates at about the level of the sternal angle, forming the right and left main bronchi (see Figure 17.2 ■). The main bronchus enters each lung at the hilus (medial depression) and maintains an oblique position in the mediastinum. The right main bronchus is shorter, wider, and more vertical than the left main bronchus; therefore, aspirated objects are more likely to enter the right lung. The bronchi continue to divide within each lobe of the lung. The terminal bronchioles are less than 0.5 mm (0.019 in.) in diameter. The bronchi and the many branches continue to warm and moisten air as it moves along the respiratory tract to the alveoli in the lungs.

Lungs

The lungs are cone-shaped, elastic, spongy, air-filled structures that are situated in the pleural cavities of the thorax on either side of the mediastinum (see Figure 17.3 ■). The apex of each lung is slightly superior to the inner third of the clavicle, and the base of each lung is at the level of the diaphragm. The left lung has two lobes (upper and lower) and tends to be longer and narrower than the right lung. The left lung accommodates the heart at the medial surface. The oblique fissure separates the two lobes of this lung.

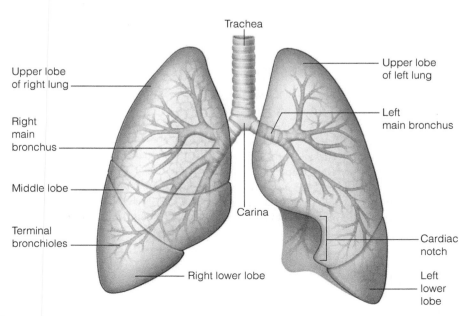

Figure 17.2 Respiratory passages.

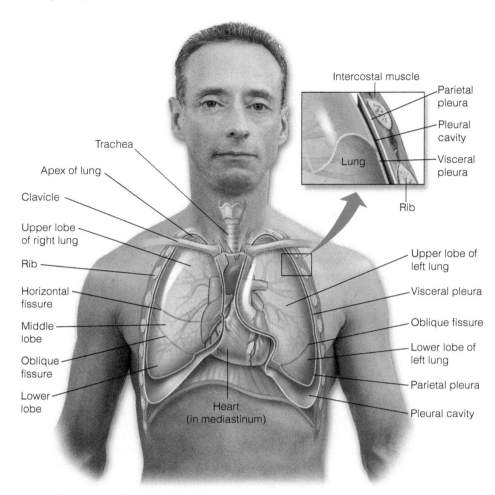

Figure 17.3 Anterior view of thorax and lungs.

The right lung has three lobes (upper, middle, and lower) and is slightly larger, wider, and shorter than the left lung. The horizontal and oblique fissures separate the lobes of the right lung. Within each lung, the numerous terminal bronchioles branch into the alveolar ducts, which lead into alveolar sacs and alveoli. The single-layered cells of the alveoli permit simple diffusion and gas exchanges to occur (see Figure 17.4 ■).

Pleural Membranes

The pleura is a thin, double-layered, serous membrane that lines each pleural cavity. The parietal membrane lines the superior aspect of the diaphragm and the thoracic wall. The visceral membrane covers the outer surface of the lung. A pleural fluid produced by these membranes acts as a lubricant, allowing the lung to glide during the respiratory cycle of inspiration and expiration. The surface tension created by the fluid and the negative pressure between the membranes helps keep the lungs expanded. As the negative pressure changes, one is able to move air into and out of the lungs.

Mediastinum

The mediastinum is the middle section of the thoracic cavity and is surrounded by the right and left pleural cavities. The mediastinum

contains the heart, the trachea, the esophagus, the proximal portion of the right and left main bronchi, and the great vessels of the body.

Respiratory Process

Respiratory process is a general term that encompasses the structures and activities of respiration. The respiratory process is dependent on the muscles of the thorax, the structures of the thoracic cage, and the ability of air to move in and out of the body.

Muscles of Respiration

The muscles of the thoracic cage (internal and external intercostal) and the diaphragm assist in the breathing process. The synergistic action of these muscle groups aids in the respiratory cycle of inspiration and expiration. The accessory muscles of the neck (trapezius, scalene, and sternocleidomastoid), abdomen (rectus), and chest (pectorals) assist the respiratory cycle as necessary. The accessory muscles play a major role in the respiratory cycle during distress and pathology.

Thoracic Cage

The thoracic cage consists of the bones, cartilage, and muscles of the thorax. The sternum (breastbone) is located in the anterior midline of the thorax. The vertebrae are located at the dorsal or posterior

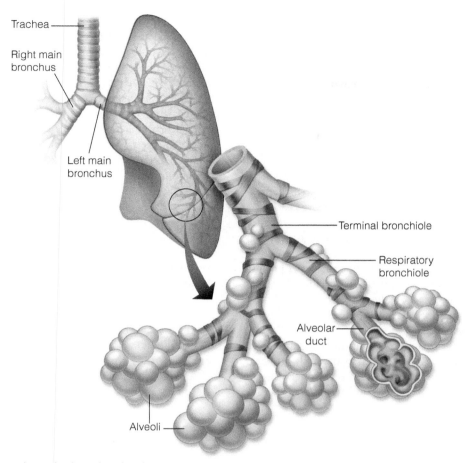

Trachea

Right main bronchus

Left main bronchus

Terminal bronchiole

Respiratory bronchiole

Alveolar duct

Alveoli

Figure 17.4 Respiratory bronchioles, alveolar ducts, and alveoli.

aspect of the thorax. The 12 pairs of ribs circle the body, form the lateral aspects of the thorax, and are attached to the vertebrae and sternum. Anteriorly, the first seven pairs of ribs articulate directly to the sternum. The cartilage of ribs 8, 9, and 10 articulates with the cartilage of rib 7, whereas the pairs of ribs 11 and 12 are free floating and do not articulate anteriorly. The costal cartilage and external intercostal muscles help to complete the thoracic cage. This bony cage helps protect the many vital organs of the pleura and mediastinum, supports the shoulders and upper extremities, and helps support many muscles of the upper part of the body.

Respiratory Cycle

Respiratory cycle, respirations, and *breathing* are terms used interchangeably to indicate the movement of air in and out of the body. Breathing consists of two phases: inspiration and expiration; thus the term *respiratory cycle.* Inspiration is considered to be the active aspect of the respiratory cycle. For air to enter the body, the respiratory muscles contract, the chest expands, alveolar pressure decreases, and the negative intrapleural pressure increases. These combined activities allow air to enter the expanded lungs. During expiration, the passive phase of the process, the activities reverse themselves: the lungs recoil, and air leaves the body. The regular, even-depth, rhythmic pattern of inspiration and expiration describes **eupnea** (normal breathing). A change in this pattern, producing shortness of breath or difficulty in breathing, is called **dyspnea.**

Landmarks

Identification and location of **landmarks** help the professional nurse develop a mental picture of the structures being assessed. Thoracic reference points and specific anatomic structures are used as landmarks (see Figure 17.5 ■). They help provide an exact location for the assessment findings and an accurate orientation for documentation of findings. Landmark identification for the thorax includes bony structures, horizontal and vertical lines, and the division of the thorax.

The thorax may be divided into two or three sections for assessment. Two sections include the anterior and posterior thorax, while three sections include the anterior, lateral, and posterior aspects. This text uses the former option: The lateral areas are incorporated into the anterior and posterior sections. The bony structures include the sternum, clavicles, ribs, and vertebrae. At the horizontal plane, the landmarks are the clavicles, the ribs, and the corresponding intercostal spaces. Anteriorly, the vertical lines start at the sternum and are strategically drawn parallel to this structure. Posteriorly, the vertical lines start at the vertebral column and additional lines are drawn parallel to this reference point.

The first bony landmark to be considered is the sternum, commonly called the breastbone. It is a flat, elongated bone located in the midline of the anterior thoracic cage and consists of three parts: the manubrium, the body, and the xiphoid process.

The clavicles and some of the pairs of ribs articulate with the sternum. The **manubrium** is the superior portion of the sternum. The depression at the superior border is called the suprasternal notch or jugular notch. This becomes a primary landmark used to identify and locate other landmarks. The manubrium joins the body of the sternum. As these structures meet, a horizontal ridge is formed, referred to as the sternal angle or **angle of Louis.** The second rib and the second intercostal space are at this level of the sternum. The sternum terminates at the xiphoid process. This process and the inferior borders of the seventh ribs form a triangle referred to as the costal angle. The inferior border of the ribs and the costal angle help identify the level of the diaphragm, the base of the lungs, and the separation of the thoracic cavity from the abdomen (see Figure 17.5A).

The clavicles are long, slender, curved bones that articulate with the manubrium at the medial aspect. The lateral aspects help form the shoulder joint with the acromion process of the scapula. The clavicles act as a shock absorber protecting the upper portion of the thoracic cage and the delicate underlying structures. Lung tissue will be assessed above and below the clavicles. Findings above the clavicle are considered supraclavicular, while findings below the clavicle are infraclavicular.

The 12 pairs of ribs are another group of bony landmarks used in respiratory assessment. The ribs circle the body and help form horizontal reference points. Posteriorly, each rib attaches to a thoracic vertebra. The ribs curve downward and forward as they become anterior (see Figure 17.5B). Bilaterally, the first seven ribs attach to the sternum and are called true ribs. Ribs 8, 9, and 10 attach to cartilage of the superior rib, while ribs 11 and 12 are free floating anteriorly. A number identifies each rib. Each intercostal space, the space between the ribs, takes the number of the superior rib. The first rib and the first intercostal space, being obscured by the clavicle, are not palpable. Anteriorly, ribs 2 to 7 and the corresponding intercostal spaces are easily palpated along the sternal border. Posteriorly, the ribs are best palpated and counted close to the vertebral column. Each rib and intercostal space form a horizontal line used as a landmark.

The vertebral column, commonly called the spine, is located at the midline of the posterior portion of the thoracic cage. Twelve vertebrae are thoracic, and a pair of ribs articulates with each. The vertebral column contributes to the vertical lines discussed later in this chapter. The seventh cervical vertebra (C7) is most visible at the base of the neck. The much larger spinous process contributes to the uniqueness of the vertebra. This prominent vertebra (C7) is used to count and locate other spinous processes. When two spinous processes are equally prominent, they are C7 and T1 (see Figure 17.6 ■).

Five imaginary vertical lines are identified on the anterior aspect of the thoracic cage (see Figure 17.7 ■). These lines are the sternal line, the right and left midclavicular lines, and the right and left anterior axillary lines. The sternal or midsternal line (SL) starts at the sternal notch and descends through the xiphoid process. It

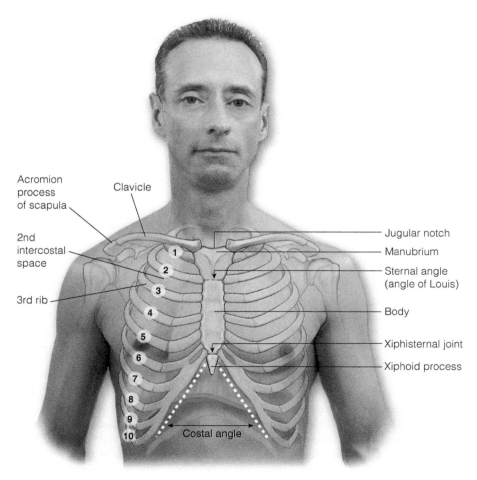

Figure 17.5A Landmarks of the anterior thorax, anterior view.

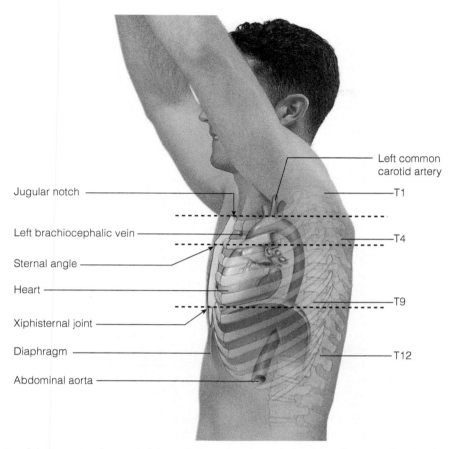

Figure 17.5B Landmarks of the anterior thorax, left lateral view, showing relationship of anterior landmarks to the vertebral column.

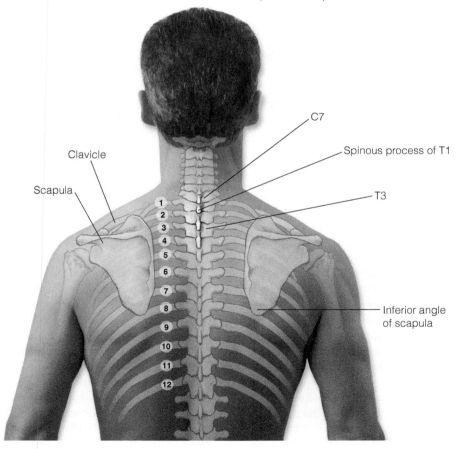

Figure 17.6 Landmarks: Posterior thorax.

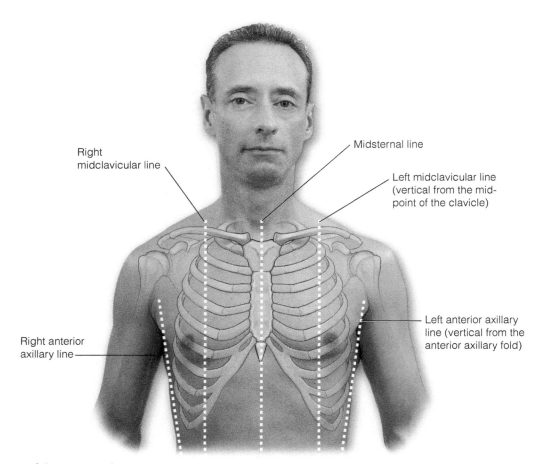

Right
midclavicular line

Midsternal line

Left midclavicular line
(vertical from the mid-
point of the clavicle)

Right anterior
axillary line

Left anterior axillary
line (vertical from the
anterior axillary fold)

Figure 17.7 Lines of the anterior thorax.

divides the sternum in half and ultimately identifies the right and left thoracic cage. The right and left midclavicular lines are parallel to the sternal line. The midclavicular line begins at the midpoint of the clavicle and descends to the level of the 12th rib. The nipples of the breast are slightly lateral to this line. This line subdivides the right and left thoracic cage into two equal parts. The anterior axillary line (AAL) is another line drawn parallel to the sternal line. It begins at the anterior fold of the axillae and descends along the anterior lateral aspect of the thoracic cage to the 12th rib.

Five imaginary lines are located on the posterior aspect of the thoracic cage (see Figure 17.8 ■). The vertebral line, the right and left scapular lines, and the right and left posterior axillary lines are used as landmarks on the posterior aspect of the thoracic cage. The vertebral or midspinous line commences at C7 and descends through the spinous process of each thoracic vertebra. It divides the vertebral column in half, forming the posterior right and left thoracic cage.

The scapular line, parallel to the vertebral line, is drawn from the inferior angle of the scapula to the level of the 12th rib. This line subdivides the right and left thoracic cage into two equal parts. The posterior axillary line (PAL) is parallel to the vertebral line. It starts at the posterior axillary fold and descends along the lateral aspect of the thoracic cage to the 12th rib.

The lateral aspect of the thoracic cage is the third section to be considered. Three imaginary lines are identified in this section (see Figure 17.9 ■). They are the anterior axillary, posterior axillary, and midaxillary lines. Two of these lines, the anterior and posterior lines,

have been described. The midaxillary line is parallel to the anterior and posterior axillary lines. This line descends from the middle of the axillae to the level of the 12th rib. It forms the frontal plane, dividing the thorax into the anterior and posterior portions.

The described landmarks serve as a reference point for internal structures of the respiratory system. Recall that the trachea bifurcates, forming the right and left main bronchi. Anteriorly, this occurs at the level of the angle of Louis or sternal angle. Posteriorly, this bifurcation occurs between the third and fifth thoracic vertebrae.

The apices of the lung extend 2 to 4 cm (0.78 to 1.57 in.) above the inner third of the clavicle anteriorly. Posteriorly, the apices of the lungs are located superior to the scapula between the vertebral line and midscapular line. The base of the lung has three reference points. The lung is cone shaped, and the base of the lung is located at the sixth intercostal space at the midclavicular line. At the midaxillary line, the base of the lung is at the eighth intercostal space. At the scapular line on the posterior thorax, the base of the lung is at the 10th intercostal space.

Using external landmarks and drawing imaginary lines can also identify the five lobes of the lungs. Remember that the right lung has three lobes and the left lung has two lobes. The right and left oblique fissure divides the lung into upper and lower lobes. Starting at C7, identify T3. Draw an imaginary line from T3 at the vertebral line to the fifth intercostal space at the midaxillary line. This line follows the border of the scapula when the arms are extended over the head. It reflects the oblique fissure on the posterior wall of the thorax (see

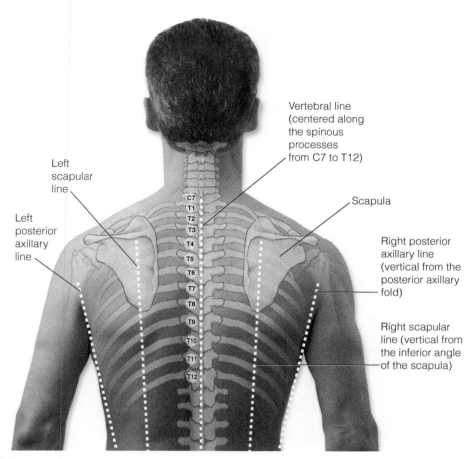

Vertebral line (centered along the spinous processes from C7 to T12)

Scapula

Right posterior axillary line (vertical from the posterior axillary fold)

Right scapular line (vertical from the inferior angle of the scapula)

Left scapular line

Left posterior axillary line

Figure 17.8 Lines of the posterior thorax.

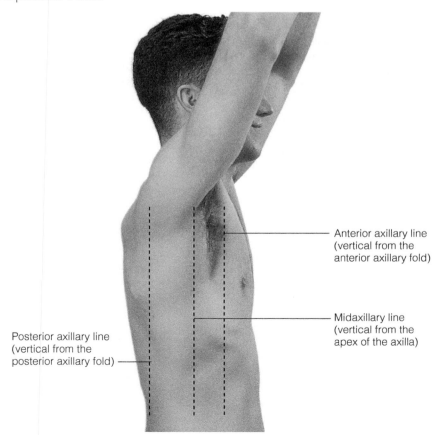

Anterior axillary line (vertical from the anterior axillary fold)

Midaxillary line (vertical from the apex of the axilla)

Posterior axillary line (vertical from the posterior axillary fold)

Figure 17.9 Lines of the lateral thorax.

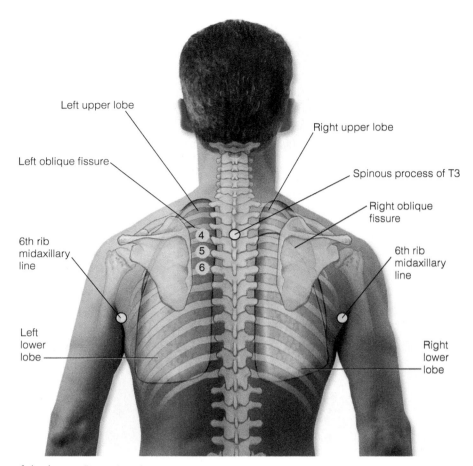

Figure 17.10 Lobes of the lungs: Posterior view.

Figure 17.10 ■). On the left side continue this line to the sixth intercostal at the left midclavicular line. The two lobes of the left lung have been identified at the posterior, lateral, and anterior aspects of the left thorax.

Anteriorly, on the right side, draw two lines from the fifth intercostal space at the midaxillary line. One line descends to the sixth intercostal space at the right midclavicular line. The second line transverses the right thorax to the sternal border inferior to the fourth rib. These lines identify the oblique fissure and the horizontal fissure, forming the three lobes of the right lung (see Figure 17.11 ■ and Figures 17.12A ■ and B ■).

The clavicle, the scapula, and the lateral base of the neck form a triangle at the superior aspect of the thorax. This triangle, also known as Kronig's area, is used for palpation of muscles and lymph nodes and for percussion and auscultation of the apex and the lungs.

Special Considerations

Throughout the assessment process the nurse gathers subjective and objective data reflecting the patient's state of health. Using critical thinking and the nursing process, the nurse identifies many factors to be considered when collecting the data. Some of these factors include but are not limited to age, developmental level, race, ethnicity, work history, living conditions, socioeconomic status, and emotional wellness.

Health Promotion Considerations

Oxygen is essential to life. Respiratory disorders and diseases include pathophysiological conditions that impair the respiratory system's ability to obtain oxygen (O_2) and expel, or get rid of, carbon dioxide (CO_2). Examples of common respiratory disorders include asthma and chronic obstructive pulmonary disease (COPD), which comprises two respiratory disorders: chronic bronchitis and emphysema.

Those objectives of *Healthy People 2020* related to the respiratory system include the prevention of asthma and COPD through reduction of exposure to known respiratory hazards. In addition, these objectives include identifying new potential threats to respiratory health. For individuals who experience asthma or COPD, *Healthy People 2020* aims to ensure the provision of effective treatment as well as to reduce the limitations caused by respiratory disease. Patient education also is a focus of objectives related to respiratory health (USDHHS, 2010). See Table 17.1 for examples of *Healthy People 2020* objectives that are designed to promote health and wellness among individuals across the life span.

Lifespan Considerations

Growth and development are dynamic processes that describe change over time. The collection of data and the interpretation of findings in relation to normative values are important. These data will reflect the growth and developmental stages of the individual.

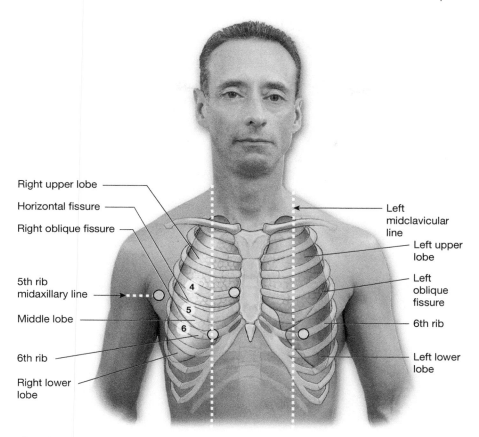

Figure 17.11 Lobes of the lungs: Anterior view.

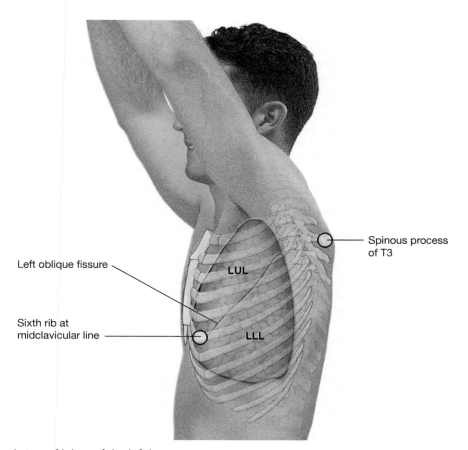

Figure 17.12A Lateral view of lobes of the left lung.

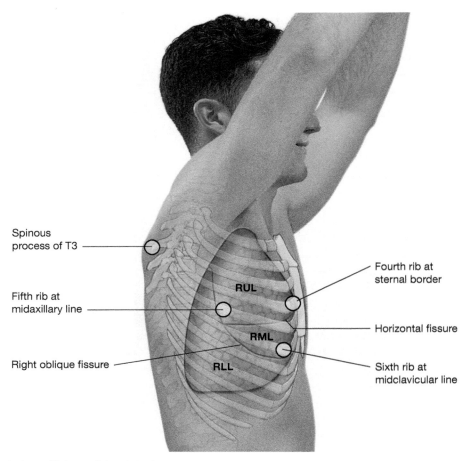

Spinous process of T3

Fifth rib at midaxillary line

Right oblique fissure

RUL

RML

RLL

Fourth rib at sternal border

Horizontal fissure

Sixth rib at midclavicular line

Figure 17.12B Lateral view of lobes of the right lung.

TABLE 17.1	Examples of *Healthy People 2020* Objectives Related to Respiratory Health
OBJECTIVE NUMBER	**DESCRIPTION**
RD-1	Reduce asthma deaths
RD-2	Reduce hospitalizations for asthma
RD-3	Reduce emergency department (ED) visits for asthma
RD-4	Reduce activity limitations among persons with current asthma
RD-5	Reduce the proportion of persons with asthma who miss school or work days
RD-6	Increase the proportion of persons with current asthma who receive formal patient education
RD-7	Increase the proportion of persons with current asthma who receive appropriate asthma care according to National Asthma Education and Prevention Program (NAEPP) guidelines
RD-8	Increase the number of States, Territories, and the District of Columbia with a comprehensive asthma surveillance system for tracking asthma cases, illness, and disability at the State level
RD-9	Reduce activity limitations among adults with chronic obstructive pulmonary disease (COPD)
RD-10	Reduce deaths from chronic obstructive pulmonary disease (COPD) among adults
RD-11	Reduce hospitalizations for chronic obstructive pulmonary disease (COPD)
RD-12	Reduce emergency department (ED) visits for chronic obstructive pulmonary disease (COPD)
RD-13	(Developmental) Increase the proportion of adults with abnormal lung function whose underlying obstructive disease has been diagnosed

Source: U.S. Department of Health and Human Services (USDHHS). (2014). *Healthy people 2020.* Retrieved from http://www.healthypeople.gov/2020/default.aspx.

The following discussion presents specific variations for different age groups.

Infants and Children

During fetal development, respirations are passive and gas exchange occurs at the placenta. At birth, rapid changes occur in the respiratory system as fetal circulation closes. One significant change that occurs is a marked increase in pulmonary blood flow. Other changes include the closure of the foramen ovale and ductus arteriosus and the increase in chest expansion. Gaseous exchanges now take place via the respiratory system and atmosphere. During the first several hours of extrauterine life, the respiratory rate of the newborn is rapid (40 to 80 per minute) and irregular. During the neonatal and infant period, the respiratory rate decreases and becomes more regular. By 5 years of age, the respiratory rate is about 35 breaths per minute.

Compared to adults, children have much smaller, more compliant airways until early adolescence. Until that time, children are more prone to airway collapse and blockage. Oxygen needs are higher in small children because their increased metabolic rates result in higher oxygen consumption. It is important to carefully assess and manage children who show signs of dyspnea and respiratory distress. The risk of respiratory failure is greatest in infants, toddlers, and preschoolers, but children of all ages experience respiratory failure much more quickly than adults.

Choanal atresia is a congenital defect that results in a thin membrane that obstructs the nasal passages. If undetected or left untreated, severe respiratory distress results. All newborns must be carefully assessed for nasal patency. **Laryngomalacia** and **tracheomalacia** are congenital defects of the cartilage in the larynx and trachea, respectively. Infants with laryngomalacia or tracheomalacia have airways that easily collapse. Parents frequently describe children with laryngomalacia or tracheomalacia as "noisy breathers." Continuous inspiratory and expiratory stridor that worsens during crying or with certain head positions and improves during the first year of life characterizes these abnormalities.

At birth, the circumference of the chest is slightly less than the circumference of the head. During childhood, chest circumference exceeds head size by about 5 to 7 cm (1.96 to 2.75 in.). The chest is usually round with the lateral and anterior–posterior diameters being almost equal. Bony structures of the chest are more prominent during infancy because skin and musculature are thin. Neonates have a respiratory rate and depth that are likely to be irregular. At this age, breathing involves use of abdominal muscles; therefore, inspection of the abdomen will yield a more accurate respiratory rate. Abdominal breathing continues during childhood until about 5 to 7 years of age. Costal breathing is the expected pattern after 7 years of age.

The Pregnant Female

The hormonal changes of pregnancy and the growing fetus produce changes in the respiratory system of the pregnant female. The ligaments of the thorax relax, the horizontal diameter expands, and the costal angle increases. At rest, the diaphragm rises into the chest to accommodate the fetus and respirations are diaphragmatic. Shortness of breath and dyspnea, especially in the last trimester, are common as the maternal and fetal demand for oxygen increases. Throughout pregnancy, the total oxygen consumption can increase by 20% and the maternal respiratory rate increases approximately two breaths per minute. Maternal hyperventilation occurs due to an increase in minute ventilation, which is the total volume of air that is inhaled and exhaled in a one-minute period (see chapter 27 ∞).

The Older Adult

As individuals age, the respiratory system becomes less efficient. The lungs lose their elasticity, the skeletal muscles begin to weaken, and bones lose their density. As a result, it becomes more difficult for the older adult to expand the thoracic cage and take a deep breath. The diameters of the thoracic cage change. The appearance of a barrel chest and calcification of cartilage contribute to the decrease in thoracic excursion. Thus, the older adult inhales and exhales smaller amounts of air. Weakening of the chest muscles hinders the older adult's ability to cough. Dry mucous membranes, decreased ciliary function, and the inability to cough compromise airway clearance.

The rate of respirations in the older adult is slightly higher than in the middle-aged adult. The older adult has a more shallow respiratory cycle because of the decreased vital capacity. Auscultatory sounds may be less audible because of the decreased pulmonary function. The trapping of air in the alveoli will produce a sound of hyperresonance upon percussion.

The number of capillaries in the pulmonary tissue decreases, and there is less blood flow available for gas exchange. Normal alveoli enlarge and their walls become thinner. Because they are less elastic, it becomes more difficult to maintain positive pressure and keep the small airways open. Gas exchange becomes compromised, especially in the bases of the lungs. Alveolar hypoventilation and carbon dioxide retention may occur.

The older person uses more accessory muscles, and, therefore, must work harder and use more energy to take in air. Older adults may tire more easily and may need frequent rest periods during the assessment process. Deep mouth breathing during auscultation may increase the fatigue of the older adult. As with any patient, the nurse must prevent hyperventilation at this time.

The older adult cannot respond well to stress. Anxiety and physical exertion can cause significant demands on the respiratory system, and infection can have devastating effects. Older adults with a long history of smoking or exposure to environmental pollutants are at increased risk for respiratory diseases. It is important for the older adult to obtain vaccinations against influenza and pneumonia.

ALERT!

Children are much more likely to die from respiratory failure than from cardiovascular collapse. Any child with altered sensorium should be immediately evaluated for respiratory compromise.

Psychosocial Considerations

Stress, anxiety, pain, and fatigue may exacerbate respiratory problems. Patients experiencing acute or chronic respiratory problems will have a physiologic alteration with gas exchange. These changes can limit or restrict the individual's ability to independently perform the activities of daily living and to participate in activities, exercise, and sports. This limitation contributes to social isolation, changes role activities, lowers self-esteem, and increases the dependency factor with support systems.

Certain drugs, such as bronchodilators, are used in the treatment of respiratory conditions and may cause the hands to tremble visibly. The nurse should not confuse this sign with nervousness. Even mild respiratory distress is frightening for the patient and family. Proceeding in a calm and reassuring manner helps reduce the patient's fear. Parents of young children who have experienced severe asthmatic attacks in the past may be extremely anxious any time the child develops a cold, seasonal allergy, or any other respiratory problem. A calm and careful assessment of the current health status helps to decrease the anxiety level of all involved individuals.

Cultural and Environmental Considerations

Culture and environment are significant factors in respiratory health. For example, with regard to cultural heritage, the prevalence of asthma is highest among individuals who are of Puerto Rican descent, followed by American Indians, Alaskan Natives, non-Hispanic Blacks, Filipinos, and non-Hispanic Whites. The lowest prevalence of asthma is found among individuals of Asian Indian descent, followed by individuals who are of Chinese or Mexican heritage (Forno & Celedon, 2009). In general, the incidence of asthma is higher among children who live in urban areas or who are of low socioeconomic status (Northridge, Ramirez, Stingone, & Claudio, 2010).

For patients of any cultural background, a thorough assessment of the respiratory system is best accomplished when the patient is disrobed and the surfaces of the anterior and posterior chest can be visualized, touched, and auscultated. However, some cultural or religious practices, including the wearing or prohibition of removal of symbolic icons, jewelry, undergarments, or clothing, may interfere with physical examination. Additionally, the requirement of a same-sex examiner or the presence of a companion during the assessment are issues that must be addressed. Careful questioning of the patient during the interview, with the assistance of a translator when necessary, will allow for clarification, negotiation, and decision making about the assessment process.

Patients with allergies or asthma should be encouraged to explore the possibility of allergens in their work or home environment. For example, pets, dust, and molds are common allergens found in the home. Secondhand smoke in the home or work environment can also lead to respiratory distress. Research has established a link between exposure to secondhand smoke and the development of lung cancer.

Workers in some industries may be exposed to substances that are hazardous to their respiratory health, such as caustic fumes, fungi, asbestos, coal tar, nickel, silver, textile fibers, chromate, and vinyl chlorides. All of these substances are known carcinogens. Exposure to large amounts of dust in a granary or mine may lead to the development of silicosis. Coal miners are susceptible to pneumoconiosis, a form of black lung disease. People working in an office building may need to be concerned with air conditioners and forced hot-air heat. The ducts of the cooling and heating systems can carry airborne organisms, increasing the risk for respiratory infections.

The geographic location of an individual's environment will also influence respiratory health. Factors to be considered are temperature, moisture, altitude, and pollution. A cold environment encourages vasoconstriction and, ultimately, a decreased need for oxygen. An environment with increased moisture or humidity has heavy air. Individuals will tire easily, increasing the need for oxygen. As the altitude increases, the partial pressure of oxygen decreases. The individual must adapt by increasing the rate and depth of the respiratory cycle. Air pollution with smog, industrial wastes, or exhaust fumes contributes to respiratory problems in all people.

Factors within the home and social environment will influence respiratory health. Forced hot air heat is very drying to the membranes of the body. Individuals are encouraged to add moisture or use a humidifier to keep the air moist and support respiratory health. In the hot, humid, hazy days of summer an air conditioner or dehumidifier may be necessary to help lessen the moisture in the air. Secondhand smoke, certain foods, dust, pets, and stress may also contribute to respiratory changes.

Gathering the Data

Respiratory health assessment includes the gathering of subjective and objective data. Recall that subjective data collection occurs during the patient interview, before the actual physical assessment. During the interview the nurse uses a variety of communication techniques to elicit general and specific information about the patient's state of respiratory health or illness. Health records, the results of laboratory tests, and x-rays are important secondary sources to be reviewed and included in the data-gathering process. In physical assessment of the respiratory system, the techniques of inspection, palpation, percussion, and auscultation will be used.

TABLE 17.2   Potential Secondary Sources for Patient Data Related to the Respiratory System

LABORATORY TESTS	NORMAL VALUES
Arterial Blood Gases (ABGs)	pH 7.35–7.45 pH units PO_2 80–100 mmHg PCO_2 35–45 mmHg HCO_3 22–26 mEq/L

Complete Blood Count (CBC)
  Red Blood Cells (RBCs)
 	
  Hemoglobin (Hgb)
 	
  Hematocrit (Hct)
	Male 4.32–5.72 million/mcL
	Female 3.90–5.03 million/mcL
	Male 13.5–17.5 g/dL
	Female 12.0–15.5 g/dL
	Male 38.8%–50.0%
	Female 34.9%–44.5%

White Blood Cells (WBCs)
  Leukocytes
  Bands
  Basophils
  Eosinophils
  Lymphocytes
  B-Lymphocytes
  T-Lymphocytes
  Monocytes
  Neutrophils
Platelets
Erythrocyte Sedimentation Rate (ESR)
	4,500–10,000/mcL
	0%–3%
	0.5%–1%
	1%–4%
	20%–40%
	4%–25%
	60%–95%
	2%–8%
	40%–60%
	150–450 billion/L
	Males less than 23 mm/hr
	Females less than 29 mm/hr

DIAGNOSTIC TESTS	
O_2 Saturation Normal Value ≥ 95% Chest x-ray Fiberoptic Bronchoscopy Pulmonary Function Testing Sputum Evaluation Tuberculin Skin Testing Ventilation Perfusion (VQ) Scan	

Before proceeding, it may be helpful to review the information about each of the data-gathering processes and practice the techniques of health assessment. See Table 17.2 for information on potential secondary sources of patient data.

Focused Interview

The focused interview for the respiratory system concerns data related to the structures and functions of that system. Subjective data related to respiratory status are gathered during the focused interview. The nurse must be prepared to observe the patient and listen for cues related to the function of the respiratory system. The nurse may use open-ended and closed questions to obtain information. Often a number of follow-up questions or requests for descriptions are required to clarify data or gather missing information. The subjective data collected and the questions asked during the health history and focused interview will provide information to help meet the objectives related to respiratory health as stated in *Healthy People 2020*. Follow-up questions are intended to identify the source of problems, the duration of difficulties, and measures taken to alleviate problems. Follow-up questions also provide clues about the patient's knowledge of his or her own health.

The focused interview guides the physical assessment of the respiratory system. The information is always considered in relation to norms and expectations about respiratory function. Therefore, the nurse must consider age, gender, race, culture, environment, health practices, past and concurrent problems, and therapies when framing questions and using techniques to elicit information. In order to address all of the factors when conducting a focused interview, categories of questions related to respiratory status and function have been developed. These categories include general questions that are asked of all patients: those questions addressing illness or infection; those related to symptoms, pain, or behaviors; those related to habits or practices; those that are specific to patients according to age; those for pregnant females; and those that address environmental concerns. One method to elicit information about symptoms is OLDCART & ICE, as described in chapter 7. ∞ See Figure 7.3 on page 120.

The nurse must consider the patient's ability to participate in the focused interview and physical assessment of the respiratory system. If a patient is experiencing dyspnea, cyanosis, difficulty with speech, and the anxiety that accompanies any of these problems, attention must focus on relief of symptoms and restoration of oxygenation.

Focused Interview Questions	Rationales and Evidence

The following sections provide sample questions and bulleted follow-up questions in each of the previously mentioned categories. A rationale for each of the questions is provided. The list of questions is not all-inclusive but rather represents the types of questions required in a comprehensive focused interview related to the respiratory system.

General Questions

1. **Describe your breathing today. Is it different from 2 months ago? From 2 years ago?**

   ▶ These questions give patients the opportunity to provide their own perceptions about breathing.

2. **Do you breathe through your mouth or through your nose?**
   - Have you always breathed through your mouth?
   - Do you have a problem with your nose?
   - How long have you had the problem?
   - Have you received any treatment for the problem?
   - Did the treatment help?

   ▶ Nose breathing allows inhaled air to be warmed, moistened, and filtered before entering the lung and is considered the norm. Patients who identify themselves as mouth breathers require follow-up. Mouth breathing is associated with problems in the nose, habit, or air hunger (Goodman, Lynm, & Livingston, 2013).

3. **Are you able to carry out all of your regular activities without a change in your breathing?**
   - Describe the change in your breathing.
   - Do you know what causes the change?
   - What do you do when this occurs?
   - How long has this been happening?
   - Have you discussed this with a healthcare professional?

   ▶ This provides an opportunity to elicit information about typical breathing patterns and changes related to normal activities of daily living. A yes would be considered the norm. Any other response requires follow-up questions to determine the type of change and factors that contribute to or predispose the patient to changes in breathing.

4. **Describe your breathing when you are engaged in exercise or vigorous activity.**
   - Describe the breathing problem that occurs when you are exercising or very active.
   - How long has this been happening?
   - What do you do when it happens?
   - Do your actions relieve the problem?

   ▶ A normal expectation is that the patient will describe his or her breathing as becoming more rapid or deeper with activity but quickly returning to normal upon completion of the exercise or activity. Follow-up is required when the patient describes dyspnea during, or slow recovery from, exercise or activity (Berman & Snyder, 2012).

5. **When you sleep do you lie down flat, prop yourself up with pillows, or sit up?**
   - Tell me why you prefer to sit up.
   - How many pillows do you use?
   - Does the position or number of pillows help with your breathing?
   - How long have you slept like this?
   - Have you discussed this with a healthcare professional?
   - What treatment was recommended?
   - Did the treatment help?

   ▶ The norm is for a patient to sleep fully reclined with a pillow. The number of pillows for propping up oneself should be determined. Patients who must prop themselves up or sit up while sleeping may have **orthopnea,** that is, dyspnea when lying down (Dumitru & Baker, 2014). It is important to determine if the propping up or sitting up is simply a preference or because of breathing problems or some other cause.

6. **Do you have any physical problems that affect your breathing?**
   - Describe the way your breathing is affected.
   - How long has this been occurring?
   - Have you sought treatment for the problem?
   - What was the treatment?
   - Did the treatment help?

   ▶ This is a general question to elicit information about respiratory or other problems that impact breathing. For example, pain from an injury to the upper body may impact breathing but not be directly related to respiratory structures. If the patient identifies any problems that affect breathing, follow-up is required. The nurse should ask for clear descriptions and details about what, when, and how problems occur and impact breathing as well as the duration of the problems.

7. **Is there anyone in your family who has or has had a respiratory disease or problem?**
   - What is/was the disease or problem?
   - Who in the family has/had the disease?
   - When was it diagnosed?
   - How has it been treated?
   - How effective is/was the treatment?

   ▶ This information may reveal information about respiratory diseases associated with familial or genetic predisposition. Follow-up is required to obtain details about specific problems and their occurrence, treatment, and outcomes.

Focused Interview Questions	**Rationales and Evidence**

Questions Related to Illness or Infection

1. **Have you ever been diagnosed with a respiratory disease?**
   - When were you diagnosed with the problem?
   - What treatment was prescribed for the problem?
   - Was the treatment helpful?
   - What kinds of things do you do to help with the problem?
   - Has the problem ever recurred (acute)?
   - How are you managing the disease now (chronic)?

   ▶ The patient has an opportunity to provide information about specific respiratory illnesses. If a diagnosed illness is identified, follow-up about the date of diagnosis, treatment, and outcomes is required. Data about each illness identified by the patient are essential to an accurate health assessment. Illnesses can be classified as acute or chronic, and follow-up regarding each classification will differ.

2. **An alternative to question 1 is to list possible respiratory illnesses, such as asthma, chronic obstructive pulmonary disease (COPD), and emphysema, and ask the patient to respond yes or no as each is stated.**

   ▶ This is a comprehensive and easy way to elicit information about all respiratory diagnoses. Follow-up would be carried out for each identified diagnosis as in question 1.

3. **Do you now have or have you had a respiratory infection?**
   - When were you diagnosed with the infection?
   - What treatment was prescribed for the problem?
   - Was the treatment helpful?
   - What kinds of things do you do to help with the problem?
   - Has the problem ever recurred (acute)?
   - How are you managing the infection now (chronic)?

   ▶ If an infection is identified, follow-up about the date of infection, treatment, and outcomes is required. Data about each infection identified by the patient are essential to an accurate health assessment. Infections can be classified as acute or chronic, and follow-up regarding each classification will differ.

4. **An alternative to question 3 is to list possible respiratory infections, such as bronchitis, pneumonia, and pleurisy, and ask the patient to respond yes or no as each is stated.**

   ▶ This is a comprehensive and easy way to elicit information about all respiratory infections. Follow-up would be carried out for each identified infection as in question 3.

Questions Related to Symptoms, Pain, and Behaviors

When gathering information about symptoms, many questions are required to elicit details and descriptions that assist in the analysis of the data. Discrimination is made in relation to the significance of a symptom, specific diseases or problems, and potential follow-up examination or referral. One rationale may be provided for a group of questions in this category.

The following questions refer to specific symptoms and behaviors associated with the respiratory system. For each symptom, questions and follow-up are required. The details to be elicited are the characteristics of the symptom; the onset, duration, and frequency of the symptom; the treatment or remedy for the symptom, including over-the-counter (OTC) and home remedies; the determination if diagnosis has been sought; the effect of treatments; and family history associated with a symptom or illness.

Questions 1 through 23 refer to coughing as a symptom associated with respiratory diseases or problems and are comprehensive enough to provide an example of the number and types of questions required in a focused interview when a symptom exists. The remaining questions refer to other symptoms associated with respiratory problems. The number and types of questions are limited to identification of the symptom. Follow-up is included only when required for clarification.

Questions Related to Symptoms

1. **Do you have a cough?**

   ▶ Question 1 identifies the existence of a symptom, and questions 2 through 7 add knowledge about the symptom.

2. **How long have you had the cough?**

   ▶ Determining the duration of symptoms is helpful in determining the significance of symptoms in relation to specific diseases and problems.

Focused Interview Questions	Rationales and Evidence
3. How often are you coughing?	
4. Do you know what causes the cough?	
5. Is there a difference in the cough at different times of the day?	
6. Describe your cough.	
7. Is it dry, hacking, hoarse, moist, or barking?	▶ The type of cough may indicate a symptom associated with a specific disease or problem. For example, wet or moist coughs are most often associated with lung infection (Chang, Redding, & Everard, 2008).
8. Are you coughing up mucus or phlegm?	
9. What does the mucus look like?	▶ The color and odor of any mucus or phlegm (sputum) is associated with specific diseases or problems. For example, pink or reddish-colored mucus is associated with tuberculosis (TB) (Yoon, Lee, & Yim, 2012), while green or yellow mucus often signals lung infection (Butler et al., 2014).
10. Does the mucus have any odor?	
11. Has the amount of mucus changed?	▶ A change in the amount or character of sputum is often a sign of a respiratory disease (Richardson, 2003).
12. Has the consistency or thickness of the mucus changed?	
13. Do you have pain when you cough? • Describe the type, severity, and location of the pain. • What do you do for the cough or the pain? • Is the remedy effective?	▶ Painful coughing may occur because of muscle pain or may be indicative of an underlying lung disease (Berman & Snyder, 2012). Follow-up elicits details that assist in data analysis.
14. Have you sought treatment for the cough?	▶ Questions 14 through 18 provide information about the need for diagnosis, referral, or continued evaluation of the symptom; information about the patient's knowledge of a current diagnosis or underlying problem; and information about the patient's response to intervention.
15. When was that treatment sought?	
16. What occurred when you sought that treatment?	
17. Was something prescribed or recommended to help with the cough?	
18. What was the effect of the remedy?	
19. Do you use OTC or home remedies for the cough?	▶ Questions 19 through 22 provide information about drugs and substances that may relieve symptoms or provide comfort. Some substances may mask symptoms, interfere with the effect of prescribed medications, or harm the patient (Wilson, Shannon, & Shields, 2013).
20. What are those OTC medications or remedies that you use?	
21. How often do you use them?	
22. How much of them do you use?	
23. Do you now have or have you ever had any wheezing?	
24. Have you had a change in your weight recently? • How much weight have you gained or lost? • Over what period of time did this change occur? • Was the change purposeful? • Can you associate the change with any event or problem?	▶ Weight loss or gain may be associated with lung or cardiac diseases (Berman & Snyder, 2012).

Focused Interview Questions	Rationales and Evidence
25. Describe your diet. Do you use any nutritional supplements?	▶ Questions about nutritional intake are important to determine the contribution to production of red blood cells (erythropoiesis) and hemoglobin, which are essential to oxygenation (Berman & Snyder, 2012).
26. Do you ever become light-headed or dizzy? • When did or does that occur? • How often? • Do you associate this with any event or activity? • What do you do when this happens?	▶ Light-headedness or dizziness may be associated with hypoxia (Berman & Snyder, 2012).

Questions Related to Pain

1. Do you have pain anywhere in your chest?	▶ Chest pain may be related to cardiac or respiratory problems (Berman & Snyder, 2012).
2. Where is the pain?	▶ Questions 2 through 6 are standard questions associated with pain to determine the location, frequency, duration, and intensity of the pain.
3. How often do you experience the pain?	
4. How long does the pain last?	
5. How long have you had the pain?	
6. How would you rate the pain on a scale of 0 to 10, with 10 being the worst?	
7. Does the pain affect your breathing? • Are you short of breath? • Are you able to take a deep breath? • What do you do when this happens?	▶ Follow-up questions would relate to the ways in which breathing is affected. ▶ Questions 7 through 11 are intended to discriminate the characteristics of pain associated with underlying acute or chronic respiratory disease from muscular pain that can occur with cough or maintaining a posture to ease breathing.
8. Does the pain occur when you are taking a breath or when you are exhaling, or both?	
9. Is there a trigger for the pain, such as a cough or movement?	
10. Can you describe the pain?	
11. Does the pain radiate to other areas?	
12. What do you do to relieve the pain?	▶ Questions 12 and 13 are intended to determine if the patient has selected a treatment based on past experience, knowledge of respiratory illness, or use of complementary care and its effectiveness.
13. Is this treatment effective?	

Questions Related to Behaviors

1. Do you now smoke or have you ever smoked tobacco products?	▶ Tobacco products include cigarettes, cigars, and pipe tobacco.
2. What type of tobacco product do/did you smoke?	
3. How much of the product do/did you smoke?	
4. When did you start smoking?	
5. When did you stop smoking?	
6. Have you tried to stop smoking?	
7. What did you do to stop smoking?	

Focused Interview Questions	Rationales and Evidence
8. Do you have any symptoms related to smoking?	▶ Smoking tobacco products is associated with respiratory diseases including emphysema and lung cancer. If the patient exhibits or affirms that respiratory symptoms exist, questions for any symptom as previously described would be asked.
9. Do you smoke or inhale marijuana, other herbal products, or chemical preparations such as glue or spray paint? Have you done so in the past? • What is the substance you inhale? • How much do you use? • How often do you inhale the substance? • For those patients who state they have inhaled substances in the past, ask: When did you stop using the substance?	▶ Inhalation of marijuana, herbal substances, and/or chemicals may result in respiratory problems associated with incidental or continuous irritation of the linings of the respiratory organs (CDC, 2013a).
10. Have you received immunization for respiratory illnesses such as flu or pneumonia? • What immunizations have you had? • When was each given? Were there any adverse effects?	▶ Immunization reduces the risk of infection from flu or pneumonia.

Questions Related to Age

The focused interview must reflect the anatomic and physiologic differences that exist along the age span. The following questions are presented as examples of those that would be specific for infants and children, the pregnant female, and older adults.

Questions Regarding Infants and Children

1. Is the child taking solid foods? • When were they started? • What types of food are taken? • Does the child have difficulty chewing or swallowing?	▶ Introduction of solid foods puts infants at risk for aspiration (Mayo Clinic, 2013a).
2. How many colds has the child had in the past 12 months? • What was the course of the cold? • Was any treatment provided? • Was medical care sought? • What was the effect of the treatment?	▶ Approximately 80% of children will experience between one and eight respiratory infections in a year (Chonmaitree et al., 2008). More than this number of complicated infections may indicate chronic disease.
3. Has the child been immunized against respiratory illnesses? • What immunization did your child have? • When was it given? • Were there any adverse effects?	▶ This question identifies risk reduction and assists in discrimination of symptoms if and when they occur. Infants are at greater risk for complications from flu and pneumonia.
4. Is your home "childproofed" in terms of small objects and toys?	▶ Small objects and toys may be put in the mouth and aspirated.

Questions for the Pregnant Female

1. Do you experience any shortness of breath or dyspnea? • When does it occur? • How long have you experienced this? • Have you sought a remedy?	▶ The enlarged uterus elevates the diaphragm and can decrease lung expansion, which may result in shortness of breath (Tan & Tan, 2013).

Questions for the Older Adult

1. Describe any changes in breathing you have experienced.	▶ Older adults may experience symptoms associated with reduced oxygenation as a result of changes in posture and muscle strength that may contribute to reduced lung expansion.

Focused Interview Questions	Rationales and Evidence

2. Have you had any difficulty performing activities that you once found easy?

3. Do you find that you are more tired than you have been in the past?

▶ Fatigue may be associated with anemia and other chronic problems such as COPD, asthma, and cancer (Osborn, Wraa, Watson, & Holleran, 2013).

4. Have you received any immunization for respiratory illnesses?
   - What immunization did you receive?
   - When was it given?
   - Were there any adverse effects?

▶ Older adults are at greater risk for flu and pneumonia (University of Maryland Medical Center [UMMC], 2012).

Questions Related to the Environment

Environment refers to both the internal and the external environments. Questions related to the internal environment include all of the previous questions and those associated with internal or physiologic responses. Questions regarding the external environment include those related to home, work, or social environments.

Internal Environment

1. Are you now experiencing or have you ever had an experience of intermittent or prolonged anxiety or emotional upset?
   - Describe the situation.
   - Can you determine precipitating factors?
   - Have you sought care or treatment for the problem?
   - What do you do when the problem arises?

▶ Anxiety, emotional situations, and stress impact the sympathetic nervous system, producing hormonal responses that affect respiratory function (Osborn et al., 2013).

2. Do you use now or have you ever used medications or devices to alter or improve your respiratory function?

▶ Medications such as inhalers and steroids for respiratory symptoms can have cascading side effects that result in exacerbation of problems or enhancement of symptoms (Wilson et al., 2013). Devices for treatment of respiratory ailments include oxygen therapy, devices to relieve sleep apnea, and others. Knowledge of the medications and devices helps the nurse to analyze patient situations and determine the significance of findings in the comprehensive assessment.

External Environment

The following questions deal with substances and irritants found in the patient's physical environment. The physical environment includes the indoor and outdoor environments of the home and the workplace, those surroundings encountered for social engagements, and any encountered during travel.

1. Have you had allergy testing?

2. Do you have any allergies?

3. Do those allergies impact respiratory function?

4. What are the allergens?

5. When were these allergies diagnosed?

6. How do you address exposure to the allergen?

7. What are the respiratory symptoms you experience?

8. What remedies do you use to take care of the symptoms?

9. Have the remedies been effective?

▶ Allergies often result in respiratory problems including asthma and bronchitis (World Allergy Organization [WAO], 2009). It is important to determine if specific allergens have been identified and determine if the patient uses appropriate measures to address the problems. Remedies may include avoidance of the allergen.

Focused Interview Questions	Rationales and Evidence
10. Are you now or have you ever been exposed to respiratory irritants (gases, fumes, dust, lint, smoke, chemical exhaust)? 11. Were the irritants identified? 12. Where are/were the irritants? In the home, in the workplace, in the community, or outside of the community? 13. What is or was your respiratory response to the irritants? 14. Have you ever experienced an illness related to exposure to an irritant? 15. How have you dealt with that illness? 16. How does the illness impact your life now? • Follow-up questions would include all of the questions previously mentioned that address symptoms and problems of the respiratory system.	▶ Irritants, pollutants, and chemicals in the environment can result in acute and/or chronic respiratory disease (i.e., mesothelioma, asbestosis, and psittacosis) (Ho & Kuschner, 2012). Acute and chronic problems with respiratory function can have devastating effects on the ability to function. Identification of the place of exposure or possible exposure through travel, military, or employment service may assist in identifying probable causes for new or ongoing respiratory problems.

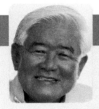

Patient-Centered Interaction

Mr. Loi is a 78-year-old with a history of COPD who recently moved from another state to live with his daughter, Anita. His daughter scheduled an appointment for Mr. Loi with her health-care group. When Anita called to arrange the appointment, she explained that her father was widowed 3 years ago and had been doing well in his own home, but he seemed lonely and was not participating in activities in his neighborhood and community as he had been. He also did not say much when she phoned. Anita stated that he has COPD. Although it did not seem to affect his activity in the past, she was concerned about him. She visited him and suggested he move in with her family and was relieved that he agreed. Since the move, he has been quiet and resting in his room most of the time. His respirations are regular and non-labored. He has had a cough once in a while, but she thought she had better get him set up with a doctor just in case something happened.

Mr. Loi completed several forms before his health interview. These forms included biographic information, personal and family health history, and information about his current diagnosis and medications.

Interview

Because Mr. Loi's only diagnosed health problem is COPD, the nurse begins the interview with questions related to his respiratory system. The nurse greets Mr. Loi, offers him a seat, and explains the interview process. Mr. Loi takes a seat, smiles, and nods.

Nurse: Tell me about your breathing.

Mr. Loi: I'm doing fine. I take all my medications.

Nurse: Has your breathing changed in the last 2 months?

Mr. Loi: Oh, I moved here to be with my daughter a month ago.

The nurse realizes that Mr. Loi has not answered the question. It is not clear if Mr. Loi did not hear the question, misunderstood the question, or is seeking an opportunity to discuss his move. The nurse uses an open-ended statement to allow him to discuss the move.

Nurse: Tell me a little about your move.

Mr. Loi leans forward and focuses on the nurse's lips while listening to the question.

Mr. Loi: Well, my daughter wanted me here. She worries that I don't get out and see people. You know I have COPD, but it's been okay as long as I take my pills.

Mr. Loi's posture and focus while the nurse spoke suggests that Mr. Loi is having difficulty hearing. Further, Mr. Loi's daughter was concerned about her father's diminished social contact and decreasing phone communication, which are additional signs of hearing deficit.

In order to complete the health assessment, the nurse will use techniques appropriate for those patients with hearing impairment.

The nurse faces Mr. Loi, uses a low-pitched voice at normal loudness, and speaks in short sentences to conduct the interview. The nurse pauses after each statement so Mr. Loi can interpret the statement.

Nurse: What do you think of the move?

Mr. Loi: So far, so good. She's been great and so has her family. It's all pretty different but I think I'll be okay. I don't want her to worry so I agreed to come and get checked out here. You know . . . my COPD and all.

Nurse: Tell me about the COPD.

Mr. Loi: Well, it started about 5 years ago. I was getting winded with just a little work around the house. Then I got bronchitis and it just took off from there.

Patient Education

The following are risk factors for physiologic, behavioral, cultural, and lifespan considerations that affect respiratory health. Several factors are cited as trends in *Healthy People 2020* documents. The nurse provides advice and education to reduce risks associated with these factors and to promote and maintain respiratory health.

LIFESPAN CONSIDERATIONS

Risk Factors	Patient Education
• Infants have small, delicate respiratory structures, leaving them susceptible to infection.	▶ Teach that immunization is important across the age span. Recommended schedules should be followed. For example: Infants should receive immunizations for DPT and *H. influenzae* type b.
• There has been an increase in the incidence of sudden infant death syndrome (SIDS), theorized to be associated with problems of the respiratory system or suffocation.	▶ Teach caregivers about guidelines to reduce the incidence of SIDS and other sleep-related deaths. Guidelines include placing infants on their back for sleep, using a firm sleep surface, avoidance of soft bedding, and others (American Academy of Pediatrics, 2011).
• The activities, environments, and hygiene practices of preschool and early school-age children put them at increased risk for respiratory infections.	▶ Teach hygiene measures, including hand hygiene, use of tissues, and cough etiquette to prevent the spread of infection.
• Suffocation and aspiration occur with greater frequency in infants and preschool children and are associated with plastic bags, toys, and household objects.	▶ Teach caregivers that toys for infants and children must be age appropriate and without small inhalable parts and that plastic bags must not be used in bedding or left within reach of children.
• Middle-aged adults are at risk from respiratory illness and problems with oxygenation because of decreased elasticity of the lung and decrease in lung capacity by 25% to 30%. • Older adults experience skeletal, muscular, and organic changes that result in decreased respiratory expansion and effectiveness, which increases the risk for respiratory problems.	▶ Teach that regular exercise strengthens the musculoskeletal system, maintains the efficiency of the respiratory system, and contributes to weight loss, all of which impact respiratory health.

CULTURAL CONSIDERATIONS

Risk Factors	Patient Education
• The incidence of TB has increased and has been attributed to existence of the disease in immigrant populations, crowded conditions in urban areas, increased international travel, and decreased immune response in individuals with AIDS.	▶ Teach travelers to update immunizations and to have TB testing. Immigrant populations require TB testing and treatment.

BEHAVIORAL CONSIDERATIONS

Risk Factors

- Smoking and experimentation with drugs (especially inhalants) are increasing, and the use of gaseous substances can result in permanent damage to the lungs.

- Experimental sexual activity, sexual activity with multiple partners, and drug use are on the rise in adolescents and young adults. These activities increase the risk of HIV transmission and development of associated respiratory diseases such as *Pneumocystis carinii* pneumonia.

- In the United States, obesity has become increasingly prevalent across the age span. Obesity can alter respiratory effort, can compromise function, and is associated with an increase in obstructive sleep apnea (OSA).

Patient Education

▶ Provide information about support for not smoking. This can be addressed within families in schools and healthcare settings.
▶ Advise parents, adolescents, and young adults about drug use in relation to respiratory health problems, how to recognize behaviors associated with drug use, and about prevention programs and addiction services that are aimed at reducing inhalation injuries and HIV transmission.

▶ Provide information about abstinence or protected sexual activity to reduce the transmission of HIV and incidence of AIDS.

▶ Teach patients that regular exercise strengthens the musculoskeletal system, maintains the efficiency of the respiratory system, and contributes to weight loss, all of which impact respiratory health.
▶ Teach that healthy eating from infancy to old age prevents obesity and contributes to improved oxygenation.

ENVIRONMENTAL CONSIDERATIONS

Risk Factors

- Asthma and other allergic and chronic respiratory diseases are increasing in all populations, but particularly among children of low socioeconomic status. The increase is attributed to urbanization and increased exposure to pollutants and chemicals in cities and rural farm areas.

Patient Education

▶ Teach patients to limit exposure to allergens, pollutants, and irritants in the home and workplace. Assist patients to identify allergens and irritants as an important first step in preventing problems and promoting respiratory health. Provide information about filters, masks, and other protective equipment for use in the home or work environments.

Physical Assessment

Assessment Techniques and Findings

Physical assessment of the respiratory system requires the use of inspection, palpation, percussion, and auscultation. During each of the procedures, the nurse is gathering data related to the patient's breathing and level of oxygenation. The nurse inspects skin color, structures of the thoracic cavity, chest configuration, and respiratory rate rhythm and effort. Knowledge of norms or expected findings is essential in determining the meaning of the data as one proceeds.

EQUIPMENT
- examination gown and drape
- examination gloves
- examination light
- stethoscope
- skin marker
- metric ruler
- tissues
- face mask for nurse, if indicated

Adults normally breathe at a rate of 12 to 20 breaths per minute. Infants and children have higher rates, up to 80 breaths per minute in newborns. The respiratory cycle includes full inspiration and expiration. The ratio of the length of inspiration to expiration is about 1:2 (I:E). Breathing should be even, regular, and coordinated. Chest movement should be uniform; the structures of the thorax should be aligned and the thorax should be symmetric. The sternum is midline and flat. The costal angle is less than 90 degrees in an adult. The vertebrae are midline and follow the pattern of cervical, thoracic, and lumbar curves. The anterior to posterior diameter of the chest should be half of the lateral diameter. Pink skin or pink undertones indicate normal oxygenation. Assessment for pink-colored tongue or oral mucous membranes may be required in dark-skinned individuals. The color of the skin of the thorax should be consistent with that of the rest of the body.

Physical assessment of the respiratory system follows an organized pattern. It begins with a patient survey followed by inspection of the anterior thorax and complete assessment of the posterior thorax. The assessment ends with palpation, percussion, and auscultation of the anterior thorax. The nurse includes the anterior, posterior, and lateral aspects of the thorax when conducting each of the assessments.

HELPFUL HINTS

- Provide an environment that is comfortable and private.
- Explain each step of the procedure.
- Provide specific instructions about what is expected of the patient, for example, whether deep or regular breathing will be required.
- Tell patient the purpose of each procedure and when and if discomfort will accompany any examination.
- Pay attention to nonverbal cues that may indicate discomfort and ask patient to indicate if he or she experiences any difficulties or discomforts.
- An organized and professional approach goes a long way toward putting the patient at ease.
- Use Standard Precautions.

Techniques and Normal Findings	Abnormal Findings / Special Considerations

Survey

A quick survey of the patient enables the nurse to identify any immediate problems as well as the patient's ability to participate in the assessment.

ALERT!

Individuals experiencing pain and dyspnea, who are restless, anxious, and unable to follow directions, may need immediate medical assistance.

Inspect the overall appearance, posture, and position of the patient. Note the skin color and respiratory effort. Observe for signs of anxiety or distress.

▶ Patients experiencing anxiety may demonstrate pallor and shallow breathing. Acknowledgment of the problem and discussion of the procedures often provide some relief. If a patient is in obvious respiratory distress, the problem must be addressed. The patient may require referral to a medical care provider or emergency care facility.

▶ Circumoral cyanosis is often an early warning sign of respiratory distress or hypoxia. Therefore, patients with circumoral cyanosis should be immediately evaluated for the source of respiratory distress and treated appropriately.

Inspection of the Anterior and Lateral Thorax

ALERT!

Be sensitive to the patient's privacy, and limit exposure of body parts.

1. **Position the patient.**
   - The patient should be in a sitting position with clothing removed except for an examination gown and drape (see Figure 17.13 ■).

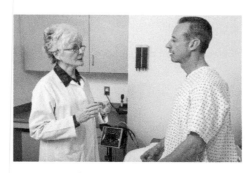

Figure 17.13 Patient positioned and gowned for assessment.

Techniques and Normal Findings	Abnormal Findings / Special Considerations

- Stand in front of the patient for anterior inspection and to the side of the patient for lateral inspection. Lighting must be adequate to detect color differences, lesions, and chest movement.

2. **Instruct the patient.**
   - Explain that you are going to be looking at the patient's chest structures. Tell the patient to breathe normally.

3. **Observe skin color.**
   - Skin color varies among individuals, but pink undertones indicate normal oxygenation. Skin color of the thorax should be consistent with that of the rest of the body.

   ▶ Pigments and levels of oxygenation influence skin color. Pallor, cyanosis, rubor, erythema, or grayness requires further evaluation.

4. **Inspect the structures of the thorax.**
   - The clavicles should be at the same height. The sternum should be midline. The costal angle should be less than 90 degrees.

   ▶ Misalignment of clavicles may be caused by deviations in the vertebral column such as scoliosis. An increase in the costal angle in an adult may indicate COPD. The thorax of children is rounder than that of adults.

5. **Inspect for symmetry.**
   - The structures of the chest and chest movement should be symmetric.

   ▶ Asymmetry may indicate postural problems or underlying respiratory dysfunction.

6. **Inspect chest configuration.**
   - The adult transverse diameter is approximately twice that of the anteroposterior diameter (AP:T = 1:2).
   - In infants, the chest circumference should measure approximately 2 to 3 cm smaller than the head circumference.

   ▶ A change in the ratio requires further evaluation. Remember: Older adults have a decreased ratio.
   ▶ Infants of diabetic mothers may have a larger chest circumference, and infants with intrauterine growth restriction will have a smaller than normal chest circumference.

7. **Count the respiratory rate.**
   - Count the number of respiratory cycles per minute. Normal adult respiratory rate is 12 to 20. Newborns have a respiratory rate of 30 to 80, and this rate gradually slows to adult rates by age 17.
     - Observe chest movement.
     - Observe the muscles of the chest and neck, including the intercostal muscles and sternocleidomastoids.
   - Do not tell the patient that you are counting respirations—it may alter the normal breathing pattern.
     - Respirations should be even and smooth. Chest movement should be symmetric.
     - Males tend to breathe abdominally.
     - Females breathe more costally.

   ▶ Infants may have an irregular respiratory rate, so count their respirations for one full minute.
   ▶ Intercostal muscle retraction and prominent sternocleidomastoids may be seen in respiratory distress.

Inspection of the Posterior Thorax

1. **Instruct the patient.**
   - Explain to the patient that you will be performing several assessments and that you will provide instructions as you move from one step to the next. Tell the patient to try to relax and breathe normally to begin the examination.

2. **Observe skin color.**
   - Skin color of the posterior thorax should be consistent with that of the rest of the body.

Techniques and Normal Findings	Abnormal Findings Special Considerations

3. **Inspect the structures of the posterior thorax.**
   - The height of the scapulae should be even; the vertebrae should be midline.

4. **Inspect for symmetry.**
   - The structures of the chest and chest movement should be symmetric.

5. **Observe respirations.**
   - Respirations should be smooth and even.

Palpation of the Posterior Thorax

1. **Instruct the patient.**
   - Explain that you will be touching the patient's back to determine if there are any areas of tenderness. Tell the patient to breathe normally during this part of the examination and to tell you if pain or discomfort is felt at any area.

2. **Lightly palpate the posterior thorax.**
   - Use the finger pads to lightly palpate symmetric areas on the posterior thorax. Include the entire thorax by starting at the areas above each scapula and move from side to side to below the 12th rib and laterally to the midaxillary line on each side (see Figure 17.14 ■).
   - Assess muscle mass.
   - Assess for growths, nodules, and masses.
   - Assess for tenderness.
   - Muscle mass should be firm and underlying tissue smooth. The chest should be free of lesions or masses. The area should be nontender to palpation.

▶ Lateral deviation of the spine and elevation of one scapula are indicative of scoliosis.

▶ Asymmetry may indicate postural problems or underlying respiratory problems.

▶ Respirations in the obese patient may be shallow and rapid.

▶ Pain may occur with inflammation of fibrous tissue or underlying structures such as the pleura. Crepitus is a crunching feeling under the skin caused by air leaking into subcutaneous tissue.

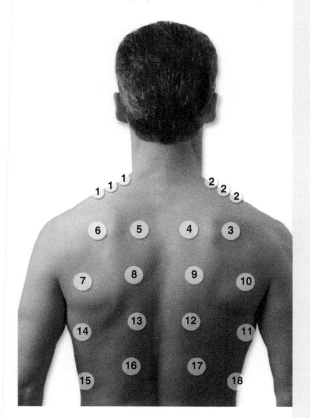

Figure 17.14 Pattern for palpating the posterior thorax.

Techniques and Normal Findings

3. **Palpate and count ribs and intercostal spaces.**
   - Instruct the patient to flex the neck, round the shoulders, and lean forward. Tell the patient you will be applying light pressure to the spine and rib areas. Instruct the patient to breathe normally and to tell you of pain or discomfort.
   - When the neck is flexed, the spinous process of C7 is most prominent. When two spinous processes are equally prominent, they are C7 and T1. Use the finger pads to palpate each spinous process. The spinous processes should form a straight line. Further assessment is discussed in chapter 25. ∞ Move to the left and right to identify ribs and intercostal spaces from C7 through T12.

4. **Palpate for respiratory expansion.**
   - Explain that you will be assessing the movement of the chest during breathing by placing your hands on the lower chest and asking the patient to take a deep breath.
   - Place the palmar surface of your hands, with thumbs close to the vertebrae, on the chest at the level of T10. Pinch up some skin between your thumbs. Ask the patient to take a deep breath (see Figure 17.15 ■).
   - The movement and pressure of the chest against your hands should feel smooth and even. Your thumbs should move away from the spine and the skin should move smoothly as the chest moves with inspiration. Your hands should lift symmetrically outward when the patient takes a deep breath.

▶ Lateral deviation of the thoracic spinous processes indicates scoliosis.

▶ Unilateral decrease or delay in expansion may indicate underlying fibrotic or obstructive lung disease or may result from splinting associated with pleural pain or pneumothorax.

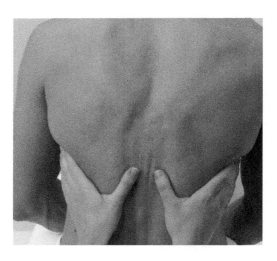

Figure 17.15 Palpation for respiratory expansion.

5. **Palpate for tactile fremitus.**
   - **Fremitus** is the palpable vibration on the chest wall when the patient speaks. Fremitus is strongest over the trachea, diminishes over the bronchi, and becomes almost nonexistent over the alveoli of the lungs.
   - Explain that you will be feeling for vibrations on the chest while the patient speaks. Tell the patient you will be placing your hands on various areas of the chest while he or she repeats "ninety-nine" or "one, two, three" in a clear, loud voice.

▶ Decreased or absent fremitus may result from a soft voice; from a very thick chest wall; from obesity; or from underlying diseases, including COPD and pleural effusion. Increased fremitus occurs with fluid in the lungs, fibrosis, tumor, or infection.

- Use the ulnar surface of the hand or the palmar surface of the hand at the base of the fingers at the metacarpophalangeal joints when palpating (see Figure 17.16 ■). Palpate and compare symmetric areas of the lungs by moving from side to side, from apices to bases. Using one hand to palpate for fremitus is believed to increase accuracy of findings. Two-handed methods may, however, increase speed and facilitate identification of asymmetry.

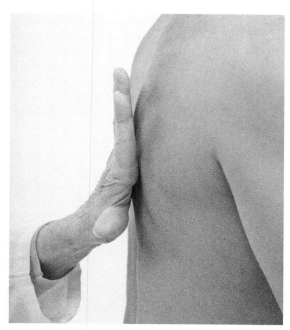

Figure 17.16 Palpation for tactile fremitus using metacarpophalangeal joint area.

Percussion of the Posterior Thorax

1. **Visualize the landmarks.**
   - Observe the posterior thorax and visualize the horizontal and vertical lines, the level of the diaphragm, and the fissures of the lungs.

2. **Recall the expected findings.**
   - Percussion allows assessment of underlying structures. The usual sound in the thorax when over lung tissue is **resonance,** a long, low-pitched hollow sound.

   ▶ An unexpected finding would be hyper-resonance, which is heard in conditions of overinflation of the lungs as in emphysema, or with pneumothorax.

3. **Instruct the patient.**
   - Explain to the patient that you will be tapping on the chest in a variety of areas.
   - Tell the patient to breathe normally through this examination. Ask the patient to lean forward and round the shoulders. This position moves the scapulae laterally, permitting more area at the upper vertebral borders, and widens the intercostal spaces for percussion.
   - Position the patient so that your arms are almost fully extended throughout the percussion.

Techniques and Normal Findings	Abnormal Findings Special Considerations

4. Percuss the lungs.

- Place the pleximeter in the intercostal space parallel to the ribs during percussion. Standing slightly to the side of the patient allows the pleximeter finger to lie more firmly on the chest as you move through all thoracic areas.
- Percuss the apex of the left lung, then the apex of the right lung. Percuss from side to side, comparing sounds, in the intercostal spaces as you percuss to the bases of the lungs and laterally to each midaxillary line (see Figure 17.17 ■).

▶ Percussion will yield dull sounds over solidified or fluid-filled areas, as may exist in pleural effusion. Percussion over bone will yield flat sounds. Be sure to check that finger placement is correct.

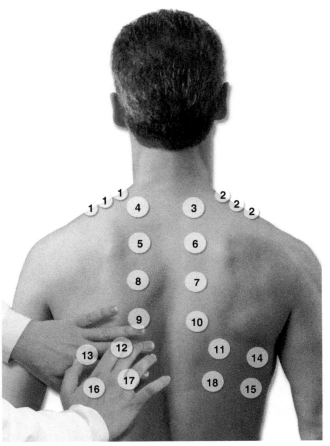

Figure 17.17 Pattern for percussion: Posterior thorax.

5. Percuss for movement of the diaphragm (Diaphragmatic excursion).

- This assessment requires the use of a skin marker and a ruler. The patient remains in the position previously described for percussion. Explain that you will be doing more tapping on the chest and at two points you will ask the patient to exhale and inhale. Determine the level of the diaphragm during quiet respiration by placing the pleximeter finger above the expected level of diaphragmatic **dullness** (T7 or T8) at the midscapular line. Percuss in steps downward until dullness replaces resonance on both sides of the chest. Mark those areas. These marks should be at approximately the level of T10.
- The marks should be parallel.

▶ An asymmetric diaphragm may indicate diaphragmatic paralysis or pleural effusion of the elevated side.
▶ Shortened excursion indicates that the lungs are not fully expanding. Pain or abdominal pressure can inhibit full expansion. Diaphragmatic movement is decreased in emphysema, atelectasis, and respiratory depression. Diaphragmatic excursion is decreased in obese patients as a result of fatty tissue on the diaphragm interfering with mechanical movement.

- Measure diaphragmatic movement by asking the patient to fully exhale. Starting at the previous skin marking on the left chest, percuss upward from dullness to resonance. Mark that area. Then ask the patient to inhale fully and hold it as you begin to percuss from the level of the diaphragm downward, moving from resonance to dullness (see Figure 17.18A ■). Mark that area and repeat on the right side of the chest. Use the ruler to measure the difference between the marks for exhalation and inhalation (see Figure 17.18B ■).

- The distance between the marks should be 3 to 5 cm (1 1/4 to 2 in.) and even on each side. The right side may be 1 to 2 cm (0.39 to 0.78 in.) higher because of the location of the liver.

- Anticipate a greater distance on a physically fit patient.

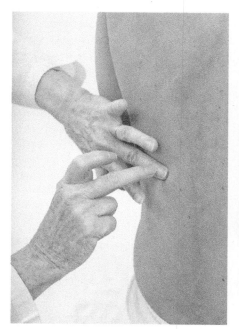

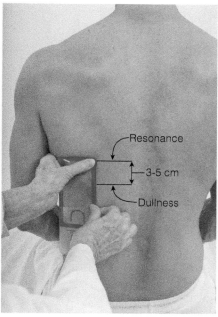

Figure 17.18A Diaphragmatic movement, percussion.

Figure 17.18B Diaphragmatic movement, measurement.

Auscultation of the Posterior Thorax

Auscultation of the respiratory system refers to listening to the sounds of breathing through the stethoscope. The sounds are produced by air moving through the airways. Sounds change as the airway size changes or with the presence of fluid or mucus.

The pattern for auscultation of the respiratory system is the same as that for percussion (see Figure 17.19 ■).

► Auscultation through clothing or coarse chest hair may produce deceptive sounds. Thick, coarse chest hair may be matted with a damp cloth or lotion to prevent interference with auscultation.

► In the obese patient the skin folds must be moved and the stethoscope placed firmly on the chest wall for auscultation. Asking overweight and obese patients to put the arm over the head and lean toward the opposite side is often helpful in accessing the chest wall during auscultation.

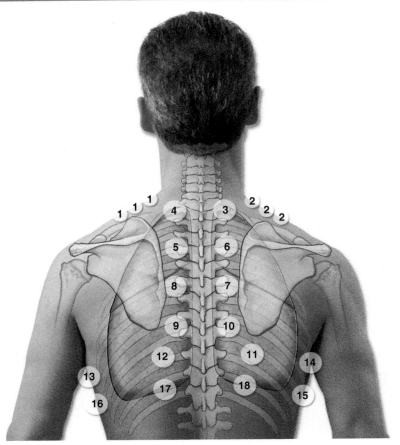

Figure 17.19 Pattern for auscultation: Posterior thorax.

Use the diaphragm of the stethoscope and listen through the full respiratory cycle. When auscultating, classify each sound according to intensity, location, pitch, duration, and characteristic.

ALERT!

It is important to monitor the patient's breathing to prevent hyperventilation.

Four normal breath sounds are heard during respiratory auscultation. **Tracheal sounds** are harsh, high-pitched sounds heard over the trachea when the patient inhales and exhales. **Bronchial sounds** are loud, high-pitched sounds heard next to the trachea and are longer on exhalation. **Bronchovesicular sounds** are medium in loudness and pitch. They are heard between the scapulae, posteriorly and next to the sternum, and anteriorly upon inhalation and exhalation. **Vesicular sounds** are soft and low pitched and heard over the remainder of the lungs. Vesicular sounds are longer on inhalation than exhalation (see Table 17.3).

| Techniques and Normal Findings | | Abnormal Findings Special Considerations |

TABLE 17.3 Normal Breath Sounds

SOUND	LOCATION	RATIO INSPIRATION TO EXPIRATION	QUALITY
Tracheal	Over trachea	I < E	Harsh, high pitched
Bronchial	Next to trachea, superior to each clavicle and in the first intercostal space	E > I	Loud, high pitched
Bronchovesicular	Over major bronchi in the second and third intercostal spaces Between scapulae	I = E	Medium loudness, medium pitch
Vesicular	Remainder of lungs	I > E	Soft, low pitched

1. **Instruct the patient.**
   - Explain that you will be listening to the patient's breathing with the stethoscope.
   - The patient will be in the same position as during percussion. Ask the patient to breathe deeply through the mouth each time the stethoscope is placed on a new spot. Tell the patient to let you know if he or she is becoming tired, short of breath, or dizzy and, if so, you will stop and allow time to rest.

2. **Visualize the landmarks.**
   - Visualize the landmarks as you did before percussing the posterior thorax.

3. **Auscultate for bronchovesicular sounds.**
   - The right and left primary bronchi are located at the level of T3 and T5. Auscultate at the right and left of the vertebrae at those levels. The breath sounds will be bronchovesicular.

4. **Auscultate for vesicular sounds.**
   - Auscultate the lungs by following the pattern used for percussion. Move the stethoscope from side to side while comparing sounds. Start at the apices and move to the bases of the lungs and laterally to the midaxillary line. The breath sounds over most of the posterior surface are vesicular.

▶ The obese patient may be unable to take deep breaths due to the weight of the chest wall and the fatty deposits in the intercostal muscles and the diaphragm.

▶ Auscultation of diminished breath sounds in both lungs may indicate emphysema, bronchospasm, or shallow breathing. Atelectasis, which is reflective of collapse or impaired expansion of one or more areas of the lung, also may produce diminished breath sounds (National Heart, Lung, & Blood Institute [NHLBI], 2013). In some cases, atelectasis will be accompanied by a faint "popping" sound at end-inspiration, if the atelectatic alveoli re-expand. Breath sounds heard in just one lung may indicate pleural effusion, pneumothorax, tumor, or mucus plugs in the airways in the other lung. Hearing bronchial or bronchovesicular sounds in areas where one would normally hear vesicular sounds may be reflective of fluid or exudate in the alveoli and small bronchioles. Fluid and exudate decrease the movement of air through small airways and result in loss of vesicular sounds.

| Techniques and Normal Findings | Abnormal Findings / Special Considerations |

TABLE 17.4   Adventitious Breath Sounds

SOUND	OCCURRENCE	QUALITY	CAUSES
Rales/ Crackles			
Fine	End inspiration, do not clear with cough	High pitched, short, crackling	Collapsed or fluid-filled alveoli open
Coarse	End inspiration, do not clear with cough	Loud, moist, low pitched, bubbling	Collapsed or fluid-filled alveoli open
Rhonchi			
Wheezes (sibilant)	Expiration/inspiration when severe	High pitched, continuous	Blocked airflow as in asthma, infection, foreign body obstruction
Rhonchi (sonorous)	Expiration/inspiration Change/disappear with cough	Low pitched, continuous, snoring, rattling	Fluid-blocked airways
Stridor	Inspiration	Loud, high-pitched crowing heard without stethoscope	Obstructed upper airway
Friction rub	Inhalation/exhalation	Low-pitched grating, rubbing	Pleural inflammation

▶ Added or **adventitious sounds** are superimposed on normal breath sounds and are often indicative of underlying airway problems or diseases of the cardiovascular or respiratory systems (see Table 17.4). Adventitious sounds are classified as discontinuous or continuous.

Discontinuous sounds are crackles, which are intermittent, nonmusical, and brief. These sounds are commonly referred to as **rales.** Fine rales are soft, high pitched, and very brief. Coarse rales/crackles are louder, lower in pitch, and longer.

Continuous sounds are musical and longer than rales but do not necessarily persist through the entire respiratory cycle. The two types are wheezes/sibilant wheezes and rhonchi (sonorous wheezes). **Wheezes** (sibilant) are high pitched with a shrill quality. **Rhonchi** are low pitched with a snoring quality.

Assessment of Voice Sounds

The spoken voice can be heard over the chest wall. The sound is produced by vibrations as the patient speaks.

1. **Instruct the patient.**
   - The patient will remain in the same position as for percussion and auscultation. Explain that you will be listening to the chest while the patient says certain words, letters, or numbers.

2. **Auscultation of voice sounds.**
   - Use the same pattern for evaluating voice sounds as for auscultation of the lungs. This sequence will be followed for three different findings.
   - **Bronchophony.** Ask the patient to say "ninety-nine" each time you place the stethoscope on the chest. In normal lung tissue the sound will be muffled.

   - **Egophony.** Ask the patient to say "E" each time you place the stethoscope on the chest. In normal lung tissue you should hear "eeeeee" through the stethoscope.
   - **Whispered pectoriloquy.** Ask the patient to whisper "one, two, three" each time you place the stethoscope on the chest. In normal lung tissue the sound will be faint, almost indistinguishable.
   - Voice sounds are heard as muffled sounds in the normal lung.

▶ The words sound loud and more distinct over areas of lung consolidation. Lung consolidation occurs when portions of the lung that are normally filled with air instead contain fluid or tissue.

▶ The "E" sounds like "aaaaay" over areas of lung consolidation.
▶ The numbers sound loud and clear over areas of lung consolidation.

Palpation of the Anterior and Lateral Thorax

1. **Position the patient.**
   - The patient is usually in a supine position for palpation, percussion, and auscultation of the anterior thorax. If the patient is experiencing discomfort or dyspnea, a sitting position may be used, or the patient may be in a Fowler's position. The breasts of female patients normally flatten when in a supine position. Large and pendulous breasts may have to be moved to perform a complete assessment. Explain this to the patient and inform her that she may move and lift her own breasts if that will make her more comfortable.

2. **Instruct the patient.**
   - Explain to the patient that you will be performing several assessments and that you will continue to provide explanations as you move from one assessment to the next. Tell the patient to breathe normally throughout this initial examination and to tell you if pain or discomfort is felt at any area.

3. **Palpate the sternum, ribs, and intercostal spaces.**
   - Locate the suprasternal notch; palpate downward to the sternal angle (angle of Louis) where the manubrium meets the body of the sternum. Palpate laterally to the left and right to locate the second rib and second intercostal space. Continue palpating the sternum to the xiphoid process and to the left and right of the sternum to count the ribs.
   - The sternum should feel flat except for the ridge of the sternal angle and should taper to the xiphoid. The ribs should feel smooth and the spacing of ribs and intercostal spaces should be symmetric.

4. **Lightly palpate the anterior and lateral thorax.**
   - Use the finger pads to lightly palpate symmetric areas of the anterior thorax. Include the entire thorax by starting at the areas above each clavicle and move from side to side to below the costal angle and laterally to the midaxillary line (see Figure 17.20 ■).

▶ The obese patient may be unable to lie flat during assessment of the anterior thorax.

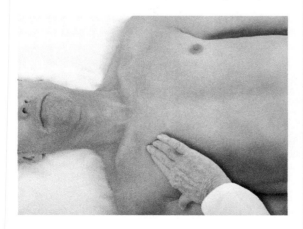

Figure 17.20 Palpation of the anterior thorax.

Techniques and Normal Findings	Abnormal Findings Special Considerations

- Assess muscle mass.
- Assess for growths, nodules, and masses.
- Assess for tenderness.
- Muscle mass should be firm and the underlying tissue should be smooth. The thorax should be free of lesions or masses. The area should be nontender to palpation.

▶ Pain may occur with inflammation of fibrous tissue or underlying structures. Crepitus may be felt if there is air in the subcutaneous tissue.

5. **Palpate for respiratory expansion.**
   - Explain that you will be assessing movement of the chest during breathing by placing your hands on the lower chest and asking the patient to take a breath.
   - Place the palmar surface of your hands along each costal margin with thumbs close to the midsternal line. Pinch up some skin between your thumbs. Ask the patient to take a deep breath (see Figure 17.21 ■).

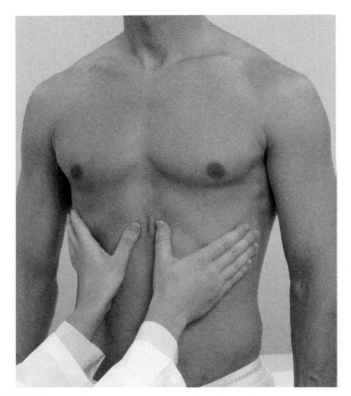

Figure 17.21 Palpation for respiratory expansion: Anterior view.

- The movement of the chest beneath your hands should feel smooth and even. Your thumbs should move apart and the skin move smoothly as the chest expands with inspiration.

▶ Unilateral decrease or delay in expansion may indicate fibrotic or obstructive lung disease or may result from splinting associated with pleural pain.

6. Palpate for tactile fremitus.

- Explain that you will be feeling for vibrations on the chest wall while the patient speaks. Explain that you will be placing your hands on various areas of the chest while the patient repeats "ninety-nine" or "one, two, three" in a clear, loud voice.

- Use the ulnar surface of the hand or the palmar surface of the hand at the base of the metacarpophalangeal joints when palpating for fremitus. Palpate and compare symmetric areas of the lungs by moving from side to side from apices to bases (see Figure 17.22 ■). Displace female breasts as required.

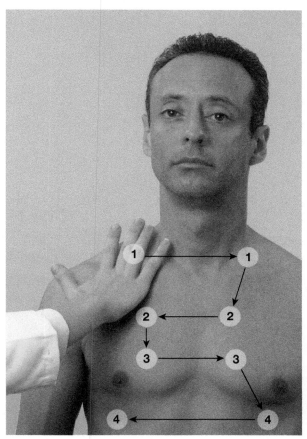

Figure 17.22 Palpation for tactile fremitus: Anterior thorax.

- Fremitus normally diminishes as you move from large to small airways and is decreased or absent over the precordium.

▶ Absent or decreased fremitus in other areas may result from underlying diseases including emphysema, pleural effusion, or fibrosis.

Percussion of the Anterior and Lateral Thorax

1. Visualize the landmarks.

- Observe the anterior thorax and visualize the horizontal and vertical lines, the level of the diaphragm, and the lobes of the lungs.

2. Recall the expected findings.

- Percussion allows assessment of underlying structures. The usual sound in the thorax, over the lung tissue, is resonance, which is a low-pitched, hollow sound.

▶ An unexpected sound would be hyperresonance, which may be heard with pneumothorax or in conditions that produce lung hyperinflation. Compared to resonance, hyperresonance is a lower-pitched, louder, longer sound.

Techniques and Normal Findings	Abnormal Findings Special Considerations

3. **Instruct the patient.**

- Explain that you will be tapping on the patient's chest in a variety of areas. Tell the patient to breathe normally throughout this examination.

4. **Percuss the lungs.**

- Begin at the apices of the lungs. Ask the patient to turn the head to the opposite side of percussion to increase the size of the surface required for placing your pleximeter finger and to avoid interference from the clavicle. Move to the chest wall and place the pleximeter in the intercostal space parallel to the ribs during percussion. Percuss the anterior chest from side to side, comparing sounds, in the intercostal spaces. Percuss to the bases and laterally to the midaxillary line (see Figure 17.23 ■).

▶ Percussion of the anterior thorax will yield dull sounds over solidified or fluid-filled areas, as may exist in pleural effusion, consolidation, or tumor.

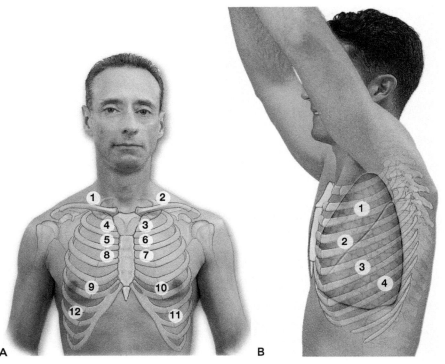

A   B

Figure 17.23 Pattern for percussion: A. Anterior thorax. B. Left lateral thorax.

- Percussion over bone or organs will yield flat or dull sounds. Avoid percussion over the clavicles, sternum, and ribs. Percussion over the heart will produce dullness to the left of the sternum from the third to fifth intercostal spaces. Percuss the left lung lateral to the midclavicular line. Percussion sounds in the lower left thorax change from resonance to tympany over the gastric air bubble. Percussion sounds in the right lower thorax change from resonance to dullness at the upper liver border.

Auscultation of the Anterior and Lateral Thorax

Auscultation is used to identify and discriminate between and among normal and adventitious breath sounds. Listen to the full respiratory cycle with each placement of the stethoscope (see Figure 17.24 ■).

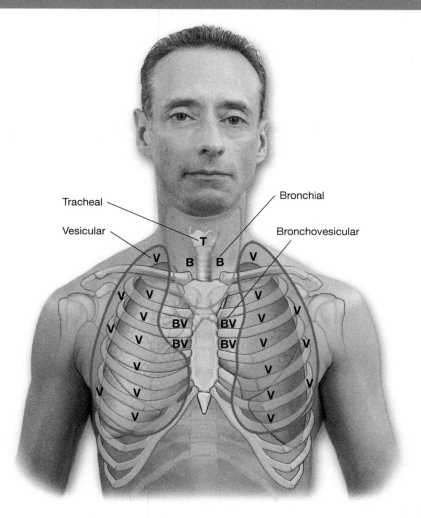

Figure 17.24 Auscultatory sounds: Anterior thorax.

1. **Instruct the patient.**
   - Explain that you will be listening to the patient's breathing with the stethoscope. Ask the patient to breathe deeply through the mouth each time the stethoscope is placed on the chest and to let you know if he or she is becoming short of breath or tired.

2. **Auscultate the trachea.**
   - Place the stethoscope over the trachea above the suprasternal notch. You will hear tracheal breath sounds. Move the stethoscope to the left, then the right side of the trachea, just above each sternoclavicular joint. You will hear bronchial breath sounds.

3. **Auscultate the apices.**
   - Place the stethoscope in the triangular areas just superior to each clavicle. You will hear bronchial sounds.

Techniques and Normal Findings	Abnormal Findings Special Considerations

4. Auscultate the bronchi.

- The bronchi are auscultated at the first intercostal space at the manubrium and left and right sternal borders. You will hear bronchial sounds. Auscultation of the major bronchi in the second and third intercostal spaces and the interscapular area will result in hearing bronchovesicular sounds.

5. Auscultate the anterior and lateral lungs.

- Auscultate the lungs by following the pattern for percussion. Move the stethoscope from side to side as you compare sounds. Move down to the sixth intercostal space and laterally to the midaxillary line. You will hear vesicular sounds. When auscultating the lateral lungs, ask the patient to sit up straight with the patient's arms raised over his or her head.

▶ Lateral auscultation of the fourth to sixth intercostal spaces is required to hear breath sounds from the right middle lobe, which is a frequent site of aspiration pneumonia.
▶ Because of the small size of the chest, breath sounds may be difficult to distinguish in newborns, especially preterm infants, as sounds may transmit to distant parts of the chest.

6. Interpret the findings.

- Refer to the descriptions and interpretations of normal and adventitious breath sounds described in auscultation of the posterior thorax.

▶ Breath sounds may be diminished in the obese patient due to poor inspiratory effort resulting from the weight of the chest and fatty deposits in the respiratory musculature.

Box 17.1 Normal and Abnormal Respiratory Rates and Patterns

Normal Findings

Eupnea

Even depth
Regular pattern
Inspiration = Expiration
Occasional sigh

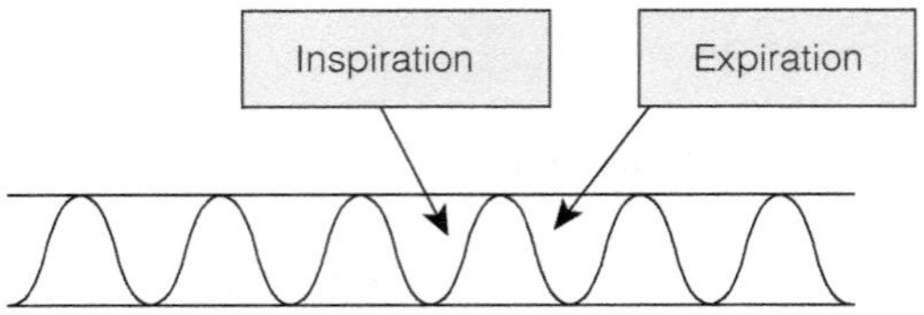

Eupnea With Sigh

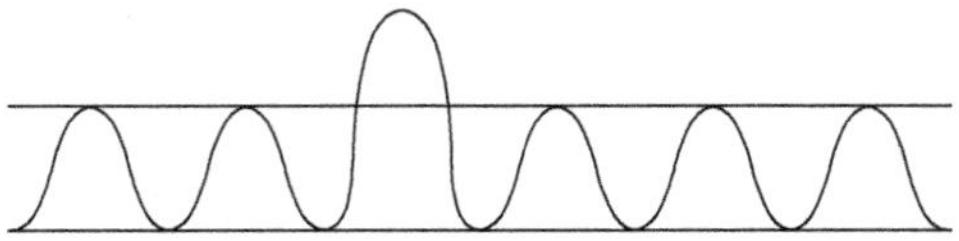

Abnormal Findings

Tachypnea

Rapid, shallow respirations
Rate > 24
Precipitating factors: fever, fear, exercise, respiratory insufficiency, pleuritic pain, alkalosis, pneumonia

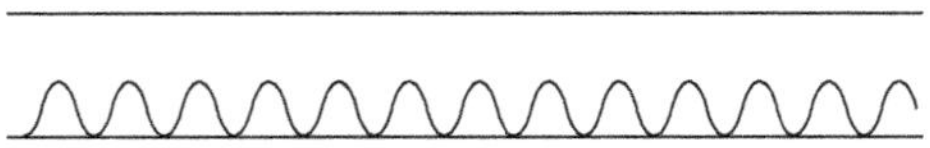

Box 17.1 Normal and Abnormal Respiratory Rates and Patterns (continued)

Bradypnea

Slow, regular respirations
Rate < 10
Precipitating factors: diabetic coma, drug-induced respiratory
depression, increased intracranial pressure

Hyperventilation

Rapid, deep respirations
Rate > 24
Precipitating factors: extreme exertion, fear, diabetic ketoacidosis
(Kussmaul's), hypoxia, salicylate overdose, hypoglycemia

Hypoventilation

Irregular, shallow respirations
Rate < 10
Precipitating factors: narcotic overdose, anesthetics, prolonged
bed rest, chest splinting

Cheyne-Stokes

Periods of deep breathing alternating with periods of apnea
Regular pattern
Precipitating factors: normal children and aging, heart failure,
uremia, brain damage, drug-induced respiratory depression

Biot's (Ataxic) Respirations

Shallow, deep respirations with periods of apnea
Irregular pattern
Precipitating factors: respiratory depression, brain damage

Sighing

Frequent sighs
Precipitating factors: hyperventilation syndrome, nervousness
Causes: dyspnea, dizziness

Obstructive Breathing

Prolonged expiration
Precipitating factors: COPD, asthma, chronic bronchitis

Expiration

Prolonged expiration

Box 17.2 Normal Chest Configurations

Adult

The adult chest is elliptical in shape with a lateral diameter that is larger than the anteroposterior diameter in a 2:1 ratio.

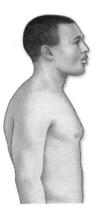
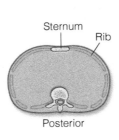

Sternum
Rib

Posterior

Child

The chest of a child is of adult proportion by age 6.

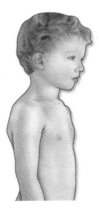
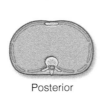

Posterior

Infant

The infant chest is rounded in shape with equal lateral and anteroposterior diameters.

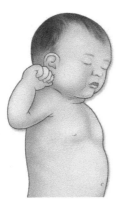

Posterior

Box 17.3 Abnormal Chest Configurations

Barrel Chest

The anteroposterior diameter is equal to the lateral diameter, and the ribs are horizontal. A barrel chest occurs normally with aging and accompanies COPD.

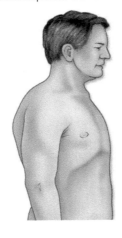
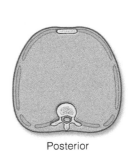

Posterior

Funnel Chest (Pectus Excavatum)

This is a congenital deformity characterized by depression of the sternum and adjacent costal cartilage. All or part of the sternum may be involved but predominant depression is at the lower portion where the body meets the xiphoid process.

If the condition is severe, chest compression may interfere with respiration. Murmurs may be present with cardiac compression.

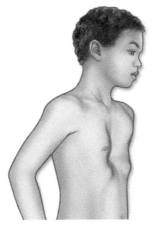
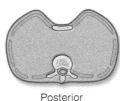

Posterior

(continued)

Box 17.3 Abnormal Chest Configurations (continued)

Scoliosis

Scoliosis is a condition in which there is lateral curvature and rotation of the thoracic and lumbar spine. It occurs more frequently in females. Scoliosis may result in elevation of the shoulder and pelvis.

Deviation greater than 45° may cause distortion of the lung, which results in decreased lung volume or difficulty in interpretation of findings from physical assessment.

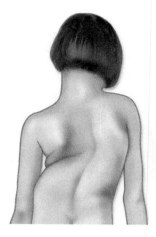
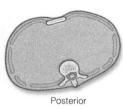

Posterior

Kyphosis

Kyphosis is exaggerated posterior curvature of the thoracic spine. It is associated with aging. Severe kyphosis may decrease lung expansion and increase cardiac problems.

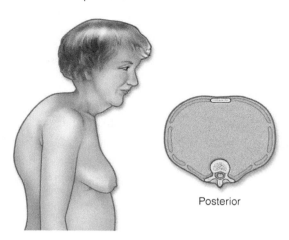

Posterior

Pigeon Chest (Pectus Carinatum)

This congenital deformity is characterized by forward displacement of the sternum with depression of the adjacent costal cartilage. This condition generally requires no treatment.

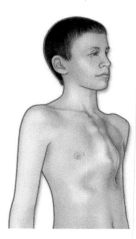
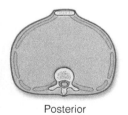

Posterior

Abnormal Findings

Respiratory Disorders

ASTHMA

A chronic hyperreactive condition resulting in bronchospasm, mucosal edema, and increased mucus secretion. This condition usually occurs in response to inhaled irritants or allergens (see Figure 17.25 ■).

Subjective findings:

- Dyspnea.
- Anxiety.
- Chest pain.

Objective findings:

- Wheezing.
- Diminished breath sounds.
- Absent breath sounds (with severe asthma).
- Increased respiratory rate.
- Increased use of accessory muscles.
- Decreased oxygen saturation.

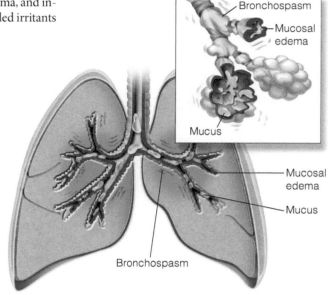

Figure 17.25 Asthma.

ATELECTASIS

A collapse or impaired inflation of one or more areas of the lung (NHLBI, 2013). The alveoli or an entire lung may collapse from airway obstruction, such as a mucus plug, lack of surfactant, or a compressed chest wall (see Figure 17.26 ■).

Subjective findings:

- Absence of symptoms, if only a small portion of the lung is affected.
- Dyspnea, if significant portions of the lung are affected.

Objective findings:

- Decreased or absent breath sounds over the affected area.
- Increased respiratory rate.
- Decreased oxygen saturation.
- Cyanosis (if severe).
- Dullness to percussion over the affected area.

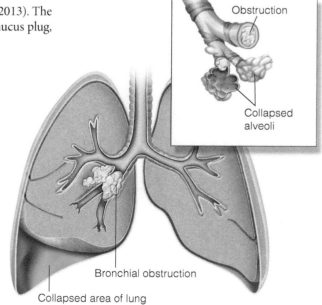

Figure 17.26 Atelectasis.

CHRONIC BRONCHITIS

Chronic inflammation of the tracheobronchial tree leads to increased mucus production and blocked airways. A productive cough is present (see Figure 17.27 ■).

Subjective findings:

- Dyspnea.
- Fatigue (related to increased work of breathing).

Objective findings:

- Chronic productive cough.
- Increased respiratory rate.
- Use of accessory muscles.
- Wheezes.
- Rhonchi.

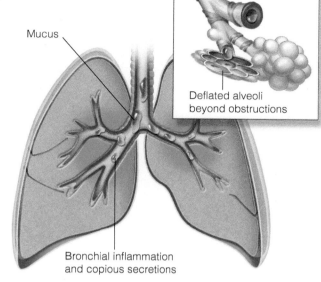

Mucus

Deflated alveoli beyond obstructions

Bronchial inflammation and copious secretions

Figure 17.27 Chronic bronchitis.

EMPHYSEMA

A condition in which chronic inflammation of the lungs leads to destruction of alveoli and decreased elasticity of the lungs. As a result, air is trapped and lungs hyperinflate (see Figure 17.28 ■).

Subjective findings:

- Shortness of breath, especially on exertion.
- Air hunger (related to hypoxemia, CO_2 retention, and air trapping).

Objective findings:

- Barrel chest and decreased chest expansion.
- Cyanosis.
- Hypercarbia (increased blood concentration of CO_2).
- Clubbing of fingers.
- Use of accessory muscles.
- Diminished breath sounds.

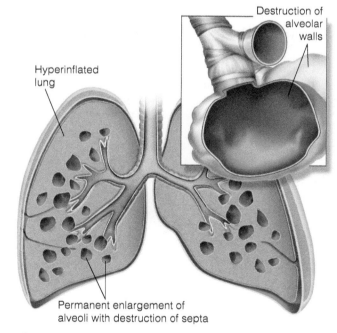

Destruction of alveolar walls

Hyperinflated lung

Permanent enlargement of alveoli with destruction of septa

Figure 17.28 Emphysema.

LOBAR PNEUMONIA

An infection that causes fluid, bacteria, and cellular debris to fill the alveoli (see Figure 17.29 ■).

Subjective findings:

- Dyspnea.
- Fatigue.
- Chills.

Objective findings:

- Increased respiratory rate.
- Fever.
- Productive cough.
- Decreased oxygen saturation.
- Bronchial breath sounds and crackles.
- Dullness to percussion over the affected area.

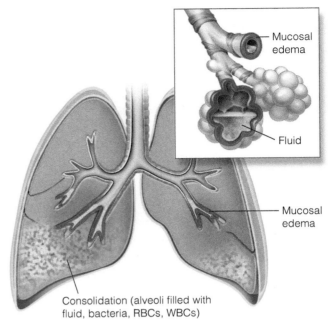

Mucosal edema

Fluid

Mucosal edema

Consolidation (alveoli filled with fluid, bacteria, RBCs, WBCs)

Figure 17.29 Lobar pneumonia.

PLEURAL EFFUSION

A fluid accumulation in the pleural space (see Figure 17.30 ■). Pleural effusion may be asymptomatic, or it could present with common signs and symptoms (Saguil, Wyrick, & Hallgren, 2014).

Subjective findings:

- Shortness of breath (dyspnea).
- Occasional sharp, nonradiating chest pain.

Objective findings:

- Cough.
- Diminished or absent breath sounds.
- Dullness to percussion over the affected area.
- Decreased or absent tactile fremitus.
- No voice transmission.

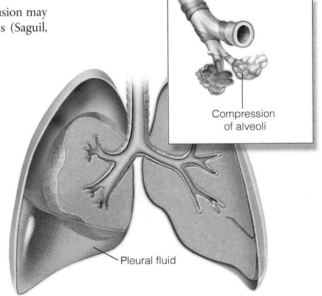

Compression of alveoli

Pleural fluid

Figure 17.30 Pleural effusion.

PNEUMOTHORAX

A condition in which air moves into the pleural space and causes partial or complete collapse of the lung. Pneumothorax can be spontaneous, traumatic, or tension (see Figure 17.31 ■).

Subjective findings:

- Shortness of breath.
- Sharp chest pain with inspiration.
- Anxiety.

Objective findings:

- Increased respiratory rate.
- Decreased oxygen saturation.
- Diminished or absent breath sounds over the affected area.
- Hyperresonance to percussion over the affected area.
- Decreased chest wall expansion on the affected side.
- Tracheal deviation to the unaffected side.

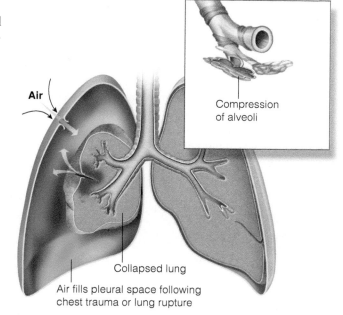

Air

Compression of alveoli

Collapsed lung

Air fills pleural space following chest trauma or lung rupture

Figure 17.31 Pneumothorax.

LEFT HEART FAILURE

Heart failure occurs when the heart is unable to effectively pump oxygen-rich blood. Heart failure may affect one or both sides of the heart. Most often, both the left and right sides of the heart are affected (NHLBI, 2014). Left heart failure typically produces respiratory symptoms as blood that is not ejected by the left ventricle backs up into the lungs. Right heart failure typically produces peripheral edema, as well as other manifestations (see chapter 19 ∞). With left heart failure, increased pressure in the pulmonary veins causes interstitial edema around the alveoli and may cause edema of the bronchial mucosa (see Figure 17.32 ■).

Subjective findings:

- Shortness of breath (especially on exertion).
- Orthopnea.
- Anxiety.

Objective findings:

- Increased respiratory rate.
- Decreased oxygen saturation.
- Pulmonary congestion with auscultation of wheezes or crackles in lung bases.
- Pallor.
- Decreased chest wall expansion on the affected side.
- Tracheal deviation to the unaffected side.

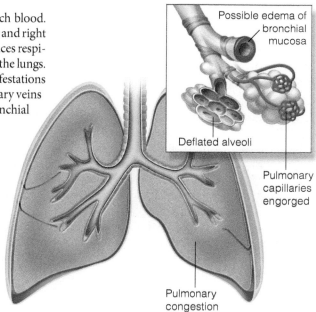

Possible edema of bronchial mucosa

Deflated alveoli

Pulmonary capillaries engorged

Pulmonary congestion

Figure 17.32 Left heart failure.

VALLEY FEVER

Valley fever is a respiratory fungal infection that occurs among populations in dry desert regions of central California, the southwestern United States, and Mexico. This disease also is prevalent among populations who live in dry areas of South and Central America (CDC, 2013b). In most cases, valley fever is asymptomatic and resolves without treatment. However, some get sick with flulike symptoms that may last for weeks or months. In rare cases, the infection can spread from the lungs to the rest of the body; this usually results in more severe consequences, such as meningitis or death. Immunosuppression (e.g., due to HIV infection or organ transplant) greatly increases the risk for developing severe complications (CDC, 2013b). Valley fever is also known as coccidioidomycosis, desert fever, desert rheumatism, and San Joaquin Valley fever.

Subjective findings:
- Chest pain.
- Chills.
- Headache.
- Fatigue.
- Joint pain.

Objective findings:
- Fever.
- Dry cough.
- Night sweats.
- Spotty red rash.

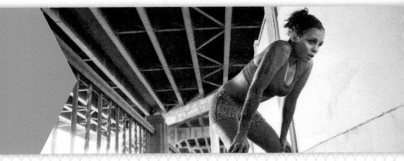

Application Through Critical Thinking

▌ Case Study

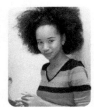

Tanisha Robinson, a 14-year-old female, has been seen regularly in the clinic for chronic asthma. Today, Tanisha's mother has accompanied her for a checkup. Tanisha has required two visits to the emergency room (ER) for severe wheezing in the month since her last clinic visit.

The physical assessment reveals that the patient is in no distress and breath sounds are clear. Her vital signs are BP 126/82—P 84—RR 20. Her skin is warm, dry, and pink in color. Tanisha can speak clearly and seems relaxed.

During the interview the nurse learns that the patient has been following her prescribed treatments and has done well except for the two ER visits.

The nurse learns that each ER visit occurred after school hours. The patient experienced severe shortness of breath and wheezing that was unrelieved by rest or use of her inhalers. ER treatment consisted of injection of epinephrine, administration of oxygen, intravenous (IV) fluids, Benadryl, and steroids. Each ER visit lasted approximately 6 hours. The patient's breathing was restored to nearly normal at discharge and she was given a prescription for a course of prednisone.

When asked if she could identify any precipitating factors, Tanisha replies, "I know they happened on days that we had gym, but I don't usually have a problem with that." The nurse asks if she had any changes in her routines, activities, or environments. She says, "No, not that I can think of." Her mother states, "We're so upset. She's been out twice this month." The patient then adds, "Yes, I hate to have to miss school and get behind and now my friend and I have to work twice as hard as before to get our project done."

The nurse asks about the project and the patient says, "We are working on an art project—collecting materials and doing a thing on textures. It's pretty cool. We collected old clothes from the Salvation Army and a garage sale and we've been cutting them up sort of in a collage." The nurse asks if the work on the project coincided with her recent attacks. The patient says, "Gee, I don't know, I never thought about it." Her mother states, "Oh, we never even thought about that, but on both days, she had been working on the project after school with her friend and really got bad as the evening wore on."

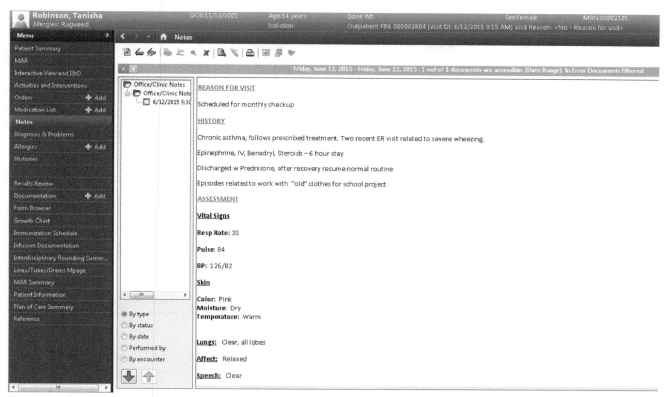

Source: From Cerner Electronic Health Record. Copyright © by Cerner Corporation. Used by permission of Cerner Corporation.

▌ Complete Documentation

The following is a sample documentation from the assessment of Tanisha Robinson.

SUBJECTIVE DATA: Visit to clinic for a checkup, 14-year-old female asthmatic. Required two ER visits for severe wheezing in month since last clinic visit. Following prescribed treatments. Doing well except ER visits. ER visits occurred on school days when patient had gym, but usually no problem with physical activity. ER visits associated with work on art project—a textile collage from old clothes. Wheezing started after work on project and increased in severity requiring epinephrine, IV, Benadryl, and steroids. Patient is discharged with course of oral steroids after each visit. Resumed normal treatment and activity after episodes.

OBJECTIVE DATA: Breath sounds clear. Skin warm, dry, and pink. Clear speech, relaxed. VS: BP 126/82—P 84—RR 20.

▌ Critical Thinking Questions

1. Describe the nurse's thoughts and actions as the nurse applies the steps of the critical thinking process in this situation.
2. In interpreting the data, how would they be clustered?

3. What are the options that could be developed for this 14-year-old and her mother?
4. Which of the *Healthy People 2020* objectives are important to Tanisha and her care?
5. What special considerations should the nurse pay attention to in this situation?

▌ Prepare Teaching Plan

LEARNING NEED: Data reveal two episodes of respiratory distress following the construction of a textile collage for a school project. Tanisha needs to learn more about environmental allergens as causing her respiratory distress.

GOAL: Tanisha will decrease the number of acute respiratory distress episodes.

OBJECTIVES: At the end of the lesson, Tanisha will be able to:

1. Identify locations of known allergens in her environment.
2. Identify strategies to decrease her exposure to allergens.

EXAMPLE OF TEACHING PLAN FOR OBJECTIVE 2: Identify strategies to decrease her exposure to allergens (cognitive)

Content	Teaching Strategy and Rationale	Evaluation

You have been able to recall your allergens and have identified environmental placement. Now you need to look for alternatives to prevent future exposure and distress.
 	
Alternative strategies could include the following:
 	
• Work in a well-ventilated area.
• Plan all activities to decrease exposure to allergens:
  • Use clean and dry materials.
  • Select other substances for texture—wood, stone, plastic.
  • Wash material before handling.
• Read all labels to be sure allergens are not in the product being used.
• Use objects that are allergen-free.
	• One-to-one discussion to provide recall and reinforcement of learner's knowledge
	• Printed material to provide review and reinforcement of material
		Name three alternative strategies to be used when completing the school project.

▶ References

American Academy of Pediatrics, Task Force on Sudden Infant Death Syndrome. (2011). SIDS and other sleep-related infant deaths: Expansion of recommendations for a safe infant sleeping environment [Policy statement]. *Pediatrics.* doi: 10.1542/peds.2011-2284.

Berman, A., & Snyder, S. J. (2012). *Kozier and Erb's fundamentals of nursing: Concepts, process and practice* (9th ed.). Upper Saddle River, NJ: Prentice Hall.

Bikley, L. S. (2008). *Bates guide to physical examination and history taking* (10th ed.). Philadelphia: Lippincott.

Butler, C. C., Kelly, M. J., Hood, K., Schaberg, T., Melbye, H., Serra-Prat, M., . . . Coenen, S. (2011). Antibiotic prescribing for discoloured sputum in acute cough/lower respiratory tract infection. *European Respiratory Journal, 38*(1), 119–125.

Centers for Disease Control and Prevention (CDC). (2013a). *Smoking & tobacco use: Hookahs.* Retrieved from http://www.cdc.gov/tobacco/data_statistics/fact_sheets/tobacco_industry/hookahs/

Centers for Disease Control and Prevention (CDC). (2013b). *Valley fever: Awareness is key.* Retrieved from http://www.cdc.gov/features/valleyfever/

Chang, A. B., Redding, G. J., & Everard, M. L. (2008). Chronic wet cough: Protracted bronchitis, chronic suppurative lung disease and bronchiectasis. *Pediatric Pulmonology, 43*(6), 519–531.

Chonmaitree, T., Revai, K., Grady, J. J., Clos, A., Patel, J. A., Nair, S., . . . Henrickson, K. J. (2008). Viral upper respiratory tract infection and otitis media complication in young children. *Clinical Infectious Diseases, 46*(6), 815–823.

Dumitru, I., & Baker, M. M. (2014). *Heart failure: Clinical presentation.* Retrieved from http://emedicine.medscape.com/article/163062-clinical

Forno, E., & Celedon, J. C. (2009). Asthma and ethnic minorities: socioeconomic status and beyond. *Current opinion in allergy and clinical immunology, 9*(2), 154–160.

Goodman, D. M., Lynm, C., & Livingston, E. L. (2013). Adult sinusitis. *Journal of the American Medical Association, 309*(8), 837–837.

Gray, H. (2010). *Gray's anatomy.* New York: Barnes & Noble Books.

Ho, L. A., & Kuschner, W. G. (2012). Respiratory health in home and leisure pursuits. *Clinics in chest medicine, 33*(4), 715–729.

Marieb, E. (2009). Essentials of human anatomy and physiology (9th ed.). Redwood City, CA: Benjamin/Cummings/Pearson Education.

Mayo Clinic. (2012). Valley fever: Symptoms. Retrieved from http://www.mayoclinic.org/diseases-conditions/valley-fever/basics/symptoms/con-20027390

Mayo Clinic. (2013b). *Tests and procedures: Sed rate (erythrocyte sedimentation rate).* Retrieved from http://www.mayoclinic.org/tests-procedures/sed-rate/basics/results/prc-20013502

Mayo Clinic. (2013a). Infant and toddler health: When's the right time to start feeding a baby solid foods? Retrieved from http://www.mayoclinic.org/healthy-living/infant-and-toddler-health/expert-answers/starting-solids/faq-20057889

Mayo Foundation for Medical Education and Research. (2014). *Rochester test catalog: 2014 online test catalog.* Available at http://www.mayomedicallaboratories.com/test-catalog/

MedlinePlus. Blood differential. (2013). Retrieved from http://www.nlm.nih.gov/medlineplus/ency/article/003657.htm

National Heart, Lung, & Blood Institute (NHLBI). (2013). *What is atelectasis?* Retrieved from http://www.nhlbi.nih.gov/health/health-topics/topics/atl/

National Heart, Lung, and Blood Institute (NHLBI). (2014). *What is heart failure?* Retrieved from http://www.nhlbi.nih.gov/health/health-topics/topics/hf/

Northridge, J., Ramirez, O. F., Stingone, J. A., & Claudio, L. (2010). The role of housing type and housing quality in urban children with asthma. *Journal of Urban Health, 87*(2), 211–224.

Osborn, K. S., Wraa, C. E., Watson, A., & Holleran, R. S. (2013). *Medical-surgical nursing: Preparation for practice* (2nd ed.). Upper Saddle River, NJ: Pearson.

Pagana, K. D. (2013). *Mosby's manual of diagnostic and laboratory tests.* (5th ed.). St. Louis, MO: Elsevier.

Richardson, M. (2003). The physiology of mucus and sputum production in the respiratory system. *Nursing Times, 99*(23), 63–64.

Saguil, A., Wyrick, K., & Hallgren, J. (2014). Diagnostic approach to pleural effusion. *American Family Physician, 90*(2), 99–104.

Seidel, H., Ball, J. W., Dains, J. E., & Benedict, W. J. (2010). *Mosby's guide to physical examination* (7th ed.). St. Louis, MO: Mosby.

Tan, E. K., & Tan, E. L. (2013). Alterations in physiology and anatomy during pregnancy. *Best Practice & Research Clinical Obstetrics & Gynaecology, 27*(6), 791–802.

Tortora, G. J., & Derrickson, B. H. (2009). *Principles of anatomy and physiology* (12th ed.). New York: John Wiley & Sons.

University of Maryland Medical Center (UMMC). (2012). *Pneumonia.* Retrieved from http://umm.edu/health/medical/reports/articles/pneumonia

U.S. Department of Health and Human Services (USDHHS). (2014). *Healthy people 2020.* Retrieved from http://www.healthypeople.gov/2020/default.aspx

Wilson, B.A., Shannon, M. T., & Shields, K.M. (2013). *Pearson nurse's drug guide.* Upper Saddle River, NJ: Pearson.

World Allergy Organization (WAO). (2009). *Chronic obstructive pulmonary disease (COPD) and asthma: Similarities and differences.* Retrieved from http://www.worldallergy.org/professional/allergic_diseases_center/copd_and_asthma/

Yoon, S. H., Lee, N. K., & Yim, J. J. (2012). Impact of sputum gross appearance and volume on smear positivity of pulmonary tuberculosis: a prospective cohort study. *BioMed Central Infectious Diseases, 12*(1), 172.

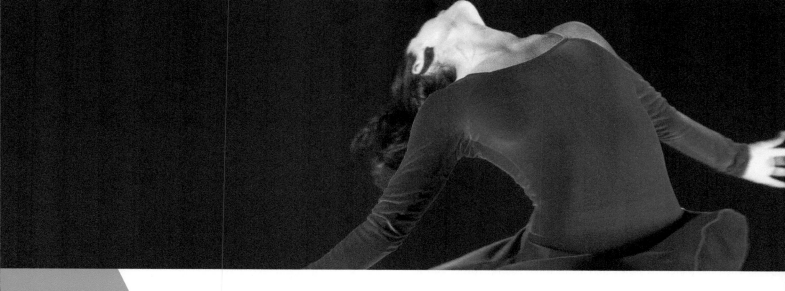

18 ▶ Breasts and Axillae

▶ Learning Outcomes

Upon completion of this chapter, you will be able to:

1. Describe the anatomy and physiology of the breasts and axillae.

2. Develop questions to be used when completing the focused interview.

3. Explain patient preparation for examination of the breasts and axillae.

4. Outline the techniques for assessment of the breasts and axillae.

5. Differentiate normal from abnormal findings in the physical assessment of the breasts and axillae.

6. Identify the anatomic, physiologic, developmental, psychosocial, and cultural variations that guide assessment.

7. Relate *Healthy People 2020* objectives to issues of the female breasts and axillae.

8. Apply critical thinking to assessment of the breasts and axillae.

Key Terms

acini cells, 423
areola, 422
axillary tail, 423
colostrum, 426
galactorrhea, 442
gynecomastia, 426
mammary ridge, 423
mastalgia, 428
Montgomery's glands, 423
peau d'orange, 437
suspensory ligaments, 423
thelarche, 426

n the United States, breast cancer is the most common type of cancer in females, except for skin cancer. Breast cancer is second only to lung cancer as a cause of cancer deaths in women. Approximately 12%, or one in eight women, will be diagnosed with breast cancer in their lifetimes. Rates of death from breast cancer are declining and are approximately 1 in 36 women (American Cancer Society [ACS], 2014a).

Assessment of the breasts and axillae begins with a thorough health history. During the focused interview, the nurse gathers additional information by asking pertinent questions relating to the patient's general health and breast and lymph nodes in particular. Physical assessment of the breasts may be incorporated into the total body assessment along with the heart and lung assessment when the patient is sitting and again when supine. Although the majority of the material in this chapter assumes that the patient is female, it is important to incorporate assessment of the male patient's breasts during the physical assessment, usually when assessing the thorax. Cancer is addressed in *Healthy People 2020*. In relation to breast health, the objectives in *Healthy People 2020* are to reduce the female breast cancer death rate and increase the proportion of women aged 40 years and older who have received a breast cancer screening based on the most recent guidelines. Therefore, the nurse must be aware of these factors as questions for the focused interview are formulated and the physical assessment is performed.

Accurate knowledge of the structure and function of the breasts and lymphatic system is necessary to carry out the assessment activities related to the breasts and axillae. It is also important that the nurse understand the interrelationships of the various body systems that contribute to this region. For example, the musculoskeletal system supports the overlying integument, and the lymphatic system drains the region. In addition, while performing the assessment, one must keep in mind the normal variations for the patient's developmental stage. An understanding and acceptance of different individuals' feelings, beliefs, and practices regarding the breasts and breast care are also essential.

Anatomy and Physiology Review

The breasts are located on the anterior chest and supported by muscles and ligaments. The breast includes the areola and nipple as well as the glandular, adipose, and fibrous tissue. A system of lymph nodes drains lymph from the breasts and axillae. These tissues and structures are described in the following paragraphs.

Breasts

The breasts are paired mammary glands located on the anterior chest wall. Breast tissue extends from the second or third rib to the sixth or seventh rib and from the sternal margin to the midaxillary line, depending on body shape and size (see Figure 18.1 ■). The breasts lie anterior to the pectoralis major and serratus anterior muscles. The nipple is centrally located within a circular pigmented field of wrinkled skin called the **areola**. The surface of the areola

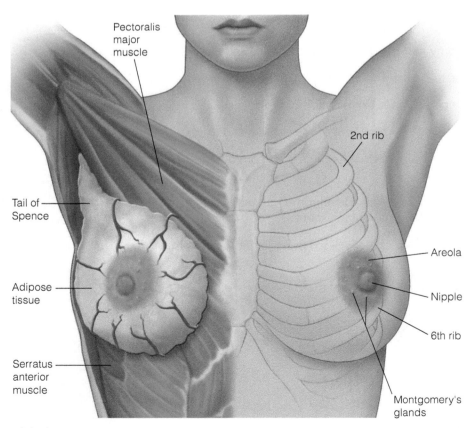

Figure 18.1 Anatomy of the breast.

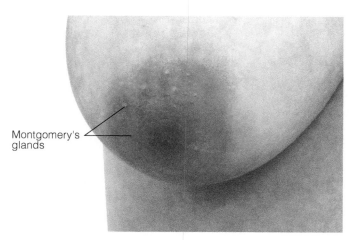

Figure 18.2 Montgomery's glands.

is speckled with tiny sebaceous glands known as **Montgomery's glands** or Montgomery's tubercles (see Figure 18.2 ■). Hair follicles are normally seen around the periphery of the areola. Commonly, breast tissue extends superiolaterally into the axilla as the **axillary**

tail (tail of Spence). The internal and lateral thoracic arteries and cutaneous branches of the posterior intercostal arteries provide an abundant supply of blood to the breasts.

Breasts are composed of glandular, fibrous, and adipose (fat) tissue. The glandular tissue is arranged into 15 to 20 lobes per breast that radiate from the nipple (see Figure 18.3 ■). Each lobe is composed of 20 to 40 lobules that contain the **acini cells** (or alveoli) that produce milk. These cells empty into the lactiferous ducts, which carry milk from each lobe to the nipple. The fibrous tissue provides support for the glandular tissue. **Suspensory ligaments** (Cooper's ligaments) extend from the connective tissue layer, through the breast, and attach to the fascia underlying the breast. Subcutaneous and retromammary adipose tissue make up the remainder of the breast. The proportions of these three components vary with age, weight, genetics, the general state of the patient's health, menstrual cycle, pregnancy, and lactation. Supernumerary nipples or breast tissue may be present along the **mammary ridge**, or "milk line," which extends from each axilla to the groin (see Figure 18.4 ■). Usually this tissue atrophies during fetal development, but occasionally a nipple persists and is visible. It needs to be differentiated from a mole (see Figure 18.5 ■).

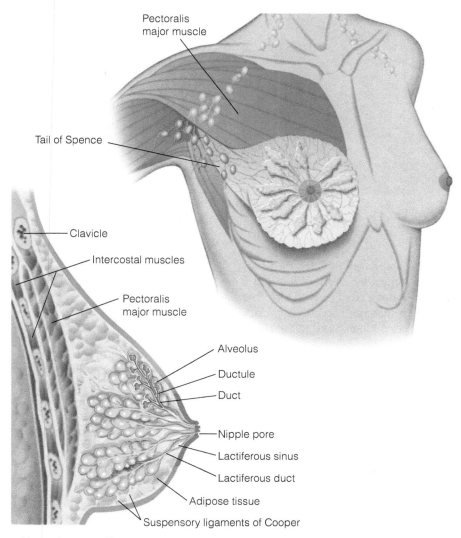

Figure 18.3 Anterior and lateral views of breast anatomy.

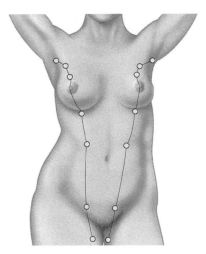

Figure 18.4 Mammary ridge.

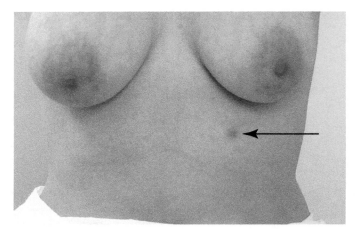

Figure 18.5 Supernumerary nipple.

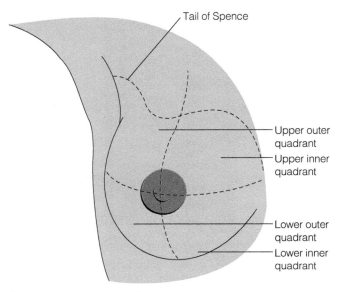

Figure 18.6 Breast quadrants.

For the purpose of documenting assessment findings, the breast is divided into four quadrants defined by a vertical line and a horizontal line that intersect at the nipple (see Figure 18.6 ■). The location of clinical findings may be described according to clock positions, for example, at the 2 o'clock position, 5 cm (1.95 in.) from the nipple. The major functions of the breasts include producing, storing, and supplying milk for the process of lactation. The male breast is composed of a small nipple and flat areola. These are superior to a thin disk of undeveloped breast tissue that may not be distinguishable from the surrounding tissues.

Breasts, in both females and males, also provide a mechanism for sexual arousal.

Axillae and Lymph Nodes

A complex system of lymph nodes drains lymph from the breasts and axillae and returns it to the blood. Superficial lymph nodes drain the skin, and deep lymph nodes drain the mammary lobules.

Figure 18.7 ■ depicts the groups of nodes that drain the breasts and axillae.

The lymph nodes are usually nonpalpable. The following nodes are palpated during the assessment:

1. Internal mammary nodes
2. Supraclavicular nodes
3. Subclavicular (infraclavicular) nodes
4. Interpectoral nodes
5. Central axillary nodes
6. Brachial (lateral axillary) nodes
7. Subscapular (posterior axillary) nodes
8. Pectoral (anterior axillary) nodes

The internal mammary nodes drain toward the abdomen and the opposite breast. Most of the lymph from the rest of the breast drains toward the axilla and subclavicular region. Thus, a cancerous lesion can spread via the lymphatic system to the subclavicular nodes, into deep channels within the chest or abdomen, and even to the opposite breast. The male breast has the same potential and needs to be examined as well. The major functions of the lymphatic system include returning water and proteins from the interstitial spaces to the blood, thus helping to maintain blood osmotic pressure and body fluid balance. It also helps filter out microorganisms and other body debris.

Muscles of the Chest Wall

The major muscles of the chest wall, which support the breast and contribute to its shape, are the pectoralis major and serratus anterior muscles (see Figure 18.1). The overall contour of the breasts is determined by the suspensory ligaments, which provide support. The major function of the muscles of the chest wall is to support breast and lymphatic tissue.

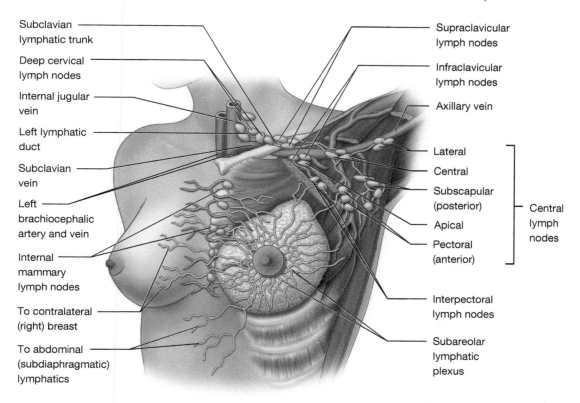

Figure 18.7 Lymphatic drainage of the breast.

Special Considerations

Age, developmental level, race, ethnicity, work history, living conditions, socioeconomics, and emotional well-being are among the factors that influence breast health. These factors must be considered when collecting subjective and objective data during the comprehensive health assessment. The nurse applies critical thinking to assess the patient's state of health and to identify the factors that may influence breast health.

Health Promotion Considerations

Breast health is included as a focus of *Healthy People 2020*. In particular, *Healthy People 2020* objectives emphasize screening for breast cancer, as well as reducing the number of deaths caused by breast cancer (USDHHS, 2010). See Table 18.1 for examples of *Healthy People 2020* objectives that are designed to promote breast health and wellness among individuals across the life span.

Lifespan Considerations

Growth and development are dynamic processes that describe change over time. The following discussion presents specific variations of the breasts for different age groups.

Infants and Children

Inverted nipples are evident at birth and common until adolescence. Because of circulating maternal estrogen and prolactin, male and female infants may have a milky white discharge from their nipples that

TABLE 18.1	Examples of *Healthy People 2020* Objectives Related to Breast Health
OBJECTIVE NUMBER	**DESCRIPTION**
C-3	Reduce the female breast cancer death rate
C-11	Reduce late-stage female breast cancer
C-17	Increase the proportion of women who receive a breast cancer screening based on the most recent guidelines

Source: U.S. Department of Health and Human Services (USDHHS). (2014). *Healthy people 2020.* Retrieved from http://www.healthypeople.gov/2020/default.aspx.

is commonly called "witch's milk." This condition will resolve within 1 to 2 weeks after birth when maternal hormone levels decrease.

Breast tissue starts to enlarge in females with the onset of puberty, usually between the ages of 9 and 13. At first there is only a bud around the nipple and areola, which may be tender initially. The ductile system matures, extensive fat deposits occur, and the areola and nipples grow and become pigmented. These changes are correlated with an increased level of estrogen and progesterone in the body as sexual maturity progresses. Growth of the breasts is not necessarily steady or symmetric. This may be frustrating or embarrassing to some girls. Because a female's primary sexual organs cannot be observed, breast development provides visual confirmation that the adolescent is becoming a woman. For the developing adolescent, her breasts are a visible symbol of her feminine identity and an important part of her body image and self-esteem. The nurse can reassure girls that the rate of breast tissue growth is dependent on changing hormone levels and is uniquely individual, as are the eventual size and shape of the breasts. **Thelarche**, or breast budding, is often the first pubertal sign in females. Breast development follows a clear pattern described by the Tanner stages as illustrated in Figure 18.8 ■.

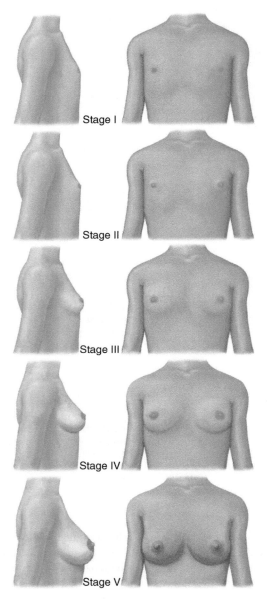

Figure 18.8 Tanner's stages of breast development: I, Preadolescent. Only the nipple is raised above the level of the breast, as in the child. II, Budding stage. Areola increased in diameter and surrounding area slightly elevated. III, Breast and areola enlarged. No contour separation. IV, Areola forms a secondary elevation above that of the breast in half of girls. V, Areola is usually part of the general breast contour and is strongly pigmented. Nipple usually projects.

Stage I

Stage II

Stage III

Stage IV

Stage V

Benign fibroadenomas in adolescent females are not uncommon. The nurse should reassure the girl and her parents or caregivers that no correlation has been established between fibroadenomas and malignant cancers. Although the American Cancer Society recommends that females be told about the advantages and disadvantages of breast self-examination (BSE) at age 20, teaching the adolescent female about examination of her breasts can help her to establish an awareness of how her own breasts feel and look and how important it can be to report changes in them to her healthcare provider.

Adolescent males may experience temporary breast enlargement, called **gynecomastia,** in one or both breasts. This condition is usually self-limiting and resolves spontaneously. Another concern to adolescent males is transient masses beneath one areola or both. These "breast buds" usually disappear within a year of onset.

The Pregnant Female

During pregnancy, breast tissue enlarges as glandular and ductal tissue increase in preparation for lactation. During the second month of pregnancy, nipples and areolae darken in color and enlarge. The degree of pigmentation varies with complexion. Nipples may leak **colostrum** in the month prior to childbirth. As breast tissue enlarges, venous networks may be more pronounced, and the breast tissue will be firmer, larger, and possibly more tender. The lobules are more distinct.

The Older Adult

More time may be required for the focused interview of an older patient. Many people have a difficult time talking about something as private as the breasts, and older adults may be even less comfortable with this topic. They may be modest and self-conscious, or they may feel that the nurse is too young to understand. There may also be cultural taboos about such private matters. The nurse should acknowledge that talking about the breasts may be somewhat uncomfortable but explain that sharing this information will promote the patient's health.

Older adults may have limited range of motion. If so, the patient should be asked to raise her arms to a height that does not cause discomfort. Because the older adult may have failing eyesight, the nurse may want to provide large mirrors, additional lighting, and a magnifying glass for close inspection when teaching BSE. Pamphlets and handouts with large print may be provided.

As menopause approaches, there is a decrease in glandular tissue, which is replaced by fatty tissue. The lobular texture of glandular tissue is replaced by a finer, granular texture. Breasts are less firm and tend to be more pendulous. As the suspensory ligaments relax, breast tissue hangs more loosely from the chest wall. The nipples become smaller and flatter and lose some erectile ability. The inframammary ridge thickens and can be palpated more easily.

Gynecomastia may occur in older adult males as a result of hormonal changes due to disease or medication. The nurse must be sensitive to possible embarrassment during the exam.

Breast cancer becomes increasingly more common as the population ages; therefore, older females must receive advice and counseling about recommended periodic breast examination and screening for breast cancer.

Psychosocial Considerations

A female patient's overall sense of self-esteem may be reflected in the way she feels about her breasts. In fact, some women may view their breasts as a badge of femininity. Media portrayal of idealized images of "perfect" breasts, especially by advertisers, may increase this feeling. Thus, patients whose breasts are smaller or larger than average, patients with asymmetric breasts, and patients who have had a mastectomy or other breast surgery or trauma are at an increased risk for body image disturbance, self-esteem disturbance, and dysfunctional grieving.

Although the U.S. Preventive Services Task Force recommends that all women between the ages of 50 and 74 receive a mammogram at least once every two years, studies indicate that just over 70% of women follow this recommendation, which is less than the *Healthy People 2020* goal of 81.1%. Factors contributing to the lack of screening include no regular health care, no health insurance, recent immigration, and lack of education (CDC, 2012). Other factors that may contribute to lack of screening may include anxiety and fear of cancer or surgery, a body image change, a change in significant relationships, denial, feelings of powerlessness, or a lack of knowledge about breast disorders. During the assessment of the breasts and axillae, the nurse needs to encourage the patient to share her fears and concerns.

Research indicates that a high-fat diet may increase a female's risk of developing breast cancer. Alcohol intake in excess of nine drinks a week has also been implicated.

Obesity has been linked with higher risks of breast cancer. However, severely obese women are less likely to comply with recommendations about breast health screening than are nonobese women. It is suggested that embarrassment in the examination room; concern about negative reactions from healthcare providers; fear of being lectured about obesity; and the small size of examination gowns, tables, and equipment are among the reasons that prevent obese women from seeking breast screening.

Although breast cancer is normally seen as a woman's disease, men can also develop breast cancer. Men should be taught the importance of reporting lumps in their breasts and seeking follow-up and treatment as needed. Men may delay reporting lumps because of social stigmas or embarrassment. Therefore, the nurse needs to encourage men to report any abnormalities they discover and discuss fears or other emotions that accompany the possible diagnosis of breast cancer.

Cultural and Environmental Considerations

The nurse must be aware of variations in breast development related to ethnicity. For example, females of African ancestry may develop secondary sexual characteristics earlier than females of European ancestry (Susman et al., 2010). The time of appearance, texture, and distribution of axillary and pubic hair also vary according to race and ethnicity (Susman et al., 2010).

Diagnosis and mortality rates related to breast cancer vary across different cultural groups. In the United States, breast cancer is more often diagnosed in White women than in women of African American, Hispanic, Latina, Asian, Pacific Islander, American Indian, or Alaskan Native heritage (National Cancer Institute [NCI], 2012a). However, in women younger than 45 years of age, breast cancer is more common among African Americans. Likewise, African American women are more likely to die of breast cancer (NCI, 2012a). Women who are of Asian, Hispanic, and Native-American heritage have a lower risk of developing and dying from breast cancer (NCI, 2012a).

Socioeconomic factors may influence a patient's access to screening mammography and regular physical examinations. As mentioned earlier, although most of the information in this chapter assumes a female patient, assessment of the male breasts and axillae is also important.

Gathering the Data

Breast health assessment includes the gathering of subjective and objective data. Subjective data collection occurs during the patient interview, before the actual physical assessment. During the interview the nurse uses a variety of communication techniques to elicit general and specific information about the patient's state of breast health or illness. Health records, the results of laboratory tests, mammography, and magnetic resonance imaging (MRI) are important secondary sources to be reviewed and included in the data-gathering process. During physical assessment of the breasts and axillae, the techniques of inspection and palpation will be used. Before proceeding, it may be helpful to review the information about each of the data-gathering processes and practice the techniques of health assessment. See Table 18.2 for information on potential secondary sources of patient data.

Focused Interview

The focused interview for the breasts and axillae concerns data related to the structures and functions of the breasts and lymphatic system. Subjective data related to breast health are gathered during the focused interview. The nurse must be prepared to observe the patient and listen for cues related to the breasts and axillae. The nurse may use open-ended and closed questions to obtain information. Often a number of follow-up questions or requests for descriptions are required to clarify data or gather missing information. Follow-up questions are aimed at identifying the source of problems, duration of difficulties, measures to alleviate problems, and clues about the patient's knowledge of his or her own health. The subjective data collected and the questions asked during the health history and focused

TABLE 18.2	Potential Secondary Sources for Patient Data Related to the Breast and Axillae

Laboratory Tests

Genetic Screen for BRCA1 and BRCA2

Diagnostic Tests

Breast Ultrasound

Excisional Biopsy

Fine-Needle Aspiration Biopsy

Mammography

MRI

Stereotactic Biopsy

TABLE 18.3	Overview of Mastalgia	
TYPE OF MASTALGIA	**DESCRIPTION**	
Cyclic	• Most common form of mastalgia	
	• Typically associated with the menstrual cycle; onset of pain occurs in the days prior to menstruation and gradually increases, then subsides once menstruation begins	
	• Most commonly affects younger women	
	• Usually occurs in both breasts (bilateral)	
	• Typically disappears after menopause.	
Noncyclic	• Not associated with the menstrual cycle	
	• Has no apparent precipitating factor, although can be related to large breasts that are not supported sufficiently	
	• Most commonly affects women 30 to 50 years of age	
	• Often occurs in one breast (unilateral)	
	• Pain is often described as sharp or burning sensation that occurs in one region of the breast	
	• Often results from changes to breast structure, including fibroadenoma, cysts, and trauma, or from pain in the chest cavity and neck that radiates to the breast	
	• May require diagnostic studies, such as mammogram or biopsy.	

Sources: Adapted from Mayo Clinic. (2013c). Breast pain. Retrieved from http://www.mayoclinic.org/diseases-conditions/breast-pain/basics/definition/con-20025541; Salzman, B., Fleegle, S., & Tully, A. S. (2012). Common breast problems. *American Family Physician, 86*(4), 343–349; WebMD. (2012). *Breast pain (mastalgia) – Topic overview: What do I need to know about breast pain?* Retrieved from http://www.webmd.com/women/tc/breast-pain-mastalgia-topic-overview; and Johns Hopkins Medicine. (n.d.). *Mastalgia (breast pain).* Retrieved from http://www.hopkinsmedicine.org/healthlibrary/conditions/breast_health/mastalgia_breast_pain_85,P00154/.

interview provide information to help meet the goals of improving breast health and preventing and controlling breast disease.

The focused interview guides physical assessment of the breasts and axillae. The information is always considered in relation to norms and expectations about breast and lymphatic function. Therefore, the nurse must consider age, gender, race, culture, environment, and health practices as well as past and concurrent problems and therapies when framing questions and using techniques to elicit information. In order to address all of the factors involved when conducting a focused interview, categories of questions related to the breasts and axillae have been developed. These categories include general questions that are asked of all patients, those addressing illness and infection, questions related to symptoms and behaviors, those related to habits or practices, questions that are specific to patients according to age, those for the pregnant female, and questions that address environmental concerns. One approach to elicit information about symptoms is the OLDCART & ICE method, which is described in chapter 7. ∞ See Figure 7.3 on page 120.

The nurse must consider the patient's ability to participate in the focused interview and physical assessment of the breasts and axillae. Patients who are experiencing breast discomfort or pain may require immediate assessment by the primary healthcare provider. Breast pain, or **mastalgia,** is most often associated with the menstrual cycle. In some cases, however, referred pain from cardiac, pulmonary, and gastrointestinal causes must be ruled out. See Table 18.3 for an overview of the two primary categories of mastalgia.

Focused Interview Questions

The following section provides sample questions and bulleted follow-up questions in each of the categories previously mentioned. A rationale for each of the questions is provided. The list of questions is not all-inclusive

Rationales and Evidence

but represents the types of questions required in a comprehensive focused interview related to the breasts and axillae.

General Questions

1. **Describe your breasts today. How do they differ, if at all, from 3 months ago? From 3 years ago?**

▶ This question gives the patient the opportunity to share her perception of her breasts and any changes she has experienced that may be related to breast health.

Focused Interview Questions	**Rationales and Evidence**

2. Are you still menstruating?
- If so, have you noticed any changes in your breasts that seem to be related to your normal menstrual cycle, such as tenderness, swelling, pain, or enlarged nodes? If so, please describe.

▶ These changes may occur with changing hormone levels, or they may be related to the use of oral, transdermal, and injectable contraceptives (Bitzer & Simon, 2011). "Lumpy breasts" occurring monthly prior to the onset of menses and resolving at the end of menstruation may be due to a benign condition called fibrocystic breasts (WebMD, 2011).

3. What was the date of your last menstrual period?

▶ This information, if applicable, helps correlate the current status of the breasts to the cycle.

Questions Related to Illness or Infection

1. Have you ever had any breast disease such as cancer, fibrocystic breast disease, benign breast disease, or fibroadenoma?

▶ A history of breast cancer poses the risk of recurrence (NCI, 2012a). Both fibroadenoma and the general lumpiness of fibrocystic breast disease need to be differentiated from cancer. Increased risk for breast cancer is associated with some benign breast lesions (NCI, 2012a). Information about these risks is available through the National Cancer Institute at www.cancer.gov/cancertopics/factsheet/detection/probability-breast-cancer.

2. Have you ever had breast surgery?
- If so, what type and when?
- How do you feel about it?
- How has it affected you?
- Has it affected your sex life? If so, how?

▶ Previous breast surgery has implications for physical and psychological well-being. Breast surgery includes lumpectomy, mastectomy, breast reconstruction, breast reduction, and breast augmentation.

3. Have you had cancer in any other region of your body such as the uterus, ovaries, or colon?

▶ A history of these cancers increases the risk for breast cancer (ACS, 2014b).

4. Has your mother or sister had breast cancer?

▶ Having a first-degree relative (mother, sister, or daughter) who has experienced breast cancer approximately doubles a woman's risk for developing the disorder. (ACS, 2014b).

5. Has one of your grandmothers or an aunt had breast cancer?

▶ While the risk is higher for women whose first-degree relative has experienced breast cancer, a history of this disorder in a second-degree relative (e.g., grandmother or aunt) also increases the risk (American Society of Clinical Oncology [ASCO], 2013).

6. Has anyone in your family been found to have a genetic mutation linked to breast cancer?

▶ BRCA1 and BRCA2, which are genetic proteins that help repair damaged DNA, are especially important in terms of cancer development. Hereditary mutations of BRCA1 and BRCA2 are associated with 20% to 25% of inherited breast cancers and 5% to 10% of all breast cancers (NCI, 2014). Further information about genetic mutation and heredity in breast cancer is available through the National Cancer Institute at www.cancer.gov/cancertopics/factsheet/risk/BRCA.

7. Have you had radiation therapy to the chest area for cancer other than breast cancer?

▶ Radiation to the chest increases the risk for breast cancer (ASCO, 2013).

Focused Interview Questions	Rationales and Evidence

Questions Related to Symptoms or Behaviors

When gathering information about symptoms, many questions are required to elicit details and descriptions that assist in analysis of the data. The questions are intended to determine the significance of a symptom in relation to specific diseases and problems and to identify the need for follow-up examination or referral.

The following questions refer to specific symptoms and behaviors associated with the breasts and axillae. For each symptom, questions and follow-up are required. The details to be elicited are the characteristics of the symptom; the onset, duration, and frequency of the symptom; the treatment or remedy for the symptom, including home remedies; the determination if a diagnosis has been sought; the effects of treatments; and family history associated with a symptom or illness.

Questions Related to Symptoms

1. **Have you noticed any changes in breast characteristics, such as size, symmetry, shape, thickening, lumps, swelling, temperature, color of skin or vessels, or sensations such as tingling or tenderness?**
   - If so, how long have you had them? Please describe them.

▶ Pain and tenderness can be caused by fibrocystic breast changes, pregnancy, lactation, cancer, or other disorders. A lump may indicate a benign cyst, a fibroadenoma, fatty necrosis, or a malignant tumor (NCI, 2012a). Skin irritation may be due to friction from a bra or to pendulous breasts. In older patients, decreased estrogen levels may cause the breasts to sag (Kam, 2011).

2. **Have you noticed any changes in nipple and areola characteristics, such as size, shape, open sores, lumps, pain, tenderness, discharge, skin changes, or retractions?**
   - If so, how long have you had them? Please describe them.

▶ Nipple discharge resulting from medication is usually clear. A bloody drainage is always a concern and needs to be further evaluated, especially in the presence of a lump. Eczematous changes of the skin of the nipples and areola may indicate Paget's disease, a rare form of breast cancer (NCI, 2012b). Dimpling of skin or retraction of the nipple also suggests cancer (MedlinePlus, 2012).

3. **Have you ever experienced any trauma or injury to your breasts?**
   - If so, please describe.

▶ Contact sports, automobile accidents, and physical abuse can cause bruising of the breast and tissue changes (WebMD, 2012).

Questions Related to Behaviors

1. **Do you exercise?**
   - If so, describe your routine.
   - What kind of bra do you wear when you exercise?

▶ Physical activity, in the form of exercise, decreases the risk for breast cancer (NCI, 2012a). Firm support is recommended during exercise to prevent loss of tissue elasticity (Kam, 2011).

2. **Have you ever had a mammogram?**
   - If so, when was your most recent one?

▶ Mammography can detect a cancer before it is detectable by palpation. The United States Preventive Services Task Force (USPSTF, 2013) has made the following recommendations: Biennial screening mammography for women aged 50 to 74 years. Decisions to start regular biennial mammography prior to age 50 years should be an individual decision and consider benefits and harms.

3. **Do you see your healthcare provider regularly for a physical examination?**

▶ Patients from lower socioeconomic brackets may have reduced access to health care (Freedman et al., 2011).
▶ Patients who see their provider regularly may have better outcomes for many diseases due to early detection (ACS, 2014d).

Focused Interview Questions	Rationales and Evidence
4. Have you ever been taught how to perform breast self-examinations (BSE)? • If so, how often do you perform them? • At what time of your menstrual cycle do you perform this exam? • If you no longer have menstrual cycles, what helps you remember to perform this exam? • Describe the procedure you use.	▶ The answer indicates the patient's knowledge level and the importance placed on BSE. Although the nurse may use this opportunity to share information about BSE, waiting for actual demonstration and teaching until after the physical examination is completed may allow for better learning.

Questions Related to Age

The following questions address breast health across the age span. Breast development begins in preadolescence, and changes continue into older adulthood.

Questions Regarding Preadolescents

1. Have you noticed any changes in the size or shape of your breasts? • If so, tell me about these changes.	▶ Growth of the breasts is not necessarily steady or symmetric. This may be frustrating or embarrassing to some girls. The nurse should reassure the patient that her breast development is normal, if appropriate. For most women, the left breast is slightly larger than the right breast (Aldersey-Williams, 2014).
2. How do you feel about your breasts and the way they are changing?	▶ Breast development provides visual confirmation that the pubescent female is becoming a woman. For the developing pubescent female, her breasts are a visible symbol of her feminine identity and an important part of her body image and self-esteem. Girls should be reassured that the rate of growth of breast tissue depends on changing hormone levels and is uniquely individual, as are the eventual size and shape of the breasts. The nurse can reassure males that breast enlargement is generally temporary and in response to hormonal changes (Berman & Snyder, 2012).

Questions for the Pregnant Female

1. What changes in your breasts have you noticed since your last examination?	▶ The breasts continue to change throughout pregnancy. Some expected changes are increased size, sense of fullness or tingling, prominent veins, darkened areolae, and a more erect nipple. A thick, yellowish discharge called colostrum may be expressed from the breasts in the final weeks of pregnancy. The patient should be reassured that all of these signs are normal (Berman & Snyder, 2012).

Questions for the Older Adult

All of the preceding questions apply to the menopausal and postmenopausal patient.	▶ It is important to obtain information from the older patient because the incidence of breast cancer and mortality rates increase with age (Simon, 2012).

Questions Related to the Environment

Environment refers to both the internal and external environments. Questions related to the internal environment include all of the previous questions and those associated with internal or physiologic responses. Questions regarding the external environment include those related to home, work, or social environments.

Focused Interview Questions	Rationales and Evidence
Internal Environment	
1. What medications are you presently taking?	▶ Hormone replacement therapy is associated with an increased risk of cancer. Females taking these drugs need to be monitored very carefully (NCI, 2012a).
2. How do you feel about your breasts?	▶ Answers to this question may reveal a body image disturbance, self-esteem disturbance, dysfunctional grieving (in a female who has had a mastectomy), or ineffective breast-feeding (in a lactating female).
3. Do you have breast implants?	▶ Breast implants do not increase the risk for breast cancer but may create difficulties in visualizing breast tissue on standard mammograms (ACS, 2014b).
4. How old were you when you started to menstruate?	▶ Patients with a history of menarche before age 12 are at greater risk for breast cancer (ASCO, 2013).
5. Do you have children? • How old were you when they were born?	▶ Females who have never had children or who had their first child after the age of 30 are at greater risk for breast cancer (NCI, 2012a).
6. Did you breast-feed your children?	▶ Breast-feeding, especially from 1.5 to 2 years, decreases the risk for breast cancer (ACS, 2014a).
7. Have you gone through menopause? • If so, at what age? • Were there any residual problems?	▶ Females who undergo menopause after the age of 55 are at greater risk for breast cancer. Postmenopausal weight gain may increase the risk of breast cancer (ACS, 2014a). After menopause, decreased estrogen levels may result in decreased firmness of breast tissue (Kam, 2011). The patient should be reassured that this is normal.
8. Have you been treated with hormone therapy during or since menopause?	▶ Combined hormone replacement therapy places patients at increased risk for breast cancer. (ACS, 2014a)
9. Describe your weight from childhood up until now. • Describe your dietary intake.	▶ Obesity is considered a predisposing factor in breast cancer (ACS, 2014a).
External Environment	
1. Have you been exposed to any environmental carcinogens such as benzene or asbestos, or to excessive radiation such as frequent, repeated x-rays?	▶ Such exposures may increase the risk of breast cancer (ACS, 2014a).
2. Have you or your mother taken diethylstilbestrol (DES)?	▶ A history of DES use is linked with increased risk for breast cancer (ACS, 2014a).
3. Do you work at night?	▶ An increased risk for breast cancer has been linked with night shift work. This may be related to disruption in melatonin, a hormone affected by light (ACS, 2014a).

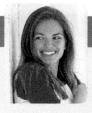

Patient-Centered Interaction

Miranda Cowan, a 22-year-old college student, makes an appointment with her gynecologist for a routine examination. Ms. Cowan indicates that she is concerned because breast cancer seems to run in her family. Following is part of the focused interview taken by the nurse working in the office.

Interview

Nurse: Hello, Ms. Cowan, I see you are here for your routine examination.

Ms. Cowan: Yes, that is correct.

Nurse: Before the physical examination, I need to get some information from you, and I will be asking you questions. You indicated a concern regarding breast cancer in your family. Would you like to begin with your concern?

Ms. Cowan No. I just don't know where to begin. You ask your questions first. I'm sure we will talk about my concerns.

Nurse: How would you describe your breasts?

Ms. Cowan: They are small and firm. My left breast is a little bigger than my right breast.

Nurse: Have your breasts changed in the past several months?

Ms. Cowan: No, I think they are the same. Maybe a little fuller before my period but that's it.

Nurse: Describe your nipples and the skin around them.

Ms. Cowan: They are small, equal in size, and stick out a little. The skin around my nipples is round and pink, almost the same color as my nipple.

Nurse: Have you noticed any changes to your nipples or areolae (the skin around the nipples)?

Ms. Cowan: No, no changes.

Nurse: Do you do breast self-examination?

Ms. Cowan: Yes, every month 5 days after my period. You taught me last year.

Nurse: Tell me about your family and breast cancer.

Ms. Cowan: My grandmother (maternal) and my aunt (paternal) both have been diagnosed and it worries me.

Nurse: What about your mother, your older sister, and your maternal aunt?

Ms. Cowan: No, they're fine. No problems.

Nurse: Your grandmother, do you know how old she was when diagnosed?

Ms. Cowan: No I don't. I guess she was in her late 60s. She was diagnosed 3 or 4 years ago and now she's 73 years old. She had surgery and seems to be doing all right.

Analysis

The nurse sets the tone and sequence of events for Ms. Cowan's visit. Ms. Cowan declines the offer from the nurse to begin with her concerns of familial cancer. The nurse knows it will be beneficial to reduce any anxiety the patient may have regarding her concern. Taking the lead from Ms. Cowan, the nurse proceeds with the focused interview using open-ended statements and introduces the family questions later in the interview.

Patient Education

The following are physiologic, behavioral, and cultural factors that influence breast health across the life span. Several factors reflect trends cited in *Healthy People 2020* documents. The nurse provides advice and education to reduce risks associated with these factors and to promote and maintain breast health.

LIFESPAN CONSIDERATIONS

Risk Factors	Patient Education
• Cyclic breast pain occurs in young females in association with the onset and continuation of the menstrual cycle.	▶ Instruct teenage girls to chart breast pain to determine if it is associated with the menstrual cycle.

LIFESPAN CONSIDERATIONS

Risk Factors	Patient Education

- Cysts are the most common breast lumps in menstruating females.
- Fibroadenomas are benign lumps found in females in the late teens and early 20s.

▶ Tell teenage and young adult females that healthcare screening is required to diagnose fibroadenomas, which are usually surgically removed.

- Fibrocystic breast changes and benign cysts occur in about 30% of females of all ages.

▶ Instruct patients that the discomfort associated with fibrocystic breast changes may be alleviated with reduction in the ingestion of caffeine, chocolate, saturated fats, and salt (WebMD, 2011). While the addition of vitamins E to one's diet is recommended by some to reduce symptoms, there is no research evidence to support the theory that vitamin E relieves breast pain (WebMD, 2011).

- The risk of breast cancer increases with aging, especially after 35 to 40 years of age.

▶ Tell all patients that the recommendations for early detection of breast cancer include biennial screening mammography for women between the ages of 50 and 74 years. Beginning biennial mammography before the age of 50 should be an individual decision and include cancer risk and values regarding benefit and harm associated with mammography (USPSTF, 2013). Additionally, the American Cancer Society (2014c) recommends completion of a clinical breast examination by a healthcare provider every 3 years for women from age 20 to 39 years. Beginning at 40 years of age, clinical breast exams should be performed annually. Further, the American Cancer Society (2014c) states that women should know how their breasts normally feel and report changes to their healthcare provider. BSE is an option for women to consider beginning at the age of 20 (ACS, 2013c). See Box 18.1 for instructions for BSE.

Box 18.1 Teaching Breast Self-Examination (BSE)

1. Teach the patient to observe her breasts in front of a mirror and in good lighting. Tell her to observe her breasts in four positions:
   - With her arms relaxed and at her sides
   - With her arms lifted over her head
   - With her hands pressed against her hips
   - With her hands pressed together at the waist, leaning forward

   Instruct her to look at each breast individually, and then to compare them. She should observe for any visible abnormalities, such as lumps, dimpling, deviation, recent nipple retraction, irregular shape, edema, discharge, or asymmetry.

2. Teach the patient to palpate both breasts while standing or sitting, with one hand behind her head (see Figure 18.9A ■). Tell her that many women palpate their breasts in the shower because water and soap make the skin slippery and easier to palpate. Show the patient how to use the pads of her fingers to palpate all areas of her breast, using the vertical strip or concentric circles techniques (see Figure 18.9B ■). Tell her to press the breast tissue with light pressure to feel the tissue closest to the skin, followed by medium pressure to feel somewhat deeper, and then with firm pressure to feel the tissue closest to the chest and ribs.

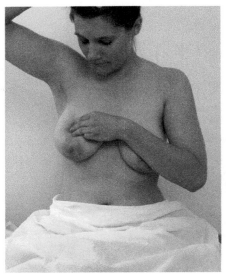

Figure 18.9A Breast self-examination. A. The female palpates her breasts while standing or sitting upright.

Box 18.1 Teaching Breast Self-Examination (BSE) (continued)

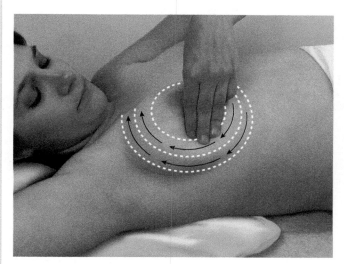

Figure 18.9B Breast self-examination. B. The concentric circles approach.

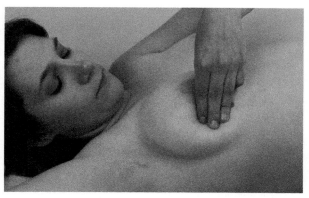

Figure 18.9C Breast self-examination. C. The female patient palpates her breasts while lying down.

3. Instruct the patient to palpate her breasts again while lying down, as described in step 2. Suggest that she place a folded towel under the shoulder and back on the side to be palpated. The arm on the examining side should be over her head, with the hand under the head (see Figure 18.9C ■). Recent studies indicate that increasing the levels of pressure for palpation in a lying-down position increases the sensitivity of BSE.

4. Teach the patient to palpate the areolae and nipples next. Show her how to palpate the nipple to check for discharge (see Figure 18.9D ■).

5. Remind the patient to use a calendar to keep a record of when she performs BSE. Teach her to perform BSE at the same time each month, usually 5 days after the onset of menses, when there is less hormonal influence on tissues.

6. Remind patients who are postmenopausal to continue monthly BSE. They should perform the exam at the same time each month.

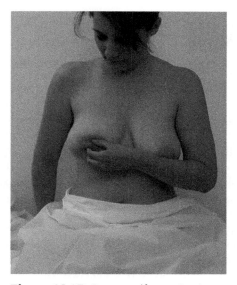

Figure 18.9D Breast self-examination. D. The woman palpates her nipples.

CULTURAL CONSIDERATIONS

Risk Factors

- Caucasian females have a higher incidence of breast cancer after age 40 than do females in other racial and ethnic groups.
- Despite their lower risk for developing breast cancer, breast cancer is the leading cause of cancer death in Hispanic females.

- Male breast cancer is rare but does occur in men with a familial history of female breast cancer in a primary relative and in men with radiation exposure, estrogen administration, and cirrhosis.

- Some Hispanic females and females from many immigrant cultures are brought up believing that looking at or touching themselves is prohibited.

Patient Education

▶ Inform all patients about the recommendations for early detection of breast cancer.

▶ Advise males with risk factors to have breast examination included as part of routine health examinations.

▶ Advise and encourage female patients who have uneasiness with touching their breasts to seek care regularly for breast examination.

ENVIRONMENTAL CONSIDERATIONS

Risk Factors

- There is a genetic predisposition to breast cancer in approximately 10% of females in Western countries, and there is a higher incidence of breast cancer in Western countries, especially in North America.

- The risk of breast cancer is increased in females with a familial history, in those who have not had children, in females who use combined estrogen and progesterone or hormone replacement therapy, in females who use alcohol, and in obese females and those with a high-fat diet.

- Low income contributes to a lack of screening for breast disease.

Patient Education

▶ Inform all patients about the recommendations for early detection of breast cancer.

▶ Refer patients to the American Cancer Society (ACS) or provide the link to the ACS breast cancer education Web site.

▶ Inform uninsured female patients of low-cost breast cancer screening available through the National Breast and Cervical Cancer Early Detection Program (NBCCEDP).

Physical Assessment

Assessment Techniques and Findings

Physical assessment of the breasts and axillae requires the use of inspection and palpation. During each of the procedures, the nurse is gathering data related to the breasts and axillae. Inspection includes looking at skin color, structures of the breast, and the appearance of the axillae. Knowledge of norms or expected findings is essential in determining the meaning of the data.

Adult breasts are generally symmetric, although one breast is typically slightly larger than the other. The areolae should be round or oval and nearly equal in size. The nipples are the same color as the areolae. The nipples are in the center of the breast, point outward and upward, and are free of discharge, ulcerations, and crust. The breasts should move away from the chest wall with ease and symmetrically. The texture of the skin is smooth and the breast tissue is slightly granular. The axillae are clean and hair is present or removed. The skin is moist. Lymph nodes are nonpalpable.

Physical assessment of the breasts and axillae follows an organized pattern. It begins with a patient survey followed by inspection of the breasts while the patient assumes a variety of positions. Palpation includes the entire surface of each breast, including the tail of Spence, and the lymph nodes of the axillae.

EQUIPMENT

- examination gown and drape
- clean, nonsterile examination gloves
- small pillow or rolled towel
- metric ruler

HELPFUL HINTS

- To relieve patient anxiety, provide an environment that is warm, comfortable, and private.
- Ask the patient if they prefer a nurse who is the same gender; some cultures only allow female healthcare workers to assess females, and some women may be uncomfortable having a male complete a breast examination.
- Provide specific instructions to the patient; state whether the patient must sit, stand, or lie down during a procedure.
- Exposure of the breasts is uncomfortable for many females. Use draping techniques to maintain the patient's dignity.
- Explore cultural and language barriers at the onset of the interaction.
- In many Hispanic cultures, touching of the breasts is considered inappropriate. Explain the reasons for the examination and provide education about BSE.
- Nonsterile examination gloves may be required to prevent infection when patients have lesions or drainage in and around the breasts.
- Use Standard Precautions.

Techniques and Normal Findings	Abnormal Findings Special Considerations

Inspection of the Breast

1. **Instruct the patient.**
   - Explain to the patient that you will be assessing her breasts in a variety of ways. First, you will have the patient sit and then assume several positions that move the breasts away from the chest wall so that differences in size, shape, symmetry, contour, and color can be detected. Inform the patient that she will then lie down and you will assess each breast by palpating the breast tissue and nipple. Also be sure to assess her axillae. Explain the purpose of each assessment in terms the patient will understand. Tell the patient that none of the assessments should be painful; however, she must inform you of any tenderness or discomfort as the examination proceeds.

2. **Position the patient.**
   - The patient should sit comfortably and erect, with the gown at the waist so both breasts are exposed (see Figure 18.10 ■).

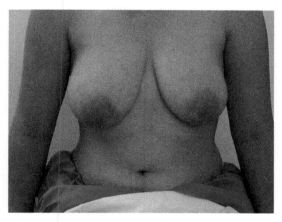

Figure 18.10 The patient is seated at the beginning of the breast examination.

3. **Inspect and compare size and symmetry of the breasts.**
   - One breast may normally be slightly larger than the other.

▶ Obvious masses, flattening of the breast in one area, dimpling, or a recent increase in the size of one breast may indicate abnormal growth or inflammation.

4. **Inspect for skin color.**
   - Color should be consistent with the rest of the body. Observe for thickening, tautness, redness, rash, or ulceration.

▶ Inflamed skin is red and warm. Edema from blocked lymphatic drainage in advanced cancer causes an "orange peel" appearance called **peau d'orange** (see Figure 18.11 ■).

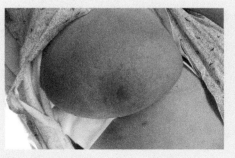

Figure 18.11 Peau d'orange sign.
Source: B. Slaven/Custom Medical Stock Photo.

Techniques and Normal Findings	Abnormal Findings Special Considerations

5. Inspect for venous patterns.

- Venous patterns are the same bilaterally. Venous patterns may be more predominant in pregnancy or obesity.

▶ Pronounced unilateral venous patterns may indicate increased blood flow to a malignancy.

6. Inspect for moles or other markings.

- Moles that are unchanged, nontender, and long-standing are of no concern. Striae that are present in pregnancy or recent weight loss or gain may appear purple in color. Striae become silvery white over time.

▶ Moles that have changed or appear suddenly require further evaluation. A mole along the milk line may be a supernumerary nipple (see Figure 18.5).

7. Inspect the areolae.

- The areolae are normally round or oval and almost equal in size. Areolae are pink in light-skinned people and brown in dark-skinned people. The areolae darken in pregnancy.

▶ Peau d'orange associated with cancer may be first seen on the areolae.
   Redness and fissures may develop with breast-feeding.

8. Inspect the nipples.

- Nipples are normally the same color as the areolae and are equal in size and shape. Nipples are generally everted but may be flat or inverted. Nipples should point in the same direction outward and slightly upward. Nipples should be free of cracks, crust, erosions, ulcerations, pigment changes, or discharge.

▶ Recent retraction or inversion of a nipple or change in the direction of the nipple is suggestive of malignancy. Discharge requires cytologic examination. A red, scaly, eczema-like area over the nipple could indicate Paget's disease, a rare type of breast cancer. The area may exude fluid, scale, or crust (see Figure 18.12 ■).

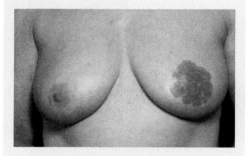

Figure 18.12 Paget's disease of the nipple.
Source: Wellcome Image Library/Custom Medical Stock Photo.

9. Observe the breasts for shape, surface characteristics, and bilateral pull of suspensory ligaments.

- Ask the patient to assume the following positions while you continue to inspect the breasts.

Techniques and Normal Findings	Abnormal Findings Special Considerations

10. **Inspect with the patient's arms over the head (see Figure 18.13 ■).**

▶ Dimpling of the skin over a mass is usually a visible sign of breast cancer. Dimpling is accentuated in this position. Variations in contour and symmetry may also indicate breast cancer (Mayo Clinic, 2013b).

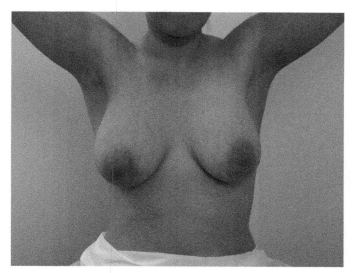

Figure 18.13 Inspection of the breasts with the patient's arms above her head.

11. **Inspect with the patient's hands pressed against her waist (see Figure 18.14 ■).**

▶ Tightening of the pectoral muscles may help to accentuate dimpling.

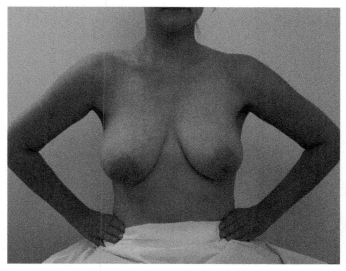

Figure 18.14 Inspection of the breasts with the patient's hands pressed against her waist.

Techniques and Normal Findings	Abnormal Findings Special Considerations

12. **Inspect with the patient's hands pressed together at the level of the waist (see Figure 18.15 ■).**

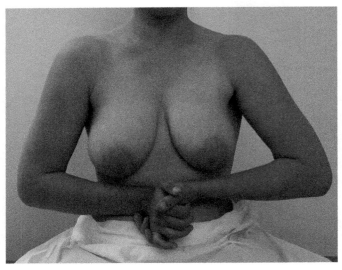

Figure 18.15 Inspection of the breasts with the patient's hands pressed together at the level of her waist.

13. **Inspect with the patient leaning forward from the waist (see Figure 18.16 ■).**
   - The breasts normally fall freely and evenly from the chest.

▶ Breast cancer should be suspected if the breasts do not fall freely from the chest.

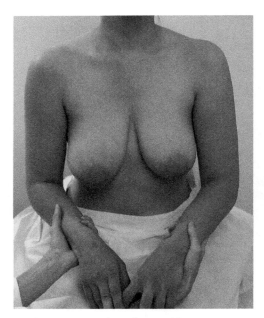

Figure 18.16 Assisting the patient to lean forward for inspection.

Techniques and Normal Findings	**Abnormal Findings** **Special Considerations**

Palpation of the Breast

1. Position the patient.

- Ask the patient to lie down. Cover the breast that is not being examined. Place a small pillow or rolled towel under the shoulder of the side to be palpated and position the patient's arm over her head. This maneuver flattens the breast tissue over the chest wall.

2. Instruct the patient.

- Explain that you will be touching the entire breast and nipple. Tell the patient to inform you of any discomfort or tenderness.

3. Palpate skin texture.

- Skin texture should be smooth with uninterrupted contour.

▶ Thickening of the skin suggests an underlying carcinoma (Mayo Clinic, 2013b).

4. Palpate the breast.

- Use the finger pads of the first three fingers in dime-sized circular motions to press the breast tissue against the chest wall (see Figure 18.17 ■). Be sure to palpate the entire breast.

▶ The incidence of breast cancers is highest in the upper outer quadrant, including the axillary tail of Spence. Masses in the tail must be distinguished from enlarged lymph nodes.

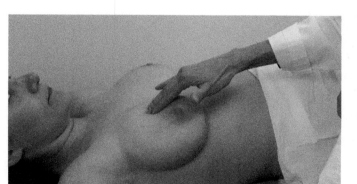

Figure 18.17 Palpating the breast.

The vertical strip pattern is the recommended method for breast palpation. (see Figure 18.18A ■).

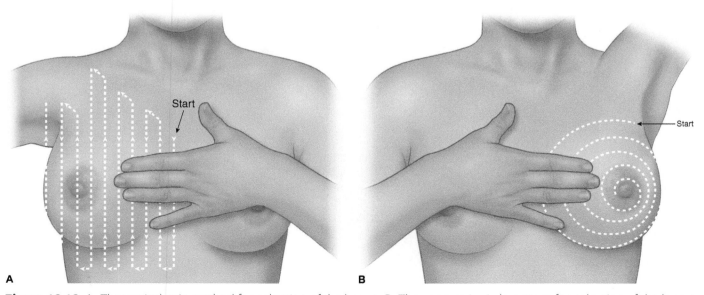

Start

Start

A

B

Figure 18.18 A. The vertical strip method for palpation of the breast. B. The concentric circle pattern for palpation of the breast.

- The following landmarks are used to be sure the entire breast is assessed: down the midaxillary line, across the inframammary ridge at the fifth or sixth rib, up at the lateral edge of the sternum, across the clavicle, and back to the midaxillary.
- As each area is examined, three levels of pressure should be applied in sequence. These are light for subcutaneous tissue, medium at the midlevel tissues, and deep to the chest wall. Pressure is adapted according to the size, shape, and consistency of the breast tissue. Additionally pressure will vary in relation to breast size and the presence of breast implants. Implants are placed behind breast tissue; therefore, the steps for breast examination are the same as for palpation of breasts in women without implants.

   Additional patterns include the concentric circles or back and forth techniques (see Figure 18.18B ■).
- In female patients with pendulous breasts, palpate with one hand under the breast to support it and the other hand pushing against breast tissue in a downward motion (see Figure 18.19 ■).

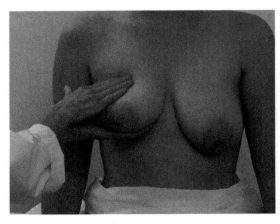

Figure 18.19 Palpating a pendulous breast.

In obese females with large breasts, palpation with two hands should be performed with the patient in the sitting and supine positions.

5. **Palpate the nipple and areolae.**
   - The area beneath and at the nipple should be palpated, not squeezed, to observe for drainage (see Figure 18.20 ■). Squeezing may result in discharge and discomfort. Confirm that the nipple is free of discharge, that it is nontender, and that the areola is free of masses.

▶ Lactation not associated with childbearing is called **galactorrhea**. It occurs most commonly with endocrine disorders or medications, including some antidepressants and antihypertensives (Wilson, Shannon, & Shields, 2013).

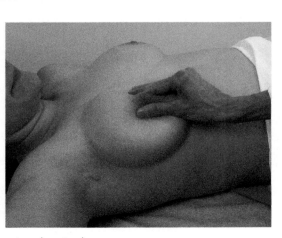

Figure 18.20 Palpating the nipple.

Techniques and Normal Findings	Abnormal Findings Special Considerations

- Repeat steps 1 through 5 on the other breast.

▶ Unilateral discharge from the nipple is suggestive of benign breast disease, an intraductal papilloma, or cancer. Spontaneous discharge from the nipple warrants further evaluation.

Examination of the Axillae

1. **Instruct the patient.**
   - Explain that you will be examining the axillae by looking and palpating. Tell the patient that she will sit for this examination and you will support the arm while palpating with the other hand. Explain that relaxation will make the examination more comfortable. Tell the patient to inform you of any discomfort.

2. **Position the patient.**
   - Ask the patient or assist the patient to assume a sitting position. Flex the arm at the elbow and support it on your arm. Note the presence of axillary hair. Confirm that the axilla is free of redness, rashes, lumps, or lesions. With the palmar surface of your fingers, reach deep into the axilla (see Figure 18.21 ■). Gently palpate the anterior border of the axilla (anterior or subpectoral nodes), the central aspect along the rib cage (central nodes), the posterior border (subscapular/posterior nodes), and along the inner aspect of the upper arm (lateral nodes).

▶ Infections of the breast, arm, and hand cause enlargement and tenderness of the axillary lymph nodes. Hard, fixed nodes are suggestive of cancer or lymphoma. Patients who have had a wide local excision (removal of tumor and narrow margin of normal tissue) or mastectomy (removal of tumor and extensive areas of surrounding tissue) need to be examined carefully. The remaining tissue on the chest wall should be palpated as it would be for nonsurgical patients.

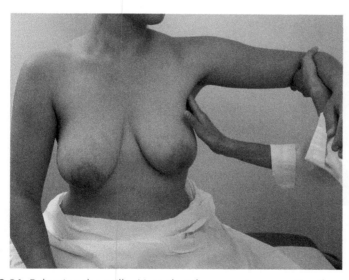

Figure 18.21 Palpating the axilla. Note that the nurse is supporting the woman's arm with her own nondominant arm.

Inspection of the Male Breast

1. **Instruct the patient.**
   - Explain all aspects of the procedure and the purpose for each part of the examination.

2. **Position the patient.**
   - The patient is in the sitting position with the gown at the waist.

3. **Inspect the male breasts.**
   - Observe that breasts are flat and free of lumps or lesions.

Techniques and Normal Findings	Abnormal Findings Special Considerations

Palpation of the Male Breast and Axillae

1. **Position the patient.**
   - Place the patient in a supine position.

2. **Instruct the patient.**
   - Explain that you will be using the pads of your fingers to gently palpate the breast area. Instruct the patient to report any discomfort.

3. **Palpate the male breasts.**
   - Using the finger pads of the first three fingers, gently palpate the breast tissue, using concentric circles until you reach the nipple (see Figure 18.22 ■). The male breast feels like a thin disk of tissue under a flat nipple and areola.

▶ Gynecomastia (breast enlargement in males) is a temporary condition seen in infants, at puberty, and in older males. In older males it may accompany hormonal treatment for prostate cancer. Breast cancer in the male is usually identified as a hard nodule fixed to the nipple and underlying tissue. Nipple discharge may be present. Pseudogynecomastia, an increase in subcutaneous fat, may occur in obese males. On palpation breast tissue is more firm than fat. A mammogram may be required to distinguish enlarged or changed breast tissue from increased subcutaneous fat.

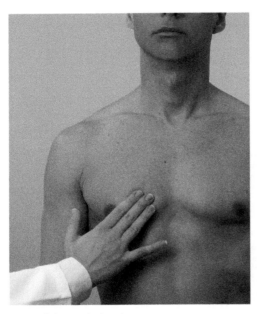

Figure 18.22 Palpation of the male breast.

4. **Palpate the nipple.**
   - Compress the nipple between your thumb and forefinger.
   - The nipple should be free of discharge.

5. **Repeat on the other breast.**

6. **Palpate the axillae.**
   - Palpate axillary nodes in the male as you would for the female.

Abnormal Findings

Some of the problems identified during the physical assessment are entirely within the realm of nursing and are addressed with appropriate nursing interventions. Some problems, however, require collaborative management.

Abnormalities of the Female Breast

Benign breast disease, fibroadenoma, intraductal papilloma, mammary duct ectasia, and breast cancer are the most common breast conditions that will challenge the nurse and the rest of the healthcare team. These common abnormalities are discussed in the following sections.

BENIGN BREAST DISEASE (FIBROCYSTIC BREAST DISEASE)

One of the most common benign breast problems, this disorder is caused by *fibrosis,* a thickening of the normal breast tissue; it is not usually clinically significant, and there is no direct link between fibrocystic tissue changes and the incidence of cancer (see Figure 18.23 ■). In some cases, it may result in ductal hyperplasia and dysplasia, which may eventually develop into noninvasive intraductal, lobular, or intraepithelial carcinoma. This can be a potential focus for invasive carcinoma. The presence of nodular breast tissue makes the early detection of malignant nodules more challenging. The physician monitors fibrocystic breast disease through periodic mammography and determines if aspiration or biopsy is necessary. This disease most often occurs among females in their 20s. After menopause, symptoms usually resolve due to lack of estrogen. Treatment may include pharmacologic agents such as hormones, diuretics, and mild analgesics. Some studies suggest that limiting caffeine may help relieve symptoms, but the evidence is inconclusive. The nurse may also suggest decreasing salt intake. Wearing a supportive bra decreases discomfort. The nurse should reinforce the need for regular BSE as well as regular mammography and physical examination.

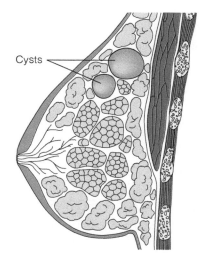

Figure 18.23 Fibrocystic breast disease.

Subjective findings

- Breast pain or tenderness that begins immediately before onset of menses.
- Resolution of pain at the end of menses.

Objective findings:

- Soft breast lumps that are well demarcated and freely movable to palpation; lumps are almost always bilateral.
- Nipple discharge (clear, straw colored, milky, or green).
- Cysts also may be present (usually located in the upper outer quadrant).

FIBROADENOMA

A benign tumor of the glandular tissue of the breast, fibroadenoma is most common in adolescent girls and women under age 30 years (Mayo Clinic, 2011) (see Figure 18.24 ■). Its development in adolescents appears to be linked to breast hypertrophy, which may occur during the growth spurt of puberty. The usual treatment is careful observation over time. Biopsy or excision of the lump is indicated if the findings are inconclusive. No relationship has been established between fibroadenomas and malignant neoplasms.

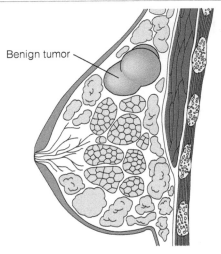

Figure 18.24 Fibroadenoma.

Subjective findings:

- None; aside from the breast mass, the individual usually is asymptomatic.
- Often discovered through BSE or during clinical breast examination.

Objective findings:

- Presence of well-defined, round, firm tumors, about 1 to 5 cm (0.39 to 1.95 in.) in diameter, that can be moved freely within the breast tissue.
- Usually involves a single tumor near the nipple or in the upper outer quadrant of the breast.

INTRADUCTAL PAPILLOMA

Intraductal papillomas are tiny growths of epithelial cells that project into the lumen of the lactiferous ducts (see Figure 18.25 ■). They are the primary cause of nipple discharge in females who are not pregnant or lactating and are more commonly found in menopausal females but may occur at any age. Treatment usually involves surgical removal (excision) and biopsy of the affected ducts.

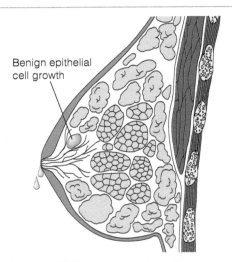

Figure 18.25 Intraductal papilloma.

Subjective findings:

- Breast enlargement.
- Breast pain (MedlinePlus, 2013).

Objective findings:

- One or more lumps in the breast.
- Nipple discharge. Because the growths are fragile, even minimal trauma causes leakage of blood or serum into the involved duct and subsequent discharge (MedlinePlus, 2013).

MAMMARY DUCT ECTASIA

Mammary duct ectasia is an inflammation of the lactiferous ducts behind the nipple. As cellular debris and fluid collect in the involved ducts, they become enlarged and can form a palpable, painful mass (see Figure 18.26 ■). Because there may be some nipple retraction, a careful assessment is required to distinguish the condition from breast cancer. Although the disorder is painful, it is not associated with cancer and usually resolves spontaneously.

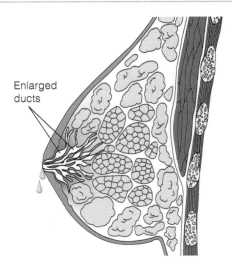

Figure 18.26 Mammary duct ectasia.

Subjective findings:

- Thick, sticky nipple discharge.
- Nipple retraction (Mayo Clinic, 2012a).

Objective findings:

- Often asymptomatic.
- Breast tenderness or inflammation of the clogged duct (periductal mastitis) may be present (Mayo Clinic, 2012a).

CARCINOMA (CANCER)

Among women in the United States, after skin cancer, carcinoma of the breast, or breast cancer, is the most commonly diagnosed form of cancer (Mayo Clinic, 2013a). While breast cancer can occur in both men and women, it is much more common in women. The screening examination and studies for breast cancer are physical examination and mammography. A positive diagnosis of cancer is made by histologic examination following an open or closed (needle) biopsy. The tumor is then staged to determine its characteristics, nodal involvement, and the presence or absence of distant metastasis (see Figure 18.27 ■). The outcome of this staging determines which protocol is used for treatment. Treatment may consist of surgery, radiation therapy, chemotherapy, or a combination of these modalities.

Subjective findings:

- Perceived change in breast size.
- Perceived change in breast shape. Irregular shape of one breast as compared to the other, such as a flattening of one quadrant.
- Breast pain or tenderness.
- Nipple pain or tenderness.
- Nipple itching (Mayo Clinic, 2013b).

Objective findings:

- Breast lump or thickening of local area of breast tissue.
- Dimpling of the skin over the tumor caused by a retraction or pulling inward of breast tissue. This results primarily from tissue fibrosis. Retraction is also caused by fat necrosis and mammary duct ectasia.
- Deviation of the breast or nipple from its normal alignment. Deviation is also caused by retraction. The nipple typically deviates toward the underlying cancer.
- Nipple retraction. The nipple flattens or even turns inward. Retraction is also caused by tissue fibrosis.
- Edema, which may result in a peau d'orange appearance, especially near the nipple. Edema is caused by blockage of the lymphatic ducts that normally drain the breast.
- Discharge, which may be bloody or clear.

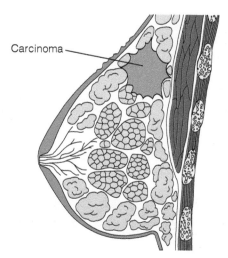

Figure 18.27 Breast cancer.

Abnormalities of the Male Breast

Male breast tissue is similar to that of the female. Therefore, changes in relation to hormone secretion and disease occur. The following sections describe abnormalities in the male breast.

GYNECOMASTIA

This enlargement of the male breast tissue can occur at birth in response to maternal hormones. Additionally, at the onset of puberty more than 30% of males have enlargement of one or both breasts in response to hormonal changes, which can be a cause of embarrassment or shame. Gynecomastia may also occur in males over 50 due to pituitary or testicular tumors and in males taking estrogenic medication for prostate cancer. It may occur in cirrhosis of the liver and with adrenal and thyroid diseases (see Figure 18.28 ■).

Subjective findings:

- Perceived swelling or increase in size of breast tissue.
- Pain or tenderness in breast tissue (Mayo Clinic, 2014).

Objective findings:

- Swelling of breast tissue.
- If gynecomastia occurs secondary to another condition, such as hyperthyroidism, manifestations also will include those related to the primary condition (Mayo Clinic, 2014).

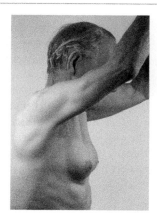

Figure 18.28 Gynecomastia.
Source: John Radcliffe/Science Source.

CARCINOMA (CANCER)

Male breast cancer is rare. Less than 1% of all breast cancer occurs in men. Predisposing factors include radiation exposure, cirrhosis, and estrogen medications. Increased rates have been seen in males with a familial history of breast cancer in primary female relatives (see Figure 18.29 ■). Men who are diagnosed with early-stage breast cancer typically have a high likelihood of being cured. However, many men delay seeking treatment for unusual signs or symptoms, such as a breast lump. As a result, for many men, breast cancer is not diagnosed until the disease is more advanced (Mayo Clinic, 2012b).

Subjective findings:

- Perceived change in breast size.
- Perceived change in breast shape.
- Pain or tenderness (Mayo Clinic, 2013b).

Objective findings:

- Breast lump or thickening of local area of breast tissue.
- Bloody or clear nipple discharge.
- Swelling of breast tissue.
- Dimpling of the breast skin.
- Nipple inversion.
- Scaling, peeling, or flaking of the nipple or breast skin.
- Redness or pitting of the breast skin, like the skin of an orange (Mayo Clinic, 2013b).

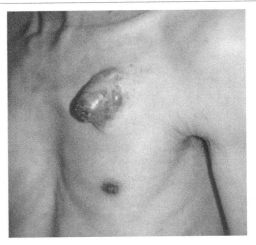

Figure 18.29 Carcinoma of the breast.
Source: JDP/Custom Medical Stock Photo.

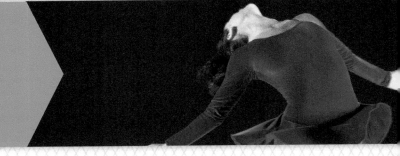

Application Through Critical Thinking

▶ Case Study

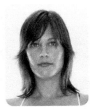

Carol Jenkins is a 29-year-old female who has come to the clinic today for complaints of increasing breast tenderness. Carol is an avid runner and has been training for a marathon but is having significant tenderness in her breasts during running. When you start to question Carol, she tells you she has had breast tenderness associated with her periods for most of her adult life. Upon further questioning you discover the tenderness has increased over the past several months and is not just associated with running. Her breasts seem swollen and heavy, and what used to hurt in the outer portion of the breast has changed to discomfort all over.

The physical assessment revealed round, tender, mobile masses with smooth borders in all quadrants. The nipples are everted, round, and free of lesions. The breasts are symmetric in shape and contour.

▶ Complete Documentation

The following is sample documentation for Carol Jenkins.

SUBJECTIVE DATA: Breast tenderness "with periods" for most of her adult life. Tenderness increasing over past several months. Breasts seem "swollen and heavy." Discomfort in outer breast now "discomfort all over."

OBJECTIVE DATA: Round, mobile masses with smooth borders in all quadrants bilaterally. Nipples everted, round, free of lesions. Breasts symmetric in shape and contour.

▶ Critical Thinking Questions

1. What is most likely the cause of the patient's symptoms?
2. Identify several differential diagnoses.
3. What information is required to validate the diagnoses?
4. What recommendations should the nurse make for this patient?
5. What do you think Carol's greatest concern was when she came to the clinic?

▶ Prepare Teaching Plan

LEARNING NEED: The data from the case study reveal that Carol Jenkins is concerned about her breast discomfort. Her symptoms indicate benign (fibrocystic) breast disease. Education about this disorder and methods to monitor breast health will be provided to this patient.

The case study provides data that are representative of concerns about breast disease, especially cancer, of many individuals. Therefore, the following teaching plan is based on the need to provide information to members of any community about measures to detect breast cancer.

GOAL: The participants in this learning program will have increased awareness of recommendations for screening for breast cancer.

OBJECTIVES: At the completion of this learning session, the participants will be able to:

1. Identify the recommended schedule for breast cancer screening.
2. Describe methods for breast cancer screening.

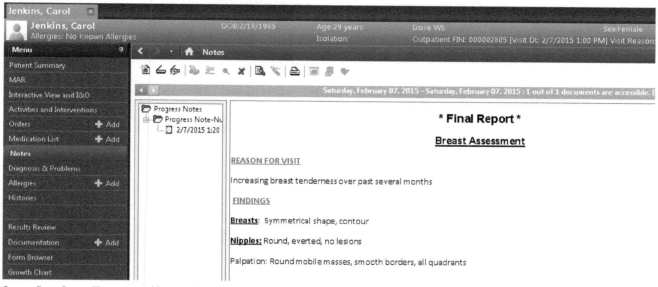

Source: From Cerner Electronic Health Record. Copyright © by Cerner Corporation. Used by permission of Cerner Corporation.

APPLICATION OF OBJECTIVE 1: Identify the recommended schedule for breast cancer screening

Content	Teaching Strategy	Evaluation
• Mammography biennial screening between the ages of 50 and 74 years.	• Lecture	• Written examination.
• Beginning biennial mammography before the age of 50 should be an individual decision and include cancer risk and values regarding benefit and harm associated with mammography (USPSTF, 2013).	• Discussion • Audiovisual materials • Printed materials Lecture is appropriate when disseminating information to large groups.	May use short answer, fill-in, or multiple-choice items, or a combination of items. If these are short and easy to evaluate, the learner receives immediate feedback.
• Annual breast examination by a healthcare provider every 3 years for women from age 20 to 39 years and annually thereafter (American Cancer Society [ACS], 2014a).	Discussion allows participants to bring up concerns and to raise questions. Audiovisual materials such as illustrations of the breast and techniques reinforce verbal presentation.	
• Breast self-examination is an option for women to consider beginning at the age of 20 (ACS, 2014c).	Printed material, especially to be taken away with learners, allows review, reinforcement, and reading at the learner's pace.	

References

Aldersey-Williams, H. (2014). *Anatomies: A cultural history of the human body.* New York, NY: W. W. Norton & Company.

American Cancer Society (ACS). (2014a). *Breast cancer: What are the key statistics about breast cancer?* Retrieved from http://www.cancer.org/cancer/breastcancer/detailedguide/breast-cancer-key-statistics

American Cancer Society (ACS). (2014b). *Breast cancer: What are the risk factors for breast cancer?* Retrieved from http://www.cancer.org/cancer/breastcancer/detailedguide/breast-cancer-risk-factors

American Cancer Society. (2014c). *Breast cancer early detection: American Cancer Society recommendations for early breast cancer detection in women without breast symptoms.* Retrieved from http://www.cancer.org/cancer/breastcancer/moreinformation/breastcancerearlydetection/breast-cancer-early-detection-acs-recs

American Cancer Society. (2014d). *Breast cancer early detection: The importance of finding breast cancer early.* Retrieved from http://www.cancer.org/acs/groups/cid/documents/webcontent/003165-pdf.pdf

American Society of Clinical Oncology (ASCO). (2013). *Breast cancer: Risk factors.* Retrieved from http://www.cancer.net/cancer-types/breast-cancer/risk-factors

Berman, A., & Snyder, S. J. (2012). *Kozier and Erb's fundamentals of nursing: Concepts, process, and practice* (9th ed.). Upper Saddle River, NJ: Prentice Hall.

Bikley, L. S. (2008). *Bates' guide to physical examination and history taking* (10th ed.). Philadelphia: Lippincott.

Bitzer, J., & Simon, J. A. (2011). Current issues and available options in combined hormonal contraception. *Contraception, 84*(4), 342–356.

Centers for Disease Control and Prevention. (2012). Cancer screening – United States, 2010. *Morbidity and Mortality Weekly Report, 61*(03), 41–45.

Freedman, R. A., Virgo, K. S., He, Y., Pavluck, A. L., Winer, E. P., Ward, E. M., & Keating, N. L. (2011). The association of race/ethnicity, insurance status, and socioeconomic factors with breast cancer care. *Cancer, 117*(1), 180–189.

Johns Hopkins Medicine. (n.d.). *Mastalgia (breast pain).* Retrieved from http://www.hopkinsmedicine.org/healthlibrary/conditions/breast_health/mastalgia_breast_pain_85,P00154/

Kam, K. (2011). *A lifetime of healthy breasts: A guide to keeping your breasts healthy now and in the years to come.* Retrieved from http://www.webmd.com/women/guide/a-lifetime-of-healthy-breasts

Mayo Clinic. (2011). *Fibroadenoma: Definition.* Retrieved from http://www.mayoclinic.org/diseases-conditions/fibroadenoma/basics/definition/con-20032223

Mayo Clinic. (2012a). *Mammary duct ectasia:Definition.* Retrieved from http://www.mayoclinic.org/diseases-conditions/mammary-duct-ectasia/basics/definition/con-20025073

Mayo Clinic. (2012b). *Male breast cancer: Definition.* Retrieved from http://www.mayoclinic.org/diseases-conditions/male-breast-cancer/basics/definition/con-20025972

Mayo Clinic. (2013a). *Breast cancer: Definition.* Retrieved from http://www.mayoclinic.org/diseases-conditions/breast-cancer/basics/definition/con-20029275

Mayo Clinic. (2013b). *Breast cancer: Symptoms.* Retrieved from http://www.mayoclinic.org/diseases-conditions/breast-cancer/basics/symptoms/con-20029275

Mayo Clinic. (2013c). *Breast pain.* Retrieved from http://www.mayoclinic.org/diseases-conditions/breast-pain/basics/definition/con-20025541

Mayo Clinic. (2014). *Gynecomastia (enlarged breasts in men): Symptoms.* Retrieved from http://www.mayoclinic.org/diseases-conditions/gynecomastia/basics/symptoms/con-20028710

MedlinePlus. (2012). *Breast skin and nipple changes.* Retrieved from http://www.nlm.nih.gov/medlineplus/ency/patientinstructions/000622.htm

MedlinePlus. (2013). *Intraductal papilloma.* Retrieved from http://www.nlm.nih.gov/medlineplus/ency/article/001238.htm

National Cancer Institute (NCI). (2012a). *National Cancer Institute fact sheet: Breast cancer risk in American women.* Retrieved from http://www.cancer.gov/cancertopics/factsheet/detection/probability-breast-cancer

National Cancer Institute (NCI). (2012b). *National Cancer Institute fact sheet: Paget disease of the breast.* Retrieved from http://www.cancer.gov/cancertopics/factsheet/Sites-Types/paget-breast

National Cancer Institute (NCI). (2014). *National Cancer Institute fact sheet: BRCA1 and BRCA2: Cancer risk and genetic testing.* Retrieved from http://www.cancer.gov/cancertopics/factsheet/Risk/BRCA

Salzman, B., Fleegle, S., & Tully, A. S. (2012). Common breast problems. *American Family Physician, 86*(4), 343–349.

Seidel, H. M., Ball, J., Dains, J., & Benedict, W. (2010). *Mosby's guide to physical examination* (7th ed.). St. Louis, MO: Mosby.

Simon, S. (2012). *Report: Breast cancer death rates down 34% since 1990.* Retrieved from http://www.cancer.org/cancer/news/report-breast-cancer-death-rates-down-34-since-1990

Susman, E. J., Houts, R. M., Steinberg, L., Belsky, J., Cauffman, E., DeHart, G., . . . Halpern-Felsher, B. L. (2010). Longitudinal development of secondary sexual characteristics in girls and boys between ages 9 1/2 and 15 1/2 years. *Archives of pediatrics & adolescent medicine, 164*(2), 166–173.

United States Department of Health and Human Services (USDHHS). (2014). *Healthy people 2020.* Retrieved from http://www.healthypeople.gov/2020/default.aspx

United States Preventive Services Task Force (USPSTF). (2013). *Screening for breast cancer.* Retrieved from http://www.uspreventiveservicestaskforce.org/uspstf14/breastcancer/breastcancerfaq.htm

WebMD. (2011). *Fibrocystic breasts: Home treatment.* Retrieved from http://www.webmd.com/women/tc/fibrocystic-breasts-home-treatment

WebMD. (2012). *Breast pain (mastalgia)—Topic overview: What do I need to know about breast pain?* Retrieved from http://www.webmd.com/women/tc/breast-pain-mastalgia-topic-overview

Wilson, B. A., Shannon, M. T., & Shields, K. M. (2013). *Pearson nurse's drug guide.* Upper Saddle River, NJ: Pearson.

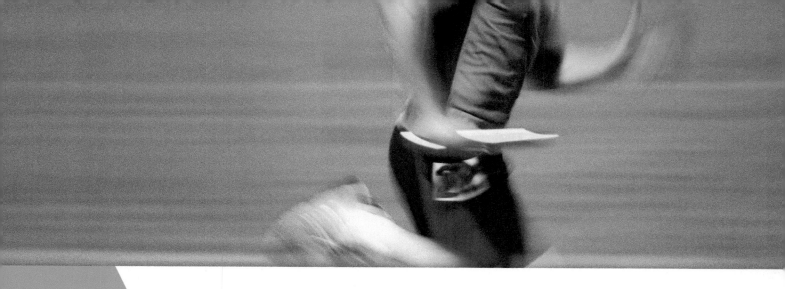

▌ Learning Outcomes

Upon completion of this chapter, you will be able to:

1. Recognize the anatomy and physiology of the cardiovascular system.

2. Recognize landmarks that guide assessment of the cardiovascular system.

3. Develop questions to be used when completing the focused interview.

4. Explain patient preparation for assessment of the cardiovascular system.

5. Outline the techniques required for assessment of the cardiovascular system.

6. Differentiate normal from abnormal findings in the physical assessment of the cardiovascular system.

7. Describe the developmental, psychosocial, cultural, and environmental variations in assessment techniques and findings.

8. Relate *Healthy People 2020* objectives to the cardiovascular system.

9. Apply critical thinking to the physical assessment of the cardiovascular system.

Key Terms

apical impulse, 453
atrioventricular (AV) node, 462
atrioventricular (AV) valves, 454
bruit, 489
bundle branches, 462
bundle of His, 462
cardiac conduction system, 462
cardiac cycle, 464
cardiac output, 466
diastole, 455
electrocardiogram (ECG), 465
endocardium, 453
epicardium, 453
heart, 453
heart murmurs, 457
infective endocarditis, 484
innocent murmurs, 481
left atrium, 454
left ventricle, 454
mediastinal space, 453
myocardium, 453
pericardium, 452
Purkinje fibers, 462

The cardiovascular system circulates blood continuously throughout the body to deliver oxygen and nutrients to the body's organs and tissues and to dispose of their excreted wastes. The health of the cardiovascular system may be promoted throughout the life span by means of self-care habits such as eating a low-fat diet, exercising, and not smoking. Still, the delicate balance of this system is vulnerable to stress, trauma, and a variety of pathologic mechanisms that may impair its ability to function. Inadequate tissue perfusion results in both a diminished supply of nutrients necessary for metabolic functions and a buildup of metabolic wastes.

To perform an accurate cardiovascular assessment, a solid understanding of cardiovascular anatomy and physiology, reviewed in the next section, is necessary. By asking appropriate questions during the focused interview, the nurse uncovers clues to the patient's health status and any cardiovascular problems. Assessment of the patient's psychosocial health, self-care habits, family, culture, and environment is a major part of the focused interview. It is important to keep these findings in mind while conducting the physical assessment and to recognize that the health of the cardiovascular system affects and is affected by the health of all other body systems.

During the physical assessment, the nurse assesses and evaluates the sometimes ambiguous cues of actual and potential cardiac disease. A plan of collaborative or independent nursing care is then developed. Finally, the nurse plays a key role in teaching the healthy patient the facts about preventing cardiovascular disease. For the patient with cardiovascular disease, the nurse provides teaching to promote optimum health according to the patient's individual needs. Nursing interventions that target the promotion of cardiovascular wellness are consistent with the objectives of *Healthy People 2020* (see Table 19.5 on page 468). Goals related to cardiovascular health are focused on prevention, early diagnosis, and reduction of risk factors.

Anatomy and Physiology Review

The cardiovascular system is composed of the heart and the vascular system. The heart includes the cardiac muscle, atria, ventricles, valves, coronary arteries, cardiac veins, electrical conducting structures, and cardiac nerves. The vascular system is composed of the blood vessels of the body: the arteries, arterioles, veins, venules, and capillaries. In this chapter, only the coronary blood vessels are considered in detail. The peripheral vascular system is discussed in chapter 20. ∞ The major functions of the cardiovascular system are transporting nutrients and oxygen to the body, removing wastes and carbon dioxide, and maintaining adequate perfusion of organs and tissues.

Pericardium

The **pericardium** is a thin sac composed of a fibroserous material that surrounds the heart (see Figure 19.1 ■). Its tougher outer layer, called the *fibrous pericardium*, protects the heart and anchors it to

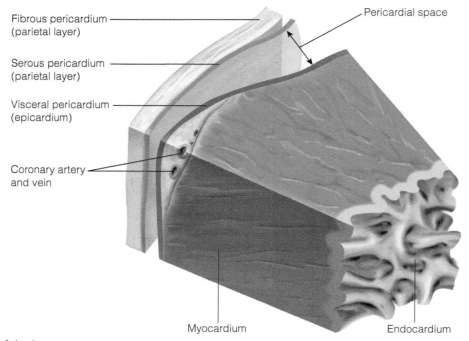

Fibrous pericardium (parietal layer)

Serous pericardium (parietal layer)

Visceral pericardium (epicardium)

Coronary artery and vein

Pericardial space

Myocardium

Endocardium

Figure 19.1 Layers of the heart.

the adjacent structures such as the diaphragm and great vessels. The inner layer is called the *serous pericardium*. The pericardium is also composed of two layers: parietal and visceral. The parietal layer is the outer layer. The **visceral layer of pericardium** is the inner layer, which lines the surface of the heart. Fluid between the fibrous and serous pericardium lubricates the layers and allows for a gliding motion between them with each heartbeat.

Heart

The **heart** is an intricately designed pump composed of a meticulous network of synchronized structures. It lies behind the sternum and typically extends from the second rib to the fifth intercostal space (see Figure 19.2 ■). The heart sits obliquely within the thoracic cavity between the lungs and above the diaphragm in an area called the **mediastinal space.** Ventrally, the right side of the heart is more forward than the left. The heartbeat is most easily palpated over the apex; thus, this point is referred to as the **apical impulse** or point of maximum impulse (PMI).

The heart is approximately 12.8 cm (5 in.) long, 9 cm (3.5 in.) across, and 6.4 cm (2.5 in.) thick. It is slightly larger than the patient's clenched fist. The heart of the female typically is smaller and weighs less than the heart of the male.

Heart Wall

The heart wall is composed of three layers: epicardium, myocardium, and endocardium (see Figure 19.1). The outer layer, called the

epicardium, is anatomically identical to the visceral pericardium. The **myocardium** is the thick, muscular layer. It is made up of bundles of cardiac muscle fibers reinforced by a branching network of connective tissue fibers called the fibrous skeleton of the heart. The innermost layer is the **endocardium**, a smooth layer that provides an inner lining for the chambers of the heart. The endocardium is continuous with the linings of the blood vessels that enter and leave the cardiac chambers.

Cardiac muscle is quite different from skeletal muscle. The muscle cells are shorter, interconnected, branched structures. Mitochondria, the cell's energy-producing organelles, compose about 25% of cardiac muscle fibers versus only about 2% of skeletal muscle fibers. This higher ratio is related to the much higher energy requirements of cardiac muscle. Unlike the independently functioning fibers of skeletal muscle, the fibers of cardiac muscle are interconnected by special junctions that provide for the conduction of impulses across the entire myocardium. This property allows the heart to contract as a single unit.

Heart Chambers

The heart is composed of four chambers: two smaller, superior chambers called atria, and two larger, inferior chambers called ventricles (see Figure 19.3 ■). One atrium is located on the right side of the heart and one on the left side. These serve as receiving chambers for blood returning to the heart from the major blood vessels of the body. The atria then pump the blood into the right and left ventricles, which lie directly below them. The ventricles also are located

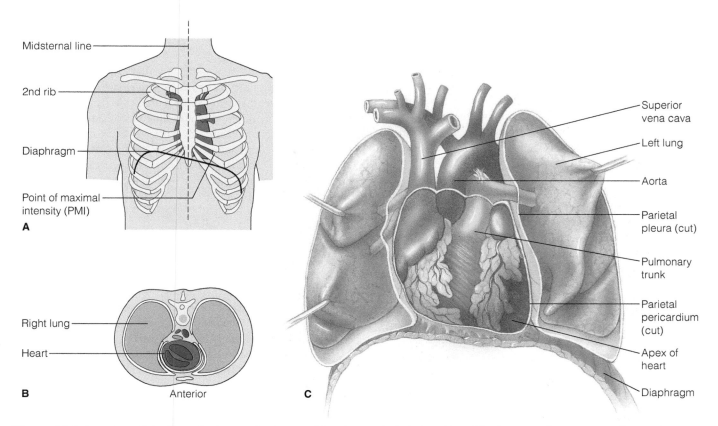

Figure 19.2 Location of the heart in the mediastinum of the thorax. A. Relationship of the heart to the sternum, ribs, and diaphragm. B. Cross-sectional view showing relative position of the heart in the thorax. C. Relationship of the heart and great vessels to the lungs.

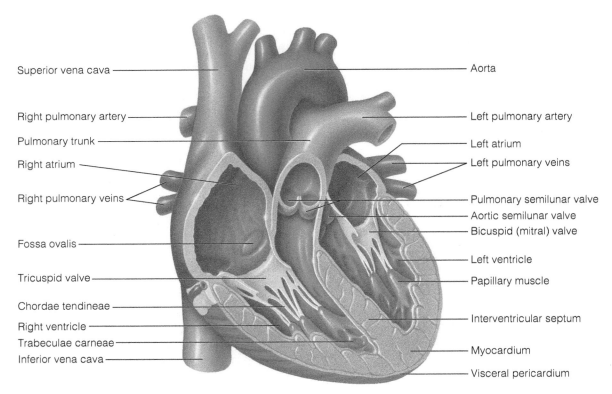

Superior vena cava

Aorta

Right pulmonary artery

Left pulmonary artery

Pulmonary trunk

Left atrium

Right atrium

Left pulmonary veins

Right pulmonary veins

Pulmonary semilunar valve

Aortic semilunar valve

Bicuspid (mitral) valve

Fossa ovalis

Left ventricle

Tricuspid valve

Papillary muscle

Chordae tendineae

Right ventricle

Interventricular septum

Trabeculae carneae

Myocardium

Inferior vena cava

Visceral pericardium

Figure 19.3 Structural components of the heart.

on each side of the heart. They eject blood into the vessels leaving the heart. A longitudinal partition separates the heart chambers. The *interatrial septum* separates the two atria, and the *interventricular septum* divides the ventricles.

RIGHT ATRIUM The **right atrium** (RA) is a thin-walled chamber located above and slightly to the right of the right ventricle. It forms the right border of the heart. Deoxygenated venous blood from the systemic circulation enters the right atrium via the inferior and superior venae cavae (two main structures of the venous system) and the coronary sinus. The blood is then ejected from the right atrium through the tricuspid valve into the right ventricle.

RIGHT VENTRICLE The **right ventricle** (RV) is formed triangularly and comprises much of the anterior or sternocostal surface of the heart. After receiving deoxygenated blood from the right atrium, the right ventricle ejects it through the pulmonary semilunar valve to the trunk of the pulmonary arteries so that the blood may be oxygenated within the lungs. Its wall is much thinner than that of the left ventricle, reflecting the relative low vascular pressure in the vessels of the lungs.

LEFT ATRIUM The **left atrium** (LA) forms the posterior aspect of the heart. Its muscular structure is slightly thicker than that of the right atrium. It receives oxygenated blood from the pulmonary vasculature via the pulmonary veins. From here, the blood is pumped through the mitral valve into the left ventricle.

LEFT VENTRICLE The **left ventricle** (LV) is located behind the right ventricle and forms the left border of the heart. The left ventricle, which is egg shaped, is the most muscular chamber of the heart. The thick wall of ventricular muscle permits the pumping of blood through the aortic semilunar valve into the aorta against high

systemic vascular resistance. This causes the left ventricle to develop more mass than the right ventricle. The left ventricle of a female has about 10% less mass compared to that of a male.

Valves

The valves of the heart are structures through which blood is ejected either from one chamber to another or from a chamber into a blood vessel. The flow of blood in a healthy individual with competent valves is mostly unidirectional. When valves are diseased, forward blood flow is restricted, resulting in regurgitation (backflow) of blood into the chambers of the heart. The regurgitation is assessed as murmurs. Valves are classified by their location as either atrioventricular or semilunar.

Atrioventricular Valves

The **atrioventricular (AV) valves** separate the atria from the ventricles. The tricuspid valve lies between the right atrium and the right ventricle, whereas the thicker mitral (bicuspid) valve lies between the left atrium and left ventricle.

The AV valves open as a direct result of atrial contraction and the concomitant buildup of pressure within the atria. This pressure forces the valvular leaflets to open. When the ventricles contract, the increased ventricular pressure forces the valvular leaflets shut, thus preventing the blood from flowing back into the atria.

Semilunar Valves

The **semilunar valves** separate the ventricles from the vascular system. The pulmonary semilunar valve separates the right ventricle from the trunk of the pulmonary arteries, whereas the aortic semilunar valve separates the left ventricle from the aorta.

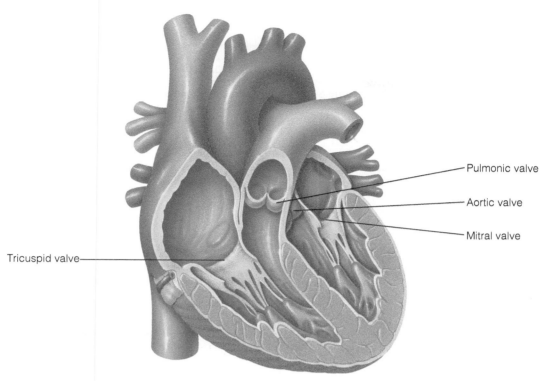

Figure 19.4 Valves of the heart.

The semilunar valves open in response to rising pressure within the contracting ventricles. When the pressure is great enough, the cusps open, allowing blood to be ejected into either the pulmonary trunk or the aorta. Upon relaxation of the ventricles, the valves close, allowing for ventricular filling and preventing backflow into the chambers.

Heart Sounds

Closure of the valves of the heart gives rise to heart sounds (see Figure 19.4 ■). Expected heart sounds include **S1** and **S2**. These are heard as the *lub-dub* of the heart when auscultated over the precordium, the area of the chest that lies over the heart. The first heart sound, S1 (*lub*), is heard when the AV valves close. Closure of these valves occurs when the ventricles have been filled. The second heart sound, S2 (*dub*), occurs when the aortic and pulmonic valves close. These semilunar valves close when the ventricles have emptied their blood into the aorta and pulmonary arteries.

The heart sounds are associated with the contraction and relaxation phases of the heart. **Systole** refers to the phase of ventricular contraction. In the systolic phase, the ventricles have been filled and then contract to expel blood into the aorta and pulmonary arteries. Systole begins with the closure of the AV valves (S1) and ends with the closure of the aortic and pulmonic valves (S2).

Diastole refers to the phase of ventricular relaxation. In the diastolic phase the ventricles relax and are filled as the atria contract. Diastole begins with the closure of the aortic and pulmonic valves (S2) and ends with the closure of the AV valves (S1) (see Figure 19.5 ■).

Splitting of S2 occurs toward the end of inspiration in some individuals. This results from a slight difference in the time in which the semilunar valves close. The increase in intrathoracic pressure during inspiration is a normal splitting of S2. The aortic valve closes

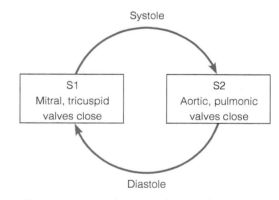

Figure 19.5 Heart sounds in systole and diastole.

just slightly faster than the pulmonic valve. As a result, a split sound is heard (instead of *dub*, one hears *t-dub*). The valves close at the same time during expiration, and the sound of S2 is *dub*.

Two other heart sounds that may be present in some healthy individuals are S3 and S4. S3 may be heard in children, in young adults, or in pregnant females in their third trimester. It is heard after S2 and is termed a *ventricular gallop*. When the AV valves open, blood flow into the ventricles may cause vibrations. These vibrations create the S3 sound during diastole. The S4 may also be heard in children, well-conditioned athletes, and even healthy elderly individuals without cardiac disease. It is caused by atrial contraction and ejection of blood into the ventricles in late diastole. S4 is heard before S1 and is termed an *atrial gallop*.

Heart sounds are interpreted according to the characteristics of pitch, duration, intensity, phase, and location on the precordium. Table 19.1 provides information about the characteristics of heart sounds.

TABLE 19.1　Characteristics of Heart Sounds

HEART SOUNDS	CARDIAC CYCLE TIMING	AUSCULTATION SITE	POSITION	PITCH
S1 (LUB — dub) — S1	Start of systole	Best at apex with diaphragm	Position does not affect the sound	High
S2 (lub — DUB) — S2	End of systole	Both at 2nd ICS; pulmonary component best at LSB; aortic component best at RSB with diaphragm	Sitting or supine	High
Split S1 (T)	Beginning of systole	If normal, at 2nd ICS, LSB; abnormal if heard at apex	Better heard in the supine position	High
Fixed Split S2	End of systole	Both at 2nd ICS; pulmonary component best at LSB; aortic component best at RSB with diaphragm	Better heard in the supine position	High
Expiration Paradoxical Split S2 (P2A2)	End of systole	Both at 2nd ICS; pulmonary component best at LSB; aortic component best at RSB with diaphragm	Better heard in the supine position	High
Expiration Wide Split S2 Inspiration	End of systole	Both at 2nd ICS; pulmonary component best at LSB; aortic component best at RSB with diaphragm	Better heard in the supine position	High
S3 (right after S2)	Early diastole right after S2	Apex with the bell	Auscultated better in left lateral position or supine	Low
S4 (right before S1)	Late diastole right before S1	Apex with the bell	Auscultated in almost a left lateral position or supine	Low

Additional Heart Sounds

Although S3 and S4 sounds are sometimes heard in healthy individuals, they are more commonly associated with pathologic conditions such as myocardial infarction (MI) or heart failure. S3 occurs when the ventricle reaches its elastic limit, causing the blood flow from the atrium to slow rapidly. This may occur in the presence of systolic or diastolic ventricular dysfunction; ischemic heart disease; tricuspid, mitral, or aortic regurgitation; volume overload; and hypertension. Patients with heart failure who have S3 sounds often have a poor prognosis. S4 sounds are associated with active atrial contractions that cause late ventricular filling, such as occurs with ventricular hypertrophy, acute MI, angina, ventricular aneurysm, and hyperkinetic states (Mangla & Gupta, 2014).

The valves of the heart open quietly and without sound unless the tissue has been damaged. Clicks and snaps may be heard in patients with valvular disease. An opening snap may be heard in mitral stenosis. Ejection clicks occur in damaged pulmonic and aortic valves, and nonejection clicks are heard in prolapse of the mitral valve.

Friction rubs result from inflammation of the pericardial sac. The surfaces of the parietal and visceral layers of the pericardium cannot slide smoothly and produce the rubbing or grating sound. Table 19.2 includes information regarding interpretation of additional heart sounds.

Heart murmurs are harsh, blowing sounds caused by disruption of blood flow into the heart, between the chambers of the heart, or from the heart into the pulmonary or aortic systems. Methods to distinguish murmurs and classification of heart murmurs are provided in Tables 19.3 and 19.4, respectively.

Coronary Arteries

The word *coronary* comes from the Latin word meaning crown, which accurately describes this extensive network of arteries supplying the heart (see Figure 19.6 ■ on page 461). The coronary arteries are visible initially on the external surface of the heart but descend deep into the myocardial tissue layers. Their function is to transport blood bringing nutrients and oxygen to the myocardial muscle. The coronary arteries fill during diastole.

The main coronary arteries are the left main coronary artery, the right coronary artery, the left anterior descending coronary artery, and the circumflex coronary artery. These arteries and those that branch from them may vary in size and configuration among individuals. The coronary arteries are located above the aortic valve. The right and left main coronary arteries originate from the aorta and then diverge to provide blood to different surfaces. Atherosclerotic plaque in these arteries as well as in their branches contributes significantly to the development of ischemic and injury processes and the potential for death.

TABLE 19.2 **Additional Heart Sounds**

CLICKS	HEART SOUNDS	CARDIAC CYCLE TIMING	AUSCULTATION SITE	POSITION	PITCH
	Aortic Click	Early systole	2nd ICS, RSB for aortic click and apex with diaphragm	Sitting or supine position may increase sound	High
	Pulmonic	Early systole	2nd ICS, LSB for pulmonic click with diaphragm	Sitting	High
	Opening Snap	Early diastole	3rd to 4th ICS, LSB with diaphragm	Sitting or supine position may increase the sound	High
	Friction Rub	Can occur at any time	Best heard with the diaphragm, location variable	May be heard in any position, but best when the patient sits forward	High, harsh in sound, grating

TABLE 19.3   Distinguishing Heart Murmurs

ASK YOURSELF	INFORMATION
1. How loud is the murmur?	Murmurs are graded on a rather subjective scale of 1–6: • Grade 1: Barely audible with stethoscope, often considered physiologic not pathologic. Requires concentration and a quiet environment. • Grade 2: Very soft but distinctly audible. • Grade 3: Moderately loud; there is no thrill or thrusting motion associated with the murmur. • Grade 4: Distinctly loud, in addition to a palpable thrill. • Grade 5: Very loud, can actually hear with part of the diaphragm of the stethoscope off the chest; palpable thrust and thrill present. • Grade 6: Loudest, can hear with the diaphragm off the chest; visible thrill and thrust.
2. Where does it occur in the cardiac cycle: systole, diastole, or both?	Location in cardiac cycle: • Systole: early systole, midsystole, late systole • Diastole: early diastole, mid-diastole, late diastole • Both
3a. Is the sound continuous throughout systole, diastole, or only heard for part of the cycle?	Duration of murmur: • Continuous through systole only • Continuous through diastole only • Continuous through systole and diastole *Systolic murmurs* may be of two types: • Midsystolic: Murmur is heard after S1 and stops before S2. • Pansystolic/holosystolic: Murmur begins with S1 and stops at S2. *Diastolic murmurs* may be one of three types: • Early diastolic: Murmur auscultated immediately after S2 and then stops. There is a gap where this murmur stops and S1 is heard. • Mid-diastolic: Murmur begins a short time after S2 and stops well before S1 is auscultated. • Late diastolic: This murmur starts well after S2 and stops immediately before S1 is heard.
3b. What does the configuration of the sound look like? *Potential configurations:* S1 [waveform] S2 **Pansystolic/holosystolic** S1 [waveform] S2 [waveform] S1 **Continuous** S2 [waveform] S1 **Crescendo (Systolic represented)**	S2 [waveform] S1 **Decrescendo (Diastolic represented)** S1 [waveform] S2 **Crescendo Decrescendo (Systole represented)** S1 [waveform] S2 **Rumble**
4. What is the quality of the sound of the murmur?	• Blowing • Harsh • Musical • Raspy • Rumbling

TABLE 19.3 Distinguishing Heart Murmurs (continued)

ASK YOURSELF	INFORMATION
5. What is the pitch or frequency of the sound?	• Low • Medium • High
6. In which landmark(s) do you best hear the murmur?	Use the five landmarks for auscultation: • Pulmonic areas 1 and 2 • Aortic area • Tricuspid area • Mitral area • Apex
7. Does it radiate?	• To the throat? • To the axilla?
8. Is there any change in pattern with respirations?	• Increases/decreases with inspiration • Increases/decreases with expiration
9. Is it associated with variations in heart sounds?	• Associated with split S1? • Associated with split S2? • Associated with S3? • Associated with S4? • Associated with a click or ejection sound?
10. Does intensity of murmur change with position?	• Increases/decreases with squatting? • Increases/decreases with patient in the left lateral position? (Do not have the patient perform the Valsalva maneuver or any abrupt positional changes, because some patients do not tolerate position changes well.)

TABLE 19.4 Classifications of Heart Murmurs

MURMUR	CARDIAC CYCLE TIMING	AUSCULTATION SITE	CONFIGURATION OF SOUND	CONTINUITY
Aortic stenosis	Midsystolic	RSB, 2nd ICS	S1 S2	Crescendo-decrescendo, continuous
Pulmonary stenosis	Midsystolic	LSB, 2nd to 3rd ICS	S1 S2	Crescendo-decrescendo, continuous
Mitral regurgitation	Systole	Apex	S1 S2	Holosystolic, continuous
Tricuspid regurgitation	Systole	4th ICS, LSB	S2 S1	Holosystolic, continuous

(continued)

TABLE 19.4 Classifications of Heart Murmurs (continued)

MURMUR	CARDIAC CYCLE TIMING	AUSCULTATION SITE	CONFIGURATION OF SOUND	CONTINUITY
Mitral stenosis	Diastole	Apical	S1 — S2	Rumble that increases in sound toward the end, continuous
Tricuspid stenosis	Diastole	Lower LSB	S2 — S1	Rumble that increases in sound toward the end, continuous
Ventricular septal defect (left-to-right shunt)	Systole	3rd, 4th, 5th ICS, LSB	S1 — S2	Holosystolic, continuous
Aortic regurgitation	Diastole (early)	3rd ICS, LSB	S2 — S1	Decrescendo, continuous
Pulmonic regurgitation	Diastole (early)	3rd ICS, LSB	S2 — S1	Decrescendo, continuous

MURMUR	QUALITY	PITCH	RADIATION	CHANGES WITH RESPIRATIONS
Aortic stenosis	Usually harsh, coarse	Medium	Most commonly into neck into carotid area and down LSB, possibly apex	Expiration may intensify the murmur
Pulmonary stenosis	Usually harsh	Medium	Toward the left upper neck and shoulder areas	Inspiration may intensify the murmur
Mitral regurgitation	Blowing and can be harsh in sound quality	High	Usually to left axilla, LSB, and base	Expiration may intensify the murmur
Tricuspid regurgitation	Blowing	High	May radiate to LSB and MCL but not to axilla	Inspiration may intensify the murmur
Mitral stenosis	Rumbling	Low and best heard with bell	Rare	Expiration may intensify the murmur
Tricuspid stenosis	Rumbling	Low	Rare	Inspiration may intensify the murmur
Ventricular septal defect (left-to-right shunt)	Harsh	High	May radiate across precordium but not to axilla	Expiration may intensify the murmur
Aortic regurgitation	Blowing	High, best auscultated with diaphragm unless patient is sitting up and leaning forward	May radiate to 2nd ICS, RSB and may proceed to apex	Expiration may intensify the murmur if the patient leans forward and sits up
Pulmonic regurgitation	Blowing	High, best auscultated with diaphragm	May radiate to 2nd ICS, RSB and may proceed to apex	Inspiration may intensify the murmur

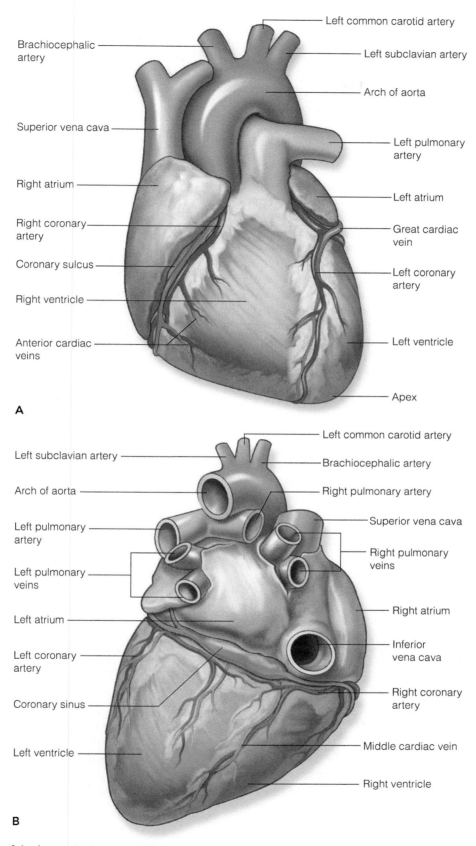

Brachiocephalic artery

Left common carotid artery

Left subclavian artery

Arch of aorta

Superior vena cava

Left pulmonary artery

Right atrium

Left atrium

Right coronary artery

Great cardiac vein

Coronary sulcus

Left coronary artery

Right ventricle

Anterior cardiac veins

Left ventricle

Apex

A

Left subclavian artery

Left common carotid artery

Brachiocephalic artery

Arch of aorta

Right pulmonary artery

Left pulmonary artery

Superior vena cava

Left pulmonary veins

Right pulmonary veins

Left atrium

Right atrium

Left coronary artery

Inferior vena cava

Coronary sinus

Right coronary artery

Left ventricle

Middle cardiac vein

Right ventricle

B

Figure 19.6 Vessels of the heart. A. Anterior. B. Posterior.

Cardiac Veins

The venous system of the heart is composed of the great cardiac vein, oblique vein, anterior cardiac vein, small cardiac vein, middle cardiac vein, cordis minimae veins, and posterior cardiac vein. The great cardiac vein serves as the tributary for the majority of venous blood drainage and empties into the coronary sinus. The small venae cordis minimae drain into the cardiac chambers.

Cardiac Conduction System

The heart has its own conduction system, which can initiate an electrical charge and transmit that charge via cardiac muscle fibers throughout the myocardial tissue. This electrical charge stimulates the heart to contract, causing the propulsion of blood throughout the heart chambers and vascular system. The main structures of the **cardiac conduction system** are the sinoatrial node (SA node), the intra-atrial conducting pathways, the atrioventricular (AV node) node, the bundle of His, the right and left bundle branches, and the Purkinje fibers (see Figure 19.7 ■). Because the cardiac conduction system relies on muscle contraction, it is very susceptible to dysregulation during electrolyte imbalances, particularly imbalances in calcium, potassium, and sodium. Therefore, electrolytes are an integral part of normal cardiac function.

Sinoatrial Node

The **sinoatrial (SA) node** initiates the electrical impulse. For this reason, it has been called the pacemaker of the heart. The SA node is located at the junction of the superior vena cava and right atrium. The autonomic nervous system feeds into the SA node and can influence it to either speed up or slow down the discharge of electrical current. In the healthy individual, the SA node discharges an average of 60 to 100 times a minute.

Intra-Atrial Conduction Pathway

These loosely organized conducting fibers assist in the propagation of the electrical current emitted from the SA node through the right and left atrium. The network is composed of three main pathways: anterior, middle, and posterior.

Atrioventricular Node and Bundle of His

The **atrioventricular (AV) node** and **bundle of His** are intricately connected and function to receive the current that has finished spreading throughout the atria. Here the impulse is slowed for about 0.1 second before it passes onto the bundle branches. The AV node is also capable of initiating electrical impulses in the event of SA node failure. The intrinsic rate of firing is slower and averages about 60 per minute.

Right and Left Bundle Branches and Purkinje Fibers

The right and left **bundle branches** are like expressways of conducting fibers that spread the electrical current through the ventricular myocardial tissue. Arising from the right and left bundle branches are the **Purkinje fibers.** These fibers fan out and penetrate into the myocardial tissue to spread the current into the tissues themselves.

The bundle branches are also capable of initiating electrical charges in case both the SA node and AV node fail. Their intrinsic rate averages 40 to 60 per minute.

Cardiac Nerves

Just as there is an extensive network of vessels transporting oxygen and nutrients to the myocardial tissue and removing waste products, an equally important network of autonomic nerves is present. Both sympathetic nervous fibers and parasympathetic nervous fibers

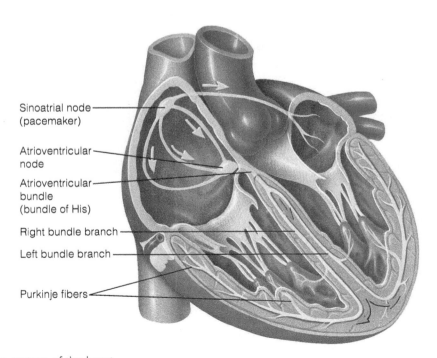

Sinoatrial node
(pacemaker)

Atrioventricular
node

Atrioventricular
bundle
(bundle of His)

Right bundle branch

Left bundle branch

Purkinje fibers

Figure 19.7 Conduction system of the heart.

interact with the myocardial tissue. The sympathetic fibers stimulate the heart, increasing the heart rate, force of contraction, and dilation of the coronary arteries. Conversely, the parasympathetic fibers, such as the vagus nerve, exercise the opposite effect. The central nervous system influences the activation and interaction of these nerves through the information supplied by the cardiac plexus.

Pulmonary Circulation

The vessels of the pulmonary circulation include arteries, veins, and an expansive network of pulmonary capillaries. This vascular system carries deoxygenated blood to the lungs, where carbon dioxide is exchanged for oxygen. Deoxygenated blood from the veins of the body enters this network by passing into the right atrium. It is then ejected through the tricuspid valve into the right ventricle and passes through the pulmonic valve into the pulmonary artery and pulmonary circulation. The pulmonary artery is the only artery to carry unoxygenated blood. After going through the pulmonary capillary network, oxygenated blood returns to the left atrium via the pulmonary veins (see Figure 19.8 ■). Pulmonary veins are the only veins to carry oxygenated blood.

Systemic Circulation

The vessels of the systemic circulation also include arteries, veins, and capillaries. This vascular system supplies freshly oxygenated blood to the body's periphery and returns deoxygenated blood to the pulmonary circuit. The arteries of the systemic circulation are composed of elastic tissue and smooth muscle, which allows their walls to stretch during systole. During systole, the elasticity of the walls propels the blood forward into the systemic circulation. The left ventricle propels freshly oxygenated blood into the aorta. As the blood moves toward the body periphery, the major arteries of the body subdivide into arterioles, which carry the nutrients and oxygen to the smallest blood vessels of the body, the capillaries. Oxygen and nutrients are exchanged in the capillaries for carbon dioxide and metabolites, which are then carried into the venules, then veins, and finally the superior and inferior venae cavae, which carry the deoxygenated blood into the right atrium of the heart (see Figure 19.8).

Landmarks for Cardiovascular Assessment

Landmarks for assessing the cardiovascular system include the sternum, clavicles, ribs, and intercostal spaces. By correlating assessment findings with the overlying body landmarks, the nurse may gain vital information concerning underlying pathologic mechanisms. Many landmarks identified during the respiratory assessment are utilized also when performing a cardiac assessment. These include but are not limited to the sternum and the second through fifth intercostal spaces. It may be helpful to review the landmarks in chapter 17 before proceeding. ∞

The **sternum** is the flat, narrow center bone of the upper anterior chest (see Figure 19.9 ■). There are three portions of the adult sternum. The upper sternum is called the manubrium, the middle part is the body, and the inferior piece is the xiphoid process. The average sternal length in an adult is 18 cm (7 in.).

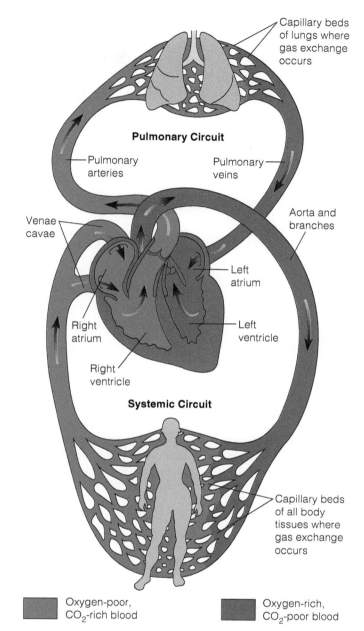

Figure 19.8 Pulmonary and systemic circulation. The left side of the heart pumps oxygenated blood (indicated in red) into the arteries of the systemic circulation, which provides oxygen and nutrients to the cells. Deoxygenated blood (indicated in blue) returns via the venous system into the right side of the heart, where it is transported to the pulmonary arterial system to be reoxygenated.

During cardiovascular assessment, the sternum is used as a vertical landmark, and the angle of Louis is used to locate the second intercostal space.

The clavicles are bones that attach at the top of the manubrium of the sternum above the first rib (see Figure 19.9). The left midclavicular line (LMCL) is used as a landmark for cardiovascular assessment.

The ribs are flat, arched bones that form the thoracic cage. There are 12 pairs of ribs. Between each rib is an intercostal space (ICS). The first ICS lies between the first and the second rib,

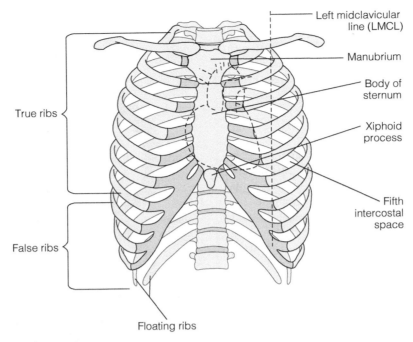

Figure 19.9 Landmarks for cardiovascular assessment.

and each remaining ICS is numbered successively (see Figure 19.9). The ICSs, horizontal landmarks for cardiac assessment, are used to locate the base of the heart and the apex of the heart and to auscultate the valvular sounds. The second ICS is located by feeling the angle of Louis, sliding the finger laterally to the second rib at the left (LSB) or right (RSB) sternal borders, and then sliding the finger down below the rib to the ICS. Each succeeding ICS is located by sliding the finger over the rib into the ICS. Additional landmarks are identified later in this chapter.

Cardiac Cycle

The **cardiac cycle** describes the events of one complete heartbeat—that is, the contraction and relaxation of the atria and ventricles. A healthy individual's heart averages about 72 beats per minute (beats/min); thus, the average time for each cardiac cycle to be completed is 0.8 second. Synchrony between the mechanical and electrical events of the cycle is imperative. Any interruption in this balance affects the ability of the heart to provide oxygen and nutrients to the body. Significant disruptions in synchrony can be fatal.

Electrical and Mechanical Events

The cardiac cycle can be divided into three periods (see Figure 19.10 ■): the period of ventricular filling, ventricular systole, and isovolumetric relaxation.

PERIOD OF VENTRICULAR FILLING This is the start of the cardiac cycle. Blood enters passively into the ventricles from the atria. About 70% of the blood that eventually ends up in the ventricles enters at this time. As this blood is entering the ventricles, the atria are stimulated to contract by the electrical current emanating from the SA node. Another 30% volume of blood exits the atria into the ventricles. This extra 30% volume is termed the *atrial kick*.

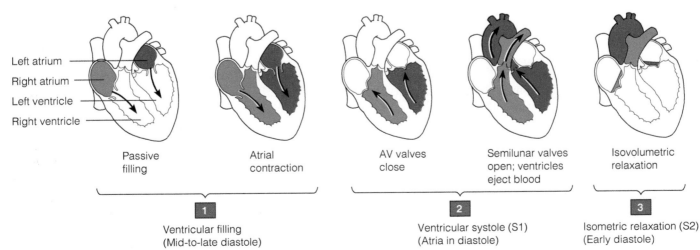

Figure 19.10 The cardiac cycle.

VENTRICULAR SYSTOLE The electrical current stimulates the ventricles, and they respond by contracting. The force of contraction increases the pressure within both ventricles. The mitral and tricuspid valves respond to this increased pressure by snapping shut (S1). The ventricular pressure continues to increase until it causes the aortic and pulmonic valves to open. Blood rushes out of the ventricles into the systemic and pulmonary circulation.

ISOVOLUMETRIC RELAXATION Once the majority of blood is ejected, the pressure in the aorta and pulmonary artery becomes higher than in the ventricles, causing the aortic and pulmonic valves to shut (S2). During ventricular systole, the atria have been filling with blood returning from the systemic and pulmonary circulation. When the pressure in the atria becomes higher than in the ventricles, the mitral and tricuspid valves open, and the cycle begins again.

Electrical Representation of the Cardiac Cycle

Electrical representations of the cardiac cycle are documented by deflections on recording paper. A straight horizontal line means the absence of electrical activity. Deflections representing the flow of electrical current toward or away from an electrode record the timing of the electrical events in the cardiac cycle. The terms describing the electrical deflections are P wave, PR interval, QRS complex, and T wave. They are recorded as an **electrocardiogram (ECG)** (see Figure 19.11 ■). When the cardiac cell is in a resting state, it is more positively charged on the outside of the cell and more negatively charged on the inside of the cell. This spread of electrical current, called *depolarization*, causes the inside of the cardiac cell to become more positively charged. Depolarization occurs when the electrical

current normally initiated in the SA node spreads across the atria. Contraction of the atria follows after stimulation by the electrical current. After contraction, the cardiac cells experience *repolarization*, during which the inside of the cell returns to its more negatively charged state. The same process occurs in the ventricles.

P WAVE The P wave represents part of atrial depolarization. The pacemaker of the heart, the SA node, emits an electrical charge that initially spreads throughout the right and left atria. As a result of the electrical stimulation, the myocardial cells contract. The initial P wave deflection is caused by the initiation of the electrical current and atrial response to the current. It lasts an average 0.08 second.

PR INTERVAL The PR interval represents the time needed for the electrical current to travel across both atria and arrive at the AV node. The normal PR interval averages 0.12 to 0.20 second.

QRS COMPLEX The QRS complex represents ventricular depolarization. Atrial repolarization is hidden in the QRS complex. The ventricular myocardial cells also respond to the spread of electrical current by becoming more positively charged. This change in polarity is ventricular depolarization. The QRS complex should range from 0.08 to 0.11 second.

T WAVE The T wave represents ventricular repolarization. Once the ventricular myocardial cells have been stimulated by the electrical current and contract, they return to their original electrical potential state. This change in polarity is repolarization. The atria also repolarize, but it is not recorded because it occurs at the same time as ventricular repolarization; therefore, the QRS complex covers it.

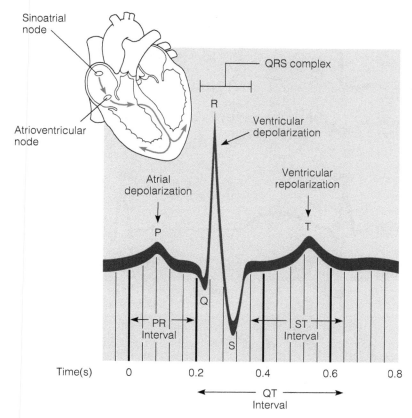

Figure 19.11 Electrocardiogram wave.

QT INTERVAL The QT interval represents the period from the beginning of ventricular depolarization to the moment of repolarization. Thus, it represents ventricular contraction. Electrical events in the heart occur slightly ahead of the mechanical events. Figure 19.12 ■ illustrates the events of the cardiac cycle in relation to heart sounds, pressure waves, and the ECG.

Measurements of Cardiac Function

When the heart is functioning at optimal level, the synchrony of the events of the cardiac cycle produces an outflow of blood with oxygen and nutrients to every cell in the body. The terms that describe the effectiveness of the action of the cardiac cycle are stroke volume, cardiac output, and cardiac index.

Stroke volume describes the amount of blood that is ejected with every heartbeat. Normal stroke volume is 55 to 100 mL/beat. The formula for calculating stroke volume is:

stroke volume = cardiac output/heart rate

Cardiac output describes the amount of blood ejected from the left ventricle over 1 minute. Normal adult cardiac output is 4 to 8 liters/minute. The formula for calculating cardiac output is:

cardiac output = stroke volume × heart rate

The cardiac index is a valuable diagnostic measurement of the effectiveness of the pumping action of the heart. The cardiac index takes into consideration the individual's weight, which is a significant factor in judging the effectiveness of the pumping action. For example, suppose a cardiac output of 4 L/min is obtained for two patients: an elderly female who weighs 60 kg (132.3 lb) and a middle-aged male who weighs 130 kg (286.6 lb). The elderly female's cardiac index is significantly higher than that of the male, whose pumping effectiveness is significantly compromised. The formula for calculating cardiac index is:

cardiac index = cardiac output/body surface area

The body surface area (BSA) measurement is obtained and determined from published tables.

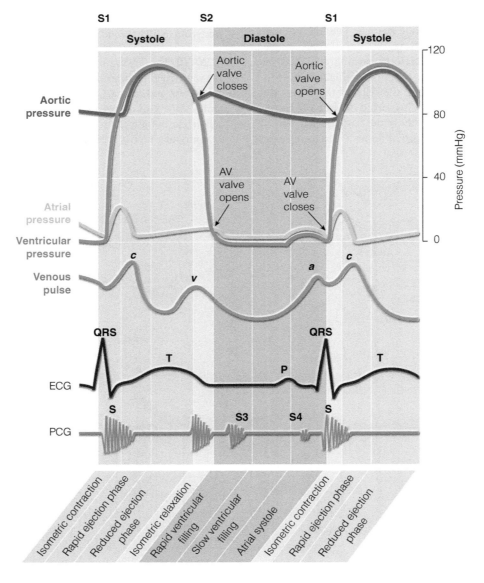

Figure 19.12 Events of the cardiac cycle.

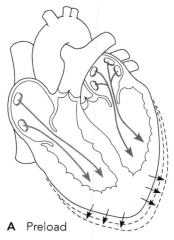

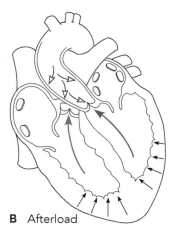

A Preload   **B** Afterload

Figure 19.13 A. Preload is related to the amount of blood and stretching of the ventricular myocardial fibers. B. Afterload is the pressure that the ventricles must overcome in order to open the aortic and pulmonic valvular cusps.

There are two strong influences on pumping action: preload and afterload. Preload is influenced by the volume of the blood in the ventricles and relates to the length of ventricular fiber stretch at the end of diastole. The Frank-Starling law states that an increasingly greater contractile ability is provided with greater stretching of the ventricular muscle fibers. Thus, the greater the stretch, the greater the contractile force, and the greater the volume of blood ejected with each contraction. Afterload is the amount of stress or tension present in the ventricular wall during systole. It is interrelated to the pressure in the aorta, because the pressure in the ventricular wall must be greater than that in the aorta and pulmonary trunk for the semilunar valves to open (see Figure 19.13 ■).

Special Considerations

Many factors influence the patient's health status. Among these are age, developmental level, race, ethnicity, work history, living conditions, socioeconomics, and emotional well-being. Each of the factors must be addressed while gathering subjective and objective data during a comprehensive health assessment.

Health Promotion Considerations

Healthy People 2020 objectives include reducing mortalities due to coronary heart disease and stroke. In addition, these national objectives emphasize promotion of cardiovascular health through enhancing public awareness of risk factors, along with increasing the use of cardiovascular screenings to identify individuals who are at risk (USDHHS, 2010). See Table 19.5 for examples of *Healthy People 2020* objectives that target the promotion of cardiovascular health and wellness among individuals across the life span.

Lifespan Considerations

Anatomy and physiology change as individuals grow and develop. It is important to understand these normal changes when interpreting findings in health assessment. Variations in the cardiovascular system for different age groups are presented in the following sections.

Infants and Children

During development, the fetus receives its nutrients and oxygen from its mother. The lungs are nonfunctional, and oxygen is carried in blood from the placenta to the right side of the heart. The majority of this blood passes through the foramen ovale to the left side of the heart, then into the aorta to enter the systemic circulation. The *foramen ovale* is a passageway for blood between the right and left atria. The rest of the blood passes through the pulmonary artery and ductus arteriosus and enters the aorta (see Figure 19.14 ■). The *ductus arteriosus* is an opening between the pulmonary artery and the descending aorta.

Inflation of the lungs at birth causes the pulmonary vasculature to dilate. Oxygenation occurs for the first time within the newborn's lungs. The foramen ovale closes shortly after birth because of increased pulmonary vascular return and decreased pressure in the right side of the heart. The ductus arteriosus closes within 24 to 48 hours in response to multiple physiologic events, including decreased pulmonary resistance and decreased pressure in the right atrium versus increased pressure in the left atrium. Murmurs may be auscultated if these openings remain patent. However, if a ventricular septal defect is present, the murmur it causes may not be auscultated until the 4th to 6th week after delivery.

The infant's arterial pressure rises at birth, and the systemic vascular resistance increases significantly when the umbilical cord is cut. Over time, the left ventricle increases in size and mass as it works to pump blood into the aorta against increasingly elevating systemic vascular resistance. The blood pressure of the full-term infant may average 70/50 mmHg, and 10 mmHg less in both systolic and diastolic readings in the preterm newborn. Weight significantly influences blood pressure.

The heart rate of the newborn initially may be as high as 160 to 180 beats/min. Over the first 6 to 8 hours, it gradually decreases to an average of 115 to 120 beats/min. Stimulation that causes crying, screaming, or coughing may cause the heart rate to rise temporarily to 180 beats/min.

A newborn's cardiovascular system undergoes tremendous changes at birth and during the first several days of life. The infant should be easily aroused and alert. The skin should demonstrate perfusion with pink quality in the nail beds, mucous membranes,

TABLE 19.5	Examples of *Healthy People 2020* Objectives Related to Cardiovascular Health
OBJECTIVE NUMBER	**DESCRIPTION**
HDS-1	(Developmental) Increase overall cardiovascular health in the U.S. population
HDS-2	Reduce coronary heart disease deaths
HDS-3	Reduce stroke deaths
HDS-15	(Developmental) Increase aspirin use as recommended among adults with no history of cardiovascular disease.
HDS-16	Increase the proportion of adults aged 20 years and older who are aware of the symptoms of and how to respond to a heart attack.
HDS-17	Increase the proportion of adults aged 20 years and older who are aware of the symptoms of and how to respond to a stroke.
HDS-18	(Developmental) Increase the proportion of out-of-hospital cardiac arrests in which appropriate bystander and emergency medical services (EMS) were administered.
HDS-19	Increase the proportion of eligible patients with heart attacks or strokes who receive timely artery-opening therapy as specified by current guidelines.
HDS-20	(Developmental) Increase the proportion of adults with coronary heart disease or stroke who have their low-density lipoprotein (LDL) cholesterol level at or below recommended levels.
HDS-21	(Developmental) Increase the proportion of adults with a history of cardiovascular disease who are using aspirin or antiplatelet therapy to prevent recurrent cardiovascular events.
HDS-22	(Developmental) Increase the proportion of adult heart attack survivors who are referred to a cardiac rehabilitation program at discharge.
HDS-23	(Developmental) Increase the proportion of adult stroke survivors who are referred to a stroke rehabilitation program at discharge.
HDS-24	Reduce hospitalizations of older adults with heart failure as the principal diagnosis.

Source: U.S. Department of Health and Human Services (USDHHS). (2014). *Healthy people 2020.* Retrieved from http://www.healthypeople.gov/2020/default.aspx.

and conjunctiva regardless of the baby's race. Precordial bulging and chest deformities such as pigeon chest and barrel chest are of concern.

The nurse should use a small diaphragm and bell with an infant or child for optimal auscultation of heart sounds. The heart is more horizontally positioned in the chest of infants; therefore, the apex is located at the fourth ICS. Pathologic murmurs of a congenital cause include patent ductus arteriosus, tetralogy of Fallot, and septal defects.

The Pregnant Female

During pregnancy, a female's body undergoes phenomenal adaptations, especially in the cardiovascular system. Usually these

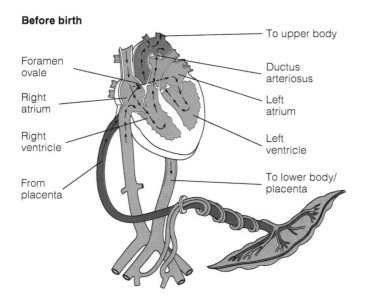

Before birth

Foramen ovale

Right atrium

Right ventricle

From placenta

To upper body

Ductus arteriosus

Left atrium

Left ventricle

To lower body/placenta

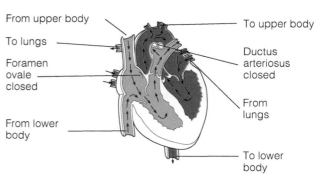

After birth

From upper body

To lungs

Foramen ovale closed

From lower body

To upper body

Ductus arteriosus closed

From lungs

To lower body

Figure 19.14 Location of the main structures and vessels present in the fetal and postpartal cardiovascular anatomy.

adaptations do not place her life at risk; however, if pre-existing cardiovascular or other disease is present, her health may be significantly compromised. The heart is displaced to the left and upward, and the apex is pushed laterally and to the left. This anatomic shift may be seen when examining the electrical axis on the female's 12-lead ECG. The axis is rotated to the left. The physical strength of the female's abdominal muscles, the shape of the fetus, the gestational age, and the structural anatomy of the uterus influence the extent of this shift.

The cardiovascular system undergoes many physiologic changes during pregnancy. Blood volume may increase as much as 30% to 50%. Red blood cell genesis is dramatically stimulated, and plasma volume increases by as much as 50%. Plasma albumin, conversely, decreases. Cardiac output increases 30% to 50% in just the first trimester. Dilation of surface veins, together with the low resistance of the uteroplacental circulation, increases the venous return to the heart. Stroke volume increases 30%. Because of the substantial increase in volume and the resultant increased workload, the heart may appear as much as 10% larger on chest radiography. Systolic blood pressure may decrease by 2 to 3 mmHg and diastolic blood pressure by 5 to 10 mmHg during the first half of the pregnancy. These values return to their previous levels as the pregnancy progresses. Last, the great vessels may become more tortuous in appearance.

There may be a slight increase in resting pulse by about 10 to 15 beats/min, although not every patient experiences this increase. Because of the increased volume, preexisting murmurs may become louder. Murmurs may even be auscultated for the first time. Systolic murmurs are the most common (90% incidence), whereas diastolic murmurs occur less frequently (20% incidence). Heart tones may also change. The S1 may split, and a prominent S3 may be heard.

The position of the patient may influence the cardiovascular dynamic state. Cardiac output may decrease when she lies on her back because of compression of the vena cava and aorta. The brachial pressure is highest when the patient is sitting, then decreases when she is supine. Pressure is lowest when she is in the lateral recumbent position. Monitoring a patient's blood pressure and pattern of the pressures is crucial. Unless a pregnant woman has preexisting uncontrolled hypertension, her blood pressure should be below 140/90; a blood pressure reading higher than this may indicate preeclampsia and needs further assessment and monitoring. If the pregnant woman does have chronic hypertension, a significant increase in blood pressure compared to her normal baseline blood pressure may be an indication of preeclampsia. For a more thorough discussion on blood pressure in pregnancy, see chapter 27. ∞

The Older Adult

The heart may stay the same size, enlarge, or atrophy. During normal aging in the absence of disease, the heart walls may thicken to some extent. The left atrium may increase in size over time. Significant enlargement of the left ventricle can be attributed to the influence of hypertension. Aging can also contribute to the loss of ventricular compliance as the cardiac valves and large vessels become more rigid. The aorta may dilate and lengthen.

Physiologically, systolic blood pressure may increase; however, there may be no significant change in resting heart rate. Diastolic filling time and pressure may increase to maintain a cardiac output adequate for physiological needs. Upon auscultation, the older patient may have an S4. Last, the electrical conduction system may experience a loss of automaticity when the SA node and conducting pathways become fibrotic and lose cellular integrity.

In the healthy older adult, cardiac output may remain stable. Stroke volume may increase just slightly when the patient is at rest. The healthy patient may tolerate exercise well. The healthy older adult may actually show a decreased heart rate, maximum oxygen consumption, and an increase in stroke volume during exercise. A patient who has been physically active most of his or her life may have twice the work capacity of a patient who has not.

The nurse should assess the older patient in a position that is comfortable and be careful not to have the patient make any sudden movements such as suddenly sitting, standing up, or lying down after standing or sitting. Orthostatic hypotension, a sudden drop in blood pressure, may occur when older adults move from lying down to sitting or standing. Systolic murmurs become more common as people age, especially because of aortic stenosis. These murmurs are usually best auscultated in the aortic area or base of the heart. Nonphysiologic murmurs are not normal findings. However, an S4 sound is a common finding in older adults who do not have identified cardiovascular disease. In individuals with preexisting heart disease, however, an S4 is a pathologic finding. The nurse must be mindful of the presence of any other heart sounds beyond S1 and S2 or any change in characteristics of preexisting heart sounds. The physician should be informed of any significant findings.

Psychosocial Considerations

Stress causes an individual to experience longer periods of sympathetic stimulation, which increases the workload on the heart. Systemic vascular resistance may be elevated for longer periods, especially in situations of excessive stress. Counseling, relaxation, yoga, meditation, and biofeedback techniques are usually helpful to reduce stress level.

Cultural and Environmental Considerations

Individuals whose blood-related parents, aunts, uncles, or siblings demonstrate atherosclerotic heart disease before the age of 50 are considered at risk for diabetes, hypertension, or high lipid levels.

In some cultures, "overfat" individuals are considered healthier than those who are leaner. The selection and preparation of food may also reflect cultural influences. African Americans have a significantly higher percentage of hypertension than Caucasians, and hypertension is a risk factor for coronary heart disease. Indeed, African American females over the age of 20 have greater risk for coronary heart disease than other female ethnic groups of the same age. High serum cholesterol is also a risk for heart disease; Caucasians have higher serum cholesterol levels than African Americans, and Caucasian females between the ages of 65 and 74 years have a higher incidence of cardiovascular disease than African American females. Cardiovascular disease contributes to a significant percentage of deaths in individuals from varied cultural backgrounds. In particular, Native Americans under the age of 35 have twice the heart disease mortality of other groups, and African Americans with heart failure have higher mortality rates than Caucasians (AHA, 2012). The correlation of diet and heritage is also significant, as demonstrated by the low incidence of heart disease in Japanese individuals adhering to a traditional Japanese diet and the increasing incidence of heart disease in Japanese individuals who have adopted the Western diet of red meat and saturated fats (Iso, 2008).

Some data suggest that a low socioeconomic bracket is correlated with a higher incidence of hypertension, especially among adult females. There may be a correlation between this situation and the effect of stress related to lower incomes, limited exercise, diets containing saturated fats, or lack of access to quality health care.

Diet is one factor that may significantly influence the development of cardiovascular disease. Intake of fat, especially saturated fat, contributes significantly to cardiovascular disease. "Couch potato" is a popular term that describes a lifestyle of inactivity. Studies on individuals who perform continuous aerobic exercise for at least 30 to 45 minutes at least three times a week have shown a significant correlation to a slower progression of atherosclerosis. Exercise also helps to diffuse the effects of stress and, in most individuals, provides a feeling of relaxation. Smoking is a well-known contributor to the development of cardiovascular disease. In fact, it is one of the most devastating. The chemicals inhaled in cigarette smoke alter and injure the linings of the arteries, especially in areas of bifurcation (division into branches). Inhalation of passive smoke is also detrimental to the cardiovascular system.

Cocaine, especially crack cocaine, causes increased oxygen demands on the heart. Ventricular ectopy, electrical impulses that originate in the ventricles and cause early contraction of the ventricles, has been linked to cocaine use. Coronary artery spasm, myocardial infarction (MI), malignant hypertension, and ruptured aorta also have been attributed to cocaine.

Alcoholism and tobacco use are associated with the development of many cardiovascular complications, such as cardiomyopathy and coronary artery disease. Alcohol consumption may also cause ventricular ectopy, which contributes to decreased cardiac output and may be life threatening.

Gathering the Data

Cardiovascular assessment includes the gathering of subjective and objective data. Subjective data collection occurs during the patient interview, before the actual physical assessment. During the interview the nurse uses a variety of communication techniques to elicit general and specific information about the patient's state of cardiovascular health or illness. Health records, the results of laboratory tests, cardiograms, and other tests are important secondary sources to be reviewed and included in the data-gathering process. In physical assessment of the cardiovascular system, the techniques of inspection, palpation, percussion, and auscultation will be used. Before proceeding, it may be helpful to review the information about each of the data-gathering processes and practice the techniques of health assessment. See Table 19.6 for information on potential secondary sources of patient data.

Focused Interview

The focused interview for the cardiovascular system concerns data related to the structures and functions of that system. Subjective data related to cardiac status are gathered during the focused interview. The nurse must be prepared to observe the patient and listen for cues related to the function of the cardiovascular system. The nurse may use open-ended and closed questions to obtain information. Often a number of follow-up questions or requests for descriptions are required to clarify data or gather missing information.

The focused interview guides the physical assessment of the cardiovascular system. The information is always considered in relation to normal parameters and expectations about cardiovascular function. Therefore, the nurse must consider age, gender, race, culture, environment, health practices, past and concurrent problems, and therapies when framing questions and using techniques to elicit information. In order to address all of the factors when conducting a focused interview, categories of questions related to cardiovascular status and function have been developed. These categories include general questions that are asked of all patients; those addressing

TABLE 19.6	Potential Secondary Sources for Patient Data Related to the Cardiovascular System
LABORATORY TESTS	**NORMAL VALUE**
Cholesterol	<200 mg/dL
Triglycerides	<150 mg/dL
HDL (high-density lipoprotein)	>60 mg/dL
LDL (low-density lipoprotein)	<50 mg/dL
CPK (creatinine phosphokinase)	Males: 52–336 Units/L Females: 38–176 Units/L
CPK-MB	0–3 mcg/mL
Myoglobin	≤ 90 mcg/mL
Troponin I	< 0.04 nanograms/mL
LDH	122–222 Units/L
SGOT	Males: 8–48 Units/L Females: 8–43 Units/L
Diagnostic Tests	
Cardiac catheterization	
Echocardiography	
Electrocardiography	
Electrophysiologic testing	
Exercise stress test	
Holter monitor	

illness and infection; questions related to symptoms, pain, and behaviors; those related to habits or practices; questions that are specific to patients according to age; those for the pregnant female; and questions that address internal and external environmental concerns. One approach to questioning about symptoms would be the OLDCART & ICE method, which is described in chapter 7. ∞ See Figure 7.3 on page 120.

As these questions are asked and subjective data are obtained during the focused interview, the data will be used to help meet the objectives for improving cardiovascular health as indicated in *Healthy People 2020*. The nurse must consider the patient's ability to participate in the focused interview and physical assessment of the cardiovascular system. If a patient is experiencing pain, dyspnea, cyanosis, difficulty with speech, and the anxiety that accompanies any of these problems, attention must focus on relief of symptoms and improvement of oxygenation.

Focused Interview Questions	Rationales and Evidence
The following section provides sample questions and bulleted follow-up questions in each of the previously mentioned categories. A rationale for each of the questions is provided. The list of questions is not all-inclusive	but represents the types of questions required in a comprehensive focused interview related to the cardiovascular system.

General Questions

1. **Describe how you are feeling. Has your sense of well-being changed in the last 2 months? Is your sense of well-being different than it was 2 years ago?**
   - Describe the change.
   - How long have you experienced the change?
   - Do you know what caused the change?
   - Have you seen a healthcare provider?
   - Was a diagnosis made?
   - Was treatment prescribed?
   - What have you done to deal with the change?

   ► This question gives patients the opportunity to provide their own perceptions about their health. Statements about fatigue, weakness, dizziness, or shortness of breath, especially after activity, may indicate problems with cardiovascular health.

2. **Are you able to perform all of the activities needed to meet your personal and work-related responsibilities?**
   - Describe the changes in your abilities.
   - Do you know what is causing the difficulty?
   - How long have you had this problem?
   - What have you done about the problem?
   - Have you discussed this with a healthcare professional?

   ► Inability to carry out or perform personal or work-related activities can be indicative of problems in the cardiovascular system.

3. **Is there anyone in your family who has had a cardiovascular problem or disease?**
   - What is the disease or problem?
   - Who in the family now has or ever had the problem?
   - When was it diagnosed?
   - How has the problem been treated?
   - What was the outcome?

   ► This may reveal information about cardiovascular diseases associated with familial predisposition. Follow-up is required to obtain details about specific problems, occurrence, treatment, and outcomes.

4. **What is your weight? Have you experienced a change in your weight?**
   - How much weight have you gained or lost?
   - Over what period of time did the change occur?
   - Do you know what caused the change?
   - Have you done anything to address the change in your weight?
   - Have you discussed the change with a healthcare provider?

   ► Obesity and high percentage of body fat are risk factors for cardiovascular disease. Weight gain or loss may accompany physical problems, including systemic diseases such as diabetes, which increases risk for cardiovascular disease. Psychosocial problems including stress can affect weight gain or loss and also contribute to cardiovascular problems (Despres, 2012).

Questions Related to Illness

1. **Have you ever been diagnosed with a cardiovascular disease?**
   - When were you diagnosed with the problem?
   - What treatment was prescribed for the problem?
   - Was the treatment helpful?
   - Describe things you have done or currently do to cope with the problem?

   ► The patient has an opportunity to provide information about specific cardiovascular illnesses. If a diagnosed illness is identified, follow-up about the date of diagnosis, treatment, and outcomes is required. Data about each illness identified by the patient are essential to an accurate health assessment.

Focused Interview Questions	Rationales and Evidence

- Has the problem ever recurred (acute)?
- How are you managing the problem now (chronic)?

▶ Illnesses can be classified as acute or chronic, and follow-up regarding each classification will differ.

2. **An alternative to question 1 is to list possible cardiovascular problems, such as MI, congestive heart failure, arteriosclerosis, coronary artery disease, angina, arrhythmia, and valvular disease, and ask the patient to respond "yes" or "no" as each is stated.**

▶ This is a comprehensive and easy way to elicit information about all diagnoses. Follow-up would be carried out for each identified diagnosis as in question 1.

3. **Do you now have or have you ever had an infection or viral illness affecting the cardiovascular system?**
   - When were you diagnosed with the infection?
   - What treatment was prescribed?
   - Has the treatment helped?
   - What kind of things do you do to help with the problem?
   - Has the infection recurred (acute)?
   - How are you managing the problem now (chronic)?

▶ If an infection is identified, follow-up about the date of infection, treatment, and outcome is required.

4. **An alternative to question 3 is to list possible infections, such as rheumatic fever, viral illness, endocarditis, and pericarditis, and ask the patient to respond "yes" or "no" as each is stated.**

▶ This is a comprehensive and easy way to elicit information about all infections related to the cardiovascular system. Follow-up would be required as in question 3.

5. **Have you ever had a diagnostic test, such as an electrocardiogram, stress test, echocardiogram, or a surgical procedure for a cardiovascular problem?**

▶ The patient has the opportunity to provide information about diagnostic testing or surgical procedures related to cardiovascular problems. If a surgical procedure is identified, follow-up about the date of surgery, outcome, and effectiveness is required.

6. **An alternative to question 5 is to list possible surgical procedures, such as coronary artery bypass graft, angioplasty, pacemaker insertion, insertion of a defibrillator, and valve replacement, and ask the patient to respond "yes" or "no" as each is stated.**

▶ This is a comprehensive and easy way to elicit information about surgeries. Follow-up would be required as in question 5.

7. **Do you have hypertension, diabetes, or thyroid disorders?**

▶ Medical conditions such as diabetes, hypertension, or thyroid dysfunction can contribute to cardiovascular problems (Berman & Snyder, 2012).

8. **Do you know your cholesterol and triglyceride levels?**

▶ Elevated cholesterol and triglyceride levels are associated with cardiovascular disease (AHA, 2011).

Questions Related to Symptoms or Behaviors

When gathering information about symptoms, many questions are required to elicit details and descriptions that assist in the analysis of the data. Discrimination is made in relation to the significance of a symptom, in relation to specific diseases or problems, and in relation to potential follow-up examination or referral. One rationale may be provided for a group of questions in this category.

The following questions refer to specific symptoms and behaviors associated with the cardiovascular system. For each symptom, questions and follow-up are required. The details to be elicited are the characteristics of the symptom; the onset, duration, and frequency of the symptom; the treatment or remedy for the symptom, including over-the-counter and home remedies; the determination if diagnosis has been sought; the effect of treatments; and family history associated with a symptom or illness.

Focused Interview Questions	**Rationales and Evidence**

Questions Related to Symptoms

1. **Have you experienced any symptoms that may suggest the presence of cardiovascular disease: activity intolerance, loss of appetite, bloody sputum (mucus), changes in sexual activities or performance, confusion or difficulty with thinking or concentrating, chest discomfort, coughing, dizziness, dyspnea (difficulty breathing), fatigue, fever, hoarseness, frequent urination at night, leg pains after activity, sleeping pattern alteration, syncope (fainting), palpitations, or swelling?**

   ▶ For any of these symptoms, the nurse should gather objective information on the specific characteristics and ask patients to describe their own subjective experience. If the nurse prompts the patient, valuable clues may be missed.

2. **Does a change in position increase, decrease, or do nothing to change the symptoms?**
   - Can you identify precipitating factors for the symptoms?

   ▶ The nurse should look for activity, emotion, stress, or drugs as a precipitating factor. However, heart symptoms may have no precipitating factors (Cleveland Clinic, n.d.).

3. **Describe the quality of the symptom.**
   - Does it feel sharp, dull, or like pressure, piercing, or ripping?

   ▶ The description of the quality offers clues to the potential origin of the disease, especially when chest discomfort is present.

4. **Does the feeling radiate to other parts of the body?**

   ▶ Radiation of pain may occur with chest discomfort.

5. **Where do you feel the symptom on the body?**

   ▶ If the symptom or one of the symptoms is chest discomfort, the patient should be asked to show the nurse the location on the body. Often, the patient identifies chest discomfort of cardiac origin by placing a clenched fist over the precordium. When the patient points one or more fingers to a limited area on the chest wall, it is generally more indicative of pain of a pulmonary or muscular origin. Females may experience less severe cardiac pain over the precordium, back pain, or fatigue. Angina pectoris, oppressive chest pain caused by decreased oxygenation of the myocardium, is typical in patients with coronary artery disease. Females with angina often experience "atypical" symptoms including burning or tenderness to touch in the back, shoulder, or jaw and may have no chest discomfort (Mayo Clinic, 2013). In MI, the loss of myocardium due to coronary artery occlusion produces the following typical symptoms in males: prolonged, dull chest pain radiating to the shoulder or jaw accompanied by diaphoresis; shortness of breath; and nausea. Females may experience nausea and vomiting, indigestion, shortness of breath or extreme fatigue, with no chest pain (Mayo Clinic, 2013).

6. **What relieves the symptoms?**

7. **Rate the severity of the symptoms on a scale of 0 to 10, with 1 being hardly noticeable and 10 being the worst discomfort you have ever experienced.**
   - What is the timing of the symptoms?
   - Is the timing predictable?
   - What is the duration of the symptoms?
   - Is it constant during that time or does it wax and wane?
   - Are the symptoms isolated or do they occur in combinations?
   - Have you seen your healthcare provider about these symptoms?
   - What is being done for these symptoms?

   ▶ This technique leaves the nurse's opinion on the degree of discomfort out of the picture.

Focused Interview Questions	Rationales and Evidence

Questions Related to Behaviors

1. Describe your diet.
- What types of food do you eat? How often? How much?

▶ Diet is one of the key interventions that a patient can control when working to minimize the effects of aging, slow the progression of disease, or maintain optimum health while experiencing cardiac disease (AHA, 2014a). Supplementing the diet with vitamins under proper supervision may be beneficial. Unfortunately, without proper supervision, the patient who is poorly informed may ingest an unbalanced proportion of supplements and compromise a healthy state. The nurse must be alert if the patient has been dieting to reduce weight. Many diets deplete valuable electrolytes and subject the patient to potential complications. Muscle wasting may occur if the diet is deficient in protein. Lack of protein may compromise cardiac function (Osborn, Wraa, Watson, & Holleran, 2013).

2. Do you keep track of the amount of fat, protein, and carbohydrates you eat?

3. Do you know the difference between saturated and unsaturated fat?
- How much daily fiber do you consume?

4. Do you add salt or other flavor enhancers to your food? If so, how much and how often?
- Do you taste the food before adding these flavor enhancers?

▶ Awareness of nutrient intake will help determine if the patient needs to alter their diet to include healthier foods. Knowledge of proper nutrition, the difference between types of fats, and the harmful effects of too much salt will determine how much patient education is needed in the area of nutrition. The nurse may need to refer the patient to a nutrition specialist or dietitian.

5. Do you eat differently when you travel, when at social functions, when under stress, or when on vacation?

6. Have you tried to lose weight? If so, describe type of diet, duration of diet, and diet supplements you take.
- Do you diet under the care of a healthcare provider?
- Do you supplement your diet with vitamins, protein supplements, or antioxidants?
- Do you use weight-loss supplements or medications?
- What type of nonalcoholic liquids do you drink? How much, and how often?
- Do you exercise to lose weight?

7. Do you smoke or are you frequently exposed to secondhand smoke?
- If you smoke, what type of product (cigarette, cigar, pipe) do you use?
- How long have you smoked?
- How many packs per day and what brand?
- If you are exposed to secondhand smoke, where and for how long each day?
- Did you ever smoke? When did you quit?

▶ Smoking has been linked to hypertension and is strongly suspected of contributing to injury in the walls of arteries, thus accelerating the development of atherosclerotic plaques. It is believed that the chemical contained in the cigarette smoke injures the inner wall of arterial vessels, thus contributing to the subsequent development of a coronary artery plaque (Talukder et al., 2011).

8. Do you take any drugs such as cocaine?
- If so, describe the type, amount, frequency, and duration of use.
- Do you drink alcohol? If so, describe the type, amount, frequency, and duration of use.

▶ Substance abuse, especially of cocaine, is associated with coronary artery spasm and potential development of ischemia or injury of myocardial tissue (Katikaneni, Akkus, Tandon, & Modi, 2013).

9. Do you exercise? What type of exercise do you perform?
- How many times a week?
- What is the duration of exercise?
- The intensity?
- What is your total exercising time?
- Is the exercise continuous or interspersed with breaks?
- What amount of aerobic exercise versus nonaerobic do you do?
- Do you exercise with a partner or alone? Is the exercise pattern regular or sporadic?
- What is your understanding about the benefits of exercise and the type of exercise selected?
- What was your reason for choosing the specific exercise routines and patterns?

▶ The benefits of exercise are well documented, yet the type, duration, and frequency of the exercise regimen produce variable results. It is important for the patient to have a basic understanding of the benefits of aerobic versus nonaerobic exercise. One is not better than the other, and, ultimately, a blending of routines is invaluable whether the patient is a well-conditioned athlete or an individual trying to stay healthy. Studies suggest that both aerobic exercise and resistance or weight training may increase high-density lipoprotein (HDL) levels in adults (Johns Hopkins Medicine, 2009).

Focused Interview Questions	**Rationales and Evidence**

- Is your exercise tolerance increasing, staying the same, or decreasing?
- If it is decreasing, how has the tolerance decreased?
- What were you able to do before versus now?
- How rapidly has this change occurred?
- What symptoms contribute to the decreased tolerance?
- Do you know the causes of the decreased tolerance?

Questions Related to Age

The focused interview must reflect the anatomic and physiologic differences that exist along the age span. The following questions are examples of those that would be specific for children, the pregnant female, and the older adult.

Questions Regarding Infants and Children

1. **What was the pregnancy with this child like?**
   - During pregnancy, did you have any complications such as fever? If so, what were they?
   - What was done about them?
   - How was the infant affected?
   - How were the infant's complications treated?
   - Have the interventions helped?

   ▶ Complications during pregnancy may contribute to malformation in the infant or child.

2. **Did you smoke, take drugs, or drink alcohol during pregnancy? If so, describe the substance, frequency, and amount.**
   - Did you take the substance early in pregnancy?
   - Did you take it right up to delivery?

   ▶ Smoking, consuming alcohol, and using recreational drugs such as cocaine may adversely affect fetal cardiovascular development, especially in the first trimester (Schmid et al., 2010).

3. **What is the child's energy level?**
   - Is the child easily fatigued?
   - Does the child's nap seem to be longer than you would expect?

   ▶ Reduced energy levels and easy fatigability may suggest underlying cardiovascular abnormalities, such as atrial septal defect and large ventricular septal defect (Cleveland Clinic, 2011; Cleveland Clinic, 2012).

4. **Does the infant take a long time to feed?**
   - Does the infant seem tired after eating?
   - Does the child ever become short of breath? If so, what causes it?

   ▶ Fatigue can be related to congenital heart disease. It is especially noticeable during feeding (Roman, 2011).

5. **Does the infant or child favor squatting rather than sitting up straight?**

   ▶ The infant or child will squat when short of breath. It is currently believed that the squatting position decreases venous return to the right atrium from the legs (Guntheroth, Mortan, Mullins, & Baum, 1968).

6. **Does the child have symptoms of joint pain, headaches, fever, or respiratory infections?**

   ▶ Rheumatic fever may follow a respiratory infection with group A beta-hemolytic *Streptococcus pyogenes* (strep throat) and produce symptoms of fever, swollen and painful joints, and headaches (Borchardt, 2013).

7. **Do you feel that the infant or child is gaining weight and growing normally?**

   ▶ Failure to grow is associated with congenital heart disease, such as ventricular septal defect.

Questions for the Pregnant Female

1. **Do you have any history of heart disease?**

   ▶ The changes of pregnancy can place the patient with preexisting heart disease at risk.

2. **Has hypertension been apparent during this pregnancy?**
   - Is there a history of hypertension?

   ▶ Hypertension is a symptom of preeclampsia and places the mother and infant at risk (Rosser & Katz, 2013).

Focused Interview Questions	Rationales and Evidence
3. **Have you observed any swelling in your face and hands?** ● Have you experienced headaches or dizziness?	► Swelling can indicate a preeclamptic condition. Headaches and dizziness are associated with hypertension and preeclampsia. Preeclampsia can also be accompanied by chest pain, visual changes, and abdominal pain (Pennington, Schlitt, Jackson, Schulz, & Schust, 2012).

Questions for the Older Adult

All of the questions listed in the general section can offer significant data. In addition to the routine questions, the nurse should ask the following ones.

1. **Have you noticed any change—no matter how subtle—in your ability to concentrate, to remember things, or to perform simple mental tasks such as writing a letter or balancing your checkbook?**	► In the older adult, a change in mentation suggests inadequate perfusion and can be seen in patients with myocardial ischemia and infarction or increasingly severe congestive heart failure (Berman & Snyder, 2012).
2. **Have you experienced reactions to any medications you are currently taking? These may include palpitations, rashes, vision changes, mentation changes, fatigue, or loss of previous sexual desire or function.**	► Many cardiovascular medications interact with medications for other diseases and may either potentiate or reduce their effects (Wilson, Shannon, & Shields, 2013).

Questions Related to the Environment

Environment refers to both the internal and external environments. Questions related to the internal environment include all of the previous questions and those associated with internal or physiologic responses. Questions regarding the external environment include those related to home, work, or social environments.

Internal Environment

1. **What medications do you take?** ● Are they prescribed or self-ordered? ● What are the dose and brand of each medication? ● How often do you take them?	► It is important to assess the patient's knowledge, compliance, and ability to administer medication accurately, whether ordered by a physician or not. Medication actions may vary depending on the mix of medications; diet; and vitamins, herbs, or dietary supplements.

2. **Why do you take these drugs?**

3. **Do you take these medications as prescribed?**
   ● If you miss a dose, do you double up the next time?

4. **Who ordered these medications?**
   ● If more than one person, does each know what the others have ordered?

5. **Do you know how the medications you are taking react with each other?**

6. **Do you know the side effects of the medications?**

7. **Are you experiencing any side effects that you think might be related to medications?**

Focused Interview Questions	Rationales and Evidence
8. How would you describe your personality? • How many hours do you work in a typical week? Do you work on weekends? • What do you do to unwind? • Describe the major stressors in your life. • What do you do to relieve stress?	▶ Having a type D (distressed) personality is often associated with heart disease (O'Dell, Masters, Spielmans, & Maisto, 2011). It is not so much the behaviors, but the effect of constant sympathetic stimulation on the cardiovascular system and the constant stress and drain on the rejuvenation process after a stressful event that may contribute to decompensation and vulnerability to disease processes. Excessive stress, no matter what the patient's personality type, is a risk factor for cardiovascular disease (AHA, 2014b).
The nurse should ask female patients the following questions. **1. Do you take oral contraceptives?**	▶ The risk of developing cardiovascular disease significantly increases in the female patient over 35 who smokes and takes oral contraceptives containing high doses of synthetic estrogen and progesterone (University of Maryland Medical Center [UMMC], 2013).
2. Are you still menstruating? • If not, at what age did menopause start? • Did you have a hysterectomy? • Were your ovaries removed?	▶ The earlier that menopause starts, the greater the risk for development of heart disease. Coronary artery disease may be increased eightfold in the patient who has had her ovaries removed before menopause (Lokkegaard et al., 2006).

External Environment

The following questions deal with substances and irritants found in the physical environment of the patient. That includes the indoor and outdoor environments of the home and the workplace, those encountered for social engagements, and any encountered during travel.

1. What is your present occupation? • What is your work environment like?	▶ Jobs with long hours, stress, deadlines, and tension are thought to contribute to the development of cardiovascular disease (Backe, Seidler, Latza, Rossnagel, & Schumann, 2012).
2. What were your previous occupations?	
3. Have you been exposed to passive smoking in your environment?	▶ Inhalation of secondhand cigarette smoke in a closed environment is currently thought to contribute to the development of coronary artery plaque (Peinemann et al., 2011).
4. Have you been exposed to chemicals or other hazardous substances?	▶ Such exposure may correlate to stress, alterations in eating habits and exercise habits, recreational drug use, and alterations in sleep patterns.

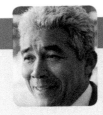

Patient-Centered Interaction

Mr. Ameen Abo-Hamzy reports to the office of his internist for his yearly physical examination. He is 53 years old and has worked for the same company for 22 years. At this time, he is part of the management team and is concerned regarding company layoffs and general downsizing. He tells the nurse, "I feel fine. I think I'm in good health. I have an occasional gas bubble or pressure right here [pointing to the xiphoid process on his chest] and then I can sometimes feel my heart beat real fast." The following is an excerpt from the focused interview with Mr. Abo-Hamzy:

Interview

Nurse: Good morning, Mr. Abo-Hamzy. I see from the record you were last here a year ago for your physical.

Mr. Abo-Hamzy: Yes, that is right.

Nurse: Let's talk about your state of health.

Mr. Abo-Hamzy: I consider myself a really healthy person. I haven't missed a day of work all year. I never got a cold when everybody at work seemed to catch one this past winter. It is just the pressure that I get right here.

Again, Mr. Abo-Hamzy points to the xiphoid process on his chest.

Nurse: Tell me more about this pressure.

Mr. Abo-Hamzy: It is just here, and not all the time.

Nurse: Does the pressure get worse before or after you eat?

Mr. Abo-Hamzy: I have not noticed any change when I eat.

Nurse: When do you notice the change?

Mr. Abo-Hamzy: I'm usually at work. I can always count on the pressure starting either during or after our management meetings.

Nurse: Do you find work stressful these days?

Mr. Abo-Hamzy: I guess you could call it that. Somebody is always getting a pink slip. You know, being let go. I don't know what I will do if it happens to me. I have a family, a mortgage, and I carry the health insurance for all of us. My wife tells me I worry too much.

Nurse: And you? Do you think you worry too much?

Analysis

Throughout the interview the nurse used open-ended and closed questions to collect detailed subjective data from Mr. Abo-Hamzy. The patient mentioned subxiphoid pressure several times. The nurse picked up on this cue, sought clarification, ruled out gastrointestinal involvement, and ascertained the source of the pressure as being stress related before discussing another concern. The nurse used open-ended statements, allowing Mr. Abo-Hamzy to discuss pertinent information about his chest discomfort. The nurse stayed with one topic before directing the response to another area of concern.

Patient Education

The following are physiologic, behavioral, and cultural factors that affect cardiovascular health across the age span. Several of these factors are cited as trends in *Healthy People 2020* documents. The nurse provides advice and education in order to reduce risks associated with these factors and to promote and maintain cardiovascular health.

LIFESPAN CONSIDERATIONS

Risk Factors	Patient Education
• Congenital heart defects occur in 1 out of every 125 to 150 infants born in the United States.	▶ Support and provide education for parents of infants with congenital defects as they make decisions about surgical and other treatments for those problems.

LIFESPAN CONSIDERATIONS

Risk Factors	Patient Education
	▶ Educate pregnant females about the role of disease, medication, and personal habits in the development of congenital heart defects. Pregnant females who have not had or been immunized against rubella must avoid contraction of the virus during the first trimester of pregnancy. The use of Accutane, lithium, and some antiseizure medications may increase the risk of congenital heart defects. Females who are planning to become pregnant must discuss the use of medications with their healthcare provider. Alcohol and cocaine have been linked with congenital heart defects, and advice about avoiding these substances during pregnancy is warranted. Females with diabetes mellitus have an increased risk of having a child with a heart defect. Careful regulation of the diabetes before and in early pregnancy can reduce the risk.
● Rheumatic fever can result in cardiac problems. Though uncommon in the United States, it occurs with the greatest frequency in school-age children. It is caused by untreated strep infection.	▶ Parents of school-age children need to be advised to seek health care for pharyngeal infections. Untreated strep throat can result in rheumatic fever.
● The incidence of cardiovascular disease increases with aging. Almost 80% of patients with coronary artery disease are 65 years of age or older.	▶ Encourage older adults to participate in regular screening for risks associated with cardiovascular disease. Explain the association of age-related changes with cardiovascular health.

CULTURAL CONSIDERATIONS

Risk Factors	Patient Education
● Hypertension is a risk factor for coronary artery disease. Hypertension occurs more frequently in African Americans and Hispanics than in other groups.	▶ Tell patients that hypertension is often referred to as the "silent killer" because it is asymptomatic in most individuals (Cleveland Clinic, n.d.). Patients need to participate in blood pressure screening, especially African Americans and Hispanics, who are at greater risk. ▶ Advise patients with a diagnosis of hypertension to be monitored regularly and to take medication as prescribed to decrease risks associated with hypertension.
● Obesity contributes to cardiovascular disease. Obesity is increasing in all age groups in the United States but occurs most frequently in Hispanic females and African American children.	▶ Provide information about diet to maintain healthy body weight and body fat percentage to patients of all ages. For obese patients, provide recommendations for weight reduction and exercise.
● Diabetes increases the risk of cardiovascular disease. The incidence of diabetes is highest in Native Americans, Hispanics, and African Americans.	▶ Provide education about diet and exercise to assist patients with diabetes to avoid the risks for cardiovascular disease.

ENVIRONMENTAL CONSIDERATIONS

Risk Factors	Patient Education
• Family history of heart disease increases the risk for developing cardiovascular disease.	▶ Provide patients who have a family history of heart disease with information about regular examinations, and encourage them to develop habits to avoid the risks. ▶ Refer patients to the American Heart Association for information and tips about heart disease and ways to reduce risks.
• Elevated cholesterol and triglyceride levels increase the risk for development of cardiovascular disease.	▶ Encourage patients to have cholesterol and triglyceride screening, explain the significance of elevated levels as risks for heart disease, educate patients about dietary habits to reduce cholesterol, and explain how to interpret the laboratory results.
• Stress is associated with the development of cardiovascular disease.	▶ Support patients in stressful events and provide information about stress reduction techniques as methods to reduce risks for cardiovascular disease.

BEHAVIORAL CONSIDERATIONS

Risk Factors	Patient Education
• Smoking is a risk factor in development of cardiovascular disease. Smokers have double the mortality rate from MI than nonsmokers.	▶ Participate in education to prevent smoking and assist patients who are looking for ways to stop smoking.
• Lack of physical activity increases the risk for developing diseases that predispose one to cardiovascular disease such as diabetes, obesity, and hypertension.	▶ Encourage regular exercise in patients of all ages. Exercise can reduce the risks for cardiovascular disease by promoting healthy weight, maintaining healthy blood pressure, and reducing the risk for development of diabetes.

Physical Assessment

Assessment Techniques and Findings

Physical assessment of the cardiovascular system requires the use of inspection, palpation, percussion, and auscultation. During each of the procedures, the nurse is gathering objective data related to the function of the heart as determined by the heart rate and the quality and characteristics of the heart sounds. In addition, the nurse observes for signs of appropriate cardiac function in relation to oxygen perfusion by assessing skin color and temperature, abnormal pulsations, and the characteristics of the patient's respiratory effort. Knowledge of normal parameters and expected findings is essential in determining the meaning of the data during a physical health assessment.

Skin is uniform in color on the face, trunk, and extremities. The eyes are symmetric. The periorbital area is flat, and the eyes do not bulge. The sclera of the eye should be white, the cornea clear, and the conjunctiva pink. The lips should be smooth and noncyanotic.

EQUIPMENT
- examination gown
- metric rulers
- examination drape
- stethoscope with bell and diaphragm
- Doppler stethoscope
- lamp

The head should be steady and the skull proportional to the face. The earlobes should be smooth and without creases. The jugular veins are not visible when the chest is upright. Further, the jugular veins distend only 3 cm (1.18 in.) above the sternal angle when the patient is at a 45-degree angle. Carotid pulsations are visible bilaterally. The fingers should be round and even with flat pink nails. The respiratory pattern is even, regular, and unlabored. ICSs and clavicles are visible; chest veins are evenly distributed and flat; and no bulges or masses are visible. Pulsations over the pericardium are absent; however, aortic pulsations in the epigastric area are visible in thin patients. The lower extremities are of uniform color and temperature with even hair distribution. The skeleton should be free of deformity and the neck and extremities in proportion to the torso. Palpation over the pericardium reveals slight vibration at the apical area only. Carotid pulses are palpable and equal in intensity. Dullness to percussion should extend to the MCL at the fifth ICS. S2 is louder than S1 at the aortic and pulmonic auscultatory areas. S1 and S2 are heard equally at Erb's point (third left ICS). S1 is louder than S2 at the tricuspid and apical areas. Murmurs are absent. The carotid pulse is synchronous with the apical pulse.

The thinner chest wall of children causes heart sounds to seem louder. Infants have a point of maximal impulse (PMI) that is difficult to assess and is located approximately one intercostal space higher than in adults. An S2 split with inspiration may be detected in children under the age of 6. The physiologic S2 split disappears with expiration. Any S2 split that persists throughout the cardiac cycle merits further evaluation. Preadolescents may have a physiologic S3 gallop that results from vibrations during rapid ventricular filling. Seventy percent of children will have a detectable innocent, or functional, murmur sometime during childhood. Any condition that increases metabolism, like fever or anemia, will make innocent murmurs more pronounced. By definition, **innocent murmurs** arise from increased blood flow across normal heart structures. Heart murmurs are graded using a scale of 1 to 6. A higher rating is reflective of greater intensity (loudness). For example, a grade 1/6 murmur is very soft and barely audible, while a grade 6/6 murmur is very loud (AHA, 2013). All innocent murmurs have the following characteristics: they are grades 1–2/6 in intensity, are systolic (with the exception of the venous hum), and are not associated with thrills or other cardiac symptoms.

Physical assessment of the cardiovascular system follows an organized pattern. It begins with inspection of the patient's head and neck, including the eyes, ears, lips, face, skull, and neck vessels. The upper extremities, chest, abdomen, and lower extremities are also inspected. Palpation includes the precordium and carotid pulses. Percussion of the chest is conducted to determine the cardiac borders. Auscultation includes the heart in five areas with the diaphragm and the bell of the stethoscope. The carotid arteries and the apical pulse are auscultated.

HELPFUL HINTS

- Provide specific instructions throughout the assessment. Explain what is expected of the patient and state that he or she will be able to breathe regularly throughout the assessment.
- Assessment of the heart will require several position changes. The nurse should assist the patient, if necessary; allow time for movement if the patient is uncomfortable; and explain the purpose of the position changes.
- The nurse's hands and the stethoscope should be warmed before beginning the assessment.
- The room should be quiet so that subtle sounds may be heard.
- Provide adequate draping to prevent unnecessary exposure of the female breasts.
- Use Standard Precautions.

Techniques and Normal Findings	Abnormal Findings Special Considerations

Inspection

1. **Instruct the patient.**
   - Explain that you will be looking at the head, neck, and extremities to provide clues to cardiac function.
   - Explain that you will ask the patient to sit up and lie down as part of the examination and that you will provide specific instructions and assistance as required throughout the examination. Explain that you will be touching the neck and chest as well as tapping on the chest and listening with the stethoscope. Tell the patient that none of the procedures should cause discomfort but assure the patient that you will stop any time if discomfort occurs or the examination is causing fatigue.

Techniques and Normal Findings	Abnormal Findings Special Considerations

2. Position the patient.

- Begin the examination with the patient seated upright with the chest exposed (see Figure 19.15 ■).

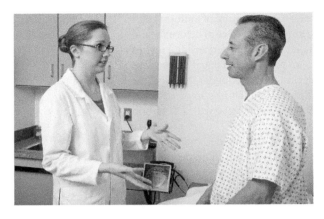

Figure 19.15
Begin the exam by having the patient sit upright.

3. Inspect the patient's face, lips, ears, and scalp.

- These structures can provide valuable clues to the patient's cardiovascular health. Begin with the facial skin. The skin color should be uniform.

▶ Flushed skin may indicate rheumatic heart disease or presence of a fever. Grayish undertones are often seen in patients with coronary artery disease or those in shock. A ruddy color may indicate *polycythemia*, a condition in which there is a significantly increased number of red blood cells, or *Cushing's syndrome*, a hormonal disorder caused by prolonged exposure of the tissues of the body to cortisol, a product of the adrenal glands.

- Examine the eyes and the tissue surrounding the eyes (periorbital area). The eyes should be uniform and not have a protruding appearance.

▶ Protruding eyes are seen in *hyperthyroidism*. In hyperthyroidism, excessive hormone secretion results in high cardiac output, a tendency toward tachycardia (rapid heart rate), and potential for congestive heart failure.

- The periorbital area should be relatively flat. No puffiness should be present.

▶ Periorbital puffiness may result from fluid retention (edema).

- The sclera should be whitish in color. The cornea should be without an *arcus*, which is a ringlike structure.

▶ A blue color in the sclera is often associated with *Marfan syndrome*, a degenerative disease of the connective tissue, which over time may cause the ascending aorta to either dilate or dissect, leading to abrupt death. An arcus in a young person may indicate hypercholesterolemia; however, in people of African descent or in adults over age 60 it may be normal.

- The conjunctiva should be clear, while underlying tissue is pinkish in color. The eyelid should be smooth. For information on how to examine the conjunctiva, see chapter 15. ∞

▶ **Xanthelasma** are yellowish cholesterol deposits seen on the eyelids and are indicative of premature atherosclerosis.

- Inspect the lips. They should be uniform in color without any underlying tinge of blueness. The buccal mucosa, gums, and tongue are also inspected for cyanosis.

▶ Blue-tinged lips may indicate cyanosis, which is often a late sign of inadequate tissue perfusion.

- Assess the general appearance of the face. It should be symmetric with uniform contours.

▶ Patients with *Down syndrome* may exhibit a large protruding tongue, low-set ears, and an underdeveloped mandible. Children with Down syndrome often have congenital heart disease. Wide-set eyes may be seen in a child with *Noonan's syndrome*, which is accompanied by pulmonic stenosis (narrowing).

Techniques and Normal Findings	Abnormal Findings Special Considerations

- Examine the head. Look first for the ability of the patient to hold the head steady. Rhythmic head bobbing should not be present.

▶ Head bobbing up and down in synchrony with the heartbeat is characteristic of severe aortic regurgitation. This bobbing is created by the pulsatile waves of regurgitated blood, which reverberate upward toward the head.

- Assess the structure of the skull and the proportion of the skull to the face.

▶ A protruding skull is seen in *Paget's disease*, a rare bone disease characterized by localized loss of calcium from the bone and replacement with a porous bone formation, which leads to distorted, thickened contours. Paget's disease is also characterized by a high cardiac output, which may lead to heart failure.

4. **Inspect the jugular veins.**
   - Examination of the jugular veins can provide essential information about the patient's central venous pressure and the heart's pumping efficiency.
   - With the patient sitting upright, adjust the gooseneck lamp to cast shadows on the patient's neck. Tangential lighting is effective in visualizing the jugular vessels.
   - Be sure that the patient's head is turned slightly away from the side you are examining. Look for the external and internal jugular veins.
   - Note that the jugular veins are not normally visible when the patient sits upright. The external jugular vein is located over the sternocleidomastoid muscle. The internal jugular vein, which is the best indicator of central venous pressure, is located behind this muscle, medial to the external jugular and lateral to the carotid artery.

   - If you are able to visualize the jugular veins, measure their distance superior to the clavicle. (Be sure not to confuse the carotid pulse with pulsations of the jugular veins.) The carotid pulse is lateral to the trachea. If jugular vein pulsations are visible, palpate the patient's radial pulse and determine whether the jugular vein pulsations coincide with the palpated radial pulse.

   ▶ Obvious pulsations that are present during both inspiration and expiration and coincide with the arterial pulse are commonly seen with severe congestive heart failure.

   - Next, have the patient lie at a 45-degree angle if the patient can tolerate this position without pain and is able to breathe comfortably.
   - Place the first of the metric rulers vertically at the angle of Louis. Place the second metric ruler horizontally at a 90-degree angle to the first ruler. One end of this ruler should be at the angle of Louis and the other end in the jugular area on the lateral aspect of the neck (see Figure 19.16 ■).

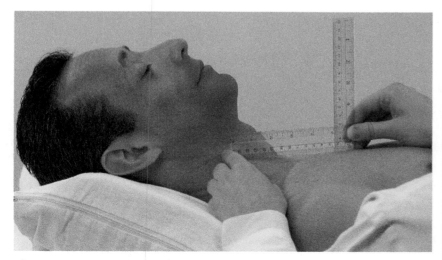

Figure 19.16 Assessment of central venous pressure.

Techniques and Normal Findings	Abnormal Findings Special Considerations

- Inspect the neck for distention of the jugular veins. Raise the lateral portion of the horizontal ruler until it is at the top of the height of the distention and assess the height in centimeters of the elevation from the vertical ruler.
- The jugular veins normally distend only 3 cm (1.18 in.) above the sternal angle when the patient is lying at a 45-degree angle (see Figure 19.16). You need to measure the distention only on one side.

▶ Distention of the neck veins indicates elevation of central venous pressure commonly seen with congestive heart failure, fluid overload, or pressure on the superior vena cava.

5. **Inspect the carotid arteries.**
   - The carotid arteries are located lateral to the patient's trachea in a groove that is medial to the sternocleidomastoid muscle.

   - With the patient still lying at a 45-degree angle, using tangential lighting, inspect the carotid arteries for pulsations. Pulsations should be visible bilaterally. Carotid pulsations may be difficult to assess in the obese patient because of the thick neck and because breathing difficulties require an upright position.

   - When you finish, help the patient back to an upright sitting position.

▶ Bounding pulses are not normal findings and may indicate fever. The absence of a pulsation may indicate an obstruction either internal or external to the artery.

6. **Inspect the patient's hands and fingers.**
   - Help the patient to resume a sitting position. Confirm that the fingertips are rounded and even. The fingernails should be relatively pink, with white crescents at the base of each nail.

▶ Fingertips and nails that are clubbed bilaterally are characteristic of congenital heart disease. Clubbing may be associated with many respiratory and cardiac disorders. Thin red lines or splinter hemorrhages in the nail beds are associated with **infective endocarditis** (see Figure 19.17 ■), a condition caused by bacterial infiltration of the lining of the heart's chambers.

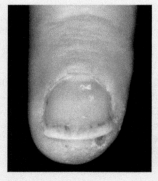

Figure 19.17 Splinter hemorrhage.
Source: Dr. P. Marazzi/Science Source.

▶ Fingernails and tips may be stained yellow when the patient is a smoker. Smoking is one of the main contributors to the development of atherosclerosis.

7. **Inspect the patient's chest.**
   - Observe the respiratory pattern, which should be even, regular, and unlabored, with no retractions.

   - Observe the veins on the chest, which should be evenly distributed and relatively flat.

   - Inspect the entire chest for bulges and masses. The ICSs and clavicles should be even.

▶ Respiratory distress may be precipitated by various disorders. Pulmonary edema is often a severe complication of cardiovascular disease.

▶ Dilated, distended veins on the chest indicate an obstructive process, as seen with obstruction of the superior vena cava.

▶ Bulges are abnormal and may indicate obstructions or aneurysms. Masses may indicate obstructions or presence of tumors.

Techniques and Normal Findings	Abnormal Findings Special Considerations

- Inspect the entire chest for pulsations. Observe the patient first in an upright position and then at a 30-degree angle, which is a low- to mid-Fowler's position. In particular, observe for pulsations over the five key landmarks (see Figure 19.18 ■).

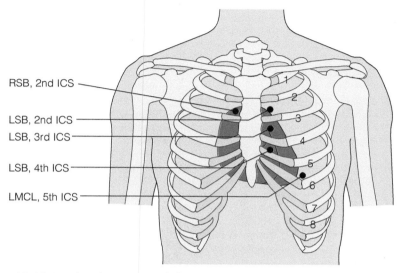

RSB, 2nd ICS

LSB, 2nd ICS
LSB, 3rd ICS

LSB, 4th ICS

LMCL, 5th ICS

Figure 19.18 Landmarks in precordial assessments.

- Start by observing the RSB, second ICS. Next, observe the LSB, second ICS. The angle of Louis can be used to mark the second ICS.

- Then observe the LSB, third to fifth ICS.
  - Move on to the apex: fifth ICS, MCL.
  - Finish with the epigastric area below the xiphoid process.

- Confirm that the apical impulse/*point of maximum impulse* (PMI) is located at the fifth ICS in the left MCL.

- Inspect the entire chest for heaves or lifts while the patient is sitting upright and again with the patient at a 30-degree angle.

- *Heaves* or *lifts* are forceful risings of the landmark area.
- In particular, make sure you observe over the five key landmarks previously listed.

8. **Inspect the patient's abdomen.**
   - Have the patient lie flat, if possible.
     - Be mindful of any discomfort or difficulty in breathing, particularly in the obese patient.

   - Look for pulsations in the abdominal area over the areas where the major arteries are located. These sites include:
     - The *aorta*, which is located superior to the umbilicus to the left of the midline.
     - The *left renal artery*, which is located to the left of the umbilicus in the left upper quadrant.
     - The *right renal artery*, which is located to the right of the umbilicus in the right upper quadrant.
     - The *right iliac artery*, which is located to the right of the umbilicus in the right lower quadrant.
     - The *left iliac artery*, which is located to the left of the umbilicus in the left lower quadrant.

▶ If the entire *precordium* (anterior chest) pulsates and shakes with every heartbeat, extreme valvular regurgitation or shunting (redirection of blood flow that does not follow the normal physiologic pathway) may be present.

▶ Pulsations present in the LSB, second ICS indicate pulmonary artery dilation or excessive blood flow.

▶ Pulsations present in the LSB, third to fifth ICS may indicate right ventricular overload.

▶ If left ventricular hypertrophy is present, the PMI is displaced laterally in the fifth ICS from the LMCL.

▶ A heave or lift found in the LSB, third to fifth ICS may indicate right ventricular hypertrophy or respiratory disease, such as pulmonary hypertension.

▶ Pulsations may be visible in lean patients. These are usually normal if seen in the epigastric area. Peristaltic waves may also be seen in thin individuals. They must not be confused with vascular pulsations. Prominent pulsations that are located in areas outside of the gastric area and are readily visible may be potentially life threatening.
▶ Abnormal pulsations usually indicate the presence of an aortic aneurysm, which is a ballooning due to a weakness in the walls of arteries. These findings require immediate physician referral.

Techniques and Normal Findings	Abnormal Findings Special Considerations

- Chapter 21 of this text reviews abdominal arteries and abdominal quadrants. ∞
- Note the pattern of fat distribution.

▶ Males usually deposit fat in the abdominal area. This distribution pattern is thought to be associated with the development of coronary artery disease. Females usually deposit fat in the buttocks and thighs.

9. **Inspect the patient's legs.**
   - Help the patient to a sitting position.
   - Inspect the legs for skin color. The skin color should be even and uniform.

▶ Patches of lighter color may indicate compromised circulation. Mottling indicates severe hemodynamic compromise.

   - Inspect the legs for hair distribution. The distribution should be even without bare patches devoid of hair.

▶ Patchy hair distribution is often a sign of circulatory compromise that has occurred over time. The patient should be asked if the hair distribution on the legs has changed over time.

10. **Inspect the patient's skeletal structure.**
   - Ask the patient to stand.
   - Observe the skeletal structure, which should be free of deformities.

▶ *Scoliosis* is associated with prolapsed mitral valve.

   - Observe the neck and extremities, which should be in proportion to the torso.

▶ A patient who is tall and thin with an elongated neck and extremities should be evaluated further for the presence of Marfan's syndrome.

Palpation

Palpate the chest in the six areas (see Figure 19.19 ■). Note that palpation may be performed with the patient sitting upright, reclining at a 45-degree or 30-degree angle, or lying flat. Start by palpating with the patient sitting upright and then in the lowest position that the patient can comfortably tolerate.

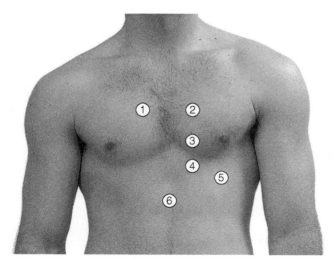

Figure 19.19 Landmarks for palpation of the chest.

1. **Palpate the chest.**
   - Place your right hand over the RSB, second ICS. Palpate with the base of your fingers.
   - You should not feel any pulsation, heave, or vibratory sensation against your palm in this location.

▶ Pulsations or heaves in the RSB, second ICS, indicate the presence of ascending aortic enlargement or aneurysm, aortic stenosis, or systemic hypertension.

Techniques and Normal Findings	Abnormal Findings Special Considerations

- Place your hand on the LSB, second ICS.
- You should not feel any pulsation, heave, or vibratory sensation against your palm in this location except in some very thin patients who are nervous about the examination.

▶ Pulsations or heaves in the LSB, second ICS, are associated with pulmonary hypertension, pulmonary stenosis, right ventricular enlargement, atrial septal defect, enlarged left atrium, and large posterior left ventricular aneurysm.

- Move your hand to the LSB, third then fourth ICS. No pulsations, heaves, or vibratory sensations should be felt.

▶ Pulsations or heaves over the LSB, third or fourth ICS, may indicate right ventricular enlargement or pressure overload on this ventricle, pulmonary stenosis, or pulmonary hypertension.

- Place your right hand over the apex: LMCL, fifth ICS.
- When palpating over the LMCL, fifth ICS, you should feel a soft vibration, a tapping sensation, with each heartbeat. The vibration felt in this location should be isolated to an area no more than 1 cm (0.39 in.) in diameter.

▶ The presence of a heave, which is a forceful thrust over the fifth ICS, LMCL, indicates the potential presence of increased right ventricular stroke volume or pressure and mild-to-moderate aortic regurgitation. If vibration is felt in a downward and lateral position from where the normal PMI should be palpated, or if it can be palpated in an area greater than 1 cm (0.39 in.) in diameter, these conditions may be present: left ventricular hypertrophy, severe left ventricular volume overload, or severe aortic regurgitation.

- Palpate the epigastric area, below the xiphoid process.

▶ The presence of heaves or thrills in the subxiphoid area suggests the presence of elevated right ventricular volume or pressure overload. **Thrills** are soft vibratory sensations best assessed with either the fingertips or the palm flattened on the chest.

- Repeat the palpation technique, with the patient at either a 30-degree angle or lying flat.

ALERT!

Some patients are unable to lie flat. The patient should be placed in the lowest angle that is comfortably tolerated. It is necessary to be alert to any physical distress experienced by the patient during examination and to stop activity immediately if distress is experienced.

- Palpation with the patient lying flat normally reveals either no pulsation or very faint taps in a very localized area. No thrills, heaves, or lifts should be palpated in any of the five locations.

2. **Palpate the patient's carotid pulses.**
   - The carotid artery is located in the groove between the trachea and sternocleidomastoid muscle beneath the angle of the jaw.
   - It is important to palpate carotid pulses to assess their presence, strength, and equality. The patient may remain supine, or you may help the patient to sit upright.

Techniques and Normal Findings	Abnormal Findings Special Considerations

- Ask the patient to look straight ahead and keep the neck straight (see Figure 19.20 ■).

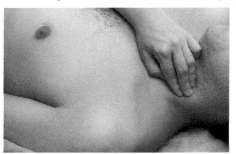

Figure 19.20 Palpating the carotid artery.
Source: Ivan Ivanov/Getty Images.

- Palpate each carotid pulse separately. Normal findings bilaterally should demonstrate equality in intensity and regular pattern. The pulses should be strong but not bounding. If the pulse is difficult to palpate, ask the patient to turn the head slightly to the examining side.

ALERT!

The carotid pulses must never be palpated simultaneously since this may obstruct blood flow to the brain, resulting in severe bradycardia *(slow heart rate) or* asystole *(absent heart rate).*

▶ Diminished or absent carotid pulses may be found in patients with carotid disease or dissecting ascending aneurysm. Absence of both pulses indicates *asystole* (absent heart rate). If the patient is in critical care and has an arterial line, a printout of the arterial waveform should be obtained.

Auscultation

The position of the patient affects objective data collected from auscultatory examination. A full examination includes auscultation with the patient sitting upright, leaning forward when upright, supine, and in the left lateral position. Have the patient breathe normally initially. If you recognize the presence of abnormal sounds, have the patient slow down the respirations so that you may listen to the effects of inspirations and expiratory efforts on the heart sounds. You may want to have some patients perform a forced expiration. When preparing to auscultate a child's chest, you may want to let the child listen to the parent's heart sounds with the stethoscope to reduce or prevent fear of this unfamiliar object. Use a stethoscope with a smaller bell and diaphragm when you examine a child. In obese patients, heart sounds are best heard at the apical area with the patient in the left lateral position and at the aortic and pulmonic areas.

1. **Auscultate the patient's chest with the diaphragm of the stethoscope.**
   - Start the auscultation with the patient sitting upright.
   - Inch the stethoscope slowly across the chest and listen over each of the five key landmarks (see Figure 19.21 ■).
   - Listen over the RSB, second ICS.
   - In this location, the S2 sound should be louder than the S1 sound, because this site is over the aortic valve.
   - Listen over the LSB, second ICS.
   - Also in this location the S2 sound should be louder than the S1 sound, because this site is over the pulmonic valve.
   - Listen over the LSB, third ICS, also called Erb's point.
   - You should hear both the S1 and S2 heart tones, relatively equal in intensity.
   - Listen at the LSB at the fourth ICS.
   - In this location the S1 sound should be louder than the S2 sound, because the closure of the tricuspid valve is best auscultated here.
   - Listen over the apex: fifth ICS, LMCL.
   - In this location the S1 sound should also be louder than the S2 sound, because the closure of the mitral valve is best auscultated here.

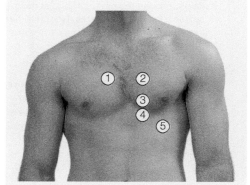

Figure 19.21 Auscultating the chest over five key landmarks.

Techniques and Normal Findings	Abnormal Findings / Special Considerations

2. Auscultate the patient's chest with the bell of the stethoscope.
- Place the bell of the stethoscope lightly on each of the five key landmark positions shown with step 1.

- Listen for softer sounds over the five key landmarks. Start with the bell and listen for the S3 and S4 sounds. Then listen for murmurs.

▶ Low-pitched sounds are best auscultated with light application of the bell. Sounds such as S3, S4, murmurs (originating from stenotic valves), and gallops are best heard with the bell.

3. Auscultate the carotid arteries.
- Listen with the diaphragm and bell of the stethoscope. Have the patient hold the breath briefly. You may hear heart tones. This finding is normal.

- You should not hear any turbulent sounds like murmurs.

▶ A **bruit,** a loud blowing sound, is an abnormal finding. It is most often associated with a narrowing or stricture of the carotid artery usually associated with atherosclerotic plaque.

4. Compare the apical pulse to a carotid pulse.
- Auscultate the apical pulse.

- Simultaneously palpate a carotid pulse.

- Compare the findings. The two pulses should be synchronous. The carotid artery is used because it is closest to the heart and most accessible (see Figure 19.22 ■).

▶ An apical pulse greater than the carotid rate indicates a pulse deficit. The rate, rhythm, and regularity must be evaluated.

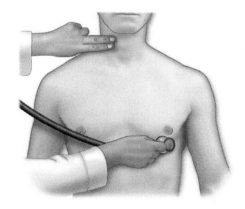

Figure 19.22 Comparing the carotid and apical pulses.

5. Repeat the auscultation of the patient's chest.
- This time have the patient lean forward, then lie supine, and finally lie in the left lateral position. Remember, not all patients will be able to tolerate all positions. In such cases, do not perform the technique (see Figures 19.23 A–C ■).

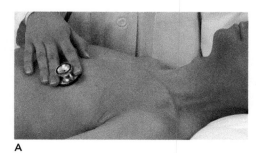

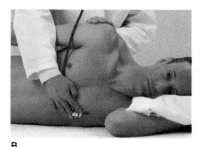

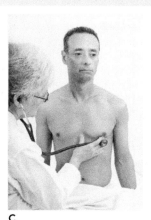

A   B   C

Figure 19.23A Positions for auscultation of the heart. A. Supine, B. Lateral, C. Sitting.

Abnormal Findings

Abnormal findings in the cardiovascular system include murmurs (see Table 19.4 on pages 459–460), diseases of the myocardium and pumping capacity, valvular heart disease, septal defects, congenital heart disease, and electrical rhythm disturbances.

Diseases of the Myocardium and Pumping Capacity of the Heart

MYOCARDIAL ISCHEMIA

Ischemia is a common problem where the oxygen needs of the body are heightened, thus increasing the work of the heart. Unfortunately, the oxygen needs of the heart are not met as it works harder, and an ischemic process ensues. Ischemia is usually due to the presence of an atherosclerotic plaque. A blood clot may be associated with the plaque.

Subjective findings:

- Pain in the chest, neck, jaw, or other region.
- Shortness of breath.
- Nausea.
- Anxiety.

Objective findings:

- Diaphoresis.
- Pallor.
- Vomiting.
- Changes or abnormalities on electrocardiogram (EKG) may or may not be present.

MYOCARDIAL INFARCTION (MI)

During infarction, there is complete disruption of oxygen and nutrient flow to the myocardial tissue in the area below a total occlusion. Infarction leads to the death of the myocardial tissue unless flow of blood is reestablished. MI is caused by ischemia to the cardiac muscle. As such, manifestations associated with myocardial infarction mirror those seen with myocardial ischemia.

Subjective findings:

- Pain in the chest, neck, jaw, or other region.
- Shortness of breath.
- Nausea.
- Anxiety.

Objective findings:

- Diaphoresis.
- Pallor.
- Vomiting.
- Changes or abnormalities on EKG may or may not be present.

Right-sided heart failure causes backup of the blood into the systemic circulation.

Subjective findings:

- Fatigue.
- Weakness.
- Mental confusion.
- Loss of appetite.

Objective findings:

- JVD.
- Hypertension.
- Liver congestion.
- Peripheral edema.

HEART FAILURE

This condition is the inability of the heart to produce a sufficient pumping effort. Most commonly, both left-sided and right-sided heart failure are present.

Left-sided heart failure causes blood to back up into the pulmonary system and results in pulmonary edema.

Subjective findings:

- Dyspnea.
- Shortness of breath.

Objective findings:

- Frothy sputum.
- Adventitious breath sounds, including rhonchi or rales (crackles).
- Decreased oxygen saturation.

VENTRICULAR HYPERTROPHY

Ventricular hypertrophy occurs in response to pumping against high pressures. Right ventricular hypertrophy occurs with pulmonary hypertension, congenital heart disease, pulmonary disease, pulmonary stenosis, and right ventricular infarction.

Left ventricular hypertrophy occurs in the presence of systemic hypertension, congenital heart disease, aortic stenosis, or MI to the left ventricle.

Subjective findings:

- Chest pain.
- Dizziness, especially after activity.
- Shortness of breath.

Objective findings:

- Cardiac dysrhythmias.
- Tachycardia.

Valvular Heart Disease

Disease of the valves denotes either narrowing (stenosis) of the valve leaflets or incompetence (regurgitation) of these same leaflets.

Valvular disease may be caused by rheumatic fever, congenital defects, MI, and normal aging. Common forms of valvular heart disease are described in Table 19.7.

| TABLE 19.7 | Overview of Valvular Heart Disease |

Mitral Stenosis

A narrowing of the left mitral valve.

Etiology: Rheumatic fever or cardiac infection.

Findings: Murmur heard at the apical area with the patient in left lateral position.

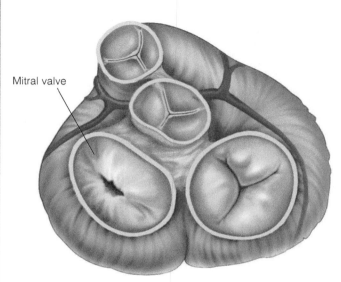

Figure 19.24 Mitral stenosis.

Aortic Stenosis

A narrowing of the aortic valve.

Etiology: Congenital bicuspid valves, rheumatic heart disease, atherosclerosis.

Findings: Murmur at aortic area, RSB, second ICS.

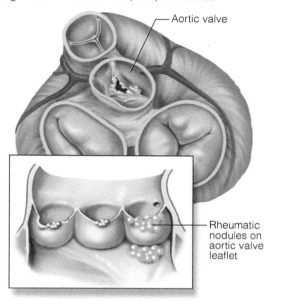

Figure 19.25 Aortic stenosis.

Mitral Regurgitation

The backflow of blood from the left ventricle into the left atrium.

Etiology: Rheumatic fever, MI, rupture of chordae tendineae.

Findings: Murmur at apex. Sound is transmitted to (L) axillae.

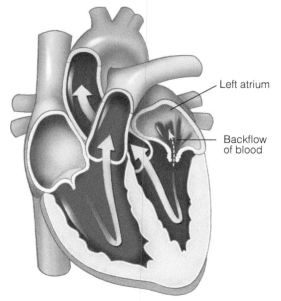

Figure 19.26 Mitral regurgitation.

Pulmonic Stenosis

The narrowing of the opening between the pulmonary artery and the right ventricle.

Etiology: Congenital.

Findings: Murmur at pulmonic area radiates to neck. Thrill in (L) second and third ICS.

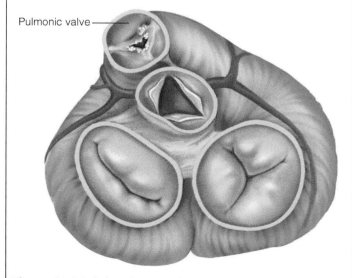

Figure 19.27 Pulmonic stenosis.

TABLE 19.7	Overview of Valvular Heart Disease (continued)

Tricuspid Stenosis

The narrowing or stricture of the tricuspid valve of the heart.

Etiology: Rheumatic heart disease, congenital defect, right atrial myxoma (tumor).

Findings: Murmur heard with the bell of the stethoscope over the tricuspid area.

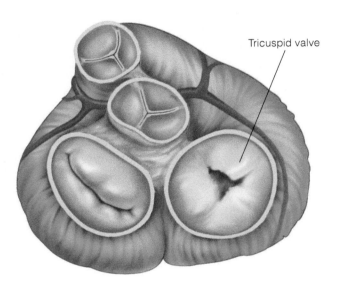

Tricuspid valve

Figure 19.28 Tricuspid stenosis.

Mitral Valve Prolapse

The mitral valve leaflets so they prolapse into the left atrium.

Etiology: May occur with pectus excavatum, often unknown.

Findings: Murmur, nonejection clicks heard (L) lower sternal border in upright position.

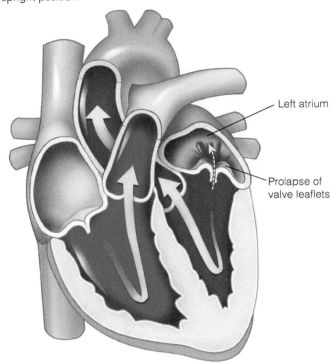

Left atrium

Prolapse of valve leaflets

Figure 19.29 Mitral valve prolapse.

Aortic Regurgitation

The backflow of blood from the aorta into the left ventricle.

Etiology: Rheumatic heart disease, endocarditis, Marfan's syndrome, syphilis.

Findings: Murmur with patient leaning forward. Click in second ICS.

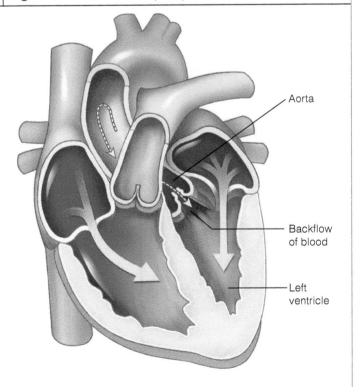

Aorta

Backflow of blood

Left ventricle

Figure 19.30 Aortic regurgitation.

Septal Defects

An atrial septal defect is an opening between the right and left atria, whereas a ventricular septal defect is an opening between the right and left ventricles. Both of these septal defects may result from congenital heart disease and MI. The two primary septal defects are described in Table 19.8.

TABLE 19.8	**Overview of Septal Defects**

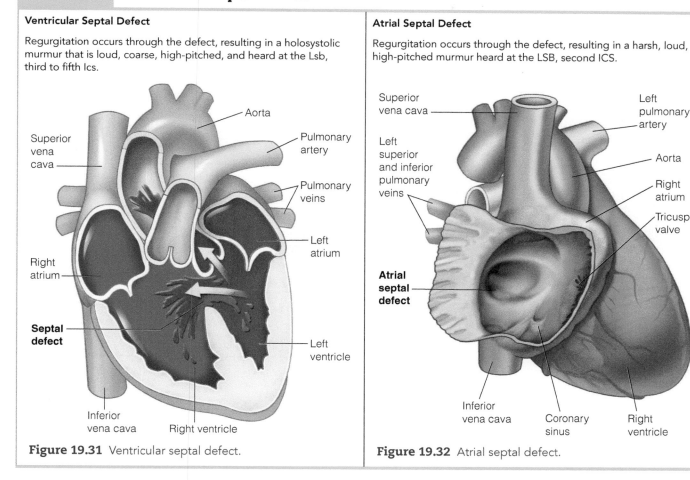

Ventricular Septal Defect

Regurgitation occurs through the defect, resulting in a holosystolic murmur that is loud, coarse, high-pitched, and heard at the Lsb, third to fifth Ics.

Figure 19.31 Ventricular septal defect.

Atrial Septal Defect

Regurgitation occurs through the defect, resulting in a harsh, loud, high-pitched murmur heard at the LSB, second ICS.

Figure 19.32 Atrial septal defect.

Congenital Heart Disease

There are many forms of congenital heart disease, which is related to developmental defects. Most often valves and septal structures are affected. An overview of congenital heart disorders is provided in Table 19.9.

TABLE 19.9	**Overview of Congenital Heart Disorders**

Coarctation of the Aorta

The aorta is severely narrowed in the region inferior to the left subclavian artery. The narrowing restricts blood flow from the left ventricle into the aorta and out into the systemic circulation, thus contributing to the development of congestive heart failure in the newborn. It can be surgically treated.

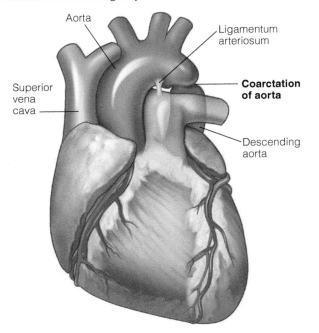

Figure 19.33 Coarctation of the aorta.

Patent Ductus Arteriosus

Occurs when the ductus arteriosus fails to close completely between 24 and 48 hours after delivery. It may be treated medically, through pharmacologic therapy, and surgically.

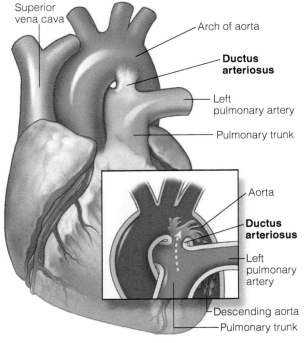

Figure 19.34 Patent ductus arteriosus.

Tetralogy of Fallot

Involves four cardiac defects: dextroposition of the aorta, pulmonary stenosis, right ventricular hypertrophy, and ventricular septal defect. This condition is life threatening for the newborn but can be treated surgically.

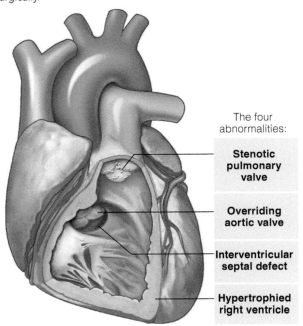

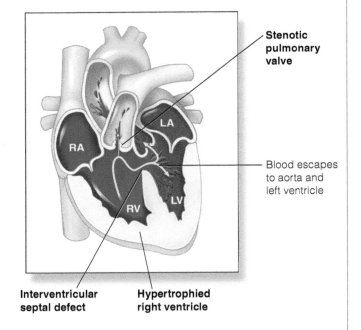

Figure 19.35 Tetralogy of Fallot.

Electrical Rhythm Disturbances

Rhythm disturbances are a common occurrence. Lethal dysrhythmias, such as ventricular tachycardia and ventricular fibrillation, are common complications of myocardial ischemia, MI, and cardiomegaly. Heart blocks, such as first-degree atrioventricular block and second-degree atrioventricular heart block type 1, rarely compromise hemodynamic stability. However, second-degree atrioventricular heart block type 2 and third-degree atrioventricular heart block can significantly compromise hemodynamic stability, especially in the presence of MI. Young individuals, mostly males, may suffer from tachycardias when extra conducting structures are present. These may be fatal in some cases. A description of common electrical rhythm disturbances is provided in Table 19.10.

TABLE 19.10 Overview of Electrical Rhythm Disturbances

Ventricular Tachycardia

Rapid, regular heartbeat as high as 200 beats/min.

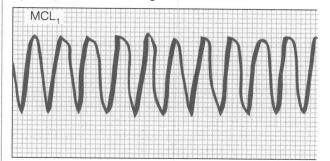

Figure 19.36 Ventricular tachycardia.

Ventricular Fibrillation

Total absence of regular heart rhythm.

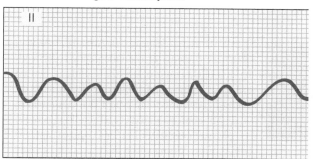

Figure 19.37 Ventricular fibrillation.

Heart Block

Slow heart rate can be as low as 20 to 40 beats/min. Conduction between the atria and ventricles is disrupted.

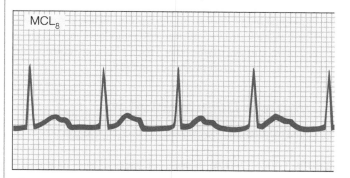

Figure 19.38 First-degree heart block.

Atrial Flutter

The atrial rate can be as high as 200 beats/min and exceeds the ventricular response and rate.

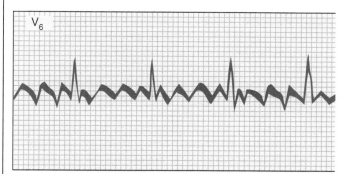

Figure 19.39 Atrial flutter.

Atrial Fibrillation

Dysrhythmic atrial contraction with no regularity or pattern.

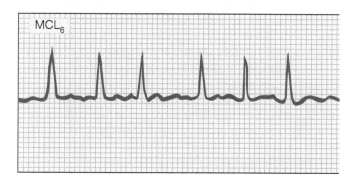

Figure 19.40 Atrial fibrillation.

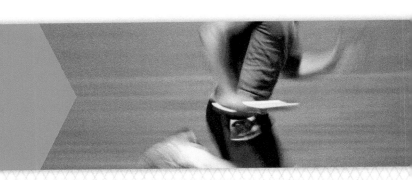

Application Through Critical Thinking

▶ Case Study

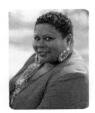

Jayla Tibbs, a 56-year-old African American female, presents to the emergency room with reports of shortness of breath, tingling in her left arm, and nausea. Mrs. Tibbs's medical history includes hypertension and type 1 diabetes mellitus, which she controls with diet and insulin injections.

Mrs. Tibbs states her signs and symptoms began this morning while she was taking a walk. Mrs. Tibbs reports that she fatigued quickly and had difficulty catching her breath. Subsequently, she felt a little nauseated and experienced a faint burning sensation in her left shoulder. Mrs. Tibbs states when she returned to her home, her husband told her she "did not look right." Mrs. Tibbs further states she felt that there was no cause for concern and told her husband, "It will go away if I rest." Despite Mrs. Tibbs's attempts to reassure her husband that she did not need medical care, her husband insisted that she go to the hospital.

First, the nurse must determine if Mrs. Tibbs is in acute distress by gathering objective and subjective data. The nurse will assess for indications of respiratory distress, chest pain, pallor or cyanosis, abnormal vital signs, and anxiety. Priorities of care include promoting adequate oxygenation and perfusion.

The nurse knows that hypertension and diabetes are risk factors for cardiovascular disease and that the symptoms of nausea, breathlessness, and unusual sensations in the shoulder may be indicators of a myocardial infarction (MI).

Using an organized approach, the nurse begins the assessment. The physical assessment reveals that Mrs. Tibbs is diaphoretic and her skin is gray-tinged, especially around the eyes. Her vital signs are B/P 144/72—P 102—RR 28. Her oxygen saturation (SaO2) is 92% on room air. Mrs. Tibbs denies chest pain or discomfort, as well as pain in any other region. She continues to report a burning sensation in her left shoulder and nausea.

Mrs. Tibbs is in acute distress. Rapid data interpretation and prompt implementation of collaborative nursing interventions are required. Her complaints include a burning sensation in her left shoulder, nausea, and shortness of breath. Her skin color suggests altered tissue perfusion. Her blood pressure is within normal limits, but her heart rate and respiratory rate are increased.

Collectively, the assessment data may be indicative of an acute cardiovascular problem. Collaborative goals of care include promoting oxygenation and perfusion, and preventing further systemic compromise.

The nurse administers O₂ via nasal cannula to Mrs. Tibbs and applies a cardiac monitor. Mrs. Tibbs's electrocardiogram (EKG) shows no obvious abnormalities; however, the nurse is aware that impaired cardiac perfusion does not always produce immediate EKG changes. Nitroglycerin sublingual (SL) as ordered by the ER physician is administered.

Two minutes after receiving nitroglycerin SL, Mrs. Tibbs's B/P is 120/64, and her heart rate (HR) is 84. Her respiratory rate is 22. She continues to receive supplemental O₂ via nasal cannula at a rate of 4 liters/minute. Her oxygen saturation has increased to 97%. Mrs. Tibbs states, "I'm not short of breath anymore and that burning in my shoulder is gone now."

Mrs. Tibbs occasionally rubs her left arm but denies tingling or pain. She continues to report mild nausea. She states, "This is all probably from something I ate or an insulin reaction. I'd like to go home."

The physician orders a 12-lead EKG and laboratory diagnostics, including cardiac enzyme tests. Mrs. Tibbs is scheduled for admission to the hospital's coronary care unit (CCU).

▶ Complete Documentation

The following is sample documentation for Jayla Tibbs.

SUBJECTIVE DATA: History of hypertension and type 1 diabetes, controlled with diet and insulin. Fatigued quickly during morning walk, shortness of breath, nausea, burning sensation in left shoulder. She felt it was nothing to worry about and stated, "it will go away if I rest." Husband stated Mrs. Tibbs "did not look right" upon returning from her morning walk.

OBJECTIVE DATA: 56-year-old African American female. Diaphoresis, gray-tinged skin, especially around eyes. VS: B/P left 144/72—P 102—RR 28—SaO2 92% on room air.

▶ Critical Thinking Questions

1. What additional information will be required to formulate a plan of care for Mrs. Tibbs in the CCU?

2. How should the nurse interpret the patient's desire "to go home" and statement that "This is all probably from something I ate or an insulin reaction"?

3. How does the absence of chest pain support or refute the possibility that Mrs. Tibbs is experiencing a myocardial infarction (MI)?

4. Explain the following conclusions about the patient's physical condition.
   a. impaired oxygenation
   b. alteration in peripheral perfusion
   c. fatigue
   d. nausea

5. What special considerations should the nurse consider when evaluating Mrs. Tibbs's situation?

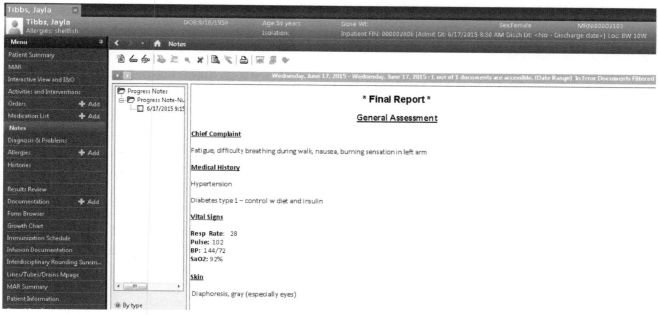

Source: From Cerner Electronic Health Record. Copyright © by Cerner Corporation. Used by permission of Cerner Corporation.

▌Prepare Teaching Plan

LEARNING NEED: Mrs. Tibbs has an increased risk for heart disease because she is African American and has been diagnosed with hypertension and diabetes. Her symptoms include some findings that may be atypical in MI, including absence of chest pain. However, in females, absence of chest pain during MI is more common. In females, less common manifestations, such as shoulder

APPLICATION OF OBJECTIVE 2: Discuss risk factors for MI

Content	Teaching Strategy	Evaluation
Risk factors: 1. Race (African Americans have higher risk.) 2. Gender (Males are at greater risk.) 3. High blood pressure 4. Diabetes 5. Family history 6. Aging 7. High cholesterol 8. Cigarette smoking 9. Stress 10. Obesity 11. Lack of exercise	• Lecture • Discussion • Slides Lecture allows information to be provided to a large group. Discussion encourages learner participation and permits for questions and answers. Audiovisual materials such as pictures and slides provide visual reinforcement of information. Printed material can be used by the learner during and after the session to review materials.	• Written examination

pain, may be associated with MI. She was reluctant to seek medical care, but at her husband's insistence, she received care shortly after the onset of symptoms.

The documentation for Mrs. Tibbs indicates that she will be admitted to the CCU for care of her acute cardiovascular problem. The signs and symptoms suggest that Mrs. Tibbs may have experienced an MI. While in the CCU, she will complete additional diagnostic testing. Prior to discharge, she will receive information about her condition and requirements for her home care regimen.

The case study provides data that are representative of risks, symptoms, and behaviors of many individuals. Therefore, the following teaching plan is based on the need to provide information to members of any community about MI and the importance of immediate care when symptoms arise.

GOAL: Participants will seek health care to promote cardiovascular health.

OBJECTIVES: Upon completion of this learning session, the participants will be able to:

1. Describe MI.
2. Discuss risk factors for MI.
3. Describe symptoms of MI.
4. Explain when to seek treatment for suspected MI.

▶ References

American Heart Association (AHA). (2011). AHA scientific statement: Triglycerides and cardiovascular disease. *Circulation, 123*, 2292–2333.

American Heart Association (AHA). (2012). AHA statistical update: Heart disease and stroke statistics—2012 update. *Circulation, 125*, e2–e220.

American Heart Association (AHA). (2013). *Heart murmurs: What causes heart murmurs?* Retrieved from http://www.heart.org/HEARTORG/Conditions/More/CardiovascularConditionsofChildhood/Heart-Murmurs_UCM_314208_Article.jsp

American Heart Association (AHA). (2014a). *The American Heart Association's diet and lifetstyle recommendations*. Retrieved from http://www.heart.org/HEARTORG/GettingHealthy/NutritionCenter/HealthyEating/The-American-Heart-Associations-Diet-and-Lifestyle-Recommendations_UCM_305855_Article.jsp

American Heart Association (AHA). (2014b). *Stress and heart health*. Retrieved from http://www.heart.org/HEARTORG/GettingHealthy/StressManagement/HowDoesStressAffectYou/Stress-and-Heart-Health_UCM_437370_Article.jsp

Backe, E-M., Seidler, A., Latza, U., Rossnagel, K., & Schumann, B. (2012). The role of psychosocial stress at work for the development of cardiovascular diseases: A systematic review. *International Archives of Occupational and Environmental Health, 85*(1), 67–69.

Berman, A., & Snyder, S. J. (2012). *Kozier and Erb's fundamentals of nursing: Concepts, process, and practice* (9th ed.). Upper Saddle River, NJ: Prentice Hall.

Bikley, L. S. (2012). *Bates' guide to physical examination and history taking* (11th ed.). Philadelphia: Lippincott.

Borchardt, R. A. (2013). Diagnosis and management of group A beta-hemolytic streptococcal pharyngitis. *Journal of the American Academy of Physician Assistants, 26*(9), 53–54.

Chwedyk, K. P. (2008, Winter). Vital signs: PAD: The health disparity nobody knows about . . . Peripheral artery disease. *Minority Nurse* (7), 94–95.

Cleveland Clinic. (n.d.). *Coronary artery disease*. Retrieved from www.clevelandclinicmeded.com/medicalpubs/diseasemanagement/cardiology/coronary-artery-disease/

Cleveland Clinic. (2011). Atrial septal defect (ASD). Retrieved from http://my.clevelandclinic.org/disorders/Atrial_Septal_Defect/hic_Atrial_Septal_Defect_ASD.aspx

Cleveland Clinic. (2012). Ventricular septal defects. Retrieved from http://my.clevelandclinic.org/heart/disorders/congenital/septal.aspx

Despres, J-P. (2012). Obesity: Body fat distribution and risk of cardiovascular disease. *Circulation, 126*, 1301–1313.

Gray, H. (2010). *Gray's anatomy*. New York: Barnes & Noble Books.

Guntheroth, W. G., Mortan, B. C., Mullins, G. L., & Baum, D. (1968). Venous return with knee-chest position and squatting in tetralogy of Fallot. *American Heart Journal, 75*(3), 313–318.

Iso, H. (2008). Heart disease in Asia: Changes in coronary heart disease risk among Japanese. *Circulation, 118*, 2725–2729.

Johns Hopkins Medicine. (2009). *Heart health special report: Ways to boost your HDL cholesterol*. Retrieved from http://www.johnshopkinshealthalerts.com/reports/heart_health/3028-1.html

Katikaneni, P. K., Akkus, N. I., Tandon, N., & Modi, K. (2013). Cocaine-induced postpartum coronary artery dissection: A case report and 80-year review of literature. *Journal of Invasive Cardiology, 25*(8), E163–E166.

Lokkegaard, E., Jovanovic, Z., Heitmann, B. L., Keiding, N., Ottesen, B., & Pedersen, A. T. (2006). The association between early menopause and risk of ischaemic heart diseaes: Influence of hormone therapy. *Maturitas, 53*(2), 226–233.

Mangla, A., & Gupta, S. (2014). *Heart sounds*. Retrieved from http://emedicine.medscape.com/article/1894036-overview#a1

Marieb, E. (2009). *Essentials of human anatomy and physiology* (9th ed.). Redwood City, CA: Benjamin/Cummings/Pearson Education.

Mayo Clinic. (2013). *Angina: Symptoms*. Retrieved from http://www.mayoclinic.org/diseases-conditions/angina/basics/symptoms/con-20031194

Mayo Foundation for Medical Education and Research. (2014). *Rochester test catalog: 2014 online test catalog*. Available at http://www.mayomedicallaboratories.com/test-catalog

O'Dell, K. R., Masters, K. S., Spielmans, G. I., & Maisto, S. A. (2011). Does type-D personality predict outcomes among patients with cardiovascular disease? A meta-analytic review. *Journal of Psychosomatic Research, 71*(4), 199–206.

Osborn, K. S., Wraa, C. E., Watson, A., & Holleran, R. S. (2013). *Medical-surgical nursing: Preparation for practice* (2nd ed.). Upper Saddle River, NJ: Pearson.

Peinemann, F., Moebus, S., Dragano, N., Möhlenkamp, S., Lehmann, N., Zeeb, H., . . . Hoffman, B. (2011). Secondhand smoke exposure and coronary artery calcification among nonsmoking participants of a population-based cohort. *Environmental Health Perspectives, 119*(11), 1556–1561.

Pennington, K. A., Schlitt, J. M., Jackson, D. L., Schulz, L. C., & Schust, D. J. (2012). Preeclampsia: Multiple approaches for a multifactorial disease. *Disease Models & Mechanisms, 5*(1), 9–18.

Roman, B. (2011). Nourishing little hearts: Nutritional implications for congenital heart defects. *Practical Gastroenterology, Vol. XXXV*, (8), 11–35.

Rosser, M. L., & Katz, N. T. (2013). Preeclampsia: An obstetrician's perspective. *Advances in Chronic Kidney Disease, 20*(3), 287–296.

Schmid, M., Kuessel, L., Klein, K., Metz, V., Fischer, G., & Krampl-Bettelheim, E. (2010). First-trimester fetal heart rate in mothers with opioid addiction. *Addiction, 105*(7), 1265–1268.

Seidel, H., Ball, J. W., Dains, J. E., & Benedict, W. J. (2010). *Mosby's guide to physical examination* (7th ed.). St. Louis, MO: Mosby.

Talukder, M. A., Johnson, W. M., Varadharaj, S., Lian, J., Kearns, P. N., El-Mahdy, M. A., . . . Zweier, J. L. (2011). Chronic cigarette smoking causes hypertension, increased oxidative stress, impaired NO bioavailability, endothelial dysfunction, and cardiac remodeling in mice. *American Journal of Physiology—Heart and Circulatory Physiology, 300*(1), H388–H396.

Tortora, G. J., & Derrickson, B. H. (2009). *Principles of anatomy and physiology* (12th ed.). New York: John Wiley & Sons.

U.S. Department of Health and Human Services (USDHHS). (2014). *Healthy people 2020*. Retrieved from http://www.healthypeople.gov/2020/default.aspx

University of Maryland Medical Center (UMMC). (2013). *Birth control options for women*. Retrieved from http://umm.edu/health/medical/reports/articles/birth-control-options-for-women

Wilson, B.A., Shannon, M.T., & Shields, K.M. (2013). *Pearson nurse's drug guide*. Upper Saddle River, NJ: Pearson.

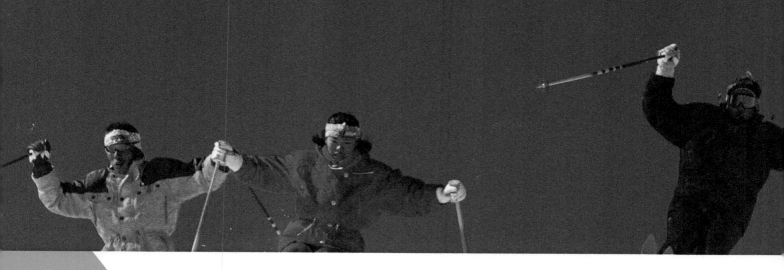

20 ▷ Peripheral Vascular System

▶ Learning Outcomes

Upon completion of this chapter, you will be able to:

1. Identify the anatomy and physiology of the peripheral vascular and lymphatic systems.

2. Develop questions that guide the focused interview.

3. Explain patient preparation for assessment of the peripheral vascular system.

4. Outline the techniques used for assessment of the peripheral vascular system.

5. Differentiate normal from abnormal findings in the physical assessment of the peripheral vascular system.

6. Describe the developmental, psychosocial, cultural, and environmental variations in assessment techniques and findings of the peripheral vascular system.

7. Relate peripheral vascular health to *Healthy People 2020* objectives.

8. Apply critical thinking to the physical assessment of the peripheral vascular system.

Key Terms

Allen's test, 511
arterial aneurysm, 525
arterial insufficiency, 525
arteries, 500
bruit, 514
capillaries, 501
claudication, 525
clubbing, 514
edema, 514
epitrochlear node, 502
hemorrhoids, 503
Homans' sign, 518
lymph, 502
lymphatic vessels, 501
lymph nodes, 502
manual compression test, 511
peripheral vascular system, 500
pulse, 500
Raynaud's disease, 527
varicosities, 517
veins, 501
venous insufficiency, 507

The **peripheral vascular system** is made up of the blood vessels of the body. Together with the heart and the lymphatic vessels, they make up the body's circulatory system, which transports blood and lymph throughout the body. This chapter discusses assessment of the 60,000-mile network of veins and arteries that make up the peripheral vascular system as well as the peripheral lymphatic vessels.

The vascular system plays a key role in the development of heart disease, one of the leading causes of death. People with high blood pressure have an increased risk of developing heart disease and stroke. Hypertension, the "silent killer," produces many physiologic changes before any symptoms are experienced. This characteristic has tended to undermine efforts at treatment. Objectives and health promotion strategies for hypertension are included in *Healthy People 2020* objectives (see Table 20.1 on page 503).

Therefore, the healthcare professional's role includes educating patients and consumers about the prevention of peripheral vascular disorders. Factors that influence a patient's vascular health include psychosocial wellness; self-care practices; and considerations related to the patient's family, culture, and environment.

Anatomy and Physiology Review

The peripheral vascular system is composed of arteries, veins, and lymphatics. Each of these is described in the following sections.

Arteries

The **arteries** of the peripheral vascular system receive oxygen-rich blood from the heart and carry it to the organs and tissues of the body. The pumping heart (ventricular systole) creates a high-pressure wave or **pulse** that causes the arteries to expand and contract. This pulse propels the blood through the vessels and is palpable in arteries near the skin or over a bony surface. The thickness and elasticity of arterial walls help them to withstand these constant waves of pressure and to propel the blood to the body periphery. The thickness or viscosity of blood, the heart rate or cardiac output, and the ability of the vessels to expand and contract influence the arterial pulse. It is described as a smooth wave with a forceful ascending portion that domes and becomes less forceful as it descends. Review chapter 19 for more detailed information. ∞

In the arm, the pulsations of the *brachial artery* can be palpated in the antecubital region. The divisions of the brachial artery, the *radial* and *ulnar arteries,* can be palpated for pulsations over the anterior wrist. The major arteries of the arm are shown in Figure 20.1 ■.

In the leg, the pulsations of the femoral artery can be palpated inferior to the inguinal ligament, about halfway between the anterior superior iliac spine and the symphysis pubis. The *femoral artery* continues down the thigh and becomes the *popliteal artery* as it passes behind the knee. Pulsations of the popliteal artery are palpable over the popliteal region. Below the knee, the popliteal artery divides into the anterior and posterior tibial arteries. The *anterior tibial artery* travels to the dorsum of the foot, and its pulsation can be felt just lateral to the prominent extensor tendon of the big toe close to the ankle. This pulse is known as the dorsalis pedis. Pulsations of the *posterior tibial artery* can be felt where it passes behind the medial

malleolus of the ankle. The major arteries of the leg are illustrated in Figure 20.2 ■.

The movement of blood through the systemic arterial system occurs in waves that cause two types of pressure. The blood pressure has

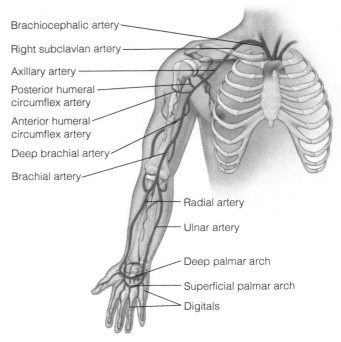

Figure 20.1 Main arteries of the arm.

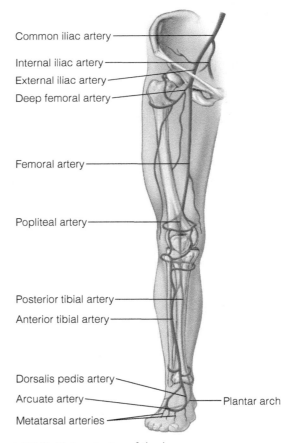

Figure 20.2 Main arteries of the leg.

two distinct parts, a systolic pressure and a diastolic pressure. The systolic pressure occurs during cardiac systole or ventricular contraction. It is the force of the blood that is exerted on the arterial wall during this cardiac action. The diastolic pressure occurs during cardiac diastole or ventricular relaxation. It is the force of the blood on the arterial wall during ventricular filling. Blood pressure is influenced by age, sympathoadrenal activity, blood volume, and ability of the vessels to contract and dilate. Blood pressure is discussed in greater detail in chapter 10. ∞

Veins

The **veins** of the systemic circulation deliver deoxygenated blood from the body periphery back to the heart. Veins have thinner walls and a larger diameter than arteries and are able to stretch and dilate to facilitate venous return. Venous return is assisted by contraction of skeletal muscles during activities such as walking and by pressure changes related to inspiration and expiration. In addition, veins have one-way intraluminal valves that close tightly when filled to prevent backflow. Thus, venous blood flows only toward the heart. Problems with the lumen or valves of the leg veins can lead to *stasis,* or pooling of blood in the veins of the lower extremities.

The femoral and the popliteal veins are deep veins of the legs and carry about 90% of the venous return from the legs. The great and small saphenous veins are superficial veins that are not as well

supported as the deep veins by surrounding tissues and, therefore, are more susceptible to venous stasis. The major veins of the leg are depicted in Figure 20.3 ■.

Capillaries

The **capillaries** are the smallest vessels of the circulatory system and where exchanges of gases and nutrients between the arterial and venous systems occur. Blood pressure in the arterial end of the capillary bed forces fluid out across the capillary membrane and into the body tissues.

Lymphatic System

The lymphatic system consists of the vast network of vessels, fluid, various tissue, and organs throughout the body. These vessels help transport escaped fluid back to the vascular system. The lymphoid organs have a major role regarding body defenses and the immune system. These structures help fight infection and provide the individual immunocompetence. The spleen, tonsils, and thymus gland are examples of lymphoid organs.

The **lymphatic vessels** form their own circulatory system in which their collected fluid flows to the heart. The vessels extend from the capillaries of their system to the two main lymphatic trunks. The *right lymphatic duct* collects lymph from the right

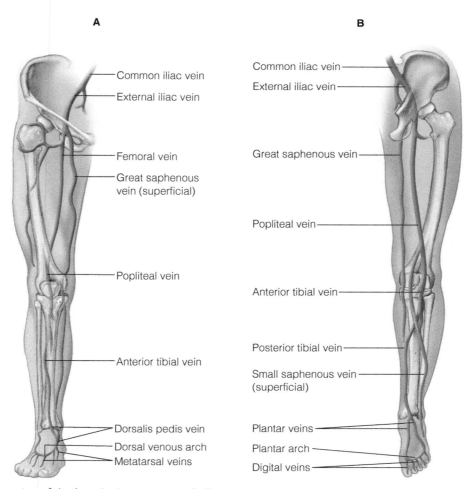

A

- Common iliac vein
- External iliac vein
- Femoral vein
- Great saphenous vein (superficial)
- Popliteal vein
- Anterior tibial vein
- Dorsalis pedis vein
- Dorsal venous arch
- Metatarsal veins

B

- Common iliac vein
- External iliac vein
- Great saphenous vein
- Popliteal vein
- Anterior tibial vein
- Posterior tibial vein
- Small saphenous vein (superficial)
- Plantar veins
- Plantar arch
- Digital veins

Figure 20.3 The main veins of the leg. A. Anterior view. B. Posterior view.

upper extremity, which is the right side of the thorax and head. The *thoracic duct* collects lymph from the remaining part of the body. The thoracic duct responds to the protein and fluid pressure at the capillary end of the vessels that help keep the lymph properly circulated. During circulation, as blood continues through the capillary bed toward the smallest veins, called *venules,* more fluid leaves the capillaries than can be absorbed by the veins. The lymphatic system retrieves this excess fluid, called **lymph,** from the tissue spaces and carries it to the lymph nodes throughout the body. **Lymph nodes** are clumps of tissue located along the lymphatic vessels either deep or superficially in the body. The lymph nodes usually are covered and protected by connective tissue and are, therefore, not palpable. Some of the more superficial nodes are located in the neck, the axillary region, and the inguinal region. Deeper clusters are located in the abdomen and thoracic cavity. The lymph nodes filter lymph fluid, removing any pathogens before the fluid is returned to the bloodstream.

The **epitrochlear node** located on the medial surface of the arm above the elbow drains the ulnar surface of the forearm and the third, fourth, and fifth digits. The nodes in the axilla of the arm drain the rest of the arm. The major lymph nodes of the arm are shown in Figure 20.4 ■.

The legs have two sets of superficial inguinal nodes, a vertical group and a horizontal group. The vertical group is located close to the saphenous vein and drains that area of the leg. The horizontal group of nodes is found below the inguinal ligament. These nodes

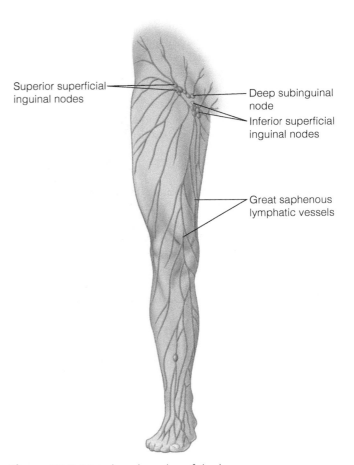

Figure 20.5 Main lymph nodes of the leg.

drain the skin of the abdominal wall, the external genitals, the anal canal, and the gluteal area. The major lymph nodes of the leg are illustrated in Figure 20.5 ■.

The functions of the peripheral vascular system are the following:

- Delivering oxygen and nutrients to tissues of the body.
- Transporting carbon dioxide and other waste products from the tissues for excretion.
- Removing pathogens from the body fluid by filtering lymph.

Special Considerations

The nurse must use critical thinking and the nursing process to identify factors to consider when conducting a comprehensive health assessment. Factors that impact the patient's health status include but are not limited to age, developmental level, race, ethnicity, work history, living conditions, socioeconomics, and emotional well-being.

Health Promotion Considerations

Healthy People 2020 objectives include promotion of peripheral vascular health. In particular, these national objectives emphasize the need for reducing the incidence of hypertension and hypercholesterolemia as well as the need for increasing public awareness and

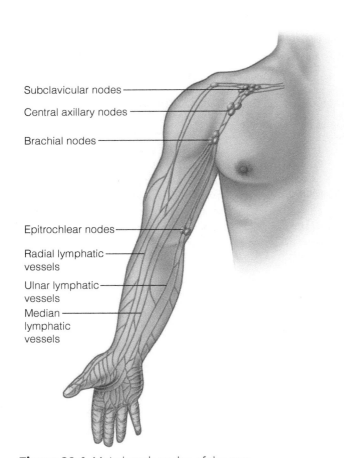

Figure 20.4 Main lymph nodes of the arm.

TABLE 20.1	Examples of *Healthy People 2020* Objectives Related to Peripheral Vascular Health
OBJECTIVE NUMBER	**DESCRIPTION**
HDS-4	Increase the proportion of adults who have had their blood pressure measured within the preceding 2 years and can state whether their blood pressure was normal or high
HDS-5	Reduce the proportion of persons in the population with hypertension
HDS-6	Increase the proportion of adults who have had their blood cholesterol checked within the preceding 5 years
HDS-7	Reduce the proportion of adults with high total blood cholesterol levels
HDS-8	Reduce the mean total blood cholesterol levels among adults
HDS-9	(Developmental) Increase the proportion of adults with prehypertension who meet the recommended guidelines
HDS-10	(Developmental) Increase the proportion of adults with hypertension who meet the recommended guidelines
HDS-11	Increase the proportion of adults with hypertension who are taking the prescribed medications to lower their blood pressure
HDS-12	Increase the proportion of adults with hypertension whose blood pressure is under control
HDS-13	(Developmental) Increase the proportion of adults with elevated LDL cholesterol who have been advised by a health-care provider regarding cholesterol-lowering management, including lifestyle changes and, if indicated, medication
HDS-14	(Developmental) Increase the proportion of adults with elevated LDL-cholesterol who adhere to the prescribed LDL-cholesterol lowering management lifestyle changes and, if indicated, medication

Source: U.S. Department of Health and Human Services (USDHHS). (2014). *Healthy people 2020.* Retrieved from http://www.healthypeople.gov/2020/default.aspx.

screening for these disorders (USDHHS, 2010). See Table 20.1 for examples of *Healthy People 2020* objectives that target the promotion of peripheral vascular health and wellness among individuals across the life span.

Lifespan Considerations

Interpretation of data from a health assessment is dependent on the ability to differentiate normal from abnormal findings. Normal variations in anatomy and physiology occur with growth and development. Specific variations associated with the peripheral vascular system for different age groups are discussed in the following sections.

Infants and Children

Assessing the blood pressure of an infant less than 1 year of age is difficult without special equipment. It is usually not necessary if the infant is moving well and the skin color is good. However, if the infant is lethargic and tires easily during feeding or if the skin becomes cyanotic when the infant cries, the blood pressure should be measured with a Doppler flowmeter. A newborn's blood pressure is much lower than that of an adult and gradually increases with age. The systolic pressure of a newborn is 60 to 76 mmHg; the diastolic pressure is 31 to 45 mmHg.

All children 3 years of age and older should have their blood pressure evaluated during their well-child examination. Children younger than 3 years of age should have their blood pressure evaluated only if they display symptoms of high blood pressure or are at risk for high blood pressure (Moyer & U.S. Preventive Services Task Force, 2013). The cuff should be no larger than two thirds of the child's arm or smaller than half of the length of the child's arm

between the elbow and the shoulder. Pediatric blood pressure cuffs are available.

In young children, the blood pressure should be measured on the thigh to rule out a significant difference between upper and lower extremity pressure. Such a difference in pressure could indicate a narrowing (coarctation) of the aorta. In a baby less than 1 year of age, the systolic pressure in the thigh should equal that of the arm. A child over 1 year of age will have a systolic pressure in the thigh that is 10 to 40 mmHg higher than that in the arm. The diastolic pressure in the thigh equals that in the arm.

The pulse increases if the child has a fever. For every degree of fever, the pulse may increase 8 to 10 beats per minute (beats/min). The lymphatic system develops rapidly from birth until puberty and then subsides in adulthood. The presence of enlarged lymph nodes in a child may not indicate illness. However, if an infection is present, the nodes may enlarge considerably.

The Pregnant Female

Blood pressure should be monitored throughout the pregnancy to test for pregnancy-induced hypertension. Blood volume during pregnancy almost doubles. In the second trimester, blood pressure may decrease because of the dilation of the peripheral vessels. However, blood pressure usually returns to the prepregnancy level by the third trimester. If the patient has a history of hypertension prior to her pregnancy, the blood pressure may increase dramatically during the third trimester, posing the threat of cerebral hemorrhage. Pressure from the uterus on the lower extremities can obstruct venous return and lead to hypotension when the patient is lying on her back, or it can cause edema, varicosities of the leg, and **hemorrhoids**. Chapter 27 describes a complete assessment of the pregnant female. ∞

The Older Adult

The aging process causes arteriosclerosis or calcification of the walls of the blood vessels. The arterial walls lose elasticity and become more rigid. This increase in peripheral vascular resistance results in increased blood pressure. Older adults are at increased risk of developing orthostatic hypotension (a drop of 20 mmHg or more when standing) as a result of medications or vascular impairment. The enlargement of calf veins can pose the risk of blood clots in leg veins. However, the amount of circulatory inadequacy at any given age is not predictable. The aging process may not cause any symptoms in some older patients.

Most hypertension is asymptomatic, but a severe elevation may produce a headache, epistaxis (nosebleed), shortness of breath, or chest pain. When evaluating the various arterial pulses, the nurse should keep in mind that the heart rate slows with the aging process. Some persons may normally have a rate of 50 beats/min; however, the patient should be evaluated if the pulse is below 60 beats/min. Likewise, it is common for older patients to manifest irregular pulses often with occasional pauses or extra beats. Again, any patient with an irregular pulse should be referred for further examination.

Psychosocial Considerations

Stress is among the factors that contribute to development of hypertension. Work-related stress has often been associated with hypertension. Stress can result from the rigors of everyday life in a complex and ever-changing world. Globalization and resulting economic fluctuations, the spread of disease, and terrorist threats have created a stressful environment. An individual's ability to cope can determine the risk of developing hypertension in response to stress.

Cultural and Environmental Considerations

There is a greater incidence of hypertension in African Americans than in Caucasians or Hispanics (National Heart, Lung, and Blood Institute [NHLBI], 2012). Obesity is a risk factor for hypertension and is increasing in the United States. The incidence of obesity is greatest in non-Hispanic Blacks and Hispanics, followed by non-Hispanic whites. In comparison, non-Hispanic Asians demonstrate the lowest incidence of obesity (Centers for Disease Control and Prevention [CDC], 2014). Diabetes, which is a significant risk factor for the development of peripheral vascular disease, is most common among non-Hispanic blacks (American Diabetes Association [ADA], 2014).

Smoking is a risk factor for hypertension and peripheral vascular disease. In the United States, smoking is most prevalent among American Indian/Alaska Natives, followed by non-Hispanic whites and non-Hispanic blacks (CDC, 2013).

Risk factors for varicose veins include Irish and German descent, family history of varicosities, a sedentary lifestyle, obesity, and multiple pregnancies. Patients whose jobs require them to stand for most of the day, such as hairdressers and cashiers, are at greater risk for developing varicose veins. Desk jobs that require sitting for prolonged periods also contribute to venous stasis and varicose veins.

Skin color variations across ethnic groups may affect assessment of circulation. The nurse must use skin temperature, capillary refill, the color of the palms of the hands and soles of the feet, the color of the oral mucosa, and pulse characteristics when pink undertones are not easily detected.

Gathering the Data

Health assessment of the peripheral vascular system includes gathering subjective and objective data. During the interview the nurse uses a variety of communication techniques to elicit general and specific information about the patient's state of health or illness. Health records and the results of laboratory tests are important secondary sources to be reviewed and included in the data-gathering process. In physical assessment of the peripheral vascular system, the techniques of inspection, palpation, and auscultation will be used. Before proceeding, it may be helpful to review the information about each of the data-gathering processes and practice the techniques of health assessment. See Table 20.2 for information on potential secondary sources of patient data.

Focused Interview

The focused interview for the peripheral vascular system concerns data related to the structures and functions of that system. Subjective data are gathered during the focused interview. The nurse must be prepared to observe the patient and listen for cues related to the functions of the systems. The nurse may use open-ended and closed questions to obtain information. Often a number of follow-up questions or requests for descriptions are required to clarify data or gather missing information.

The focused interview guides the physical assessment of the peripheral vascular system. The information is always considered in relation to normal parameters and expectations. Therefore, the

TABLE 20.2	**Potential Secondary Sources for Patient Data Related to the Peripheral Vascular System**

LABORATORY TESTS	NORMAL VALUES
PT (prothrombin time)	10–12 seconds
Platelets	150,000–300,000/mm^3
Thrombin Time	15–23 seconds
ACT (activated clotting time)	90–130 seconds
aPTT (activated partial thromboplastin time)	28–38 seconds
INR (international normalized ratio)	0.8–1.2 (if not taking warfarin)
	2.5–3.5 (if taking warfarin)

DIAGNOSTIC TESTS
Arterial Blood Flow Studies
Doppler Ultrasonography
Venous Ultrasonography
Ankle Brachial Index (ABI)

nurse must consider age, gender, race, culture, environment, health practices, past and concurrent problems, and therapies when framing questions and using techniques to elicit information. In order to address all of the factors when conducting a focused interview, categories of questions related to the peripheral vascular system status and function have been developed. These categories include general questions that are asked of all patients; those addressing illness and infection; questions related to symptoms, pain, and behaviors; those related to habits or practices; questions that are specific to patients according to age; those for the pregnant female; and questions that address environmental concerns. One approach to eliciting information about symptoms is the OLDCART & ICE method as described in chapter 7 ∞. See Figure 7.3. The data will be used to help meet the objectives for improving peripheral vascular health as indicated in *Healthy People 2020*.

The nurse must consider the patient's ability to participate in the focused interview and physical assessment. If a patient is experiencing pain or anxiety, attention must focus on relief of symptoms.

Focused Interview Questions

The following section provides sample questions and bulleted follow-up questions in each of the previously mentioned categories. A rationale for each of the questions is provided. The list of questions is not all-inclusive

Rationales and Evidence

but represents the types of questions required in a comprehensive focused interview related to the peripheral vascular and lymphatic systems.

General Questions

1. **Describe your circulation.**
   - Have you felt cold or hot?
   - Have you had numbness anywhere?
   - Has your skin been pale or blue?
   - Has your circulation changed in the last 2 months or 2 years?

   ▶ This gives patients the opportunity to provide subjective data about circulatory status.

2. **Have you or any member of your family ever had heart problems, respiratory disease, diabetes, varicose veins, or blood clots?**

   ▶ These problems can damage the peripheral circulation, and they tend to be hereditary (American Heart Association [AHA], 2013; Wedro, Schiffman, & Stöppler, 2012).

Questions Related to Illness

1. **Have you ever been diagnosed with a disease of your circulatory or lymphatic system?**
   - When were you diagnosed with the problem?
   - What treatment was prescribed for the problem?
   - Was the treatment helpful?
   - Describe things you have done or currently do to cope with this problem.
   - Has the problem ever recurred (acute)?
   - How are you managing the disease now (chronic)?

   ▶ The patient has an opportunity to provide information about specific illnesses. If a diagnosed illness is identified, follow-up about the date of diagnosis, treatment, and outcomes is required. Data about each illness identified by the patient are essential to an accurate health assessment. Illnesses can be classified as acute or chronic, and follow-up regarding each classification will differ.

Focused Interview Questions	Rationales and Evidence

2. **An alternative to question 1 is to list possible illnesses, such as hypertension, arteriosclerosis, Raynaud's disease, varicose veins, thrombophlebitis, and aneurysms, and ask the patient to respond "yes" or "no" as each is stated.**

▶ This is a comprehensive and easy way to elicit information about all diagnoses. Follow-up would be carried out for each identified diagnosis as in question 1.

Questions Related to Symptoms, Pain, and Behaviors

When gathering information about symptoms, many questions are required to elicit details and descriptions that assist in the analysis of the data. Discrimination is made in relation to the significance of a symptom, in relation to specific diseases or problems, and in relation to potential follow-up examination or referral. One rationale may be provided for a group of questions in this category.

The following questions refer to specific symptoms and behaviors associated with the peripheral vascular and lymphatic systems. For each symptom, questions and follow-up are required. The details to be elicited are the characteristics of the symptom; the onset, duration, and frequency of the symptom; the treatment or remedy for the symptom, including over-the-counter and home remedies; the determination if diagnosis has been sought; the effect of treatments; and family history associated with a symptom or illness.

Questions Related to Symptoms

1. **Have you noticed any skin changes on your arms, hands, fingers, legs, feet, or toes?**
   - If so, describe the changes.
   - Have you noticed any swelling or shiny skin, particularly on your legs?

▶ Shiny skin and swelling is sometimes caused by fluid leaking into tissue spaces because of incompetent valves in the veins (University of Rochester Medical Center [URMC], 2014).
▶ Peripheral arterial insufficiency can result in hair loss or skin changes (Johns Hopkins University, n.d.).

2. **If the patient reports swelling: Is the swelling in one leg or both legs?**
   - When did this swelling start?
   - Is the swelling worse in the morning or at the end of the day, or is the swelling constant?
   - What relieves the swelling?

▶ Answers to these questions may help the nurse collect data that will be useful in determining the reason for the swelling.

3. **Have you noticed any changes in temperature in your arms or legs, such as extreme coolness or heat?**

▶ Extreme coolness may indicate arterial insufficiency (URMC, 2014).

4. **Have you noticed any skin changes such as sores or ulcers on your legs?**
   - If so, is there any pain associated with the sores?

▶ Leg ulcers can be an indication of chronic arterial or venous problems (Markova & Mostow, 2012).

5. **Have you noticed any changes in the feeling in your legs, such as numbness or tingling?**

▶ Decreased circulation in the lower extremities can cause a loss of sensation, particularly in persons with diabetes (URMC, 2014).

6. **Have you noticed a change in the growth of hair on your legs?**

▶ Hair loss or slowed hair growth on the legs may be a manifestation of peripheral vascular disease (URMC, 2014).

7. **Do you have any swollen glands? If so, where are they in your body?**
   - How long have they been swollen?
   - Is there any pain or redness associated with these swollen glands?
   - Have you had any other symptoms such as fever, fatigue, or bleeding?

▶ Enlarged lymph glands usually are associated with an infectious process in the body. Older adults have fewer and smaller lymph glands as a result of a decrease in lymphatic tissue (Hadamitzky et al., 2010).

8. **For male patients: Have you experienced any difficulty in achieving an erection?**

▶ Impotence may occur as a result of a diminished arterial flow to the pelvic arteries (URMC, 2014). This condition is a common finding in peripheral vascular disease and is not always reported because of patient embarrassment.

Focused Interview Questions	Rationales and Evidence
Questions Related to Pain	
1. Do you ever have pains in your legs or leg cramps? Is the sensation in one or both legs? • If so, please describe the pain or cramp, the location, and the time it most often occurs.	▶ Pain associated with arterial insufficiency is usually described as gnawing, sharp, or stabbing and increases with exercise (Woo, Abbott, & Libroch, 2013). Pain is relieved with the cessation of movement and when legs are dangling. The pain is most commonly in the calf of the leg but it may also be in the lower leg or top of the foot. **Venous insufficiency** is described as aching or a feeling of fullness. It intensifies with prolonged standing or sitting in one position. Swelling and varicosities in the legs may also be present. The condition is relieved by elevating the legs or by walking.
Questions Related to Behaviors	
1. Do you smoke? Do you use smokeless tobacco? • If so, how long have you smoked? • How many cigarettes, cigars, or pipes of tobacco do you smoke per day? How much smokeless tobacco do you use?	▶ Nicotine is a vasoconstrictor and aggravates peripheral vascular disease.
2. Do you exercise regularly? • If so, describe your exercise routine. • How often do you exercise? • For how long?	▶ Exercise not only helps to prevent vascular disease but also improves the survival rate of people who have already suffered a heart attack and reduces the likelihood of their suffering a second attack. Even modest levels of physical activity are beneficial, according to the American Heart Association (AHA, 2014).

Questions Related to Age

The focused interview must reflect the anatomic and physiologic differences that exist along the age span. The following questions are presented as examples of those that would be specific for children, the pregnant female, and older adults.

Questions Regarding Infants and Children

1. Has the infant become lethargic? • Does the infant tire during feeding or become cyanotic when crying?	▶ These are signs of hypotension or hypoxemia associated with vascular disease.
2. Has the child had a blood pressure screening?	▶ It is recommended that blood pressure screening begin at age 3 years (NHLBI, 2014).
3. Does the child have any enlarged lymph nodes?	▶ Enlarged lymph nodes in a child may not indicate illness. However, in infection considerable enlargement is found (American Cancer Society [ACS], 2014).

Questions for the Pregnant Female

1. Have you had your blood pressure monitored?	▶ Monitoring can reduce risks for pregnancy-induced hypertension.
2. Are you experiencing swelling of the face, hands, or legs?	▶ Edema in the lower extremities is common in pregnancy, especially at the end of the day and into the third trimester (Mayo Clinic, 2014).

Questions for the Older Adult

No additional questions for the older adult are required.

Focused Interview Questions	Rationales and Evidence

Questions Related to the Environment

Environment refers to both the internal and external environments. Questions related to the internal environment include all of the previous questions and those associated with internal or physiologic responses. Questions regarding the external environment include those related to home, work, or social environments.

Internal Environment

1. **Are you now experiencing or have you ever had an experience of intermittent or prolonged anxiety or emotional upset?**
   - Describe the situation.
   - Can you determine precipitating factors?
   - Have you sought care or treatment for the problem?
   - What do you do when the problem arises?

   ▶ Anxiety and situations of emotion impact the sympathetic nervous system, producing hormonal responses that affect vascular function.

2. **What medications are you taking, either over the counter or prescription?**

   ▶ Contraceptive medications have been associated with blood clots in the peripheral vascular system (Wilson, Shannon, & Shields, 2013). Aspirin is an anticoagulant.

External Environment

The following questions deal with the physical environment of the patient. That includes the indoor and outdoor environments of the home and the workplace, those encountered for social engagements, and any encountered during travel.

1. **Describe your daily activities.**

   ▶ Sedentary activities and prolonged periods of sitting and standing at work or in the home can promote peripheral vascular problems, varicosities, or problems associated with venous stasis.

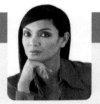

Patient-Centered Interaction

Ms. Mercedes Carlos, age 35, is an accountant at a local firm. She is married and has two children, 6 and 4 years of age. They recently returned from a 10-day vacation in Florida where they visited many of the theme parks. The flight home was delayed 2 hours, and they were seated on the plane for more than 4 hours. Ms. C. reports to the employee health office complaining of right leg pain and edema of the right ankle and foot that seems to be worse when standing or sitting at the desk. Following is an excerpt of the nurse–patient interaction.

Interview

Nurse: Good morning Ms. Carlos. What brings you here?

Ms. Carlos: I've been having some trouble with my leg. I just got back from vacation at a theme park in Florida. Our trip was great. Some of the lines at the parks were long. We did a lot of standing, walking, and sitting.

Nurse: How long was your trip?

Ms. Carlos: We were away for 10 days. We got home Saturday night, and here I am Tuesday morning seeing you.

Nurse: Tell me about the pain and swelling in your right leg.

Ms. Carlos: The pain started in my lower right leg about the fifth day of our trip. When I got back to the hotel, I would rest with my legs up and the pain seemed to go away.

Nurse: Did you have pain every day thereafter?

Ms. Carlos: Yes, and then after our flight home I noticed my foot was swollen. That was the first I noticed any swelling.

Nurse: Have you ever had a problem like this before?

Ms. Carlos: During my last pregnancy I had a problem like this. The doctor told me I could be developing varicose veins. After the delivery I never had a problem until now. I'm too young to have varicose veins.

Analysis

Throughout the interview, the nurse uses open-ended and closed questions to obtain information. The opening question by the nurse was to determine the patient's problem or chief complaint. Additional statements by the nurse give direction to the patient to provide specific subjective data.

Patient Education

The following are physiologic, behavioral, and cultural factors that affect the health of the peripheral vascular system across the age span. Several of these factors are cited as trends in *Healthy People 2020* documents. The nurse provides advice and education to reduce risks associated with these factors and to promote and maintain health of the peripheral vascular and lymphatic systems.

LIFESPAN CONSIDERATIONS

Risk Factors	Patient Education
• Palpable lymph nodes often occur in healthy infants and children.	▶ Advise parents that lymph nodes enlarge during infection but may remain enlarged even when the child is well. Abdominal pain may be a result of enlarged mesenteric lymph nodes that accompany an upper respiratory infection. Parents should be encouraged to seek care when lymph node enlargement is unaccounted for and they should be supported when seeking advice about the discomfort associated with expected lymph involvement.
• The hormonal changes of pregnancy cause vascular changes and increased blood volume, which can result in hypo- or hypertension. As the pregnancy progresses, drainage of the iliac veins and inferior vena cava is obstructed. As a result, venous pressure increases, causing edema, varicosities, and hemorrhoids.	▶ Provide prenatal education and care to reduce risk for and associated with hypertension and vascular changes.
• Obesity is increasingly prevalent across the age span. Obesity increases the risk for diabetes, hypertension, and cardiac disease.	▶ Provide education about healthy eating and exercising regularly to prevent obesity and the associated vascular problems.
• Varicose veins occur in both sexes and are associated with enlargement of calf veins in aging as well as with prolonged standing or sitting in one position and constrictive clothing.	▶ Provide education and encouragement to prevent varicosities with elevation of legs and by avoidance of tight clothing such as socks or garters to reduce the risk of hypertension and varicosities.

CULTURAL CONSIDERATIONS

Risk Factors	Patient Education
• African Americans are at greater risk for developing hypertension than other groups.	▶ Advise all patients to have blood pressure screening. African Americans and those in the prehypertensive category must receive information about blood pressure monitoring and activities to reduce risks including healthy dietary practices, weight reduction, and exercise.
• Guidelines for hypertension include a "prehypertensive" category for those with a systolic blood pressure between 120 and 139 and diastolic between 80 and 89. Those with prehypertension are at risk for progression to hypertension.	

ENVIRONMENTAL CONSIDERATIONS

Risk Factors

- Diabetes increases the risk for vascular diseases including hypertension, arterial or venous insufficiency, and coronary artery disease (CAD).

- The use of oral contraceptives increases the risk for development of thrombosis, especially in females who smoke.

- Peripheral vascular disease (PVD) can result in slow-healing ulcers. Risks for PVD include obesity, family history, diabetes, CAD, aging, and high cholesterol.

- Medications for hypertension may have side effects including nausea, headache, dizziness, decreased sex drive, and impotence in males. Noncompliance with treatment increases the risks for complications of hypertension.

Patient Education

► Advise those with a family history of diabetes about screening. Early diagnosis can reduce risks for complications.

► Explain the risks of oral contraceptives to female patients, provide information about the signs of thrombosis, and advise them to seek health care if symptoms arise.

► Educate patients with diabetes or PVD about skin assessment and care, particularly of the feet.

► Educate patients about the importance of following recommended treatment for hypertension. Advise patients to discuss side effects with their healthcare provider so that effective treatment can be provided.

BEHAVIORAL CONSIDERATIONS

Risk Factors

- Hypertension increases the risk for cardiac disease and stroke. Risk factors for hypertension include obesity, lack of exercise, alcohol consumption, smoking, and stress.

- Prolonged immobility is a risk factor for development of deep vein thrombosis (DVT), which can occur in those who are severely ill, postsurgery, involved in prolonged sitting at work, or in travel.

- Smoking is associated with increased risk for PVD and hypertension.

Patient Education

► Advise all patients to have blood pressure screening. African Americans and those in the prehypertensive category must receive information about blood pressure monitoring and activities to reduce risks including healthy dietary practices, weight reduction, and exercise.

► Provide general education about immobility as a risk for DVT, especially to older patients and those who are involved in air or other travel. Include advice to get up and walk and to increase intake of water when traveling.

► Educate patients about the risks of smoking and encourage them to join a cessation program.

Physical Assessment

Assessment Techniques and Findings

Physical assessment of the peripheral vascular and lymphatic systems requires the use of inspection, palpation, auscultation, and assessment of blood pressure. During each aspect of the assessment, the nurse is gathering objective data about circulation. Inspection includes looking at skin color, appearance of superficial vasculature, and shape and size of the extremities and nails. Palpation of pulses and auscultation of blood pressure and arteries provide information about vascular status. Knowledge of normal parameters and expected

EQUIPMENT

- examination gown
- sphygmomanometer
- stethoscope
- Doppler stethoscope

findings is essential in determining the meaning of the data as the physical assessment is performed.

The adult has a normal systolic blood pressure of less than 120 and normal diastolic blood pressure below 80. Normal pediatric blood pressure ranges are listed in Table 10.2 on page 165. ∞ The carotid pulses are palpable, symmetric, and synchronous with S1 of the heart. Auscultation of carotid arteries yields a soft sound, occasionally with transmission of heart sounds, but absence of bruits. The upper extremities should be of equal size and warm with pink undertones and no edema. Capillary refill should occur in less than 2 seconds. The brachial and radial arteries should be equal in rate and symmetric in amplitude. The epitrochlear nodes are not palpable. The lower extremities are warm and equal in size and the color is consistent with the rest of the body; hair is evenly distributed; and the extremities have no edema, lesions, or varicosities. The inguinal nodes are nonpalpable. The femoral, popliteal, posterior tibial, and dorsalis pedis pulses are equal and symmetric in rate and amplitude. The toes have hair and the toenails are pink and without clubbing.

Physical assessment of the peripheral vascular and lymphatic systems proceeds in an organized pattern. Blood pressure is assessed in upper and lower extremities. A cephalocaudal pattern for assessment of the vascular and lymphatic system begins with the carotid arteries and follows through inspection of the upper and lower extremities and palpation of pulses and lymph nodes within them. Additional assessment techniques include **Allen's test** to determine patency of the radial and ulnar arteries and the **manual compression test** to determine the length of varicose veins. Trendelenburg's test, which is an advanced test, may be performed by the primary care provider to evaluate valve competence when varicosities are present.

Techniques and Normal Findings	Abnormal Findings Special Considerations

Blood Pressure

1. **Instruct the patient.**
   - Explain that you will be assessing blood pressure in the arms and legs. Tell the patient you will inflate the cuff twice for each location. The first time you will only touch a pulse area, and the second time you will use the stethoscope. Tell the patient to breathe normally and relax the extremity. The only discomfort should occur when the cuff is fully inflated and will be relieved as the cuff deflates. Tell the patient to report any other problems.
   - Ask the patient to remain still and not to speak during the auscultation because you will not hear well when the stethoscope is in place for the blood pressure reading.
   - Explain that you will take the blood pressure while the patient is sitting and then when lying down. The readings will be compared.

2. **Position the patient.**
   - Place the patient in a sitting position on the examination table (see Figure 20.6 ■).

▶ Be sure to select the correct cuff size, especially for children or for obese patients. Inappropriate cuff size can alter the blood pressure reading.

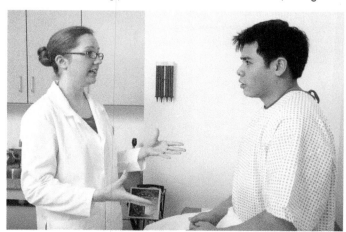

Figure 20.6 The patient is positioned for the examination.

Techniques and Normal Findings

Abnormal Findings
Special Considerations

- Take the blood pressure in both arms. Assess the palpable systolic pressure (see Figure 20.7A ■).
- Auscultate the blood pressure (see Figure 20.7B ■).

▶ Assessing the palpable systolic pressure helps to avoid an inaccuracy due to auscultatory gap when auscultating blood pressure.

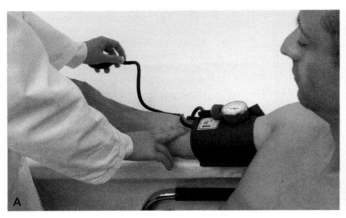 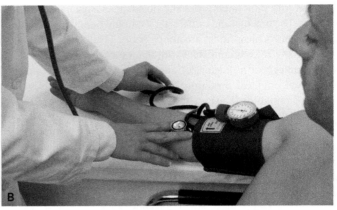

Figure 20.7 Blood pressure measurements. A. Palpable blood pressure. B. Auscultation of blood pressure.

- The blood pressure normally does not vary more than 5 to 10 mmHg in each arm.

▶ A difference of 10 mmHg or more between the arms may indicate an obstruction of arterial flow to one arm (Clark, Taylor, Shore, Ukoumunne, & Campbell, 2012).

- Table 20.3 includes current guidelines regarding interpretation of blood pressure readings for individuals age 18 and older.

▶ A systolic reading below 90 or a diastolic reading under 60 may be an early indication of shock, which requires immediate medical attention.

TABLE 20.3 **Classification of Blood Pressure for Adults 18 Years and Older**

CLASSIFICATION	SYSTOLIC		DIASTOLIC
Normal	Less than 120	and	Less than 80
Prehypertension	120–139	or	80–89
Hypertension (Stage 1)	140–159	or	90–99
Hypertension (Stage 2)	160 or higher	or	100 or higher
Hypertensive Crisis	Higher than 180	or	Higher than 110

Source: Based on American Heart Association (AHA). (2012). *Understanding blood pressure readings.* Retrieved from http://www.heart.org/HEARTORG/Conditions/HighBloodPressure/AboutHighBloodPressure/Understanding-Blood-Pressure-Readings_UCM_301764_Article.jsp.

3. **Assist the patient to a supine position.**

ALERT!

When caring for older adults, it is important to assist the patient to a sitting or standing position before retaking the blood pressure and to be cautious that the patient does not fall.

4. **Take the blood pressure in both arms.**
   - Pressures are lower when taken in the supine position.
   - Standards for blood pressure are set for patients in the sitting position.

▶ It is important to document the patient's position for each assessment of blood pressure.

Techniques and Normal Findings	Abnormal Findings Special Considerations

5. **Take the blood pressure in both legs.**
   - The blood pressure in the popliteal artery is usually 10 to 40 mmHg higher than that in the brachial artery.

Carotid Arteries

1. **Inspect the neck for carotid pulsations.**
   - With the patient in a supine or sitting position, inspect the neck from the hyoid bone to the clavicles. Bilateral pulsations will be seen between the trachea and sternocleidomastoid muscle.

   ▶ The absence of pulsation may indicate internal or external obstruction.

2. **Palpate the carotid pulses.**
   - Place the pads of your first two or three fingers on the patient's neck between the trachea and the sternocleidomastoid muscle below the angle of the jaw (see Figure 20.8 ■).

   ▶ Assessment of the carotid pulses may be difficult in obese patients with short, thick necks.

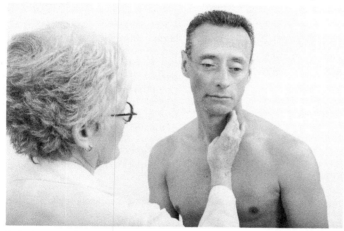

Figure 20.8 Palpating the carotid artery.

   - Ask the patient to turn the head slightly toward your hand to relax the sternocleidomastoid muscle.

   - Palpate firmly but not so hard that you occlude the artery.
   - Palpate one side of the neck at a time. If you are having difficulty finding the pulse, try varying the pressure of your fingers, feeling carefully below the angle.

   ▶ If both carotid arteries are palpated at the same time, the result can be a drop in blood pressure or a reduction in the pulse rate from the stimulation of baroreceptors (Berman & Snyder, 2012).

   - Note the rate, rhythm, amplitude, and symmetry of the carotid pulses. Compare this rate to the apical pulse.

   ▶ A rate over 90 beats/min is considered abnormal unless the patient is anxious or has recently been exercising or smoking. A rate below 60 is also considered abnormal.
   ▶ Some athletes have a resting pulse as low as 50 beats/min. An irregular rhythm or a pulse with extra beats or missed beats is considered abnormal. An exaggerated pulse or a weak, thready pulse is abnormal. A discrepancy between the two carotid pulses is abnormal.

3. **Auscultate the carotid pulses.**
   - Using the diaphragm and bell of the stethoscope, auscultate each carotid artery inferior to the angle of the jaw and medial to the sternocleidomastoid muscle. Ask the patient to hold his or her breath for several seconds to decrease tracheal sounds. You may need to have the patient turn the head slightly to the side not being examined.
   - Repeat the procedure using the bell of the stethoscope.

Techniques and Normal Findings	Abnormal Findings / Special Considerations

ALERT!

It is important not to put pressure on the bell of the stethoscope because this may occlude the sounds in the blood vessel.

- While auscultating, you should hear a very quiet sound. Normal heart sounds could be transmitted to the neck, but there should be no swishing sounds.

▶ A swishing sound indicates the presence of a **bruit,** an obstruction causing turbulence, such as a narrowing of the vessel due to the buildup of cholesterol.
▶ An increased cardiac output such as that seen in hyperthyroidism or anemia also will produce a bruit.

Arms

1. **Assess the hands.**
   - Take the patient's hands in your hands. Note the color of skin and nail beds, the temperature and texture of the skin, and the presence of any lesions or swelling. Look at the fingers and nails from the side and observe the angle of the nail base. The angle should be about 160 degrees.

▶ Flattening of the angle of the nail and enlargement of the tips of the fingers (**clubbing**) is a sign of oxygen deprivation in the extremities. In patients with chronic hypoxia (oxygen deprivation), there may be a rounding of the tip of the finger described as "turkey drumsticks." The nail may feel spongy instead of firm, and there may be a blue discoloration of the nail.

2. **Observe for capillary refill in both hands.**
   - Holding one of the patient's hands in your hand, apply pressure to one of the patient's fingernails for 5 seconds.
   - The area under pressure should turn pale. Release the pressure and note how rapidly the normal color returns.
   - In a healthy patient, the color should return in less than 1 to 2 seconds.
   - Repeat the procedure for the other hand.

▶ A delayed capillary refill could indicate decreased cardiac output or constriction of the peripheral vessels. However, cigarette smoking, anemia, or cold temperatures can also cause delayed capillary refill.

3. **Place both arms together and compare their size.**
   - They should be nearly equal in size.

▶ **Edema** (increased accumulation of fluid) in the arms could indicate an obstruction of the lymphatic system.

4. **Palpate the radial pulse.**
   - The radial pulses are found on the ventral and medial side of each wrist. Ask the patient to extend one hand, palm up.
   - Palpate with two fingers over the radial bone (see Figure 20.9 ▪).

▶ You may need to add more pressure to palpate if the patient is obese and has thick wrists.

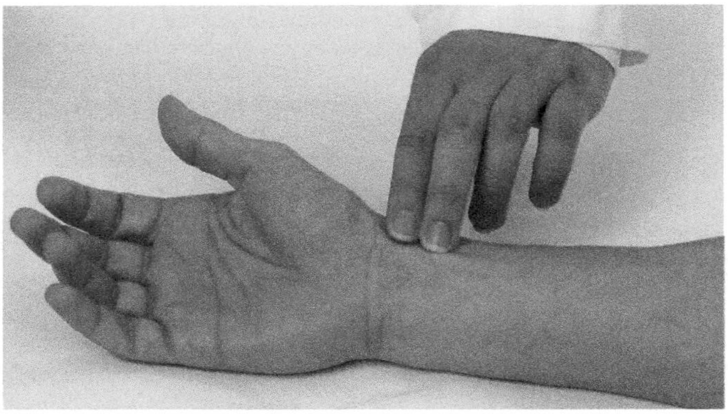

Figure 20.9 Palpating the radial pulse.

Techniques and Normal Findings	**Abnormal Findings Special Considerations**

- Repeat the procedure for the other arm. Note the rate, rhythm, amplitude, and symmetry of the pulses.
- Characteristics of peripheral pulse are included in Box 20.1.

> ► It is not necessary to palpate the ulnar pulses, located medial to the ulna on the flexor surface of the wrist. They are deeper than the radial pulses and are difficult to palpate.

Box 20.1 Assessing Peripheral Pulses

Assess peripheral pulses by palpating with gentle pressure over the artery. Use the pads of your first three fingers.

Note the following characteristics:

- Rate—the number of beats per minute
- Rhythm—the regularity of the beats
- Symmetry—pulses on both sides of body should be similar
- Amplitude—the strength of the beat, assessed on a scale of 0 to 4:

  0 = Absent or nonpalpable

  1 = Weak

  2 = Normal

  3 = Increased

  4 = Bounding

5. Palpate both brachial pulses.

- The brachial pulses are found just medial to the biceps tendon.
- Ask the patient to extend the arm.
- Palpate over the brachial artery just superior to the antecubital region (see Figure 20.10 ■).
- Repeat the procedure for the other arm.
- Note the rate, rhythm, amplitude, and symmetry of the pulses.
- Grade the amplitude on the 4-point scale as before.

> ► If any pulses are difficult to palpate, a Doppler flowmeter should be used. When positioned over a patent artery, this device emits sound waves as the blood moves through the artery. Peripheral pulses may be difficult to assess in obese patients.

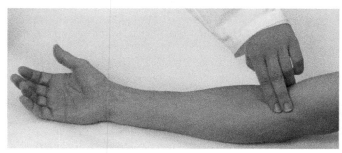

Figure 20.10 Palpating the brachial pulse.

6. Perform Allen's test.

- If you suspect an obstruction or insufficiency of an artery in the arm, Allen's test may determine the patency of the radial and ulnar arteries.
- Ask the patient to place the hands on the knees with palms up.
- Compress the radial arteries of both wrists with your thumbs.
- Ask the patient to open and close his or her fist several times.
- While you are still compressing the radial arteries, ask the patient to open his or her hands.
- The palms should become pink immediately, indicating patent ulnar arteries.

> ► If normal color does not return, the ulnar arteries may be occluded (Allen, 1929).

- Next, occlude the ulnar arteries and repeat the same procedure to test the patency of the radial arteries (see Figure 20.11 ■).

▶ If normal color does not return, the radial arteries may be occluded (Allen, 1929).

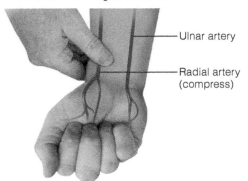

Ulnar artery

Radial artery (compress)

A   Open and close fist

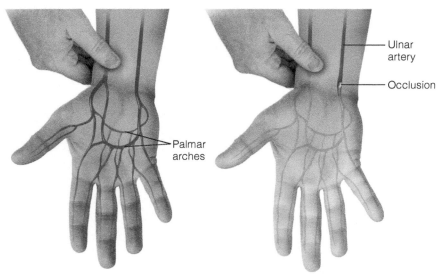

Palmar arches

Ulnar artery

Occlusion

B   Blood returns via ulnar artery

C   No blood returns

Figure 20.11 Allen's test.

7. **Palpate the epitrochlear lymph nodes in each arm.**
   - The epitrochlear node drains the forearm and the third, fourth, and fifth fingers.
   - Hold the patient's right hand in your right hand. With your left hand, reach behind the elbow to the groove between the biceps and triceps muscles (see Figure 20.12 ■).

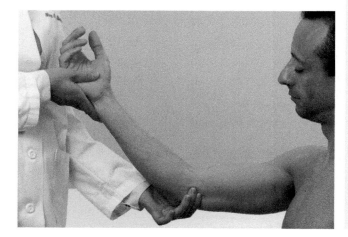

Figure 20.12
Palpating the epitrochlear lymph nodes.

Techniques and Normal Findings	Abnormal Findings Special Considerations

- Note the size and consistency of the node. Normally, it is not palpable or is barely palpable.
- Repeat the procedure for the left arm.

▶ An enlarged node may indicate an infection in the hand or forearm (Catalano, Nunziata, Saturnino, & Siani, 2010).

8. Palpate the axillary lymph nodes.
- With the palmar surface of your fingers, reach deep into the axilla. Gently palpate the anterior border of the axilla (anterior or subpectoral nodes), the central aspect along the rib cage (central nodes), the posterior border (subscapular/posterior nodes), and along the inner aspect of the upper arm (lateral nodes). Palpation of the axillary nodes is often part of the breast examination. Refer to Figure 18.21 on page 443 for a depiction of palpating the axillary lymph nodes.

Legs

1. Inspect both legs.
- Observe skin color, hair distribution, and any skin lesions.
- Skin color should match the skin tone of the rest of the body. Hair is normally present on the legs.

- If the hair has been removed, there is still usually hair on the dorsal surface of the great toes. Hair growth should be symmetric. The skin should be intact with no lesions.

▶ If peripheral vessels are constricted, the skin will be paler than the rest of the body. If the vessels are dilated, the skin will have a reddish tone.

▶ A rusty discoloration over the anterior tibial surface with the skin intact is associated with venous disease. The characteristic color stems from blood leaking out of a vessel with decreased capacity for it to be reabsorbed. Unintentional absence of hair on the legs may be a manifestation of peripheral vascular disease (URMC, 2014).
▶ If skin lesions or ulcerations are present, the size and location should be noted. Ulcers occurring as a result of arterial deficit tend to occur on pressure points, such as tips of toes and lateral malleoli. Venous ulcers occur at medial malleoli because of fragile tissue with poor drainage.
▶ If any blackened tissue is discovered, the patient must be referred to a physician immediately. The presence of blackened tissue can indicate tissue death (necrosis).

2. Compare the size of both legs.
- Both legs should be symmetric in size. If the legs are unequal in size, measure the circumference of each leg at the widest point. It is important to measure each leg at the same point.

▶ A discrepancy in the size of the legs could indicate an accumulation of fluid (edema) resulting from increased pressure in the capillaries or an obstruction of a lymph vessel. Unequal size of the legs could also indicate a blood clot in the deep vessels of the leg.

3. Palpate the legs for temperature.
- Palpate from the feet up the legs, using the dorsal surface of your hands.
- Note any discrepancies.
- The skin should be the same temperature on both legs.

▶ If the peripheral vessels are constricted, the skin will feel cool. If the peripheral vessels are dilated, the skin will feel warm. A difference in the temperature of the feet may be a sign of arterial insufficiency.

4. Assess the legs for the presence of superficial veins.
- With the patient in a sitting position and legs dangling from the examination table, inspect the legs.
- Now ask the patient to elevate the legs.
- The veins may appear as nodular bulges when the legs are in the dependent position, but any bulges should disappear when the legs are elevated.
- Palpate the veins for tenderness or inflammation (phlebitis).

▶ **Varicosities** (distended veins) frequently occur in the anterolateral aspect of the thigh and lower leg or on the posterolateral aspect of the calf. These bulging veins do not disappear when legs are elevated. Varicose veins are dilated but have a diminished blood flow and an increased intravenous pressure. An incompetent valve, a weakness in the vein wall, or an obstruction in a proximal vein causes varicosities (Franceschi, 2013).

Techniques and Normal Findings	Abnormal Findings Special Considerations

5. Perform the manual compression test.

- If varicose veins are present, you can determine the length of the varicose vein and the competency of its valves with the manual compression test.
- Ask the patient to stand.
- With the fingers of one hand, palpate the lower part of the varicose vein.
- Keeping that hand on the vein, compress the vein firmly at least 15 to 20 cm higher with the fingers of your other hand (see Figure 20.13 ■).

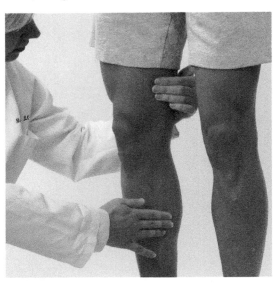

Figure 20.13 Performing the manual compression test.

- You will not feel any pulsation beneath your lower fingers if the valves of the varicose vein are still competent.

▶ If the valves are incompetent, an impulse in the vein will be felt between your two hands.

6. Test for Homans' sign.

- Assist the patient to a supine position.
- Flex the patient's knee about 5 degrees.
- Now sharply dorsiflex the patient's foot (see Figure 20.14 ■).
- Ask whether the patient feels calf pain.
- This maneuver exerts pressure on the posterior tibial vein and should not cause pain.

▶ A positive **Homans' sign** could indicate a blood clot in one of the deep veins of the leg. However, a positive Homans' sign could also indicate an inflammation of one of the superficial leg veins or an inflammation of one of the tendons of the leg. The reliability of Homans' sign in indicating disease has been shown to be inconsistent (Koepplinger & Jaeblon, 2010). Follow-up studies such as a venous Doppler examination may be required to identify the presence of a clot in the deep veins of the leg.

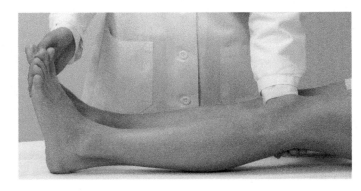

Figure 20.14 Testing for Homans' sign.

7. Palpate the inguinal lymph nodes.

- Move the patient's gown aside over the inguinal region. Palpate over the top of the medial thigh (see Figure 20.15 ■).

Techniques and Normal Findings	Abnormal Findings Special Considerations

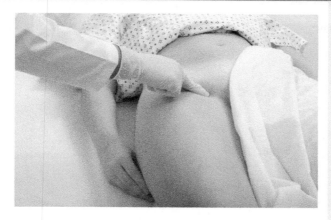

Figure 20.15
Palpating the inguinal lymph nodes.

- If the nodes can be palpated, they should be movable and not tender.
- Repeat the procedure for the other leg.

► Generally, lymph nodes that are larger than 1 cm (0.39 in.) or tender are considered to be abnormal and may be an indication of an infection in the legs or a sexually transmitted infection (Cleveland Clinic, 2013).

8. **Palpate both femoral pulses.**
   - The femoral pulses are inferior and medial to the inguinal ligament.
   - Ask the patient to flex the knee and externally rotate the hip. Palpate over the femoral artery (see Figure 20.16 ■).

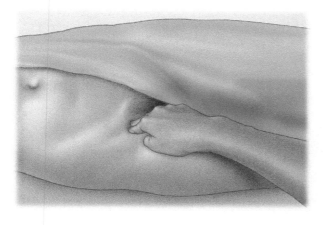

Figure 20.16
Palpating the femoral artery.

- The femoral artery is deep, and you may need to place one hand on top of the other to locate the pulse. Repeat the procedure for the other leg.
- Note the rate, rhythm, amplitude, and symmetry of the pulses.
- Grade the amplitude on the 4-point scale.

► If it is not possible to palpate the femoral pulse, an artery may be occluded.

9. **Palpate both popliteal pulses.**
   - The pulsations of the popliteal artery can be palpated deep in the popliteal fossa lateral to the midline.
   - Ask the patient to flex the knee and relax the leg.
   - Palpate the popliteal pulse.
   - If you cannot locate the pulse, ask the patient to roll onto the abdomen and flex the knee (see Figure 20.17 ■).

► If the popliteal pulse cannot be palpated, an artery may be occluded.
► A Doppler ultrasound may be required to assess popliteal pulses.

Techniques and Normal Findings

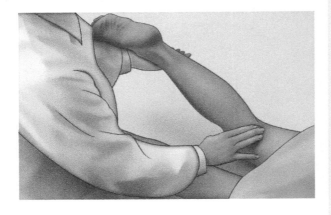

Figure 20.17
Palpating the popliteal
pulse.

- Palpate deeply for the pulse.
- Repeat the procedure for the other leg.
- Note the rate, rhythm, amplitude, and symmetry of the pulses.
- Grade the amplitude on the 4-point scale.

10. Palpate both dorsalis pedis pulses.
- The dorsalis pedis pulses may be felt on the medial side of the dorsum of the foot.
- Palpate the pulse lateral to the extensor tendon of the great toe (see Figure 20.18 ■).
- Use light pressure.
- Repeat the procedure for the other foot.
- Note the rate, rhythm, amplitude, and symmetry of the pulses.
- Grade the amplitude on the 4-point scale.

▶ The absence of a dorsalis pedis pulse may
not be indicative of occlusion because another
artery may be supplying blood to this area of
the foot. Edema in the foot will make palpation difficult. A Doppler ultrasound device may
be used to assess the pulse in an obese or
edematous area.

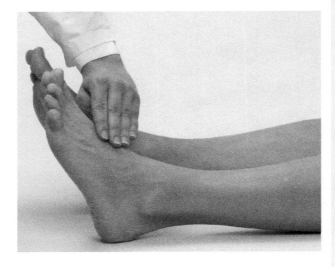

Figure 20.18
Palpating the dorsalis
pedis pulse.

11. Palpate both posterior tibial pulses.
- The posterior tibial pulses may be palpated behind and slightly inferior to the medial
malleolus of the ankle, in the groove between the malleolus and the Achilles tendon.

▶ If it is not possible to palpate the posterior
tibial pulse, an artery may be occluded. If the
patient has edematous ankles, this pulse may
be difficult to palpate.

- Palpate the pulse by curving your fingers around the medial malleolus (see Figure 20.19 ■).

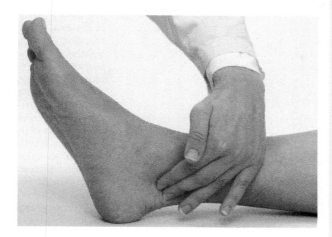

Figure 20.19
Palpating the posterior
tibial pulse.

- Repeat the procedure for the other foot. Note the rate, rhythm, amplitude, and symmetry of the pulses.
- Grade the amplitude on the 4-point scale.

12. **Assess for arterial supply to the lower legs and feet.**
    - If you suspect an arterial deficiency, test for arterial supply to the lower extremities. Ask the patient to remain supine.
    - Elevate the patient's legs 12 inches above the heart (see Figure 20.20 ■).
    - Ask the patient to move the feet up and down at the ankles for 60 seconds to drain the venous blood.
    - The skin will be blanched in color because only arterial blood is present.
    - Now ask the patient to sit up and dangle the feet.
    - Compare the color of both feet.
    - The original color should return in about 10 seconds.

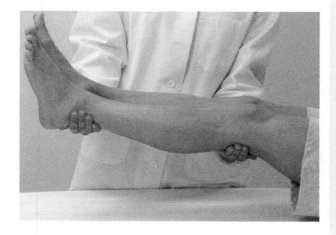

Figure 20.20 Testing
the arterial supply to
the lower extremities.

- The superficial veins in the feet should fill in about 15 seconds.

▶ Marked pallor of the elevated extremities may indicate arterial insufficiency.

Techniques and Normal Findings	Abnormal Findings / Special Considerations
• The feet of a dark-skinned person may be difficult to evaluate, but the soles of the feet should reflect a change in color.	▶ A marked bluish red color of the dependent feet occurs with severe arterial insufficiency. This color is due to a lack of oxygenated blood to the area, which leads to a loss of vasomotor tone and venous stasis. ▶ Delayed filling of the superficial veins of the feet also could indicate arterial insufficiency. Motor loss may occur with arterial insufficiency. ▶ Sensory loss may occur with arterial insufficiency. ▶ Pitting edema can be related to a failure of the right side of the heart or an obstruction of the lymphatic system. Edema in only one leg may indicate an occlusion of a large vein in the leg. Diminished arterial flow thickens toenails, which often become yellow and loosely attached to the nail bed. Patients with diabetes often acquire fungal and bacterial infections of the nail because of increased glucose collecting in the skin under the nail. Careful examination of the feet is essential in the patient with diabetes because of the potential decrease in sensitivity to pain or injury and altered capacity for healing.

13. Test the lower legs for muscle strength.

- With the patient in a sitting position, instruct the patient to extend each knee while you apply opposing force. Instruct the patient to flex the knees again. The patient should be able to perform the movement against resistance. The strength of the muscles in both legs is equal. Testing of muscle strength is discussed in greater detail in chapter 25. ∞

14. Test the lower legs for sensation.

- Use a cotton wisp, lightly applied to symmetric areas on each lower extremity to assess light touch. The rounded end and the sharp end of a safety pin are used to assess pain sensation. The ends are applied to symmetric areas of the lower legs in a random pattern of sharp and dull to assess sensation. The patient should have eyes closed during the assessment. Ask the patient to state "now" when the cotton wisp is felt, and "sharp" or "dull" when the ends of the safety pin are applied.
- The patient should sense touch and pain. Testing for the perception of sensation is discussed in greater detail in chapter 26. ∞

15. Check for edema of the legs.

- Press the skin for at least 5 seconds over the tibia, behind the medial malleolus, and over the dorsum of each foot (see Figure 20.21 ■).

▶ Edema can be localized or generalized. It refers to a collection of fluid in the body tissues. It is classified as pitting or nonpitting. Edema can result from cardiac, vascular, or lymphatic problems; fluid and electrolyte disturbances; nutritional disturbances; renal failure; and in response to toxins and chemicals (Trayes, Studdiford, Pickle, & Tully, 2013).

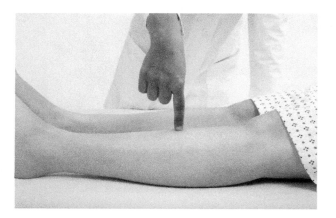

Figure 20.21
Palpating for edema over the tibia.

| **Techniques and Normal Findings** | **Abnormal Findings Special Considerations** |

- Look for a depression in the skin (called pitting edema) caused by the pressure of your fingers (see Figure 20.22 ■).

▶ Pitting edema usually occurs in the extremities.

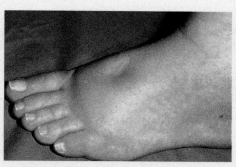

Figure 20.22 Pitting edema of the lower extremities.
Source: Dr. P. Marazzi/Science Photo Library.

- If edema is present, you should grade it on a scale of 1+ (mild) to 4+ (severe) as shown in Figure 20.23 ■.

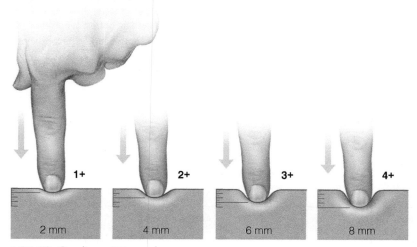

| 1+ | 2+ | 3+ | 4+ |
| 2 mm | 4 mm | 6 mm | 8 mm |

Figure 20.23 Grading pitting edema.

16. **Inspect the toenails for color and thickness.**
- Nails should be pink and not thickened. Clubbing should not be present.

Abnormal Findings

Findings from physical assessment of the peripheral vascular and lymphatic systems include normal and abnormal pulses (Table 20.4) and common alterations of the peripheral vascular and lymphatic systems as discussed in the following pages.

TABLE 20.4 **Normal and Abnormal Pulses**

NAME OF PULSE	CHARACTERISTICS	ARTERIAL WAVEFORM PATTERN	CONTRIBUTING CONDITIONS
Normal	• Regular, even in intensity		• Normal
Absent	• No palpable pulse, no waveform		• Arterial line disconnected • Cardiac arrest
Weak/Thready	• Intensity of pulse is +1 • May wax and wane • May be difficult to find		• Shock • Severe peripheral vascular disease
Bounding	• Intensity of pulse is +4 • Very easy to observe in arterial locations near surface of skin • Very easy to palpate and difficult to obliterate with pressure from fingertips		• Hyperdynamic states such as seen with hyperthyroidism, exercise, anxiety, vasodilation seen in high cardiac output syndromes • May be due to normal aging secondary to arterial wall stiffening • Aortic regurgitation • Anemia
Biferiens	• Has two systolic peaks with a dip in between • Easier to detect in the carotid location • In the case of hypertrophic obstructive cardiomyopathy only one systolic peak palpated, but waveform demonstrates double systolic peak		• Aortic regurgitation • Combination of aortic regurgitation and stenosis • Hypertrophic obstructive cardiomyopathy
Pulsus Alternans	• Alternating strong and weak pulses • Equal interval between each pulse		• Aortic regurgitation • Terminal left ventricular heart failure • Systemic hypertension
Pulsus Bigeminus	• Alternating strong and weak pulses, but the weak pulse comes in *early* after the strong pulse		• Regular bigeminal dysrhythmias such as premature ventricular contractions (PVCs) and premature atrial contractions (PACs)
Pulsus Paradoxus	• Reduced intensity of pulse during inspiration versus expiration	Expiration Inspiration	• Cardiac tamponade • Acute pulmonary embolus • Pericarditis • May be present in patients with chronic lung disease • Hypovolemic shock • Pregnancy
Water-Hammer, Corrigan's Pulse	• Rapid systolic upstroke and no dicrotic notch secondary to rapid collapse		• Aortic regurgitation
Unequal	• Difference in intensity or amplitude between right and left pulses	Right femoral Left femoral	• Dissecting aneurysm (location of aneurysm determines where the difference in amplitude is felt)

Arterial Insufficiency

Arterial insufficiency is inadequate circulation in the arterial system, usually due to the buildup of fatty plaque or calcification of the arterial wall. Narrowing or obstruction of the arteries in the legs, aorta, or both regions causes a reduction in blood flow to specific muscle groups. When arterial insufficiency causes pain in the thigh, calf, or buttocks, this condition is referred to as **claudication**, which may be a symptom of peripheral arterial disease (PAD). In most cases, pain related to claudication is triggered by walking and resolves with rest (Johns Hopkins University, n.d.). Ulcers due to arterial insufficiency are usually seen on the toes or areas of trauma of the feet or lateral malleolus (see Figure 20.24 ■). The ulcer is pale in color with well-defined edges and no bleeding.

Subjective findings:

- Pain, aching, burning, or discomfort in the feet, calves, or thighs.
- Numbness in legs or feet when at rest.
- Appearance of symptoms only when walking uphill, walking at a brisk pace, or walking for extended periods (MedlinePlus, 2014).

Objective findings:

- Diminished pulses.
- Cool, shiny skin.
- Absence of hair on toes.
- Pallor of lower extremities on elevation.
- Red color (rubor) of lower extremities when dependent.

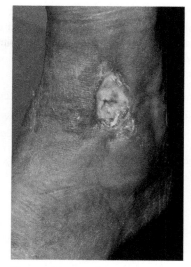

Figure 20.24 Ulcer due to arterial insufficiency.
Source: Science Photo Library/Science Source.

Arterial Aneurysm

Arterial aneurysm is a bulging or dilation caused by a weakness in the wall of an artery (see Figure 20.25 ■). It can occur in the aorta and abdominal, renal, or femoral arteries. Aneurysms can sometimes be detected by a characteristic bruit over the artery; however, if they are located deep in the abdomen, they can be difficult to discover. Note that both the subjective and objective findings vary greatly depending on the location of the aneurysm; some aneurysms are not discovered prior to rupturing.

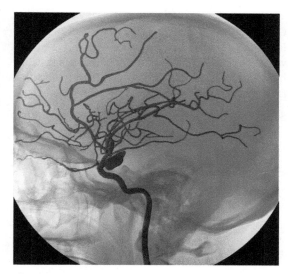

Figure 20.25 Arterial aneurysm.
Source: Simon Fraser/RNC, Newcastle/Science Source.

Venous Insufficiency

Venous insufficiency is inadequate circulation in the venous system usually due to incompetent valves in deep veins or a blood clot in the veins. Ulcers related to venous insufficiency are often found on the medial malleolus and are characterized by bleeding and uneven edges (see Figure 20.26 ■). There is minimal pain associated with the ulcer, and the skin surrounding the ulcer is coarse.

Subjective findings:

- Feeling of fullness or discomfort in the legs.
- Exacerbation of leg discomfort due to prolonged standing or sitting.
- Discomfort relieved by several hours of rest.

Objective findings:

- Normal skin temperature.
- Edema is usually present.
- Thickening and brown discoloration of skin around the ankles.

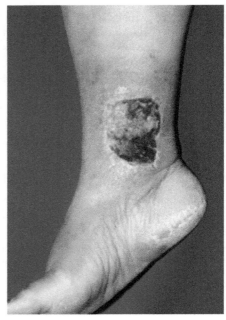

Figure 20.26 Ulcer related to venous insufficiency.
Source: Ribotsky D.P.M/Custom Medical Stock Photo.

Orthostatic Hypotension

Orthostatic hypotension is a temporary drop in blood pressure that occurs after standing up rapidly from a sitting or lying down position. This is due to abrupt peripheral vasodilation without a compensatory increase in cardiac output. Causes of orthostatic hypotension include dehydration; decrease in blood volume; neurologic, cardiovascular, or endocrine disorders; and some medications.

Subjective findings:

- Dizziness or lightheadedness.
- Blurred vision.
- Weakness.
- Nausea.
- Headache or chest, neck, or shoulder pain.

Objective findings:

- A decrease in systolic blood pressure of 20 mmHg or more or a decrease in diastolic blood pressure of 10 mmHg or more within three minutes of standing.
- Palpitations.
- Syncope (Lanier, Mote, & Clay, 2011).

Varicose Veins

Varicose veins are veins that have become dilated and have a diminished rate of blood flow and increased intravenous pressure (see Figure 20.27 ■). The condition may be the result of incompetent valves that permit the reflux of blood or an obstruction of a proximal vein.

Subjective findings:

- Aching, burning. heaviness, tiredness, or pain in legs.
- Exacerbation of symptoms due to extended periods of sitting or standing.
- Burning or itching over affected veins.

Objective findings:

- Distended, twisted veins near the skin's surface.
- Edema in feet or ankles.
- Skin changes, including discoloration, dryness, or scaling.
- Skin ulceration.
- Bleeding after minor trauma.

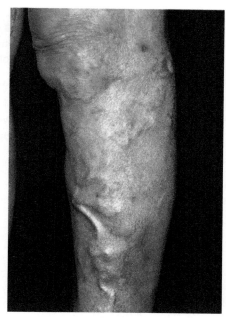

Figure 20.27 Varicose veins.
Source: Dr. P. Marazzi/Science Source.

Raynaud's Disease

Raynaud's disease is a condition in which the arterioles in the fingers develop spasms, causing intermittent skin pallor or cyanosis and then rubor (red color). This condition is seen most commonly in young, otherwise healthy females, frequently secondary to connective tissue disease, drug intoxication, pulmonary hypertension, or trauma (see Figure 20.28 ■).

Subjective findings:

- Bilateral spasms lasting from minutes to hours.
- Numbness or pain during the pallor or cyanotic state.
- Burning or throbbing pain during the rubor (Mayo Clinic, 2011a).

Objective findings:

- Skin pallor or cyanosis that may progress to rubor.
- Swelling of affected digits or areas (Mayo Clinic, 2011a).

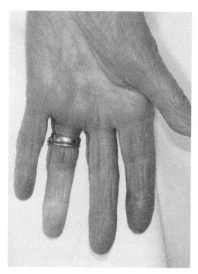

Figure 20.28 Raynaud's disease.
Source: Dr. P. Marazzi/Science Source.

Deep Vein Thrombosis

Deep vein thrombosis (DVT) is the occlusion of a deep vein, such as in the femoral or pelvic circulation, by a blood clot (see Figure 20.29 ■). This condition requires immediate referral because of the danger of the clot becoming a venous thromboembolism (VTE) and migrating to the lung, resulting in a pulmonary embolism (PE).

Subjective findings:

- Absence of symptoms, or the patient may describe intense, sharp pain along the iliac vessels, in the popliteal space, or in the calf muscles.
- Increased pain with sharp dorsiflexion of the foot (Homans' sign), though this maneuver is not absolutely reliable for diagnosis.

Objective findings:

- Unilateral edema.
- Low-grade fever.
- Tachycardia (rapid heartbeat).

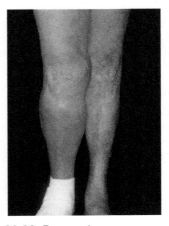

Figure 20.29 Deep vein thrombosis.
Source: Dr. P. Marazzi/Science Source.

Arteriovenous Fistula

An arteriovenous (AV) fistula is an abnormal connection between an artery and vein. This is commonly caused by piercing injuries, such as stab or gunshot wounds that occur in a location where a vein and artery lie close together. However, it can also be congenital, genetic, or as the result of a procedure such as cardiac catheterization. An AV fistula may be surgically formed if needed for kidney dialysis.

Subjective findings:

- Fatigue.
- Difficulty breathing.
- Dizziness.
- Lightheadedness.

Objective findings:

- Machinery murmur (a sound like the clicking or humming of machinery) when auscultated.
- Bulging veins near the surface of the skin.
- Decreased blood pressure, increased heart rate, and heart failure.
- Cyanosis.
- Clubbing of fingers (Mayo Clinic, 2012).

Lymphedema

Lymphedema is unilateral swelling associated with an obstruction in lymph nodes (see Figure 20.30 ■).

Subjective findings:

- Sensation of heaviness or tightness in the associated limb.
- Discomfort or aching in the associated limb (Mayo Clinic, 2011b).

Objective findings:

- Limited range of motion in the associated limb.
- Swelling of all or part of the associated arm or leg, including fingers or toes.
- Chronic, recurrent infections in the associated limb.
- Thickening and hardening of the skin of the associated limb (Mayo Clinic, 2011b).

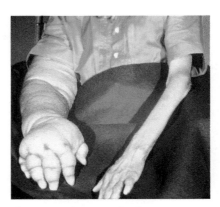

Figure 20.30 Lymphedema.
Source: O.J. Staats MD/Custom Medical Stock Photo.

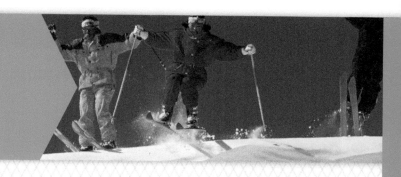

Application Through Critical Thinking

▌ Case Study

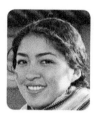

Jenny Battaglia, a 26-year-old female, is seen in the emergency department (ED) for pain in her lower legs. The patient states that she has had pain in her calves for about 48 hours, starting when she got home from vacation. She does not recall any injury. She says it started like cramping but has not improved with rest or taking Tylenol. She thinks there is a little swelling and some tenderness.

The nurse knows that an organized approach to data collection is essential. Further, every effort must be made to get a comprehensive picture of the situation and to avoid missing pieces of information that will guide decision making for the patient.

The approach to care of the patient will be determined by the patient's condition. When a patient is in acute distress—for example, with dyspnea, with a bleeding injury, in shock, or in severe pain—data gathering focuses on the immediate problem and its resolution.

Ms. Battaglia is uncomfortable but does not appear to be in acute distress and denies severe discomfort. She states, "I'm a little nervous. I've never really been sick and have only been in the emergency department once before for a couple of stitches when I was 10." The nurse tells Ms. Battaglia that they will begin an examination to determine the cause of her problem.

The assessment reveals the following: A thin female. The patient is suntanned, and without pink undertone to her skin. B/P 116/64 (R) arm, sitting, pulse 88, 3+, RR 16, temperature 99.2°F. Upper extremities symmetric in size, no edema, radial and brachial pulses equal, regular; lower extremities, edema, rubor (redness) bilateral posterior lower legs, warm and tender to touch. Radial and pedal pulses present, equal, 3+. Bilateral positive Homans' signs.

The nurse considers the data and determines that Ms. Battaglia is not in acute distress. However, pallor, edema in lower extremities, and the positive Homans' sign suggest a vascular problem. The nurse decides to continue the health assessment by further interview for missing subjective information.

The interview reveals that Ms. Battaglia has no personal or family history of vascular problems, cardiovascular disease, or diabetes. She is not married and lives with her boyfriend. She takes aspirin or Tylenol occasionally for headaches or menstrual cramps. She has no allergies. She is para 0 gravida 0, LMP 2 weeks prior to ED visit, regular menses, has taken birth control pills for 3 years.

The nurse asks Ms. Battaglia several questions about the leg pain. The patient states it is 5 to 7 on a scale of 1 to 10 and continuous. Nothing she has done has relieved the pain. It started 48 hours ago "at the end of my vacation" and wakes her at night.

The nurse asks if travel was involved in the vacation. Ms. Battaglia says, "Yes, we flew to Aruba for 6 days. That's how I got a tan. We had a great time and I was feeling rested, ready to go back to work, and looked forward to seeing family and friends." Further questions reveal that the flight was 6 hours and Ms. Battaglia "slept almost all the way back, I never really moved."

The data suggest to the nurse that Ms. Battaglia has deep vein thrombosis. Ms. Battaglia is admitted to a medical unit. She will be on bed rest and receive anticoagulation therapy.

▌ Complete Documentation

The following is a sample narrative complete documentation for Jenny Battaglia.

SUBJECTIVE DATA: Pain in lower legs for about 48 hr. Started when she got home from vacation. No recall of injury. Started as cramping, no improvement with rest or Tylenol. She thinks there is some swelling and tenderness. "A little nervous." No personal or family history of vascular problems, cardiac disease, or diabetes. Single, lives with boyfriend. Tylenol or aspirin occasionally for headache or menstrual cramps. No allergies. Gravida 0, Para 0, LMP 2 weeks prior to ED visit, regular menses. Oral contraceptives for 3 years. Air travel—flight of 6 hr—Jenny slept almost all the time.

OBJECTIVE DATA: Suntanned, without pink undertone. Vital signs: B/P 116/64 right, sitting. Radial pulse 88, 3+, RR 16, temperature 99.2°F. Pain: 5 to 7 on a scale of 1 to 10, continuous, wakes at night. Upper extremities symmetric in size, no edema, warm, brachial and radial pulses = regular. Cap refill < 2 sec L & R. Extremities—below knees, posterior bilateral rubor, edema 1+, warm, tender to touch. Pulses present, 3+. Bilateral positive Homan's signs. No lesions, no visible superficial vessels. Feet warm, no edema. Toenails—polish—unable to assess.

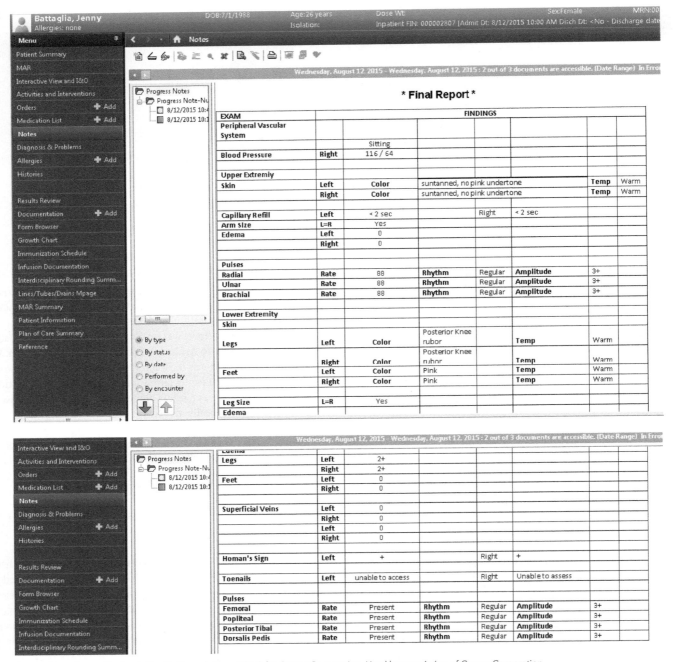

Source: From Cerner Electronic Health Record. Copyright © by Cerner Corporation. Used by permission of Cerner Corporation.

▶ Critical Thinking Questions

1. Identify the data that suggest the presence of DVT.

2. How would the data be clustered?

3. Describe the areas for patient education derived from this case study.

4. What would you recommend the patient do to prevent a future occurance?

5. What additional factors would put the patient at even greater risk for DVT?

▶ Prepare Teaching Plan

LEARNING NEED: The data in the case study reveal that Ms. Battaglia is at risk for development of DVT because she is using oral contraceptives and has experienced recent air travel. Her symptoms are typical for DVT. She will be admitted for treatment of DVT and will receive education regarding her treatment regimen and follow-up care.

The case study provides data that are representative of risks, symptoms, and behaviors of many individuals. Therefore, the following teaching plan is based on the need to provide information to members of any community about DVT.

GOAL: The participants in this learning program will have increased awareness of risk factors and strategies to prevent DVT.

OBJECTIVES: At the completion of this learning session, the participants will be able to:

1. Describe DVT.
2. Identify risk factors associated with DVT.
3. List the symptoms of DVT.
4. Discuss strategies to prevent DVT.

APPLICATION OF OBJECTIVE 2: Identify risk factors associated with DVT

Content	Teaching Strategy	Evaluation

• Age—over 40 years of age
• Family history of clotting disorder or DVT
• Circulation problems
• Obesity
• Cancer treatment
• Pregnancy or recent birth
• Oral contraception or hormonal therapy
• Immobility:
  1. Sitting for long periods during auto or air travel
  2. Surgery or illness
  3. Recent surgery
  4. Trauma
• Smoking
• Dehydration
	• Lecture
	• Discussion
	• Audiovisual materials
	• Printed materials
	
	Lecture is appropriate when disseminating information to large groups.
	
	Discussion allows participants to bring up concerns and to raise questions.
	
	Audiovisual materials reinforce verbal presentation.
	
	Printed material, especially to be taken away with learners, allows review, reinforcement, and repeated reading at the learner's pace.
		• Written examination.
		
		May use short answer, fill-in, or multiple-choice items or a combination of items.
		
		If these are short and easy to evaluate, the learner receives immediate feedback.

▶ References

Allen, E. V. (1929). Thromboangiitis obliterans (methods of diagnosis of chronic occlusive arterial lesions distal to the wrist with illustrative cases). *American Journal of the Medical Sciences, 2,* 1–8.

American Cancer Society (ACS). (2014). *How is non-Hodgkin lymphoma diagnosed in children?* Retrieved from http://www.cancer.org/cancer/non-hodgkinlymphomainchildren/detailedguide/non-hodgkin-lymphoma-in-children-diagnosis

American Diabetes Association. (2014). *Statistics about diabetes.* Retrieved from http://www.diabetes.org/diabetes-basics/statistics/

American Heart Association (AHA). (2012). *Understanding blood pressure readings.* Retrieved from http://www.heart.org/HEARTORG/Conditions/HighBloodPressure/AboutHighBloodPressure/Understanding-Blood-Pressure-Readings_UCM_301764_Article.jsp

American Heart Association (AHA). (2013). *Family history and heart disease, stroke.* Retrieved from http://www.heart.org/HEARTORG/Conditions/More/MyHeartandStrokeNews/Family-History-and-Heart-Disease-Stroke_UCM_442849_Article.jsp

American Heart Association (AHA). (2014). *AHA/ASA guideline: Guidelines for the prevention of stroke in patients with stroke and transient ischemic attack.* Retrieved from http://stroke.ahajournals.org/content/early/2014/04/30/STR.0000000000000024.short

Berman, A., & Snyder, S. (2012). *Kozier and Erb's fundamentals of nursing: Concepts, process, and practice* (9th ed.). Upper Saddle River, NJ: Prentice Hall.

Bikley, L. S. (2012). *Bates' guide to physical examination and history taking* (11th ed.). Philadelphia: Lippincott.

Catalano, O., Nunziata, A., Saturnino, P. P., & Siani, A. (2010). Epitrochlear lymph nodes: Anatomy, clinical aspects, and sonography features. Pictorial essay. *Journal of Ultrasound, 13*(4), 168–174.

Centers for Disease Control and Prevention (CDC). (2013). *Cigarette smoking in the United States: Current cigarette smoking among U.S. adults aged 18 years and older.* Retrieved from http://www.cdc.gov/tobacco/campaign/tips/resources/data/cigarette-smoking-in-united-states.html

Centers for Disease Control and Prevention (CDC). (2014). *Overweight and obesity: Adult obesity facts.* Retrieved from http://www.cdc.gov/obesity/data/adult.html

Clark, C. E., Taylor, R. S., Shore, A. C., Ukoumunne, O. C., & Campbell, J. L. (2012). Association of a difference in systolic blood pressure between arms with vascular disease and mortality: A systematic review and meta-analysis. *The Lancet, 379*(9819), 905–914.

Cleveland Clinic. (2013). *Diseases & conditions: Swollen lymph nodes.* Retrieved from http://my.clevelandclinic.org/disorders/lymph-nodes/hic-swollen-lymph-nodes.aspx

Franceschi, C. (2013). Definition of the venous hemodynamics parameters and concepts. *Veins and Lymphatics, 2*(4), 1.

Gray, H. (2010). *Gray's anatomy.* New York: Barnes & Noble Books.

Hadamitzky, C., Spohr, H., Debertin, A. S., Guddat, S., Tsokos, M., & Pabst, R. (2010). Age-dependent histoarchitectural changes in human lymph nodes: An underestimated process with clinical relevance? *Journal of Anatomy, 216*(5), 556–562.

Johns Hopkins University. (n.d.). *Claudication: What is claudication?* Retrieved from http://www.hopkinsmedicine.org/healthlibrary/conditions/cardiovascular_diseases/claudication_85,P08251/

Koepplinger, M. E., & Jaeblon, T. D. (2010). Venous thromboembolism diagnosis and prophylaxis in the trauma population. *Current Orthopaedic Practice, 21*(3), 301–305.

Lanier, J. B., Mote, M. B., & Clay, E. C. (2011). Evaluation and management of orthostatic hypotension. *American Family Physician, 84*(5), 527–536.

Marieb, E. (2009). *Essentials of human anatomy and physiology* (9th ed.). San Francisco: Benjamin/Cummings/Pearson Education.

Markova, A., & Mostow, E. N. (2012). US skin disease assessment: Ulcer and wound care. *Dermatologic Clinics, 30*(1), 107–111.

Mayo Clinic. (2011a). *Raynaud's disease: Symptoms.* Retrieved from http://www.mayoclinic.org/diseases-conditions/raynauds-disease/basics/symptoms/con-20022916

Mayo Clinic. (2011b). *Lymphedema: Symptoms.* Retrieved from http://www.mayoclinic.org/diseases-conditions/lymphedema/basics/symptoms/con-20025603

Mayo Clinic. (2012). *Arteriovenous fistula.* Retrieved from http://www.mayoclinic.org/diseases-conditions/arteriovenous-fistula/basics/definition/con-20034876

Mayo Clinic. (2014). *Third trimester pregnancy: What to expect.* Retrieved from http://www.mayoclinic.org/healthy-living/pregnancy-week-by-week/in-depth/pregnancy/art-20046767

Mayo Foundation for Medical Education and Research. (2014). *Rochester test catalog: 2014 online test catalog.* Available at http://www.mayomedicallaboratories.com/test-catalog/

MedlinePlus. (2014). *Peripheral artery disease – Legs.* Retrieved from http://www.nlm.nih.gov/medlineplus/ency/article/000170.htm

Moyer, V. A., & U.S. Preventive Services Task Force. (2013). Screening for primary hypertension in children and adolescents: U.S. Preventive Services Task Force recommendation statement. *Pediatrics, 132*(5), 907–914.

National Heart, Lung, and Blood Institute (NHLBI). (2012). *Who is at risk for high blood pressure?* Retrieved from http://www.nhlbi.nih.gov/health/health-topics/topics/hbp/atrisk.html

National Heart, Lung, and Blood Institute (NHLBI). (2014). *Expert panel on integrated guidelines for cardiovascular health and risk reduction in children and adolescents: Summary report.* Retrieved from http://www.nhlbi.nih.gov/guidelines/cvd_ped/summary.htm#chap8

Seidel, H., Ball, J. W., Dains, J. E., & Benedict, W. J. (2010). *Mosby's guide to physical examination* (7th ed.). St. Louis, MO: Mosby.

Trayes, K. P., Studdiford, J. S., Pickle, S., & Tully, A. S. (2013). Edema: Diagnosis and management. *American Family Physician, 88*(2), 102–110.

U.S. Department of Health and Human Services (USDHHS). (2014). *Healthy people 2020.* Retrieved from http://www.healthypeople.gov/2020/default.aspx

University of Rochester Medical Center (URMC). (2014). *Peripheral vascular disease: What is peripheral vascular disease (PVD)?* Retrieved from http://www.urmc.rochester.edu/Encyclopedia/Content.aspx?ContentTypeID=85&ContentID=P00

Wedro, B., Schiffman, G., & Stöppler, M. C. (2012). *Pulmonary embolism.* Retrieved from http://www.medicinenet.com/pulmonary_embolism/page2.htm

Wilson, B. A., Shannon, M. T., & Shields, K. M. (2013). *Pearson nurse's drug guide.* Upper Saddle River, NJ: Pearson.

Woo, K. Y., Abbott, L. K., & Librach, L. (2013). Evidence-based approach to manage persistent wound-related pain. *Current Opinion in Supportive and Palliative Care, 7*(1), 86–94.

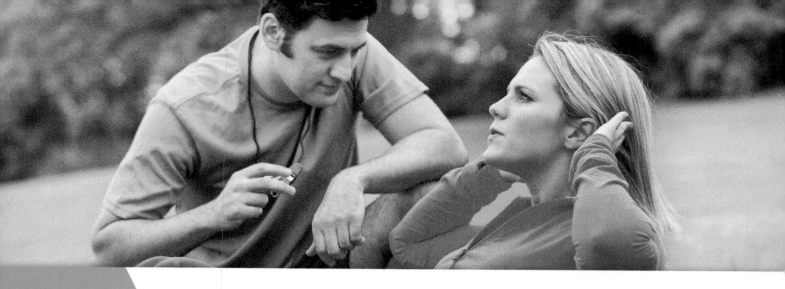

21 Abdomen

▶ Learning Outcomes

Upon completion of this chapter, you will be able to:

1. Describe the anatomy and physiology of the abdomen.

2. Identify landmarks that guide assessment of the abdomen.

3. Develop questions to be used when completing the focused interview.

4. Explain patient preparation for assessment of the abdomen.

5. Differentiate normal from abnormal findings in the physical assessment of the abdomen.

6. Describe developmental, psychosocial, cultural, and environmental variations in assessment techniques and findings related to the abdomen.

7. Describe the variation in techniques required for assessment of the abdomen.

8. Relate *Healthy People 2020* objectives to issues of the abdomen and gastrointestinal system.

9. Apply critical thinking to the physical assessment of the abdomen.

Key Terms

abdomen, 534
accessory digestive organs, 536
alimentary canal, 534
ascites, 542
Blumberg's sign, 565
borborygmi, 542
dysphagia, 571
esophagitis, 572
friction rub, 557
hepatitis, 572
hernia, 570
mapping, 537
peritoneum, 535
peritonitis, 572
referred pain, 569
striae, 556
ulcerative colitis, 572
umbilical hernia, 541

The **abdomen** is not a system unto itself. It is the largest cavity of the body and contains many organs and structures that belong to various systems of the body. For example, the liver, gallbladder, and stomach belong to the digestive system. The kidneys, ureters, and bladder belong to the urinary system. These structures and many other structures are assessed when performing an abdominal assessment. The primary focus of this chapter is the assessment of the structures of the digestive system.

The primary responsibility of the digestive system is to take in, break down, and absorb nutrients to be used by all cells of the body. The ability to perform these functions is influenced by the health of many other body systems. The parasympathetic fibers of the nervous system increase digestion, while the sympathetic fibers inhibit the process. The respiratory system provides oxygen needed for the metabolic processes and removes the carbon dioxide created by metabolism. The hormones of the endocrine system help regulate digestion and the metabolic processes.

Abnormalities of the gastrointestinal system include colorectal cancer, hepatitis, and foodborne illnesses, all of which are addressed in the U.S. Department of Health and Human Services (USDHHS) publication, *Healthy People 2020*. Health-related objectives are intended to reduce deaths from colorectal cancer; to decrease the number of foodborne infections; to decrease anaphylaxis from foods; and to reduce the number of cases of hepatitis A, B, and C, as illustrated in Table 21.1 on page 540.

Anatomy and Physiology Review

The abdomen is composed of the alimentary canal, the intestines, the accessory digestive organs, the urinary system, the spleen, and the reproductive organs. Each of these structures or systems is discussed in the following sections.

Abdomen

The abdomen is situated in the anterior region of the body. It is inferior to the diaphragm of the respiratory system and superior to the pelvic floor. The abdominal muscles, the intercostal margins, and the pelvis form the anterior borders of the abdomen. The vertebral column and the lumbar muscles form the posterior borders of the abdomen.

The anatomy and physiology review of the abdomen has a two-point focus. The primary focus is the gastrointestinal system, and the secondary focus is the abdominal structures of other systems. The gastrointestinal system consists of the alimentary canal and the accessory organs of the digestive system. The **alimentary canal**, a continuous, hollow, muscular tube, begins at the mouth and terminates at the anus. The accessory organs include the teeth, salivary glands, liver, gallbladder, and pancreas (see Figure 21.1 ■).

The anatomy, physiology, and assessment of the mouth, teeth, tongue, salivary glands, and pharynx are discussed in chapter 16 of this text. ∞ Before proceeding with the assessment of the abdomen, it may be helpful to review the information in that chapter.

Alimentary Canal

The alimentary canal is the continuous hollow tube extending from the mouth to the anus. The boundaries include the mouth, pharynx, esophagus, stomach, small and large intestines, rectum, and anus.

Esophagus

The esophagus, a collapsible tube, connects the pharynx to the stomach. Approximately 25 cm (10 in.) in length, it passes through the mediastinum and diaphragm to meet the stomach at the cardiac sphincter. The primary function of the esophagus is to propel food and fluid from the mouth to the stomach.

Stomach

The stomach extends from the esophagus at the cardiac sphincter to the duodenum at the pyloric sphincter. Located in the left side of the upper abdomen, the stomach is directly inferior to the diaphragm. The diameter and volume of the stomach are directly related to the food it contains. Food mixes with digestive juices in the stomach and becomes chyme before entering the small intestine. The primary function of the stomach is the chemical and mechanical breakdown of food.

Small Intestine

The small intestine is the body's primary digestive and absorptive organ. Approximately 6 m (18 to 21 ft) in length, it has three subdivisions. The first segment, the duodenum, meets the stomach at the pyloric sphincter and extends to the middle region, called the jejunum. The ileum extends from the jejunum to the ileocecal valve at the cecum of the large intestine. Intestinal juices, bile from the liver and gallbladder, and pancreatic enzymes mix with the chyme to promote digestion and facilitate the absorption of nutrients. The primary functions of the small intestine are the continuing chemical breakdown of food and the absorption of digested foods.

Large Intestine

The last portion of the alimentary canal is the large intestine, which extends from the ileocecal valve to the anus. The large intestine is approximately 1.5 m (5 to 5.5 ft) in length. It consists of the cecum, ascending colon, transverse colon, descending colon, sigmoid colon, rectum, and anus. The vermiform appendix is attached to the large intestine at the cecum. The appendix contains masses of lymphoid tissue that make only a minor contribution to immunity; however, when inflamed, the appendix causes significant health problems. The large intestine is wider and shorter than the small intestine. It is on the periphery of the abdominal cavity, surrounding the small intestine and other structures. The main functions of the large intestine are absorbing water from indigestible food residue and eliminating the residue in the form of feces.

Accessory Digestive Organs

The **accessory digestive organs**—the liver, gallbladder, and pancreas—contribute to the digestive process of foods. These structures connect to the alimentary canal by ducts.

Liver

The largest gland of the body, the liver is located in the right upper portion of the abdominal cavity directly inferior to the diaphragm to just below the costal margin and extends into the left side of the abdomen. The lower portion of the rib cage, which makes only the lower border of the liver palpable, protects the liver. The only

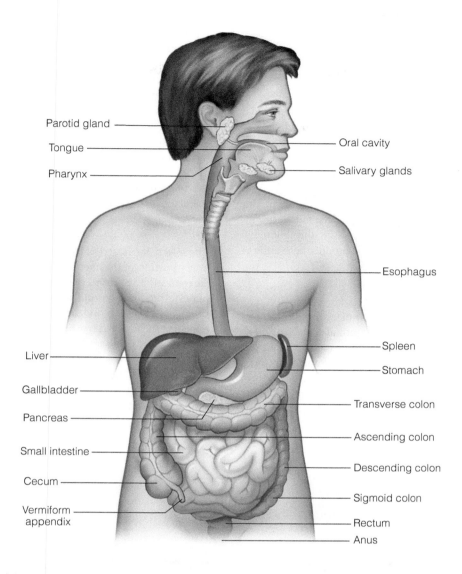

Parotid gland

Tongue

Pharynx

Oral cavity

Salivary glands

Esophagus

Liver

Gallbladder

Pancreas

Small intestine

Cecum

Vermiform appendix

Spleen

Stomach

Transverse colon

Ascending colon

Descending colon

Sigmoid colon

Rectum

Anus

Figure 21.1 Organs of the alimentary canal and related accessory organs.

digestive function of the liver is the production and secretion of bile for fat emulsification. It has a major role in the metabolism of proteins, fats, and carbohydrates. The liver has the ability to store some vitamins, produce substances for coagulation of blood, produce antibodies, and detoxify harmful substances.

Gallbladder

Chiefly a storage organ for bile, the gallbladder, a thin-walled sac, is nestled in a shallow depression on the ventral surface of the liver. The main functions of the gallbladder are storing of bile and assisting in the digestion of fats. The gallbladder releases stored bile into the duodenum when stimulated and thus promotes the emulsification of fats.

Pancreas

An accessory digestive organ, the pancreas is a triangular-shaped gland located in the left upper portion of the abdomen. The head of the pancreas is nestled in the C curve of the duodenum, and the

body and tail of the pancreas lie deep to the left of the stomach and extend toward the spleen at the lateral aspect of the abdomen. The pancreas is an endocrine and exocrine gland. As an endocrine gland, it secretes insulin, an important factor in carbohydrate metabolism. As an exocrine gland, it releases pancreatic juice, which contains a broad spectrum of enzymes that mixes with bile in the duodenum. The main function of the pancreas is assisting with the digestion of proteins, fats, and carbohydrates.

Other Related Structures

Some structures located in the abdomen have no connection to the digestive process. They are part of other systems and are considered with the general assessment of the abdomen.

Peritoneum

The **peritoneum** is a thin, double layer of serous membrane in the abdominal cavity. The visceral peritoneum covers the external surface of most digestive organs. The parietal peritoneum lines the walls of the abdominal cavity. The serous fluid secreted by the membranes helps lubricate the surface of the organs, allowing motion of structures without friction.

Muscles of the Abdominal Wall

Having no bony reinforcements, the anterior and lateral abdominal walls depend on the musculature for support and protection. The four pairs of abdominal muscles, when well toned, support and protect the abdominal viscera most effectively (see Figure 21.2 ■). The muscle groups include the rectus abdominis, external oblique, internal oblique, and transverse abdominis. Secondary functions of these muscle groups include lateral flexion, rotation, and anterior flexion of the trunk. Simultaneous contraction of the muscle groups increases intra-abdominal pressure by compressing the abdominal wall. Weakness in the muscular structure will produce herniation of structures.

Aorta

As the descending aorta passes through the diaphragm and enters the abdominal cavity, it becomes the abdominal aorta. This penetration occurs at the T12 level of the vertebral column slightly to the left of the midline of the body. The abdominal aorta continues to the L4 level of the vertebral column, where it bifurcates to form the right and left common iliac arteries. The many branches of the abdominal aorta serve all the parietal and visceral structures (see Figure 21.3 ■).

Kidneys, Ureters, and Bladder

The kidneys are located in the posterior abdomen on either side of the spine, protected by the lower ribs. Besides filtering nitrogenous wastes from blood and producing urine, the kidneys produce a biologically active form of vitamin D. The kidneys also secrete erythropoietin and renin. The slender tubelike structures that carry the urine from the kidneys to the bladder are the ureters. The urinary bladder, a smooth, collapsible muscular sac, is located in the pelvis of the abdominal cavity. The primary function of the bladder is to store urine until it can be released. As the bladder fills with urine, it may rise above the symphysis pubis into the abdominal cavity. Assessment of the kidneys, ureters, and bladder is discussed in chapter 22 of this text. ∞

Spleen

The spleen, the largest of the lymphoid organs, is located in the left upper portion of the abdomen directly inferior to the diaphragm. Surrounded by a fibrous capsule, the spleen provides a site for lymphocyte proliferation and immune surveillance and response. It filters and cleanses blood, destroying worn-out red blood cells and returning their breakdown products to the liver.

Reproductive Organs

In the female, the uterus, fallopian tubes, and ovaries are in the pelvic portion of the abdominal cavity. In the male, the prostate gland surrounds the urethra just below the bladder. The assessment of these structures is discussed in chapters 23 and 24 of this text. ∞

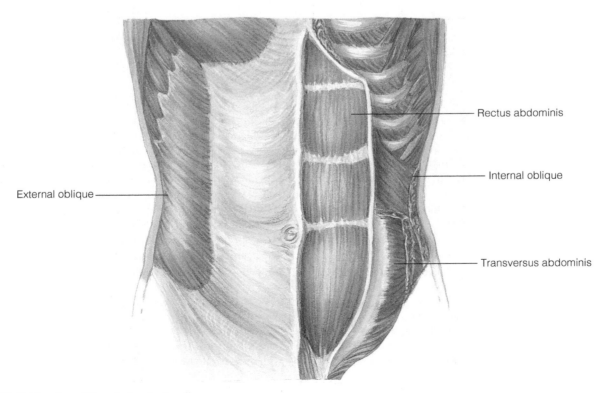

Figure 21.2 Muscles of the abdominal wall.

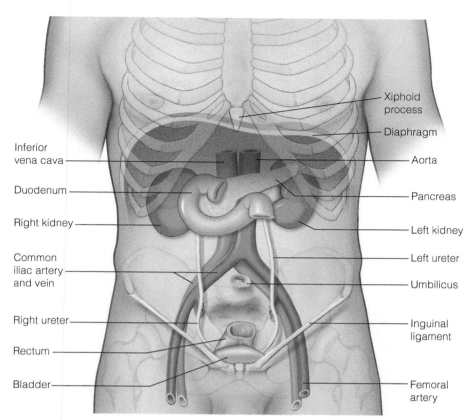

Inferior vena cava

Duodenum

Right kidney

Common iliac artery and vein

Right ureter

Rectum

Bladder

Xiphoid process

Diaphragm

Aorta

Pancreas

Left kidney

Left ureter

Umbilicus

Inguinal ligament

Femoral artery

Figure 21.3 Abdominal vasculature and deep structures.

Landmarks

Reference points and anatomic structures need to be identified when assessing the abdomen. Defined landmarks help to identify specific underlying structures and provide a source for description and recording of findings. Landmarks for the abdomen include the xiphoid process, umbilicus, costal margin, iliac crests, and pubic bone.

Mapping is the process of dividing the abdomen into quadrants or regions for the purpose of examination. To obtain the four quadrants, the nurse extends the midsternal line from the xiphoid process through the umbilicus to the pubic bone and then draws a horizontal line perpendicular to the first line through the umbilicus. These two perpendicular lines form four equal quadrants of the abdomen, as illustrated in Figure 21.4 ■. The quadrants are simply named right upper quadrant (RUQ), right lower quadrant (RLQ), left upper quadrant (LUQ), and left lower quadrant (LLQ).

The second mapping method divides the abdomen into nine regions. To obtain these abdominal regions, one extends the right and left midclavicular lines to the groin and then draws a horizontal line across the lowest edge of the costal margin. The final step is to draw another horizontal line at the level of the iliac crests.

The abdomen has now been divided into nine regions as shown in Figure 21.5 ■. The names of the regions are right hypochondriac, epigastric, left hypochondriac, right lumbar, umbilical, left lumbar, right inguinal, hypogastric or pubic, and left inguinal.

Of the two methods described, the quadrant method is more commonly used. When using the quadrant method, it is important to pay attention to structures that are in the midline of the abdomen and do not belong to any specific quadrant. These structures include the abdominal aorta, urinary bladder, and uterus.

The nurse should select one mapping method and use it consistently. Once a method has been selected, the nurse visualizes the underlying structures before proceeding (see Figure 21.6 ■). The gallbladder sits in the upper right quadrant of the abdomen inferior to the liver and lateral to the right midclavicular line (RMCL). The kidneys are posterior to the abdominal contents and situated in the retroperitoneal space, protected by the 11th and 12th pairs of ribs. The costovertebral angle is formed as the ribs articulate with the vertebra. The liver displaces the right kidney, thus making the lower pole palpable. The spleen, part of the lymphatic system, is at the level of the 10th rib lateral to the left midaxillary line (LMAL). The lower pole of the spleen moves into the abdomen toward the midline when enlarged.

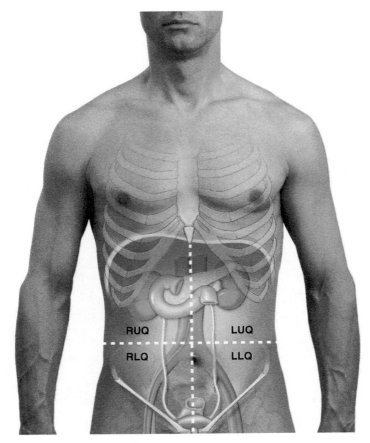

Figure 21.4 Mapping of the abdomen into four quadrants.

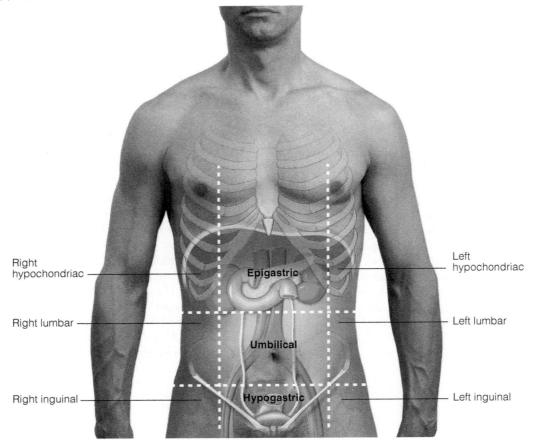

Figure 21.5 Mapping of the abdomen into nine regions.

FOUR ABDOMINAL QUADRANTS

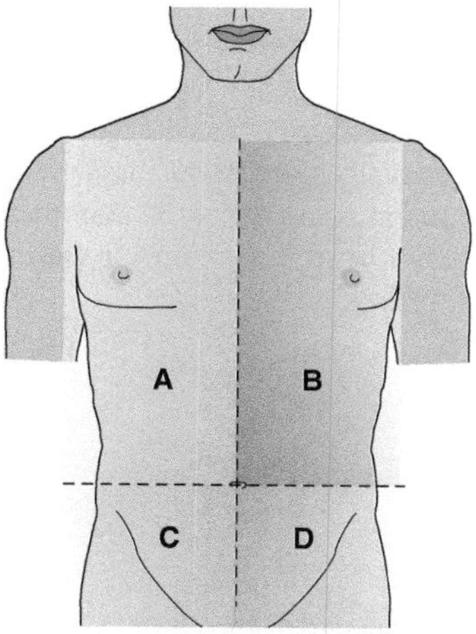

Midline
Aorta
Bladder
Uterus

◯ = Umbilicus

A
Right Upper Quadrant
Liver and gallbladder
Pyloric sphincter
Duodenum
Head of pancreas
Right adrenal gland
Portion of right kidney
Hepatic flexure of colon
Portions of ascending and
  transverse colon

B
Left Upper Quadrant
Left lobe of liver
Spleen
Stomach
Body of pancreas
Left adrenal gland
Portion of left kidney
Splenic flexure of colon
Portions of transverse and
  descending colon

C
Right Lower Quadrant
Lower pole of right kidney
Cecum and appendix
Portion of ascending colon
Ovary and uterine tube
Right spermatic cord
Right ureter

D
Left Lower Quadrant
Lower pole of left kidney
Sigmoid colon
Portion of descending colon
Ovary and uterine tube
Left spermatic cord
Left ureter

NINE ABDOMINAL REGIONS

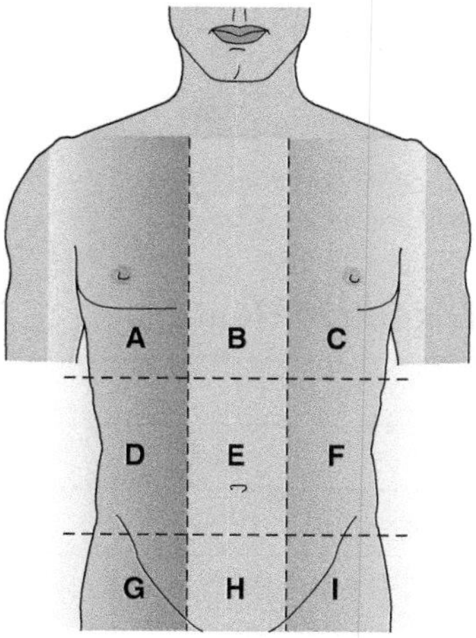

A
Right Hypochondriac
Right lobe of liver
Gallbladder
Portion of duodenum
Hepatic flexure of colon
Portion of right kidney
Right adrenal gland

B
Epigastric
Pyloric sphincter
Duodenum
Pancreas
Portion of liver
Aorta

C
Left Hypochondriac
Stomach
Spleen
Tail of pancreas
Splenic flexure of colon
Upper pole of left kidney
Left adrenal gland

D
Right Lumbar
Ascending colon
Lower half of right kidney
Portion of duodenum
  and jejunum

E
Umbilical
Lower part of duodenum
Jejunum and ileum

F
Left Lumbar
Descending colon
Lower half of left kidney
Portions of jejunum
  and ileum

G
Right Inguinal
Cecum
Appendix
Lower end of ileum
Right ureter
Right spermatic cord
Right ovary and uterine tube

H
Hypogastric (Pubic)
Ileum
Bladder
Uterus (in pregnancy)

I
Left Inguinal
Sigmoid colon
Left ureter
Left spermatic cord
Left ovary and uterine tube

Figure 21.6 Upper torso: Organs of the four abdominal quadrants. Lower torso: Organs of the nine abdominal regions.

Special Considerations

Subjective and objective data inform the nurse about the patient's health status. A variety of factors may influence health and include age, developmental level, race, ethnicity, work history, living conditions, socioeconomics, and emotional well-being. These factors are discussed in the following sections.

Health Promotion Considerations

A healthy digestive system promotes efficient nutrient absorption, which is essential for healthy growth and development. Digestive health also allows for adequate elimination of wastes and toxins from the body. Objectives of *Healthy People 2020* related to digestive health include reducing the incidence of colorectal cancer, which in 2010 was the second-leading cause of cancer-related deaths in the United States (Centers for Disease Control and Prevention [CDC], 2013a). In addition, national objectives include increasing food safety measures and reducing the incidence of foodborne illnesses. Prevention of various forms of hepatitis, as well as education about this illness, also are included as *Healthy People 2020* priorities (USDHHS, 2010).

See Table 21.1 for examples of *Healthy People 2020* objectives that are designed to promote health and wellness among individuals across the life span.

Lifespan Considerations

Data collection and interpretation of findings in relation to changes that accompany growth and development are important. Expected variations in the abdomen for different age groups are discussed in the following sections.

Infants and Children

The abdomen of the newborn and infant is round. The umbilical cord, containing two arteries and one vein, is ligated at the time of delivery. The stump dries and ultimately forms the umbilicus.

Typically, the umbilical cord will dry and fall off 10 to 14 after birth. The toddler has a characteristic "potbelly" appearance as depicted in Figure 21.7 ■. Respirations are abdominal; therefore, movement of the abdomen is seen with breathing. This breathing pattern is evident until about the sixth year, at which age respirations become thoracic.

Peristaltic waves are usually more visible in infants and children than in adults because the muscle wall of the abdomen is thinner. Children have the tendency to swallow more air than adults when

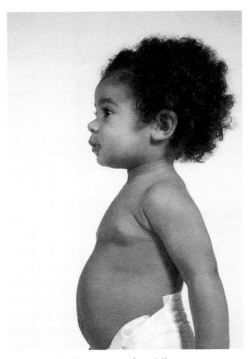

Figure 21.7 Potbelly stance of toddler.
Source: Alex Cao/Photodisc/Getty Images.

| TABLE 21.1 | Examples of *Healthy People 2020* Objectives Related to Digestive Health |

OBJECTIVE NUMBER	DESCRIPTION
C-9	Reduce invasive colorectal cancer
FS-1	Reduce infections caused by key pathogens transmitted commonly through food
FS-2	Reduce the number of outbreak-associated infections due to Shiga toxin-producing *E. coli* O157, or *Campylobacter*, *Listeria*, or *Salmonella* species associated with food commodity groups
FS-5	Increase the proportion of consumers who follow key food safety practices
IID-15	(Developmental) Increase hepatitis B vaccine coverage among high-risk populations
IID-23	Reduce hepatitis A
IID-24	Reduce chronic hepatitis B virus infections in infants and young children (perinatal infections)
IID-26	Reduce new hepatitis C infections
IID-27	Increase the proportion of persons aware they have a hepatitis C infection
IID-28	(Developmental) Increase the proportion of persons who have been tested for hepatitis B virus within minority communities experiencing health disparities

Source: U.S. Department of Health and Human Services (USDHHS). (2014). *Healthy people 2020.* Retrieved from http://www.healthypeople.gov/2020/default.aspx.

eating, thus creating a greater sound of tympany, a loud, high-pitched, drumlike tone, when percussion is performed. The area of tympany on the right side of the abdomen is smaller because the liver is larger in children.

Congenital defects such as cleft lip, cleft palate, esophageal atresia, pyloric stenosis, and hernias influence the nutritional status, growth, and development of the child and, therefore, must be assessed with care.

The size of the abdomen at all ages is an indication of the nutritional state of the child. For children of all ages, the nurse should ascertain feeding and eating habits and food tolerance. The child's symptoms such as nausea, vomiting, and skin rashes, as well as the actions taken by the parent, are important.

The liver edge may be palpable at the right lower costal margin because the thoracic cage of young children is smaller. The lower liver edge is palpable 1 to 2 cm (0.39 to 0.78 in.) below the costal margin in most infants. Any liver edge that is palpable more than 2 cm below the costal margin indicates hepatomegaly and should be evaluated. Detect the presence of tenderness or masses. Stop palpation if a mass is suspected. Wilms' tumor is a malignancy of the kidney commonly diagnosed in infants and toddlers. The most common presentation of Wilms' tumor is parental history of feeling an abdominal mass during bathing or diaper changes. Refer children with suspected Wilms' tumor for immediate evaluation. Palpation of the tumor will disseminate the tumor seeds into the abdomen. Do not palpate the abdomen if Wilms' tumor, or mass, is suspected. Constipation may result in a palpable cigar-shaped mass in the left lower quadrant.

Umbilical hernias cause a protrusion at the umbilicus and are visible at birth (see Figure 21.29 on page 571). Umbilical hernias are more common in African American children and among infants who are born prematurely (Johns Hopkins Medicine, n.d.a). The majority of umbilical hernias close before 5 years of age. Umbilical hernias require no medical intervention unless they incarcerate, cause symptoms, enlarge, or persist after age 5 years (Johns Hopkins Medicine, n.d.a).

Infectious mononucleosis is most common in school-age children. Splenomegaly occurs in up to 65% of acute mononucleosis cases (Luzuriaga & Sullivan, 2010). Enlarged spleens are vulnerable to trauma because they no longer fit completely behind the thoracic cage. Careful abdominal assessment is indicated in any child with suspected mononucleosis. Splenomegaly is common in young children with sickle cell disease (SCD) (Swarnkar, Kale, & Lakhkar, 2010). All children with SCD should be assessed for this complication.

Acute gastroenteritis (AGE) is an acute, common diarrhea disease that may or may not be accompanied by vomiting. Additional symptoms include abdominal pain, cramping, and fever. Pertinent history findings include frequency and amount of diarrhea, vomiting, magnitude and duration of fever, and presence and location of abdominal pain. Exposure to infectious substances (*Salmonella*, *Shigella*, etc.) and people with similar symptoms, as well as questions regarding hydration status, are important parts of the history. Abdominal examination may reveal hyperactive bowel sounds. Assessment of hydration status is essential and should include documentation of level of consciousness, presence of thirst, time and amount of last urination, vital signs (heart rate and blood pressure), skin turgor, and capillary perfusion of less than 2 seconds. Fontanelles should be assessed, and depressed or sunken fontanelles should be further evaluated.

> **ALERT!**
>
> *In children, decreased level of consciousness, weight loss, and decreased urine output are the most accurate indicators of dehydration. Vital sign, skin turgor, and capillary perfusion changes will be present only with moderate to severe dehydration and indicate risk of cardiovascular collapse.*

The Pregnant Female

During pregnancy, the abdomen undergoes many changes. As the pregnancy progresses, the uterus enlarges and moves into the abdominal cavity. The height of the fundus should be measured and compared against predictable levels based on the gestational week. By the 14th week of the pregnancy, the fundus should be above the pubic bone and easily palpable. By the 36th week, the fundus is high in the abdomen, close to the diaphragm, and compresses many abdominal structures (see Figure 21.8 ■). Constipation, flatulence, hemorrhoids, and frequent voiding are common problems resulting from the displacement of abdominal organs and pressure from the uterus. Changing levels of hormones decrease peristaltic activity, leading to a decrease in bowel sounds. Acid indigestion or heartburn, nausea, vomiting, and constipation are additional problems with the gastrointestinal system during pregnancy.

The skin of the abdomen undergoes some characteristic changes. Striae gravidarum (stretch marks) become most visible during the second half of the pregnancy (see chapter 27 ∞). Linea nigra, a dark line, extends from the umbilicus to the pubic bone along the midline of the abdomen (see Figure 13.7 on page 215 ∞). The muscles of the abdominal wall are stretched and may lose tone.

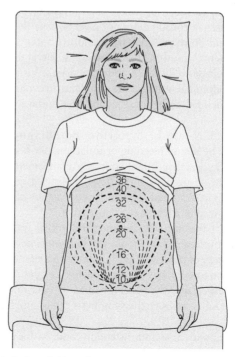

Figure 21.8 Fundal height measurements during specific gestational weeks.

The Older Adult

The digestive system of the older adult undergoes characteristic changes; however, these may not be as pronounced as changes in other body systems. There is a gradual decrease in secretion of saliva, digestive enzymes, peristalsis, intestinal absorption, and intestinal activity. These changes may lead to indigestion, constipation, and gastroesophageal reflux and could exacerbate any preexisting changes or disease.

Constipation is a common problem with older adults. Mostly, constipation in older adults is a product of many factors including decreased gastrointestinal motility; impaired physical mobility; medications such as opioids, anticholinergics, calcium suppliments, and NSAIDs; and cognitive disorders (Mayo Clinic, n.d.). Periodontal disease, with the subsequent loss of natural teeth, is also another factor because the inability to chew foods results in a diet of soft, nonfibrous foods. The loss of teeth makes chewing and swallowing of food difficult. Ill-fitting, broken, or lost dentures also alter nutritional status. Lack of fresh fruits and vegetables or other sources of bulk or fiber contributes to the pattern of constipation, as well. To decrease the frequency of urination, the older adult may self-limit daily fluid intake, especially water, which increases the potential for constipation. Other changes the nurse should anticipate with this age group are dry mouth, delayed esophageal and gastric emptying, decreased gastric acid production, and decreased liver size.

The appearance of the abdomen changes with the aging process. In the older adult, the abdomen may be more rounded or protuberant due to increased adipose tissue distribution, decreased muscle tone, and reduced fibroconnective tissue. The abdomen tends to be softer and more relaxed than in the younger adult. A scaphoid and flaccid abdomen is seen in the very old with additional fat loss, but this may also be a sign of rapid weight loss accompanying malnutrition or cancer. A distended abdomen is often seen with fluid in the peritoneal cavity (**ascites**) or excessive gas. Asymmetry may indicate tumors, hernia, constipation, or bowel obstruction. Although the slight up-and-down pulsation from a normal aorta is more readily seen in patients with thin abdominal walls, lateral pulsations or soft, pulsatile masses indicate an aortic aneurysm. Visible tortuous veins on the abdominal wall near the umbilicus, in conjunction with a firm and distended abdomen, may indicate portal hypertension with ascites.

Bowel sounds may be hypoactive. **Borborygmi** (stomach growling) may be due to bleeding or inflammatory bowel disease. High-pitched hyperactive bowel sounds accompanied by colicky pain and distention are signs of small bowel obstruction, which occurs most often in older males. Bruits heard over any of the arteries are signs of stenosis or aneurysms.

Because of the normally thinner abdominal wall, tympany may be more noticeable but should still be within normal ranges. Areas of dullness in the lower left quadrant and sigmoid area are probably related to stool, but it is essential to rule out tumors. Shifting dullness, especially when accompanied by firm dullness, suggests ascites. Dullness above the symphysis pubis could indicate a full bladder.

Tenderness with moderate distention could be due to flatus but could also indicate irritation of the stomach or bowel. The thinner abdominal wall of the older adult makes it easier to feel the underlying bowel. A soft mass or small firm masses felt in the left lower quadrant may be stool, especially because constipation is common. Firmness is associated with fluid or excessive gas, but rigidity is a sign of peritoneal inflammation. Distention just above the symphysis pubis may be caused by bladder distention due to prostatic hypertrophy or incomplete emptying. If the liver can be palpated below the costal margins, the liver is probably enlarged. Enlargement may reflect passive congestion due to congestive heart failure or liver disease, especially if the liver feels nodular.

Psychosocial Considerations

High stress levels may cause or aggravate abdominal problems. Gastritis, gastric or duodenal ulcers, and ulcerative colitis are several examples of stress-related problems.

Self-perception may have a subtle influence on the patient's weight. Patients who perceive themselves as naturally thin may show greater dedication to restricting their caloric intake and exercising to maintain that self-image. Conversely, patients who perceive themselves as naturally fat may overeat and avoid exercise, feeling that there is nothing they can do to alter their weight.

Surgical scars may alter an individual's body image. Gastrointestinal surgery may require a colostomy, which might be a temporary or permanent change. Many adults consider "wearing a bag" a significant limitation, causing embarrassment and anxiety. This often leads to depression and withdrawal.

Cultural and Environmental Considerations

Culture, customs, family, and religious practices influence the foods patients choose to eat. Certain foods may be prescribed or avoided in certain cultures or religions; however, a healthy diet usually can be achieved even with significant food restrictions. Patients used to a diet of meat and potatoes may not fully appreciate the value of fresh fruits and vegetables. For example, Seventh Day Adventists do not consume alcohol and caffeine or eat meat; Navajo indians do not eat fish; Muslims do not eat pork and during Ramadan do not eat, drink, or smoke between sunrise and sunset; Hindus may abstain from eating meat and fish; and Buddhists are often vegetarians.

The financial security of the patient also has an impact on eating habits. In some areas, certain foods may not be available year-round or may be much more costly than in other areas. For example, fresh fruits and vegetables typically increase in price in many regions in winter months. Unfortunately, highly processed foods are often lower in fiber than their fresh counterparts.

Cultural factors also may affect the incidence of gastrointestinal disorders. For example, African Americans experience a higher rate of colorectal cancer in comparison to White, Asian/Pacific Islander, American Indian/Alaskan Native, or Hispanic individuals (Centers for Disease Control and Prevention [CDC], 2013a). Likewise, the incidence of infection by *Helicobacter pylori*, which is a major cause of peptic ulcer disease, is highest among individuals of African American heritage (Epplein et al., 2011).

Gathering the Data

Health assessment of the abdomen includes the gathering of subjective and objective data. Subjective data collection occurs during the patient interview, before the actual physical assessment. During the interview the nurse uses a variety of communication techniques to elicit general and specific information about the patient's state of abdominal health or illness. Health records, the results of laboratory tests, and radiologic studies are important secondary sources to be reviewed and included in the data-gathering process.

During physical assessment of the abdomen, four techniques of physical assessment will be used. However, the order of the techniques changes to inspection, auscultation, percussion, and palpation. Auscultation is performed after inspection. This order prevents augmentation or disturbance of abdominal sounds that could occur from percussion and palpation. Percussion and palpation could influence peristaltic activity, thereby changing the findings upon auscultation. The diaphragm of the stethoscope should be used when auscultating for bowel sounds. The nurse should not apply heavy pressure to the diaphragm because this could influence peristaltic activity and, ultimately, the natural sounds of the intestinal activity. The bell is used when auscultating the aorta and other arteries. See Table 21.2 for information on potential secondary sources of patient data.

TABLE 21.2 **Potential Secondary Sources for Patient Data Related to the Digestive System**

LABORATORY TESTS		NORMAL VALUES
Stomach		
Helicobacter Pylori		Negative for antibody, antigen
Liver		
ALT (alanine aminotransferase)		Males: 7-55 Units/L
		Females: 7-45 Units/L
AST (aspartate aminotransferase)		Males: 8-48 Units/L
		Females: 8-43 Units/L
ALP (alkaline phosphatase)		44–147 Units/L
LDH (lactic dehydrogenase)		122–222 Units/L
Hepatic antigens		Negative
Serum vitamin B12		180–914 nanograms/L
Serum total bilirubin		$\leq$ 1.2 mg/dL
Serum ammonia		15–45 mcg/dL
Serum albumin		3.5–5 g/dL
Pancreas		
Amylase		26–102 Units/L
Lipase		10–73 Units/L
Glucose		70–140 mg/dL
Calcium		8.9–10.1 mg/dL
Diagnostic Tests		
Abdominal X-ray		
Barium Swallow		
Colonoscopy		
Computed Tomography (CT)		
Endoscopic Retrograde Cholangiography (ECP)		
Esophagoscopy		
Fecal Occult Blood Testing		
Gallbladder Ultrasonography		
Gastric Analysis		
Gastroscopy		
Liver Biopsy		
Magnetic Resonance Imaging (MRI)		
Percutaneous Transhepatic Cholangiography (PTCA)		

Focused Interview

The focused interview for assessment of the abdomen concerns data related to the structures and functions of organs within the abdomen. Subjective data related to the status and function of the structures within the abdomen are gathered during the focused interview. The nurse must be prepared to observe the patient and listen for cues related to the function of the organs and systems within the abdomen. The nurse may use open-ended and closed questions to obtain information. Often a number of follow-up questions or requests for descriptions are required to clarify data or gather missing information.

The focused interview guides the physical assessment of the abdomen. The information is always considered in relation to norms and expectations about the function of organs and systems within the abdomen. Therefore, the nurse must consider age, gender, race, culture, environment, health practices, past and concurrent problems, and therapies when framing questions and using techniques to elicit information. In order to address all of the factors when conducting a focused interview, categories of questions related to status and function of organs and systems within the abdomen have been developed. These categories include general questions that are asked of all patients, those addressing illness and infection, questions related to symptoms and behaviors, those related to habits or practices, questions that are specific to patients according to age, those for the pregnant female, and questions that address environmental concerns. One method to elicit information about symptoms is OLDCART & ICE as described in chapter 7. ∞ See Figure 7.3 on page 120.

The nurse must consider the patient's ability to participate in the focused interview and physical assessment of the abdomen. If a patient is experiencing pain, cramping, problems with elimination (including frequency or urgency), difficulty swallowing, nausea and vomiting, or the anxiety that accompanies any of these problems, attention must focus on identification of immediate problems and relief of symptoms.

Focused Interview Questions	Rationales and Evidence

The following section provides sample questions and bulleted follow-up questions in each of the previously mentioned categories. A rationale for each of the questions is provided. The list of questions is not all-inclusive but represents the types of questions required in a comprehensive focused

interview related to the abdomen. Subjective data collected and questions asked during the health history and focused interview provide information to help meet the objectives for gastrointestinal health described in Healthy People 2020.

General Questions

1. **Describe your appetite. Has it changed in the last 24 hours? In the last month? In the last year?**
   - What do you believe has caused the change in your appetite?
   - Have you done anything to address the change?
   - Have you spoken to a healthcare professional about the change?
   - Has anything else occurred with the change in appetite?

▶ These questions elicit basic information about the patient's eating. In addition, appetite change can be indicative of underlying physical and emotional problems. If a change has occurred, it is important to elicit the patient's perception of the change and to identify factors that may have contributed to the change.

2. **What is your weight? Has your weight changed?**
   - Over what period of time did the weight change occur?
   - What do you believe has contributed to your weight change?
   - Have any problems or symptoms accompanied the weight change?
   - Have you discussed this with a healthcare professional?

▶ Weight loss or gain can accompany physical and emotional problems. Dietary consumption is one of the leading factors in weight control. The nurse should determine if weight gain is associated with decrease in activity, changes in metabolic rates, hormonal factors, or fluid retention. Emotional problems may cause an individual to over- or underconsume foods. Weight loss may be an appropriate or desired outcome for some individuals. The nurse must determine if the weight loss was purposeful. Weight loss can accompany problems associated with diabetes, hyperthyroidism, and some cancers (Berman & Snyder, 2012).

   - Questions about dietary intake can be included in the follow-up about weight or may be included in questions about behaviors. These questions would include the following: Tell me what you have had to eat and drink in the last 24 hours. Be sure to include snacks. How much of each item did you consume? Is this a typical eating pattern for you?

▶ In addition to obtaining data about weight, the nurse is building on the nutritional data already collected. The nurse is establishing the patient's dietary patterns, paying special attention to overconsumption and underconsumption.

Focused Interview Questions	Rationales and Evidence

3. Describe your bowel habits. Describe the color and consistency of your stool.
- Have you experienced any changes in your elimination pattern or in your stool?
- What kind of change has occurred in your elimination pattern or stool?
- When did the change begin?
- Can you identify anything you believe may have caused the change?
- What have you done about the problem?
- Have you discussed the changes with a healthcare professional?
- Questions about the use of medications such as laxatives or antidiarrheals may be included as follow-up questions here. However, this information may have been obtained in the health history or can be included in questions about behaviors.

► These questions provide initial information about bowel functioning. The nurse determines if the patient has an established pattern for bowel elimination. If the patient indicates that there has been a change in the pattern of elimination or in the characteristics of the stool, follow-up questions are indicated. Tarry stool indicates bleeding in the upper part of the gastrointestinal tract. A clay color may indicate lack of bile in the stool (Sira, Salem, & Sira, 2013).

4. Do you have feelings of bloating or increased gas?
- What do you think causes this? Have any changes been made in your diet or medications?
- What do you do to decrease these feelings?
- What do you do to relieve the symptoms?
- Do you use antacids?
- Do you increase water intake?
- Do you exercise?

► Some foods (broccoli, cauliflower, figs) and intolerance to lactose will cause this feeling. Some medications are constipating (Wilson, Shannon, & Shields, 2013). Severe bloating and gas can be indicative of abdominal pathology.

5. Do you have any physical problems that affect your appetite, affect your bowel functioning, or contribute to abdominal problems?
- Describe the way your abdominal function is affected.
- How long has this been occurring?
- Have you sought relief for the problem?
- What have you done to relieve the problem?
- Did the remedy help?
- Have you sought advice from a healthcare professional?

► This question is used to elicit information about abdominal or other problems that may impact the structures and functions within the abdomen. For example, pain from any source may diminish appetite, and intake of medications for nonabdominal problems may affect digestion and abdominal comfort. If the patient identifies any problems that affect abdominal functions, follow-up is required for clear descriptions and details about what, when, and how problems occur; how abdominal function is impacted; and the duration of the problem.

6. Is there anyone in your family who has had an abdominal disease or problem?
- What is the disease or problem?
- Who in the family now has or has had the disease?
- When was it diagnosed?
- Describe the treatment.
- How effective was the treatment?

► This may reveal information about abdominal diseases associated with familial or genetic predisposition.
► Follow-up is required to obtain details about specific problems as well as their occurrence, treatment, and outcomes.

Questions Related to Illness or Infection

1. Have you ever been diagnosed with an abdominal disease?
- When were you diagnosed with the problem?
- What treatment was prescribed for the problem?
- Was the treatment helpful?
- What kinds of things do you do to help with the problem?
- Has the problem ever recurred (acute)?
- How are you managing the disease now (chronic)?

► The patient has an opportunity to provide information about specific abdominal diseases. If a diagnosed illness is identified, follow-up about the date of diagnosis, treatment, and outcomes is required. Data about each illness identified by the patient are essential to an accurate health assessment. Illness can be classified as acute or chronic, and follow-up regarding each classification will differ.

2. An alternative to question 1 is to list possible abdominal illnesses, such as cholecystitis, cholelithiasis, ulcers, diverticulosis, and cirrhosis, and ask the patient to respond "yes" or "no" as each is stated.
- Follow-up would be carried out for each identified diagnosis as in question 1.

► This is a comprehensive and easy way to elicit information about all abdominal diagnoses.

Focused Interview Questions	Rationales and Evidence

3. Do you now have or have you ever had an infection within the abdomen?
- When were you diagnosed with the infection?
- What treatment was prescribed for the problem?
- Was the treatment helpful?
- What kinds of things do you do to help with the problem?
- Has the problem ever recurred (acute)?
- How are you managing the infection now (chronic)?

▶ If an infection is identified, follow-up about the date of the infection, treatment, and outcomes is required. Data about each infection identified by the patient are essential to an accurate health assessment. Infections can be classified as acute or chronic, and follow-up regarding each classification will differ.

4. An alternative to question 3 is to list possible abdominal disorders, such as hepatitis, cholecystitis, and diverticulitis, and ask the patient to respond "yes" or "no" as each is stated.

▶ This is a comprehensive and easy way to elicit information about all abdominal disorders. Follow-up would be carried out for each identified diagnosis as in question 3.

Questions Related to Symptoms, Pain, and Behaviors

When gathering information about symptoms, many questions are required to elicit details and descriptions that assist in the analysis of the data. Discrimination is made in relation to the significance of a symptom, in relation to specific diseases or problems, and in relation to potential follow-up examination or referral. One rationale may be provided for a group of questions in this category.

The following questions refer to specific symptoms and behaviors associated with the organs and structures within the abdomen. For each symptom, questions and follow-up are required. The details to be elicited are the characteristics of the symptom; the onset, duration, and frequency of the symptom; the treatment or remedy for the symptom, including over-the-counter (OTC) and home remedies; the determination if a diagnosis has been sought; the effect of treatments; and family history associated with a symptom or illness.

Questions Related to Symptoms

Questions 1 through 20 refer to nausea as a symptom associated with abdominal problems and are comprehensive enough to provide an example of the number and types of questions required in a focused interview when a symptom exists. The remaining questions refer to other symptoms associated with abdominal problems. The number and types of questions are limited to identification of the symptom. Follow-up is included only when required for clarification.

1. Do you have nausea?

▶ Question 1 identifies the existence of a symptom, and questions 2 through 5 add knowledge about the symptom.

2. How long have you had the nausea?

▶ Determining the duration of symptoms is helpful in determining the significance of symptoms in relation to specific diseases and problems.

3. How often are you nauseated?

4. Do you know what is causing the nausea?

5. Is there a difference in the nausea at different times of the day?

6. Describe your nausea.

Focused Interview Questions	Rationales and Evidence
7. Is the nausea accompanied by burning, indigestion, or bloating?	▶ The description of the nausea may indicate a symptom associated with a specific disease or problem.
8. Do you vomit when you experience the nausea?	
9. What does the vomitus look like?	
10. Does the vomitus have any odor?	▶ The color and odor of vomitus may be associated with specific diseases or problems. For example, brown vomitus with a fecal odor can indicate an intestinal obstruction (Durston, 2009).
11. What was the cause, in your opinion?	
12. How frequently do you have this experience?	
13. What do you do to relieve the symptoms?	
14. When you vomit, describe what comes up and the amount.	▶ Vomiting can be related to a variety of pathologic conditions, such as food poisoning, ulcers, varices of the esophagus, hepatitis, and beginning of an intestinal obstruction (Mahadevan & Garmel, 2012). Medications, prescribed and OTC, may contribute to or cause vomiting (Wilson, et al., 2013).

15. Do you have pain with the nausea?
  • Describe the type, severity, and location of the pain.
  • What do you do for the pain?
  • Is the remedy effective?
	▶ Pain associated with nausea and vomiting may be indicative of an underlying abdominal disease. Follow-up elicits details that assist in the data analysis.

16. Have you sought treatment for the nausea?	▶ These questions provide information about the need for diagnosis, referral, or continued evaluation of the symptom. They also provide information about the patient's knowledge of a current diagnosis or problem, and his or her response to intervention.
17. When was the treatment sought?	
18. What occurred when you sought that treatment?	
19. Was something prescribed or recommended for the nausea?	
20. What was the effect of the remedy?	
21. Do you use OTC or home remedies for the nausea?	▶ Questions 21 through 24 provide information about drugs and substances that may relieve symptoms or provide comfort. Some substances may mask symptoms, interfere with the effect of prescribed medications, or harm the patient.
22. What are the OTC or home remedies that you use?	
23. How often do you use them?	
24. How much of them do you use?	
25. Do you have any difficulty chewing or swallowing your food?	▶ Ill-fitting dentures, failure to wear them, and missing or diseased teeth make chewing and swallowing difficult (Berman & Snyder, 2012). Disorders of the throat and esophagus can also make swallowing difficult.
26. Do you wear dentures?	
27. Do you have any crowns?	

Focused Interview Questions	Rationales and Evidence
28. Do your gums bleed easily?	▶ Chronic dry mouth, peridontal disease, anticoagulant use, and decreased platelets can cause an older adult's gums to bleed easily. If an anticoagulant dosing is too high, such as with coumadin, bleeding of the mucous membranes may occur (MedlinePlus, 2013). Bacterial growth from plaque can cause periodontal disease, which may not be easily diagnosed due to being painless until its late stages (American Dental Association, 2013).
29. Do you have indigestion? • Questions would include onset, frequency, and duration as well as knowledge about causative factors including food intolerance and discomfort associated with medications or treatments for other problems. For example, when did the indigestion start?	
30. Do you suffer from diarrhea or constipation?	
31. What do you think is the cause?	
32. What have you done to correct the situation?	
33. Have these measures helped the situation?	
34. Do you experience any rectal itching or bleeding?	▶ Dark, tarry stool indicates bleeding, usually in the upper or middle part of the intestinal tract. Bright red (frank) blood usually indicates lower tract bleeding (Berman & Snyder, 2012).

Questions Related to Pain

1. Are you having any abdominal pain at this time?
2. Where is the pain?
3. How often do you experience the pain?
4. How long does the pain last?
5. How long have you had the pain?
6. How would you rate the pain on a scale of 0 to 10, with 10 being the worst pain?
7. Does the pain radiate?
8. Where does the pain radiate?
9. Is there a trigger for the pain?
10. Does the pain affect your breathing or any other functions?
11. What do you think is causing the pain?
12. What do you do to relieve the pain?

▶ Questions 2 through 12 are standard questions associated with pain to determine the location, frequency, duration, and intensity of the pain.
▶ Pain could indicate cardiac disease, ulcers, cholecystitis, renal calculi, diverticulitis, urinary cystitis, or ectopic pregnancy (Mahadevan & Garmel, 2012).

Questions Related to Behaviors

1. What have you had to eat and drink in the last 24 hours?
2. What snacks do you have in a 24-hour period?
3. What size portions do you eat?

Focused Interview Questions	Rationales and Evidence
4. Is the 24-hour pattern you described typical for the way you eat?	▶ This provides input about diet and nutrition, which may contribute to obesity or problems with weight loss. This also provides information about meeting nutritional requirements.
5. How much coffee, tea, cola, alcoholic beverages, or chocolate do you consume in a 24-hour period?	▶ Caffeine and alcohol irritate the gastrointestinal system and can contribute to ulcers and irritable bowel syndrome (Johns Hopkins Medicine, n.d.b).

Questions Related to Age

The focused interview must reflect the anatomic and physiologic differences that exist along the age span. The following questions are examples of those that would be specific for infants and children, the pregnant female, and the older adult.

Questions Regarding Infants and Children

1. Is the baby breast fed or bottle fed?	▶ These questions assist in evaluation of gastrointestinal function by the baby's ability to take in nutrients, digest them, and eliminate waste products. The types of formula and food consumed influence color, consistency, amount, and frequency of the stool (Westerbeek et al., 2011).
2. Does the baby tolerate the feeding?	
3. How frequently does the baby eat?	
4. Have you recently started the baby on any new foods?	
5. Is the baby colicky? What do you do to relieve the colic?	
6. How much water does the baby drink?	
7. Does the toddler eat at regular times?	▶ Eating habits, patterns, and preferences established in the early years of life are likely to have a lasting effect.
8. What and how much does the toddler eat?	
9. Is the toddler able to feed himself or herself?	
10. What type of snacks does the toddler eat?	
11. Does the toddler experience restlessness at night related to rectal itching?	▶ Toddlers and school-aged children are at an increased risk of accquiring pinworms because they are spread by the fecal-oral route (CDC, 2013b).
12. Is the child toilet trained?	
13. Describe how toilet training is taught to the child.	
14. Have there been any lapses in toilet training?	
15. If so, how frequently? How recently?	
16. How do you typically respond to these lapses?	▶ As the nervous system matures, the child gradually achieves control of the anal sphincter (Berman & Snyder, 2012). The nurse should explore the developmental level and readiness of the child.
17. What does the child eat?	
18. Does the child bring a lunch and snack to school or buy it at school?	
19. When at home, how often does the child snack, and what are the snacks?	
20. Does the family have one meal a day together?	
21. What kind of food do you eat at this meal?	

Focused Interview Questions	Rationales and Evidence
22. Describe the atmosphere at this meal.	▶ The quality of the food is more important than the quantity of food. Mealtime should be enjoyable. Often this is the only time the family is together.

Questions for the Pregnant Female

1. Are you experiencing any nausea or vomiting?

▶ Nausea is common during early pregnancy and may be due to changing hormone levels and changes in carbohydrate metabolism. Fatigue is also a factor. Vomiting is less common. If it occurs more than once a day or for a prolonged period, the patient should be referred to a physician.

2. Are you experiencing any elimination problems such as constipation?

▶ A number of factors increase the likelihood of constipation during pregnancy. Among these are displacement of the intestines by the growing uterus, bowel sluggishness caused by increased progesterone and steroid metabolism, and the use of oral iron supplements, which are prescribed for many patients during pregnancy (Berman & Snyder, 2012; Wilson, Shannon, & Shields, 2013).

3. Are you experiencing heartburn or flatulence?

▶ Heartburn (regurgitation of gastric contents into the esophagus) is primarily caused by displacement of the stomach by the enlarging uterus. Flatulence results from decreased gastrointestinal motility, which is common during pregnancy, and from pressure on the large intestine from the growing uterus (Berman & Snyder, 2012).

Questions for the Older Adult

1. Are you ever incontinent of feces?

▶ Muscle tone decreases with age, and the older adult may lose sphincter control (Berman & Snyder, 2012).

2. How often are you constipated?

3. Do you take laxatives?

4. How often?

5. Which laxative do you take?

▶ Constipation is a common problem with older adults. Influencing factors include decreased peristaltic activity, decreased desire to eat, and self-limited fluid intake. To help relieve the problem, some older patients take OTC laxatives. With prolonged use, laxatives can become habit forming (Mohamed & Hanafy, 2013).

6. How many foods containing fiber or roughage do you eat during a typical day?

▶ Older adults tend to have diets low in fiber or roughage. Loss of natural teeth and ill-fitting dentures make chewing difficult (Berman & Snyder, 2012).

7. Are you able to get to the store for groceries?

8. Do you eat alone? With someone?

▶ Responses to questions 7 and 8 help determine mobility patterns, availability of food, and social isolation at mealtimes.

Focused Interview Questions	Rationales and Evidence

Questions Related to the Environment

Environment refers to both the internal and external environments. Questions related to the internal environment include all of the previous questions and those associated with internal or physiologic responses. Questions regarding the external environment include those related to home, work, or social environments.

Internal Environment

9. **How would you describe your stress level?**

10. **Do you think you are coping well?**

11. **Could your coping skills be better?**

▶ Prolonged stress is linked to gastrointestinal disease (Konturek, Brzozowski, & Konturek, 2011).

External Environment

1. **Do you work with any chemical irritants?**

▶ Exposure to benzol, lead, or nickel may lead to gastric irritation (Cherian, Mulky, & Menon, 2014). Excessive exposure to chemical hepatotoxins such as carbon tetrachloride may lead to postnecrotic cirrhosis (Muriel & Escobar, 2003).

2. **Have you recently done any traveling?**

3. **Where did you travel?**

▶ Water purification and food storage methods vary in different regions and different countries. Exposure to food- or waterborne microorganisms can lead to gastroenteritis, hepatitis, diarrhea, or parasite infestation.
▶ Follow-up questions would include all of the questions mentioned above that address symptoms and problems.

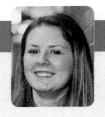

Patient-Centered Interaction

Ms. Emily Zabriski is a 20-year-old college student living on campus. She has purchased the 7-day meal plan and has lunch and dinner in the student dining room. Breakfast is usually one cup of coffee and one glass of orange juice "to go." This is determined by the time of her first class and how late she gets up.

Not having slept last night, Ms. Zabriski reports to the health center on campus early in the morning with complaints of nausea, vomiting, diarrhea, abdominal pain, and cramping in the right and left lower quadrants. She has experienced these symptoms for approximately 18 hours. The following is an excerpt of the focused interview.

Interview

Nurse: Good morning, Ms. Zabriski. I see by your report you have had nausea, vomiting, diarrhea, lower abdominal pain, and cramping for about 18 hours.

Ms. Zabriski: Yes, that is correct.

Nurse: First, I want you to rate and describe your pain. On a scale of 0 to 10, with 0 being no pain and 10 being the most severe pain ever, choose a number that matches your pain.

Ms. Zabriski: Oh, it is a 2 to 3 right now. When I vomit or have diarrhea it goes up, maybe to 8, then comes down. I have a lot of cramps.

Nurse: With your pain at a 2 to 3 level, do you think you could answer a few questions?

Ms. Zabriski: Oh, that won't be a problem. It is only a problem when I'm going to vomit or have diarrhea. Right now I'm OK.

Nurse: These symptoms could occur for any number of reasons. What do you think is causing your problem?

Ms. Zabriski: I don't understand what you mean.

Nurse: These symptoms could be caused by stress, food allergies, an intestinal disease such as Crohn's disease, or pregnancy, just to mention a few.

Ms. Zabriski: It could be something I ate, or maybe it is a stomach virus. Five dorm mates on my floor have the same thing.

Nurse: Let's talk about you. Since you indicated maybe it was something you ate, tell me about your eating prior to getting sick.

Ms. Zabriski: I had lunch in the student dining room. I had a glass of ice tea, cottage cheese with fruit salad, and a small bag of chips.

Nurse: What have you had to eat since lunch yesterday?

Ms. Zabriski: Well, I started to vomit and have cramps about 1½ hours after I ate. Now even crackers won't stay down.

Nurse: When was the last time you drank something?

Ms. Zabriski: I tried some diet cola after I vomited the first time and that came up.

Nurse: What have you taken to try to stop the nausea, vomiting, and diarrhea?

Ms. Zabriski: Nothing, I thought it would stop and go away, but it hasn't. That's why I'm here.

Analysis

The nurse used several communication strategies to obtain information from Ms. Zabriski. First, the nurse determined Ms. Zabriski's level of pain and discomfort and ability to participate in the interview. When asked what could be causing the symptoms, Ms. Zabriski responded with uncertainty. The nurse provided clarity with some diagnoses that could contribute to the symptoms. Following the response by Ms. Zabriski, the nurse brought the focus to Ms. Zabriski and not the dorm mates. The interview continued with the nurse obtaining specific subjective data using open-ended questions.

Patient Education

The following are physiologic, behavioral, and cultural factors that affect the health of the gastrointestinal system and abdominal structures across the life span. Several factors reflect trends cited in *Healthy People 2020* documents. The nurse provides advice and education to promote and maintain health and reduce risks associated with the aforementioned factors.

LIFESPAN CONSIDERATIONS

Risk Factors

Patient Education

- Congenital defects such as cleft lip, cleft palate, esophageal atresia, pyloric stenosis, and hernias affect the nutritional status as well as the growth and development of infants and children.

▶ Educate parents of children with congenital defects about alterations in foods and feeding patterns.

- Pregnant females experience hormonal shifts that result in nausea, vomiting, and constipation.

▶ Tell pregnant patients that dietary changes including small, frequent meals of dry foods are helpful in relieving the nausea and vomiting in early pregnancy.
▶ Inform patients that increased fluid intake, fruits, and high-fiber foods increase regularity in bowel elimination in pregnant females and in older adults.

- A decrease in digestive enzymes and decreased peristalsis occur in older adults.

▶ Tell patients that regular exercise promotes and maintains the efficiency of gastrointestinal function.

- Obesity has become increasingly prevalent across the age span in the United States.

▶ Provide information about healthy eating from infancy to old age to prevent obesity and contribute to improved gastrointestinal function.

- Dental diseases occur at all ages and impact nutrition by affecting the desire for food and the ability to chew foods.

▶ Advise patients about regular dental hygiene and care to reduce risks for malnutrition.

- Foodborne illness occurs in all age groups; however, children, older adults, and those with immunosuppression are at greatest risk.

▶ Provide information about hand hygiene and safe food preparation, handling, and storage because it is important in reducing the incidence of foodborne illnesses and hepatitis.

- Hepatitis infections can be acute or chronic and occur in all ages. Hepatitis A occurs most frequently in children and young adults. Hepatitis can be an acute self-limiting illness or a chronic debilitating disease. It can result in liver necrosis and death. Individuals who travel to India, Asia, Africa, and Central America are at risk for hepatitis E.

▶ Tell patients that immunization for hepatitis is important across the age span. Recommended schedules should be followed.

CULTURAL CONSIDERATIONS

Risk Factor

Patient Education

- The types of foods one eats and the ways in which foods are prepared are influenced by culture. Frequent ingestion of fried foods can result in obesity and health problems associated with high cholesterol.

▶ Discuss alternative methods of food preparation and seasoning to decrease the incidence of obesity and gastrointestinal disorders that occur with greater frequency in cultural groups who prepare spicy and fried foods.

ENVIRONMENTAL CONSIDERATIONS

Risk Factors

Patient Education

- Medications can impact the function and integrity of the gastrointestinal system. For example, aspirin and nonsteroidal anti-inflammatory drugs (NSAIDs) can irritate the mucosa of the gastrointestinal tract. Pain medications often slow the peristaltic process.

▶ Provide instruction about prescribed and OTC medications to reduce the risks of side effects that impact gastrointestinal health and other physiologic functions or systems.

- Stress is associated with increased frequency, duration, and acuity of gastrointestinal and abdominal problems including ulcerative diseases and eating disorders.

▶ Provide information about stress reduction techniques, support groups, and resources in the community to assist with crisis management and ongoing stressful situations.

Risk Factor	Patient Education
• Alcohol abuse is associated with gastritis and liver disease. The number of adolescents who abuse alcohol is on the rise. Alcohol use is greater in Caucasians and Hispanics than in African Americans.	▶ Advise adolescents, parents, and adults about alcohol abuse in relation to gastrointestinal and liver diseases. Teach patients how to recognize behaviors associated with alcohol abuse, and about prevention programs and addiction services to reduce the incidence of physical and emotional problems associated with alcohol abuse.

Physical Assessment

Assessment Techniques and Findings

Physical assessment of the abdomen requires the use of inspection, auscultation, percussion, and palpation. This order differs from that of physical assessment of other systems. The nurse should remember to auscultate after inspection. Delaying percussion and palpation prevents disturbance of the normal bowel sounds. During each of the procedures, the nurse is gathering data related to problems with underlying abdominal organs and structures. Inspection includes looking at skin color, structures of the abdomen, abdominal contour, pulsations, and abdominal movements. Knowledge of normative values or expected findings is essential in determining the meaning of the data as the physical assessment is performed.

The skin of the abdomen should be consistent with the skin of the rest of the body. The umbilicus should be midline in an abdomen that may be round, flat, convex, or protuberant. The abdomen should be symmetric and free of bulges. Pulsations and wavelike movements below the xiphoid process are normal in thin adults.

Physical assessment of the abdomen follows an organized pattern. It begins with a patient survey followed by inspection, auscultation, percussion, and palpation of the abdomen. The lateral aspects of the abdomen are included when conducting each of the assessments.

Techniques and Normal Findings	**Abnormal Findings Special Considerations**

Survey

A quick survey of the patient enables the nurse to identify any immediate problems as well as the patient's ability to participate in the assessment.

Inspect the overall appearance, posture, and position of the patient. Observe for signs of pain or discomfort and signs of anxiety or distress.

▶ Patients experiencing anxiety may demonstrate pallor and shallow breathing. They may be diaphoretic and use their hands to guard their abdomen.

▶ Acknowledgment of the problem and a discussion of the procedures often provide some relief. If the patient is experiencing severe pain or discomfort, the problem must be addressed and a complete abdominal assessment may need to be delayed.

Inspection of the Abdomen

1. **Position the patient.**
   - The patient should be in a supine position with a small pillow placed beneath the head and knees. Drape the examination gown over the chest, exposing the abdomen. Place the drape at the symphysis pubis, covering the patient's pubic area and legs (see Figure 21.9 ■).

▶ These measures relax the abdominal musculature and prevent unnecessary exposure of the patient.

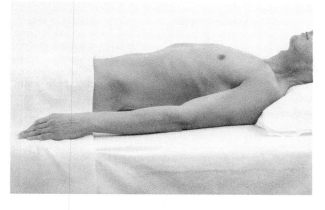

Figure 21.9
Patient positioned and draped.

   - Stand at the right side of the patient. Lighting must be adequate to detect color differences, lesions, and movements of the abdomen.

2. **Instruct the patient.**
   - Explain that you will be looking at the patient's abdomen. Tell the patient to breathe normally.

▶ If the patient is guarding the abdomen, demonstrated by posture or breathing, ask the patient to take several deep breaths. This assists in relaxation of abdominal musculature.

3. **Map the abdomen.**
   - Visualize the imaginary horizontal and vertical lines delineating the abdominal quadrants and regions as identified in Figures 21.5 and 21.6.
   - Visualize the underlying structures as identified in Figure 21.6.

4. **Determine the contour of the abdomen.**
   - Observe the profile of the abdomen between the costal margins and the symphysis pubis.
   - The abdominal profile should be viewed at eye level. You may need to sit or kneel to observe the abdominal profile.
   - Normal findings include flat, rounded, or scaphoid contours (see Figure 21.10 ■).

▶ A protuberant abdomen is normal in toddlers and in pregnancy. It may indicate obesity or ascites in a nonpregnant patient.

Techniques and Normal Findings

Abnormal Findings Special Considerations

Flat. A straight horizontal line is observed from the costal margin to the symphysis pubis. This contour is common in a thin person.

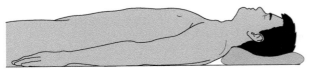

Rounded. Sometimes called a convex abdomen. The horizontal line now curves outward, indicating an increase in abdominal fat or a decrease in muscle tone. This contour is considered a normal variation in the toddler and the pregnant female.

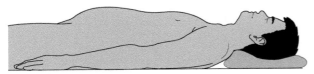

Figure 21.10 Contour of the abdomen.

Protuberant. Similar to the rounded abdomen, only greater. This contour is anticipated in pregnancy. It is also seen in the adult with obesity, ascites, and other conditions.

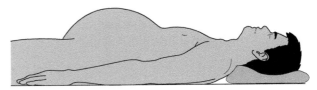

Scaphoid. Sometimes called a concave abdomen. The horizontal line now curves inward toward the vertebral column, giving the abdomen a sunken appearance. In the adult, this contour is seen in the very thin person.

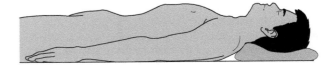

5. **Observe the position of the umbilicus.**
   - The umbilicus is normally in the center of the abdomen. It may be inverted or protruding. The umbilicus should be clean and free of inflammation or drainage.

> **ALERT!**
>
> *A patient with drainage from the umbilicus following laparoscopic surgery should be referred to the physician immediately. If a bowel diversion ostomy (e.g., gastrostomy, colonostomy, jejunostomy, or ileostomy) is present, the nurse should assess the patient's stoma for color and presence of drainage. Usually, the stoma is red, moist, and free from drainage (Berman & Snyder, 2012).*

6. **Observe skin color.**
   - The abdominal skin should be consistent in color and luster with the skin of the rest of the body. The skin is smooth, moist, and free of lesions.

7. **Observe the location and characteristics of lesions, scars, and abdominal markings.**
   - Lesions such as macules, moles, and freckles are considered normal findings.

8. **Observe the abdomen for symmetry, bulging, or masses.**
   - First, observe the abdomen while standing at the patient's side. Second, observe the abdomen while standing at the foot of the examination table. Compare the right and left sides. The sides should appear symmetric in shape, size, and contour.
   - Third, return to the patient's side and use a tangential light across the abdomen. No shadows should appear.

▶ A protruding or displaced umbilicus is a normal variation in pregnant females. In the nonpregnant adult, it could indicate an abdominal mass or distended urinary bladder. Inflammation or drainage may indicate an infection or complication from recent laparoscopic surgery. A displaced or protruding umbilicus may be a sign of a hernia in a child.

▶ Taut, glistening skin could indicate ascites.

▶ **Striae,** commonly called stretch marks, are silvery, shiny, irregular markings on the skin. These are seen in obesity, pregnancy, and ascites (refer to Figure 27.8A on page 803 ∞).
▶ Scars indicate previous surgery or trauma and the possibility of underlying adhesions. The location of all lesions must be documented as baseline data and for determination of change in future assessment.

▶ Asymmetry may indicate masses, adhesions, or strictures of underlying structures.

▶ Shadows may indicate bulges or masses.

Techniques and Normal Findings	Abnormal Findings / Special Considerations

- Observe the abdomen from eye level, by sitting or kneeling, and shine the light across the abdomen. The abdomen should appear symmetric without bulges or masses.
- You may repeat all of the assessments above while asking the patient to take a deep breath and raise the head off the pillow.

▶ Bulges could indicate tumors, cysts, or hernias.
▶ Deep breathing and head raising accentuate masses.

9. Observe the abdominal wall for movement.
- Movements can include pulsations or peristaltic waves. In thin patients it is normal to observe a pulsation of the abdominal aorta below the xiphoid process. The observation of peristaltic waves in thin patients is normal.

▶ Marked pulsations could indicate aortic aneurysm or increased pulse pressure. Increased peristaltic activity could indicate gastroenteritis or an obstructive process.

Auscultation of the Abdomen

Auscultation of the abdomen refers to listening to bowel sounds, vascular sounds, and friction rubs through the stethoscope.

> **ALERT!**
> It is important to auscultate before percussing and palpating, because the latter techniques could alter peristaltic action.

The pattern for auscultation of bowel sounds is to begin in the RLQ and then proceed through each of the remaining quadrants. The diaphragm of the stethoscope is used to auscultate bowel sounds. The pattern for auscultation of vascular sounds is to begin at the midline below the xiphoid process for the aorta and to proceed from side to side over renal, iliac, and femoral arteries. The bell of the stethoscope is used to auscultate vascular sounds.

The pattern for auscultation for friction rubs is to begin in the RLQ and proceed through each of the remaining quadrants and to listen over the liver and spleen.

The normal bowel sounds heard upon auscultation of the abdomen are irregular, high-pitched, gurgling sounds.

Normal bowel sounds occur from 5 to 30 times per minute. Borborygmi typically refers to more frequent sounds heard in patients who have not eaten in a few hours.

Auscultation of the normal abdomen will not produce vascular sounds or friction rubs.

▶ Hyperactive bowel sounds are loud, high-pitched, and rushing. They may occur more frequently with gastroenteritis or diarrhea.
▶ Hypoactive sounds that are slow and sluggish are common following abdominal surgery or bowel obstruction.
▶ Absent bowel sounds may be indicative of paralytic ileus.
▶ Vascular sounds include bruits and venous hum. A bruit is pulsatile and blowing. A venous hum is soft, continuous, and low-pitched.
Friction rub refers to a rough, grating sound caused by the rubbing together of organs or an organ rubbing on the peritoneum.

1. Instruct the patient.
- Explain that you will be listening to the patient's abdomen with the stethoscope. The patient will be in the supine position. Tell the patient to breathe normally. Explain that you will be moving the stethoscope around the patient's abdomen and stopping to listen when the stethoscope is placed down. Inform the patient that this will cause no discomfort.

Techniques and Normal Findings	Abnormal Findings Special Considerations

2. Auscultate for bowel sounds.

- Use the diaphragm of the stethoscope. Start in the RLQ and move through the other quadrants. Note the character and frequency of the sounds. Count the sounds for at least 60 seconds (see Figure 21.11 ■).

▶ Hyperactive sounds are common in gastroenteritis and diarrhea.
▶ Hypoactive sounds are common following abdominal surgery and occur in end-stage intestinal obstruction.
▶ Absence of bowel sounds may indicate paralytic ileus or intestinal obstruction.

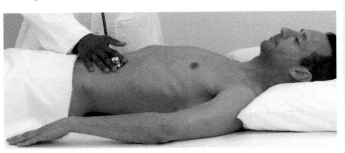

Figure 21.11
Auscultating the abdomen for bowel sounds.

- Normal bowel sounds are irregular, gurgling, and high-pitched. They occur from 5 to 30 times per minute. Borborygmi is a normal finding.

▶ Patients with paralytic ileus or intestinal obstruction require immediate attention.

> **ALERT!**
>
> *It may be difficult for the novice nurse to hear bowel sounds in some patients. Bowel sounds may be difficult to hear in obese patients with large amounts of adipose tissue in the abdomen. All four quadrants are auscultated for a total of at least 5 minutes before documenting absent bowel sounds.*

3. Auscultate for vascular sounds.

- Use the bell of the stethoscope. Listen at the midline below the xiphoid process for aortic sounds. Move the stethoscope from side to side as you listen over the renal, iliac, and femoral arteries (see Figure 21.12 ■).

▶ Bruits heard during systole and diastole may indicate arterial occlusion.
   A venous hum usually indicates increased portal tension.

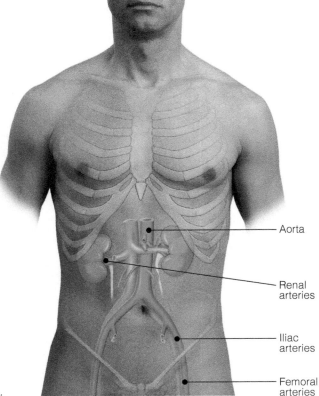

Aorta

Renal arteries

Iliac arteries

Femoral arteries

Figure 21.12
Auscultatory areas for vascular sounds.

Techniques and Normal Findings	Abnormal Findings Special Considerations

4. Auscultate for friction rubs.

- Auscultate the abdomen, listening for a coarse, grating sound. Listen carefully over the liver and spleen. Friction rubs are not normally heard.

Percussion of the Abdomen

1. Visualize the landmarks.

- Observe the abdomen and visualize the horizontal and vertical lines. Visualize the organs and underlying structures of the abdomen.

2. Recall the expected findings.

- Percussion allows you to assess underlying structures. The normal sounds heard over the abdomen are tympany, a loud hollow sound, and dullness, a short high-pitched sound heard over solid organs and the distended bladder.

▶ Hyperresonance is louder than tympany and is heard over air-filled or distended intestines. Flat sounds are short and abrupt and heard over bone. Correct placement of the fingers is important.

3. Instruct the patient.

- Explain that you will be tapping on the patient's abdomen in a variety of areas.
- Tell the patient to breathe normally through this examination. If muscle tension is detected, ask the patient to take several deep breaths.

4. Percuss the abdomen.

- Place your pleximeter finger on the abdomen during the examination. Review the technique of percussion in chapter 9. ∞ Start in the RLQ and percuss through all of the remaining quadrants (see Figure 21.13 ■).

Figure 21.13 Percussion pattern for abdomen.

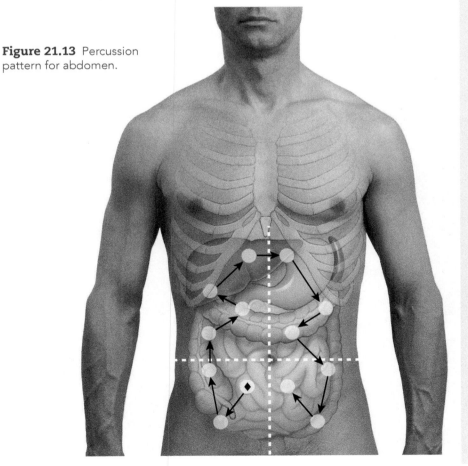

Techniques and Normal Findings	Abnormal Findings Special Considerations

- Percussion over the abdomen produces tympany. Tympany is more pronounced over the gastric bubble. Dullness is heard over the liver and spleen.

▶ Dullness may indicate an enlarged uterus, distended urinary bladder, or ascites. Dullness in the LLQ may indicate the presence of stool in the colon. It is important to ask when the patient last had a bowel movement.

ADVANCED SKILL

PERCUSSION OF THE LIVER

Percuss the liver to determine the upper and lower borders at the anterior axillary line, MCL, and midsternal line. Measure the distance between marks drawn to identify the borders.

1. **Instruct the patient.**
   - Explain that you will be tapping the patient's abdomen and chest on the right side. Explain that you will be making marks on the abdomen and using a ruler to measure the marks in order to evaluate the size of the liver. Tell the patient to remain relaxed and that there should be no discomfort during this assessment.

2. **Percuss the liver.**
   - Begin percussion at the level of the umbilicus and move toward the rib cage along the extended right MCL (see Figure 21.14 ■).

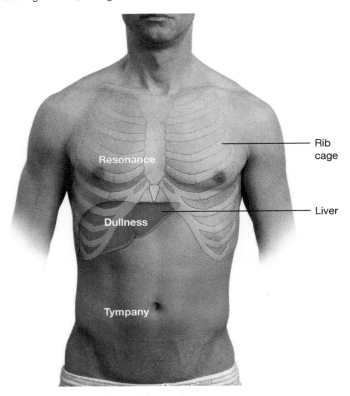

Figure 21.14 Normal tones elicited during liver percussion.

- The first sound you should hear is tympany. When the sound changes to dullness, you have identified the lower border of the liver. Mark the point with a skin-marking pen. The lower border is normally at the costal margin.

▶ Tympany often is heard over the lower abdomen due to the presence of gas in the gastrointestinal tract. Dullness below the costal margin suggests liver enlargement or downward displacement due to respiratory disease. Dullness above the fifth or sixth intercostal space could indicate an enlarged liver (hepatomegaly) or displacement upward due to ascites or a mass.

- Percuss downward from the fourth intercostal space along the right MCL. The first sound you should hear is resonance because you are over the lung. Percuss downward until the sound changes to dullness. This is the upper border of the liver. Mark the point with a pen. The upper border should be at the level of the sixth intercostal space.

▶ Movement of the liver is diminished when atelectasis or pneumothorax of the right lung exists.

- Measure the distance between the two points. The distance should be approximately 5 to 10 cm (2 to 4 in.). This distance is called the *liver span*.
- Percuss along the midsternal line, using the same technique as before. The liver size at the midsternal line should be approximately 4 to 9 cm (1.5 to 3 in.).
- To determine the movement of the liver with breathing, ask the patient to take a deep breath and hold it. Percuss upward along the extended MCL.
- The lower liver border should descend about 2.54 cm (1 in.). Remember, liver size is influenced by age, gender, height, and disease process.

ADVANCED SKILL

PERCUSSION OF THE SPLEEN

The spleen is located in the left side of the abdomen. Percussion is conducted to identify enlargement of the organ.

1. **Instruct the patient.**
   - Explain that you will be tapping on the left side of the patient's abdomen to examine the spleen. Tell the patient to continue to relax, taking deep breaths if required.

2. **Percuss the spleen.**
   - Percuss the abdomen on the left side posterior to the midaxillary line (see Figure 21.15 ■).

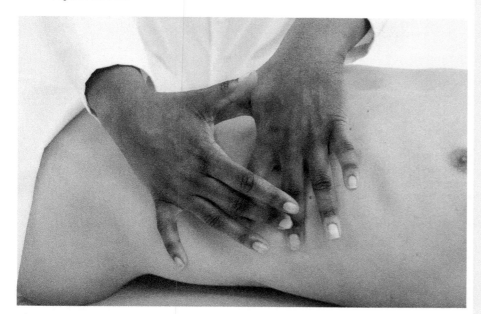

Figure 21.15 Percussing the spleen.

Techniques and Normal Findings	Abnormal Findings Special Considerations

- A small area of splenic dullness will usually be heard from the 6th to 10th intercostal spaces.

▶ Splenic dullness at the left anterior axillary line indicates splenomegaly, an enlarged spleen. The dull percussion sound is identifiable before an enlarged spleen is palpable. The spleen enlarges anteriorly and inferiorly (see Figure 21.16 ■).

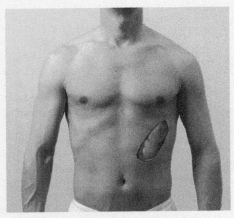

Figure 21.16 Splenic enlargement.

Percussion of the Gastric Bubble

Percussion of the gastric bubble is conducted to determine the area occupied by the stomach.

1. **Instruct the patient.**
   - Explain that you will be tapping on the patient's abdomen over the stomach area. Repeat the explanation about relaxation, if required.

2. **Percuss the gastric bubble.**
   - Percuss the abdomen in the area between the left costal margin and the midsternal line extended below the xiphoid process.
   - The percussion sound will be tympany.
   - The sound is influenced by the stomach contents.

▶ A dull percussion sound suggests a stomach mass. Dull percussion sounds may occur after a meal.
▶ A very loud sound and an increased area suggest gastric dilation.

Palpation of the Abdomen

Palpation of the abdomen is conducted to determine organ size and placement, muscle tightness or guarding, masses, tenderness, and the presence of fluid. This is performed after auscultation to avoid changing the natural sounds and movements of the abdomen. Identify painful areas and palpate these areas last.

You will use both light and deep palpation.

▶ Muscle tightness or guarding may indicate abdominal pain. Guarding is involuntary contraction of abdominal muscles associated with peritonitis.
▶ Abdominal pain from an organ is often experienced as referred pain—that is, felt on the surface of the abdomen or back.

ALERT!

Palpation of the abdomen is contraindicated in the following conditions: suspected appendicitis or dissecting abdominal aortic aneurysm, polycystic kidneys, and transplanted organs.

1. **Instruct the patient.**
   - Explain that you will be touching the patient's abdomen with your hands. Explain that you are going to use light touch and then slight pressure to explore the abdomen. Instruct the patient to inform you of any discomfort. Observe the patient's facial expression for signs of pain. Also watch for the tendency to guard the abdomen with the hands or to flex the knees.
   - Instruct the patient to take several deep breaths to relax the muscles of the abdomen.

Techniques and Normal Findings	Abnormal Findings Special Considerations

2. Lightly palpate the abdomen.

- Place the palmar surface of your hand on the abdomen and extend your fingers. Lightly press into the abdomen with your fingers (see Figure 21.17 ■).

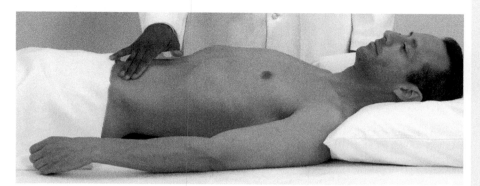

Figure 21.17 Light palpation of abdomen.

- Move your hand over the four quadrants by lifting your hand and then placing it in another area. Do not drag or slide your hand over the surface of the skin.
- The abdomen should be soft, smooth, nontender, and pain free.

3. Deeply palpate the abdomen.

- Proceed as for light palpation, described in the previous step. Exert pressure with your hand to depress the abdomen about 5 cm (2 in.).

- Palpate all four quadrants in an organized sequence.

▶ Masses, tumors, or obstructions may be palpated.

- In an obese patient or a patient with an enlarged abdomen, use a bimanual technique. Place the fingers of your nondominant hand over your dominant hand (see Figure 21.18 ■).

▶ In the pregnant female the uterus is palpable. The height of the fundus varies according to the week of gestation.

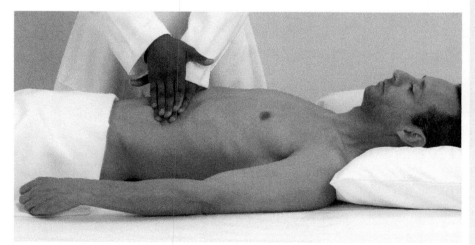

Figure 21.18 Deep palpation of abdomen using a bimanual technique.

- Identify the size of the underlying organs and any masses for tenderness. The pancreas is nonpalpable because of its size and location.

▶ A mass in the LLQ may be stool in the colon.
▶ A vaguely palpable sensation of fullness in the epigastric region may be pancreatic in origin.

Techniques and Normal Findings	Abnormal Findings Special Considerations

ADVANCED SKILL

PALPATION OF THE LIVER

The liver is palpated to detect enlargement, pain, and consistency.

1. **Instruct the patient.**
   - Explain that you will be using your hands to palpate the patient's liver. Explain that you will place one hand under the ribs in the back and ask the patient to take a deep breath while you apply slight pressure in an upward motion under the ribs on the patient's right side. Instruct the patient to tell you of any pain and observe the patient for cues of discomfort.

2. **Palpate the liver.**
   - Stand on the right side of the patient. Place your left hand under the lower portion of the ribs (ribs 11 and 12). Tell the patient to relax into your left hand. Lift the rib cage with your left hand.

   - Place your right hand into the abdomen using an inward and upward thrust at the costal margin (see Figure 21.19 ■). Ask the patient to take a deep breath. The descent of the diaphragm will cause the liver to descend, and the lower border will meet your right hand.

▶ Pain on palpation indicates gallbladder disease, hepatitis, or enlargement of the liver (hepatomegaly) associated with congestive heart failure.

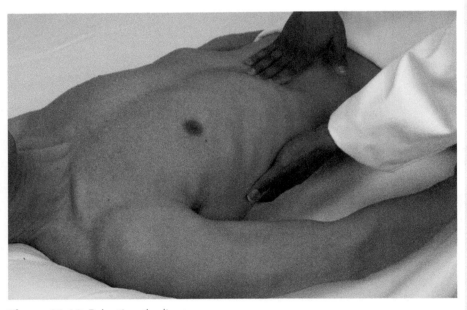

Figure 21.19 Palpating the liver.

   - Normally, the liver is nonpalpable, except in thin patients. If you feel the lower border of the liver it will be smooth, firm, and nontender.

▶ Nodules occur with cirrhosis or metastatic carcinoma.

Techniques and Normal Findings	Abnormal Findings Special Considerations

ADVANCED SKILL

PALPATION OF THE SPLEEN

The spleen is palpated to detect enlargement. Careful palpation is required because the spleen is fragile and sensitive.

1. Instruct the patient.
- Explain that you will be touching the patient with both hands to palpate the spleen. Explain that you will be lifting the patient slightly with your left hand while applying slight pressure with your fingers under the ribs on the left side. Instruct the patient to inform you of any pain or discomfort.

2. Palpate the spleen.
- Stand on the patient's right side. Place your left hand under the lower border of the rib cage on the left side and elevate the rib cage. This moves the spleen anteriorly. Press the fingers of your right hand into the left costal margin area of the patient (see Figure 21.20 ■).

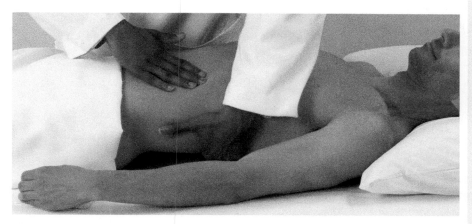

Figure 21.20 Palpating the spleen.

- Ask the patient to take a slow deep breath. As the diaphragm descends, the spleen moves forward to the fingertips of your right hand. The spleen is normally not palpable.

► Splenomegaly, enlargement of the spleen, occurs in acute infections such as mononucleosis. The enlarged spleen is palpable.

ADDITIONAL PROCEDURES

1. Palpate the aorta for pulsations.
- Using your fingertips, press deeply and firmly in the upper abdomen to the left of midline below the xiphoid process.

► Obesity and masses make palpation of the aorta difficult.

- The average adult aorta is 3 cm (1.17 in.) wide.

► The widened aorta may indicate aneurysm.

2. Palpate for rebound tenderness.
- With the patient in a supine position, hold your hand at a 90-degree angle to the abdominal wall in an area of no pain or discomfort. Press deeply into the abdomen, using a slow steady movement.
- Rapidly remove your fingers from the patient's abdomen (see Figure 21.21 ■).
- Ask if the patient feels any pain. Normally, the patient feels the pressure but no pain.

► The experience of sharp stabbing pain as the compressed area returns to a noncompressed state is known as **Blumberg's sign.** This finding occurs in peritoneal irritation and requires immediate medical attention.
► Pain referred to McBurney's point (2.5 to 5.1 cm [1 to 2 in.] above the anterosuperior iliac spine, on a line between the ileum and the umbilicus) on palpation of the left lower abdomen is Rovsing's sign, suggestive of peritoneal irritation in appendicitis.

Techniques and Normal Findings	Abnormal Findings Special Considerations

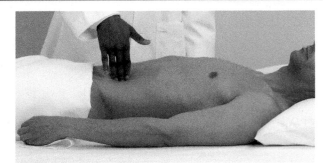

A

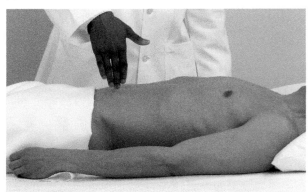

B

Figure 21.21 Palpating for rebound tenderness. A. Applying pressure. B. Rapid release of pressure.

> **ALERT!**
>
> *To avoid causing unnecessary pain or discomfort, abdominal palpation for rebound tenderness should not be performed when assessing patients whose current subjective reports include abdominal pain or tenderness.*

3. **Percuss the abdomen for ascites.**
   - Ascites is an abnormal collection of fluid in the peritoneal cavity. With the patient in a supine position, percuss at the midline to elicit tympany. Continue to percuss in lateral directions away from the midline and listen for dullness (see Figure 21.22 ■).

▶ Ascites is found in congestive heart failure, cirrhosis, and renal failure and in many types of cancer. Ascites may occur in morbid obesity due to portal hypertension resulting from pressure on the abdominal blood vessels.

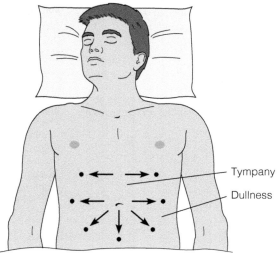

Tympany

Dullness

Figure 21.22 Percussion pattern for ascites.

Techniques and Normal Findings	**Abnormal Findings** **Special Considerations**

- Mark the skin, identifying possible levels of fluid.
- An alternative method, called *shifting dullness,* is to position the patient on the right or left side. Percuss the abdomen. Because fluid settles, anticipate tympany at a superior level and dullness at lower levels (see Figure 21.23 ■).
- If ascites is suspected, measure the abdominal girth with a tape measure.

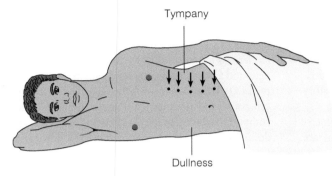

Tympany

Dullness

Figure 21.23 Percussion pattern for ascites, alternative method.

4. **Test for psoas sign.**
   - Perform this test when lower abdominal pain is present and you suspect appendicitis.
   - With the patient in a supine position, place your left hand just above the level of the patient's right knee. Ask the patient to raise the leg to meet your hand. Flexion of the hip causes contraction of the psoas muscle (see Figure 21.24 ■).

   ▶ Pain during this maneuver is indicative of irritation of the psoas muscle associated with the peritoneal inflammation or appendicitis.

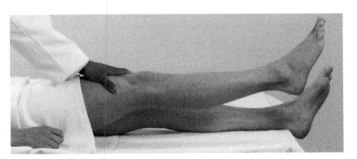

Figure 21.24 Psoas sign.

   - Normally there is no abdominal pain associated with this maneuver.

5. **Test for Murphy's sign.**
   - While palpating the liver, ask the patient to take a deep breath. The diaphragm descends, pushing the liver and gallbladder toward your hand.
   - In a healthy patient, liver palpation is painless.

   ▶ Sharp abdominal pain and the need to halt the examination is a positive Murphy's sign. This occurs in patients with cholecystitis.

Abnormal Findings

Abnormal findings in the abdomen occur in association with general health and in illness. For example, protrusion of the abdomen is seen in obese individuals and in pregnancy. Abdominal hernias are often seen in otherwise healthy adults and children. Untreated hernias, however, can lead to obstructive intestinal complications that give rise to acute symptoms and serious health problems. Further, alterations of the gastrointestinal tract include nutritional problems, eating disorders, cancers, ulcers, and inflammatory and infectious processes.

For accurate diagnosis in many abdominal and gastrointestinal problems, the health history and physical assessment are accompanied by observations of products of elimination and require diagnostic testing. Diagnostic testing includes laboratory studies of blood, urine, and feces as well as radiographic and magnetic resonance imaging (MRI). In appendicitis, for example, physical findings include facial expressions demonstrating pain, abdominal guarding, tenderness to palpation at McBurney's point, RLQ rebound tenderness, and a positive *Rovsing's sign* (pain in the RLQ upon palpation of the LLQ). Diagnosis is confirmed by an elevation in the white blood cell count and findings from an abdominal X-ray, ultrasound, or computerized tomography (CT) scan. Abnormal findings from abdominal assessment are presented in the following section.

Abnormal Abdominal Sounds

When conducting an abdominal assessment, the nurse auscultates for bowel sounds and for vascular sounds. Table 21.3 includes information for interpretation of abnormal abdominal sounds.

TABLE 21.3 **Abnormal Abdominal Sounds**

SOUND	LOCATION	CAUSATIVE FACTORS
Bowel Sounds		
Hyperactive sounds	Any quadrant	Gastroenteritis, diarrhea
Hyperactive sounds followed by absence of sound	Any quadrant	Paralytic ileus
High-pitched sounds with cramping	Any quadrant	Intestinal obstruction
Vascular Sounds		
Systolic bruit (blowing)	Midline below xiphoid	Aortic arterial obstruction
	Left and right lower costal borders at midclavicular line	Stenosis of renal arteries
	Left and right abdomen at midclavicular line between umbilicus and anterior iliac spine	Stenosis of iliac arteries
Venous hum (continuous tone)	Epigastrium and around umbilicus	Portal hypertension
Rubbing		
Friction rub (harsh, grating)	Left and right upper quadrants, over liver and spleen	Tumor or inflammation of organ

Abdominal Pain

Pain is associated with acute and chronic conditions that affect the digestive organs and abdominal structures. Table 21.4 provides information about several disorders that cause abdominal pain. Disruption of function of the abdominal structures may result in referred pain. **Referred pain** is pain or discomfort that is perceived in an area of the body other than the region or point from which the pain originates. For example, pain related to pancreatitis may be perceived in the individual's back. See Figure 11.5 on page 177 for an illustration of common sites of referred pain and their origins.

TABLE 21.4	**Pain in Common Abdominal Disorders**		
DISORDER	**DEFINITION**	**PAIN CHARACTERISTICS**	**PRECIPITATING FACTORS**
Appendicitis	Acute inflammation of vermiform appendix	Epigastric and periumbilical Localizes to RLQ Sudden onset	Obstruction (fecal stone, adhesions)
Cholecystitis	Acute or chronic inflammation of wall of gallbladder	RUQ, radiates to right scapula Sudden onset	Fatty meals, obstruction of duct in cholelithiasis
Diverticulitis	Inflammation of diverticula (outpouches of mucosa through intestinal wall)	Cramping LLQ Radiates to back	Ingestion of fiber-rich diet, stress
Duodenal Ulcer	Breaks in mucosa of duodenum	Aching, gnawing, epigastric	Stress, use of nonsteroidal anti-inflammatory drugs (NSAIDs)
Ectopic Pregnancy	Implantation of blastocyte outside of the uterus, generally in the fallopian tube	Fullness in the rectal area Abdominal cramping, unilateral pain	Tubal damage, pelvic infection, hormonal disorders, lifting, bowel movements
Gastritis	Inflammation of mucosal lining of the stomach (acute and chronic)	Epigastric pain	Acute: NSAIDs, alcohol abuse, stress, infection Chronic: *H. pylori* Autoimmune responses
Gastroesophageal Reflux Disorder (GERD)	Backflow of gastric acid to the esophagus	Heartburn, chest pain	Food intake, lying down after meals
Intestinal Obstruction	Blockage of normal movement of bowel contents	*Small intestine*: aching *Large intestine*: spasmodic pain *Neurogenic*: diffuse abdominal discomfort *Mechanical*: colicky pain associated with distention	*Mechanical*: physical block from impaction, hernia, volvulus *Neurogenic*: manipulation of bowel during surgery, peritoneal irritation
Irritable Bowel Syndrome (Spastic Colon)	Problems with gastrointestinal (GI) motility	LLQ accompanied by diarrhea and/or constipation Pain increases after eating and decreases after bowel movement	Stress, intolerated foods, caffeine, lactose intolerance, alcohol, familial linkage
Pancreatitis	Inflammation of the pancreas	Upper abdominal, knifelike, deep epigastric or umbilical area pain	Ductal obstruction, alcohol abuse, use of acetaminophen, infection

Abdominal Distention

Abdominal distention occurs for a variety of reasons including obesity, gaseous distention, and ascites. Each of these conditions is described in Table 21.5.

TABLE 21.5 Selected Causes of Abdominal Distention

Obesity

Distention or protuberance of the abdomen. Abdomen's increased size is caused by a thickened abdominal wall and fat deposited in the mesentery and omentum.

Percussion produces normal tympanic sounds.

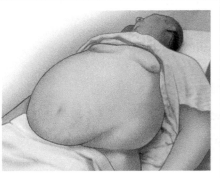

Figure 21.25 Obesity.

Gaseous Distention

A result of increased production of gas in the intestines, which occurs with the ingestion of some foods. In paralytic ileus and intestinal obstruction, it is also associated with altered peristalsis in which gas cannot move through the intestines. Can be localized or generalized. Percussion produces tympany over a large area.

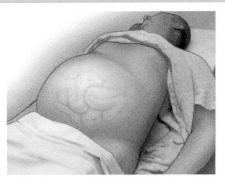

Figure 21.26 Distended abdomen.

Abdominal Tumor

Tumor produces abdominal distention. The abdomen is firm to palpation and dull to percussion. This type of distention is common in ovarian and uterine tumors.

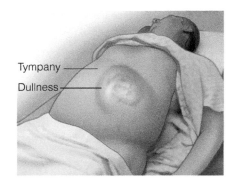

Tympany

Dullness

Figure 21.27 Abdominal tumor.

Ascites

The accumulation of fluid in the abdomen in which the abdomen becomes protuberant like bulging flasks. Fluid descends with gravity, resulting in dullness to percussion in the lower abdomen. May also be assessed by placing the patient in a lateral position and observing fluid shift to the dependent side. Occurs in cirrhosis, congestive heart failure (CHF), nephrosis, peritonitis, and neoplastic diseases.

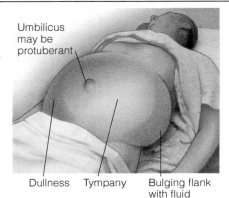

Umbilicus may be protuberant

Dullness   Tympany   Bulging flank with fluid

Fluid level   Tympany   Dullness

Figure 21.28 Ascites.

Abdominal Hernias

A **hernia**, commonly called a rupture, is a protrusion of an organ or structure through an abnormal opening or weakened area in a body wall. The abdominal wall is the most common site of hernias. This weakening could be congenital or acquired. If the protruding or displaced abdominal contents return to their normal position when the patient relaxes, the hernia is said to be reducible or reduced. When the displaced or protruding structures do not return to their normal position, the hernia is said to be incarcerated or nonreducible. An incarcerated hernia can become strangulated. In strangulated hernias, the blood supply to the displaced abdominal contents is compromised. The strangulated visceral contents can become gangrenous. Overstretched rectus muscles with weakened fascia cause an umbilical hernia. An overview of common types of hernias is presented in Table 21.6.

TABLE 21.6 Overview of Common Types of Hernias

Umbilical Hernia

Occurs when the abdominal rectus muscle separates or weakens, allowing abdominal structures, usually the intestines, to push through and come closer to the skin. More common in children than in adults.

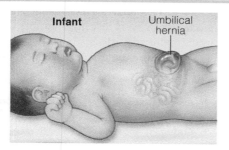

Figure 21.29 Umbilical hernia.

Ventral (Incisional) Hernias

Occurs at the site of an incision when the incision weakens the muscle, and the abdominal structures move closer to the skin. Causes include obesity, repeated surgeries, postoperative infection, impaired wound healing, and poor nutrition.

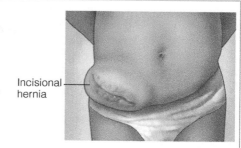

Figure 21.30 Ventral hernia.

Hiatal Hernia

Weakening in the diaphragm allows a portion of the stomach and esophagus to move into the thoracic cavity. Classified as sliding or rolling; more common in adults than children.

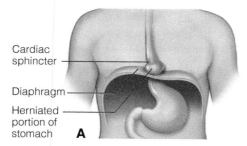
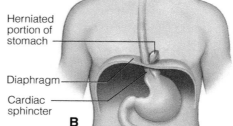

Figure 21.31 Abdominal hernias. A. Sliding hiatal hernia. B. Rolling hiatal hernia.

Alterations of the Gastrointestinal Tract

Alterations of the gastrointestinal tract include cancers and inflammatory diseases. These alterations are described in the following sections.

CANCERS

Cancer of the esophagus is a malignant growth of the esophagus, most common in males over 50 years of age. The lower third of the esophagus is most commonly involved. Patients commonly complain of weight loss, **dysphagia** (difficulty swallowing), and odynophagia (pain on swallowing). Alcohol abuse, smoking, and poor oral hygiene appear to be predisposing factors.

Hepatic Cancer

Hepatic cancer is a malignant growth of the liver. Often, this type of cancer is proceeded by the onset of cirrhosis related to alcohol abuse, autoimmune diseases of the liver, or hepatitis B and C infections. The use of the liver in the metabolism of drugs leads to limited treatment options.

Subjective findings:

- Upper right quadrant abdominal pain.
- Bruising or bleeding easily.
- Nausea.
- Fatigue.

Objective findings:

- Acities or fluid accumulation in the abdomen.
- Jaundicing (yellowing) of the skin, eye sclera, and or mucous membranes.
- Vomiting.
- Pale or white stools.

Pancreatic Cancer

Pancreatic cancer is a malignant growth of the pancreas. Because it metastasizes very rapidly, pancreatic cancer offers a poor prognosis. The pancreas helps contribute to digestion, produces insulin, and produces hormones. Though smoking is a major risk factor in pancreatic cancer, age, race, and genetic disposition are also risk factors.

Subjective findings:

- Upper middle to left quadrant abdominal pain that radiates to the back.
- Nausea.
- Pruritis (itching) (American Cancer Society [ACS], 2014a).

Objective findings:

- Extreme weight loss.
- Jaundicing of the skin, eyes, or mucous membranes.
- Dark-colored urine.
- Diarrhea.
- Greasy, pale-colored stools (ACS, 2014a).

Stomach Cancer

Cancer of the stomach is a malignant growth of the stomach. The disease is often in the advanced stages before a diagnosis is made. Dietary habits seem to be an influencing factor.

Subjective findings:

- Indigestion.
- Loss of appetite.
- Sense of abdominal bloating after eating.
- Nausea.
- Abdominal pain.

Objective findings:

- Weight loss.
- Vomiting.
- Abdominal distention.
- Gastrointestinal bleeding.
- Cancerous lesions, most frequently located in the distal third of the stomach.

Colorectal Cancer

Colorectal cancer is a malignant lesion involving any part of the large intestine, sigmoid colon, or rectum. Predisposing factors include poor dietary habits and chronic constipation. Signs and symptoms vary according to the location of the growth. Risk factors include age over 50, family history, preexisting disorder of the GI tract, diabetes, history of tobacco use, history of moderate alcohol use, obesity, diet high in red and/or processed meats, and lack of physical activity (ACS, 2014b).

Subjective findings:

- Variation in bowel habits or elimination patterns.
- Abdominal cramping or pain.
- Increased production of intestinal gas.
- Fatigue.

Objective findings:

- Rectal bleeding (occult or overt).
- Unexplained weight loss.
- Intestinal obstruction, which requires surgical intervention and may necessitate permanent colostomy.

INFLAMMATORY PROCESSES

Inflammatory processes may affect any organ in the digestive tract. Common gastrointestinal inflammatory processes include ulcerative colitis, esophagitis, peritonitis, hepatitis and Crohn's disease.

Ulcerative Colitis

Ulcerative colitis is a recurrent inflammatory process causing ulcer formation in the lower portions of the large intestine and rectum. This condition is common in adolescents and young adults. The distribution of the inflammatory process is diffuse. The ulcerative areas abscess and later become necrotic. Manifestations vary depending on the location of the inflammation.

Subjective findings:

- Rectal pain.
- Urgency to move bowels without or without ability to pass stool.
- Abdominal pain and cramping.

Objective findings:

- Weight loss.
- Diarrhea (which may be bloody).
- Fever.

Esophagitis

Esophagitis is an inflammatory process of the esophagus. It is caused by a variety of irritants. The more common causes include smoking, alcohol abuse, reflux of gastric contents, and ingestion of extremely hot or cold foods and liquids.

Subjective findings:

- Dysphagia (difficulty swallowing).
- Chest pain.
- Nausea.

Objective findings:

- Vomiting.
- Weight loss.
- Esophageal obstruction (Mayo Clinic, 2011a).

Peritonitis

Peritonitis is a local or generalized inflammatory process of the peritoneal membrane of the abdomen. The precipitant can be an infectious process (pelvic inflammatory disease), perforation of an organ (ruptured duodenal ulcer), internal bleeding (ruptured ectopic pregnancy), or trauma (stab wound to abdomen).

Subjective findings:

- Abdominal pain or tenderness.
- Abdominal bloating.
- Nausea.
- Decreased appetitite.

Objective findings:

- Abdominal distention.
- Vomiting.
- Decreased urine output.
- Fever (Mayo Clinic, 2011b).

Hepatitis

Hepatitis is an inflammatory process of the liver. Manifestations of hepatitis vary, depending on the form of hepatitis that is contracted. Its causes include viruses, bacteria, chemicals, and drugs. Types of hepatitis include the following:

- **Hepatitis A virus** (HAV), infectious hepatitis, is transmitted via enteric routes (feces or oral routes).
- **Hepatitis B virus** (HBV) is transmitted parenterally, sexually, or perinatally.
- **Hepatitis C virus** (HCV) is transmitted via blood and blood products, parenterally, and through unknown factors.
- **Hepatitis D virus** (HDV) is the same as HBV and requires HBV to replicate.
- **Hepatitis E virus** (HEV) is a non-A, non-B type transmitted enterically. HEV is most common in those who travel to India, Africa, Asia, and Central America.

Crohn's Disease

Crohn's disease is a chronic inflammatory process of the intestine. It is sometimes called regional ileitis, which is a misnomer because it can involve any part of the lower intestinal tract. Crohn's disease is characterized by "skipped" sections of involvement. It is most common in young adults and usually has an insidious onset. The inflammation involves all layers of the intestinal mucosa. Transverse fissures develop in the bowel, producing a characteristic cobblestone appearance.

Subjective findings:

- Abdominal pain or cramping.
- Fatigue.
- Decreased appetite.

Objective findings:

- Diarrhea (which may be bloody).
- Weight loss.
- Fever (Mayo Clinic, 2011c).

Application Through Critical Thinking

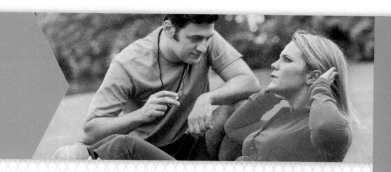

▌ Case Study

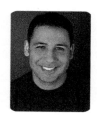

Luiz Hernandez, a 28-year-old Hispanic male, is seeking care in the neighborhood clinic for abdominal pain and weight loss. He has been seen here previously for employment physicals, which revealed no acute or chronic health problems.

During the interview the nurse learns that the patient has had abdominal pain, on and off, for a couple of months and that the pain is getting worse. The pain is in the middle of his stomach and is like an ache. Mr. Hernandez says he has also had no interest in food, feels gassy, and has lost about 10 lb.

When asked about factors that precipitate or affect the pain, the patient reveals that the pain occurs most frequently late in the morning and afternoon and that he wakes up at night with the pain. When asked if he has tried any remedy for the pain, Mr. Hernandez states that he uses an antacid once in a while and it helps, and that he takes mint because that is what his mother gave to the family members when they had stomach troubles.

In response to questions about weight loss, Mr. Hernandez says that he thinks he has been losing weight because he just hasn't been feeling hungry and many of the foods he is used to eating do not appeal to him. He also states that he is starting to get nervous about the pain, and when he is nervous he never feels like eating. The nurse asks if he is nervous about this clinic visit. The patient replies that he was really nervous when he arrived but is feeling a little better now that he is talking about what is going on. He further states, "I am still scared about what might be causing this."

The nurse continues the interview with questions about the patient's past and family history. No acute or chronic problems are revealed. The nurse asks the patient about use of medications and his habits. Mr. Hernandez states that he uses Tylenol occasionally for a headache. He does not smoke and uses alcohol socially, mostly on weekends.

The physical assessment reveals vital signs of B/P 132/84, P 88, RR 22. The skin is cool, dry, and pale. The abdomen is soft and not distended, bowel sounds are present in all quadrants, and there is no tenderness on palpation.

The plan for this patient is to begin antacids three times a day, after meals and at bedtime; schedule an endoscopy; obtain cultures for *H. pylori*; and arrange for a follow-up visit in 1 week.

▌ Complete Documentation

The following is sample documentation for Luis Hernandez.

SUBJECTIVE DATA: Aching midabdominal pain for several months, getting worse. Feels "gassy." No interest in food. Weight loss 10 lb. Pain occurs late in a.m. and p.m., wakes at night. Antacid used infrequently with relief. Uses mint for symptoms. Nervous about pain and what it might mean.

OBJECTIVE DATA: Skin pale, cool, dry. Abdomen soft, nontender. BS + 4Qs. VS: B/P 132/84 Left, B/P 130/83 Right—P 88—RR 22.

▌ Critical Thinking Questions

1. What data suggest the need for *H. pylori* cultures?
2. How would data be clustered to formulate nursing diagnoses?
3. What would be included in an educational plan for this patient?
4. Which psychosical considerations would be important to evaluate?
5. What cultural considerations should be addressed?

▌ Prepare Teaching Plan

LEARNING NEED: Mr. Hernandez sought health care for abdominal pain and weight loss. The data reveal that he experiences pain late in the morning and afternoon and that he often wakes at night with pain. He uses antacids with some relief. He admits to being nervous about the problem. Following the interview and physical examination, the plan of care includes antacids and a scheduled diagnostic test for *H. pylori*.

The case study provides data that are representative of symptoms and behaviors associated with *H. pylori* and peptic ulcer disease. Individuals and community groups could benefit from education about *H. pylori*. The following teaching plan is intended for a group of learners and focuses on *H. pylori* and ulcers.

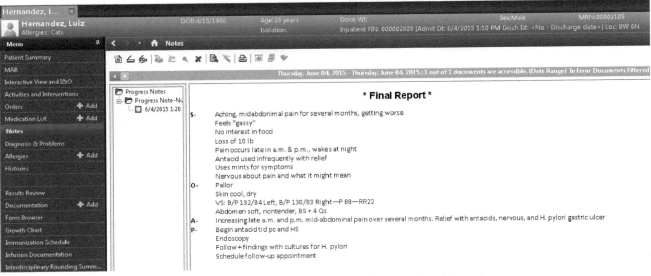

Source: From Cerner Electronic Health Record. Copyright © by Cerner Corporation. Used by permission of Cerner Corporation.

GOAL: The participants will have increased awareness of ulcers and *H. pylori* infection.

OBJECTIVES: Upon completion of this educational session, the participants will be able to:

1. Define peptic ulcer.
2. Discuss causes of peptic ulcer disease.
3. Describe symptoms of peptic ulcer.
4. Identify diagnostic tests for peptic ulcer.
5. List treatments for peptic ulcer.

APPLICATION OF OBJECTIVE 2: Discuss causes of peptic ulcer disease

Content	Teaching Strategy	Evaluation
• In the past it was believed that ulcers were caused by stress or eating too much acidic food. Now it is known that this is not true. • Most stomach ulcers are caused by infection. • The infection is caused by a bacteria named *Helicobacter pylori* or *H. pylori*. • *H. pylori* causes more than 90% of peptic ulcers. • *H. pylori* infects almost two thirds of the world's population. • In the United States, *H. pylori* is more prevalent in older adults, African Americans, Hispanics, and those in lower socioeconomic groups. • Most people with *H. pylori* never have symptoms. • *H. pylori* can be transmitted from person to person. Always wash hands after using bathroom and before eating. • Peptic ulcers are also caused by long-term use of nonsteroidal anti-inflammatory drugs (NSAIDs) such as ibuprofen and aspirin. • Peptic ulcers can be caused by tumors in the stomach or pancreas.	• Lecture • Discussion • Audiovisual materials such as illustrations of the gastrointestinal system These reinforce verbal presentation. Printed materials allow review and reinforcement at the learner's own pace.	• Written examination. May use short answer, fill-in, or multiple-choice items or a combination of items. If these are short and easy to evaluate, the learner receives immediate feedback. • Question-and-answer period. With small groups, can prompt discussion. Provides immediate feedback.

▶ References

American Cancer Society (ACS). (2014a). *Signs and symptoms of pancreatic cancer.* Retrieved from http://www.cancer.org/cancer/pancreaticcancer/detailedguide/pancreatic-cancer-signs-and-symptoms

American Cancer Society (ACS). (2014b). *What are the risk factors for colorectal cancer?* Retrieved from http://www.cancer.org/cancer/colonandrectumcancer/detailedguide/colorectal-cancer-risk-factors

American Dental Association. (2013). *Adults over 60: Concerns.* Retrieved from http://www.mouthhealthy.org/en/adults-over-60/concerns

Berman, A., & Snyder, S. J. (2012). *Kozier and Erb's fundamentals of nursing: Concepts, process, and practice* (9th ed.). Upper Saddle River, NJ: Prentice Hall.

Centers for Disease Control and Prevention (CDC). (2013a). *Colorectal cancer rates by race and ethnicity.* Retrieved from http://www.cdc.gov/cancer/colorectal/statistics/race.htm

Centers for Disease Control and Prevention. (2013b). *Pinworm infection FAQs.* Retrieved from http://www.cdc.gov/parasites/pinworm/gen_info/faqs.html

Cherian, K. M., Mulky, M. J., & Menon, K. K. G. (2014). Toxicological considerations in the use of consumer products. *Defence Science Journal, 37*(2), 143–159.

Durston, S. (2009). Bowel obstruction: Backup along the 750. *Nursing Made Incredibly Easy, 7*(2), 40–52.

Epplein, M., Signorello, L. B., Zheng, W., Peek, R. M., Michel, A., Williams, S. M., . . . Blot, W. J. (2011). Race, African ancestry, and Helicobacter pylori infection in a low-income United States population. *Cancer Epidemiology Biomarkers & Prevention, 20*(5), 826–834.

Johns Hopkins Medicine. (n.d.a). *Inguinal and umbilical hernia.* Retrieved from http://www.hopkinsmedicine.org/healthlibrary/conditions/adult/pediatrics/inguinal_and_umbilical_hernia_90,P01998/

Johns Hopkins Medicine. (n.d.b). *Stomach and duodenal ulcers: Peptic ulcers.* Retrieved from http://www.hopkinsmedicine.org/healthlibrary/conditions/digestive_disorders/stomach_and_duodenal_ulcers_peptic_ulcers_85,P00394/

Konturek, P. C., Brzozowski, T., & Konturek, S. J. (2011). Stress and the gut: pathophysiology, clinical consequences, diagnostic approach and treatment options. *Journal of Physiology and Pharmacology, 62*(6), 591–599.

Luzuriaga, K., & Sullivan, J. L. (2010). Infectious mononucleosis. *New England Journal of Medicine, 362*(21), 1993–2000.

Mahadevan, S. V., & Garmel, G. M. (Eds.). (2012). *An introduction to clinical emergency medicine* (2nd ed.). New York, NY: Cambridge University Press.

Marieb, E. N. (2009). *Essentials of human anatomy and physiology* (9th ed.). Redwood City, CA: Benjamin/Cummings.

Mayo Clinic. (n.d.). *Chronic constipation in older patients.* Retrieved from http://www.mayoclinic.org/medical-professionals/clinical-updates/digestive-diseases/chronic-constipation-older-patients-educational-approach

Mayo Clinic. (2011a). *Esophagitis: Symptoms.* Retrieved from http://www.mayoclinic.org/diseases-conditions/esophagitis/basics/symptoms/con-20034313

Mayo Clinic. (2011b). *Peritonitis: Symptoms.* Retrieved from http://www.mayoclinic.org/diseases-conditions/peritonitis/basics/symptoms/con-20032165

Mayo Clinic. (2011c). *Crohn's disease: Symptoms.* Retrieved from: http://www.mayoclinic.org/diseases-conditions/crohns-disease/basics/symptoms/con-20032061

Mayo Foundation for Medical Education and Research. (2014). *Rochester test catalog: 2014 online test catalog.* Available at http://www.mayomedicallaboratories.com/test-catalog/

MedlinePlus. (2013). *Warfarin.* Retrieved from http://www.nlm.nih.gov/medlineplus/druginfo/meds/a682277.html

Mohamed, L. A. E. K., & Hanafy, N. F. (2013). Hydrotherapy versus laxative for treatment of postoperative constipation among orthopedic patients. *Advances in Life Science and Technology, 14*(1), 50–63.

Muriel, P., & Escobar, Y. (2003). Kupffer cells are responsible for liver cirrhosis induced by carbon tetrachloride. *Journal of Applied Toxicology, 23*(2), 103–108.

Murray, R. B., & Zentner, J. P. (2009). *Health assessment and promotion strategies through the life span* (8th ed.). Upper Saddle River, NJ: Prentice Hall.

Sira, M. M., Salem, T. A. H., & Sira, A. M. (2013). Biliary atresia: A challenging diagnosis. *Global Journal of Gastroenterology & Hepatology, 1*(1), 34–45.

Swarnkar, K., Kale, A., & Lakhkar, B. (2010). Clinico-epidemiological and hematological profile of sickle cell anemia with special reference to penicillin prophylaxis in a rural hospital of central India. *The Internet Journal of Epidemiology. 9*(2).

U.S. Department of Health and Human Services (USDHHS). (2014). *Healthy people 2020.* Retrieved from http://www.healthypeople.gov/2020/default.aspx

Westerbeek, E. A. M., Hensgens, R. L., Mihatsch, W. A., Boehm, G., Lafeber, H. N., & Van Elburg, R. M. (2011). The effect of neutral and acidic oligosaccharides on stool viscosity, stool frequency and stool pH in preterm infants. *Acta Paediatrica, 100*(11), 1426–1431.

Wilson, B. A., Shannon, M. T., & Shields, K. M. (2013). *Pearson nurse's drug guide.* Upper Saddle River, NJ: Pearson.

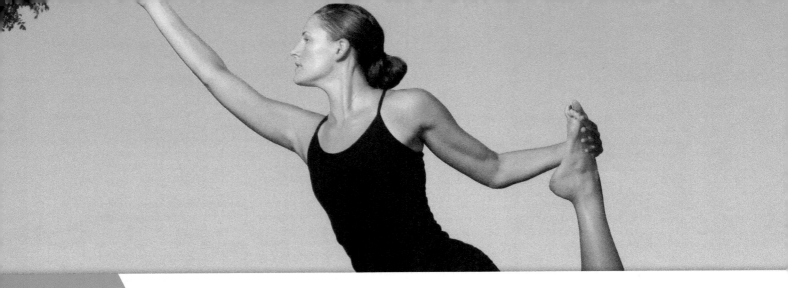

▶ Learning Outcomes

Upon completion of this chapter, you will be able to:

1. Describe the anatomy and physiology of the urinary system.

2. Identify landmarks that guide assessment of the urinary system.

3. Develop questions to be used when completing the focused interview.

4. Explain patient preparation for assessment of the urinary system.

5. Outline the techniques required for assessment of the urinary system.

6. Differentiate normal from abnormal findings in the physical assessment of the urinary system.

7. Identify the developmental, psychosocial, cultural, and environmental variations in assessment techniques and findings.

8. Relate *Healthy People 2020* objectives to issues of the urinary system.

9. Apply critical thinking to the physical assessment of the urinary system.

The urinary system is composed of the kidneys, ureters, bladder, and urethra. The **glomeruli** (tufts of capillaries) of the kidneys filter more than 1 liter (L) of fluid each minute. As a result, wastes, toxins, and foreign matter are removed from the blood. The urinary system acts through the kidneys to prevent the accumulation of nitrogenous wastes, promotes fluid and electrolyte balance, assists in maintenance of blood pressure, and contributes to *erythropoiesis* (development of mature red blood cells).

The organs of the urinary system are distributed among the retroperitoneal space, abdomen, and genitals. Assessment of the urinary system is incorporated into assessment of the abdomen and reproductive systems. Urinary function is interdependent with other body systems. In addition, psychosocial and developmental factors impact the function of the urinary system.

Chronic kidney disease is one of the topics addressed in *Healthy People 2020*. Objectives have been developed to reduce the number of new cases; the many complications, disabilities, and deaths; and, ultimately, the cost for treatment, as described in Table 22.1 on page 582.

Anatomy and Physiology Review

The structures of the urinary system include the kidneys, ureters, urinary bladder, urethra, and renal vasculature (blood vessels). Each of the structures is described in the following sections.

Kidneys

The **kidneys** are bean-shaped organs located in the retroperitoneal space on either side of the vertebral column. Extending from the level of the 12th thoracic vertebra to the 3rd lumbar vertebra, the upper portion of the kidneys is protected by the lower rib cage. The right kidney is displaced downward by the liver and sits slightly lower than the left kidney. A layer of fat cushions each kidney, and the kidney itself is surrounded by tissue called the renal capsule (see Figure 22.1 ■). The renal fascia connects the kidney and fatty layer to the posterior wall of the abdomen. Each adult kidney weighs approximately 150 g (5 oz) and is 11 to 13 cm (4 to 5 in.) long, 5 to 7 cm (2 to 3 in.) wide, and 2.5 to 3 cm (1 in.) thick. The lateral surface of the kidney is convex. The medial surface is concave and contains

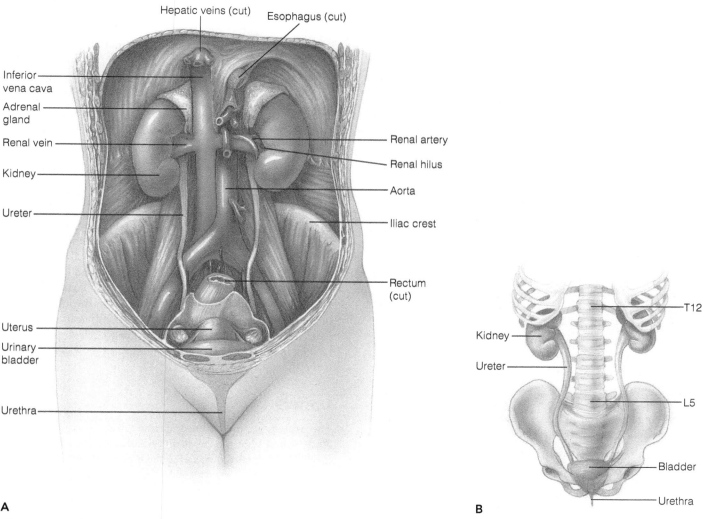

Figure 22.1 The urinary system. A. Anterior view of the urinary organs of a female. B. Relationship of the kidneys to the vertebrae.

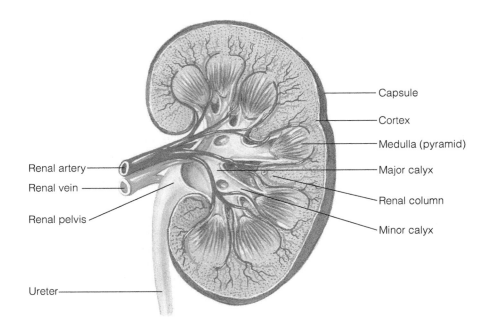

Figure 22.2 Internal anatomy of the kidney.

the hilus, a vertical cleft that opens into a space within the kidney referred to as the renal sinus. The ureters, renal blood vessels, nerves, and lymphatic vessels pass through the hilus into the renal sinus. The superior part of the kidney is referred to as the upper pole, whereas the inferior surface is called the lower pole.

The inner portion of the kidney is called the *renal medulla.* The renal **medulla** is composed of structures called pyramids and calyces. The pyramids are wedgelike structures made up of bundles of urine-collecting tubules. At their apex, the pyramids have papillae that are enclosed by cuplike structures called calyces. The calyces collect urine and transport it into the renal pelvis, which is the funnel-shaped superior end of the ureter (see Figure 22.2 ■).

The outer portion of each kidney is called the renal **cortex.** It is composed of over 1 million nephrons, which form urine. The first part of each nephron is the renal corpuscle, which consists of a tuft of capillaries called a glomerulus. These glomeruli begin the filtration of the blood. Larger blood components, such as red blood cells and larger proteins, are separated from most of the fluid, which passes into the glomerular capsule (or Bowman's capsule). The filtrate then moves into a proximal convoluted tubule, then into the loop of Henle, and finally into a distal convoluted tubule, from which it is collected as urine by a collecting tubule. Along the way, some of the filtrate is resorbed along with electrolytes and chemicals such as glucose, potassium, phosphate, and sodium. Each collecting tubule guides the urine from several nephrons out into the renal pyramids and calyces and from there through the renal pelvis and into the ureters.

The major functions of the kidneys are the following:

- Eliminating nitrogenous waste products, toxins, excess ions, and drugs through urine.
- Regulating volume and chemical makeup of the blood.
- Maintaining balance between water and salts and acids and bases.
- Producing renin, an enzyme that assists in the regulation of blood pressure.
- Producing erythropoietin, a hormone that stimulates production of red blood cells in the bone marrow.
- Assisting in the metabolism of vitamin D.

Renal Arteries

The kidneys require a tremendous amount of oxygen and nutrients and receive about 25% of the cardiac output. Although not part of the urinary system, an extensive network of arteries intertwines within the renal network. These arteries include renal arteries, arcuate arteries, interlobular arteries, afferent arteries, and efferent arterioles. The vasa recta are looping capillaries that connect with the juxtamedullary nephrons and continue into the medulla alongside the loop of Henle. The vasa recta help to concentrate urine. The major function of the renal arteries is providing a rich supply of blood (approximately 1,200 mL per minute when an individual is at rest) to the kidneys.

Ureters

The **ureters** are mucus-lined narrow tubes approximately 25 to 30 cm (10 to 12 in.) in length and 6 to 12 mm (0.25 to 0.5 in.) in diameter. The major function of the ureters is transporting urine from the kidney to the urinary bladder. As the ureter leaves the kidney, it travels downward behind the peritoneum to the posterior wall of the urinary bladder. The middle layer of the ureters contains smooth muscle that is stimulated by transmission of electric impulses from the autonomic nervous system. Their peristaltic action propels urine downward to the urinary bladder. The major function of the ureters is transporting urine from the kidney to the urinary bladder.

Urinary Bladder

The urinary bladder is a hollow, muscular, collapsible pouch that acts as a reservoir for urine. It lies on the pelvic floor in the retroperitoneal space. The bladder is composed of two parts: the rounded muscular sac made up of the detrusor muscle, and the portion between the body of the bladder and the urethra known as the neck. In males, the bladder lies anterior to the rectum, and the neck of the bladder is encircled by the prostate gland of the male reproductive system. In females, the bladder lies anterior to the vagina and uterus. The detrusor muscle allows the bladder to expand as it fills with urine and to contract to release urine to the outside of the body during micturition (voiding). When empty, the bladder collapses upon itself, forming a thick-walled, pyramidal organ that lies low in the pelvis behind the symphysis pubis. As urine accumulates, the fundus, the superior wall of the bladder, ascends in the abdominal cavity and assumes a rounded shape that is palpable. When moderately filled (500 mL), the bladder is approximately 12.5 cm (5 in.) long. When larger amounts of urine are present, the bladder becomes distended and rises above the symphysis pubis.

The major functions of the urinary bladder are the following:

- Storing urine temporarily.
- Contracting to release urine during micturition.

Urethra

The **urethra** is a mucus-lined tube that transports urine from the urinary bladder to the exterior. In females, the urethra is approximately 3 to 4 cm (1.5 in.) long and lies along the anterior wall of the vagina. The female urethra terminates in the external urethral orifice or meatus, which lies between the clitoris and the vagina. The male urethra is approximately 20 cm (8 in.) long and runs the length of the penis. It terminates in the external urethral orifice in the glans penis. In addition to providing a passageway for urine, the male urethra also carries semen outside of the body. Because the female urethra is short and its meatus lies close to the anus, it can become contaminated with bacteria more readily than the male urethra. A more detailed review of the penis, prostate gland, and male and female external genitalia is presented in chapters 23 and 24. ∞ The major function of the urethra is providing a passage for the elimination of urine.

Landmarks

During assessment of the urinary system, the nurse uses three landmarks to locate and palpate the kidneys and urinary bladder. These landmarks are the costovertebral angle, the rectus abdominis muscle, and the symphysis pubis. The **costovertebral angle (CVA)** is the area on the lower back formed by the vertebral column and the downward curve of the last posterior rib, as depicted in Figure 22.3A ■. It is an important anatomic landmark because the lower poles of the kidney and ureter lie below this surface. The

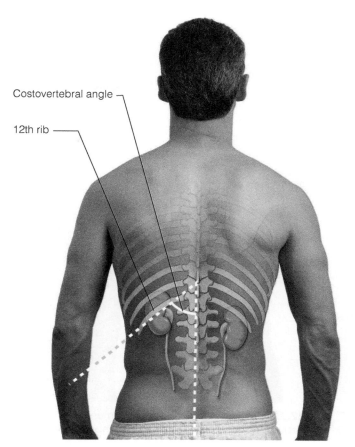

Figure 22.3A Landmarks for urinary assessment. A. The costovertebral angle.

rectus abdominis muscles are a longitudinal pair of muscles that extend from the pubis to the rib cage on either side of the midline, as illustrated in Figure 22.3B ■. These muscles are used as guidelines for positioning the hands when palpating the kidneys through the abdominal wall. The symphysis pubis is the joint formed by the union of the two pubic bones by cartilage at the midline of the body (see Figure 22.3B). The bladder is cradled under the symphysis pubis. When the bladder is full, the nurse is able to palpate it as it rises above the symphysis pubis.

Special Considerations

The patient's health status is influenced by a number of factors, including age, developmental level, race, ethnicity, work history, living conditions, socioeconomics, and emotional health. During a comprehensive health assessment, effective communication and critical thinking enable the nurse to identify the ways in which one or more factors influence the patient's health, beliefs, and practices.

Health Promotion Considerations

Healthy People 2020 objectives target the promotion of a variety of aspects of urinary system health. For example, this national initiative emphasizes reducing the incidence of chronic kidney disease

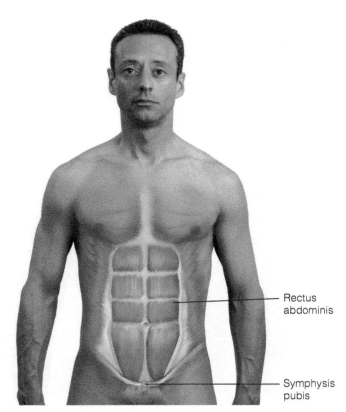

Rectus
abdominis

Symphysis
pubis

Figure 22.3B Landmarks for urinary assessment.
B. The rectus abdominis muscles and the symphysis pubis.

(CKD) while increasing awareness of this disorder—especially among individuals who have unknowingly developed it. In addition, *Healthy People 2020* objectives include reducing the incidence of end-stage renal disease (ESRD) as well as identifying individuals who are at risk for ESRD in order to facilitate early treatment and preventative measures (USDHHS, 2010). See Table 22.1 for examples of *Healthy People 2020* objectives that target the promotion of urinary system health and wellness among individuals across the life span.

Lifespan Considerations

Changes in anatomic structures and functions occur as a normal part of growth and development. Knowledge of normal, age-related variations in findings from health assessment is essential in interpreting data and planning care for patients. Specific variations in the urinary system for different age groups are presented in the following sections.

Infants and Children

Renal blood flow increases with a significant allotment to the renal medulla at birth. The glomerular filtration rate also increases at birth compared to the fetal filtration rate and continues to increase until the first or second year of life. The fluid and electrolyte balance in an infant or child is fragile. Illnesses that cause dehydration, loss of fluids, or lack of fluid intake may rapidly lead to metabolic acidosis and fluid imbalance. Serious, chronic dysfunction of this system may impair the child's growth and development.

Children do not have adult bladder capacities (approximately 700 mL) until adolescence. A quick way to estimate a child's bladder capacity is to use the following formula: the child's age (in years) plus or minus 2 oz. For example, a 4-year-old child has a bladder capacity of 2 to 6 oz:

$$\text{Age in years} \pm 2 \text{ oz} = 4 \pm 2 = 2 \text{ to } 6 \text{ oz}$$

On average, children attain bladder sphincter control at approximately 3 years for females and age 3 ½ years for males. Bladder training requires bladder sphincter control. Normal urine output for children is at least 1 to 2 mL/kg/hr.

Minimal genital growth occurs prior to puberty. The onset of genital development is expected by age 11 in females and age 13 in males. Refer to the Tanner stages, Figure 23.4, page 611, for males and Figure 24.3, page 648, for females.

The nurse examines infants for anomalies such as scrotal edema, undescended testes, and noncentral placement of the urinary meatus. Uncircumcised males have unretractile foreskins until 2 to 3 years of age. **Cryptorchidism** is the failure of one or both testicles to descend through the inguinal canal during the final stages of fetal development. This condition is more common in premature infants and is detectable at birth. Males with undescended testicles should be referred for surgical evaluation by 9 to 12 months of age, because there is an increased risk of testicular cancer in retained testicles, and spontaneous descent is rare after this age.

Infant females may have a bloody vaginal discharge during the first 2 weeks of life. This "false menses" is the result of exposure to maternal estrogen and progesterone. **Labial adhesions** occur when the labia minora fuse together. They are common in preadolescent females because decreased estrogen levels result in labial and genital atrophy. When present, labial adhesions extend from the posterior fourchette and look like a skin covering of all or part of the introitus. They are of medical concern if there is blockage of urinary flow or if they result in recurrent urinary tract infections.

It is important to consider the health practices of the family when the genital areas are unclean in infants or children of any age. Presence of a diaper rash is a clue that the nurse should explore the family's hygiene practices; however, diaper rash is often difficult to control, and supportive teaching is indicated. Bed-wetting is a difficult problem for both the child and the family and may influence the child's relationship with the family. The child's confidence and social development may also be affected by bed-wetting. Bed-wetting is not generally considered problematic unless the child has no daytime dryness after 4 years of age or nighttime dryness after 6 years of age.

The Pregnant Female

During the first trimester, the enlarging uterus presses against the bladder, increasing the frequency of urination. Frequency decreases during the second trimester and then recurs during the third trimester as the presenting part of the fetus descends into the pelvis and again presses on the bladder.

During pregnancy, the amount of urine produced increases, causing the patient to feel the need to urinate more frequently. For reasons that are not completely understood, tubular reabsorption of glucose is impaired during pregnancy. Therefore, glucosuria (glucose in urine) can be present in normal pregnancies. In the

TABLE 22.1	Examples of *Healthy People 2020* Objectives Related to Urinary System Health
OBJECTIVE NUMBER	**DESCRIPTION**
CKD-1	Reduce the proportion of the U.S. population with chronic kidney disease
CKD-2	Increase the proportion of persons with chronic kidney disease (CKD) who know they have impaired renal function
CKD-3	Increase the proportion of hospital patients who incurred acute kidney injury who have follow up renal evaluation in 6 months post discharge
CKD-4	Increase the proportion of persons with diabetes and chronic kidney disease who receive recommended medical evaluation
CKD-5	Increase the proportion of persons with diabetes and chronic kidney disease who receive recommended medical treatment with angiotensin-converting enzyme (ACE) inhibitors or angiotensin II receptor blockers (ARBS)
CKD-6	Improve cardiovascular care in persons with chronic kidney disease
CKD-7	Reduce the number of deaths among persons with chronic kidney disease
CKD-8	Reduce the number of new cases of end-stage renal disease (ESRD)
CKD-9	Reduce kidney failure due to diabetes
CKD-10	Increase the proportion of chronic kidney disease patients receiving care from a nephrologist at least 12 months before the start of renal replacement therapy
CKD-11	Improve vascular access for hemodialysis patients
CKD-12	Increase the proportion of dialysis patients waitlisted and/or receiving a deceased donor kidney transplant within 1 year of end-stage renal disease (ESRD) start (among patients under 70 years of age).
CKD-13	Increase the proportion of patients with treated chronic kidney failure who receive a transplant
CKD-14	Reduce deaths in persons with end-stage renal disease (ESRD)

Source: U.S. Department of Health and Human Services (USDHHS). (2014). *Healthy people 2020.* Retrieved from http://www.healthypeople.gov/2020/default.aspx

postpartum period, edema and hyperemia of the bladder mucosa cause decreased sensation and contribute to overdistention of the bladder. Incomplete emptying of the bladder often accompanies this condition, increasing the patient's susceptibility to urinary tract infection (UTI).

The Older Adult

The effects of aging take their toll on the kidneys. The weight of the kidneys may drop by as much as 30%, particularly in the renal cortex. Renal blood flow and perfusion gradually decrease. The capillary system in the glomeruli atrophies. Although the vasculature in the renal medulla remains relatively well preserved, the arcuate and interlobular arteries may become distorted, resulting in a tortuous configuration. All structures of the renal cortex and the renal medulla experience some degree of decline, especially the nephrons. By ages 75 to 80, a 50% loss of nephrons has occurred; thus, glomerular filtering is decreased. This has major implications for increased susceptibility for drug toxicity in older adults. Atherosclerosis of renal arteries can decrease renal blood flow and may lead to atrophy of the kidneys. Tubular function also diminishes, and urine is not as effectively concentrated as at a younger age; maximum specific gravity may be only 1.024. About 30% to 50% of the glomeruli degenerate because of fibrosis, hyalinization, and fat deposition. All of these factors contribute to the loss of filtration surface area in the glomerular capillary tufts by the age of 75. Creatinine clearance decreases slowly after 40 years of age, as does the ability to concentrate and dilute urine.

The older patient's decreased sensation of thirst and resultant decreased intake of water relates directly to the body's compensatory response of concentrating urine. However, antidiuretic hormone is not as effective as in a younger patient; thus, concentrations and activity of renin and aldosterone are reduced with advanced age by as much as 30% to 50%. This combination of circumstances places the older patient at risk for hyperkalemia.

The older adult also has a reduced capacity to produce ammonia, which interacts with acids. Reduced ability to clear medications and acids, along with reduced ability to resorb bicarbonate and glucose, makes the older patient more susceptible to toxicity related to medications, the effects of respiratory or metabolic acidosis, increased concentrations of glucose in the urine, and the loss of fluids.

Urinary elimination becomes a major concern as an individual advances in age and significant changes in urinary and bladder function begin to occur. Major changes in both males and females include urinary retention leading to increased urinary infections; involuntary bladder contractions resulting in urgency, frequency, and incontinence; decreased bladder capacity causing frequent voiding; and weakening of the urinary sphincters, causing urgency and incontinence.

Nocturia (nighttime urination) is another major concern of older persons, especially males. When an older person is at rest in a horizontal position, the heart is able to pump blood through the kidneys more efficiently, facilitating the excretion of urine. This factor, combined with weakened bladder and urethral muscles, contributes to nocturnal micturition. Other causes of nocturia, such as urinary infection, hyperglycemia, medication use, and stool impactions, should be considered.

Benign prostatic hypertrophy (hyperplasia) is a common cause of urinary retention and obstruction in males. As males age, the prostate gland enlarges, encroaching on the urethra. Prostatic enlargement, which occurs in 95% of all males by age 85, results in problems of urinary retention with frequent overflow voiding, especially during the night. Unrecognized urinary tract obstruction from an enlarged prostate results in damage to the upper urinary tract.

The nurse should allow older patients with urinary tract problems extra time to explain their concerns. Quite often, older adults have difficulty talking about bladder or bowel concerns because they consider the subject too personal. Additionally, some patients may find it distasteful to discuss elimination with anyone of the opposite sex. It is helpful to use the terms with which the patient is comfortable and familiar.

Urinary incontinence can cause embarrassment and lead to social isolation, infection, and skin breakdown. It is the leading cause of institutionalization into long-term care facilities. It is related to diminished bladder elasticity, bladder capacity, and sphincter control as well as to cognitive impairment. Stretching of perineal muscles due to childbirth and obesity further contributes to stress incontinence in females. When assessing an individual who experiences incontinence, the nurse should ask about the patient's ability to get to the bathroom. Many patients who are diagnosed as incontinent simply cannot get to the bathroom on time because of other age-related conditions such as arthritis, strokes, or blindness. Whenever possible, the nurse should observe patients in their own settings to determine what disabilities or environmental barriers (e.g., stairs, distance) hinder the ability to function.

Endocrine changes affect size, lubrication, and function of genital structures in both men and women. Decreased hormone production affects both libido and performance. Postmenopausal females experience a decrease in estrogen that affects the strength of the pubic muscles and may lead to urine leakage, reduced acidity in the lower urinary tract, and UTI.

The physical assessment of the older person is similar to that of any other adult. Because the abdominal musculature of older persons tends to be more flaccid than that of younger adults, less pressure is used during deep palpation. The kidneys of the older patient are more difficult to palpate abdominally because the mass of the adrenal cortex decreases with age. The nurse should omit blunt percussion in a frail older person. Palpation of the costovertebral angles and flanks can be used instead to reveal any pain or tenderness. A digital examination of the prostate gland is generally included as part of the urinary assessment in older males. Palpation of the urethra through the anterior vaginal wall is recommended for all older females.

Psychosocial Considerations

Patients suffering from incontinence are at increased risk for social isolation, self-esteem disturbance, and other psychosocial problems. Increasing body mass index (BMI) has been associated with stress and urge incontinence. In addition, the increased weight of adipose tissue in obesity impacts the function of the muscles of the bladder and rectal sphincters, resulting in incontinence. Incontinence in combination with decreased mobility in obese patients may result in problems with perineal and rectal hygiene, leading to odor, greater risk of urinary infection, and skin irritation. A stressful lifestyle may contribute to chronic UTIs. Stasis of urine and resultant infection may occur when a patient feels "too busy" to empty the bladder as needed. Urinary tract infections in females may also result from sexual trauma, sexual intercourse with a new partner, or coital frequency. The nurse should consider the possibility of sexual abuse in a child or adolescent who presents with a UTI.

Cultural and Environmental Considerations

When considering the influence of culture on a patient's healthcare practices, the nurse must be open-minded and sensitive to the specific values and beliefs of the patient without passing judgment. Not all individuals adhere to the norms, values, and practices of their culture. Consideration for the patient's privacy and modesty is essential when obtaining subjective and objective data regarding urinary elimination. Though not every patient is embarrassed by these components of assessment, many individuals experience considerable uneasiness. It is essential to afford the patient as much privacy and dignity as possible. Some individuals will not disrobe or allow a physical examination by anyone of the opposite sex. Other patients will not allow a sample of their body fluids to be taken and examined by strangers.

Patients with hypertension or diabetes mellitus are especially vulnerable to kidney damage if they do not follow a strict medication and diet regimen. Hispanics and African Americans experience higher rates of hypertension and diabetes mellitus (Office of Minority Health [OMH], 2014); however, these conditions are not limited to these populations. The nurse can help all patients maintain optimal health by providing information on diet, prevention of hypertension, and the importance of compliance with medication regimens.

Renal **calculi** (stones) occur with greater frequency in Caucasians than in Hispanic, African American or Asian American populations (Romero, Akpinar, & Assimos, 2010). Obesity and weight gain increase the risk for development of kidney stones. Also, people who live in the southeastern United States appear to be more susceptible to renal calculi (Willard & Nguyen, 2013).

Information obtained during the focused interview may identify whether the patient is taking herbs prescribed by a healer. The nurse should obtain as complete information about the herbal remedies as possible.

Gathering the Data

Assessment of the health of the urinary system includes gathering subjective and objective data. Subjective data collection occurs during the patient interview, before the actual physical assessment. During the interview the nurse uses a variety of communication techniques to elicit general and specific information about the patient's state of health or illness. Health records and the results of laboratory tests are important secondary sources to be reviewed and included in the data-gathering process. During physical assessment of the urinary system, the techniques of inspection, palpation, percussion, and auscultation will be used to collect objective data. Before proceeding, it may be helpful to review the information about each of the data-gathering processes and practice the techniques of health assessment. See Table 22.2 for information on potential secondary sources of patient data.

TABLE 22.2 | **Potential Secondary Sources for Patient Data Related to the Urinary System**

TESTS	NORMAL VALUES
Blood Chemistry	
Albumin	3.5–5 g/dL
Ammonia	15–45 mcg/dL
Blood Urea Nitrogen (BUN)	6–23 mg/dL
Creatinine	Male 0.7–1.3 mg/dL Female 0.6–1.1 mg/dL
Urinalysis	
Color	Yellow-straw
Specific Gravity	1.005–1.030
pH	5–8
Glucose	Negative
Sodium	10–40 mEq/L
Potassium	<8 mEq/L
Chloride	25–40 mEq/L
Protein	negative–trace
Osmolality	500–800 mOsm/L
Urine Culture, Colony Count, Sensitivity	
Diagnostic Tests	
Angiography	
Computed Tomography (CT)	
Cystoscopy	
Cystourethography	
Intravenous Urography	
Magnetic Resonance Imaging (MRI)	
Radionuclide Scanning	
Tissue and Cell Sampling—Kidney Biopsy	
Ultrasonography	
Urine Cytology	

Focused Interview

The focused interview for the urinary system concerns data related to the structures and functions of that system. Subjective data are gathered during the focused interview. The nurse must be prepared to observe the patient and listen for cues related to the functions of the urinary system. The nurse may use open-ended and closed questions to obtain information. Often a number of follow-up questions or requests for descriptions are required to clarify data or gather missing information. Follow-up questions are aimed at identifying the source of problems, duration of difficulties, measures to alleviate problems, and clues about the patient's knowledge of his or her own health.

Discussion of urinary system function may be difficult for some patients because it is considered a private matter. The nurse should try to determine and use the terms used by the patient in referring to parts of the body and urination.

The focused interview guides the physical assessment of the urinary system. The information is always considered in relation to norms and expectations about the function of the urinary system. Therefore, the nurse must consider age, gender, race, culture, environment, health practices, past and concurrent problems, and therapies when framing questions and using techniques to elicit information. In order to address all of the factors when conducting a focused interview, categories of questions have been developed. These categories include general questions that are asked of all patients; those addressing illness and infection; questions related to symptoms, pain, and behaviors; those related to habits or practices; questions that are specific to patients according to age; those for the pregnant female; and questions that address internal and external environmental concerns. One approach to questioning about symptoms would be the OLDCART & ICE method, described in detail in chapter 7 (see Figure 7.3 on page 120). ∞

The nurse must consider the patient's ability to participate in the focused interview and physical assessment of the urinary system. If a patient is experiencing pain, urgency, incontinence, or the anxiety that accompanies any of these problems, attention must focus on relief of symptoms.

Focused Interview Questions	Rationales and Evidence

The following section provides sample questions and follow-up questions in each of the categories previously mentioned. A rationale for questions is provided. The list of questions is not all-inclusive but rather represents the types of questions required in a comprehensive focused interview related to the urinary system. The follow-up bulleted questions are asked to seek clarification with additional information from *the patient to enhance the subjective database. The subjective data collected and the questions asked during the health history and focused interview will provide data to help meet the objectives related to decreasing new cases of chronic kidney disease and promoting health as stated in* Healthy People 2020.

General Questions

1. **What are your normal patterns when you urinate?**
   - How often do you urinate each day?
   - How much do you pass each time you urinate? (Note: The nurse may use terms familiar to the patient, such as "pass water," when asking about urination.)

   ▶ Many factors influence the number of times and amount that a patient voids. Among these are size of the bladder, amount of fluid intake, type of fluid or solid intake, medications, amount of perspiration, and the patient's temperature. The adult may void five or six times per day in amounts averaging 100 to 400 mL. For adults, daily urine output typically averages 1,500 mL (Berman & Snyder, 2012). However, adults may urinate as much as 2 L of fluid. At minimum, the adult patient should produce urine at a rate of 30 mL/kg/hour. The child may void more frequently in smaller amounts. The key point is to determine the patient's normal patterns and to identify excess or insufficient urine output.

2. **Have you noticed any change from your normal urination patterns?**
   - Have you noticed any changes in your pattern recently?
   - Have you had any of these changes: urinating more often, urinating less often, urinating more fluid, or urinating less fluid?

   ▶ Changes in urinary elimination patterns signal fluid retention, which may indicate heart failure, kidney failure, or improper nutritional intake. Other considerations include obstructions, infections, and endocrine alterations (Devarajan, 2014).

Focused Interview Questions	Rationales and Evidence
3. **When you urinate, do you feel you are able to empty your bladder completely?** • If not, describe your feeling.	▶ The feeling of being unable to empty the bladder may indicate the patient is retaining urine or developing increased residual urine, which may contribute to the development of infection (Moore & Spence, 2014).
4. **Are you always able to control when you are going to urinate?** • If not, do you have to hurry to the bathroom as soon as you feel the urge to urinate? • When you feel the urge to urinate, are you able to get to the toilet? • Have you ever had an "accident" and wet yourself? • Have you ever urinated by accident when you have coughed, sneezed, or lifted a heavy object?	▶ Urgency and stress incontinence may be caused by an infection, an inflammatory process, or the loss of muscle control over urination (for example, after the vaginal delivery of a child or vaginal hysterectomy) (Forsgren et al., 2012).
5. **Do you ever have to get up at night to urinate?** • If so, can you describe why? • Is there any predictable pattern? • How many times per night? • Describe your fluid intake for a day.	▶ Nocturia may indicate the presence of aging changes in the older adult, cardiovascular changes, diuretic therapy, or habit. Nocturia can be influenced by the amount and timing of fluid intake.
6. **Do you have difficulty starting the flow of the stream?** • Does the stream flow continuously, or does it start and stop? • Do you need to strain or push during urination to empty your bladder completely?	▶ Difficulties of this sort may signify the presence of prostate disease in the male.
7. **If you have urinary problems, have they caused you embarrassment or anxiety?** • Have your urinary problems affected your social, personal, or sexual relationships?	▶ These are important considerations because they may affect patients' abilities to function in other parts of their lives.
8. **Has anyone in your family had a kidney disease or urinary problem?** • If so, when did they have it? • How was it treated? • Do they still have it?	▶ A family history of kidney disease may signify a genetic predisposition to the development of renal disorders in some individuals (Chambers et al., 2010).
9. **Have you had a recent urine analysis or blood work evaluating your kidneys?** • If so, do you know the results?	▶ It is valuable for patients to know the results of laboratory work and to provide the healthcare professional with their impression of the results.

Questions Related to Illness or Infection

1. **Have you ever been diagnosed with a disease of the kidney or bladder?** • When were you diagnosed with the problem? • What treatment was prescribed for the problem? • Was the treatment helpful? • What kinds of things do you do to help with the problem? • Has the problem ever recurred (acute)? • How are you managing the disease now (chronic)?	▶ The patient has an opportunity to provide information about specific urinary illnesses. If a diagnosed illness is identified, follow-up about the date of diagnosis, treatment, and outcomes is required. Data about each illness identified by the patient are essential to an accurate health assessment. Illnesses can be classified as acute or chronic, and follow-up regarding each classification will differ.
2. **An alternative to question 1 is to list possible illnesses of the urinary system, such as renal calculi, nephrosis, and renal failure, and ask the patient to respond "yes" or "no" as each is stated.**	▶ This is a comprehensive and easy way to elicit information about all diagnoses. Follow-up would be carried out for each identified diagnosis as in question 1.
3. **Do you now have or have you had an infection in the urinary system?** • When were you diagnosed with the infection? • What treatment was prescribed for the problem? • Was the treatment helpful? • What kinds of things do you do to help with the problem? • Has the problem ever recurred (acute)? • How are you managing the infection now (chronic)?	▶ If an infection is identified, follow-up about the date of infection, treatment, and outcomes is required. Data about each infection identified by the patient are essential to an accurate health assessment. Infections can be classified as acute or chronic, and follow-up regarding each classification will differ.

Focused Interview Questions	Rationales and Evidence

4. **An alternative to question 3 is to list possible urinary system infections, such as cystitis, pyelonephritis, and prostatitis, and ask the patient to respond "yes" or "no" as each is stated.**

▶ This is a comprehensive and easy way to elicit information about all urinary system infections. Follow-up would be carried out for each identified infection as in question 2.

5. **Have you ever had surgery on the urinary system?**
   - If so, describe the procedure. How long ago did you have it done? Is the problem corrected?
   - If not, describe it.
   - Has anyone in your family ever had surgery on the urinary system?
   - If so, please describe the procedures.
   - How long ago was the surgery?
   - Is the problem corrected?
   - If not, describe it.

▶ Previous surgeries help provide insight as to the patient's history of urological problems. Some urinary problems, such as overflow incontinence, are more common among patients who have had urological surgery (Urology Care Foundation, 2011).

6. **Do you have any of these problems: high blood pressure, diabetes, frequent bladder infections, kidney stones?**
   - If so, how has the problem been treated?
   - Describe any associated symptoms.
   - Do you still have problems with this condition?
   - Do you have any idea what causes this problem?

▶ High blood pressure may contribute to the development of renal disease (Centers for Disease Control and Prevention [CDC], 2014). Diabetes may significantly contribute to the development of renal disease (CDC, 2014). Infections may be caused by inadequate fluid intake, inadequate hygiene, and structural anomalies (Berman & Snyder, 2012). In some patients this is an infrequent situation; in others it is a common malady. Kidney stones may be an isolated event or a recurring condition. Parathyroid disorders and any condition that causes an increase in calcium may contribute to the formation of kidney stones (NEMDIS, 2012).

7. **Do you have any of these neurologic diseases: multiple sclerosis, Parkinson's disease, spinal cord injury, or stroke?**
   - If so, which one?
   - When was it diagnosed? How are you being treated?

▶ These conditions contribute to the retention and stasis of urine, thus placing the patient at risk for chronic urinary infections (Moore & Spence, 2014).

8. **Do you have any type of cardiovascular disease?**
   - If so, what was the diagnosis?
   - When was it diagnosed?
   - How are you being treated?

▶ Hypertension in particular may significantly contribute to the development of renal failure (CDC, 2014).

9. **Have you had influenza, a skin infection, a respiratory tract infection, or other infection recently?**
   - If so, what was it?
   - What medication did the physician prescribe?
   - Did you take all of the medication?
   - Is this a recurrent problem?

▶ If the infection was untreated, the patient may be at risk for developing a renal infection (Wong & Stevens, 2013).

Questions Related to Symptoms, Pain, and Behaviors

When gathering information about symptoms, many questions are required to elicit details and descriptions that assist in the analysis of the data. Discrimination is made in relation to the significance of a symptom, in relation to specific diseases or problems, and in relation to potential follow-up examination or referral. One rationale may be provided for a group of questions in this category.

The following questions refer to specific symptoms and behaviors associated with the urinary system. For each symptom, questions and follow-up are required. The details to be elicited are the characteristics of the symptom; the onset, duration, and frequency of the symptom; the treatment or remedy for the symptom, including over-the-counter (OTC) and home remedies; the determination if diagnosis has been sought; the effect of treatments; and family history associated with a symptom or illness.

Focused Interview Questions	**Rationales and Evidence**

Questions Related to Symptoms

1. Have you noticed any changes in the quality of the urine?
- If so, describe the change.
- Has your urine been cloudy?
- Does it have an odor?
- Has the color changed?
- If there has been a color change, what is it?
- Does the color change happen each time you urinate?
- Is there a pattern?
- Can you predict the color change?

▶ Color changes offer clues to the presence of infection, kidney stones, or neoplasm. The quantity of urine may indicate the presence of renal failure or may reflect hydration status (Berman & Snyder, 2012).

2. If the urine is bloody (hematuria), the nurse should ask these questions:
- Have you fallen recently?
- Do you experience burning when the blood is present? Have you seen clots in the urine?
- Have you noticed any stones or other material in the urine?
- Have you noticed any granular material on the toilet paper after you wipe?

▶ The patient may offer valuable information about the source and characteristics of bleeding, because this symptom is present in a wide variety of conditions. Hematuria is a serious finding and warrants additional follow-up (Berman & Snyder, 2012).

3. Is your urine foamy and amber in color?

▶ This finding may indicate the presence of kidney dysfunction or other illnesses (Stöppler, 2012).

4. Have you had any weight gain recently?
- If so, describe it.
- Are you retaining fluid?
- Are your rings, clothing, or shoes becoming tighter?
- Has this change been gradual or did it come on suddenly?

▶ This may alert the nurse to the presence of hypertension, associated heart failure, or endocrine problems. These ultimately affect the renal circulation and function of the kidneys.

5. Have you noticed any discharge from the urethra?
- If so, describe the color, odor, amount, and frequency.
- When did it start?
- Is this a recurrent problem? If so, what was the diagnosis?
- How was it treated?
- Did you follow the treatment as prescribed by the physician?

▶ Discharge signals the potential presence of an infective process.

6. Have you noticed any redness or other discoloration in the urethral area or penis? If so, describe the characteristics.

▶ Redness may indicate the presence of inflammation, irritation, or infection.

7. *For male patients:* Do you have prostate problems?
- If so, describe the symptoms and treatment.
- When was your last prostate exam?

▶ Enlargement of the prostate gland contributes to problems in urination, including frequency, difficulty starting a stream, or incomplete emptying of the bladder (Berman & Snyder, 2012).

8. Has your skin changed recently?
- Describe the change.
- Has the color changed?
- Is it itchy all the time?

▶ Patients with chronic renal failure have itchy skin (pruritus), and lichenification (a thickening of the skin) may develop (Kuypers, 2009).

9. Have you recently had nausea, vomiting, diarrhea, or chills?
- If so, which one? Describe it.
- How was it treated?
- Has it recurred?

▶ These conditions may indicate the presence of infection or recurring infection.

10. Have you had any shortness of breath or difficulty breathing lately? If so, describe it.

▶ This may alert the nurse to the presence of hypertension and associated heart failure. These ultimately affect the renal circulation and function of the kidneys.

Focused Interview Questions	Rationales and Evidence

11. Do you have difficulty concentrating, reading, or remembering things?

▶ Difficulty remembering may be associated with azotemia (a buildup of wastes in the bloodstream due to renal dysfunction) (Toor, Liptzin, & Fischel, 2013). There are many conditions that contribute to memory disturbances.

Questions Related to Pain

When assessing pain the nurse needs to gather information about the characteristics of the pain, which include quality, severity, location, duration, predictability, onset, relief, and radiation.

1. Do you ever have pain, burning, or other discomfort before, during, or after urination?
- If so, describe the discomfort, location, and timing.
- Do you have symptoms all of the time or some of the time?
- Is the discomfort predictable? For instance, is it related to time of the day, or certain foods or beverages?
- Do you feel it after sexual intercourse?

▶ Painful urination may indicate the presence of an infective process (Berman & Snyder, 2012).

2. Do you have any pain or discomfort in your back, sides, or abdomen?
- If so, show me where the pain or discomfort is located.
- Describe the pain.
- What aggravates or alleviates the symptoms?

▶ Back or abdominal pain often accompanies renal disease (Berman & Snyder, 2012).

3. Have you noticed any pain or discomfort when your urine is bloody?
- If so, describe the type, location, and timing of the discomfort.

▶ Hematuria without pain is often associated with cancer (Ozkanli, Girgin, Kosemetin, & Zemheri, 2014).

Questions Related to Behaviors

1. Describe your diet.
- Describe what you have eaten and drunk over the last week.
- How is your appetite?
- On a typical day, how much do you eat and drink?
- Do you drink alcoholic beverages?
- How many glasses of water do you drink a day?
- Are there any foods or beverages that bother you?
- Do any foods or beverages cause you discomfort either before or upon urination?
- Do any foods or beverages cause you to feel bloated or gassy?
- Do any foods or beverages affect the color, clarity, or smell of your urine?
- How much salt do you use?
- Do you retain fluid after consuming certain foods or beverages?

▶ Questions such as these may provide information regarding the patient's hydration status, potential allergic reaction to foods, and retention of fluid.

2. Do you smoke or are you exposed to passive smoke?
- If so, what type of smoking (cigarette, cigar, pipe)?
- For how long?
- How many packs per day?

▶ Smoking has been linked to hypertension, which over time may contribute to the development of renal failure. Smoking also significantly increases an individual's risk for developing bladder cancer (Freedman, Silverman, Hollenbeck, Schatzkin, & Abnet, 2011).

3. Do you use any recreational drugs?
- If so, describe the type, amount, and frequency.
- How long have you been using these drugs?

▶ Abuse of certain drugs over time may lead to kidney failure (National Institute on Drug Abuse [NIDA], 2012), potential for inadequate nutrition and hydration, and susceptibility to infection.

4. How often do you have intercourse?
- Do you urinate after intercourse?
- Are you aware of any sexual partners who may have sexually transmitted diseases?

▶ Some patients may have a tendency to develop UTIs if they do not urinate after intercourse (University of Maryland Medical Center [UMMC], 2013).

Focused Interview Questions	Rationales and Evidence

5. *For female patients:* **How do you cleanse yourself after urination or bowel movement?**
   - Do you use bubble bath?
   - Do you use sprays, powders, or feminine hygiene products?

▶ Cleansing materials such as bubble bath, sprays, and powders may increase the incidence of UTIs. Improper cleansing methods after elimination may also lead to infection (UMMC, 2013).

Questions Related to Age

The focused interview must reflect the anatomic and physiologic differences that exist along the age span. The following questions are examples of those that would be specific for infants and children, the pregnant female, and the older adult.

Questions Regarding Infants and Children

1. **Have you ever been told that the child has a kidney that has failed to grow?**

▶ Renal agenesis may involve one or both kidneys. A genetic factor may be associated with the development of this condition in some cases. Bilateral renal agenesis is invariably fatal. Unilateral renal agenesis may be asymptomatic and is often incidentally diagnosed by abdominal ultrasound or computed tomography (CT) scan secondary to another condition. In infants with unilateral renal agenesis, the remaining kidney may be enlarged, and there is increased risk of problems with the remaining kidney (Westland, Schreuder, Ket, & van Wijk, 2013).

2. **Has the child ever been diagnosed with a kidney disorder?**
   - If so, what is it called, what were the symptoms, and how was it treated?
   - Is it still being treated?

▶ Some disorders, such as infections, are easily treated and do not recur; others, such as glomerulonephritis, may be chronic.

3. **Has the child had hearing problems?**

▶ The ears and kidneys develop at the same time in utero. Congenital deafness is associated with renal disease (Weber, 2012).

4. **Have you ever observed any unusual shape or structure in the child's genital anatomy?**

▶ Parents may report abnormally shaped external genitals, as seen in hypospadias and epispadias. In children with exstrophy of the bladder, the lower urinary tract is visible.

5. **Has the child ever had problems with involuntary urination?**
   - If so, what are the characteristics?
   - What was the diagnosis?
   - How was it treated?
   - Is it still occurring?

▶ **Enuresis** is the medical term for involuntary urination after age 4. If it occurs at night, it is termed nocturnal enuresis after age 6. This condition may have extensive impact on the social, mental, and physical well-being of the family and child.

6. **Have you started toilet training with the child?**
   - If yes, how successful has it been?
   - Are there any current problems with toilet training?
   - What method are you using for toilet training?

▶ These questions elicit information about maturity of the neurologic and urinary systems.

7. **Has the child decreased play activity?**

▶ Loss of interest in play may signal fatigue, which may be associated with renal failure.

8. **Are you changing the baby's diaper more or less than you were?**

▶ There are a variety of contributors to changes in elimination patterns, but renal failure, dehydration, overhydration, diet changes, obstruction, and stress may contribute to a change in normal pattern.

Focused Interview Questions	Rationales and Evidence

Questions for the Pregnant Female

1. **Have you noticed any changes in your urinary pattern?**

▶ Often, the developing fetus places increasing pressure on the mother's bladder, causing urinary urgency. As a result, the patient voids more often in smaller amounts (Berman & Snyder, 2012).

2. **Have you noticed unusual swelling in your ankles, feet, fingers, or wrists?**
   - Have you noticed any headaches?

▶ These signs may be associated with pregnancy-induced hypertension and preeclampsia (Berman & Snyder, 2012).

Questions for the Older Adult

1. **Have you noticed any unusual swelling in your ankles, feet, fingers, or wrists?**

▶ Swelling may be indicative of congestive heart failure. Associated with the swelling can be weight gain, fatigue, activity intolerance, and shortness of breath.

2. *For male patients:* **Have you noticed difficulty initiating the stream of urine, voiding in small amounts, and feeling the need to void more frequently than in the past?**

▶ These symptoms may be due to an enlarged prostate.

Questions Related to the Environment

Environment refers to both the internal and external environments. Questions related to the internal environment include all of the previous questions and those associated with internal or physiologic responses. Questions regarding the external environment include those related to home, work, or social environments.

Internal Environment

1. **What medications do you currently take?**
   - What medications have you been taking in the last several months?
   - Describe the type, the dose, and the reason why you are taking the medication.
   - How often do you take it?
   - Every day, as needed, or only when you remember?

▶ It is important to know the patient's compliance with the medication regimen. If the patient has not completed a regimen of antibiotic therapy to clear a UTI, kidney infection, or sexually transmitted disease, the infection may persist (Wong & Stevens, 2013).

2. **Do you take any vitamins, protein powders, or dietary supplements?**
   - If so, which ones?
   - How much do you take?
   - How many days a week do you take it?
   - How many times a day?
   - Why do you take it?

▶ Excessive ingestion of certain nutritional supplements or herbal agents may contribute to the development of renal disorders (Shaw, Graeme, Pierre, Elizabeth, & Kelvin, 2012).

External Environment

The following questions deal with substances and irritants found in the physical environment of the patient. The physical environment includes the indoor and outdoor environments of the home and workplace, those encountered for social engagements, and any encountered during travel.

1. **Do you live in an environment or work in an industry that exposes you to toxic chemicals?**

▶ These may contribute to the development of cancer of the urinary system (Soderland, Lovekar, Weiner, Brooks, & Kaufman, 2010).

2. **Have you traveled recently to a foreign country or any unfamiliar place?**

▶ The patient may have been exposed to bacterial, viral, or fungal agents that affect renal function.

Patient-Centered Interaction

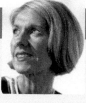

Ms. Angela Carbone, age 55, comes to the Medi-Center at 10:30 a.m. with the chief complaint of left back pain. She has some nausea and no vomiting. She complains of dysuria and gross hematuria and indicates she had a kidney stone on the right side several years ago. The following is an excerpt from the focused interview with Ms. Carbone.

Interview

Nurse: Good morning. Ms. Carbone. Are you having pain now?

Ms. Carbone: Yes, I am.

Nurse: On a scale of 0 to 10 with 10 being the highest, how do you rate your pain?

Ms. Carbone: Now it is about 4 but I'm afraid it will become 10 or 12 like the last time.

Nurse: I need to ask you some questions to get information from you. Will you be able to talk to me for a few minutes?

Ms. Carbone: I think so! I'll try. I'll let you know if I can't sit any more.

Nurse: Tell me about the pain.

Ms. Carbone: I have back pain on my left side, right here (pointing to the left costovertebral area). It feels like it moves down my back but not all the time. It really hurts and is getting worse each day.

Nurse: When did the pain start?

Ms. Carbone: It started about 5 days ago. That's when I noticed my urine was darker than usual.

Nurse: Did you do anything to help reduce the pain?

Ms. Carbone: Not really. At first I thought I slept funny. Then my urine got darker. I tried to drink three glasses of water a day, but I became nauseated and had to stop drinking.

Nurse: Earlier you commented that you are afraid the pain will become 10 or 12 like the last time. Tell me more.

Ms. Carbone: I had a kidney stone about 3 years ago on my right side. Now the pain is similar on the left side.

Analysis

The nurse immediately asked Ms. Carbone about her current pain status to determine her ability to participate in the interview. Throughout the interview, the nurse used open-ended questions and leading statements. These statements encouraged verbalization by the patient to explore and describe actions and feelings in detail. The open-ended questions and leading statements permitted the patient to provide detail, thereby eliminating the need for multiple closed questions.

Patient Education

The following are physiologic, behavioral, and cultural factors that affect the health of the urinary system across the age span. Several factors reflect trends cited in *Healthy People 2020* documents. The nurse provides advice and education to reduce risks associated with these factors and to promote and maintain urinary health.

LIFESPAN CONSIDERATIONS

Risk Factors	Patient Education
• Structure or functional abnormalities in infants may cause urinary obstruction, hydronephrosis, and reflux diseases.	▶ Tell parents that hydronephrosis can be diagnosed antenatally by ultrasound. Parents then need support and counseling about treatment. UTI in infants is usually the first sign of reflux disorders. Parents need guidance regarding health care of infants when symptoms arise. Reflux disorders generally resolve without treatment. Parents need support and guidance regarding prevention of further infection and long-term care recommendations when problems do not resolve or result in chronic renal disorders.
• Bed-wetting (enuresis) is common in children, especially males.	▶ Inform parents that most bed-wetting ceases by the age of 4 or 5. Parents should be encouraged to seek health care if the problem persists at ages 6 and 7. Limiting fluid intake before bedtime or waking the child to void are some methods to address the problem.
• Prostate enlargement occurs in aging and can lead to problems with urinary elimination.	▶ Encourage males over 40 years of age to have regular prostate examinations.

CULTURAL CONSIDERATIONS

Risk Factors	Patient Education
• Hypertension is a risk factor for chronic kidney disease. African Americans have increased incidence of hypertension.	▶ Advise patients to discuss all medications—including OTC, herbal, and folk medications—with their healthcare provider.

ENVIRONMENTAL CONSIDERATIONS

Risk Factors	Patient Education
• UTIs can occur at any age. Females are more susceptible because of the short urethra.	▶ Inform patients that UTIs are generally caused by bacteria and treated with antibiotics. Inform patients of the importance of taking all of the medication, even when symptoms subside. ▶ Provide information, especially to females, about methods to prevent UTI.
• Renal calculi occur more frequently in individuals with a family history of calculi. Calculi can develop following UTI and in patients with parathyroid disorders and hypercalcemia.	▶ Tell patients that renal calculi are caused by a variety of problems. Guidance for reducing the risk for development of stones in those with a family history includes drinking enough fluid in a 24-hour period to produce 2 quarts of urine. Dietary changes and medications may be prescribed for patients with renal calculi. Support and encouragement to follow guidelines is an important role of the nurse.
• Patients with diabetes are at increased risk for problems in the urinary system.	▶ Advise patients with diabetes to follow their prescribed regimen and to schedule urinary and renal function screenings with their healthcare provider.

BEHAVIORAL CONSIDERATIONS

Risk Factors

- The use of analgesics, both prescribed and OTC medications for pain, has been linked with renal disease.

- Cigarette smoking has been linked with bladder cancer and renal tumors.

Patient Education

▶ Instruct about the proper use of analgesics, especially OTC medications, to prevent renal disease. Patients should be advised to follow the instructions on the label, avoid prolonged use of combination ingredients (those with aspirin, acetaminophen, and caffeine in one pill), and drink six to eight glasses of water a day when using analgesics.

▶ Advise patients to discuss all medications—including OTC, herbal, and folk medications—with their healthcare provider.

▶ Educate patients to prevent the start of smoking and provide advice and support to foster smoking cessation.

Physical Assessment

Assessment Techniques and Findings

Physical assessment of the urinary system includes the use of inspection, palpation, percussion, and auscultation. The skills are used to gather information about the function of the urinary system. Knowledge of normal parameters and expected findings is essential in determining the meaning of the data as the nurse performs the physical assessment.

Skin is moist and supple with pink undertones. The abdomen is symmetric and free of lesions, bruises, and swelling. The renal arteries are without bruits. The costovertebral angle and flanks are symmetric, even in color, and nontender to palpation and percussion. The kidneys are not enlarged; they are rounded, smooth, firm, and nontender. The bladder is nonpalpable, and percussion reveals tympany above the symphysis pubis.

Physical assessment of the urinary system follows an organized pattern. It begins with a survey of the patient's general appearance followed by inspection of the abdomen. The renal arteries are auscultated and then the costovertebral angles and flank areas are inspected, palpated, and percussed. The kidneys are palpated. Bladder fullness is determined by palpation and percussion of the lower abdomen.

EQUIPMENT

- examination gown and drape
- clean, nonsterile examination gloves
- stethoscope
- specimen container

HELPFUL HINTS

- Have the patient empty the bladder before the examination and collect a urine specimen at that time.
- Provide clear instructions for specimen collection and provide privacy.
- Males and females respond in a variety of ways when exposed for examination of private areas. Use appropriate draping to maintain the dignity of the patient.
- Explain each step of the procedures and tell the patient to report any discomfort or difficulty.
- Use Standard Precautions.

Techniques and Normal Findings	Abnormal Findings Special Considerations

General Survey

A quick survey of the patient enables the nurse to identify any immediate problem as well as the patient's ability to participate in the assessment.

1. **Instruct the patient.**
   - Explain that you will be looking, listening, touching, and tapping on parts of the abdomen. Tell the patient you will explain each procedure as it occurs. Tell the patient to report any discomfort and that you will stop the examination if the procedure is uncomfortable.

2. **Position the patient.**
   - Begin the examination with the patient in a supine position with the abdomen exposed from the nipple line to the pubis (see Figure 22.4 ■).

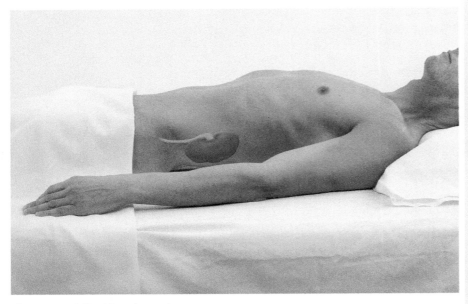

Figure 22.4 Position the patient.

3. **Assess the general appearance.**
   - Assess general appearance and inspect the patient's skin for color, hydration status, scales, masses, indentations, or scars.
   - The patient should not show signs of acute distress and should be mentally alert and oriented.

▶ Patients with kidney disorders frequently look tired and complain of fatigue. If a kidney disorder is suspected, it is important to look for signs of circulatory overload (pulmonary edema) or peripheral edema (puffy face or fingers) or indications of pruritus (scratch marks on the skin).

▶ Elevated nitrogenous wastes (azotemia) in the blood contribute to mental confusion.

Techniques and Normal Findings	Abnormal Findings Special Considerations

4. Inspect the abdomen for color, contour, symmetry, and distention.

- It may be helpful to stand at the foot of the examination table and inspect the abdomen from there (see Figure 22.5 ■).

▶ A distended bladder may be visible in the suprapubic area, indicating the need to void and perhaps the inability to do so.

▶ The increased adipose tissue in the abdomen of the obese patient may inhibit visualization of underlying structures.

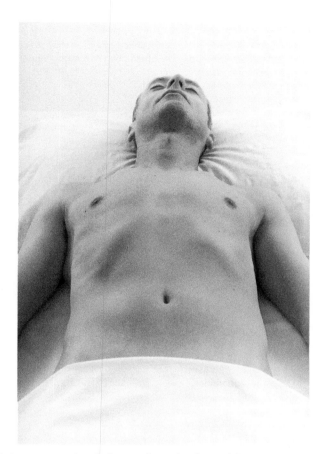

Figure 22.5 Inspecting the abdomen from the foot of the bed.

- Note that visual inspection of the suprapubic area may confirm the presence or absence of a distended bladder.
- Normally, the patient's abdomen is not distended; is relatively symmetric; and is free of bruises, masses, and swellings. (A complete discussion of abdominal assessment is provided in chapter 21.) ∞

▶ Many diseases may contribute to abdominal distention. These include renal conditions such as polycystic kidney disease; enlarged kidneys, as seen in acute pyelonephritis; ascites (accumulation of fluid) due to hepatic disease; and displacement of abdominal organs. Pressure from the abdominal contents on the diaphragm may alter the patient's breathing pattern.

Techniques and Normal Findings	Abnormal Findings Special Considerations

5. Auscultate the right and left renal arteries to assess circulatory sounds.

- Gently place the bell of the stethoscope over the extended midclavicular line (MCL) on either side of the abdominal aorta, which is located above the level of the umbilicus (see Figure 22.6 ■).
- Be sure to auscultate both the right and left sides, and over the epigastric and umbilical areas.
- In most cases, no sounds are heard; however, an upper abdominal bruit, a swishing or murmur-like sound, is occasionally heard in young adults and is considered normal. On a thin adult, renal artery pulsation may be auscultated.

▶ Presence of a bruit may indicate narrowing or obstruction of a blood vessel.

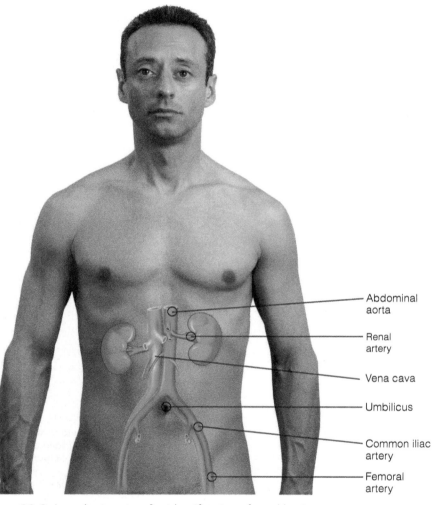

- Abdominal aorta
- Renal artery
- Vena cava
- Umbilicus
- Common iliac artery
- Femoral artery

Figure 22.6 Auscultation sites for identification of renal bruits.

6. For patients with a urinary catheter, inspect the catheter for signs of infection, correct placement, and urinary outflow.

- Patients with limited mobility, such as patients with paralysis, recent surgery, or a fractured hip, will likely use an indwelling catheter or undergo intermittent catheterization.
- Inspect the urine and urethral meatus for signs of infection, irritation, tenderness, and cleanliness.
- Inspect the collection bag for fullness, and empty if needed; also inspect the bag and tubing for possible obstructions.
- Inspect the bag for correct placement on the leg and ensure that the bag is lower than the bladder at all times.
- Record urine outflow and fluid intake to ensure that the urinary drainage system is working properly.

▶ Because of the high risk of infection, the need for a catheter shoud be assessed at every interaction. Signs of infection include hematuria, foul-smelling or cloudy urine, and lower back pain.
▶ Improper drainage of the catheter may result in urinary backflow into the bladder, which is a major cause of infection.

| **Techniques and Normal Findings** | **Abnormal Findings Special Considerations** |

The Kidneys and Flanks

1. Position the patient.
- Place the patient in a sitting position facing away from you with the patient's back exposed.

2. Inspect the left and right costovertebral angles for color and symmetry.
- The color should be consistent with the rest of the back.

▶ A protrusion or elevation over a costovertebral angle occurs when the kidney is grossly enlarged or when a mass is present.

3. Inspect the flanks (the side areas between the hips and the ribs) for color and symmetry.
- The costovertebral angles and flanks should be symmetric and even in color.

▶ This finding must be carefully correlated to other diagnostic cues as the assessment proceeds. If ecchymosis is present (Grey Turner's sign), there may be other signs of trauma such as blunt, penetrating wounds or lacerations.
▶ Pain, discomfort, or tenderness from an enlarged or diseased kidney may occur over the costovertebral angle, flank, and abdomen. When questioned, the patient complains of a dull, steady ache. This type of pain is associated with polycystic formation, pyelonephritis, and other disorders that cause kidney enlargement. In the patient with polycystic kidney disease, a sharp, sudden, intermittent pain may mean that a cyst in the kidney has ruptured. If the costovertebral angle is tender, red, and warm, and if the patient is experiencing chills, fever, nausea, and vomiting, the underlying kidney could be inflamed or infected.

> **ALERT!**
>
> *Do not percuss or palpate the patient who reports pain or discomfort in the pelvic region. Do not percuss or palpate the kidney if a tumor of the kidney is suspected, such as a neuroblastoma or Wilms' tumor. Palpation increases intra-abdominal pressure, which may contribute to intraperitoneal spreading of this neuroblastoma. Deep palpation should be performed only by experienced practitioners.*

4. Gently palpate the area over the left costovertebral angle (see Figure 22.7 ■).
- Watch the reaction and ask the patient to describe any sensation the palpation causes. Normally, the patient expresses no discomfort.

▶ The pain caused by calculi (stones) in the kidney or upper ureter is unique and different in character, severity, and duration than that caused by kidney enlargement. This pain occurs as calculi travel from the kidney to the ureters and the urinary bladder.
▶ Some patients experience no pain, and others feel excruciating pain. A stationary stone causes a dull, aching pain. As stones travel down the urinary tract, spasms occur. These spasms produce sharp, intermittent, colicky pain (often accompanied by chills, fever, nausea, and vomiting) that radiates from the flanks to the lower quadrants of the abdomen and, in some cases, the upper thigh and scrotum or labium.
▶ If the patient reports severe pain, **hematuria** (blood in the urine) or **oliguria** (diminished volume of urine), and nausea and vomiting, it is important to be alert for hydroureter, a frequent complication that occurs when a renal calculus moves into the ureter. The calculus blocks and dilates the ureter, causing spasms and severe pain. Hydroureter can lead to shock, infection, and impaired renal function. If the nurse suspects hydroureter or obstruction at any point in the urinary tract, medical collaboration must be sought immediately.

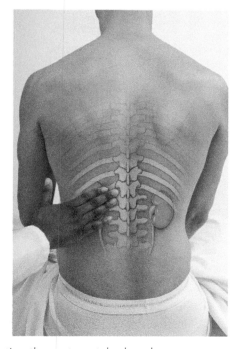

Figure 22.7 Palpating the costovertebral angle.

Techniques and Normal Findings	Abnormal Findings Special Considerations

5. Use blunt or indirect percussion to further assess the kidneys.
- Place your left palm flat over the left costovertebral angle.
- Thump the back of your left hand with the ulnar surface of your right fist, causing a gentle thud over the costovertebral angle (see Figure 22.8 ■).

▶ Pain or discomfort during and after blunt percussion suggests kidney disease. This finding is correlated with other assessment findings.

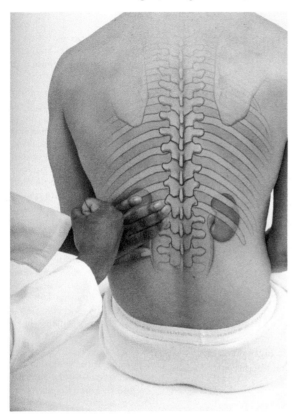

Figure 22.8 Blunt percussion over the left costovertebral angle.

6. Repeat the procedure on the right side. Ask the patient to describe the sensation as you examine each side.
- The patient should feel no pain or tenderness with pressure or percussion.

ADVANCED SKILL

THE LEFT KIDNEY

1. Attempt to palpate the lower pole of the left kidney.
- Although it is not usually palpable, attempt to palpate the lower pole of the kidney for size, contour, consistency, and sensation. Note that the rib cage obscures the upper poles.

▶ When enlargement occurs in the presence of conditions such as neoplasms and polycystic disease, the kidneys may be palpable. Otherwise, they are rarely palpable.

ALERT!

Because deep kidney palpation can cause tissue trauma, novice nurses should not attempt either deep palpation or capture of the kidney unless supervised by an experienced nurse or nurse practitioner. Deep kidney palpation should not be done in patients who have had a recent kidney transplant or an abdominal aortic aneurysm.

Techniques and Normal Findings	Abnormal Findings Special Considerations

- Position the patient in a supine position. All palpation should be performed from the patient's right side.
- While standing on the patient's right side, reach over the patient and place your left hand between the posterior rib cage and the iliac crest (the left flank).
- Place your right hand on the left upper quadrant of the abdomen lateral and parallel to the left rectus muscle just below the costal margin.
- Instruct the patient to take a deep breath. As the patient inhales, lift the patient's left flank with your left hand and press deeply with your right hand (approximately 4 cm) to attempt to palpate the lower pole of the kidney (see Figure 22.9 ■).

▶ Care must be taken not to mistake an enlarged spleen for an enlarged left kidney. An enlarged kidney feels smooth and rounded, whereas an enlarged spleen feels sharper with a more delineated edge.

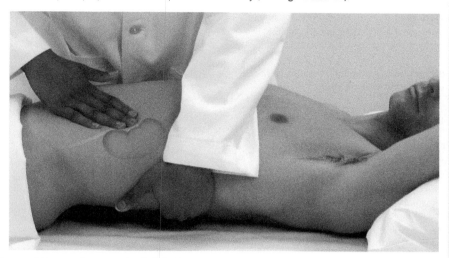

Figure 22.9   Palpating the left kidney.

2. **Attempt to capture the left kidney.**
   - Because of its position deep in the retroperitoneal space, the left kidney is not normally palpable. The capture maneuver may enable you to palpate it. This maneuver is possible because the kidneys descend during inspiration and slide back into their normal position during exhalation.
   - Standing on the patient's right side, place your left hand under the patient's back to elevate the flank as before. Place your right hand on the left upper quadrant of the abdomen lateral and parallel to the left rectus muscle with the fingertips just below the left costal margin. Instruct the patient to take a deep breath and hold it. As the patient inhales, attempt to capture the kidney between your two hands. Ask the patient to exhale slowly and then to briefly hold the breath. At the same time, slowly release the pressure of your fingers.
   - As the patient exhales, you will feel the captured kidney move back into its previous position. The kidney surface should be rounded, smooth, firm, and nontender.

▶ An enlarged palpable kidney could be painful for the patient. This suggests tumor, cyst, or hydronephrosis.

ADVANCED SKILL

THE RIGHT KIDNEY

1. **Attempt to palpate the lower pole of the right kidney.**
   - Standing on the patient's right side, place your left hand under the back parallel to the right 12th rib (about halfway between the costal margin and iliac crest) with your fingertips reaching for the costovertebral angle. Place your right hand on the right upper quadrant of the abdomen lateral to the right rectus muscle and just below the right costal margin.
   - Instruct the patient to take a deep breath. As the patient inhales, lift the flank with your left hand and use deep palpation to feel for the lower pole of the kidney.

Techniques and Normal Findings	Abnormal Findings Special Considerations

2. Attempt to capture the right kidney.

- Place your left hand under the patient's right flank.
- Place your right hand on the right upper quadrant of the abdomen with the fingertips lateral and parallel to the right rectus muscle just below the right costal margin.
- Instruct the patient to take a deep breath and hold it. As the patient inhales, attempt to capture the kidney between your two hands.
- Ask the patient to exhale slowly and then to briefly hold the breath. At the same time, slowly release the pressure of your fingers.
- As the patient exhales you will feel the captured kidney move back into its previous position. The kidney surface should be rounded, smooth, firm, and nontender.
- The lower pole of the right kidney is palpable in some individuals, especially in thin, relaxed females. If palpable, the lower pole of the kidney has a smooth, firm, uninterrupted surface.
- During the capture maneuver, some patients describe a nonpainful sensation as the kidney slides between the nurse's fingers back into its normal position.

▶ It is important not to mistake an enlarged liver for an enlarged right kidney. An enlarged kidney feels smooth and rounded, whereas an enlarged liver is closer to the midline and has a more distinct border.
▶ Polycystic kidney disease or carcinoma should be suspected when there is gross enlargement of the kidney. The kidneys may be two or three times their normal size in patients with polycystic disease.

The Urinary Bladder

1. Palpate the bladder to determine symmetry, location, size, and sensation.

- Use light palpation over the lower portion of the abdomen. The abdomen should be soft.
- Use deep palpation to locate the fundus (base) of the bladder, approximately 5 to 7 cm (2 to 2.5 in.) below the umbilicus in the lower abdomen. Once you have located the fundus of the bladder, continue to palpate, outlining the shape and contour (see Figure 22.10 ■). Bimanual palpation may be required in the obese patient.
- Slide your fingers over the surface of the bladder and continue palpating to determine smoothness and continuity.
- The surface of the bladder should feel smooth and uninterrupted. An empty bladder is usually not palpable. When the bladder is moderately full, it should be firm, smooth, symmetric, and nontender. As the bladder fills, the fundus can reach the level of the umbilicus. A full bladder is firm and buoyant.

▶ A distended bladder feels smooth, round, and taut. An asymmetric contour or nodular surface suggests abnormal growth that should be correlated with other findings.
▶ In males with urethral obstruction due to hypertrophy or hyperplasia of the prostate, the bladder is enlarged.

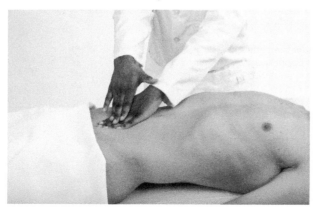

Figure 22.10 Palpating the bladder.

2. Percuss the bladder to determine its location and degree of fullness.

- Begin with indirect percussion in the midline of the abdomen at the level of the umbilicus.
- Move your fingers downward as you continue to percuss toward the suprapubic area. Continue percussing downward until tympanic tones change to dull tones. A full bladder produces a dull sound. The point at which tympanic tones cease is the upper margin of the bladder.
- Some practitioners conclude the assessment of the urinary system with the inspection and palpation of the penis and urethral meatus in the male patient or the inspection of the urethral meatus in the female patient. Other practitioners consider these structures with the assessment of the genitalia. These techniques are discussed in chapters 23 and 24.∞

▶ Bladder scanning or bedside bladder ultrasonography is a safe, noninvasive technique to assess bladder fullness in suspected urinary retention.

Abnormal Findings

Common alterations of the urinary system include bladder cancer, kidney and urinary tract infections, calculi, tumors, renal failure, and changes in urinary elimination. Each of these alterations is discussed in the following section.

Bladder Cancer

Seen later in life, bladder cancer occurs more frequently in males than in females. Smoking has been linked to this disease. In some cases, the patient who experiences bladder cancer is asymptomatic.

If signs and symptoms are present,

Subjective findings:

- Flank pain.
- Dysuria.

Objective findings:

- Hematuria.
- Frequent urination.
- Edema in lower extremities.
- Pelvic mass.

Glomerulonephritis

This condition is an inflammation of the glomerulus.

Subjective findings:

- Fatigue.
- Changes in urinary patterns.

Objective findings:

- Hypertension.
- Generalized edema.
- Hematuria.
- Proteinuria.

Renal Calculi

Calculi are stones that block the urinary tract. They are usually composed of calcium; struvite; or a combination of magnesium, ammonium, phosphate, and uric acid (see Figure 22.11 ■).

Subjective findings:

- Radiating pain that is variable in location and severity.
- Ureteral spasms.
- Nausea.
- Dysuria.
- Increased urinary urgency.

Objective findings:

- Vomiting.
- Increased urinary frequency.
- Gross hematuria.

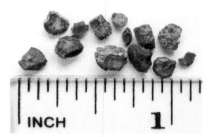

Figure 22.11   Renal calculi.
Source: iStock.

Renal Tumor

Renal tumors may be either benign or malignant, with malignant being more common. Research has shown that there is an association with renal tumors and smoking.

Subjective findings:

- Flank pain.
- Lethargy.

Objective findings:

- Hematuria.
- Weight loss.
- Palpable flank mass.

Renal Failure

Renal failure may be acute or it may progress to a chronic state. Acute renal failure that does not progress to a chronic state includes three stages: oliguria, diuresis, and recovery. Signs and symptoms of uremia, which is the hallmark of chronic renal failure, may include anorexia, nausea, vomiting, altered mentation, uremic frost, weight loss, fatigue, and edema.

Subjective findings:

- Anorexia.
- Nausea.
- Pruritus.
- Fatigue.

Objective findings:

- Fluid retention.
- Electrolyte imbalances (such as hyperkalemia and hyperphosphatemia).
- Vomiting.
- Uremia.
- Changes in mentation.

Urinary Tract Infection

Bacteria cause urinary tract infections (UTIs). The bladder is the most common site of the infection, which results in inflammation of the bladder (cystitis); however, infection may include the kidneys. UTIs are common with catheter use for urinary retention or incontinence. Therefore, patients with catheters should be assessed regularly for UTIs. Patients may be asymptomatic.

Subjective findings:

- Increased urinary urgency.
- Dysuria.
- Suprapubic or lower back pain.

Objective findings:

- Increased urinary frequency.
- Hematuria.
- Cloudy, foul-smelling urine.

Changes in Urinary Elimination

The following are examples of alterations in urinary elimination:

Dysreflexia affects patients with spinal cord injuries at level T7 or higher. Bladder distention causes a sympathetic response that can trigger a potentially life-threatening hypertensive crisis.

Incontinence is the inability to retain urine. If this is the patient's problem, the nurse must determine which of the five types of incontinence is present.

- *Functional incontinence* occurs when the patient is unable to reach the toilet in time because of environmental, psychosocial, or physical factors.
- *Reflex incontinence* occurs in patients with spinal cord damage when urine is involuntarily lost.
- *Stress incontinence,* involuntary urination, occurs when intra-abdominal pressure is increased during coughing, sneezing, or straining. Aging changes may also contribute to stress incontinence.
- *Urge incontinence* may be caused by consuming a significant volume of fluids over a relatively short period. Urge incontinence may also be due to diminished bladder capacity.
- *Total incontinence* is related to a neurologic condition.

Urinary retention is a chronic state in which the patient cannot empty the bladder. In most cases, the patient voids small amounts of overflow urine when the bladder reaches its greatest capacity.

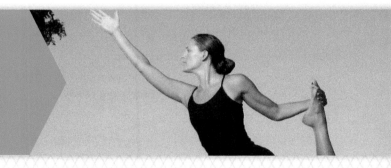

Application Through Critical Thinking

▶ Case Study

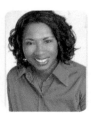

Ms. Sadie Basset is a 52-year-old African American female who arrives at the Metropolitan Women's Clinic complaining of itching, burning, and frequency of urination. She tells Louise Lo, RN, "I feel like I have to go to the bathroom every 10 minutes. I'm just miserable. I'm burning all the time, and I have tenderness here." (She points to her lower abdominal area.) Ms. Basset states that sometimes she feels a sharp abdominal pain and a sudden urge to urinate. On a few of these occasions, she has had difficulty getting to the bathroom on time and has even had a few "accidents." Ms. Lo asks if Ms. Basset has any illnesses. Ms. Basset reports that she was diagnosed with diabetes mellitus a few weeks ago.

After the interview, Ms. Lo performs a physical assessment. Blood pressure is 106/82, pulse 68, respirations 20, and temperature 101.2°F. Abdomen is flat and soft. Bowel sounds are active and present in all four quadrants. The patient complains of tenderness over the suprapubic area on palpation. The urinary meatus is red and edematous with no apparent discharge. Induration of the urinary meatus is noted on palpation of the anterior vaginal wall. The urinary stream is strong and steady. The urine is dark yellow with a hint of blood. It is cloudy and has a strong, foul odor.

Ms. Lo determines that there are four targets of concern for Ms. Basset: urge incontinence, pain, elevated temperature, and lack of knowledge.

Complete Documentation

The following is sample documentation for Sadie Basset.

SUBJECTIVE DATA: Complains of itching, burning, and frequency of urination. "I feel like I'm going to the bathroom every 10 minutes. I'm just miserable. I'm burning all the time and I have tenderness here" (points to lower abdomen). Sometimes feels a sharp abdominal pain and sudden urge to urinate. Occasional difficulty getting to bathroom and few "accidents." Diagnosed with diabetes 2 weeks ago.

OBJECTIVE DATA: VS: B/P Left 106/82, Right 110/80. Temperature 101.2°F. Abdomen flat, soft. Bowel sounds present all quadrants. Tenderness over suprapubic area on palpation. Urinary meatus red, edematous, no discharge. Induration of meatus. Urinary stream strong, steady. Urine dark yellow, cloudy, strong, foul odor, Hematest positive.

Critical Thinking Questions

1. Identify the data that support Ms. Lo's targets of concern.
2. What additional missing data are required to determine treatment for this patient?
3. Describe a plan of nursing care for Ms. Basset.

4. What additional factors would put the patient at risk for urinary infections if the patient were older?
5. Why is it important for the nurse to address the issue of urinary incontinence?

Prepare Teaching Plan

LEARNING NEED: Sadie Basset is a patient newly diagnosed with diabetes with frequent, painful urination and lower abdominal pain. Her urine is dark, cloudy, and foul smelling with a hint of blood. The data indicate that she has a UTI. Diabetes increases the risk for development of UTI. Therefore, the nurse has a twofold responsibility. First, the nurse must ascertain Ms. Basset's ability to adhere to the prescribed regimen for diabetes. Second, in the presence of this acute problem, the nurse must address this patient's need to learn about UTI.

GOAL: Sadie Basset will reduce her risk for further episodes of UTI.

OBJECTIVES: Upon completion of this learning experience, Sadie Basset will be able to:

1. Describe UTI.
2. Identify factors that contribute to the development of UTI.
3. Describe measures to prevent UTI.

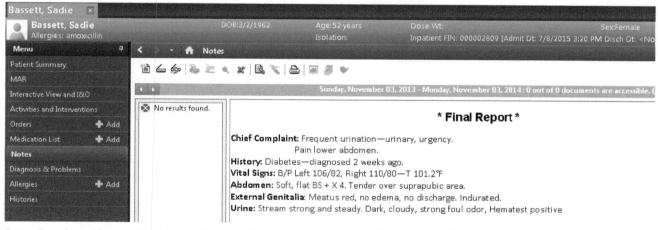

Source: From Cerner Electronic Health Record. Copyright © by Cerner Corporation. Used by permission of Cerner Corporation.

APPLICATION OF OBJECTIVE 3: Describe measures to prevent UTI

Content	Teaching Strategy	Evaluation
• Follow the prescribed diabetic regimen.	One-on-one discussion.	Verbal questioning in which Ms. Basset describes the eight measures to prevent UTI.
• Report changes in blood glucose readings.	Permits repetition and introduction of sensitive information.	
• Drink six to eight glasses of water daily.		
• Urinate as soon as you feel the urge. Do not wait.		
• Cleanse the genital area from front to back to prevent organisms from the rectal area from entering the vagina or urethra.		
• Shower rather than bathe in a tub.		
• Avoid irritation of the urethra that can occur with douching, vaginal sprays, perfumed soaps, and bubble bath. Avoid wet clothing.		
• Avoid tight clothing and pantyhose without cotton linings.		
• Cleanse the genital area before and after intercourse.		
• Urinate after intercourse.		

▶ References

Berman, A., & Snyder, S. J. (2012). *Kozier and Erb's fundamentals of nursing: Concepts, process, and practice* (9th ed.). Upper Saddle River, NJ: Prentice Hall.

Centers for Disease Control and Prevention (CDC). (2014). *Diabetes, high blood pressure raise kidney risk.* Retrieved from http://www.cdc.gov/features/worldkidneyday/

Chambers, J. C., Zhang, W., Lord, G. M., van der Harst, P., Lawlor, D. A., Sehmi, J. S., ... Melander, O. (2010). Genetic loci influencing kidney function and chronic kidney disease. *Nature Genetics, 42*(5), 373–375.

Devarajan, P. (2014). *Oliguria.* Retrieved from http://emedicine.medscape.com/article/983156-overview#aw2aab6b2b2

Forsgren, C., Lundholm, C., Johansson, A. L., Cnattingius, S., Zetterström, J., & Altman, D. (2012). Vaginal hysterectomy and risk of pelvic organ prolapse and stress urinary incontinence surgery. *International Urogynecology Journal, 23*(1), 43–48.

Freedman, N. D., Silverman, D. T., Hollenbeck, A. R., Schatzkin, A., & Abnet, C. C. (2011). Association between smoking and risk of bladder cancer among men and women. *Journal of the American Medical Association, 306*(7), 737–745.

Gray, H. (2010). *Gray's anatomy.* London: Arcturus.

Kuypers, D. R. (2009). Skin problems in chronic kidney disease. *Nature Clinical Practice Nephrology, 5*(3), 157–170.

Marieb, E. (2009). *Essentials of human anatomy and physiology* (9th ed.). Redwood City, CA: Benjamin/Cummings.

Mayo Foundation for Medical Education and Research. (2014). *Rochester test catalog: 2014 online test catalog.* Available at http://www.mayomedicallaboratories.com/test-catalog/

Moore, K., & Spence, K. (2014). Urinary tract infection. *Hospital Medicine Clinics, 3*(1), e93–e110.

National Endocrine and Metabolic Diseases Information Service (NEMDIS). 2012. *Primary hyperparathyroidism.* Retrieved from http://www.endocrine.niddk.nih.gov/pubs/hyper/

National Institute on Drug Abuse (NIDA). (2012). *Medical consequences of drug abuse: Kidney damage.* Retrieved from http://www.drugabuse.gov/publications/medical-consequences-drug-abuse/kidney-damage

Office of Minority Health (OMH). (2014). *Diabetes data/statistics.* Retrieved from http://minorityhealth.hhs.gov/templates/browse.aspx?lvl=3&lvlid=62

Ozkanli, S., Girgin, B., Kosemetin, D., & Zemheri, E. (2014). Case report – Hemangioma of the urinary bladder. *Science, 3*(1), 15–16.

Romero, V., Akpinar, H., & Assimos, D. G. (2010). Kidney stones: A global picture of prevalence, incidence, and associated risk factors. *Reviews in Urology, 12*(2–3), e86–e96.

Shaw, D., Graeme, L., Pierre, D., Elizabeth, W., & Kelvin, C. (2012). Pharmacovigilance of herbal medicine. *Journal of Ethnopharmacology, 140*(3), 513–518.

Soderland, P., Lovekar, S., Weiner, D. E., Brooks, D. R., & Kaufman, J. S. (2010). Chronic kidney disease associated with environmental toxins and exposures. *Advances in Chronic Kidney Disease, 17*(3), 254–264.

Stöppler, M. C. (2012). *Cloudy urine.* Retrieved from http://www.medicinenet.com/cloudy_urine/symptoms.htm

Toor, R., Liptzin, B., & Fischel, S. V. (2013). Hospitalized, elderly, and delirious: What should you do for these patients? *Current Psychiatry, 12*(8), 10–18.

University of Maryland Medical Center (UMMC). (2013). *Urinary tract infection.* Retrieved from http://umm.edu/health/medical/reports/articles/urinary-tract-infection

University of Rochester Medical Center. (n.d.). *Health encyclopedia: Chloride (urine).* Retrieved from http://www.urmc.rochester.edu/encyclopedia/content.aspx?ContentTypeID=167&ContentID=chloride_urine

Urological Care Foundation. (2011). *Incontinence: Surgical management.* Retrieved from: http://www.urologyhealth.org/urology/index.cfm?article=33

U.S. Department of Health and Human Services (USDHHS). (2014). *Healthy people 2020.* Retrieved from http://www.healthypeople.gov/2020/default.aspx

Weber, S. (2012). Novel genetic aspects of congenital anomalies of kidney and urinary tract. *Current Opinion in Pediatrics, 24*(2), 212–218.

Westland, R., Schreuder, M. F., Ket, J. C., & van Wijk, J. A. (2013). Unilateral renal agenesis: A systematic review on associated anomalies and renal injury. *Nephrology Dialysis Transplantation, 28*(7), 1844–1855.

Willard, S. D., & Nguyen, M. M. (2013). Internet search trends analysis tools can provide real-time data on kidney stone disease in the United States. *Urology, 81*(1), 37–42.

Wong, C. J., & Stevens, D. L. (2013). Serious Group A Streptococcal infections. *Medical Clinics of North America, 97*(4), 721–736.

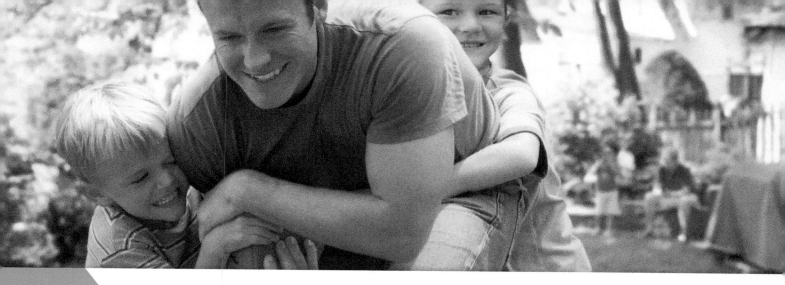

CHAPTER

23 ▶ Male Reproductive System

Learning Outcomes

Upon completion of this chapter, you will be able to:

1. Describe the anatomy and physiology of the male reproductive system.

2. Develop questions to be used when completing the focused interview.

3. Describe techniques required for assessment of the male reproductive system.

4. Differentiate normal from abnormal findings in the physical assessment of the male reproductive system.

5. Describe developmental, psychosocial, cultural, and environmental variations in assessment techniques and findings of the male reproductive system.

6. Discuss the objectives for the male reproductive system as presented in *Healthy People 2020*.

7. Apply critical thinking to the physical assessment of the male reproductive system.

Key Terms

anus, 609
bulbourethral glands, 608
cremasteric reflex, 629
epididymis, 608
epididymitis, 618
epispadias, 610
hypospadias, 610
inguinal hernia, 609
orchitis, 627
penis, 608
perineum, 610
Peyronie's disease, 615
phimosis, 610
prostate gland, 608
scrotum, 606
seminal vesicles, 608
smegma, 625
spermatic cord, 608
spermatocele, 627
testes, 608
urethra, 608
urethral stricture, 626
varicocele, 629

The male reproductive system produces hormones, which impact physical development and sexual behavior. The reproductive organs in males provide for sexual pleasure and producing offspring. The structures of the male reproductive system produce and transport sperm (the male reproductive cells) and protective fluid (semen) for the deposition of sperm within the female reproductive tract and produce the male sex hormones. Many factors including psychosocial health, self-care habits, family, culture, and environment impact reproductive health. Therefore, the nurse must consider these factors while conducting the interview and physical assessment. The nurse must have a thorough understanding of the constituents of a healthy reproductive system and consider the relationship of other body systems to the reproductive system.

During the physical assessment, the nurse will assess and evaluate the occasional ambiguous cues of actual and potential reproductive disease and the variety of contributors to the development of pathology. The nurse documents and communicates the findings to the other members of the healthcare team. Additionally, the nurse has a key role in teaching the patient how to establish and maintain reproductive wellness. The goal of patient education is the promotion of optimum health according to the patient's individual needs. Reproductive health is reflected in *Healthy People 2020*. Objectives related to sexually transmitted diseases and prostate cancer are included in Table 23.2 on page 610.

Anatomy and Physiology Review

The male reproductive system is divided anatomically into external and internal genital organs. The penis and scrotum, the two external organs, are easily inspected and palpated. The internal organs include the testes, spermatic cord, duct system, accessory glands, and inguinal and perianal areas. Only some of the internal structures are palpable. A basic understanding of anatomic structure and function is fundamental to performing assessment techniques correctly and

safely. Figure 23.1 ■ illustrates the gross anatomy of the male reproductive system.

Some of the male reproductive organs serve dual roles as part of the reproductive system and the urinary system. As part of the urinary system, the male genitals serve as a passageway for expelling urine. The functions of the male reproductive system are manufacturing and protecting sperm for fertilization, transporting sperm to the female vagina, regulating hormonal production of and secretion of male sex hormones, and providing sexual pleasure. Each component of the male reproductive system is described in the following sections.

Scrotum

The **scrotum** is a loosely hanging, pliable, pear-shaped pouch of darkly pigmented skin that is located behind the penis. It houses the testes, which produce sperm. Spermatogenesis (sperm production) requires an environment in which the temperature is slightly lower than core body temperature; thus, the scrotum hangs outside of the abdominopelvic cavity and maintains a surface temperature of about 34 °C (93.2 °F), which is approximately 3 °C cooler than core body temperature (Agarwal, Aitken, & Alvarez, p. 169, 2012). A vertical septum within the scrotum divides it into two sections, each containing a testis, epididymis, vas deferens, and spermatic cord as well as other functional structures (see Figures 23.2 ■ and 23.3 ■).

Pubic hair scantily covers the scrotum. It is visibly asymmetric, with the left side extending lower than the right, because the left spermatic cord is longer.

Below the scrotal surface lie two muscles, the cremaster muscle and the dartos muscle, which play a protective role in sperm production and viability. In cold temperatures, the dartos muscle wrinkles the scrotal skin, whereas the cremaster muscle contracts, causing the testes to elevate toward the body. Warmer temperatures cause the reverse reaction. The testes also become more wrinkled and contract toward the body during sexual arousal.

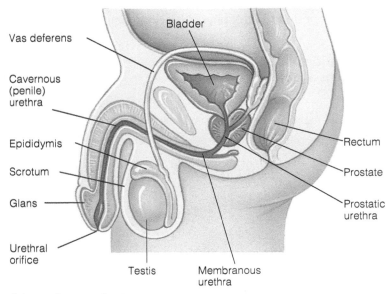

Figure 23.1 Gross anatomy of the male reproductive organs.

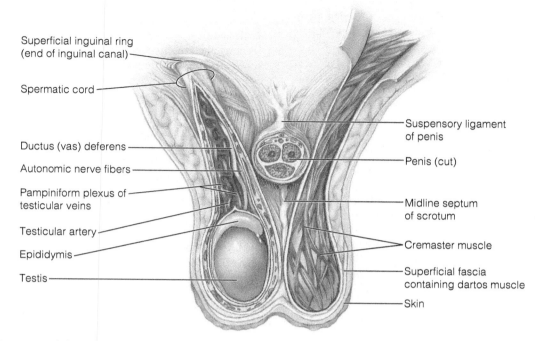

Figure 23.2 Contents of the scrotum, anterior view.

Superficial inguinal ring
(end of inguinal canal)

Spermatic cord

Ductus (vas) deferens

Autonomic nerve fibers

Pampiniform plexus of
testicular veins

Testicular artery

Epididymis

Testis

Suspensory ligament
of penis

Penis (cut)

Midline septum
of scrotum

Cremaster muscle

Superficial fascia
containing dartos muscle

Skin

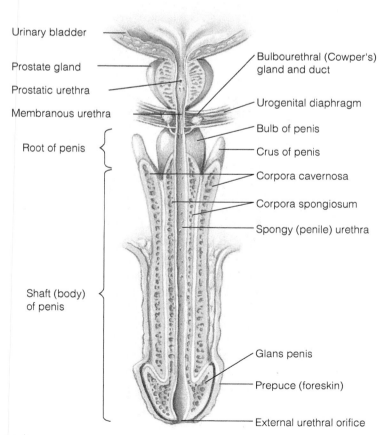

Figure 23.3 Structure of the penis.

Urinary bladder

Prostate gland

Prostatic urethra

Membranous urethra

Root of penis

Shaft (body)
of penis

Bulbourethral (Cowper's)
gland and duct

Urogenital diaphragm

Bulb of penis

Crus of penis

Corpora cavernosa

Corpora spongiosum

Spongy (penile) urethra

Glans penis

Prepuce (foreskin)

External urethral orifice

The major functions of the scrotum are protecting the testes, epididymides, and part of the spermatic cord and protecting sperm production and viability through the maintenance of an appropriate surface temperature.

Testes

The **testes** are two firm, rubbery, olive-shaped structures that measure 4 to 5 cm (1.57 to 1.96 in.) long and 2 to 2.5 cm (0.78 to 0.98 in.) wide. They manufacture sperm and are, thus, the primary male sex organs. Each testis has two coats, the outer tunica vaginalis and the inner tunica albuginea, that separate it from the scrotal wall. Within each testis are the seminiferous tubules that produce sperm and Leydig's cells that produce testosterone. Testosterone plays a significant role in sperm production and the development of male sexual characteristics. The testes receive their blood supply from the testicular arteries. The testicular veins not only remove deoxygenated blood from the testes, but also form a network called the pampiniform plexus (see Figure 23.2). This plays a crucial supportive role in regulating the temperature in the testes by cooling arterial blood before it passes into the testes. The major functions of the testes are producing spermatozoa and secreting testosterone.

Spermatic Cord

The **spermatic cord** is composed of fibrous connective tissue. Its purpose is to form a protective sheath around the nerves, blood vessels, lymphatic structures, and muscle fibers associated with the scrotum (see Figure 23.2).

Duct System

The duct system plays a crucial role in the transportation of sperm. The three structures comprising the duct system are the epididymis, the ductus deferens, and the urethra (see Figures 23.2 and 23.3).

Epididymis

Positioned on top of and just posterior to each testicle is a comma- or crescent-shaped **epididymis**, which is palpable upon physical examination. It is actually a long, coiled tube, about 18 to 20 ft (5.5 to 6 meters) in length, which forms the beginning of the male duct system. Once the immature sperm have been produced in the testes, they are transported into the epididymis where they mature and become mobile. During orgasm, forceful contraction of muscles in this structure propels the sperm into the ductus deferens. The major functions of the epididymis are storing sperm as they mature and transporting sperm to the ductus deferens.

Ductus Deferens

Also known as the vas deferens, this tubular structure stretches from the end of the epididymis to the ejaculatory duct. Extending about 46.15 cm (18 in.) long, the tube runs through the inguinal canal, on the backside of the bladder, and to the ejaculatory duct as it enters into the prostate gland. Mature sperm remain in the ductus deferens until ready for transport. The major functions of the ductus deferens are serving as an excretory duct in the transport of sperm and serving as a reservoir for mature sperm.

Urethra

The **urethra** serves as a conduit for the transportation of both urine and semen to the outside of the body. It is composed of three sections: the prostatic urethra, the membranous urethra, and the spongy (penile) urethra (see Figure 23.3).

Accessory Glands

The accessory glands play a crucial role in the formation of semen. These glands include the seminal vesicles, the prostate gland, and the bulbourethral gland.

Seminal Vesicles

The **seminal vesicles** are a pair of saclike glands, 7.5 cm (2.95 in.) long, located between the bladder and rectum. These vesicles are the source of 60% of the semen produced. Semen, a thick yellow fluid, is composed of a high concentration of fructose, amino acids, prostaglandins, ascorbic acid, and fibrinogen. It is secreted into the ejaculatory duct, where it mixes with sperm, which has been propelled from the ductus deferens. Semen nourishes and dilutes the sperm, enhancing its motility. Seminal fluid is propelled from the ejaculatory duct into the prostatic urethra.

Prostate Gland

The **prostate gland** borders the urethra near the lower part of the bladder. About the size of a chestnut (2 cm or 0.784 in.), it is partially palpable through the front wall of the rectum because it lies just anterior to the rectum (see Figure 23.1). The prostate is composed of glandular structures that continuously secrete a milky, alkaline solution. During sexual intercourse, glandular activity increases, and the alkaline secretions flow into the urethra. Because sperm motility is reduced in an acidic environment, these secretions aid sperm transport. Additionally, the prostate gland produces about one third of all semen.

Bulbourethral Glands

Also referred to as Cowper's glands, the **bulbourethral glands** are located below the prostate within the urethral sphincter (see Figure 23.3). These glands are small (4.5 to 5 mm [0.17 to 0.19 in.]) and round. Just before ejaculation, the bulbourethral glands secrete a clear mucus into the urethra that lubricates the urethra and increases its alkaline environment.

Penis

The **penis** is centrally located between the left and right groin areas and lies directly in front of the scrotum. Internally, the penile shaft consists of the penile urethra and three columns of highly vascular, erectile tissue: the two dorsolateral columns (corpora cavernosa) and the midventral column surrounding or encasing the urethra (see Figure 23.3). The penis contracts and elongates during sexual arousal when its vasculature dilates as it fills with blood. This process allows the penis to become firm and erect so that it can deposit sperm into the female vagina. The distal end of the urethra (the external meatus) appears as a small opening centrally located on the glans of the penis, the cone-shaped distal end of the organ. In uncircumcised males, the glans is covered by a layer of skin called the foreskin. The major functions of the penis are serving as an exit for

TABLE 23.1 Inguinal Hernias

TYPE OF HERNIA	CHARACTERISTICS	SIGNS AND SYMPTOMS
Direct Hernia	Extrusion of abdominal intestine into inguinal ring. Bulging occurs in the area around the pubis. Abdominal intestine may remain within the inguinal canal or extrude past the external ring.	Most often is painless. Appears as a swelling. During palpation, have the patient cough. You will feel pressure against the side of your finger.
Indirect Hernia	Abdominal intestine may remain within the inguinal canal or extrude past the external ring. Most common type of hernia. Located within the femoral canal.	Appears as a swelling. During palpation, have the patient cough. You will feel pressure against your fingertip. Palpate soft mass.
Femoral Hernia	Bulge occurs over the area of the femoral artery. The right femoral artery is affected more frequently than the left. Lowest incidence of all three hernias.	May not be painful; however, once strangulation occurs, pain is severe.

urine and as a passageway for sperm to exit and be deposited into the vagina during sexual intercourse.

Inguinal Areas

The inguinal areas are located laterally to the pubic region over the iliac region or the upper part of the hip bone. Within this area are the inguinal ligaments and the inguinal canals, which lie above the inguinal ligaments. The inguinal canals are associated with the abdominal muscles and actually represent a potential weak link in the abdominopelvic wall. When a separation of the abdominal muscle exists, the weak points of these canals afford an area for the

protrusion of the intestine into the groin region. This is called an **inguinal hernia.** Table 23.1 describes types, characteristics, and signs and symptoms of inguinal hernias.

Perianal Area

The **anus** is the terminal end of the gastrointestinal system. The anal canal is between 2 and 4 cm (0.78 to 1.57 in.) long, opens onto the perineum at the midpoint of the gluteal folds, and has internal and external muscles. The external muscles are skeletal muscles, which form the part of the anal sphincter that voluntarily controls evacuation of stool. Above the anus is the rectum with the prostate gland in close proximity to the anterior surface of the rectum. Mucosa of the anus is moist, darkly pigmented, and hairless. Lying between the scrotum and the anus is the **perineum**, which has a smooth surface and is free of lesions.

Special Considerations

The nurse uses effective communication, critical thinking, the nursing process, and appropriate assessment techniques throughout a comprehensive assessment process to determine the patient's health status. Health status is influenced by a number of factors including age, developmental level, race, ethnicity, work history, living conditions, socioeconomics, and emotional well-being. These factors are described in the following sections.

Health Promotion Considerations

Diseases that affect the reproductive system have a national impact. Objectives of *Healthy People 2020* related to the reproductive system include improving reproductive health among individuals in the United States by reducing the incidence and prevalence of sexually transmitted diseases (STDs). For males, goals of this national initiative target the effective implementation of screening and preventative measures related to infectious diseases such as chlamydia, syphilis, and gonorrhea (U.S. Department of Health and Human Services [USDHHS], 2014). Central to the initiative is decreasing the transmission rate of human immunodeficiency virus (HIV) infection, as well as preventing the development of acquired immunodeficiency syndrome (AIDS) and HIV-related deaths (USDHHS, 2014). See Table 23.2 for examples of *Healthy People 2020* objectives that are designed to promote reproductive health and wellness among individuals across the life span.

Lifespan Considerations

Changes in anatomy and physiologic function occur as normal parts of growth and development. The accurate interpretation of findings from assessment is dependent on knowledge of the expected variations across the age span. The following sections address specific age-related variations in the male reproductive system.

Infants and Children

The male newborn's genitals should be clearly evident and not ambiguous. If there is ambiguity, referral for genetic counseling is indicated. The penis may vary in size but averages about 2.5 cm (0.98 in.) in length and is slender. The urethral meatus should be in the center of the glans. If the opening is located on the underside of the glans, **hypospadias** is present. If the opening is on the superior aspect of the glans, **epispadias** exists. *Chordee*, a tight band of skin, causes bowing of the penis. The penis appears to have a C shape. This is associated with epispadias and hypospadias. The foreskin may be somewhat tight and not retractable until 2 or 3 years of age. By 3 years of age, penile foreskin is retractable in approximately 90% of male children (Modgil, Rai, & Anderson, 2014). If it is still tight after this time, **phimosis** exists. Cultural values and religious beliefs determine whether the family or caregiver circumcises the child. The family requires teaching about either maintaining the cleanliness of the uncircumcised penis or caring for the penis in the days following a circumcision.

TABLE 23.2	Examples of *Healthy People* 2020 Objectives Related to Male Reproductive Health

OBJECTIVE NUMBER	DESCRIPTION
STD-1	Reduce the proportion of adolescents and young adults with *Chlamydia trachomatis* infections
STD-6	Reduce gonorrhea rates
STD-7	Reduce sustained domestic transmission of primary and secondary syphilis
STD-8	Reduce congenital syphilis
STD-10	Reduce the proportion of young adults with genital herpes infection due to herpes simplex type 2
C-10	Reduce the prostate cancer death rate
HIV-6	Reduce new AIDS cases among adolescent and adult men who have sex with men.
HIV-13	Increase the proportion of persons living with HIV who know their serostatus.
HIV-18	Reduce the proportion of men who have sex with men (MSM) who reported unprotected anal intercourse with a partner of discordant or unknown status during their last sexual encounter.

Source: U.S. Department of Health and Human Services (USDHHS). (2014). *Healthy people 2020.* Retrieved from http://www.healthypeople.gov/2020/default.aspx

ALERT!

The foreskin of uncircumcised males will not retract until the child is between 2 and 4 years old. Do not forcefully retract the foreskin of infants and toddlers. In older children with retractile foreskins, always return the foreskin to the natural position after urethral or glans examination.

The male infant's scrotum should be consistent in color with other body parts. It should seem oversized in comparison with the penis. This proportion changes as the infant grows. If the scrotum is enlarged and filled with fluid, a hydrocele may be present. The testes should be palpable and are about 2 cm (0.78 in.) in diameter at birth. Undescended testes, called cryptorchidism, is a common finding, especially if the infant is preterm. The testes should descend spontaneously within the first year of life. If both testes do not descend, the male will be infertile and will be at a greater risk for the development of testicular cancer. Enlargement of the testes in adolescence indicates the presence of a tumor. Testes smaller than 1.5 to 2 cm (0.59 to 0.78 in.) may indicate adrenal hyperplasia.

The onset of puberty in the male child occurs between 10 and 15 years of age. At this time, under the influence of elevating levels of testosterone, the male child begins to develop adult sexual characteristics. The testes and scrotum enlarge. Pubic, facial, and axillary hair develops. The penis begins to elongate, and the testes begin to produce mature sperm. The male child will experience unexpected erections and nocturnal emissions (wet dreams). Open, supportive communication is essential at this time. The nurse can show male children pictures of the sexual maturation of genitals to demonstrate that their development is normal. Figure 23.4 ■ includes Tanner's staging for evaluating sexual maturity. The male child often displays a fascination with his genitals. Masturbation and exploration of the genitals are usual practices in infants, toddlers, and preschoolers. Males may express curiosity in comparing their genitals with those of other children, both male and female, in preschool and school ages.

Precocious puberty is an endocrine disorder characterized by the development of adult male characteristics in males under age 10. It includes dense pubic hair, penile enlargement, and enlargement of the testes. Precocious puberty may be idiopathic or caused by a genetic trait, lesions in the pituitary gland or hypothalamus, or testicular tumors. Referral to an endocrinologist may be required for definitive diagnosis.

It is important to assess not only the physical development of the male child's sexual organs but also the presence of abnormalities such as infection, tumors, and hernias. Assessment is completed using the same methods as described for the adult male.

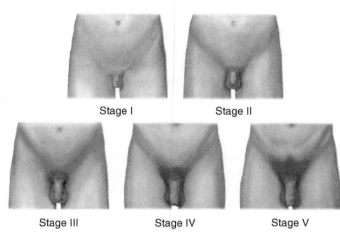

Stage I   Stage II

Stage III   Stage IV   Stage V

Figure 23.4 The Tanner stages of male pubic hair and external genital development with sexual maturation. Stage I, Preadolescent, hair present is no different than that on the abdomen. Testes, scrotum, and penis are the same size and shape as in a young child. Stage II, pubic hair is slightly pigmented, longer, straight, often still downy, usually at base of penis, sometimes on scrotum; enlargement of scrotum and testes. Stage III, pubic hair is dark, definitely pigmented, curly pubic hair appears around base of penis; enlargement of penis, especially in length, further enlargement of testes, descent of scrotum. Stage IV, pubic hair is definitely adult in type but not in extent, spreads no further than inguinal fold. Continued enlargement of penis and sculpturing of glans, increased pigmentation of scrotum. Stage V, hair spreads to medial surface of thighs in adult distribution. Adult stage, scrotum ample, penis reaching nearly to bottom of scrotum.

It is essential to assess for sexual molestation in male children. Some signs of sexual molestation are trauma, depression, eating disorders, bruising, swelling, and inflammation in the genital and anal areas. Additionally, the male child may appear withdrawn. Often the male child will deny the experience.

Adolescents often express interest in the changes related to puberty. The desire to explore sexual relationships and sexual contact, from kissing and fondling to intercourse, may be intense. Thus, adolescents need counseling on relationship issues, birth control, protection against sexually transmitted diseases (STDs; may also be called sexually transmitted infections, or STIs), and delaying sexual activity. An adolescent may be concerned about or confused by an attraction to individuals of the same sex. It is important to provide open communication so that the adolescent may express concerns.

The Older Adult

The older male patient experiences the following changes to the external genitals. Pubic hair thins and grays, the prostate gland enlarges, the size of the penis and testes may diminish, the scrotum hangs lower, and the testes are softer to palpation. Sperm production decreases in middle age; however, the older male may remain able to contribute viable sperm and father children throughout his life span.

Sexual function and ability change as well. Testosterone production decreases, resulting in diminished libido. Sexual response is often slower and not as intense. The older male may be slower to achieve erection, yet may be able to maintain the erection longer. Ejaculation can be less forceful and last for a shorter time, and less semen may be ejaculated.

Even though older male adults can achieve sexual gratification and participate in a satisfying sexual relationship, a decrease in sexual drive may contribute to the patient's withdrawing from sexual experiences and relationships. The following factors are known to influence sexual drive:

- Chronic or acute diseases
- Certain medications
- Loss of spouse or significant other
- Loss of privacy
- Depression
- Fatigue
- Any stressful situation
- Use of alcohol or illicit drugs

Psychosocial Considerations

Fatigue, depression, and stress can decrease sexual desire in a patient of any age. Grief over the loss of a relationship, whether because of separation, divorce, or death, can have long-term effects on a patient's willingness to seek new relationships. Feelings of betrayal—for example, when a partner becomes intimate with another person—can have the same effect.

Past or recent trauma, as from childhood abuse, physical assault, and sexual assault, whether or not penetration occurred, may have a significant impact on a patient's ability to enjoy a sexual relationship. This may be true even if the trauma is completely repressed.

A male's body image may be affected by his perception of his penis size in relation to that of other males. Some males fear that they are "too small" to satisfy a female sexually. Caring and sensitive teaching are needed to help the patient understand that variations in penis size are normal and that there is little correlation between penis size and a partner's sexual satisfaction.

Males who have had a surgical sterilization procedure may feel suddenly freed from the worry of unwanted pregnancy and experience an increase in sexual desire, or they may suddenly feel less masculine than before the surgery and withdraw from sexual relationships.

Cultural and Environmental Considerations

Religious and cultural beliefs may influence multiple aspects of reproductive health and sexuality, including the patient's preference for a same-gender examiner. Prior to assessment, the nurse should determine the patient's preference in this regard. Although general awareness of cultural influences is essential to patient care, the nurse should be careful to avoid making assumptions, including that all patients of a given cultural background share every belief or follow all practices of their religious or cultural group.

Some cultures and religions have specific beliefs or encourage specific behaviors related to circumcision and sexual practices. For example, male circumcision is required in some religions, such as Judaism and Islam. In many cultures, this practice is preferred as a means of hygiene promotion. Circumcision is least common among Hispanic males (Castro, Jones, Lopez, Barradas, & Weiss, 2010).

Testicular cancer is the most common type of cancer in males between the ages of 20 and 34 (National Cancer Institute [NCI], 2014); thus, even adolescent males should perform a monthly testicular self-examination (see Box 23.1). Testicular cancer is most common among White males (NCI, 2014).

Among all races, prostate cancer is most common in African American males and in Carribean males of African ancestry

(American Cancer Society [ACS], 2014a). The signs of the condition are not usually noticeable until the prostatic cancer is advanced. The signs are usually confounding because benign prostatic disease presents with similar symptoms. These signs are dribbling, retention of urine, difficulty initiating the urinary stream, and cystitis. Risk factors include a family history of prostatic cancer and smoking. For males who are at average risk of developing this disease, annual prostate examination is recommended after the age of 50. Men who are at higher risk, including those whose first-degree relative (e.g., brother, father, or son) was diagnosed with prostate cancer before age 65, are encouraged to begin screenings at age 45. If two or more first-degree relatives are diagnosed with prostate cancer at an early age, the man is encouraged to begin screenings by age 40 (ACS, 2014b). Due to the uncertainty related to the diagnosis of prostate cancer based on prostate specific antigen (PSA), primary care providers may vary with regard to their approaches to caring for patients whose PSA is elevated. Additionally, healthcare providers vary with regard to what constitutes an elevated blood PSA level. In general, a normal PSA is considered to be <4 ng/mL. However, some healthcare providers consider a PSA of >2.5 ng/mL to be elevated. For men in whom PSA elevation is noted, risk factors (including race, age, and family history) are taken into consideration when planning further assessment, such as prostate biopsy (ACS, 2014b).

Penile cancer, which is rare among men in the United States, accounts for less than 1% of cancers in this country. However, in some parts of South America, Asia, and Africa, this disease accounts for up to 10% of all forms of cancer among men (ACS, 2014c).

Adults living in overcrowded conditions may feel that their lack of privacy inhibits their ability to experience sexual gratification. Today, one or more grandparents or older relatives may live with their adult child, and sexual expression and gratification may be compromised for all of the adults in the family.

Sexual, physical, or verbal abuse among family members may cause significant sexual dysfunction. Some family members may be aware of the experience but are unwilling or unable to stop the perpetrators or help the victims.

Negative family reactions to an individual's sexual orientation and lifestyle choices can constrain a person's ability and willingness to find a sexual partner and maintain a satisfying sexual relationship. The family's influence may be so strong that individuals choose partners acceptable to the family who do not meet their own needs or desires. This can have a negative emotional and physical impact on the individuals. Homosexual experimentation is common in adolescence and may not signify homosexuality or bisexuality.

Males who work in the microelectronics industry—in which the design and production of semiconductors, circuit boards, and other components of high-speed electronic equipment occur—may be exposed to arsenic, glycol ethers, lead, and radiation. These substances have been linked to birth defects. Lead is also still present in some homes, especially those built before 1979. Males who have been exposed to lead may experience decreased libido, diminished sperm count, and abnormal sperm morphology. Exposure to vinyl chloride, a gas used in the manufacture of building and construction materials, wire and cable insulation, glass, paper, household goods, and medical supplies, may increase the risk for chromosomal changes in the male germ cells. Federal regulations regarding exposure to vinyl chloride have been adopted to prevent known health risks.

Box 23.1 Testicular Self-Examination

Testicular cancer has no early warning signs. Thus, males should perform a testicular self-exam monthly, beginning in adolescence. Describe to the patient how to perform the exam:

- The best time to perform the exam is in the shower or bath, since the heat and steam will warm your hands and the water will help your hands to glide over the skin surface. If your hands are cold, a reflex response will occur, causing your testicles to move up against your body. They will then be more difficult for you to feel.

- Feel each testicle by applying gentle pressure with your thumb, index, and middle fingers. If your testicle hurts while you feel it, you are pressing too hard.

- The contour of the testicle should be smooth, rounded, and firm.

- You will feel the epididymis on top of and behind each testicle.

- You should not feel any distinct lumps or areas of hardness, nor should your testicle be enlarged. If any of these signs are present, make an appointment with your healthcare provider immediately.

Gathering the Data

Health assessment of the male reproductive system includes gathering subjective and objective data. Subjective data collection occurs during the patient interview, before the actual physical assessment. During the interview the nurse uses a variety of communication techniques to elicit general and specific information about the patient's state of health or illness. Health records, the results of laboratory tests, and X-rays are important secondary sources to be reviewed and included in the data-gathering process (see Table 23.3). During physical assessment of the male reproductive system, the techniques of inspection and palpation will be used.

Focused Interview

The focused interview for the male reproductive system concerns data related to the structures and functions of this body system. Subjective data related to the status of the reproductive system are gathered during the focused interview. The nurse must be prepared to observe the patient and listen for cues related to the function of this body system. The nurse may use open-ended and closed questions to obtain information. Often a number of follow-up questions or requests for descriptions are required to clarify data or gather missing information. Follow-up questions are aimed at identifying the source of problems, duration of difficulties, measures to alleviate problems, and clues about the patient's knowledge of his own health.

Because of the dual functions of some of the male reproductive structures, some of the data gathered during the focused interview will relate to the status of the urinary system as well as the

TABLE 23.3	**Potential Secondary Sources for Patient Data Related to the Male Reproductive System**
LABORATORY TESTS	**NORMAL VALUES**
Prostate Specific Antigen (PSA)	0–4 ng/dL
Testosterone	300–1,000 ng/dL
Serum Studies for Tumor Markers	
Serum Studies for STDs	
Urethral Discharge Smears	
Diagnostic Tests	
Residual Post-void Urine Ultrasonography	0 mL
Transrectal Ultrasound and Biopsy of the Prostate	
Uroflometry	Normal 14 mL/second

reproductive system. Some commonly reported problems are those related to altered patterns of voiding, the presence of masses or lesions, unusual discharge, pain and tenderness, changes in sexual functioning, suspected contact with a sexual partner who may have an STD, and infertility. Examination of the anus and rectum is included in examination of the male reproductive system. Related problems include hemorrhoids, fissures, and infectious processes.

Nurses need to understand their own feelings and comfort about various aspects of sexuality to be efficient in gathering data. It is essential for the nurse to put aside personal beliefs and values about sexual practices and focus in a culturally competent and nonjudgmental manner on gathering data to determine the health status of the male patient.

During the focused interview, the nurse will need to create an atmosphere that facilitates open communication and comfort for the patient. Male patients commonly experience anxiety, fear, and embarrassment when the nurse requests information about a topic that, in most patients' minds, is very personal. These emotions may be expressed either verbally or nonverbally. With this in mind, the nurse should approach the patient in as nonthreatening a manner as possible and assure the male patient that the information provided and the results of the physical examination will remain confidential. Furthermore, the nurse should be aware of personal behaviors that may serve as a hindrance to effective communication. The nurse should sit down with the male patient to convey that it is important to spend time discussing the patient's concerns. The nurse's verbal and nonverbal communication should convey a nonjudgmental attitude while requesting only the information needed to assess the patient's health status. It is a good idea to begin with questions that are the least threatening and have the least sexual connotation because the information the nurse gathers may reveal some abnormality that may threaten sexual activity and health. A conversational approach with the use of open-ended statements may be helpful, especially with male adolescents. As the patient provides information, the male patient's choice of terminology can serve as a guide in deciding which terms would be most appropriate to use. When discussing any sensitive or controversial topic, it is always best to start with a general statement that opens the door for male patients to express their thoughts.

The focused interview guides the physical assessment of the male reproductive system. The information is always considered in relation to normal parameters and expectations about the function of the system. Therefore, the nurse must consider age, gender, race, culture, environment, health practices, past and concurrent problems, and therapies when framing questions and using techniques to elicit information. In order to address all of the factors when conducting a focused interview, categories of questions related to reproductive status and function have been developed. These categories include general questions that are asked of all patients, those addressing illness and infection, questions related to symptoms and behaviors, those related to habits or practices, questions that are specific to patients according to age, and questions that address environmental concerns. One approach to elicit data about symptoms is the OLDCART & ICE method, described in chapter 7. See Figure 7.3 on page 120. ∞

The nurse must consider the patient's ability to participate in the focused interview and physical assessment of the male reproductive system. If a patient is experiencing discomfort or anxiety, the nurse should focus on relief of symptoms.

Focused Interview Questions	Rationales and Evidence

The following section provides sample questions and bulleted follow-up questions in each of the categories previously mentioned. A rationale for each of the questions is provided. The list of questions is not all-inclusive but does represent the types of questions required in a comprehensive focused interview related to the male reproductive system. The subjective

data collected and questions asked during the health history and focused interview will provide information to help meet the objectives related to promoting reproductive health and preventing STDs as described in Table 23.2 on page 610.

General Questions

1. **Do you have any concerns about your sexual health?**
   - Have you had concerns in the past? If so, please tell me about those concerns.

   ► These questions may prompt the male patient to discuss any concerns about reproductive health.

2. **Are you sexually active? If so, how would you describe your sexual relationship(s)?**

   ► The male patient may feel pressured to be in a sexual relationship. These pressures may be external (expectations of family, friends, or work associates) or internal (fear of being viewed by others as less than desirable or not of an accepted sexual orientation, fear of being alone, or fear of not being loved and accepted).

3. **Are there any obstacles to your ability to achieve sexual satisfaction?**

   ► Causes of inability to achieve sexual satisfaction include fear of acquiring an STD, fear of being unable to satisfy the partner, fear of pregnancy, confusion regarding sexual preference, unwillingness to participate in sexual activities enjoyed by the partner, job stress, financial considerations, crowded living conditions, loss of partner, attraction to or sexual involvement with individuals that the partner does not know about, criticism of sexual performance by the partner, or history of sexual trauma.

4. **Have you noticed a change in your sex drive recently?**

   ► This may be indicative of some physical or psychologic problems that need follow-up (Smith et al., 2011). If the patient answers "yes," the nurse should ask the following question.

5. **Can you associate the change with anything in particular?**

   ► Often patients can relate a decrease in sex drive with stress, illness, drug therapy, or some other factor (Basson, Rees, Wang, Montejo, & Incrocci, 2010).

6. **For patients who are sexually active:**
   - What type of contraception do you use?
   - What kind of sexual activities do you engage in?

   ► Questions about types of sexual activities provide information related to risk for STDs.

7. **Do your family and friends support your relationship with your sexual partner?**

   ► The patient's family and friends can influence the patient's sexual relationship in a variety of ways. The patient may feel tension if the partner is not accepted.

8. **Are you able to talk to your partner about your sexual needs?**
   - Does your partner accept your needs and help you fulfill them?
   - Are you able to do the same for your partner?

   ► Communication with a sexual partner helps in establishing a fulfilling relationship (Montesi, Fauber, Gordon, & Heimberg, 2011).

Focused Interview Questions	Rationales and Evidence
9. Some patients come to a healthcare provider to discuss sexual abuse. • Have you ever been forced to have sexual intercourse or other sexual contact against your will? • Have you ever been molested or raped?	▶ The opening statement lets the patient know that sexual abuse is a topic that can be addressed in this encounter. The questions allow the patient to describe abusive encounters in some detail.
10. *If the patient answers "yes," the nurse should ask the following questions:* • When did the abuse occur? • Who abused you? • What was the experience? • How often did this happen? • What was done about the situation and for you?	
11. *For patients who are sexually active:* • Are you in a relationship with one partner? • If not, how many sexual partners have you or your partner had over the last year?	▶ Sexual activity with many different partners increases the risk of acquiring STDs (Mayo Clinic, 2014a).
12. Do you have children? • If so, how many? • *If the patient answers "no":* Have you tried to have children? • *If the patient answers "yes":* How long have you been trying to have a child?	▶ The couple is not considered potentially infertile unless they have been unable to conceive for a year (World Health Organization [WHO], n.d.).
13. *If the patient indicates that his partner has shown inability to conceive after 1 year:* **How often do you and your partner have intercourse?**	▶ For couples attempting to have a child, it is important to engage in intercourse routinely, two to three times a week (Mayo Clinic, 2014b). Although nurses do not treat infertility, they may be involved in teaching the patient about certain measures that may be helpful, such as temperature tracking in the female partner, to determine the optimal time for intercourse. Concerns about infertility can produce great anxiety for many couples.
14. Have you ever had mumps?	▶ Mumps occurring after puberty has been linked to sterility in males (Johns Hopkins Medicine, n.d.).
15. Have you ever sought professional help for fertility problems? If so, describe this experience.	▶ This provides the opportunity to identify diagnostic testing and procedures for infertility. In addition, the patient can describe psychosocial or emotional issues surrounding the fertility problem.
16. Has an inability for your partner to conceive placed a strain on your relationship? • How has this problem affected your relationship? • How are you feeling about this?	▶ The patient has the opportunity to express emotional or psychosocial concerns surrounding a partner's infertility.
17. Are you able to be sexually aroused? • Has this ability changed over time or recently?	▶ A variety of factors may influence an individual's ability to become sexually aroused. These include use of prescribed or illicit drugs; disorders of the nervous system; diabetes; stress; and fear (e.g., of intimacy, inability to satisfy a partner, or acquiring an STD) (Byun et al., 2013).
18. Are you able to achieve and maintain an erection? • Have any aspects in your ability to achieve an erection changed? • Are you satisfied with the length of time it takes to achieve and maintain an erection?	▶ The ability to achieve an erection depends on both physiologic factors and state of mind (Byun et al., 2013).
19. When you have an erection, is the shaft of the penis straight or crooked?	▶ **Peyronie's disease** causes the shaft of the penis to be crooked during an erection (Mayo Clinic, 2011).

Focused Interview Questions	Rationales and Evidence

20. Are you able to achieve orgasm?
- Are you satisfied with your ability to control the timing of your orgasms?

▶ Premature ejaculation is defined by some researchers as orgasm immediately after, or even before, penetration. It may also be defined as ejaculation before the male's sexual partner reaches orgasm in more than half of the male's sexual experiences. It is often a devastating disorder that may severely compromise sexual relationships. The patient can learn techniques to delay ejaculation (Mayo Clinic, 2014c).

Questions Related to Illness or Infection

1. Have you ever been diagnosed with an illness or disease of the reproductive organs?
- When were you diagnosed with the problem?
- What treatment was prescribed for the problem?
- Was the treatment helpful?
- What kinds of things do you do to help with the problem?
- Has the problem ever recurred (acute)?
- How are you managing the disease now (chronic)?

▶ The patient has an opportunity to provide information about specific illnesses. If a diagnosed illness is identified, follow-up about the date of diagnosis, treatment, and outcomes is required. Data about each illness identified by the patient are essential to an accurate health assessment. Illnesses can be classified as acute or chronic, and follow-up regarding each classification will differ.

2. An alternative to question 1 is to list possible disorders of the male reproductive system—such as benign prostatic disease; erectile dysfunction; and cancer of the penis, prostate, or testicles—and ask the patient to respond "yes" or "no" as each is stated.

▶ This is a comprehensive and easy way to elicit information about illnesses of the reproductive system. Follow-up would be required for each diagnosis as in question 1.

3. Have you ever had a sexually transmitted disease (such as herpes, gonorrhea, syphilis, or chlamydia)?
- *If the patient answers "yes":* Was it treated?
- Did you inform your partner?
- Did you have sexual relations with your partner while you were infected?
- *If the patient answers "yes":* Did you use condoms?
- What treatment did you receive?

▶ Serious, sometimes fatal, complications can develop if treatment is delayed. For example, untreated syphilis can eventually involve the cardiovascular and central nervous systems, and genital herpes is contagious and may infect partners with every sexual encounter (Centers for Disease Control and Prevention [CDC], 2013a).
▶ The nurse should educate the patient regarding the risks and methods of STD transmission, as well as strategies for prevention of STD transmission.

4. Are you aware of having had any exposure to HIV?
- *If the patient answers "yes":* Describe the situation and how you feel you were exposed.

▶ This question helps to determine at-risk practices and knowledge of the transmission of HIV.

5. What are your views on sexual relations and the potential for acquiring HIV?
- Have you ever been tested for HIV?
- What were the results?

▶ Further information about at-risk sexual activity and the determination of HIV status or transmissibility is obtained.

6. Do you have sexual intercourse without condoms?
- *If the patient answers "yes":* On one occasion or routinely?

▶ Consistent, correct use of latex condoms by males is a highly effective means by which to prevent the transmission of HIV, as well as for preventing the spread of numerous other STDs (CDC, 2013c).

7. Have you had surgery on any of your reproductive organs?
- If so, what was the surgery?

▶ Some surgeries, such as penile implants, require periodic follow-up for problems, including possible infection. Surgeries such as prostatectomy (removal of the prostate) or surgeries that alter body image, such as colostomy, may have bearing on sexual function as well as attitude about oneself in relation to sexuality.

Focused Interview Questions	Rationales and Evidence

Questions Related to Symptoms, Pain, and Behaviors

When gathering information about symptoms, many questions are required to elicit details and descriptions that assist in the analysis of the data. Discrimination is made in relation to the significance of a symptom, in relation to specific diseases or problems, and in relation to potential follow-up examination or referral. One rationale is provided for a group of questions in this category.

The following questions refer to specific symptoms and behaviors associated with the male reproductive system. For each symptom, questions and follow-up are required. The details to be elicited are the characteristics of the symptom; the onset, duration, and frequency of the symptom; the treatment or remedy for the symptom, including over-the-counter (OTC) and home remedies; the determination if diagnosis has been sought; the effect of treatments; and family history associated with a symptom or illness.

Questions Related to Symptoms

1. **Have you felt any lumps or masses on your penis, scrotum, or surrounding areas? If so, describe the mass.**
   - Exactly where is it?
   - Describe the size.
   - Is it soft or hard?
   - Is it movable?
   - When did you first notice the mass?
   - Is it painful?
   - Has there been any pattern to the swelling: an increase, decrease, or unchanged pattern?
   - What treatments have you tried?

   ▶ This information helps the nurse to understand the nature of the mass or lump.

2. **Have you noticed any swelling of your scrotum, penis, or surrounding areas?**
   - If so, when did it start?
   - Is it painful?
   - Has there been any pattern to the swelling: an increase, decrease, or unchanged pattern?
   - What treatments have you tried?

   ▶ This information could help identify problems of rapid onset, which sometimes have the potential to be more detrimental. Swelling in the inguinal area may signal the presence of a hernia. Sources of swelling in the scrotal area include an acute or chronic inflammatory process, a hydrocele, scrotal edema, or scrotal hernia (University of Rochester Medical Center [URMC], n.d.).

3. **Have you noticed any unusual discharge from your penis?**
   - If so, of what color?
   - Is there any odor to the discharge?
   - Is it a small, moderate, or large amount?
   - When did you first notice the discharge?
   - Is there any burning or pain with the discharge?

   ▶ Discharge characteristics may indicate whether an infectious process is occurring (Berman & Snyder, 2012).

4. **Have you noticed any change in color of your penis or scrotum?**
   - If so, describe the change and the location.

   ▶ Inflammatory processes may cause redness in the affected area (Berman & Snyder, 2012).

5. **Have you had any unusual itching in your genital area?**
   - If so, where? Have you noticed any rash, scaling, or lumps?

   ▶ Causes may include environmental allergens, soaps, lotions, and the presence of pubic lice (crabs).

6. **Have you had any problems with your rectal area such as pain, itching, bruising, burning, or bleeding?**
   - When did the problem begin?
   - Do you know the cause of the problem?
   - Have you sought health care for the problem?
   - Was a diagnosis made?
   - What treatment was prescribed?
   - What do you do to help with the problem?
   - Has the treatment helped?

   ▶ Pain, itching, bleeding, or burning may indicate the presence of infection, irritation, or injury to the anus or rectum. Bleeding, pain, and irritation may result from passing hard stools, from hemorrhoids, from injuries, or from trauma including anal sex. Fungal infection may result in chronic pruritus or irritation of the perianal area (Klein, 2014).
   ▶ When symptoms involving the anorectal area are associated with hemorrhoids or hard stool, follow-up would include information about diet and bowel habits (Berman & Snyder, 2012).

Focused Interview Questions	Rationales and Evidence
	▶ Irritation or injury to the perianal area can occur as a result of sexual practices or sexual abuse (Berkowitz, 2011). Sensitive questioning about these topics is required when sexual activity is described or when abuse is suspected or disclosed.

Questions Related to Pain

1. **Have you noticed any pain, tenderness, or soreness in the areas of your penis or scrotum?**
   - If so, describe the pain.
   - Is it dull? Sharp? Radiating? Intermittent? Continuous?
   - Does anything make the pain better or worse?

▶ Testicular torsion may cause excruciating acute pain in the testicular area. Often, the affected testicle will be higher in the scrotal sac than the nonaffected testicle. A dull, aching pain is a common symptom of **epididymitis**, which is swelling of the epididymus. This condition is most often caused by infection (Shridharani, Lockwood, & Sandlow, 2012).

2. **Are you having any pain in the area now?**

▶ This question helps the nurse determine if the problem is current, experienced in the past only, or chronic.

Questions Related to Behaviors

1. **Do you check your genitals on a routine basis?**
   - Do you know how to perform testicular self-exam?
   - How often do you perform this exam?
   - What technique do you use?

▶ Self-examination of the genitals should be performed at least monthly for early detection of changes that need follow-up. Teaching may be indicated if the patient is not performing self-examination. Refer to Box 23.1.

2. **How often do you get physical examinations?**

▶ Screening for problems such as prostate or testicular cancer usually is performed during a routine physical.

3. **Are you circumcised? If not, have you had any difficulty keeping this area clean?**

▶ If the patient is having problems with maintaining hygiene of the area, patient teaching may be necessary.

4. **Do you have any genital or body piercings? If so, are you aware of any problems or changes at the piercing site(s)?**

▶ Common complications of genital piercings include scar tissue formation and infection (Dalke, Fein, Jenkins, Caso, & Salgado, 2013).

5. **Are you and your partner using contraception?**
   - If so, what kind?
   - Are you using it consistently?

▶ This helps to determine knowledge of the product being used and practice of contraception.

6. **Would you like to know more about the use of birth control?**

▶ This is a very important question to ask adolescents who shy away from talking about sexual practices but have verbalized that they are sexually active.

7. **How do you protect yourself from sexually transmitted diseases, including HIV?**

▶ Abstinence is the only 100% effective protection against STDs. Latex condoms offer significant protection, especially when treated with spermicide; however, they are not 100% effective (CDC, 2013c).

8. **Do you drink alcohol? If so, how many drinks per week do you consume?**

▶ Chronic alcoholism has been linked to impotence (Cioe, Anderson, & Stein, 2013). Additionally, intake of alcoholic beverages can contribute to an individual "taking chances," such as failing to use condoms, and can impact fertility.

Focused Interview Questions	Rationales and Evidence
9. **Do you use recreational drugs? If so, what type and how much?**	▶ Taken in sufficient amounts, some drugs, such as marijuana and opiates, may decrease libido and lead to impotence (Cioe et al., 2013). Drug use may also contribute to failure to use protection against STDs.

Questions Related to Age

The focused interview must reflect the anatomic and physiologic differences that exist along the age span. The following questions are examples of those that would be specific for children and older adults.

Questions Regarding Infants and Children

1. **Have you noticed any redness, swelling, or discharge that is discolored or foul smelling in the child's genital areas?**	▶ These may indicate inflammatory processes or infection.
2. **Have you noticed any asymmetry, lumps, or masses in the infant's genitals?** *If the parent or caregiver answers "yes":* • Where are they? • Are they movable? • Are they hard or soft? • Does touching the mass elicit a pain response from the child?	▶ These symptoms may indicate the development of an obstructive process, hydrocele, or inguinal hernia.
3. **Has the child complained of itching, burning, or swelling in the genital area?**	▶ These symptoms may indicate the presence of pinworms or infections such as yeast infections (Dennie & Grover, 2013).

The nurse should ask the preschool child, school-age child, or adolescent the following questions:

1. **Has anyone ever touched you when you didn't want him or her to? Where? (The nurse may want to have the child point to a picture.)**	▶ The nurse must try to determine exactly what the person did to the child. Has there been more than touching? Has any other form of sexual contact occurred? The child may feel responsible for the situation and not wish to discuss it, particularly if the abuser is a parent or relative (Leander, 2010). The nurse should assure the child that he has not been bad and that it helps to talk to an adult about it. Referral should be made to a specialist immediately for sexual abuse examination. Careful documentation is required. Information may be considered forensic evidence.

2. **Has anyone ever asked you to touch him or her when you didn't want to? (If the child answers "yes," the child may be sexually abused. The nurse should try to obtain additional information by asking the following questions, but must remember to be sensitive.)**

3. **Where did he or she ask you to touch him or her?**

4. **Who touched you? How many times did this happen? Who knows about this?**

Many of the questions the nurse asks adolescents are similar to those the nurse would ask male adults. It is important to explore adolescents' feelings and concerns regarding their sexual development—for instance, concerns about wet dreams. The male adolescent should be reassured that these changes are normal. Some adolescents may be confused about their feelings of sexual attraction to the opposite or same sex. The nurse should ask open-ended questions and assure the male adolescent that such feelings are normal.

Focused Interview Questions	Rationales and Evidence

Whether or not a male adolescent admits to being sexually active, the nurse should offer information on teenage pregnancy, birth control, and protection against STDs. While many males have had the vaccine series for hepatitis B by adolescence, many have not received Gardasil, which is recommended for protection from human papillomavirus (HPV) in males 11–12 years old (CDC, 2013b). Some teenagers may be fearful that the nurse will relay this information to their parents. The nurse should reinforce that all information is confidential except in situations of sexual abuse.

Use of gender-neutral terms prevents value judgments about sexual orientation. This question allows patients to define what they think sex is. Many teens consider anything not involving vaginal penetration as not being sex.

Questions for the Older Adult

The questions for older male adults are the same as those for younger male adults. In addition, the nurse should explore whether older patients perceive any changes in their sexuality related to advancing age. For example, an older male may find he needs more time to achieve erection. The older adult can be reassured that these changes are normal and do not necessarily indicate disease.

Questions Related to the Environment

Environment refers to both the internal and external environments. Questions related to the internal environment include all of the previous questions and those associated with internal or physiologic responses. Questions regarding the external environment include those related to home, work, or social environments.

Internal Environment

1. **Do you know if your mother received diethylstilbestrol (DES) treatment during pregnancy?**

   ▶ Some reports indicate that sons of mothers who received DES have higher than average rates of genitourinary problems such as hypospadias, infertility, and undescended or enlarged testicles. They may be at risk for testicular cancer and have low sperm counts (Olsen & Ramlau-Hansen, 2014). Physician referral is indicated if the patient's response is "yes."

2. **Do you take any prescribed or OTC medications, home remedies, herbal or cultural medicines, or dietary supplements?**

   ▶ Medications, herbs, dietary supplements, and home remedies can alter, enhance, or interfere with one another in terms of therapeutics and can result in side effects affecting reproductive functioning (Wilson, Shannon, & Shields, 2013).

External Environment

The following questions deal with substances and irritants found in the physical environment of the patient. The physical environment includes the indoor and outdoor environments of the home and workplace, those encountered for social engagements, and any encountered during travel.

1. **Have you been exposed to lead, chemicals, or toxins in the environment?**

   ▶ Lead exposure may result in decreased libido and sperm abnormalities (Karavolos, Stewart, Evbuomwan, McEleny, & Aird, 2013).

2. **Do you use protective equipment when engaged in work or athletic activities?**

   ▶ The use of protective equipment including athletic supports and cups reduces the incidence of testicular damage.

Patient-Centered Interaction

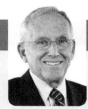

Mr. Edward O'Reilly, age 71, comes to the Urgi-Medi Center at 8:00 p.m. accompanied by his son. He tells the clerk at the reception desk that he needs to see Nurse Jack, stating, "I haven't passed my water since yesterday afternoon." His son tells the clerk his father called him about 5:00 p.m. just as he was leaving work, screaming, "I can't go! I'm going to burst. I have a lot of pressure down there." Mr. O'Reilly is observed pacing in the reception area waiting for the nurse. His chart indicates he came to the center 2 weeks ago with a similar complaint. At that time a diagnosis of benign prostatic hypertrophy was made, along with a recommendation for a transurethral resection of the prostate (TURP). The patient was obviously uncomfortable and was quickly escorted to an examination room. During the walk to the room the nurse began to question the patient. The following is an excerpt from the focused interview.

Interview

Nurse: Good evening, Mr. O'Reilly. I see by the report you are having trouble voiding again.

Mr. O'Reilly: Oh, I'm glad you are here tonight. I can't talk to Ms. Pat about my problem.

Nurse: Tell me about the problem.

Mr. O'Reilly: I have not passed any water since yesterday afternoon, not even a few drops. I have to go really bad. The pressure down there really hurts. I need the tube again.

Nurse: The last time you were able to pass your water, did you have trouble starting the stream?

Mr. O'Reilly: Oh, yes. That's been getting worse. I need to push very hard to start and then I leak when I'm finished.

Nurse: You leak?

Mr. O'Reilly: Yes, I'm like my grandson; I always have wet briefs. I leak and it never stops. I'm so embarrassed.

Nurse: When was the last time you tried to pass your water?

Mr. O'Reilly: I didn't sleep much last night. I'm always trying. I tried before I left the house, nothing, and then when I was waiting for you, and nothing. Nothing, don't you understand me?

Analysis

The patient was clearly uncomfortable and was quickly brought to an examination room. In this clinical example, the nurse used several strategies while assisting the patient to the room. First, the patient's request to see a male nurse was honored. The nurse used open-ended statements and reflection and sought clarification as needed. The use of patient terminology was employed to put the patient at ease.

Patient Education

The following are physiologic, behavioral, and cultural factors that affect the health of the male reproductive system across the age span. Several factors reflect trends cited in *Healthy People 2020* documents. The nurse provides advice and education to reduce risks associated with the aforementioned factors and to promote and maintain the health of the male reproductive system.

LIFESPAN CONSIDERATIONS

Risk Factors	Patient Education
• Infants may be born with ambiguous external genital organs.	▶ Counsel and support parents when making decisions about intervention for ambiguous external genitalia. ▶ Advise parents that surgery to correct cryptorchidism should occur before age 1 to decrease the risk of testicular cancer.

LIFESPAN CONSIDERATIONS

Risk Factors

- Approximately 3% of males are born with cryptorchidism (undescended testicles). Cryptorchidism is a risk factor for testicular cancer.

- Adolescents are interested in exploring their sexuality, and the number of sexually active teenagers is increasing.

- The occurrence of an STD in infants and children often indicates sexual abuse.

- Changes in reproductive organs and sexual drive occur with aging.

Patient Education

▶ Inform males from adolescence through the middle adult years about testicular self-examination (see Box 23.1).

▶ Instruct parents and guardians to observe and seek treatment for their adolescent child's problems with external genitalia that may signal the presence of an STD (drainage, itching, painful urination).

▶ Advise parents to observe for changes in behavior, appetite, activity in school, and friends that can signal problems associated with sexual activity, concern about sexual identity, or abuse.

▶ Advise older males that changes in external genitalia are a normal part of aging.

CULTURAL CONSIDERATIONS

Risk Factors

- Prostate cancer occurs more frequently in African American males than in other ethnic groups.

Patient Education

▶ Most major U.S. medical organizations recommend that clinicians discuss with patients the benefits and harms of PSA screening, consider patient preferences, and individualize the decision to screen. Generally, the most appropriate candidates for screening include men older than 50 years of age and younger men at increased risk for prostate cancer, but that screening is unlikely to benefit men who have a life expectancy of fewer than 10 years. Men from 50 to 70 years of age at average risk and men older than 45 years of age with increased risk, such as African Americans and men with a first-degree relative with prostate cancer, are most likely to benefit from screening (ACS, 2014d).

▶ Males should be informed of symptoms of prostate enlargement, which require follow-up. These include frequent urination; dysuria; difficulty initiating or stopping urination; a change in the urine stream; and pain in the back, hips, or upper thighs.

ENVIRONMENTAL CONSIDERATIONS

Risk Factors

- Uncircumcised males are at greater risk of irritation to the penis and possibly penile cancer.

Patient Education

▶ Instruct patients and parents of uncircumcised infant males regarding retraction of the foreskin when cleaning the penis.

BEHAVIORAL CONSIDERATIONS

Risk Factors

- Human papillomavirus (HPV) increases the risk for penile cancer. The risk for HPV is increased in males who begin sexual relations at an early age, have multiple partners, have sexual relations with a female who has had multiple partners, and have unprotected sexual activity.

- Smoking increases the risk for penile cancer. Uncircumcised males may be at increased risk for penile cancer as well.

- Psychosocial factors including anxiety, stress, and grief can affect sexual behavior across the age span.

Patient Education

▶ Provide information about safe sex practices to all males to reduce risk of all STDs. The CDC (2013b) recommends providing an HPV vaccine for boys age 11–12, young men who have not previously received the vaccine up to age 21, and immunocompromised males through the age of 26.

▶ Inform patients about smoking cessation programs and, as appropriate, provide information about circumcision.

▶ Provide counseling when patients experience a decrease in sexual desire or ability to perform. Explore the reason for the problems. Physiologic changes may be involved and include the effects of some medications and treatments. Psychosocial problems including stress, anxiety, or grief may contribute to the problem and warrant counseling.

Physical Assessment

Assessment Techniques and Findings

The adult male has clean, evenly distributed pubic hair in a diamond pattern thinning as it extends toward the umbilicus. The penis is free of hair and of a size appropriate to the stage of development. The skin is of darker pigment than the rest of the body and loose over a flaccid penis. The dorsal vein is midline on the shaft of the penis. The glans penis is smooth and free of lesions or discharge. The urinary meatus is in the center of the tip of the penis. The scrotum is pear-shaped with wrinkled, loose skin, and is lower on the left side. The inguinal areas are flat. The penis and scrotum are nontender to palpation. The testes are mobile, smooth, elastic, and solid. The spermatic cord is palpable, smooth, and resilient. The inguinal canal is free of masses or lumps. The anus is darkly pigmented and the perianal area is smooth. The bulbourethral gland is smooth and lesion-free, and the prostate gland is nontender, smooth, and firm.

Physical assessment of the male reproductive system follows an organized pattern. It begins with inspection and palpation of the external genitalia. This is followed by inspection of the perianal area, palpation of the bulbourethral and prostate glands via rectal examination, and examination of stool for occult blood.

EQUIPMENT

- examination gown and drape
- clean, nonsterile examination gloves
- examination light
- flashlight
- lubricant
- slides and swabs to obtain a specimen of abnormal discharge

HELPFUL HINTS

- Provide an environment that is warm and private.
- Explain each step in the procedure and provide specific instructions about what is expected of the patient. For example, the nurse should state whether the patient will be expected to sit, stand, or bear down during an assessment.
- Males from puberty through adulthood respond in a variety of ways when the genitals are exposed for examination. It is imperative to maintain the patient's dignity throughout the assessment.
- Explore cultural issues and seek remedies for concerns at the onset of the interaction.
- Use Standard Precautions.

Techniques and Normal Findings	Abnormal Findings Special Considerations

Inspection

1. **Instruct the patient.**
    - Have the male patient empty his bladder and bowel before the examination.
    - Explain to the patient that you will be looking at and touching his genitals and pubic area. Tell him that the assessment should not cause physical discomfort. However, he must tell you of pain or discomfort at any point during the examination.
    - Reassure the patient that anxiety and embarrassment are normal. Explain that relaxation and focusing on instructions will make the assessment easier. If the patient experiences an erection during the examination, explain that this is normal and has no sexual connotation.

2. **Position the patient.**
    - The patient stands in front of the examiner for the first part of the assessment.

3. **Position yourself on a stool, sitting in front of the patient.**

4. **Inspect the pubic hair.**
    - Observe the pubic hair for normal distribution, amount, texture, and cleanliness (see Figure 23.5 ▪).

▶ The amount, distribution, and texture of pubic hair vary according to the patient's age and race. Absent or extremely sparse hair in the pubic area may be indicative of sexual underdevelopment. The pubic hair of elderly males may be gray and thinning.

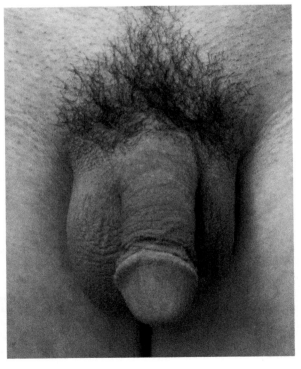

Figure 23.5 Inspecting the pubic hair.

- Confirm that pubic hair is distributed heavily at the symphysis pubis in a diamond- or triangular-shaped pattern, thinning out as it extends toward the umbilicus. The hair will thin as it reaches the inner thigh area and over the scrotum. Hair should be absent on the penis.
- If the patient has complained of itching in his pubic area, comb through the pubic hair with two or three fingers.
- Confirm the absence of small bluish gray spots, or nits (eggs), at the base of the pubic hairs.

▶ These signs indicate the presence of crabs or pubic lice. Marks may be visible from persistent scratching to relieve the intense itching crabs cause.

Techniques and Normal Findings	Abnormal Findings Special Considerations

5. **Inspect the penis.**

- Inspect the penis size, pigmentation, glans, location of the dorsal vein, and the urethral meatus.
- Start by confirming that the penis size is appropriate for the stage of development of the patient. In adult males, penis size varies.

▶ Penis size varies according to the developmental stage of the patient (see Figure 23.4). The penis appears small in obese males due to the development of a pad of fat at the base of the penis.

- Note the pigmentation of the penis.
- Pigmentation should be evenly distributed over the penis. The color depends on the patient's race but will be slightly darker than the color of the skin over the rest of his body.

▶ Pigmentation of the penis of males with lighter complexions ranges from pink to light brown. In dark-skinned patients, the penis is light-to-dark brown.

- Assess the looseness of the skin over the shaft of the penis. The skin should be loose over the flaccid penis.
- Confirm that the dorsal vein is midline on the shaft.
- Inspect the glans penis. It should be smooth and free of lesions or discharge. No redness or inflammation should be present. **Smegma,** a white, cheesy substance, may be present. This finding is considered normal.

▶ Urethral discharge (see Figure 23.6 ■) or lesions may indicate the presence of infective diseases such as *herpes, genital warts, gonorrhea,* or *syphilis,* or may indicate cancer. If discharge is present, the substance should be cultured. Consistency, color, and odor are noted.

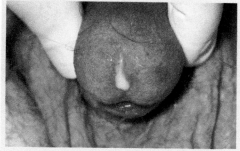

Figure 23.6 Urethral discharge caused by the sexually transmitted disease gonorrhea.
Source: SPL/Custom Medical Stock Photo.

- If the patient is uncircumcised, either ask the patient to pull the foreskin back or do so yourself. To retract the foreskin, gently pull the skin down over the penile shaft from the side of the glans using the thumb and first two fingers or forefinger (see Figure 23.7 ■).

▶ Phimosis is a condition in which the foreskin is so tight that it cannot be retracted.
▶ Paraphimosis describes a condition in which the foreskin, once retracted, becomes so tight that it cannot be moved back over the glans.

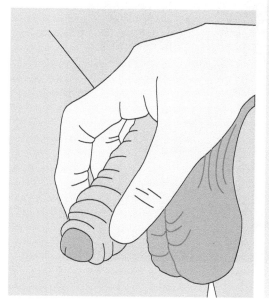

Figure 23.7 Retracting the foreskin.

Techniques and Normal Findings

Abnormal Findings
Special Considerations

- Gently move the foreskin back into place over the glans. The foreskin should move smoothly.

6. Assess the position of the urinary meatus.
- The meatus should be located in the center of the tip of the penis (see Figure 23.8 ■).

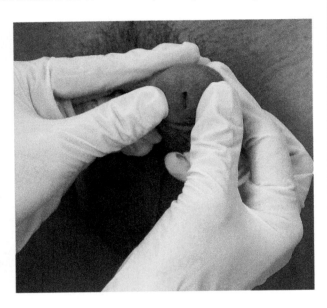

Figure 23.8 Assessing the position of the urinary meatus.

7. Inspect the scrotum.
- Ask the patient to hold his penis up so that the scrotum is fully exposed (see Figure 23.9 ■). Optionally, you may hold the penis up by letting it rest on the back of your nondominant hand.

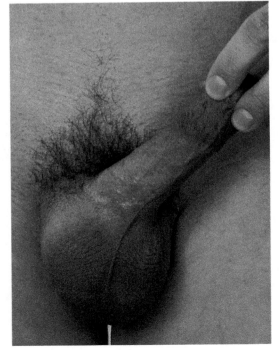

Figure 23.9 Inspecting the scrotum.

▶ Immediate assistance must be sought if the foreskin cannot be retracted. Prolonged constriction of the vessels can obstruct blood flow and lead to tissue damage or necrosis.

▶ In rare cases, the urinary meatus is located on the upper side of the glans (*epispadias*) or the under side of the glans (*hypospadias*). These conditions are usually corrected surgically shortly after birth.
▶ A pinpoint appearance of the urinary meatus is indicative of **urethral stricture.**

- While the patient is standing, observe the shape of the scrotum and how it hangs unsupported. It should be pear shaped, with the left side hanging lower than the right.

- Inspect the front and back of the scrotum. The skin should be wrinkled, loosely fitting over its internal structures. Note any swelling, redness, distended veins, and lesions. If swelling is present, note if it is unilateral or bilateral.

- If you detect a mass, transillumination may be indicated. While not all nurses will be required to perform this assessment skill, the nurse should be familiar with the basic steps involved, as well as its purpose.
- In a darkened room, place a lighted flashlight behind the area in which the abnormal mass was palpated (see Figure 23.10 ■).

▶ An appearance of flatness could suggest testicular abnormality. Elderly males may have a pendulous, sagging scrotal sac.

▶ Scrotal swelling and inflammation could suggest problems such as **orchitis** (inflammation of the testicles), *epididymitis* (inflammation of the epididymis), *scrotal edema* (an accumulation of fluid in the scrotum), *scrotal hernia*, or *testicular torsion* (twisting of the testicle onto the spermatic cord). Swelling and inflammation may also be seen in renal, cardiovascular, and other systemic disorders. Edema of the genitalia can occur in obesity as a result of increased pressure on the groin from the enlarged abdomen.

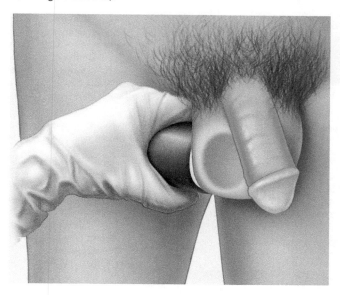

Figure 23.10
Transilluminating the scrotum.

- Note that the light shines through the scrotum with a red glow. The testicle shows up as a nontransparent oval structure.
- Repeat these steps on the other side and compare the results.

▶ Note any area where the light does not transilluminate. Light will not penetrate a mass. Masses may indicate *testicular tumor*, **spermatocele** (a cyst located in the epididymis), or other conditions.

8. **Inspect the inguinal area.**
   - The inguinal area should be flat. This may be difficult to confirm if the patient is overweight. Even in the presence of adipose tissue, the contour of the inguinal area should be consistent with the rest of the body. Lymph nodes are present in this location, but not normally visible.
   - Inspect both the right and left inguinal areas with the patient breathing normally.
   - Have the patient hold his breath and bear down as if having a bowel movement.
   - Observe for any evidence of lumps or masses. The contour of the inguinal areas should remain even.

▶ Masses or lumps may be related to the presence of an inguinal hernia or cancer within the reproductive, abdominal, urinary, lymphatic, and other systems.

Techniques and Normal Findings

Abnormal Findings
Special Considerations

Palpation

1. **Palpate the penis.**
   - Place the glans between your thumb and forefinger (see Figure 23.11 ■).
   - Gently compress the glans, allowing the meatus to gape open. The meatus should be pink, patent, and free of discharge.

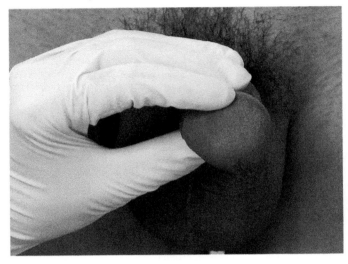

Figure 23.11
Palpating the penis.

   - Note any discharge or tenderness.

   - Continue gentle palpation and compression up the entire shaft of the penis.

2. **Palpate the scrotum.**
   - Ask the patient to hold his penis up to expose the scrotum.
   - Gently palpate the left and then the right scrotal sacs (see Figure 23.12 ■). Each scrotal sac should be nontender, soft, and boggy. The structures within the sacs should move easily with your palpation.
   - Note any tenderness, swelling, masses, lesions, or nodules.

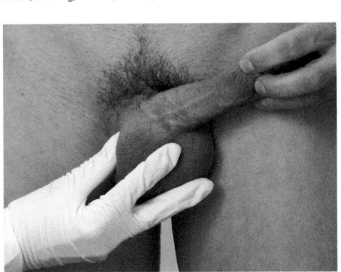

Figure 23.12
Palpating the scrotum.

▶ The patient may be hesitant to verbalize pain when palpation is performed. It is important to watch for nonverbal facial and body gestures.

▶ A *urethral stricture* is suspected if the meatus is only about the size of a pinpoint.

▶ Signs of *urethritis* include redness and edema around the glans and foreskin, eversion of urethral mucosa, and drainage. If urethritis is suspected, the patient should be asked if he experiences itching and tenderness around the meatus and painful urination. If drainage is present, observe for color, consistency, odor, and amount. Obtain a specimen if indicated. Suspect a gonococcal infection (gonorrhea) if the drainage is profuse and thick, purulent, and greenish yellow (see Figure 23.6).

▶ Consider inflammation or infection higher up in the urinary tract if redness, edema, and discharge are visible around the urethral opening, because the mucous membrane in the urethra is continuous with the mucous membrane in the rest of the tract.

▶ Be alert for any lesions, masses, swelling, or nodules.

▶ Note characteristics of any abnormal findings. Culture any discharge.

▶ Assess shape, size, consistency, location, and mobility of any masses. If the patient expresses pain, lift the scrotum. If the pain is relieved, the patient may have epididymitis, inflammation of the epididymis.

Techniques and Normal Findings	**Abnormal Findings / Special Considerations**

3. Palpate the testes.

- Be sure that your hands are warm.
- Approach each testis from the bottom of the scrotal sac and gently rotate it between your thumb and fingertips (see Figure 23.13 ■). Each testis should be nontender, oval shaped, walnut-sized, smooth, elastic, and solid.

▶ The **cremasteric reflex** may cause the testicles to migrate upward temporarily. Cold hands, a cold room, or the stimulus of touch could cause this response. To prevent this reflexive action when examining a child, have him sit tailor style. Gentle pressure over the canal with the nondominant hand can reduce this response.

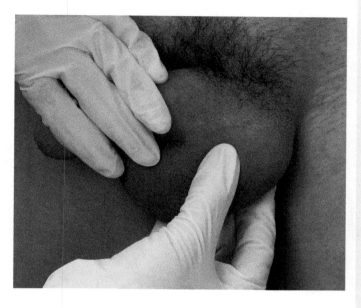

Figure 23.13
Palpating the testes.

4. Palpate the epididymis.

- Slide your fingertips around to the posterior side of each testicle to find the epididymis, a small, crescent-shaped structure.

▶ In some patients, the epididymis may be palpated on the front surface of each testis.

5. Palpate the spermatic cord.

- Slide your fingers up just above the testicle, feeling for a vertical, ropelike structure about 3 mm (0.12 in.) wide.
- Gently grasp the cord between your thumb and index finger (see Figure 23.14 ■).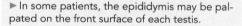
- Do not squeeze or pinch. Trace the cord up to the external inguinal ring using a gentle rotating motion.
- The cord should feel thin, smooth, nontender to palpation, and resilient.

▶ A cord that is hard, beaded, or nodular could indicate the presence of a varicosity or varicocele. A **varicocele** is a distended cord and is a common cause of male infertility. Upon palpation, it may feel like a "bag of worms."

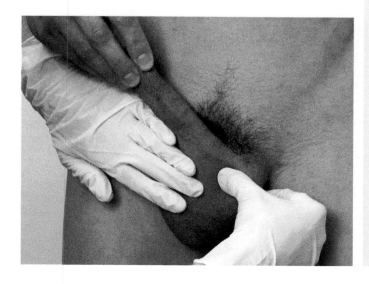

Figure 23.14
Palpating the spermatic cord.

Techniques and Normal Findings	Abnormal Findings Special Considerations

6. Palpate the inguinal region.

- Start by preparing the patient for palpation in the right inguinal area.
- Ask the patient to shift his balance so that his weight is on his left leg.
- Place your right index finger in the upper corner of the right scrotum.
- Slowly palpate the spermatic cord up and slightly to the patient's left.
- Allow the patient's scrotal skin to fold over your index finger as you palpate.
- Proceed until you feel an opening that feels like a triangular slit. This is the external ring of the inguinal canal. Attempt to gently glide your finger into this opening (see Figure 23.15 ■).

ALERT!

If you cannot insert your finger with gentle pressure, do not force your finger into the opening.

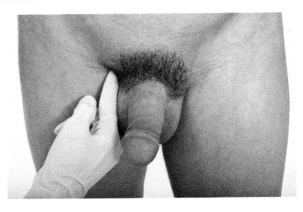

Figure 23.15 Palpating the inguinal canal.

- If the opening has admitted your finger, ask the patient to either cough or bear down.
- Palpate for masses or lumps.

ALERT!

Do not pinch or squeeze any mass, lesion, or other structure.

- Repeat this procedure by palpating the patient's left inguinal area. Use your left index finger when performing the palpation.

▶ An *inguinal hernia* feels like a bulge or mass.

▶ A *direct inguinal hernia* can be palpated in the area of the external ring of the inguinal ligament. It will be felt either right at the external ring opening or just behind it.

▶ An *indirect inguinal hernia* is more common, especially in younger males. It is located deeper in the inguinal canal than the direct inguinal hernia. It can pass into the scrotum, whereas a direct inguinal hernia rarely protrudes into the scrotum.

▶ It is also possible that a *femoral hernia* may be present. It is more commonly found in the right inguinal area and near the inguinal ligament.

▶ Table 23.1 illustrates these three types of hernias.

ALERT!

An acute inguinal bulge with tenderness, pain, nausea, or vomiting, may be manifestations of a strangulated hernia, which is a medical emergency and may require surgical intervention. Should a strangulated hernia be suspected, the patient's primary care provider should be notified immediately.

7. **Palpate the inguinal lymph chain.**
   - Using the pads of your first three fingers, palpate the inguinal lymph nodes.
   - Confirm that nodes are nonpalpable and the area is nontender (Figure 23.16 ■).
   - Occasionally some of the inguinal lymph nodes are palpable. They are usually less than 0.5 cm (0.197 in.) in size, spongy, movable, and nontender.

▶ It is important to assess if a node is larger than 0.5 cm (0.197 in.) or if multiple nodes are present. Tenderness in this area suggests infection of the scrotum, penis, or groin area.

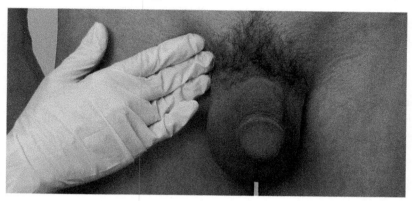

Figure 23.16 Palpating the inguinal lymph nodes.

8. **Inspect the perianal area.**
   - Reposition the patient. Ask the patient to turn and face the table and bend over at the waist. The patient can rest his arms on the table (see Figure 23.17 ■).

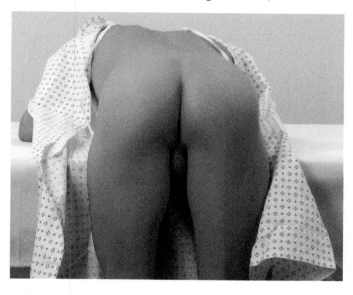

Figure 23.17
Positioning for
assessment
of internal
structures.

   - If the patient is unable to tolerate this position, he may lie on his left side on the examination table with both knees flexed.
   - Inspect the sacrococcygeal and perianal areas. The skin should be smooth and without lesions.

▶ Tufts of hair or dimpling at the sacrococcygeal area are associated with pilonidal cysts. Rashes, redness, excoriation, or inflammation in the perianal area can signal infection or parasitic infestation. Obese males may have fecal incontinence due to pressure of the enlarged abdomen on the bowel and sphincter. This may result in rashes, excoriation, or lesions.

Techniques and Normal Findings	Abnormal Findings Special Considerations

9. Palpate the sacrococcygeal and perianal areas.

- The areas should be nontender and without palpable masses.

▶ Tenderness, mass, or inflammation may indicate pilonidal cyst, anal abscess, fissure, or pruritus.

10. Inspect the anus.

- Spread the buttocks apart. Visualize the anus. The skin is darker and coarse. The area should be free of lesions.
- Ask the patient to bear down. The tissue stretches, but there are no bulges or discharge.

▶ Lesions may include skin tags, warts, hemorrhoids, or fissures.
▶ Fistulas, fissures, internal hemorrhoids, or rectal prolapse are more easily detected when the patient bears down.

11. Palpate the bulbourethral gland and the prostate gland.

- Lubricate your right index finger with lubricating gel.
- Tell the patient that you are going to insert your finger into his rectum in order to palpate his prostate gland. Explain that the insertion may cause him to feel as if he needs to have a bowel movement. Tell him that this technique should not cause pain but to inform you immediately if it does.
- Place the index finger of your dominant hand against the anal opening (see Figure 23.18 ■). Be sure that your finger is slightly bent and not forming a right angle to the buttocks. If you insert your index finger at a right angle to the buttocks, the patient may experience pain.
- Apply gentle pressure as you insert your bent finger into the anus (see Figure 23.19 ■).
- As the sphincter muscle tightens, stop inserting your finger.
- Resume as the sphincter muscle relaxes.
- Press your right thumb gently against the perianal area.

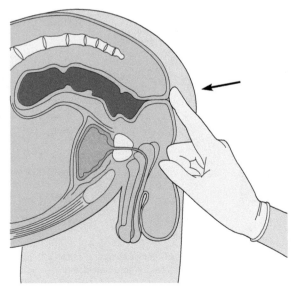

Figure 23.18 Placing the finger against the anal opening.

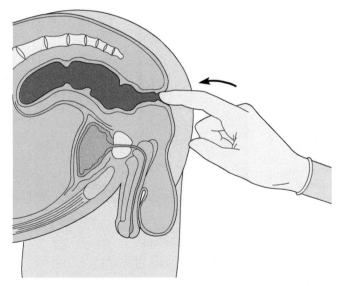

Figure 23.19 Inserting the finger into the anus.

Techniques and Normal Findings	Abnormal Findings Special Considerations

- Palpate the bulbourethral gland by pressing your index finger gently toward your thumb (see Figure 23.20 ■). This should not cause the patient to feel pain or tenderness. No swelling or masses should be felt.

▶ If the bulbourethral gland is inflamed, the patient may feel pain upon palpation. Pain, masses, or abnormalities should be reported to the primary healthcare provider. Referral for further examination, which may include ultrasound of the affected area, is warranted.

- Release the pressure between your index finger and thumb. Continue to insert your index finger gently.

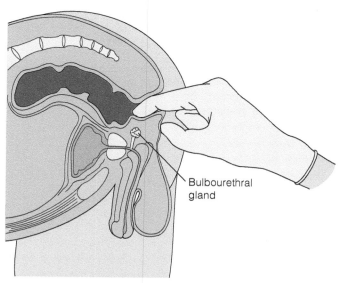

Figure 23.20 Palpating the bulbourethral gland.

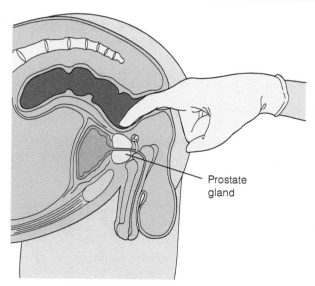

Figure 23.21 Palpating the prostate gland.

- Palpate the posterior surface of the prostate gland (see Figure 23.21 ■).
- Confirm that it is smooth, firm, even somewhat rubbery, nontender, and extends out no more than 1 cm (0.39 in.) into the rectal area.
- Remove your finger slowly and gently.
- Remove your gloves.
- Help the patient to a standing position.
- Wash your hands.
- Give the patient tissues to wipe the perianal area.

▶ Note tenderness, masses, nodules, hardness, or softness. Nodules are characteristic of *prostate cancer*. Tenderness indicates inflammation.

12. **Stool examination.**
- Inspect feces remaining on the gloved finger. Feces are normally brown and soft.

▶ Rectal bleeding is suspected when bright red blood is on the surface of the stool. Feces mixed with bright red blood is associated with bleeding above the rectum. Black, tarry stool is associated with upper gastrointestinal tract bleeding.

- Test feces for occult blood. Normally, the test is negative. A positive test may signal the presence of occult blood but may occur if red meat was eaten within 3 days of the test.

Abnormal Findings

Abnormal findings of the male reproductive system include direct, indirect, and femoral hernias, as previously discussed (see Table 23.1). In addition, reproductive dysfunction may involve disorders of the penis (Table 23.4), abnormalities of the scrotum (Table 23.5), and problems in the perianal area (Table 23.6). These conditions are described on the following pages.

TABLE 23.4	**Abnormalities of the Penis**
Hypospadias	**Peyronie's Disease**
The congenital displacement of the meatus to the inferior surface of the penis, most commonly near the tip of the penis. The opening may also appear in the midline or base of the penis, or behind the scrotum.	Hard plaques are found along the dorsum and are palpable under the skin that result in pain and bending of the penis during erection.

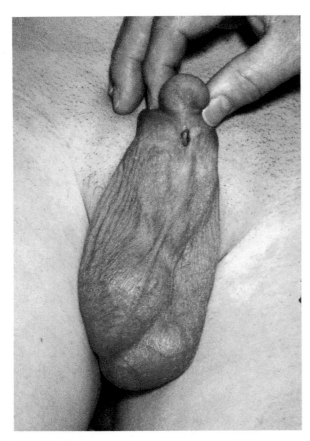

Figure 23.22 Hypospadias.
Source: Centers for Disease Control and Prevention (CDC).

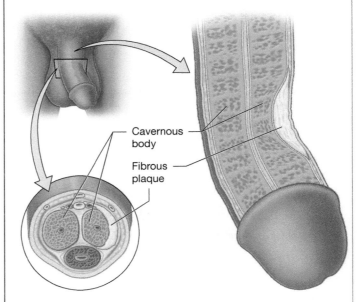

Cavernous body

Fibrous plaque

Figure 23.23 Peyronie's disease.

TABLE 23.4   Abnormalities of the Penis (continued)

Carcinoma

Carcinoma of the penis usually occurs in the glans. It appears as a reddened nodule growth, or ulcer-like lesion.

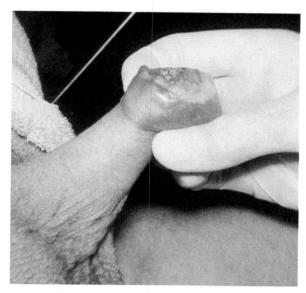

Figure 23.24 Carcinoma.
Source: O.J. Staats MD/Custom Medical Stock Photo.

Genital Warts

A sexually transmitted disease that is caused by human papillomavirus (HPV), genital warts are rapidly growing papular lesions.

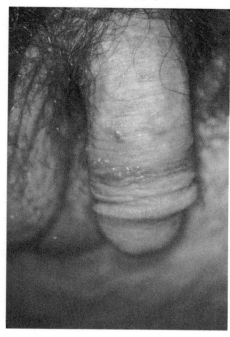

Figure 23.25 Genital warts.
Source: Dr. M. F. Rein/Centers for Disease Control and Prevention (CDC).

Syphilitic Chancre

These nontender lesions appear as round or oval reddened ulcers. A chancre often is the first symptom of primary syphilis, a sexually transmitted disease. Lymphadenopathy is present.

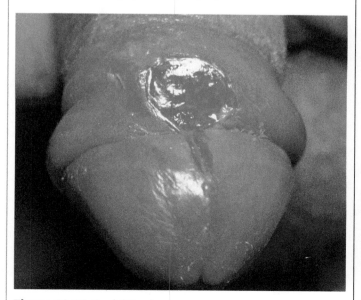

Figure 23.26 Syphilitic chancre.
Source: Science Source.

Genital Herpes

A sexually transmitted disease caused by the herpes simplex virus (HSV), these painful, small vesicles appear in clusters on any part of the surface of the penis. The area around the vesicles is erythematous.

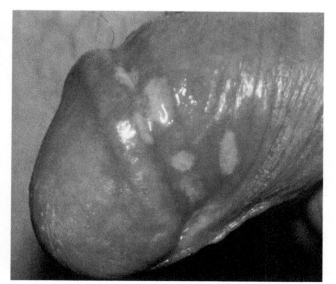

Figure 23.27 Genital herpes.
Source: Biophoto Associates/Science Source.

TABLE 23.5	**Abnormalities of the Scrotum**

Hydrocele

A fluid-filled, nontender mass that occurs within the tunica vaginalis.

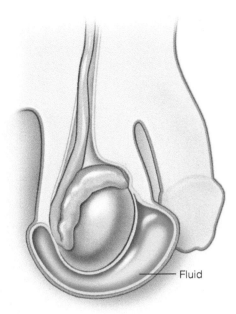

Fluid

Figure 23.28 Hydrocele.

Scrotal Hernia

An indirect inguinal hernia located within the scrotum.

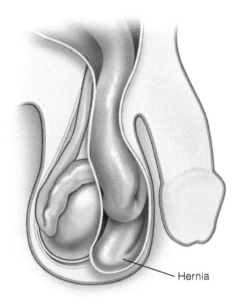

Hernia

Figure 23.29 Scrotal hernia.

Testicular Tumor

A painless nodule on the testes. As it grows, the entire testicle seems to be overtaken.

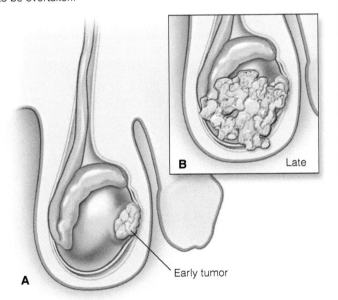

B   Late

A

Early tumor

Figure 23.30 Testicular tumor. A. Early. B. Late.

Orchitis

This inflammatory process results in painful, tender, and swollen testes.

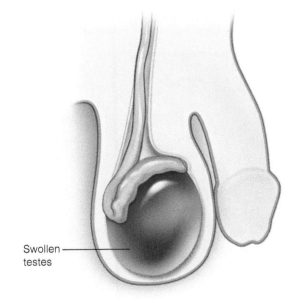

Swollen testes

Figure 23.31 Orchitis.

TABLE 23.5   **Abnormalities of the Scrotum** (continued)

Epididymitis

The epididymis is inflamed and tender. This condition, which can occur in adult males of any age, is most commonly caused by a bacterial infection.

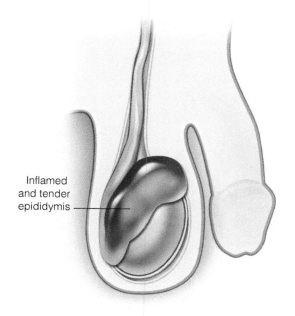

Inflamed and tender epididymis

Figure 23.32 Epididymitis.

Torsion of the Spermatic Cord

Torsion occurs with greatest frequency in adolescents. The twisting of the testicle or the spermatic cord creates edema and pain, requiring immediate surgical intervention.

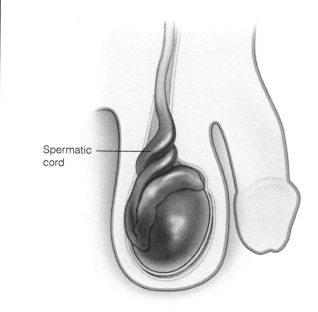

Spermatic cord

Figure 23.33 Torsion of the spermatic cord.

Small Testes

Testes are considered small when they are less than 2 cm (0.78 in.) long. Atrophy may occur in liver disease, in orchitis, and with estrogen administration.

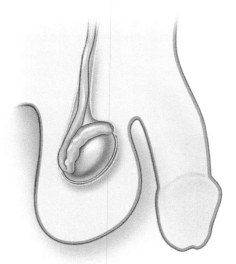

Figure 23.34 Small testes.

Cryptorchidism

Absence of a testicle in the scrotal sac. This condition may result from an undescended testicle.

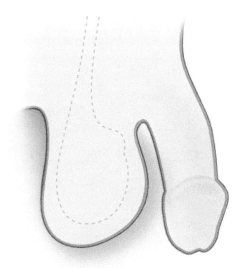

Figure 23.35 Cryptorchidism.

(continued)

TABLE 23.5 **Abnormalities of the Scrotum** (continued)

Scrotal Edema

Edema of the scrotum is seen in conditions causing edema of the lower body, including renal disease and heart failure. Scrotal edema, which may or may not be painful, can occur in males of any age. The edema may be unilateral or bilateral. The testicles and penis also may be edematous, though this is not always the case. Causes include conditions that produce edema of the lower body, such as renal disease and heart failure. Localized conditions also can cause scrotal edema; for example, epididymitis, testicular cancer, testicular torsion, and hydrocele.

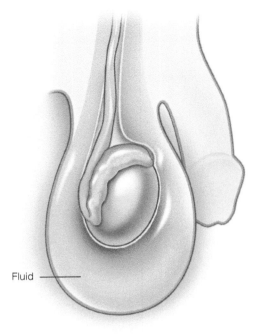

Fluid

Figure 23.36 Scrotal edema.

TABLE 23.6 **Abnormalities of the Perianal Area**

Pilonidal Cyst

Seen as dimpling in the sacrococcygeal area at the midline. An opening is visible and may reveal a tuft of hair. Usually asymptomatic, these cysts may become acutely abscessed or drain chronically.

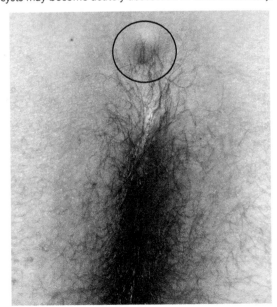

Figure 23.37 Pilonidal cyst.
Source: M. English/Custom Medical Stock Photo.

Anal Fissure

Tears or splits in the anal mucosa that are usually seen in the posterior anal area and most frequently associated with the passage of hard stools or prolonged diarrhea. They are most common in young infants.

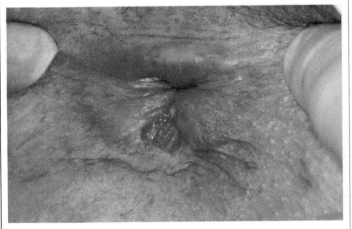

Figure 23.38 Anal fissure.
Source: BSIP/Getty Images.

TABLE 23.6   **Abnormalities of the Perianal Area** (continued)

Hemorrhoids (Internal)

Varicosities of the hemorrhoidal veins of the anus or lower rectum.

Internally, they occur in the venous plexus superior to the mucocutaneous junction of the anus and are rarely painful. Identified by bright red bleeding that is unmixed with stool.

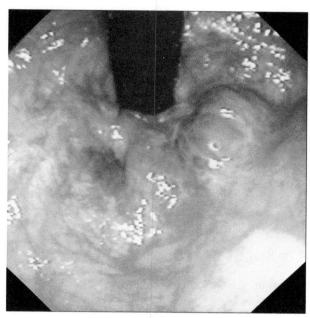

Figure 23.39 Hemorrhoids, internal.
Source: M. D. David M. Martin/Science Source.

Hemorrhoids (External)

Externally, they occur in the inferior venous plexus inferior to the mucocutaneous junction. Rarely bleed; cause anal irritation and create difficulty with cleansing the area.

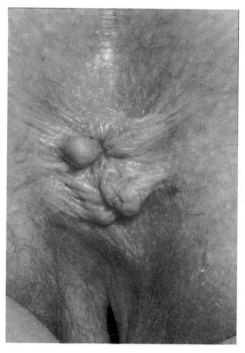

Figure 23.40 Hemorrhoids, external.
Source: M. English/Custom Medical Stock Photo.

Perianal Perirectal Abscess

Painful and tender abscesses with perianal erythema; generally caused by infection of an anal gland. Can lead to fistulas (openings between the anal canal and outside skin).

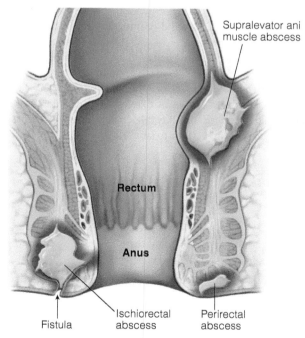

Figure 23.41 Perianal perirectal abscess.

Prolapse of the Rectum

Occurs when the rectal mucosa, with or without the muscle, protrudes through the anus. In mucosal prolapse, a round or oval pink protrusion is seen outside the anus. When the muscular wall is involved, a large red protrusion is visible.

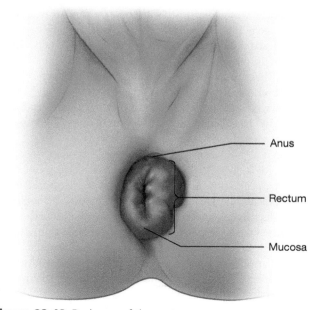

Figure 23.42 Prolapse of the rectum.

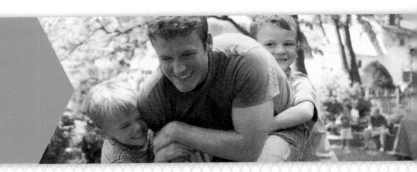

Application Through Critical Thinking

▶ Case Study

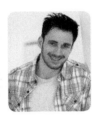

James Lewis is a 24-year-old male who is seen in the clinic for "pain in the groin." During the interview the patient states, "I have a soreness in my groin area on both sides." Mr. Lewis denies any trauma to the area, states he has not done any heavy lifting, nor has he been involved in athletic activities or "working out." He reports that he is in good health. He does not take any medications except vitamins and, occasionally, some nonaspirin product for a headache. He denies nausea, vomiting, diarrhea, or fever. He has no pain in his legs or back. He tells the nurse his appetite is okay but he is tired. He thinks his fatigue is because he's been "a little worried about this problem and really having a hard time deciding to come in for help."

When asked about the onset of the problem, Mr. Lewis explains that he "started feeling some achiness about a week ago." When asked if he has ever experienced these feelings before, he replies, "No." He is then asked to describe or discuss any other symptoms. He looks away, shifts in his chair, and then says, "Well, I have had some burning when I pass urine and it's kind of cloudy."

When asked if he has ever had a problem like this before, he replies, "Yes, about 2 months ago." With further questioning, the nurse learns that Mr. Lewis was diagnosed with gonorrhea and treated with an injection and pills he was supposed to take for a week. He says he was not supposed to have sex until he finished the pills. When asked if he followed the prescribed treatment, he reluctantly responds that he finished all but a couple of pills and he did have sex with one of his girlfriends about 4 or 5 days after he got the injection.

Mr. Lewis tells the nurse he did not inform his girlfriends of his problem and he generally avoids condoms because "I've known these girls for a long time."

The physical assessment yields the following information: B/P 128/86, P 96, RR 20, T 98.6. His color is pale, and the skin is moist and warm. External genitalia are intact, without lesions or erythema. There is lymphadenopathy in bilateral groin areas. Compression of the glans yields milky discharge. A smear of urethral discharge is obtained.

The nurse knows that Mr. Lewis's original gonococcal infection was treated with an injection, most likely ceftriaxone. The nurse also knows that chlamydia is present in almost half of the patients with gonorrhea and is treated with a 7-day regimen of oral antibiotics. Between 40% and 60% of patients with gonorrhea have lymphadenopathy.

Based on the data, the nurse suspects that Mr. Lewis has a reinfection with gonorrhea and may have a concomitant chlamydial infection.

The nurse recommends single-injection treatment for gonorrhea and a new oral regimen for chlamydia. A urine specimen will be obtained and submitted with the urethral discharge smear. The patient will be scheduled for a follow-up phone conference about the laboratory results in 48 hours and a return visit in 7 days. The nurse conducts an information, education, and advice session prior to discharge from the clinic.

▶ Complete Documentation

The following is sample documentation for James Lewis.

SUBJECTIVE DATA: Seeking care for "pain in groin." Pain in groin bilateral. Denies trauma, heavy lifting, athletic activity, or "working out." Reports he is in "good health." Takes no medications except vitamins and nonaspirin product for a headache. Denies nausea, vomiting, diarrhea, or fever. No pain in back or legs. Reports "okay" appetite. Reports fatigue. "Became a little worried about this problem and decided to come in for help." Achiness 1 week ago. Burning on urination, cloudy urine. Gonorrhea diagnosis 2 months ago, treated with injection and oral meds. Did not complete prescription and had intercourse "4 or 5 days after injection." Did not inform partners of diagnosis, generally avoids condoms.

OBJECTIVE DATA: VS: B/P 128/86, P 96, RR 20, T 98.6°F. Color pale, skin moist and warm. External genitalia intact, no lesions or erythema. Lymphadenopathy bilateral groin. Milky discharge on compression of glans. Culture to lab.

▶ Critical Thinking Questions

1. Describe the critical thinking process as applied by the nurse to direct the care of this patient.

2. What additional data should the nurse seek when conducting the health assessment for this patient?

3. What data informed the nurse of a need to provide education for the patient?

4. What data will the nurse seek upon the return visit with Mr. Lewis?

5. What *Healthy People 2020* objectives are related to this scenario?

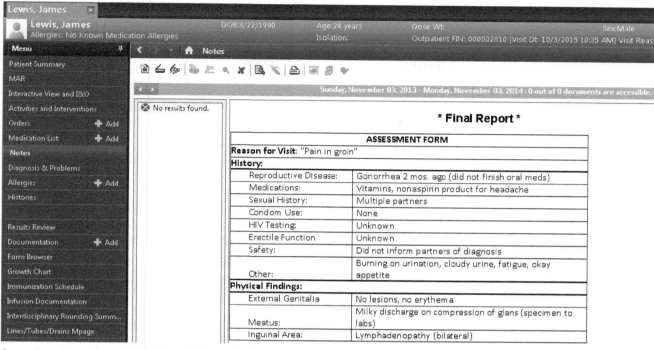

Source: From Cerner Electronic Health Record. Copyright © by Cerner Corporation. Used by permission of Cerner Corporation.

◗ Prepare Teaching Plan

LEARNING NEED: The data from the case study reveal that James Lewis has an ongoing problem with STDs, particularly gonorrhea. The data reveal that Mr. Lewis has not followed recommendations for a previous infection. Education and counseling will be provided for this patient.

The case study provides data that are representative of concerns about STDs, especially gonorrhea, of many individuals. Therefore, the following teaching plan is based on the need to provide information to members of any community about gonorrhea.

GOAL: The participants in this learning program will have the knowledge to prevent contraction and transmission of gonorrhea.

OBJECTIVES: At the completion of this learning session the participants will be able to:

1. Describe gonorrhea.
2. Identify symptoms of gonorrhea.
3. Discuss treatment strategies.
4. Describe methods to prevent contraction and transmission of gonorrhea.

APPLICATION OF OBJECTIVE 4: Describe methods to prevent contraction and transmission of gonorrhea		
Content	**Teaching Strategy**	**Evaluation**
• Avoid sexual partners whose health status is unclear. • Use condoms correctly and consistently during sexual intercourse. • When infected, notify all sexual contacts so they can be treated. Refrain from sexual contact for 1 week after treatment is completed. Take all prescribed medications exactly as ordered until they are gone.	• Lecture • Discussion • Audiovisual materials • Printed materials Lecture is appropriate when disseminating information to large groups. Discussion allows participants to bring up concerns and to raise questions. Audiovisual materials such as illustrations of the genitals and reproductive structures reinforce verbal presentation. Printed material allows review, reinforcement, and reading at the learner's pace.	• Written examination. May use short answer, fill-in-the-blank, multiple-choice items, or a combination of items. If these are short and easy to evaluate, the learner receives immediate feedback.

▶ References

Agarwal, A., Aitken, R. J., & Alvarez, J. G. (Eds.). (2012). *Studies on men's health and fertility*. New York, NY: Humana Press.

American Cancer Society (ACS). (2014a). *Prostate cancer: What are the risk factors for prostate cancer?* Retrieved from http://www.cancer.org/cancer/prostatecancer/detailedguide/prostate-cancer-risk-factors

American Cancer Society (ACS). (2014b). *Prostate cancer: Can prostate cancer be found early?* Retrieved from http://www.cancer.org/cancer/prostatecancer/detailedguide/prostate-cancer-detection

American Cancer Society (ACS). (2014c). *Penile cancer: What are the key statistics about penile cancer?* Retrieved from http://www.cancer.org/cancer/penilecancer/detailedguide/penile-cancer-key-statistics

American Cancer Society (ACS). (2014d). *Prostate cancer early detection: American Cancer Society recommendations for prostate cancer early detection.* Retrieved from http://www.cancer.org/cancer/prostatecancer/moreinformation/prostatecancerearlydetection/prostate-cancer-early-detection-acs-recommendations

Basson, R., Rees, P., Wang, R., Montejo, A. L., & Incrocci, L. (2010). Sexual function in chronic illness. *The Journal of Sexual Medicine, 7*, 374–388.

Berkowitz, C. D. (2011). Healing of genital injuries. *Journal of Child Sexual Abuse, 20*(5), 537–547.

Berman, A., & Snyder, S. J. (2012). *Kozier and Erb's fundamentals of nursing: Concepts, process, and practice* (9th ed.). Upper Saddle River, NJ: Prentice Hall.

Bikley, L. S. (2008). *Bates' guide to physical examination and history taking* (10th ed.). Philadelphia, PA: Lippincott.

Byun, J. S., Lyu, S. W., Seok, H. H., Kim, W. J., Shim, S. H., & Bak, C. W. (2013). Sexual dysfunctions induced by stress of timed intercourse and medical treatment. *British Journal of Urology International, 111*(4b), E227–E234.

Cancer reference information. (2008). Retrieved from http://www.cancer.org/docroot/home/index.asp

Castro, J. G., Jones, D. L., Lopez, M., Barradas, I., & Weiss, S. M. (2010). Making the case for circumcision as a public health strategy: Opening the dialogue. *AIDS Patient Care and STDs, 24*(6), 367–372.

Centers for Disease Control and Prevention (CDC). (2013a). *Herpes: Genital herpes – CDC fact sheet.* Retrieved from http://www.cdc.gov/std/herpes/stdfact-herpes-detailed.htm

Centers for Disease Control and Prevention (CDC). (2013b). *HPV vaccines.* Retrieved from http://www.cdc.gov/hpv/vaccine.html

Centers for Disease Control and Prevention (CDC). (2013c). *Male latex condoms and sexually transmitted diseases: Condoms and STDs: Fact sheet for public health personnel.* Retrieved from http://www.cdc.gov/condomeffectiveness/latex.htm

Cioe, P. A., Anderson, B. J., & Stein, M. D. (2013). Change in symptoms of erectile dysfunction in depressed men initiating buprenorphine therapy. *Journal of Substance Abuse Treatment, 45*(5), 451–456.

Dalke, K. A., Fein, L., Jenkins, L. C., Caso, J. R., & Salgado, C. J. (2013). Complications of Genital Piercings. *Anaplastology, 2*(122). doi: 10.4172/2161-1173.1000122

Dennie, J., & Grover, S. R. (2013). Distressing perineal and vaginal pain in prepubescent girls: An aetiology. *Journal of Paediatrics and Child Health, 49*(2), 138–140.

Gray, H. (2010). *Gray's anatomy.* New York: Barnes & Noble Books.

Johns Hopkins Medicine. (n.d.). *Male factor infertility: What is infertility?* Retrieved from http://www.hopkinsmedicine.org/healthlibrary/conditions/mens_health/male_factor_infertility_85,P01484/

Karavolos, S., Stewart, J., Evbuomwan, I., McEleny, K., & Aird, I. (2013). Assessment of the infertile male. *The Obstetrician & Gynaecologist, 15*(1), 1–9.

Klein, J. W. (2014). Common Anal Problems. *Medical Clinics of North America, 98*(3), 609–623.

Leander, L. (2010). Police interviews with child sexual abuse victims: Patterns of reporting, avoidance and denial. *Child Abuse & Neglect, 34*(3), 192–205.

Marieb, E. (2009). *Essentials of human anatomy and physiology* (9th ed.). Redwood City, CA: Benjamin/Cummings.

Mayo Clinic. (2011). *Peyronie's disease: Definition.* Retrieved from http://www.mayoclinic.org/diseases-conditions/peyronies-disease/basics/definition/con-20028765

Mayo Clinic. (2014a). *Sexually transmitted diseases (STDs): Risk factors.* Retrieved from http://www.mayoclinic.org/diseases-conditions/sexually-transmitted-diseases-stds/basics/risk-factors/con-20034128

Mayo Clinic. (2014b). *Getting pregnant: How to get pregnant.* Retrieved from http://www.mayoclinic.org/healthy-living/getting-pregnant/in-depth/how-to-get-pregnant/art-20047611

Mayo Clinic. (2014c). *Premature ejaculation: Treatments and drugs.* Retrieved from http://www.mayoclinic.org/diseases-conditions/premature-ejaculation/basics/treatment/con-20031160

Mayo Foundation for Medical Education and Research. (2014). *Rochester test catalog: 2014 online test catalog.* Available at http://www.mayomedicallaboratories.com/test-catalog

Modgil, V., Rai, S., & Anderson, P. C. (2014). Male circumcision: Summary of current clinical practice. *Trends in Urology & Men's Health, 5*(3), 21–24.

Montesi, J. L., Fauber, R. L., Gordon, E. A., & Heimberg, R. G. (2011). The specific importance of communicating about sex to couples' sexual and overall relationship satisfaction. *Journal of Social and Personal Relationships, 28*(5), 591–609.

Murray, R. B., & Zentner, J. P. (2009). *Health promotion strategies through the life span* (8th ed.). Upper Saddle River, NJ: Prentice Hall.

National Cancer Institute (NCI). (2014). *Testicular cancer screening (PDQ®): Description of the evidence.* Retrieved from http://www.cancer.gov/cancertopics/pdq/screening/testicular/HealthProfessional/page2

Olsen, J., & Ramlau-Hansen, C. H. (2014). Epidemiologic methods for investigating male fecundity. *Asian Journal of Andrology, 16*(1), 17–22.

Shridharani, A., Lockwood, G., & Sandlow, J. (2012). Varicocelectomy in the treatment of testicular pain: A review. *Current Opinion in Urology, 22*(6), 499–506.

Smith, A., Lyons, A., Ferris, J., Richters, J., Pitts, M., Shelley, J., & Simpson, J. M. (2011). Sexual and relationship satisfaction among heterosexual men and women: The importance of desired frequency of sex. *Journal of Sex & Marital Therapy, 37*(2), 104–115.

Tortora, G. J., & Derrickson, B. H. (2009). *Principles of anatomy and physiology* (12th ed.). New York: John Wiley & Sons.

University of Rochester Medical Center (URMC). (n.d.). *Scrotal swelling in children.* Retrieved from http://www.urmc.rochester.edu/encyclopedia/content.aspx?ContentTypeID=160&ContentID=59

U.S. Department of Health and Human Services (USDHHS). (2014). *Healthy people 2020.* Retrieved from http://www.healthypeople.gov/2020/default.aspx

Wilson, B.A., Shannon, M.T., & Shields, K.M. (2013). *Pearson nurse's drug guide.* Upper Saddle River, NJ: Pearson.

World Health Organization (WHO). (n.d.). *Sexual and reproductive health: Infertility definitions and terminology.* Retrieved from http://www.who.int/reproductivehealth/topics/infertility/definitions/en/

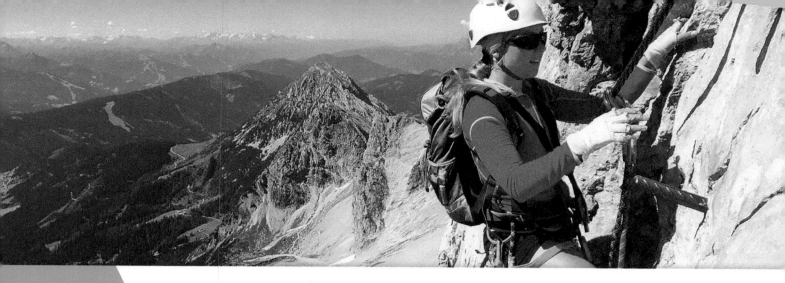

Learning Outcomes

Upon completion of this chapter, you will be able to:

1. Describe the anatomy and physiology of the female reproductive system.

2. Explain patient preparation for the assessment of the female reproductive system.

3. Develop questions to be used when conducting the focused interview.

4. Describe techniques required for assessment of the female reproductive system.

5. Differentiate normal from abnormal findings in the physical assessment of the female reproductive system.

6. Describe developmental, cultural, psychosocial, and environmental variations in assessment and findings of the female reproductive system.

7. Discuss the objectives related to women's health as stated in *Healthy People 2020.*

8. Apply critical thinking to the physical assessment of the female reproductive system.

Key Terms

The female reproductive system provides for both human reproduction and sexual gratification. Many factors influence the female patient's reproductive health on both physiologic and psychologic levels. Assessment of the patient's psychosocial health, self-care habits, family, culture, and environment is an important part of the focused interview. The nurse must keep these findings in mind when conducting the physical assessment. The nurse also must have a thorough understanding of the constituents of a healthy reproductive system and be able to consider the relationship of other body systems to the reproductive system.

Throughout assessment of the female reproductive system, the nurse considers not only the function of the reproductive system but also the patient's sexual fulfillment on both a physical and psychologic basis. Reproductive health is reflected in *Healthy People 2020*. Objectives concerning unintended pregnancy, maternal deaths, and sexually transmitted diseases (STDs) are included in Table 24.1 on page 647.

To be efficient in gathering data, nurses need to understand their own feelings and comfort about various aspects of sexuality. They must put aside personal beliefs and values about sexual practices and focus in a nonjudgmental manner on gathering data to determine the health status of the patient.

It is essential to create an atmosphere that facilitates open communication and comfort for the patient. Patients commonly experience anxiety, fear, and embarrassment when requested for information about a topic that, in most patients' minds, is very personal. These emotions may be expressed either verbally or nonverbally. The nurse should approach the patient in as nonthreatening a manner as possible and assure the patient that the information provided and the results of the physical assessment will remain confidential.

Anatomy and Physiology Review

The female reproductive system is unique in that it experiences cyclic changes in direct response to hormonal levels of estrogen and progesterone during the childbearing years. The uterus changes throughout the ovarian cycle during which the ova (eggs) are prepared for fertilization with sperm. During the menstrual cycle, the uterine lining is prepared for the development of a fetus. The onset of menopause represents the end of the childbearing years.

Unlike the male reproductive system, the female reproductive tract is completely separate from the urinary tract. However, structures of the two tracts lie within close proximity.

The functions of the female reproductive system are the following:

- Manufacturing and protecting ova for fertilization.
- Transporting the fertilized ovum for implantation and embryonic/fetal development.
- Regulating hormonal production and secretion of several sex hormones.
- Providing sexual stimulation and pleasure.

External Genitalia

Female external genitalia include the mons pubis, labia, glands, clitoris, and perianal area. These are described in the following sections.

Mons Pubis

The mons pubis is the mound of adipose tissue overlying the symphysis pubis (see Figure 24.1 ■). In the mature female, it is thickly covered with hair and provides protection to the underlying reproductive structures.

Labia Majora and Labia Minora

The **labia** are a dual set of liplike structures lying on either side of the vagina (see Figure 24.1). The exterior labia majora are two thick, elongated pads of tissue that become fuller toward the center. An extension of the external skin surface, the labia majora are covered with coarse hair extending from the mons pubis. The enclosed

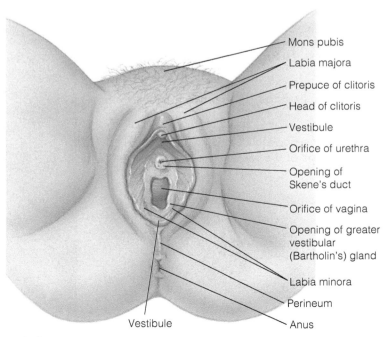

Mons pubis
Labia majora
Prepuce of clitoris
Head of clitoris
Vestibule
Orifice of urethra
Opening of Skene's duct
Orifice of vagina
Opening of greater vestibular (Bartholin's) gland
Labia minora
Perineum
Anus

Vestibule

Figure 24.1 External female genitalia.

labia minora are two thin, elongated pads of tissue that overlie the vaginal and urethral openings as well as several glandular openings. Anteriorly, the labia minora join to form the prepuce, which covers the clitoris. Posteriorly, the labia join to form the *fourchette* (small fold of membrane). The labia minora border an almond-shaped area of tissue known as the *vestibule*. It extends from the clitoris to the fourchette. The urethral meatus, vaginal opening (**introitus**), Skene's glands, and Bartholin's glands lie within the vestibule. The major function of the labia is providing protection from infection and physical injury to the urethra and vagina and, ultimately, other urinary and reproductive structures.

Skene's and Bartholin's Glands

The Skene's glands, also called **paraurethral glands**, are located just posterior to the urethra (see Figure 24.1). They open into the urethra and secrete a fluid that lubricates the vaginal vestibule during sexual intercourse. The **Bartholin's glands**, or greater vestibular glands, are located posteriorly at the base of the vestibule and produce mucus, which is released into the vestibule (see Figure 24.1). This mucus actively promotes sperm motility and viability.

Clitoris

Located at the anterior of the vestibule is the **clitoris**, a small, elongated mound of erectile tissue (see Figure 24.1). As the labia minora merge together anteriorly, a small hoodlike covering is formed that lies over the top of the clitoris. The clitoris is homologous with the penis. It is permeated with numerous nerve fibers responsive to touch. When stimulated, the clitoris becomes erect as its underlying corpus cavernosa become vasocongested. The major function of the clitoris is serving as the primary organ of sexual stimulation.

Perianal Area

The perianal area is bordered anteriorly by the top of the labial folds, laterally by the ischial tuberosities, and posteriorly by the anus (see Figure 24.1). The anus is the terminal end of the gastrointestinal system. The anal canal opens onto the perineum at the midpoint of the gluteal folds. The external muscles of the anal canal are skeletal muscles, which form the part of the anal sphincter that voluntarily controls stool evacuation. The anal mucosa is smooth, moist, hairless, and darkly pigmented.

Internal Reproductive Organs

The internal female reproductive organs are the vagina, uterus, cervix, fallopian tubes, and ovaries. These organs are described in the following paragraphs.

Vagina

The **vagina** is a long, tubular, muscular canal (approximately 9 to 15 cm [3.5 to 5.9 in.] in length) that extends from the vestibule to the cervix at the inferior end of the uterus (see Figure 24.2A ■). The muscularity of the vaginal wall and its thick, transverse rugae (ridges) allow it to dilate widely to accommodate the erect penis and, during childbirth, the head of the fetus. At the point of juncture with the cervix, a continuous circular cleft called the *fornix* is formed. The major functions of the vagina are serving as the female organ of copulation, the birth canal, and the channel for the exit of menstrual flow.

Uterus

The **uterus** is a pear-shaped, hollow, muscular organ that is located centrally in the pelvis between the neck of the bladder and the rectal wall (see Figure 24.2A). The body of the uterus is about 4 cm (1.56 in.) wide and 6 to 8 cm (2.34 to 3.12 in.) in length. Its walls are 2 to 2.5 cm (0.78 to 0.94 in.) thick and are composed of serosal, muscular, and mucosal layers. Anatomically, the uterus is divided into three segments. These segments are the fundus, the corpus, and the cervix. The **cervix** projects into the vagina about 2.5 cm and is about 2.5 cm (0.98 in.) round. A small central canal connects the vagina to the inside of the uterus. The *external* **cervical os** is the inferior opening (the vaginal end of the canal), and the *internal cervical os* opens directly into the uterine chamber. The uterus has two adnexal, or accessory structures, the fallopian (uterine) tubes and the ovaries.

The uterus is easily moved within the pelvic cavity, but its basic position is secured with several ligaments that attach it to the pelvic floor. The ligaments also prevent the uterus from dropping into the vaginal canal. The major functions of the uterus are serving as the site of implantation of the fertilized ovum and as a protective sac for the developing embryo and fetus.

Uterine Tubes

The **uterine tubes** (or fallopian tubes) are two ducts on either side of the fundus of the uterus (see Figure 24.2B ■). They are about 7 to 10 cm (2.75 to 3.9 in.) in length and extend from the uterus almost to the ovaries. An ovum released by an ovary travels to the uterus within the uterine tubes. Normally fertilization takes place within the uterine tubes. The major functions of the fallopian tubes include serving as the site of fertilization and providing a passageway for unfertilized and fertilized ova to travel to the uterus.

Ovaries

Lying close to the distal end of either side of the uterine tubes are the **ovaries** (see Figure 24.2B). These almond-shaped glandular structures produce ova as well as estrogen and progesterone. They are about 3 cm (1.17 in.) long and 2 cm (0.78 in.) wide. The ovarian ligaments and suspensory ligaments hold the ovaries in place. The ovaries become fully developed after puberty and atrophy after menopause. The major functions of the ovaries are producing ova for fertilization by sperm and producing estrogen and progesterone.

Special Considerations

Throughout the assessment process, the nurse gathers subjective and objective data reflecting the patient's state of health. Using critical thinking and the nursing process, the nurse identifies many factors to be considered when collecting the data. The subjective and objective data gathered throughout the assessment process inform the nurse about the patient's state of health. A variety of factors including age, developmental level, race, ethnicity, work history, living conditions, socioeconomics, and emotional well-being influence health and must be considered during assessment. The impact of these factors is discussed in the following sections.

Health Promotion Considerations

Reproductive system diseases and disorders significantly impact female health and wellness. Objectives of *Healthy People 2020*

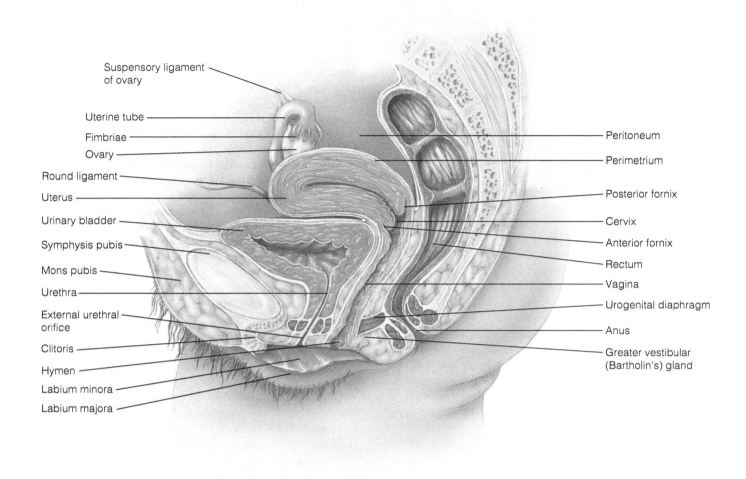

Figure 24.2A Internal organs of the female reproductive system within the pelvis.

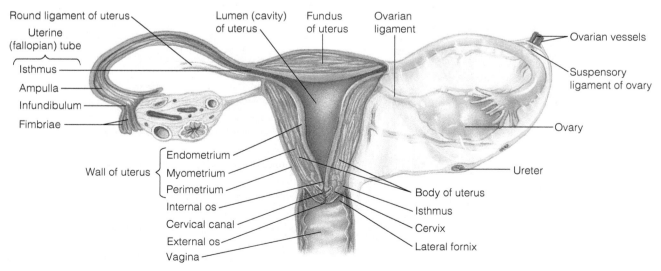

Figure 24.2B Cross section of the anterior view of the female pelvis.

related to the reproductive system include improving reproductive health among individuals in the United States by reducing the incidence and prevalence of sexually transmitted diseases (STDs). For both women and men, goals of this national initiative target the effective implementation of screening and preventative measures related to infectious diseases such as chlamydia, syphilis, and gonorrhea (USDHHS, 2014). A primary focus is decreasing the transmission rate of human immunodeficiency virus (HIV) infection, as well as preventing the development of acquired immunodeficiency syndrome (AIDS) and HIV-related deaths. For females, pelvic inflammatory disease and invasive uterine cervical cancer are additional topics of concern (USDHHS, 2014). See Table 24.1 for examples of *Healthy People 2020* objectives that are designed to promote reproductive health and wellness among individuals across the life span.

Lifespan Considerations

Anatomy and physiology change with growth and development. The nurse must be aware of expected changes as data are gathered and findings are interpreted. The following sections describe specific variations in the female reproductive system across the age span.

Infants and Children

The female infant's labia majora will be enlarged at birth in response to maternal hormones. The labia majora should cover the labia minora. The urinary meatus and vaginal orifice should be visible. No inflammation should be present. Bloody and mucoid discharge (false menses) is commonly seen in newborns due to exposure to maternal hormones in utero.

The female child reaches puberty a few years before the male. Changes begin to occur at any time from 8 to 13 years of age; most commonly, breast changes begin at age 9 and menstruation at age 12. Release of estrogen initiates the changes, which are first demonstrated in the development of breast buds and growth of pubic hair, followed several years later by menstruation. Figure 24.3 ■ describes Tanner's stages of maturation in girls.

The female child may experience a precocious puberty. These children develop the adult female sex characteristics of dense pubic and axillary hair, breasts, and menstrual bleeding before 8 years of age. Early maturation may be caused by hypothalamic tumor. Further, the early development of sexual characteristics allows for pregnancy before the child is intellectually or emotionally prepared for the experience. Early maturation can also lead to anemia related to menstrual bleeding and to emotional difficulties.

TABLE 24.1	Examples of *Healthy People 2020* Objectives Related to Female Reproductive Health
OBJECTIVE NUMBER	**DESCRIPTION**
STD-1	Reduce the proportion of adolescents and young adults with *Chlamydia trachomatis* infections
STD-3	Increase the proportion of sexually active females aged 24 years and under enrolled in Medicaid plans who are screened for genital Chlamydia infections during the measurement year
STD-4	Increase the proportion of sexually active females aged 24 years and under enrolled in commercial health insurance plans who are screened for genital Chlamydia infections during the measurement year
STD-5	Reduce the proportion of females aged 15 to 44 years who have ever required treatment for pelvic inflammatory disease (PID)
STD-6	Reduce gonorrhea rates
STD-7	Reduce sustained domestic transmission of primary and secondary syphilis
STD-8	Reduce congenital syphilis
STD-9	Reduce the proportion of females with human papillomavirus (HPV) infection
STD-10	Reduce the proportion of young adults with genital herpes infection due to herpes simplex type 2
HIV-2	Reduce the number of new HIV infections among adolescents and adults
HIV-3	Reduce the rate of HIV transmission among adolescents and adults
HIV-8	Reduce perinatally acquired HIV and AIDS cases
HIV-9	Reduce the proportion of persons with a diagnosis of Stage 3 HIV (AIDS) within 3 months of diagnosis of HIV infection
HIV-13	Increase the proportion of persons living with HIV who know their serostatus
HIV-14	Increase the proportion of adolescents and adults who have been tested for HIV in the past 12 months
C-10	Reduce invasive uterine cervical cancer

Source: U.S. Department of Health and Human Services (USDHHS). (2014). *Healthy people 2020.* Retrieved from http://www.healthypeople.gov/2020/default.aspx.

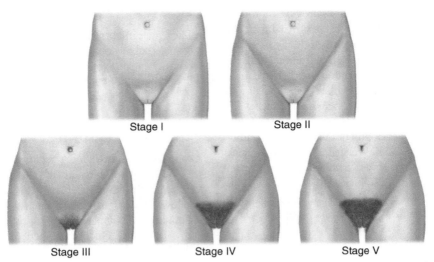

Figure 24.3 The Tanner stages of female pubic hair development with sexual maturation. Stage I: Preadolescent—no growth of pubic hair. Stage II: Soft downy straight hair along the labia majora is an indication that sexual maturation is beginning. Stage III: Sparse, dark, visibly pigmented curly pubic hair on labia. Stage IV: Hair coarse and curly, abundant but less than adults. Stage V: Lateral spreading in triangle shape to medial surface of thighs.

It is essential to assess for sexual molestation with female children. Some signs of sexual molestation are trauma; depression; eating disorders; bruising; swelling; and inflammation in the vaginal, perineal, and anal areas. Foreign bodies commonly cause malodorous, blood-tinged vaginal discharge. Vaginal foreign bodies, with the exception of those caused by retained toilet paper, are suspicious for sexual abuse. The child may appear withdrawn and, in many cases, may deny the experience. Adolescents often express interest in the changes related to puberty. The desire to explore sexual relationships and sexual contact, from kissing and fondling to intercourse, may be intense. Thus, adolescents need counseling on relationship issues, birth control, protection against STDs, and delaying sexual activity. A female adolescent may be concerned about or confused by an attraction to individuals of the same sex. Lesbian experimentation is developmentally normal in adolescents. It does not mean they are definitively lesbian or bisexual. The nurse should provide open communication so that the adolescent may ask questions and express her feelings and concerns.

The Pregnant Female

Pregnancy brings a multitude of changes to the female reproductive organs. The uterus, cervix, ovaries, and vagina undergo significant structural changes related to the pregnancy and the influence of hormones.

The uterus becomes hypertrophied and weighs about 1 kg (2.2 lb) by the end of pregnancy. Its capacity increases to about 5 L (5.2 qt). The growth of the uterus during pregnancy causes it to push up into the abdominal cavity and displace the liver and intestines from their normal positions. Contractions of the uterus occur. Throughout the pregnancy, the female may have irregular Braxton Hicks contractions, which are usually not painful. However, by the end of the pregnancy, these contractions may become more intense and cause pain.

During pregnancy, the vascularity of the cervix increases and contributes to the softening of the cervix. This softening is called **Goodell's sign**. The vascular congestion creates a blue-purple blemish or change in cervical coloration. This change is considered normal and is referred to as **Chadwick's sign**. Estrogen causes the glandular cervical tissue to produce thick mucus, which builds up and forms a mucous plug at the endocervical canal. The mucous plug prevents the introduction of any foreign matter into the uterus. At the initiation of labor, this plug is expelled. This expulsion is called the "bloody show."

The vagina undergoes changes similar to those of the uterus during pregnancy. Hypertrophy of the vaginal epithelium occurs. The vaginal wall softens and relaxes to accommodate the movement of the infant during birth. The vagina also displays Chadwick's sign. A thorough discussion of the pregnant female is found in chapter 27. ∞

The Older Adult

Reproductive ability in the female usually peaks in her late 20s. Over time, estrogen levels begin to decline. Between the ages of 46 and 55, menstrual periods become shorter and less frequent until they stop entirely. Menopause is said to have occurred when the female has not experienced a menstrual period in over a year. Other symptoms of menopause include mood changes and unpredictable episodes of sweating or hot flashes.

As the female progresses into older age, her sexual organs atrophy. Vaginal secretions are not as plentiful, and she may experience pain during intercourse. Intercourse may produce vaginal infections. The clitoris becomes smaller.

Even though older adults can achieve sexual gratification and participate in a satisfying sexual relationship, a decrease in sexual drive may contribute to the patient's withdrawing from sexual experiences and relationships. Chronic or acute disease, medications, loss of a spouse or significant other, loss of privacy, depression, fatigue, stress, and use of alcohol and illicit drugs are factors known to influence sexual drive.

Psychosocial Considerations

Fatigue, depression, and stress can decrease sexual desire in a female patient of any age. Grief over the loss of a relationship, whether because of separation, divorce, or death, can have long-term effects on a patient's willingness to seek new relationships. Feelings of betrayal—for example, when a partner becomes intimate with another person—can have the same effect.

Past or recent trauma, as from childhood abuse, physical assault, and sexual assault, whether or not penetration occurred, may have a significant impact on a female patient's ability to enjoy a sexual relationship. This may be true even if the trauma is unremembered.

Some females may fear sexual intimacy because of an altered body image related to their weight, body type, breast size, or other factors. Reproductive surgeries can affect a female patient's self-image and sexual expression. For example, patients who have had a hysterectomy may feel free from the worry of unwanted pregnancy and experience an increase in sexual desire, or they may feel less feminine than before the surgery and withdraw from sexual relationships.

Cultural and Environmental Considerations

Some cultures and religions have specific beliefs or encourage specific behaviors related to sexual practices. For example, many religions forbid premarital sex. Likewise, among certain cultures, female genital mutilation (FGM) is a common practice. Believed to affect as many as 140 million women worldwide, FGM involves partial or total excision of the external female genitalia for non-medical reasons (Simpson, Robinson, Creighton, & Hodes, 2012). FGM constitutes a breach of human rights law. In many parts of the world—including Africa, where FGM is commonly performed—FGM is illegal. FGM also is prevalent in Asia and the Middle East (Simpson et al., 2012). When assessing patients, the nurse should be aware of the individual's potential cultural practices, while at the same time avoiding making assumptions about the patient's beliefs or experiences.

In any culture, environmental influences also can significantly impact sexual health. Sexual dysfunction can result from sexual, physical, or verbal abuse among family members. Negative family reactions to an individual's sexual orientation and lifestyle choices may impact the individual's ability to find a sexual partner and maintain a satisfying sexual relationship. Because of family pressures, females may choose partners who do not meet their own needs or desires. This can have a negative emotional and physical impact, especially among female adolescents.

Females who work in the microelectronics industry (i.e., high-speed electronics, such as circuit boards) may be exposed to arsenic, glycol ethers, lead, and radiation. These substances have been linked to birth defects and spontaneous abortions. Lead is also still present in some homes. Exposure to vinyl chloride (used in construction and building materials) may increase the risk for stillbirths and premature births. Exposure to high concentrations of halogenated hydrocarbons, such as polychlorinated biphenyls (PCBs), found in plastics manufacturing and in the electrical industries, is associated with low birth weight, spontaneous abortion, hyperpigmentation of infants, and microcephaly (abnormally small head size). Oncology nurses exposed to antineoplastic drugs may have spontaneous abortions, fetal anomalies, changes in the regularity of their menstrual cycle, or even cessation of their menstrual cycle.

Maintaining the cleanliness of the female genitalia requires daily washing and changing of underclothes. Douching is not only unnecessary, but may even be harmful. Douching has been shown to promote irritation, rashes, and infection in some females. The likelihood of rashes or infections can be reduced by keeping the genitals dry by changing sweaty underclothes after physical exercise, changing into dry clothes immediately after bathing or swimming, and changing an infant's diaper immediately after it is wet.

Although research has shown that infections can be transmitted sexually even when the partners are using a latex condom, its use significantly lowers the incidence of transmission. A history of human papillomavirus (HPV) and more than four sexual partners in a lifetime increases a female patient's risk for cervical cancer. According to the Centers for Disease Control and Prevention (CDC, 2012), the vaccine Gardasil can protect against most cervical cancers related to HPV. CDC's Advisory Committee on Immunization Practices (ACIP) recommends routine 3-dose vaccination of girls aged 11 and 12 years. The vaccine is also recommended for girls and women ages 13 through 26 years who have not yet been vaccinated or who have not received all 3 doses. A history of STDs in children may indicate sexual abuse. The risk for cervical cancer is increased in those females who participate in early (before age 18) and frequent sexual activity and have a history of many sexual partners. Obesity is a risk factor for uterine cancer.

Gathering the Data

Health assessment of the female reproductive system includes gathering subjective and objective data. Collection of subjective data occurs during the patient interview, before the physical assessment. The nurse uses a variety of communication techniques to elicit general and specific information about the health of the reproductive system. Health records and the results of laboratory and clinical examinations are important secondary sources to be reviewed and included in the data-gathering process (see Table 24.2). Physical assessment of the female reproductive system includes the techniques of inspection and palpation as well as the use of equipment and techniques specific to the assessment of the female reproductive system.

TABLE 24.2   **Potential Secondary Sources for Patient Data Related to the Female Reproductive System**

LABORATORY TESTS	NORMAL VALUES
Follicle Stimulating Hormone (FSH)	Before puberty: 0–4 mIU/mL
	During puberty: 0.3–10 mIU/mL
	Women who are menstruating: 4.7–21.5 mIU/mL
	Postmenopausal: 25.8–134.8 mIU/mL
	Pregnant women: too low to measure
Luteinizing Hormone (LH)	5 to 25 International units/L
Progesterone	Female (preovulation): less than 1 ng/mL
	Female (midcycle): 5 to 20 ng/mL
	Postmenopausal: less than 1 ng/mL
Estradiol	Female (premenopausal): 30–300 pg/mL
	Female (postmenopausal): <15 pg/mL
Pap Smear	Normal
Serum Studies for STDs	
Diagnostic Tests Endometrial Biopsy Hysterosalpingogram Hysteroscopy Laparoscopy Pelvic/Transvaginal Ultrasonography	

Focused Interview

The focused interview of the female concerns data related to the structures and functions of the reproductive system. Subjective data related to that system are gathered during the focused interview. The nurse should be prepared to observe the patient and listen for cues related to the function of this body system. Open-ended and closed questions are used to obtain information. Often a number of follow-up questions or requests for descriptions are required to clarify data or gather missing information. Follow-up questions are aimed at identifying the source of problems, duration of difficulties, measures to alleviate problems, and clues about the patient's knowledge of her own health.

Information about the genital areas, reproduction, and sexual activity is generally considered very private. The nurse must be sensitive to the patient's need for privacy and carefully explain that all information is confidential. A conversational approach with the use of open-ended statements is often helpful in a situation that promotes anxiety and embarrassment. The patient's terminology about body parts and functions should guide the nurse's questions.

The focused interview guides the physical assessment of the female reproductive system. The information is always considered in relation to normal parameters and expectations about the health of the system. Therefore, the nurse must consider age, gender, race, culture, environment, health practices, past and concurrent problems,

and therapies when framing questions and using techniques to elicit information. In order to address all of the factors when conducting a focused interview, categories of questions related to status and function of the reproductive system have been developed. These categories include general questions that are asked of all patients; those addressing illness and infection; questions related to symptoms, pain, and behaviors; those related to habits or practices; questions that are specific to patients according to age; and questions that address environmental concerns. One approach to elicit information about symptoms is the OLDCART & ICE method as described in chapter 7. ∞ See Figure 7.3 on page 120.

The nurse must consider the patient's ability to participate in the focused interview and physical assessment of the reproductive system. If a patient is experiencing pain or anxiety, attention must focus on relief of these symptoms. Because of the close proximity of some of the female reproductive structures to the urethra, data gathered during the focused interview will relate to the status of the urinary system as well. Questions related to the health and function of the female urinary system are discussed in chapter 22. ∞

Abnormal vaginal discharge, pelvic pain, inflammation, infection, and suspicion of contracting an STD are some of the more frequent problems that the female reports. Examination of the perianal area is included in assessment of the female reproductive system. Related problems include hemorrhoids, fissures, and infectious processes.

Focused Interview Questions	**Rationales and Evidence**

The following section provides sample questions and bulleted follow-up questions in each of the previously mentioned categories. A rationale for the questions is provided. The list of questions is not all-inclusive but represents the types of questions required in a comprehensive focused — *interview related to the female reproductive system. The subjective data from questions asked during the health history and focused interview will provide information to meet the objectives related to reproductive health and preventing STDs as described in* Healthy People 2020.

General Questions

1. **Do you have any concerns about your reproductive health? Have you had concerns in the past? If so, please tell me about those concerns.**

   ▶ This question may prompt the patient to discuss any concerns about reproductive health.

2. **How old were you when you had your first menstrual period?**

   ▶ Onset of menses is influenced by a variety of factors including percent of body fat. Menarche (onset of menstruation) between the ages of 11 and 14 indicates normal development. Late onset is associated with endocrine problems (Lee, Oh, Yoon, & Choi, 2012).

3. **What was the first day of your last menstrual period?**

   ▶ This establishes a pattern for the patient and has significance for physical assessment in relation to physical changes that occur at points throughout the cycle.

4. **How many days does your cycle usually last?**
   - Is this consistent with each period?
   - How many days does bleeding occur?

   ▶ A cycle is defined as the first day of one period to the first day of the next. These questions establish the pattern for the patient.

5. **Describe your menstrual flow.**
   - Is this consistent each period?
   - How many tampons or pads do you use each day?
   - For how many days?

   ▶ Clotting and excessive bleeding warrant additional follow-up. Any uterine bleeding that the patient views as unusual warrants additional follow-up. The patient's assessment of her menstrual flow is subjective. Generally, an excessively heavy flow is characterized by use of more than one pad or tampon per hour (Mayo Clinic, 2011).

6. **How do you usually feel during your period? Is this a pattern for you?**

   ▶ This may provide clues as to whether discomfort is occurring. Dysmenorrhea (painful or difficult menstruation) is a common gynecologic disorder (Ju, Jones, & Mishra, 2013).

7. **How do you usually feel just before your period?**
   - Has this gotten worse or better?
   - Do you use any self-care remedies?

   ▶ Premenstrual syndrome (PMS) presents with a variety of signs and symptoms including irritability, headache, cramping, and breast engorgement. PMS usually occurs a few days before menstruation. Typically, sudden relief occurs with the onset of full menstrual flow.

8. **Do you take any medications for cramps?**
   - If so, what do you take and how much?
   - If not, how do you relieve your cramps?

   ▶ This helps to determine if the female is able to continue with her daily routine.

9. **Have you ever been pregnant? If so, how many times?**

   ▶ Questions 9 through 11 provide information about significant obstetric history, which impacts current status and anticipated physical findings.

10. **Did you have any problems during pregnancy, the delivery, or postpartum?** *If the patient answers "yes":* Describe the problem(s).

11. **Was delivery vaginal or by cesarean section?**

12. **Have you ever had a miscarriage?**
    - What were you told was the cause?
    - Was surgery required?
    - Have you ever had an abortion?
    - At how many weeks, and by what method?
    - How has it been emotionally since the abortion or miscarriage?

    ▶ Strong emotions often accompany the issue of termination of a pregnancy by either spontaneous or surgical abortion. The nurse may want to follow up.

Focused Interview Questions	Rationales and Evidence
13. Do you have children? • If so, how many? • *If the patient answers "no":* Have you tried to have children? • *If the patient answers "yes":* How long have you been trying to have a child?	▶ The couple is not considered potentially infertile unless they have been unable to conceive for a year (World Health Organization [WHO], n.d.).
14. *If the patient indicates inability to conceive after 1 year:* **How often do you and your partner have intercourse?**	▶ For couples attempting to have a child, it is important to engage in intercourse routinely, such as two to three times a week (Mayo Clinic, 2014a). Although nurses do not treat infertility, they may be involved in teaching the patient about certain measures that may be helpful, such as temperature tracking to determine the optimal time for intercourse. Concerns about infertility can produce great anxiety and depression for many females.
15. Have you ever sought professional help for fertility problems? If so, describe this experience.	▶ The patient can explain and describe specific diagnostic procedures and treatments for infertility as well as the emotional response to the processes and procedures.
16. Has an inability to conceive placed a strain on your relationship with your partner? • How has this problem affected your relationship? • How are you feeling about this?	▶ Specific questions enable the patient to affirm or deny relationship problems, to discuss changes in the relationship, and to discuss feelings about the partnership.
17. Are you sexually active?	▶ The patient may feel pressured to be in a sexual relationship. These pressures may be external (expectations of family, friends, or work associates) or internal (fear of being viewed by others as less than desirable or not of an accepted sexual orientation, fear of being alone, or fear of not being loved and accepted).
18. Are there any obstacles to your ability to achieve sexual satisfaction?	▶ Causes of inability to achieve sexual satisfaction include fear of acquiring an STD, fear of being unable to satisfy the partner, fear of pregnancy, confusion regarding sexual preference, unwillingness to participate in sexual activities enjoyed by the partner, job stress, financial considerations, crowded living conditions, loss of partner, attraction to or sexual involvement with individuals that the partner does not know about, criticism of sexual performance by the partner, or history of sexual trauma.
19. Have you noticed a change in your sex drive recently?	▶ This may be indicative of some physical or psychologic problems that need follow-up.
20. *If the patient answers "yes" to question 19:* **Can you associate the change with anything in particular?**	▶ Often patients can relate a decrease in sex drive with stress, illness, drug therapy, or some other factor (Basson, Reese, Wang, Montejo, & Incrocci, 2010).
21. Do you use contraceptives? • Which type of contraceptives do you use? • How long have you been using contraceptives? • Do you take oral contraceptives for a reason other than preventing pregnancy? • Have you ever had any adverse effects from using contraceptives?	▶ This question provides information about the patient's knowledge about contraception, at-risk behaviors, and specific contraceptive devices or medications. ▶ In addition to preventing pregnancy, some women take oral contraceptives to regulate hormones and menstrual flow or to control symptoms of diseases such as polycystic ovarian syndrome. Discussing contraception use may provide insight into the patient's medical history.

Focused Interview Questions	Rationales and Evidence

Questions Related to Illness or Infection

1. **Do you now have or have you ever had an illness associated with the female reproductive system?**
   - When were you diagnosed with the problem?
   - What was the treatment for the illness?
   - Was the treatment helpful?
   - What kinds of things do you do to help with the problem?
   - Has the problem ever recurred?
   - How are you managing the problem now?

   ► This allows the patient to provide her own perceptions about problems with her reproductive system.

2. **An alternative to question 1 is to list common problems with the reproductive system such as dysmenorrhea; uterine fibroids; and uterine, ovarian, or vulvar cancer and ask the patient to respond "yes" or "no" as each is stated.**

   ► This is a comprehensive and easy way to elicit information about illnesses associated with the female reproductive system. Follow-up would be carried out for each identified diagnosis as in question 1.

3. **Do you now have or have you ever had an infection of the reproductive system?**
   - When were you diagnosed with the infection?
   - What treatment was prescribed for the problem?
   - Was the treatment helpful?
   - What kinds of things do you do to help with the problem?
   - Has the problem ever recurred (acute)?
   - How are you managing the infection now (chronic)?

   ► If an infection is identified, follow-up about the date of infection, treatment, and outcomes is required. Data about each infection identified by the patient are essential to an accurate health assessment. Infections can be classified as acute or chronic, and follow-up regarding each classification will differ.

4. **An alternative to question 3 is to list possible infections, such as vaginitis, cystitis, and pelvic inflammatory disease (PID), and ask the patient to respond "yes" or "no" as each is stated.**

   ► This is a comprehensive and easy way to elicit information about all reproductive system infections. Follow-up would be carried out for each identified infection as in question 3.

5. **Have you ever had any surgery of the reproductive system?**
   - If so, what was it? When? Where?
   - What was the outcome?

   ► Questions 5 and 6 provide information about patient knowledge in regard to pathologies and treatments. This establishes variations in expected findings in physical examination.

6. **Have you ever had an abnormal Pap smear?**
   - If so, how long ago was this?
   - What treatment, if any, did you receive?
   - Have you had follow-up Pap smears? When? What were the results?

7. **Have you ever had an STD such as herpes, gonorrhea, syphilis, HPV, or chlamydia?**
   - *If the patient answers "yes":* Was it treated?
   - Did you inform your partner?
   - Was your partner treated?
   - Did you have sexual relations with your partner while you were infected?
   - *If the patient answers "yes":* Did you use condoms?
   - What treatment did you receive?

   ► Serious, sometimes fatal, complications can develop if treatment is delayed. STDs can be detected only by testing. If untreated, STDs can cause sterility and problems with the reproductive and other body systems (CDC, 2013a).

8. **Are you aware of having had any exposure to HIV?**
   - *If the patient answers "yes":* Describe the situation and how you believe you were exposed.
   - What are your views on sexual relations and the potential for acquiring HIV?

   ► The incidence of HIV is still greatly on the rise. Despite the wide availability of information on the risk and methods of protection for sexually active individuals, many females continue to have unprotected sex.

9. **Have you ever been tested for HIV?**
   - *If the patient answers "yes":* On one occasion or routinely?
   - What were the results of the test?

Focused Interview Questions	Rationales and Evidence

Questions Related to Symptoms, Pain, and Behaviors

When gathering information about symptoms, many questions are required to elicit details and descriptions that assist in the analysis of the data. Discrimination is made in relation to the significance of a symptom, in relation to specific diseases or problems, and in relation to potential follow-up examination or referral. One rationale may be provided for a group of questions in this category.

The following questions refer to specific symptoms and behaviors associated with the female reproductive system. For each symptom, questions and follow-up are required. The details to be elicited are the characteristics of the symptom; the onset, duration, and frequency of the symptom; the treatment or remedy for the symptom, including over-the-counter and home remedies; the determination if diagnosis has been sought; the effect of treatments; and family history associated with a symptom or illness.

Questions Related to Symptoms

1. **Have you noticed any rashes, blisters, ulcers, sores, or warts on your genital area or surrounding areas?**

   ▶ Rashes may occur with yeast infections, which are the most common female genital infection. Yeast infections generally produce redness, pruritus (itching), and cheeselike discharge. Herpes infection causes small painful ulcerations, whereas syphilitic chancres are not painful. In the older patient, a raised, reddened lesion may indicate carcinoma of the vulva. Reddened lesions that eventually weep and form crusts characterize contact dermatitis. Venereal warts are cauliflower shaped (Osborn, Wraa, Watson, & Holleran, 2013).

2. **Have you felt any lumps or masses in your genital area or surrounding areas?**
   - If so, describe the mass. Exactly where is it?
   - About what size?
   - Is it soft or hard?
   - Is it movable?
   - When did you first notice the mass?
   - Is it painful?
   - Have you noticed any change in it since it developed?
   - Have you used any remedies such as ice, heat, or creams?

   ▶ Sebaceous cysts can be noted in the labial area. A lump created by an abscess of the Bartholin's gland causes localized pain. An abscess of the Bartholin's gland may indicate the presence of gonorrhea (Kessous et al., 2013).

3. **Have you noticed any swelling or redness of your genitals?**

   ▶ Vulvovaginitis may cause edema in the genital and perineal area, including the vulva. Redness and swelling may indicate an alteration in health such as an abscess of the Bartholin's gland, which may be caused by gonorrhea. Bruising may indicate sexual trauma.

4. **Have you noticed any changes in the appearance of your vaginal opening?**
   - Have you felt any pressure from your vagina?
   - Have you felt bulging or masses from within your vagina?

   ▶ Uterine prolapse may be so severe that the uterus protrudes into and at times out of the vagina. Surgery may be indicated.

5. **Have you experienced any itching in your labia or vaginal area?**
   - If so, when did it start?
   - Has it been treated and, if so, how?
   - Have there been any associated urinary symptoms?

   ▶ Crab lice, atrophic vaginitis, candidiasis, and contact dermatitis may cause intense itching.

6. **Have you noticed any discharge from your vagina?**
   - If so, what color is it?
   - Is there any odor to it?
   - Is it a small, moderate, or large amount?
   - When did you first notice the discharge?

   ▶ Vaginal discharge is a typical complaint of patients with vaginitis. The most common presenting symptom in females with STDs is vaginal discharge; however, the patient may have no symptoms (Xu et al., 2013).

Focused Interview Questions	Rationales and Evidence
7. **Have you had any vaginal bleeding outside the time of your normal menstrual period?**	▶ Abnormal bleeding may be related to hormonal influences and may be easily corrected. Conditions such as uterine fibroids and several forms of cancer can also cause abnormal bleeding patterns (Mayo Clinic, 2014b).
8. *If the patient answers "yes" to question 7:* **When did it occur? How much bleeding was there?**	▶ The nurse should obtain quantitative data by asking whether panties were saturated or how many pads or tampons were saturated in 24 hours. A calendar should be used to determine the number of days since the patient's last menstrual period.
9. **Have you had any problems in and around your rectal area, such as pain, itching, burning, or bleeding?** • When did the problem begin? • Do you know the cause of the problem? • Have you sought health care for the problem? • Was a diagnosis made? • What treatment was prescribed? • What do you do to help with the problem? • Has the treatment helped?	▶ Pain, itching, bleeding, or burning may indicate the presence of abuse; infection; irritation; or injury to the anus, rectum, or perineum. Rectal bleeding, pain, and irritation may result from passing hard stools, from hemorrhoids, or from injuries. Fungal infection may result in pruritus or irritation of the perianal area (Osborn et al., 2013). ▶ When symptoms in the perianal area are associated with hemorrhoids or hard stool, follow-up would include questions about diet, exercise, and bowel habits. ▶ Irritation or injury to the perianal area can occur as a result of sexual practices or sexual abuse. Sensitive questioning about these topics is required when sexual activity is described or when sexual abuse is suspected or disclosed.

Questions Related to Pain

1. **Do you have any pain, tenderness, or soreness in your pelvic area?** • If so, describe the pain. • Is it dull? Sharp? Radiating? Intermittent? Continuous? • When did it start? • Are you having any pain in the area now? • What makes the pain better or worse? • Do you have associated symptoms of headache, vomiting, or diarrhea?	▶ Common causes of gynecologic pain include infection, menstrual difficulties, endometriosis (abnormal condition involving the endometrial lining of the uterus), ectopic pregnancy (fetus implanted in abnormal location), threatened abortion, pelvic masses, uterine fibroids, and ovarian cancer (Osborn et al., 2013).

Questions Related to Behaviors

1. **Do you check your genitals on a routine basis?** *If the patient answers "yes":* **How often?**	▶ Self-examination of the genitals should be performed at least monthly for early detection of changes that need follow-up. Teaching may be indicated if the patient is not performing self-examination.
2. **How often do you get physical examinations?**	▶ Screening for problems such as cervical or endometrial cancer is typically performed during routine physical or gynecologic examinations.
3. **Do you use tampons?** • If so, how frequently do you change the tampons? • Are you aware of the risk for toxic shock syndrome with the use of tampons? • Are you aware of the signs of toxic shock?	▶ Tampons, when not used cautiously (for example, lack of frequent changes), have been linked with toxic shock syndrome (MacPhee et al., 2013).
4. **What kinds of products do you use for hygiene in the genital area?**	▶ Use of soap, sprays, powders, and douche products can irritate the tissues of the reproductive system. Some studies suggest that females who have used talc in the genital area for many years may be at increased risk of developing ovarian cancer.

Focused Interview Questions	Rationales and Evidence
5. *If the patient is sexually active:* **Are you in a mutually monogamous relationship? If not, how many sexual partners have you or your partner had over the last year? Do you or your partner regularly use protection during sexual intercourse?**	▶ Sexual activity with many different partners increases the risk of acquiring STDs and, possibly, certain gynecologic cancers. ▶ Use of protection (e.g., male or female condoms) can reduce the risk of acquiring STDs.
6. **Are you able to be sexually aroused?** • Has this ability changed over time or recently?	▶ A variety of factors may interfere with a female's ability to be sexually aroused. These factors include prescribed or illicit drug use, disorders of the nervous or endocrine systems, stress, and fear (e.g., of intimacy, inability to satisfy a partner, acquiring an STD, or becoming pregnant).
7. **Are you satisfied with your sexual experiences?** • *If the patient expresses dissatisfaction:* Are you able to achieve orgasm? • Have you noticed a change in your ability to have an orgasm?	▶ A variety of factors may interfere with a female's ability to experience orgasm.
8. **Are you using contraception?** • If so, what kind? • Are you using it consistently?	▶ This provides information about knowledge of contraception in general and regarding the products indicated by the patient.
9. **Would you like to know more about the use of birth control?**	▶ This is a very important question to ask adolescents who shy away from talking about sexual practices but have verbalized that they are sexually active.
10. **How do you protect yourself from sexually transmitted diseases, including HIV?**	▶ Abstinence is the only 100% effective protection against STDs. Latex condoms offer significant protection, especially when treated with spermicide; however, they are not 100% effective (CDC, 2013b).

Questions Related to Age

The focused interview must reflect the anatomic and physiologic differences that exist along the life span. The following questions are examples of those that would be specific for infants and children, adolescents, the pregnant female, and the older adult.

Questions Regarding Infants and Children

1. **Have you noticed any redness, swelling, or discharge that is discolored or foul smelling in the child's genital areas?**	▶ These may indicate inflammatory processes or infection.
2. **Has the child complained of itching, burning, or swelling in the genital area?**	▶ These symptoms may indicate the presence of pinworms, yeast infections and other infections, trauma, or sexual abuse (Dei, Di Maggio, Di Paolo, & Bruni, 2010).

The nurse should ask the preschool or school-age child the following questions:

3. **Has anyone ever touched you when you didn't want him or her to?** • Where? (*The nurse may want to have the child point to a picture or doll.*) • Has anyone ever asked you to touch him or her when you didn't want to? • Where did he or she ask you to touch him or her? • *If the child answers "yes," the child may be experiencing sexual abuse. The nurse should try to obtain additional information by asking the following questions, but must remember to be sensitive:* • Who touched you? • How many times did this happen? • Who knows about this?	▶ The nurse must try to determine exactly what the person did to the child. Has there been more than touching? Has any other form of sexual contact occurred? The child may feel responsible for the situation and not wish to discuss it. The abuser may be a parent or relative. The nurse should assure the child that she has not been bad and that it helps to talk to an adult about it. Referral should be made to a specialist immediately for sexual abuse assessment.

| Focused Interview Questions | Rationales and Evidence |

Questions Regarding Adolescents

Many of the questions nurses ask adolescents are similar to questions they ask adults. It is important to explore adolescents' feelings and concerns regarding their sexual development. The nurse can reassure the adolescent that these changes are normal. Some adolescents may be confused about their feelings of sexual attraction to the opposite or same sex. The nurse should ask open-ended questions and assure the adolescent that such feelings are normal.

Whether or not an adolescent admits to being sexually active, it is important to offer information on teenage pregnancy, birth control, and protection against STDs. Some teenagers may be fearful that the nurse will relay this information to their parents. The nurse should reinforce that all information is confidential unless sexual abuse is reported.

1. **Are you having sex with anyone now?**

   ► Use of gender-neutral terms prevents value judgments about sexual orientation. This question allows patients to define what they think sex is. Many teens consider anything not involving vaginal penetration as not being sex. The nurse must stress that oral sex is indeed sexual activity.

2. **Have you been taught that sexual intercourse can lead to pregnancy?**

   ► Despite the prevalence of sexual references in the media and the sexual activity of many adolescents, many teenage girls do not know why they got pregnant. Providing teaching about sex and pregnancy may help reduce teenage pregnancies.

3. **Do you understand that sexual intercourse can lead to STDs?**

   ► If sex education is not provided by the schools or if the patient is too young to have received sex education at school, they may be unaware that serious STDs, including HIV/AIDS, can result from unprotected sex. Adolescents need to understand the risks of acquiring STDs from sexual activity, regardless of the number of partners or the use of protection. However, if they must be sexually active, they should be taught the importance of limiting the number of sexual partners and consistently using protection during vaginal, oral, and anal sex.

Questions for the Pregnant Female

Questions for the pregnant female would include menstrual, obstetric, gynecologic, family, and partner histories.

This information would provide data about the patient and her partner and identify risk factors. Specific questions for the pregnant female are included in chapter 27 of this text. ∞

Questions for the Older Adult

The questions for aging female adults are the same as those for younger adults. In addition, the nurse should explore whether older patients perceive any changes in their sexuality related to advancing age. For example, an older female may notice a decrease in vaginal lubrication even when she is fully aroused. The female older adult can be reassured that these changes are normal and do not indicate disease.

1. **When did menopause begin for you?**

   ► This information establishes a reference for the onset of physiologic changes that accompany menopause.

2. **Tell me about physical changes you have noticed since menopause.**

   ► It is common for aging females to experience a variety of symptoms, including mood changes and "hot flashes." Vaginal dryness causes dyspareunia (painful intercourse).

Focused Interview Questions	Rationales and Evidence
3. Have you had any vaginal bleeding since starting menopause?	▶ Some females assume that postmenopausal bleeding is normal and tend to ignore it. Post-menopausal bleeding may be suggestive of inadequate estrogen therapy and endometrial cancer (Colombo et al., 2011). It could also be indicative of serious problems such as genital tract cancer.

Questions Related to the Environment

Environment refers to both the internal and external environments. Questions related to the internal environment include all of the previous questions and those associated with internal or physiologic responses. Questions regarding the external environment include those related to home, work, or social environments.

Internal Environment

1. Do you know if your mother received diethylstilbestrol (DES) treatment during pregnancy with you?	▶ Studies indicate that daughters of mothers who received DES during pregnancy have a significantly higher number of reproductive tract problems, including cervical cancer, infertility, and ectopic pregnancy (Laronda, Unno, Butler, & Kurita, 2012). This may have some bearing on the current problem. If the patient answers "yes" to this question, the nurse should refer her to a physician.
2. Do you drink alcohol? How many drinks per week?	▶ Intake of alcoholic beverages can contribute to an individual "taking chances" such as failing to ask the partner to use condoms.
3. Do you use illicit drugs? If so, what type and how much?	▶ Taken in sufficient amounts, some drugs, such as marijuana and opiates, may decrease libido. Drug use may also contribute to failure to use protection against STDs.

External Environment

The following questions deal with substances and irritants found in the physical environment of the patient. The physical environment includes the indoor and outdoor environments of the home and the workplace, those encountered for social engagements, and any encountered during travel.

1. Do your family and friends support your relationship with your sexual partner?	▶ The patient's family and friends can influence the patient's sexual relationship in a variety of ways. The patient may feel tension if the partner is not accepted.
2. Are you able to talk to your partner about your sexual needs? ● Does your partner accept your needs and help you fulfill them? ● Are you able to do the same for your partner?	▶ The ability to openly discuss sexual needs and preferences fosters strong and lasting relationships.
3. Some patients come to a healthcare provider to discuss sexual abuse. ● Have you ever been forced to have sexual intercourse or other sexual contact against your will? ● Have you ever been molested or raped? ● If the patient answers "yes": When was this? ● Who abused you? ● What was the experience? ● What was done about the situation and for you?	

Patient-Centered Interaction

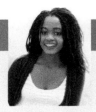

Ms. Tanya Jacobs comes to the clinic and tells the admission clerk she needs help and needs to see a female nurse. She further indicates she would like to see Mary Bart, RN, again today if she is working. When asked why she is seeking health care, Ms. Jacobs responds, "I have a bad itch down there." About 5 minutes later Mary Bart greets Ms. Jacobs. Part of the focused interview follows.

Interview

Nurse: Tell me about the problem.

Ms. Jacobs: I don't know where or how to begin. I'm so embarrassed.

Nurse: First, we need to address your feelings of embarrassment, and then it might be easier for you to talk about your problem. I understand that discussion of problems with your genitals is embarrassing. These are difficult issues to discuss. I will keep all that is said here confidential. I will let you take your time as you tell me about the problem. Your discussion will help to determine the cause of the problem and the best way to take care of it.

Ms. Jacobs: I just don't know how this could happen. I haven't seen my boyfriend in 2 weeks. He is away, and I get this itch. What did I do wrong?

Nurse: As we discuss your symptoms, the cause of the itch will become more clear. Let's first talk about the itch. Try to be as specific as possible. Where is it?

Ms. Jacobs: You know, in my private area.

Nurse: On the outside or inside?

Ms. Jacobs: The outside.

Nurse: When did you first notice the itch?

Ms. Jacobs: I noticed it 2 days ago.

Nurse: Do you have a rash?

Ms. Jacobs: No.

Nurse: Is your private area red?

Ms. Jacobs: Yes.

Nurse: What have you done to relieve the itch and redness?

Ms. Jacobs: I try not to scratch, but that is why I'm here. I can't stand it. It seems to be getting worse.

Analysis

The nurse realized that discussing matters related to the reproductive system and genitalia might be very difficult for the patient. Ms. Jacobs' stated embarrassment and her verbal burst of information were verbal and nonverbal cues interpreted by the nurse to set the tone for the interview. The interview began with an open-ended statement. This allowed the patient to respond within the area of greatest comfort. The nurse recognized the emotional aspect of this situation and addressed this before seeking more information. Closed statements were used to obtain specific subjective data. The nurse listened to the patient and did not impose judgment.

Patient Education

The following are physiologic, behavioral, and cultural risk factors that affect female reproductive health across the age span. Several factors are cited as trends in *Healthy People 2020* documents. The nurse provides advice and education to reduce risks associated with these factors and to promote and maintain reproductive health.

LIFESPAN CONSIDERATIONS

Risk Factors	Patient Education
• Infants may be born with ambiguous external genitalia.	▶ Counsel and advise parents about decisions regarding ambiguous genitalia, including genetic testing.
• Young females experience changes associated with puberty between the ages of 8 and 13 years.	▶ Provide information to young females and parents regarding the changes that accompany the onset of puberty, including menstruation.

LIFESPAN CONSIDERATIONS

Risk Factors

- Adolescents are interested in exploring their sexual identity and may engage in sexual contact with others.

- Changes in the reproductive system occur with aging and include physiologic changes as well as changes in sexual activity.

Patient Education

▶ Advise and counsel adolescents regarding sexual activity. Information should include the risks associated with sexual activity including STDs, HIV, and pregnancy. Teaching should also include the importance of the proper and consistent use of protection during sex as well as the early signs of pregnancy.

▶ Provide aging females with information about changes that accompany menopause. Aging females should be advised that atrophy of the reproductive organs occurs, vaginal lubrication diminishes, and sexual intercourse may be painful. Lubricants are available to decrease discomfort.

CULTURAL CONSIDERATIONS

Risk Factors

- Culture and language influence knowledge and practices related to the reproductive system.

Patient Education

▶ Be sensitive to cultural differences regarding discussion of reproductive function. In addition, information regarding hygiene, risk, and treatments should be provided in the native language of the patient. Obtain a translator if needed.

ENVIRONMENTAL CONSIDERATIONS

Risk Factors

- The proximity of the urinary tract to genitalia and the perianal area requires the need for careful hygiene.

- Psychologic and physical problems may be a result of sexual trauma or abuse.

- Females with a family history of reproductive cancer are at greater risk for the disease.

Patient Education

▶ Inform females of all ages about cleansing of the genitoperineal area to decrease risk of urinary tract infections. The use of bubble baths, perfumed soaps, antiseptics, and douche solutions may promote local irritation to the genitalia. Advise about avoidance of those hygiene products.
▶ Provide information about the safe use of tampons to all females to reduce risks of infection and toxic shock syndrome.

▶ Tell parents or caregivers that behavioral and physical changes may signal abuse. Withdrawal, changes in grades or participation in activities, changes in physical appearance, sleeplessness, or appetite change are among the behaviors that warrant follow-up. Encourage all females to report inappropriate sexual advances or abuse.

▶ Inform adult females of recommendations for Pap smears for cervical cancer screening. These recommendations include having the first Pap smear by age 21 or within 3 years of initiating vaginal intercourse. Annual Pap tests are recommended. At age 30, Pap testing may occur every 2 to 3 years in females who have had three normal tests. At 70 years, females with three or more normal tests may discontinue Pap tests. Advise patients to reduce their risk for cervical cancer by delaying initial sexual encounters until adulthood, limiting the number of partners (thereby reducing exposure to HPV), and not smoking. Inform patients with a first-degree relative with ovarian cancer that the cancer antigen (CA) 125 assay is used to measure the level of CA 125, which is a tumor marker.

ENVIRONMENTAL CONSIDERATIONS

Risk Factors

- Psychosocial factors influence sexual desire and enjoyment.

Patient Education

▶ Provide patients with information about the actions and interactions of medications in relation to health and function of the reproductive and other systems and sexual activity. For example, antibodies can alter the vaginal flora and lead to vaginal yeast infections. Eating active culture yogurt while on antibiotics can reduce this risk. Some medications for cardiovascular problems diminish sexual desire. The use of oral contraceptives increases the risk for thrombosis, especially in smokers. Therefore, smoking cessation and precautions regarding periods of prolonged immobility, such as air flights, are important aspects of education about medications.

BEHAVIORAL CONSIDERATIONS

Risk Factor

- Risks for problems with the female reproductive system correlate to the numbers and types of sexual contacts.

Patient Education

▶ Discuss the risks associated with multiple sexual partners, including HPV, HIV, other STDs, and hepatitis C. Discuss safe sex practices.

Physical Assessment

Assessment Techniques and Findings

Physical assessment of the female reproductive system includes the techniques of inspection and palpation. In addition, the speculum is used to visualize the vagina and cervix. During each of the procedures, the nurse is gathering data related to the health and function of the reproductive system. Knowledge of normal or expected findings is essential in determining the meaning of the data as the nurse conducts the physical assessment.

The adult female has pubic hair that is distributed in an even, inverted triangular pattern over the mons pubis. Hair distribution is less dense over the labia, perineum, and inner thighs. The labia majora are symmetric, smooth, and without lesions. The labia minora are smooth, pink, and moist. The clitoris is smooth, midline, and about 1 cm (0.39 in.) in length. The urethra is slitlike, midline, smooth, pink, and patent. The vaginal opening is pink and round. On bearing down, there should be no urine leakage at the meatus or protrusions from the vagina. The perineum is smooth and firm. The anus is intact, moist, darkly pigmented, and without lesions. Upon palpation the vaginal wall is rugated and soft; the Skene's glands and Bartholin's glands are nontender and without discharge. The examination with the speculum reveals a pink, moist, round, and centrally positioned cervix. The cervix is free of lesions with clear, odorless secretions present. Palpation of the cervix reveals it as firm, smooth, and mobile like the tip of the nose. The fornices are smooth and nontender. The uterus is palpated and found tilted upward above the bladder with the cervix tilted forward. Variations in uterine position may be anteverted, midline, or retroverted.

EQUIPMENT

- examination gown and examination drape
- clean, nonsterile examination gloves
- lubricant
- Pap smear equipment
- speculum
- handheld mirror

When ovaries are palpable, they are smooth, firm, mobile, and almond shaped. They may be slightly tender. The uterine tubes are nonpalpable. The rectovaginal system is thin, smooth, and nontender.

Physical assessment of the female reproductive system follows an organized pattern. It begins with inspection of the external genitalia and perianal area, palpation of the vagina and glands, and speculum examination and specimen collection. This is followed by palpation of the cervix, fornices, uterus, uterine tubes, and ovaries. The assessment ends with the rectovaginal examination. An internal pelvic examination is not recommended for healthy, asymptomatic females below the age of 21. Annual pelvic examination (both internal and external) should be performed on all patients age 21 and older (ACOG, 2014).

Techniques and Normal Findings	Abnormal Findings Special Considerations

Inspection

1. Instruct the patient.

- Explain to the patient that you will be looking at and touching her external genital area. Tell her that it should not cause discomfort, but if pain occurs she should tell you and you will stop. Explain that deep breathing is a good way to relax during the examination.
- Tell the patient you will provide instructions and explanations at each point in the assessment.

2. Position the patient.

- Ask the patient to lie down on the examination table.
- Assist her into the lithotomy position (supine with knees and hips flexed so that feet rest flat on the examination table), and then have her slide her hips as close to the end of the table as possible.
- Place her feet in the stirrups (see Figure 24.4 ■).

▶ In the obese patient, the presence of large thighs and extra adipose tissue in the perineal area may require having an assistant to hold thighs apart or to move extra tissue during the examination. It may be necessary to raise the hips and increase flexion of the hips to visualize genital structures.

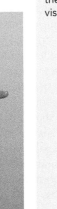

Figure 24.4
Positioning the patient.

Techniques and Normal Findings	**Abnormal Findings / Special Considerations**

3. Inspect the pubic hair.

- Confirm that the hair grows in an inverted triangle and is scattered heavily over the mons pubis. It should become sparse over the labia majora, perineum, and inner thighs (see Figure 24.5 ■).

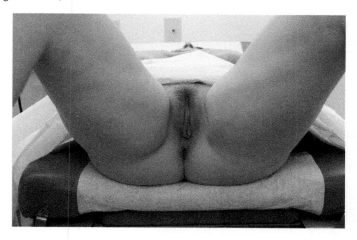

Figure 24.5
Inspecting the pubic hair.

▶ A sparse hair pattern may be indicative of delayed puberty. It is also a common and normal finding in females of Asian ancestry. The elderly patient's pubic hair will become sparse, scattered, and gray. Figure 24.3 depicts Tanner's stages of female development.

- If the patient has complained of itching in the pubic area, comb through the pubic hair with two or three fingers.
- Confirm the absence of small, bluish gray spots, or nits (eggs), at the base of the pubic hairs.

▶ These signs indicate pubic lice (crabs). Marks may be visible from persistent scratching to relieve the intense itching caused by the lice.

4. Inspect the labia majora.

- Confirm that the labia majora are fuller and rounder in the center of the structure and that the skin is smooth and intact.
- Compare the right and left labia majora for symmetry.
- Observe for any lesions, warts, vesicles, rashes, or ulcerations. If you notice drainage, note the color, distribution, location, and characteristics.

▶ The labia majora of older females may be thinner and wrinkled.

▶ These findings may signal a variety of conditions. *Contact dermatitis* appears as a red rash with associated lesions that are weepy and crusty. There often are scratches due to intense itching.

▶ **Genital warts** are raised, moist, cauliflower-shaped papules.

▶ The herpes simplex virus (HSV) may produce red, painful vesicles accompanied by localized swelling of the genitals and surrounding areas. Genital herpes is usually caused by herpes simplex type 2 (HSV-2).

- Remember to change gloves as needed during the exam to prevent cross-contamination. Also remember to culture any abnormal discharge.

- Confirm the absence of any swelling or inflammation in the area of the labia majora.

▶ Swelling over red, inflamed skin that is tender and warm to palpation may indicate an abscess in the Bartholin's gland. The abscess may be caused by gonorrhea. Labia and other structures in the perineum may be edematous in the obese patient as a result of pressure in the groin from the enlarged abdomen.

5. Inspect the labia minora.

- Confirm that the labia minora are smooth, pink, and moist.
- Observe for any redness or swelling. Note any bruising or tearing of the skin.

▶ The older female may have drier, thinner labia minora.

▶ Redness and swelling indicate the presence of an infective or inflammatory process. Bruising or tearing of the skin may suggest forceful intercourse or sexual abuse, especially in the case of adolescents and children.

Techniques and Normal Findings	Abnormal Findings Special Considerations

6. Inspect the clitoris.

- Place your right or left hand over the labia majora and separate these structures with your thumb and index finger.
- The clitoris should be midline, about 1 cm (0.39 in.) in length, with more fullness in the center. It should be smooth

- Observe for any redness, lesions, or tears in the tissue.

▶ An elongated clitoris may signal elevated levels of testosterone and warrants further investigation and referral to a physician.

7. Inspect the urethral orifice.

- Confirm that the urethral opening is midline, pink, smooth, slitlike, and patent (see Figure 24.6 ■).

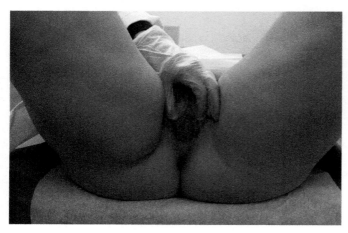

Figure 24.6
Inspection of the urethra.

- Ask the patient to cough. No urine should leak from the urethral opening.

- Inspect for any redness, inflammation, or discharge.

▶ Urine leakage indicates stress incontinence and weakening of the pelvic musculature.

▶ These symptoms indicate urinary tract infection. Pressure of the enlarged abdomen in the obese patient may lead to urinary incontinence resulting in redness and excoriation.

8. Inspect the vaginal opening, perineum, and anal area.

- Confirm that the vaginal opening or introitus is pink and round. It may be either smooth or irregular.
- Locate the **hymen**, which is a thin layer of skin within the vagina. It may be present in females who have never had sexual intercourse; however, certain activities, including tampon usage or vigorous exercise, may result in hymen rupture despite the absence of sexual activity (Hegazy & Al-Rukban, 2012).
- Inspect for tears, bruising, or lacerations.

▶ Tears, bruising, or lacerations could be due to forceful, consensual sex or rape. Additional follow-up is needed after examination. It is important not to ask any questions that the patient may interpret as probing or threatening during the physical assessment.

- The **perineum**, the space between the vaginal opening and anal area, should be smooth and firm.
- Scars from episiotomy procedures may be observed in parous females. These are normal.
- The anus should be intact, moist, and darkly pigmented. There should be no lesions.

▶ Fecal incontinence is common in the obese patient due to increased abdominal pressure on the bowel and anal sphincter. This may result in redness, or excoriation.

Techniques and Normal Findings	Abnormal Findings Special Considerations

- Have the patient bear down.

- Inspect for any protrusions from the vagina.

▶ Thin, fragile perineal tissues indicate atrophy. Tears and fissures may indicate trauma.

▶ A **prolapsed uterus** may protrude right at the vaginal wall with straining, or it may hang outside of the vaginal wall without any straining (see Figure 24.7 ■).

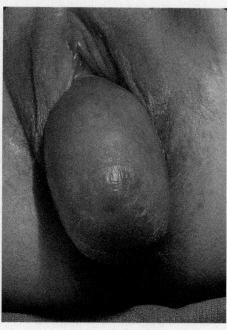

Figure 24.7 Prolapsed uterus.
Source: M. English/Custom Medical Stock Photo.

▶ A **cystocele** is a hernia that is formed when the urinary bladder is pushed into the anterior vaginal wall.
▶ A **rectocele** is a hernia that is formed when the rectum pushes into the posterior vaginal wall.

Palpation

1. **Palpate the vaginal walls.**
   - Explain to the patient that you are going to palpate the vaginal walls. Tell her that she will feel you insert a finger into the vagina.
   - Place your left hand above the labia majora and spread the labia minora apart with your thumb and index finger.
   - With your right palm facing toward the ceiling, gently place your right index finger at the vaginal opening.
   - Insert your right index finger gently into the vagina.
   - Gently rotate the right index finger counterclockwise. The vaginal wall should feel rugated, consistent in texture, and soft.
   - Ask the patient to bear down or cough.
   - Note any bulging in this area.

▶ Bulging may occur with uterine prolapse, cystocele, or rectocele.

2. **Palpate the urethra and Skene's glands.**
   - Explain to the patient that you are going to palpate her urethra. Tell her that she will again feel pressure against her vaginal wall.
   - Your left hand should still be above the labia majora and you should still be spreading the labia minora apart with your thumb and index finger.
   - Your right index finger should still be inserted in the patient's vagina.
   - With your right index finger, apply very gentle pressure upward against the vaginal wall.
   - Milk the Skene's glands by stroking outward (see Figure 24.8 ■).

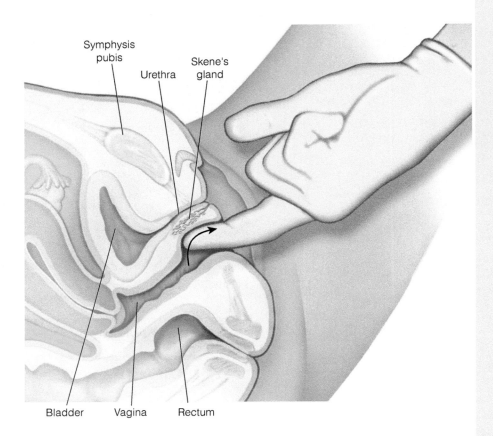

Figure 24.8 Palpating Skene's glands.

   - Now apply the same upward and outward pressure on both sides of the urethra.
   - No pain or discharge should be elicited.

▶ Discharge from the urethra or Skene's glands may indicate an infection such as gonorrhea. A culture must be obtained.

3. **Palpate the Bartholin's glands.**
   - With your right index finger still inserted in the patient's vagina, gently squeeze the posterior region of the labia majora between your right index finger and right thumb (see Figure 24.9 ■).

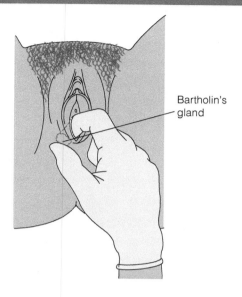

Bartholin's gland

Figure 24.9 Palpating Bartholin's glands.

- Perform this maneuver bilaterally, palpating both Bartholin's glands.
- No lump or hardness should be felt. No pain response should be elicited. No discharge should be produced.

▶ Lumps, hardness, pain, or discharge suggest the presence of an abscess and infective process. Often the source is a gonorrheal infection. A culture should be obtained of any discharge.

Inspection With a Speculum

Speculum examination is most often performed by a physician or an advanced practice nurse. Prior to this examination, patients should be advised to avoid douching for up to three days, because douching prior to a Pap test can wash away surface cells and affect the examination results (Johns Hopkins Medicine, n.d.).

1. **Select the speculum.**
   - The speculum should be the proper size for the patient.
   - Use a speculum that has been prewarmed with a heating pad. Do not prewarm a speculum with warm water, because it is not desirable to introduce water into the vagina. To promote patient comfort, a water-based gel lubricant may be used during the exam (Pawlik & Martin, 2009).

2. **Hold the speculum in your dominant hand.**
   - Place the index finger on top of the blades, the third finger on the bottom of the blades, and be sure to move the thumb just underneath the thumbscrew before inserting (see Figure 24.10 ■).

▶ For patients who experience vaginitis, speculum examination may be performed to evaluate complaints related to symptomatic vaginal discharge (Singh et al., 2012). In the obese patient, the sidewalls of the vagina have increased loose connective tissue, resulting in inward collapse of the vaginal walls when using a standard "duckbill" speculum.

Examination may require two examiners, one to insert the standard speculum and the second to insert another speculum to open laterally. This permits full visualization of the cervix and enables the examiner to obtain scrapings for slides. This is uncomfortable for the patient.

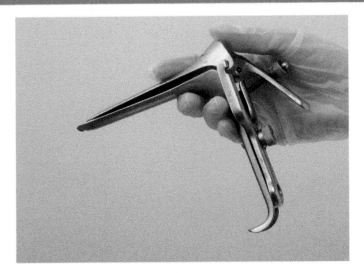

Figure 24.10 Holding the speculum.

3. **Insert the speculum.**

   - Tell the patient that you are going to examine her cervix, and that to do so, you are going to insert a speculum. If this is the patient's first vaginal examination, show her the speculum, and briefly demonstrate how you will use it to visualize her cervix. Have a mirror available to share findings with the patient. Also explain that she will feel pressure, first of your fingers, and then of the speculum. You may also want to show her a booklet with a picture demonstrating the technique.
   - With your nondominant hand, place your index and middle fingers on the posterior vaginal opening and apply pressure gently downward.
   - Turn the speculum blades obliquely.
   - Place the blades over your fingers at the vaginal opening and slowly insert the closed speculum at a 45-degree downward angle (see Figure 24.11 ■). This angle matches the downward slope of the vagina when the patient is in the lithotomy position.

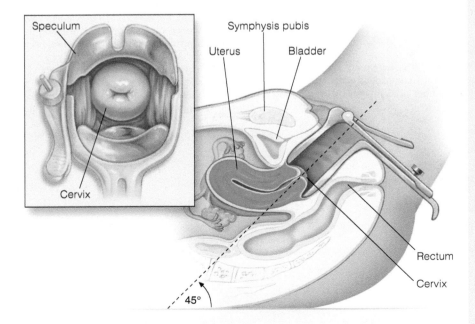

Figure 24.11 Speculum inserted into vagina.

Techniques and Normal Findings	Abnormal Findings Special Considerations

- Ask the patient to bear down as you insert the speculum. It is normal for the patient to tense as the speculum is inserted, and bearing down helps to relax the muscles.
- Once the speculum is inserted, withdraw your fingers and turn the speculum clockwise until the blades are in a horizontal plane.
- Advance the blades at a downward 45-degree angle until they are completely inserted.
- This maneuver should not cause the patient pain.
- Avoid pinching the labia or pulling on the patient's pubic hair. If insertion of the speculum causes the patient pain, stop immediately and reevaluate your technique.
- To open the speculum blades, squeeze the speculum handle.
- Sweep the speculum blades upward until the cervix comes into view.
- Adjust the speculum blades as needed until the cervix is fully exposed between them.
- Tighten the thumbscrew to stabilize the spread of the blades.

▶ Prior to insertion, apply lubricating gel to the speculum. Lubricating gel is superior to water for reducing pain associated with speculum insertion (VandenBerg & Prasad, 2012).

4. Visualize the cervix.
- Confirm that the cervix is pink, moist, round, and centrally positioned, and that it has a small opening in the center called the os.
- Note any bluish coloring.

▶ A bluish coloring is seen during the second month of pregnancy and is called *Chadwick's sign*. Otherwise, a bluish color is indicative of cyanosis.

- Confirm that any secretions are clear or white and without odor.

▶ Green discharge that has a foul smell is associated with gonorrhea. Thick discharge is seen in *candidiasis*. Frothy, yellow-green discharge is seen in *trichomoniasis*. A yellow discharge can also be visualized in chlamydial infection. *Bacterial vaginitis* presents with a creamy-gray to white discharge that has a fishy odor.

- Confirm that the cervix is free from erosions, ulcerations, lacerations, and polyps.

▶ Erosions are associated with carcinoma or infections. Ulcerations can be due to carcinoma, syphilis, and tuberculosis. Yellow cysts or nodules are *nabothian cysts*, benign cysts that may appear after childbirth.

Obtaining the Pap Smear and Gonorrhea Culture

The Pap (Papanicolaou) smear consists of three specimens: an endocervical swab, a cervical scrape, and a vaginal pool sample.

Have ready prelabeled slides for specimens, either (a) one labeled *endocervical*, one labeled *vaginal*, and one labeled *cervical* or (b) one slide that has sections for each sample.

1. Perform an endocervical swab.
- Carefully insert a saline-moistened, cotton-tipped applicator or Cytobrush®GT into the vagina and into the cervical os.

▶ Moistening the applicator with saline prevents the cells from being absorbed into the cotton.
   The cytobrush is recommended over the cotton-tipped applicator because more endocervical cells adhere to it, thus yielding more accurate results.

- Do not force insertion of the applicator.

▶ If the applicator cannot be slipped into the cervical os, a tumor may be blocking the opening.

Techniques and Normal Findings	Abnormal Findings Special Considerations

- Rotate the applicator in a complete circle (see Figure 24.12 ■).

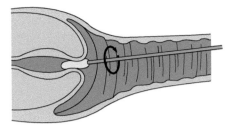

Figure 24.12 The endocervical swab.

- Roll a thin coat across the slide labeled *endocervical*.
- Spray fixative on the slide immediately or place it in a container filled with fixative.

▶ A thin coat is preferred because a thick coat may be difficult to assess under the microscope.

2. **Obtain a cervical scrape.**
   - Insert the longer end of a bifid spatula into the patient's vagina.
   - Advance the fingerlike projection of the bifid end gently into the cervical os.
   - Allow the shorter end to rest on the outer ridge of the cervix.
   - Rotate the applicator one full 360-degree turn clockwise to scrape cells from the cervix (see Figure 24.13 ■).

▶ If the patient has had a hysterectomy, obtain the scrape from the surgical stump.

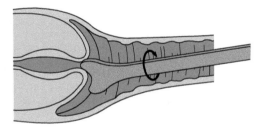

Figure 24.13 The cervical scrape.

- Do not rotate the applicator more than once or turn it in a counterclockwise manner.
- Spread a thin smear across the slide labeled *cervical* from each side of the applicator.
- Spray fixative on the slide immediately or place in a container filled with fixative.

3. **Obtain a vaginal pool sample.**
   - Insert the paddle end of the spatula into the vaginal recess area (fornix). Alternatively, you may use a saline-moistened cotton-tipped applicator.
   - Gently rotate the spatula back and forth to obtain a sample (see Figure 24.14 ■).

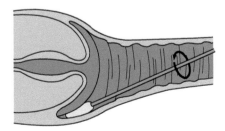

Figure 24.14 The vaginal pool sample.

- Apply the specimen to the slide labeled *vaginal*.
- Spray fixative on the slide immediately.

Techniques and Normal Findings	Abnormal Findings Special Considerations

4. Obtain a gonorrhea culture.

- Obtain a gonorrhea culture if the assessment findings indicate.
- Insert a saline-moistened cotton-tipped applicator into the cervical os.
- Leave the applicator in place for 20 seconds to allow full saturation of the cotton.
- Using a Z-shaped pattern, roll a thin coat of the secretions onto a Thayer-Martin culture plate labeled *cervical*.

▶ Nurses must be sure to check with the laboratory in their institution because techniques and protocols may differ.

5. Remove the speculum.

- Gently loosen the thumbscrew on the speculum while holding the handles securely.

▶ The infections that contribute to the development of discolored or foul-smelling vaginal discharge are the same as those listed in the previous section on identifying cervical discharge.

- Slant the speculum from side to side as you slide it from the vaginal canal.
- While you withdraw the speculum, note that the vaginal mucosa is pink, consistent in texture, rugated, and nontender. Discharge is thin or stringy and clear or opaque.
- Close the speculum blades before complete removal.

Bimanual Palpation

Stand at the end of the examination table. The patient remains in the lithotomy position.

1. Palpate the cervix.

- Lubricate the index and middle fingers of your gloved dominant hand.
- Inform the patient that you are going to palpate her cervix.
- Place your nondominant hand against the patient's thigh, then insert your lubricated index and middle fingers into her vaginal opening.
- Proceed downward at a 45-degree angle until you reach the cervix.
- Keep the other fingers of that hand rounded inward toward the palm and put the thumb against the mons pubis away from the clitoris.

▶ Pressure on the clitoris may be painful for the patient.

Techniques and Normal Findings

Abnormal Findings
Special Considerations

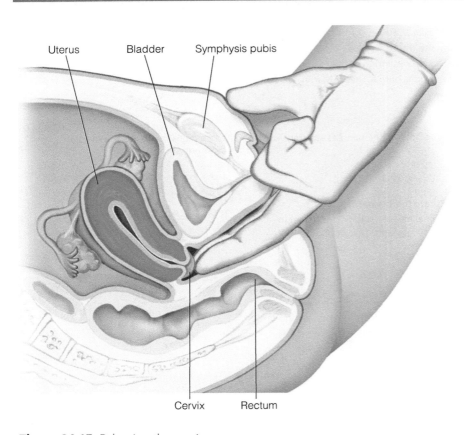

Uterus   Bladder   Symphysis pubis

Cervix   Rectum

Figure 24.15 Palpating the cervix.

- Palpate the cervix. It should feel firm and smooth, somewhat like the tip of a nose (see Figure 24.15 ■).

- Gently try to move it. It should move easily about 1 to 2 cm (0.39 to 0.78 in.) in either direction.

▶ Nodules, hardness, or lack of mobility suggest a tumor.

▶ If the woman is pregnant, the cervix will be soft. This is a normal finding and is called Goodell's sign.

2. **Palpate the fornices.**
   - Slip your fingers into the vaginal recess areas, called the fornices.
   - Palpate around the grooves.
   - Confirm that the mucosa of the vagina and cervix in these areas is smooth and nontender.
   - Leave your fingers in the anterior fornix when you have checked all sides.

▶ Note any tenderness, which could be indicative of inflammation.

3. **Palpate the uterus.**
   - Place the fingers of your nondominant hand on the patient's abdomen.

Techniques and Normal Findings	Abnormal Findings Special Considerations

- Invaginate the abdomen midway between the umbilicus and the symphysis pubis by pushing with your fingertips downward toward the cervix (see Figure 24.16 ■).

▶ Note tenderness, masses, nodules, or bulging. These findings may indicate inflammation, infection, cysts, tumors, or wall prolapse. Note size, shape, consistency, and mobility of nodules and masses.

▶ In the obese female, it may be difficult to clearly differentiate the uterine structures, and an ultrasound study may be needed.

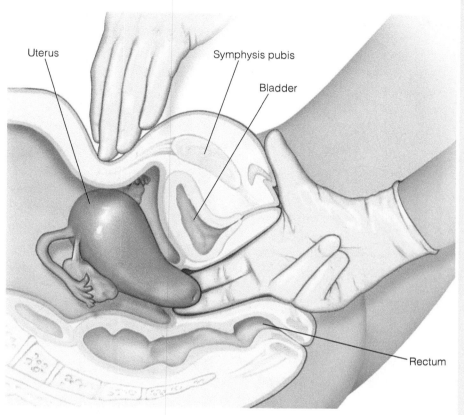

Uterus
Symphysis pubis
Bladder
Rectum

Figure 24.16 Palpating the uterus.

- Palpate the front wall of the uterus with the hand that is inside the vagina.
- As you palpate, note the position of the uterine body to determine that the uterus is in a normal position. When in a normal position, the uterus is tilted slightly upward above the bladder, and the cervix is tilted slightly forward.

Techniques and Normal Findings	Abnormal Findings Special Considerations

- Normal variations of uterine position are:
  - **Anteversion** uterus tilted forward, cervix tilted downward (see Figure 24.17A ■)
  - **Midposition** uterus lies parallel to tailbone, cervix pointed straight (see Figure 24.17B)
  - **Retroversion** uterus tilted backward, cervix tilted upward (see Figure 24.17C)

▶ Abnormal variations of uterine position are:
- **Anteflexion** uterus folded forward at about a 90-degree angle, and cervix tilted downward (see Figure 24.17D)
- **Retroflexion** uterus folded backward at about a 90-degree angle, cervix tilted upward (see Figure 24.17E).

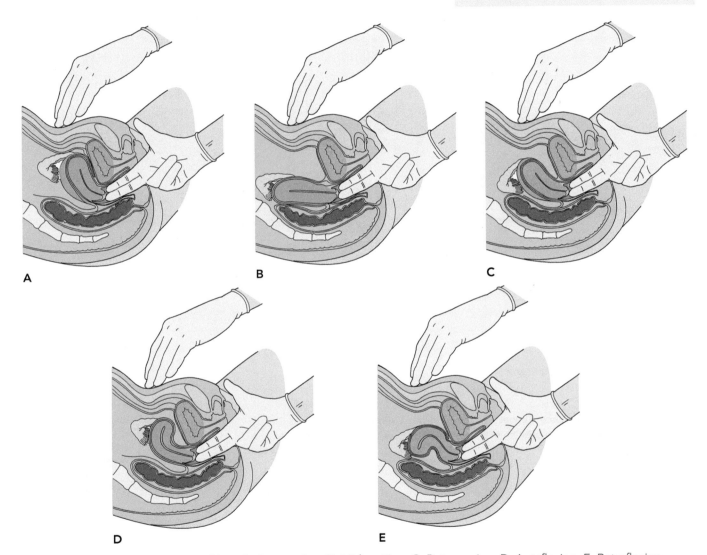

Figure 24.17 Variations in uterine position. A. Anteversion. B. Midposition. C. Retroversion. D. Anteflexion. E. Retroflexion.

- Move the inner fingers to the posterior fornix, and gently raise the cervix up toward your outer hand.
- Palpate the front and back walls of the uterus as it is sandwiched between the two hands.

▶ Masses, tenderness, nodules, or bulging require further evaluation.

4. **Palpate the ovaries.**
   - While positioning the outer hand on the left lower abdominal quadrant, slip the vaginal fingers into the left lateral fornix.

▶ Extreme tenderness; nodularity; and masses are suggestive of inflammation, infection, cysts, malignancies, or tubal pregnancy.

Techniques and Normal Findings	Abnormal Findings Special Considerations

- Push the opposing fingers and hand toward one another, and then use small circular motions to palpate the left ovary with your intravaginal fingers (see Figure 24.18 ■).

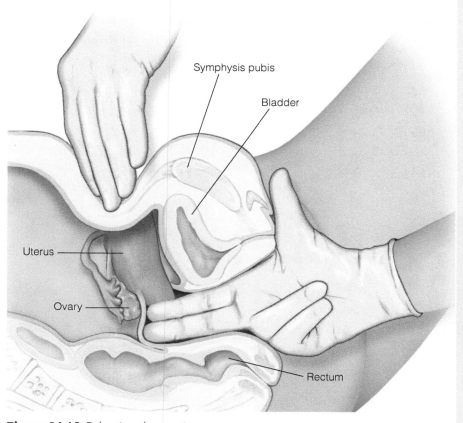

Symphysis pubis

Bladder

Uterus

Ovary

Rectum

Figure 24.18 Palpating the ovaries.

- If you are able to palpate the ovary, it will feel mobile, almond shaped, smooth, firm, and nontender to slightly tender. Often you will be unable to palpate the ovaries, especially the right ovary.

- Slide your vaginal fingers around to the right lateral fornix and your outer hand to the lower right quadrant to palpate the right ovary.
- Confirm that the uterine tubes are not palpable.

- Remove your hand from the vagina and put on new gloves.

5. **Perform the rectovaginal exam.**
- Tell the patient that you are going to insert one finger into her vagina and one finger into her rectum in order to perform a rectovaginal exam. Tell her that this maneuver may make her feel as though she needs to have a bowel movement.
- Lubricate the gloved index and middle fingers of the dominant hand.
- Ask the patient to bear down.
- Touch the patient's thigh with your nondominant hand to prepare her for the insertion.

▶ In obese females, it may not be possible to palpate the ovaries. In the female patient who has been postmenopausal for more than 2 ½ years, palpable ovaries are considered abnormal because the ovaries usually atrophy with the postmenopausal decrease in estrogen.

▶ If the uterine tubes are palpable, an inflammation or some other disease process such as salpingitis or ectopic pregnancy may be present.

▶ This prevents cross-contamination from the vagina to the rectum.

▶ Note tenderness, masses, nodules, bulging, and thickened areas.

Techniques and Normal Findings	Abnormal Findings / Special Considerations

- Insert the index finger into the vagina (at a 45-degree downward slope) and the middle finger into the rectum.
- Compress the rectovaginal septum between your index and middle fingers.
- Confirm that it is thin, smooth, and nontender.
- Place your nondominant hand on the patient's abdomen.
- While maintaining the position of your intravaginal hand, press your outer hand inward and downward on the abdomen over the symphysis pubis.
- Palpate the posterior side of the uterus with the pad of the rectal finger while continuing to press down on the abdomen (see Figure 24.19 ■).

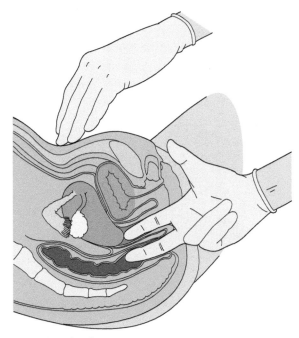

Figure 24.19 Rectovaginal palpation.

- Confirm that the uterine wall is smooth and nontender.
- If the ovaries are palpable, note that they are normal in size and contour.
- Remove your fingers from the vagina and rectum slowly and gently.

▶ Tenderness, masses, nodules, bulging, or thickened areas require further evaluation.

6. Examine the stool.
- Remove your gloves.
- Assist the patient into a comfortable position.
- Inspect feces remaining on the glove. Feces is normally brown and soft. Test feces for occult blood. Normally the test is negative.

▶ Rectal bleeding is suspected when bright red blood is on the surface of the stool. Feces mixed with blood signals bleeding above the rectum.
▶ Black, tarry stool indicates upper gastrointestinal tract bleeding.

- Wash your hands.
- Give the patient tissues to wipe the perineal area. Some patients may need a perineal pad.
- Inform the patient that she may have a small amount of spotting for a few hours after the speculum examination.

Abnormal Findings

Abnormal findings from assessment of the female reproductive system include but are not limited to problems with the external genitalia, perianal area, cervix, internal reproductive organs, and inflammatory processes. Problems in the perianal area are described in this chapter. Abnormal findings of the external genitalia are depicted and described in Table 24.3. Abnormal findings of the cervix are illustrated and described in Table 24.4. Common inflammatory processes in the female reproductive system are depicted and described in Table 24.5. Abnormal findings of the internal reproductive organs include myomas/fibroids, ovarian cancer, and ovarian cysts, which are discussed in the following section.

TABLE 24.3	**Abnormal Findings of the External Genitalia**

Pediculosis Pubis	**Herpes Simplex**
Nits and lice are on and around roots of pubic hair and cause itching. The area is reddened and excoriated.	A sexually transmitted disease caused by the herpes simplex virus (HSV), these small vesicles appear on the genitalia and may spread to the inner thigh. Ulcers are painful and may rupture. The virus may be dormant for long periods.

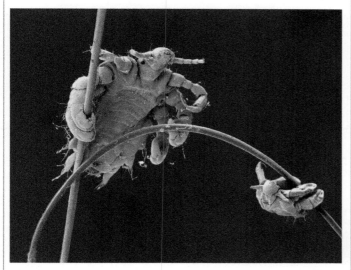

Figure 24.20 Pediculosis pubis (crab lice; magnification 40X).

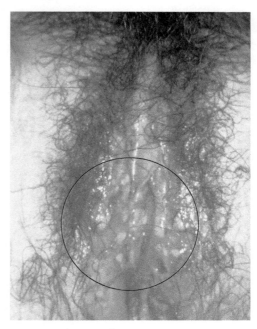

Figure 24.21 Herpes simplex.
Source: Lester V. Bergman/Corbis.

(continued)

TABLE 24.3 **Abnormal Findings of the External Genitalia** (continued)

Syphilitic Lesion

A nontender solitary papule that gradually changes to a draining ulcer. A rash of syphilitic lesions typically develops during the second stage of symptoms associated with syphilis. In most cases, the first stage of syphilis presents as a single chancre (CDC, 2014a).

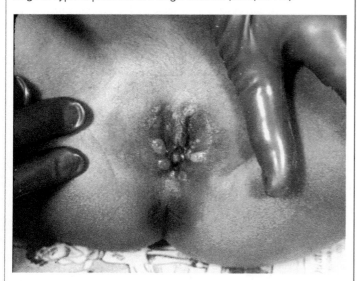

Figure 24.22 Syphilitic lesions.
Source: Centers for Disease Control and Prevention (CDC).

Human Papillomavirus (HPV)

Infection with this sexually transmitted disease causes wartlike, painless growths that appear in clusters. These are seen on the vulva, inner vagina, cervix, or anal area.

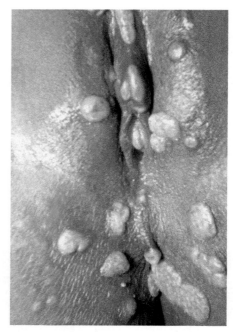

Figure 24.23 Human papillomavirus (genital warts).
Source: Centers for Disease Control and Prevention (CDC).

Abscess of Bartholin's Gland

The Bartholin's gland may become obstructed, causing fluid to back up and form a cyst. Cysts range in size from 1-3 cm or larger. If infected, a cyst develops into an abscess that includes labial edema and erythema with a palpable mass. There is purulent drainage from the duct.

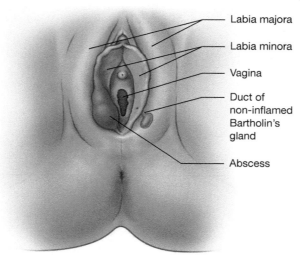

Labia majora

Labia minora

Vagina

Duct of non-inflamed Bartholin's gland

Abscess

Figure 24.24 Abscess of Bartholin's gland.

TABLE 24.4   Abnormal Findings of the Cervix

Cyanosis

Cyanosis of the cervix is associated with hypoxic conditions such as congestive heart failure (CHF). Blue coloring of the cervix is normal in pregnancy.

Diethylstilbestrol (DES) Syndrome

Abnormalities of the cervix arise in females who had prenatal exposure to DES. Epithelial abnormalities occur as granular patchiness extending from the cervix to the vaginal walls.

Carcinoma

Ulcerations with vaginal discharge, postmenopausal bleeding or spotting, or bleeding between menstrual periods are characteristics of cervical carcinoma. Diagnosis is confirmed by Pap smear.

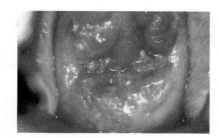

Figure 24.25 Cervical carcinoma.
Source: Centers for Disease Control and Prevention (CDC).

Erosion

Inflammation and erosion are visible on the surface of the cervix. It is difficult to distinguish erosion from carcinoma without a biopsy.

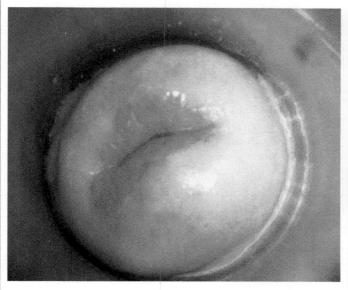

Figure 24.26 Erosion of the cervix.
Source: Centers for Disease Control and Prevention (CDC).

Polyp

A soft, fingerlike growth extends from the cervical os. A polyp is usually bright red and may bleed. Polyps are usually benign.

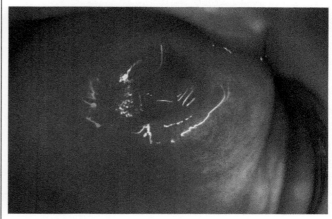

Figure 24.27 Cervical polyp.
Source: Dr. P. Marazzi/Science Source.

TABLE 24.5	Common Inflammatory Processes in the Female Reproductive System

Atrophic Vaginitis	**Chlamydia**	**Pelvic Inflammatory Disease (PID)**
Estrogen deficiency in postmenopausal females results in dryness, itching, and burning sensations in the vagina. The vaginal mucosa may appear pale with mucousy discharge.	A sexually transmitted disease (STD) that is often asymptomatic, characterized by purulent discharge with tenderness to movement of the cervix. Chlamydia can cause sterility if untreated.	An infection of a woman's reproductive organs. PID may cause lower abdominal pain, fever, malodorous discharge from the vagina, painful intercourse or urination, or irregular menstrual bleeding (CDC, 2014b).

Candidiasis	**Gonorrhea**
Alteration of the pH of the vagina or antibiotic use predispose the female to this condition. The vulva and vagina are erythematous. Thick, cheesy white discharge is seen.	This sexually transmitted disease is caused by a bacterial infection. One may see vaginal discharge or bleeding and abscesses in Bartholin's or Skene's glands; generally asymptomatic.

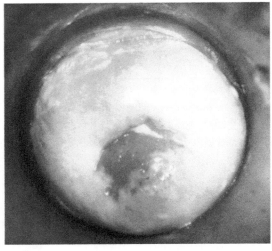

Figure 24.29 Gonorrhea.
Source: Centers for Disease Control and Prevention (CDC).

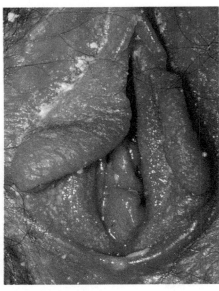

Figure 24.28 Candidiasis (yeast infection).
Source: Wellcome Image Library/Custom Medical Stock Photo.

Trichomoniasis

This is a sexually transmitted disease that causes painful urination, vulvular itching, and purulent vaginal discharge. The vagina and vulva are reddened and the discharge is yellow and foul smelling.

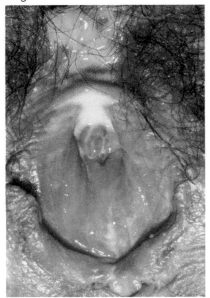

Figure 24.30 Trichomoniasis.
Source: Wellcome Image Library/Custom Medical Stock Photo.

Disorders of the Internal Reproductive Organs

MYOMAS/FIBROIDS

Myomas, or uterine fibroids, are tumors that consist of smooth muscle tissue. They may form in several locations, including the uterine cavity or the uterine muscles (see Figure 24.31 ■). While the exact cause is unknown, estrogen is believed to influence their development (Osborn et al., 2013). Some patients who experience this disorder will be asymptomatic.

Subjective findings:

- Abdominal pain.
- Constipation.
- Frequent urination.
- Excessive menstrual bleeding.

Objective findings:

- Uterine enlargement.
- Abdominal distention.
- Intestinal obstruction.

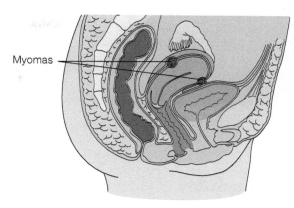

Figure 24.31 Myomas/fibroids.

OVARIAN CANCER

Ovarian cancer (see Figure 24.32 ■) is a type of cancer that begins in the cells of the ovaries and includes the epithelial and germ cells. Although this form of cancer may occur in women of any age, it is most common among women who are 50–60 years old. Factors that increase the risk for development of ovarian cancer include estrogen hormone replacement therapy, smoking, and never being pregnant (Mayo Clinic, 2014b). In early stages, patients who experience ovarian cancer may be asymptomatic.

Subjective findings:

- Abdominal pressure or cramping.
- Unexplained weight loss.
- Changes in bowel habits.
- Loss of appetite.
- Pain in the calves or lower back.

Objective findings:

- Abdominal bloating.
- Ascites.
- Abnormal vaginal bleeding.

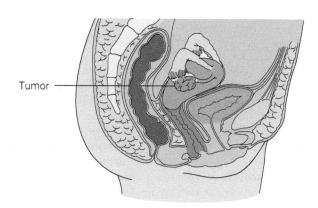

Figure 24.32 Ovarian cancer.

OVARIAN CYSTS

Ovarian cysts are nonmalignant vesicles that may develop at any point between puberty and menopause. These fluid-filled sacs form within the ovary or on the ovarian surface (see Figure 24.33 ■). Some patients who experience ovarian cysts may be asymptomatic.

Subjective findings:

- Pelvic pain.
- Lower back pain.
- Pain during intercourse.

Objective findings:

- Abdominal distention.
- Vomiting.
- Increased urination.
- Menstrual irregularities.

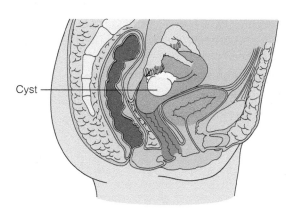

Figure 24.33 Ovarian cysts.

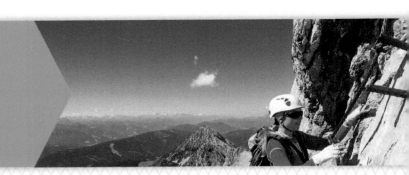

Application Through Critical Thinking

▌ Case Study

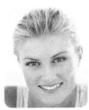

Jessica Johnson, a 24-year-old Caucasian female, arrives in the clinic with lower abdominal pain and nausea. She states, "I've had this throbbing pain for 3 days and it kept getting worse." She further states, "I haven't been able to eat. I feel awful. You have to do something for the pain."

The nurse explains that more information is needed so that the proper treatment can be initiated. In further interview the following information is obtained. Ms. Johnson's last menstrual period was 1 week ago and she had more crampiness than usual. She has had brownish, thick vaginal discharge on and off since then. She has had some itchiness in the vaginal area and burning when she voids. She states she has to go to the bathroom all the time: "All I did was pee little bits, until this pain got to me. I have hardly gone since last night."

When asked about the pain, Ms. Johnson says it is mostly 8 on a scale of 1 to 10 and getting pretty constant. "Nothing I do helps, except it helps a little if I curl up and hold still."

Physical assessment reveals a thin, pale female.

VS: B/P 108/64, P 92, RR 20, T 101.4°F.	Skin is hot, dry, poor turgor.

Mucous membranes dry. Posture—abdominal guarding.

Abdomen BS × 4, tender in RLQ & LLQ to palpation. Vulvar pruritus, thick purulent vaginal drainage, pain upon cervical and uterine movement.

Cultures from vaginal secretions obtained	To lab
Blood drawn for CBC	To lab
Urine specimen obtained—clear, yellow	To lab

The patient's clinic record reveals that she has been sexually active since age 16. She has had multiple partners and one abortion. She has been treated for an STD three times, most recently 2 months prior to this visit. The patient is on birth control pills. She has no allergies to medications, and no family history of cardiovascular, abdominal, neurologic, urologic, endocrine, or reproductive disease.

Interpretation of the data suggests a diagnosis of PID. The options are outpatient treatment with antibiotics and education about limitations in activity and sexual practices, or inpatient treatment with intravenous fluids, antibiotics, analgesia, and bed rest.

Because Ms. Johnson is acutely ill, with pain and dehydration, she is admitted to the acute care facility with a diagnosis of PID.

▌ Complete Documentation

The following is sample documentation for Jessica Johnson.

SUBJECTIVE DATA: Throbbing abdominal pain for 3 days and getting worse. Rated 8 on scale of 1 to 10 with slight relief when "curled up and still." Nausea, unable to eat. LMP 1 week ago with increased crampiness. Brownish thick vaginal discharge. Vaginal itchiness. Urgent, burning urination of small amounts until past 12 hours. Sexually active with history of multiple partners, recent STD. No family history of disease, no allergies to medication.

OBJECTIVE DATA: Thin, pale female. Dry mucous membranes, skin hot, dry, poor turgor. Abdominal guarding, BS present × 4, tender RLQ, LLQ to light palpation. Vulvar pruritus, purulent vaginal discharge, adnexal tenderness with vaginal and bimanual examination.

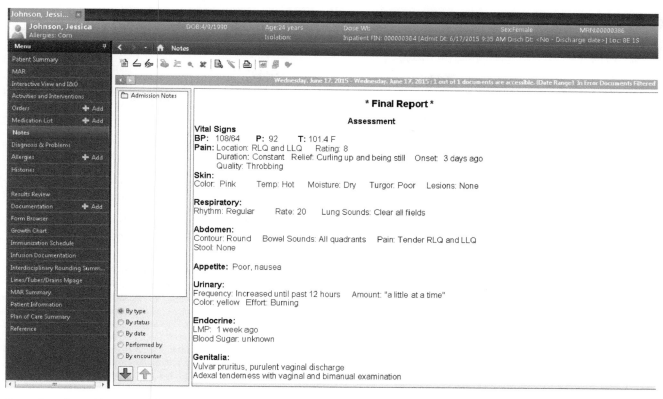

Source: From Cerner Electronic Health Record. Copyright © by Cerner Corporation. Used by permission of Cerner Corporation.

▌ Critical Thinking Questions

1. What clusters of information suggest the diagnosis of PID?
2. What additional information is required to develop a plan of care for Jessica Johnson?
3. What would discharge planning for Ms. Johnson include?
4. Which *Healthy People 2020* objectives are related to this scenario?
5. What environmental considerations should you screen for in a young female of childbearing age during the patient interview?

▌ Prepare Teaching Plan

LEARNING NEED: Jessica Johnson initiated sexual activity at 16 years of age. She has had multiple partners and frequent episodes of STD. These data indicate a need to learn about PID and to discuss this infection with her partner.

GOAL: Jessica Johnson will decrease her risk for repeated episodes of PID.

OBJECTIVES: Jessica Johnson will be able to:

1. Describe PID.
2. Relate personal practices to the occurrence of PID.
3. Describe treatment modalities for PID.

APPLICATION OF OBJECTIVE 2: Relate personal practices to the occurrence of PID (Cognitive)

Content	Teaching Strategy	Evaluation
• Frequent douching will mask symptoms or push organisms internally. • Sexual activity before age 25. • Multiple partners. • Partner with multiple partners. • Use of IUD. • Not practicing safe sex—use of condoms will help decrease risk. • Untreated STD.	One-on-one discussion encourages learner participation, permits reinforcement of content, and is appropriate for sensitive subject matter.	Jessica relates her personal practices to the occurrence of PID.

▶ References

The American College of Obstetricians and Gynecologists (ACOG). (2014). *Committee opinion: Well-woman visit.* Retrieved from http://www.acog.org/Resources-And-Publications/Committee-Opinions/Committee-on-Gynecologic-Practice/Well-Woman-Visit

Basson, R., Rees, P., Wang, R., Montejo, A. L., & Incrocci, L. (2010). Sexual function in chronic illness. *The Journal of Sexual Medicine, 7,* 374–388.

Berman, A., & Snyder, S. J. (2012). *Kozier and Erb's fundamentals of nursing: Concepts, process, and practice* (9th ed.). Upper Saddle River, NJ: Prentice Hall.

Bikley, L. S. (2008). *Bates' guide to physical examination and history taking* (10th ed.). Philadelphia, PA: Lippincott.

Centers for Disease Control and Prevention (CDC). (2012). *Human papillomavirus: HPV vaccines.* Retrieved from http://www.cdc.gov/hpv/vaccine.html

Centers for Disease Control and Prevention (CDC). (2013a). *Sexually transmitted diseases (STDs): STDs & infertility.* Retrieved from http://www.cdc.gov/STD/infertility/default.htm

Centers for Disease Control and Prevention (CDC). (2013b). Condoms and STDs: fact sheet for public health personnel. Retrieved from http://www.cdc.gov/condomeffectiveness/docs/condoms_and_stds.pdf

Centers for Disease Control and Prevention (CDC). (2014a). *Syphilis: CDC fact sheet.* Retrieved from http://www.cdc.gov/std/syphilis/stdfact-syphilis-detailed.htm

Centers for Disease Control and Prevention (CDC). (2014b). *Pelvic inflammatory disease (PID).* Retrieved from http://www.cdc.gov/std/pid/stdfact-pid.htm

Colombo, N., Preti, E., Landoni, F., Carinelli, S., Colombo, A., Marini, C., & Sessa, C. (2011). Endometrial cancer: ESMO Clinical Practice Guidelines for diagnosis, treatment and follow-up. *Annals of Oncology, 22*(Suppl 6), vi35–vi39.

Dei, M., Di Maggio, F., Di Paolo, G., & Bruni, V. (2010). Vulvovaginitis in childhood. *Best Practice & Research Clinical Obstetrics & Gynaecology, 24*(2), 129–137.

Gray, H. (2010). *Gray's anatomy.* New York: Barnes & Noble Books.

Hegazy, A. A., & Al-Rukban, M. O. (2012). Hymen: facts and conceptions. *The Health, 3,* 109–115.

Ignatavicus, D., & Workman, M. L. (2008). *Medical-surgical nursing: Critical thinking for collaborative care* (5th ed.). St. Louis, MO: Elsevier/Saunders.

Johns Hopkins Medicine. (n.d.). *Pap test: Procedure overview.* Retrieved from http://www.hopkinsmedicine.org/healthlibrary/test_procedures/gynecology/pap_test_procedure_92,P07783/

Ju, H., Jones, M., & Mishra, G. (2013). The prevalence and risk factors of dysmenorrhea. *Epidemiologic reviews, 36*(1), 104–113.

Kessous, R., Aricha-Tamir, B., Sheizaf, B., Steiner, N., Moran-Gilad, J., & Weintraub, A. Y. (2013). Clinical and microbiological characteristics of Bartholin gland abscesses. *Obstetrics & Gynecology, 122*(4), 794–799.

Laronda, M. M., Unno, K., Butler, L. M., & Kurita, T. (2012). The development of cervical and vaginal adenosis as a result of diethylstilbestrol exposure in utero. *Differentiation, 84*(3), 252–260.

Lee, D. Y., Oh, Y. K., Yoon, B. K., & Choi, D. (2012). Prevalence of hyperprolactinemia in adolescents and young women with menstruation-related problems. *American Journal of Obstetrics and Gynecology, 206*(3), 213,e1–213.e5.

MacPhee, R. A., Miller, W. L., Gloor, G. B., McCormick, J. K., Hammond, J. A., Burton, J. P., & Reid, G. (2013). Influence of the vaginal microbiota on toxic shock syndrome toxin 1 production by Staphylococcus aureus. *Applied and Environmental Microbiology, 79*(6), 1835–1842.

Marieb, E. (2009). *Essentials of human anatomy and physiology* (9th ed.). Redwood City, CA: Benjamin/Cummings.

Mayo Clinic. (2011). *Menorrhagia (heavy menstrual bleeding): Symptoms.* Retrieved from http://www.mayoclinic.org/diseases-conditions/menorrhagia/basics/symptoms/con-20021959

Mayo Clinic. (2014a). *Getting pregnant: How to get pregnant.* Retrieved from http://www.mayoclinic.org/healthy-living/getting-pregnant/in-depth/how-to-get-pregnant/art-20047611

Mayo Clinic. (2014b). *Ovarian cancer: Risk factors.* Retrieved from http://www.mayoclinic.org/diseases-conditions/ovarian-cancer/basics/risk-factors/con-20028096

Mayo Foundation for Medical Education and Research. (2014). *Rochester test catalog: 2014 online test catalog.* Available at http://www.mayomedicallaboratories.com/test-catalog/

Osborn, K. S., Wraa, C. E., Watson, A., & Holleran, R. S. (2013). *Medical-surgical nursing: Preparation for practice.* (2nd ed.). Upper Saddle River, NJ: Pearson.

Pawlik, M., & Martin, F. J. (2009). Does a water-based lubricant affect Pap smear and cervical microbiology results? *Canadian Family Physician, 55*(4), 376–377.

Simpson, J., Robinson, K., Creighton, S. M., & Hodes, D. (2012). Female genital mutilation: The role of health professionals in prevention, assessment, and management. *BMJ, 344,* e1361: 1–7.

Singh, R. H., Zenilman, J. M., Brown, K. M., Madden, T., Gaydos, C., & Ghanem, K. G. (2012). The role of physical examination in diagnosing common causes of vaginitis: A prospective study. *Sexually Transmitted Infections, 89*(3), 185–190.

U.S. Department of Health and Human Services (USDHHS). (2014). *Healthy people 2020.* Retrieved from http://www.healthypeople.gov/2020/default.aspx

VandenBerg, N., & Prasad, S. (2012). Easing the discomfort of a speculum exam. *Journal of Family Practice, 61*(9): E1–E3.

World Health Organization (WHO). (n.d.). *Sexual and reproductive health: Infertility definitions and terminology.* Retrieved from http://www.who.int/reproductivehealth/topics/infertility/definitions/en/

Xu, F., Stoner, B. P., Taylor, S. N., Mena, L., Martin, D. H., Powell, S., & Markowitz, L. E. (2013). "Testing-only" visits: An assessment of missed diagnoses in patients attending sexually transmitted disease clinics. *Sexually Transmitted Diseases, 40*(1), 64–69.

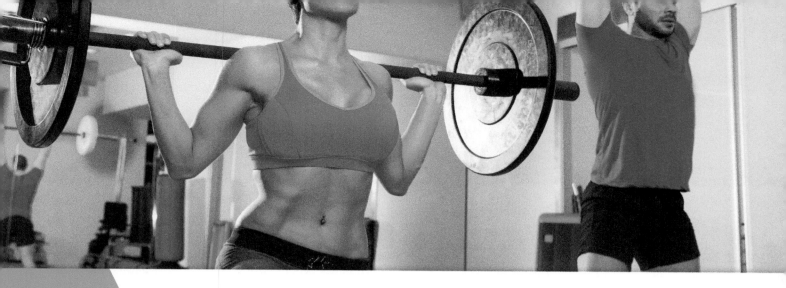

▌ Learning Outcomes

Upon completion of this chapter, you will be able to:

1. Describe the anatomy and physiology of the bones, muscles, and joints.

2. Discuss the directional movements of the joints.

3. Develop questions to be used when completing the focused interview.

4. Outline techniques used for assessment of the musculoskeletal system.

5. Differentiate normal from abnormal findings of the musculoskeletal system.

6. Describe the developmental, cultural, psychosocial, and environmental variations in assessment and findings of the musculoskeletal system.

7. Relate musculoskeletal health to *Healthy People 2020* objectives.

8. Apply critical thinking to the physical assessment of the musculoskeletal system.

Key Terms

abduction, 691
acetabulum, 694
adduction, 691
ballottement, 727
bursae, 686
calcaneus, 694
cartilaginous joint, 686
circumduction, 691
depression, 692
developmental dysplasia
   of the hip, 725
dorsiflexion, 691
elevation, 692
eversion, 692
extension, 691
fibrous joint, 686
flexion, 691
fracture, 736
gliding, 691
hallux valgus, 729
hyperextension, 691
inversion, 692
joint, 686
kyphosis, 731
lordosis, 731

The primary function of the musculoskeletal system is to provide structure and movement for the human body. The 206 bones of the musculoskeletal system and accompanying skeletal muscles allow the body to stand erect and move, and they support and protect body organs. This system produces red blood cells, stores fat and minerals, and generates body heat.

A thorough assessment of the musculoskeletal system provides data relevant to activity, exercise, nutrition, and metabolism. The physical assessment of the musculoskeletal system is extensive, requiring a head-to-toe approach because it extends throughout the body. Musculoskeletal assessment could be combined with assessment of other body systems to obtain data reflecting the patient's total health status, because every other body system is affected by or affects this body system. For example, should the patient have difficulty moving a specific part of the body, the nurse will need to collect data that is useful in determining whether the origin of the problem is neurologic or musculoskeletal. Bone density and curvatures vary widely among people of different cultural groups. Working conditions that require heavy lifting, repetitive motions, or substantial physical activity present potential risks to this system. Participation in hobbies and athletic activities can contribute to "wear and tear" damage to joints and create risks for trauma to bones, muscles, and joints. Changes in bone density and injury to bone and muscle are factors in health promotion as discussed in *Healthy People 2020*. Actions to achieve the objectives are included in Table 25.3 on page 697.

Anatomy and Physiology Review

The musculoskeletal system consists of the bones, skeletal muscles, and joints. A thorough discussion of these anatomic structures is included in the following sections.

Bones

The bones support and provide a framework for the soft tissues and organs of the body. They are classified according to shape and composition. Bone shapes include *long bones* (femur, humerus); *short bones* (carpals, tarsals); *flat bones* (the parietal bone of the skull, the sternum, ribs); and *irregular bones* (vertebrae, hip bones) as shown in Figure 25.1 ■. Bones are composed of osseous tissue that is arranged in either a dense, smooth, compact structure, or a cancellous, spongy structure with many small open spaces (see Figure 25.2 ■). The bones of the human skeleton are illustrated in Figure 25.3 ■.

The major functions of the bones include providing a framework for the body, protecting structures, acting as levers for movement, storing fat and minerals, and producing blood cells.

Skeletal Muscles

A skeletal muscle is composed of hundreds of thousands of elongated muscle cells or fibers arranged in striated bands that attach to skeletal bones (see Figure 25.4 ■ on page 689). Although some skeletal muscles react by reflex, most skeletal muscles are voluntary and are under an individual's conscious control. Figure 25.5 ■ on page 689 illustrates the muscles of the human body. The major functions of the skeletal muscles include providing for movement, maintaining posture, and generating body heat.

Joints

A **joint** (or *articulation*) is the point where two or more bones in the body meet. Joints may be classified structurally as fibrous, cartilaginous, or synovial. Bones joined by fibrous tissue, such as the sutures joining the bones of the skull, are called **fibrous joints.** Bones joined by cartilage, such as the vertebrae, are called **cartilaginous joints.** Bones separated by a fluid-filled joint cavity are called **synovial joints**. The structure of synovial joints allows tremendous freedom of movement, and all joints of the limbs are synovial joints. Most synovial joints are reinforced and strengthened by a system of *ligaments,* which are bands of flexible tissue that attach bone to bone. Some ligaments are protected from friction by small, synovial fluid–filled sacs called **bursae. Tendons** are tough fibrous bands that attach muscle to bone, or muscle to muscle. Tendons, subjected to continuous friction, develop fluid-filled bursae called *tendon sheaths* to protect the joint from damage.

During the assessment of the musculoskeletal system, the nurse assesses the joint; its range of motion; and its surrounding structures of muscles, ligaments, tendons, and bursae. Table 25.1 on page 690 describes the classification of synovial joints, and Table 25.2 on page 691 describes the movements of the joints. A description of selected joints to be examined during the physical assessment of the musculoskeletal system follows. Information about terminology used to describe anatomic planes and positions is provided in Table 1.1 (see page 6). ∞

Temporomandibular Joint

The temporomandibular joint (TMJ) permits articulation between the mandible and the temporal bone of the skull (see Figure 25.6 ■ on page 693). Lying just anterior to the external auditory meatus, at the level of the tragus of the ear, the temporomandibular joint allows an individual to speak and chew. Temporomandibular joint movements include the following:

- Opening and closing of the lower jaw
- Protraction and retraction of the lower jaw
- Side-to-side movement of the lower jaw

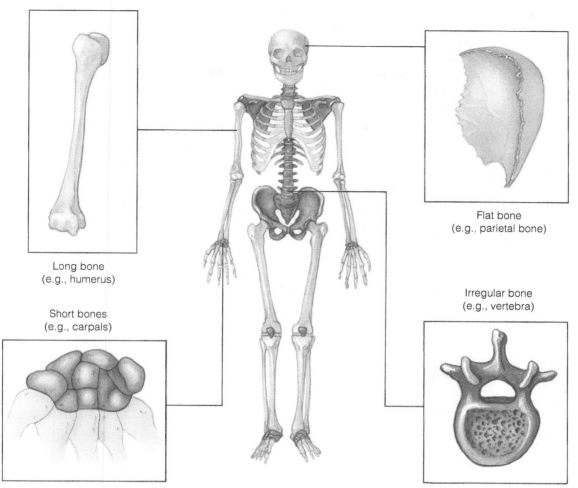

Long bone
(e.g., humerus)

Short bones
(e.g., carpals)

Flat bone
(e.g., parietal bone)

Irregular bone
(e.g., vertebra)

Figure 25.1 Classification of bones according to shape.

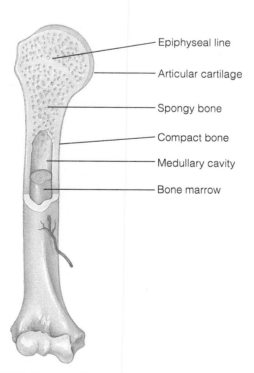

- Epiphyseal line
- Articular cartilage
- Spongy bone
- Compact bone
- Medullary cavity
- Bone marrow

Figure 25.2 Composition of a long bone.

Shoulder

The shoulder joint is a ball-and-socket joint in which the head of the humerus articulates in the shallow glenoid cavity of the scapula (see Table 25.1). The shoulder is supported by the rotator cuff, a sturdy network of tendons and muscles, as well as a series of ligaments (see Figure 25.7 ■ on page 693). The major landmarks of the shoulder include the scapula, the acromion process, the greater tubercle of the humerus, and the coracoid process. The subacromial bursa, which allows the arm to abduct smoothly and with ease, lies just below the acromion process. Movements of the shoulder include the following:

- Abduction (180 degrees)
- Adduction (50 degrees)
- Horizontal forward flexion (180 degrees)
- Horizontal backward extension (50 degrees)
- Circumduction (360 degrees)
- External rotation (90 degrees)
- Internal rotation (90 degrees)

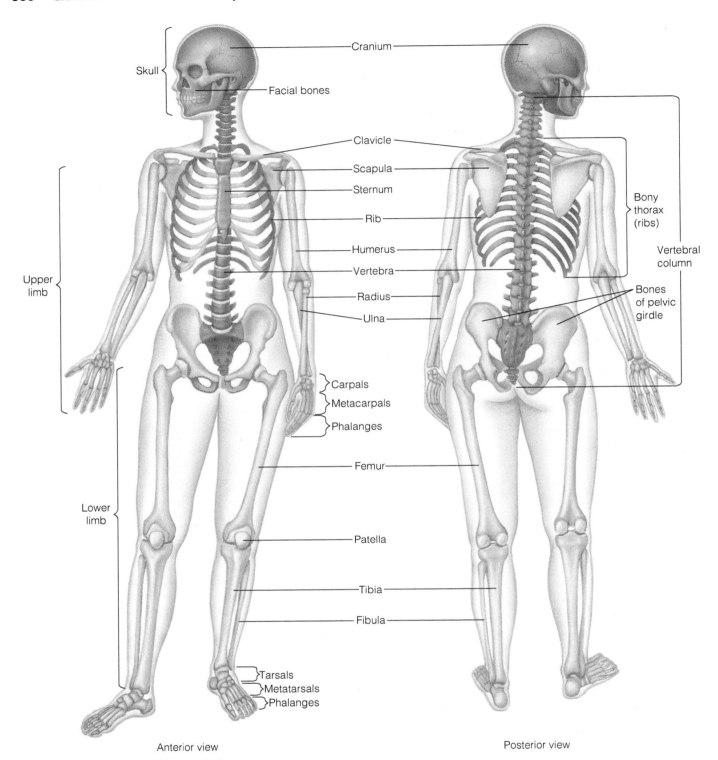

Figure 25.3 Bones of the human skeleton.

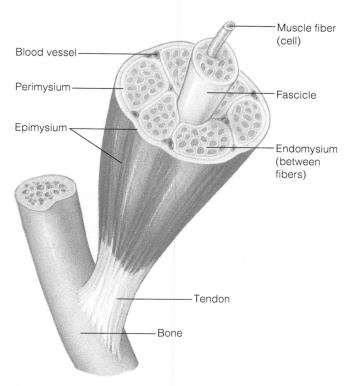

Figure 25.4 Composition of a skeletal muscle.

Elbow

The elbow is a hinge joint that allows articulation between the humerus of the upper arm and the radius and ulna of the forearm (see Figure 25.8 ■ on page 693). Landmarks include the lateral and medial epicondyles on either side of the distal end of the humerus and the olecranon process of the ulna. The olecranon bursa sits between the olecranon process and the skin. The ulnar nerve travels between the medial epicondyle and the olecranon process. When inflamed, the synovial membrane is palpable between the epicondyles and the olecranon process. Elbow movements include the following:

- Flexion of the forearm (160 degrees)
- Extension of the forearm (160 degrees)
- Supination of the forearm and hand (90 degrees)
- Pronation of the forearm and hand (90 degrees)

Wrist and Hand

The wrist (or *carpus*) consists of two rows of eight short carpal bones connected by ligaments as illustrated in Figure 25.9 ■ (see page 694). The distal row articulates with the metacarpals of the hand. The proximal row includes the scaphoid and lunate bones,

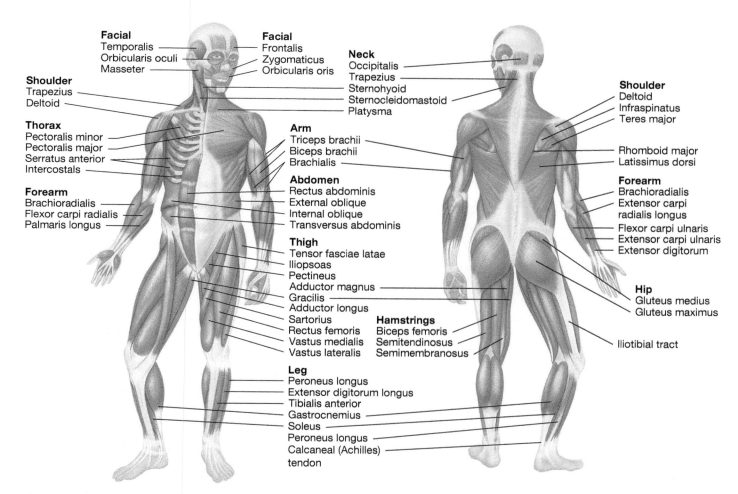

Figure 25.5 Anterior and posterior views of the muscles of the human body.

TABLE 25.1	Classification of Synovial Joints
TYPE OF JOINT	
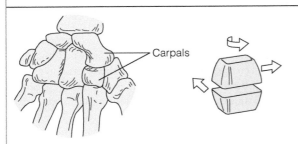 **A** Plane joint	In *plane joints*, the articular surfaces are flat, allowing only slipping or gliding movements. Examples include the intercarpal and intertarsal joints and the joints between the articular processes of the ribs.
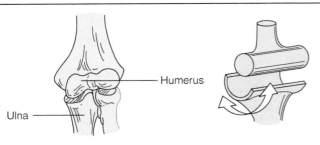 **B** Hinge joint	In *hinge joints*, a convex projection of one bone fits into a concave depression in another. Motion is similar to that of a mechanical hinge. These joints permit flexion and extension only. Examples include the elbow and knee joints.
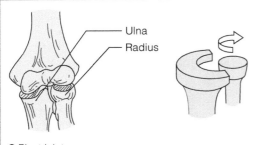 **C** Pivot joint	In *pivot joints*, the rounded end of one bone protrudes into a ring of bone (and possibly ligaments). The only movement allowed is rotation of the bone around its own long axis or against the other bone. An example is the joint between the atlas and axis of the neck.
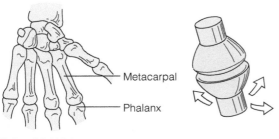 **D** Condyloid joint	In *condyloid joints*, the oval surfaces of two bones fit together. Movements allowed are flexion and extension, abduction, adduction, and circumduction. An example is the radiocarpal (wrist) joints.
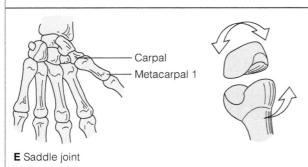 **E** Saddle joint	In *saddle joints*, each articulating bone has both concave and convex areas (resembling a saddle). The opposing surfaces fit together. The movements allowed are the same as for condyloid joints, but the freedom of motion is greater. The carpometacarpal joints of the thumbs are an example.

TABLE 25.1	**Classification of Synovial Joints** (continued)

TYPE OF JOINT	
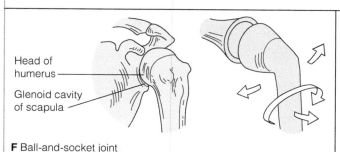 Head of humerus Glenoid cavity of scapula **F** Ball-and-socket joint	In *ball-and-socket joints,* the ball-shaped head of one bone fits into the concave socket of another. These joints allow movement in all axes and planes, including rotation. The shoulder and hip joints are the only examples in the body.

TABLE 25.2	**Joint Movement**

TYPE OF MOVEMENT	
	Gliding movements are the simplest type of joint movements. One flat bone surface glides or slips over another similar surface. The bones are merely displaced in relation to one another.
	Flexion is a bending movement that decreases the angle of the joint and brings the articulating bones closer together. **Extension** increases the angle between the articulating bones. (**Hyperextension** is a bending of a joint beyond 180 degrees.)
	Flexion of the ankle so that the superior aspect of the foot approaches the shin is called **dorsiflexion.** Extension of the ankle (pointing the toes) is called **plantar flexion.**
	Abduction is movement of a limb away from the midline or median plane of the body, along the frontal plane. When the term is used to describe movement of the fingers or toes, it means spreading them apart. **Adduction** is the movement of a limb toward the body midline. Bringing the fingers close together is adduction.
	Circumduction is the movement in which the limb describes a cone in space: While the distal end of the limb moves in a circle, the joint itself moves only slightly in the joint cavity.

(continued)

TABLE 25.2   Joint Movement (continued)

TYPE OF MOVEMENT

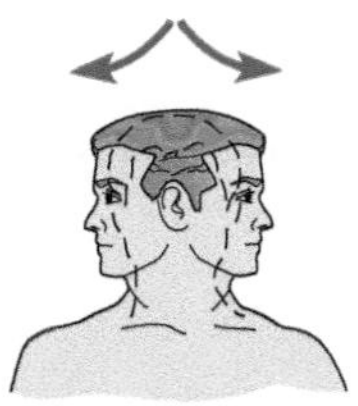	**Rotation** is the turning movement of a bone around its own long axis. Rotation may occur toward the body midline or away from it.
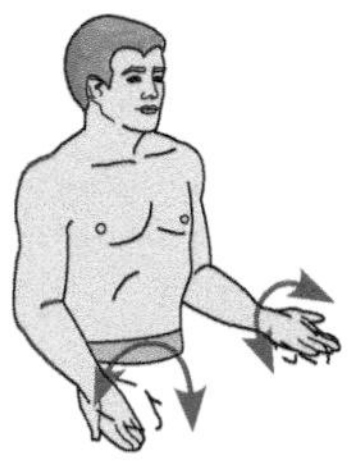	The terms **supination** and **pronation** refer only to the movements of the radius around the ulna. Movement of the forearm so that the palm faces anteriorly or superiorly is called *supination*. In *pronation*, the palm moves to face posteriorly or inferiorly.
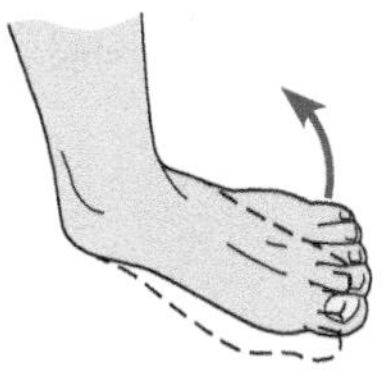	The terms **inversion** and **eversion** refer to movements of the foot. In *inversion*, the sole of the foot is turned medially. In *eversion*, the sole faces laterally.
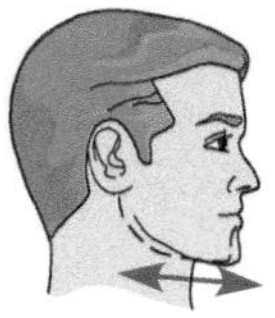	**Protraction** is a nonangular anterior movement in a transverse plane. **Retraction** is a nonangular posterior movement in a transverse plane.
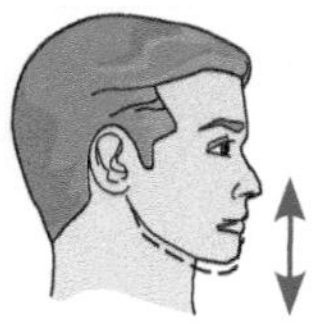	**Elevation** is a lifting or moving superiorly along a frontal plane. When the elevated part is moved downward to its original position, the movement is called **depression.** Shrugging the shoulders and chewing are examples of alternating elevation and depression.
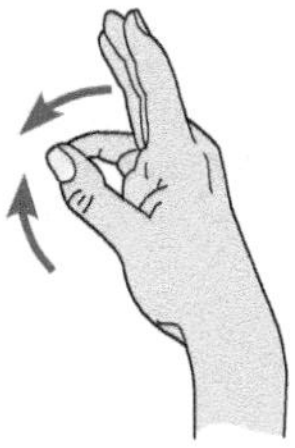	**Opposition** *of the thumb* is only allowed at the saddle joint between metacarpal 1 and the carpals. It is the movement of touching the thumb to the tips of the other fingers of the same hand.

which articulate with the distal end of the radius to form the wrist joint. Wrist movements include the following:

- Extension (70 degrees)
- Flexion (90 degrees)
- Hyperextension (30 degrees)
- Radial deviation (20 degrees)
- Ulnar deviation (55 degrees)

Each hand has metacarpophalangeal joints, and each finger has interphalangeal joints. Finger movements include the following:

- Abduction (20 degrees)
- Extension
- Hyperextension (30 degrees)
- Flexion (90 degrees)
- Circumduction

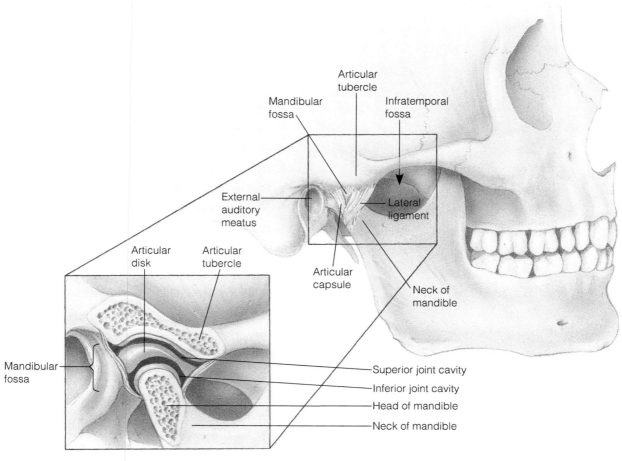

Figure 25.6 Temporomandibular joint. The enlargement shows a sagittal section through the joint.

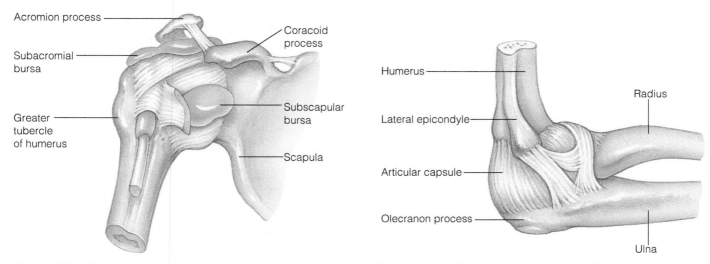

Figure 25.7 Shoulder joint.

Figure 25.8 Elbow joint. Lateral view of the right elbow.

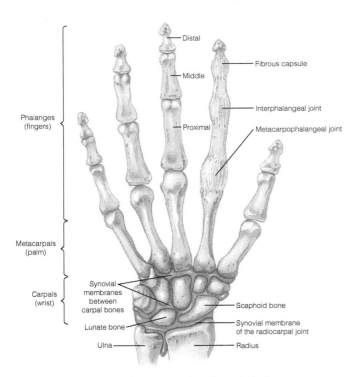

Figure 25.9 Bones of the wrist, hand, and phalanges.

Thumb movements include the following:

- Extension
- Flexion (80 degrees)
- Opposition

Hip

The hip joint is a ball-and-socket joint composed of the rounded head of the femur as it fits deep into the **acetabulum**, a rounded cavity on the right and left lateral sides of the pelvic bone (see Figure 25.10 ■). Although not as mobile as the shoulder, the hip is surrounded by a system of cartilage, ligaments, tendons, and muscles that contribute to its strength and stability. Landmarks include the iliac crest (not shown), the greater trochanter of the femur, and the anterior inferior iliac spine. Hip movements include the following:

- Extension (90 degrees)
- Hyperextension (15 degrees)
- Flexion with knee flexed (120 degrees)
- Flexion with knee extended (90 degrees)
- Internal rotation (40 degrees)
- External rotation (45 degrees)
- Abduction (45 degrees)
- Adduction (30 degrees)

Knee

The knee is a complex joint consisting of the patella (knee cap), femur, and tibia (see Figure 25.11 ■). It is supported and stabilized by the cruciate and collateral ligaments, which have a stabilizing effect on the knee and prevent dislocation. The landmarks of the knee include the tibial tuberosity and the medial and lateral condyles of the tibia. Knee movements include the following:

- Extension (0 degree)
- Flexion (130 degrees)
- Hyperextension (15 degrees)

Ankle and Foot

The ankle is a hinge joint that accommodates articulation between the tibia, fibula, and *talus*, a large, posterior tarsal of the foot (see Figure 25.12 ■). The **calcaneus** (heel bone) is just inferior to the talus. It is stabilized by a set of taut ligaments that are anchored from bony prominences at the distal ends of the tibia and fibula (the

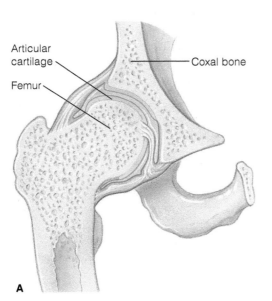

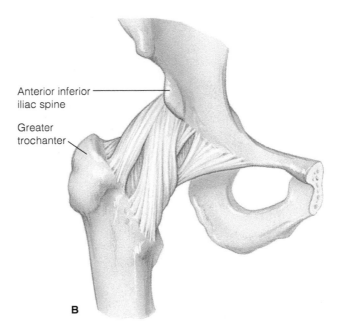

Figure 25.10 Hip joint. A. Cross section. B. Anterior view.

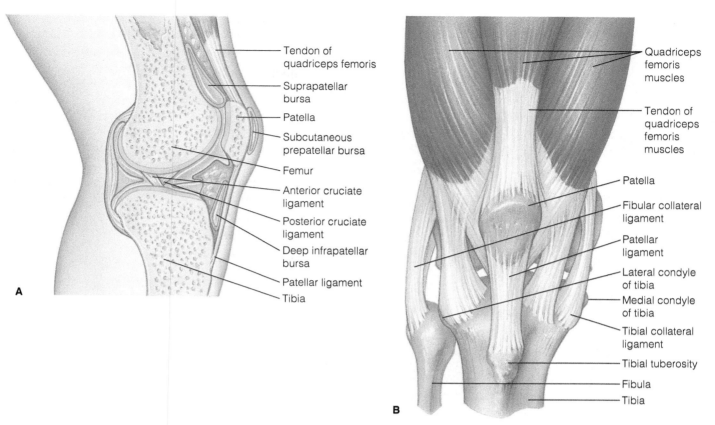

Figure 25.11 Knee joint. A. Sagittal section through the right knee. B. Anterior view.

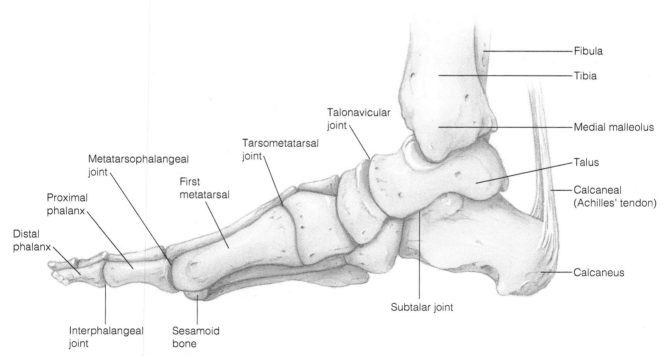

Figure 25.12 Medial view of joints of right ankle and foot.

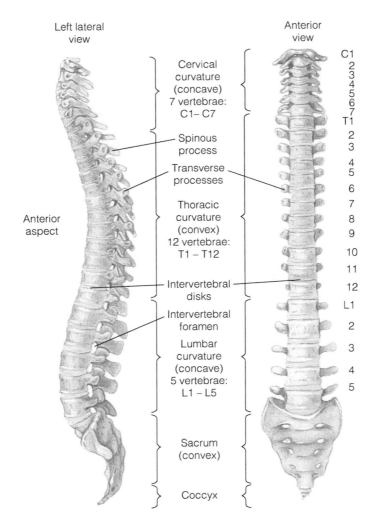

Left lateral view

Anterior view

Cervical curvature (concave) 7 vertebrae: C1– C7

Spinous process

Transverse processes

Thoracic curvature (convex) 12 vertebrae: T1 – T12

Anterior aspect

Intervertebral disks

Intervertebral foramen

Lumbar curvature (concave) 5 vertebrae: L1 – L5

Sacrum (convex)

Coccyx

C1
2
3
4
5
6
7
T1
2
3
4
5
6
7
8
9
10
11
12
L1
2
3
4
5

Figure 25.13 The spine.

lateral and medial malleoli), and then extend and attach to the foot. Movements of the ankle and foot include the following:

- Dorsiflexion of ankle (20 degrees)
- Plantar flexion of ankle (45 degrees)
- Inversion of foot (30 degrees)
- Eversion of foot (20 degrees)

Movements of the toes include the following:

- Extension
- Flexion
- Abduction (10 degrees)
- Adduction (20 degrees)

Spine

The spine is composed of 26 irregular bones called vertebrae (see Figure 25.13 ■). There are 7 *cervical vertebrae*, which support the base of the skull and the neck. All 12 of the *thoracic vertebrae* articulate with the ribs. The 5 *lumbar vertebrae* support the lower back. They are heavier and denser than the other vertebrae, reflecting their weight-bearing function. The *sacrum* shapes the posterior wall of the pelvis, offering strength and stability. The *coccyx* is a small, triangular tailbone at the base of the spine.

Viewed laterally, the spine has cervical and lumbar concavities and a thoracic convexity. As a person bends forward, the normal concavity should flatten, and there should be a single convex C-shaped curve. Figure 25.5B shows the main muscles of the neck and the spine. Movements of the neck include the following:

- Flexion (45 degrees)
- Extension (55 degrees)
- Hyperextension (10 degrees)
- Lateral flexion (bending) (40 degrees)
- Rotation (70 degrees)

Movements of the spine include the following:

- Lateral flexion (35 degrees)
- Extension (30 degrees)
- Flexion (90 degrees)
- Rotation (30 degrees)

Special Considerations

There are a variety of factors or special considerations that contribute to health status. Among these are age, developmental level, race,

TABLE 25.3	Examples of *Healthy People 2020* Objectives Related to the Musculoskeletal System
OBJECTIVE NUMBER	**DESCRIPTION**
AOCBC-1	Reduce the mean level of joint pain among adults with doctor-diagnosed arthritis
AOCBC-2	Reduce the proportion of adults with doctor-diagnosed arthritis who experience a limitation in activity due to arthritis or joint symptoms
AOCBC-3	Reduce the proportion of adults with doctor-diagnosed arthritis who find it "very difficult" to perform specific joint-related activities
AOCBC-4	Reduce the proportion of adults with doctor-diagnosed arthritis who have difficulty in performing two or more personal care activities, thereby preserving independence
AOCBC-5	Reduce the proportion of adults with doctor-diagnosed arthritis who report serious psychological distress
AOCBC-6	Reduce the impact of doctor-diagnosed arthritis on employment in the working-age population
AOCBC-7	Increase the proportion of adults with doctor-diagnosed arthritis who receive healthcare provider counseling
AOCBC-8	Increase the proportion of adults with doctor-diagnosed arthritis who have had effective, evidence-based arthritis education as an integral part of the management of their condition
AOCBC-9	Increase the proportion of adults with chronic joint symptoms who have seen a healthcare provider for their symptoms
AOCBC-10	Reduce the proportion of adults with osteoporosis
AOCBC-11	Reduce hip fractures among older adults
AOCBC-12	Reduce activity limitation due to chronic back conditions

Source: U.S. Department of Health and Human Services (USDHHS). (2014). *Healthy people 2020.* Retrieved from http://www.healthypeople.gov/2020/default.aspx.

ethnicity, work history, living conditions, socioeconomics, and emotional well-being. The following sections describe special considerations to include when gathering subjective and objective data.

Health Promotion Considerations

Healthy People 2020 objectives related to musculoskeletal health include prevention of illness and disability due to disorders including arthritis, osteoporosis, and chronic back conditions. See Table 25.3 for an overview of *Healthy People 2020* objectives that are designed to promote musculoskeletal health and wellness among individuals across the life span.

Lifespan Considerations

Accurate interpretation of findings requires knowledge of the variations in anatomy and physiology that occur with growth and development. Specific variations in the musculoskeletal system across the age span are described in the following sections.

Infants and Children

Fetal positioning and the delivery process may cause musculoskeletal anomalies in the infant. These include *tibial torsion,* a curving apart of the tibias, and *metatarsus adductus,* a tendency of the forefoot to turn inward. Many such anomalies correct themselves spontaneously as the child grows and walks.

Newborns normally have flat feet; arches develop gradually during the preschool years. Before learning to walk, infants tend to exhibit genu varum (bowlegs). Then, as the child begins to walk,

this tendency gradually reverses. By the age of 4, most children tend to exhibit genu valgum (knock knees). This condition also resolves spontaneously, usually by late childhood or early adolescence.

The nurse should inspect the newborn's spine. During fetal development and in the early stages of infancy, a baby's spine is C-shaped, or kyphotic. With development of muscles that allow for lifting of the head and walking, the infant's body weight shifts to the spine. Over time, curvatures in the cervical and lumbar regions develop, forming lordotic curves. Normal development of these curvatures, which produces a slight S shape, continues until growth ceases. Inspection of the spine also includes assessing for tufts of hair, cysts, or masses, which may indicate abnormalities such as spina bifida or a congenital neural tube defect. All known or suspected abnormalities require further evaluation by a primary care provider.

The nurse also palpates the length of the clavicles at each office visit, noting any lumps or irregularities and observing the range of motion of the arms. The clavicle is frequently fractured during birth, and the fracture often goes unnoticed until a callus forms at the fracture site.

The infant is assessed for congenital hip dislocation at every office visit until 1 year of age. Additionally, *Allis' sign* is used to detect unequal leg length. The nurse is positioned at the child's feet. With the infant supine, the nurse flexes the infant's knees, keeping the femurs aligned, and compares the height of the knees. An uneven height indicates unequal leg length, as depicted in Figure 25.14 ■.

While holding the infant, the nurse's hands should be beneath the infant's axillae. Shoulder muscle strength is present if the infant remains upright between the nurse's hands. Muscle weakness is indicated if the infant begins to slip through the hands.

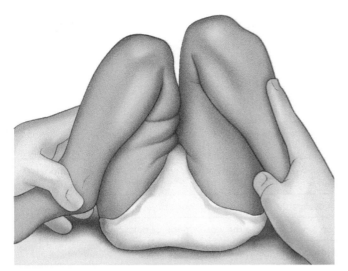

Figure 25.14 Allis' sign—demonstration of unequal knee height.

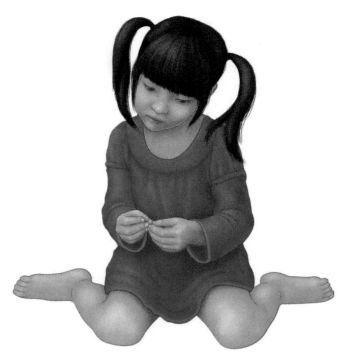

Figure 25.15 Reverse tailor position.

Bone growth is rapid during infancy and continues at a steady rate during childhood until adolescence, at which time both girls and boys experience a growth spurt. Long bones increase in width because of the deposition of new bony tissue around the diaphysis (shaft). Long bones also increase in length because of a proliferation of cartilage at the growth plates at the epiphyses (ends) of the long bones. Longitudinal growth ends at about 21 years of age, when the epiphyses fuse with the diaphysis. Throughout childhood, ligaments are stronger than bones. Therefore, childhood injuries to the long bones and joints tend to result in fractures instead of sprains. Individual muscle fibers grow throughout childhood, but growth is especially increased during the adolescent growth spurt. Muscles vary in size and strength due to genetics, exercise, and diet.

Much of the examination of the child and adolescent includes the same techniques of inspection, palpation, and assessment of range of motion and muscle strength used in the examination of the adult. However, children also have unique assessment needs. Children present wonderful opportunities for assessing range of motion and muscle strength as they play with toys in the waiting area or examination room. The nurse should encourage children to jump, hop, skip, and climb. Most children are eager to show off their abilities.

At each office visit, the nurse should ask children to demonstrate their favorite sitting position. If a child assumes the reverse tailor position (see Figure 25.15 ■), common when watching television, the nurse should encourage the child to try other sitting positions. Parents should be told that the reverse tailor position stresses the hip, knee, and ankle joints of the growing child.

The nurse should ask the child to lie supine, then to rise to a standing position. Normally, the child rises without using the arms for support. Generalized muscle weakness may be indicated if the child places the hands on the knees and pushes the trunk up (Gowers' sign).

The child's spine is assessed for scoliosis at each office visit. It is also important to inspect the child's shoes for signs of abnormal wear, and assess the child's gait. Before age 3, the gait of the child is normally broad based. After age 3, the child's gait narrows. At each visit, the nurse assesses the range of motion of each arm. **Subluxation** of the head of the radius occurs commonly when adults dangle children from their hands or remove their clothing forcibly.

The nurse must obtain complete information on any sports activity the child or adolescent engages in, because participation in these can indicate the need for special assessments or preventive teaching such as the use of helmets and other safety equipment.

The Pregnant Female

Estrogen and other hormones soften the cartilage in the pelvis and increase the mobility of the joints, especially the sacroiliac, sacrococcygeal, and symphysis pubis joints. As the pregnancy progresses, lordosis (exaggeration of the lumbar spinal curve) compensates for the enlarging fetus. The female's center of gravity shifts forward, and she shifts her weight farther back on her lower extremities (see Figure 25.16 ■). This shift strains the lower spine, causing the lower back pain that is so common during late pregnancy. As the pregnancy progresses, she may develop a waddling gait because of her enlarged abdomen and the relaxed mobility in her joints. Typically, a female resumes her normal posture and gait shortly after the pregnancy.

The Older Adult

As individuals age, physiologic changes take place in the bones, muscles, connective tissue, and joints. These changes may affect the individual's mobility and endurance. Bone changes include decreased calcium absorption and reduced osteoblast production. If the older adult has a chronic illness, such as chronic obstructive lung disease or hyperthyroidism, or takes medications containing glucocorticoids, thyroid hormone preparation, or anticonvulsants, bone strength may be greatly compromised because of decrease in the bone density. Elderly persons who are housebound and immobile or whose dietary intake of calcium and vitamin D is low may also experience reduced bone mass and strength. During aging, bone

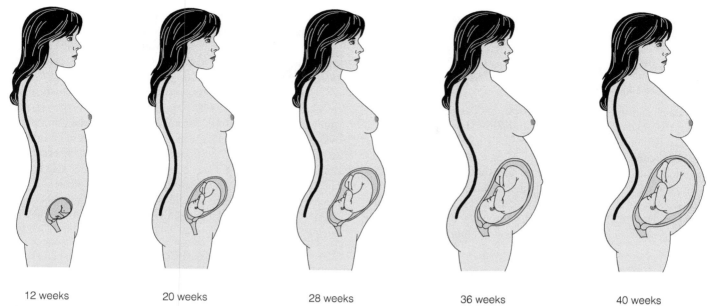

| 12 weeks | 20 weeks | 28 weeks | 36 weeks | 40 weeks |

Figure 25.16 Postural changes with pregnancy.

resorption occurs more rapidly than new bone growth, resulting in the loss of bone density typical of osteoporosis. The entire skeleton is affected, but the vertebrae and long bones are especially vulnerable. Most aging adults develop some degree of osteoporosis, but it is more marked in Caucasian females, especially those of Scandinavian ancestry.

The decreased height of the aging adult occurs because of a shortening of the vertebral column. Thinning of the intervertebral disks during middle age and an erosion of individual vertebrae due to osteoporosis contribute to this shortening. There is an average decrease in height of 1 to 2 inches from the 20s through the 70s, and a further decrease in the 80s and 90s because of additional collapse of the vertebrae. Kyphosis, an exaggerated convexity of the thoracic region of the spine, is common. When the older adult is standing, the nurse may notice a slight flexion of the hips and knees. These changes in the vertebral column may cause a shift in the individual's center of gravity, which in turn may put the older adult at an increased risk for falls.

The size and quantity of muscle fibers tend to decrease by as much as 30% by the 80th year of life. The amount of connective tissue in the muscles increases, and they become fibrous or stringy. Tendons become less elastic. As a result, the older patient experiences a progressive decrease in reaction time, speed of movements, agility, and endurance.

Degeneration of the joints causes thickening and decreased viscosity of the synovial fluid, fragmentation of connective tissue, and scarring and calcification in the joint capsules. In addition, the cartilage becomes frayed, thin, and cracked, allowing the underlying bone to become eroded. Because of these changes, the joints of older people are less shock absorbent and have decreased range of motion and flexibility. These normal degenerative joint changes that occur from aging and use are referred to as *osteoarthrosis*. In some individuals, *Heberden's nodes*—hard, typically painless, bony enlargements associated with osteoarthritis—may occur in the distal interphalangeal joints. Others may develop Bouchard's nodes, enlargement of proximal interphalangeal joints.

The gait of an older patient alters as the bones, muscles, and joints change with advancing age. Both males and females tend to walk slower; some support themselves as they move. Elderly males tend to walk with the head and trunk in a flexed position, using short, high steps, a wide gait, and a smaller arm swing. The bowlegged stance that is observed in older females is due to reduced muscular control, thus altering the normal angle of the hip and leading to increased susceptibility to falls and subsequent fractures.

As individuals age, there is a general decrease in reaction time and speed of performance of tasks. This can affect mobility and safety, especially with unexpected environmental stimuli (for example, objects on the floor, loose carpeting, or wet surfaces). In addition, any health problem that contributes to decreased physical activity tends to increase the chance of alterations in the health of the musculoskeletal system. A well-balanced diet and regular exercise help to slow the progression of these musculoskeletal changes.

The physical assessment of the musculoskeletal system of the elderly person is similar to that of any other adult. When testing range of motion, the nurse must be careful not to cause pain, discomfort, or damage to the joint. The musculoskeletal exam is conducted at a slower pace when necessary because older patients often have health problems that affect endurance.

Psychosocial Considerations

Psychosocial problems such as anxiety, depression, fear, altered body image, or a disturbance in self-esteem may promote inactivity or isolation, which in turn may lead to musculoskeletal degeneration. By the same token, any health problem that contributes to inactivity may trigger or contribute to psychosocial disturbances. Impaired physical mobility may lead to stress, hopelessness, ineffective coping, social isolation, or other problems.

Physical abuse should be considered if a patient has a history of frequent fractures, sprains, or other musculoskeletal trauma.

The nurse must follow the state's guidelines for referring the patient to social or protective services.

Cultural and Environmental Considerations

The bone density of people of African ancestry is significantly higher than that of people of other ethnicities (May, Pettifor, Norris, Ramsay, & Lombard, 2013). Asians typically have lower bone density than people of European descent (Kruger et al., 2013). The risk for developing osteoporosis is greater for women, and Asians and Caucasians tend to experience a higher incidence of osteoporosis than do African Americans (Mayo Clinic, 2013). The curvature of long bones varies widely among cultural groups and seems to be related to genetics and body weight. Weight also impacts the incidence of lower back problems; obesity is linked to an increased risk for lumbar back pain (Lidar et al., 2012).

The number and distribution of vertebrae vary. While 24 vertebrae is the average (present in about 85% to 90% of all people), 23 or 25 vertebrae are not uncommon.

Certain working conditions present potential risks to the musculoskeletal system. Workers required to lift heavy objects may strain and injure their back. Jobs requiring substantial physical activity, such as those of construction workers, firefighters, or athletes, increase the likelihood of musculoskeletal injuries such as sprains, strains, and fractures. Frequent repetitive movements may lead to misuse disorders such as carpal tunnel syndrome, pitcher's elbow, or vertebral degeneration. Musculoskeletal injuries may also arise when individuals sit for long periods at desks with poor ergonomic design.

Gathering the Data

Health assessment of the musculoskeletal system includes gathering subjective and objective data. Subjective data collection occurs during the patient interview, before the physical assessment. During the interview, various communication techniques are used to elicit general and specific information about the status of the patient's musculoskeletal system and ability to function. Health records, the results of laboratory tests, X-rays, and imaging reports are important secondary sources to be included in the data-gathering process. During the physical assessment of the musculoskeletal system, the techniques of inspection and palpation will be used to gather objective data. See Table 25.4 for information on potential secondary sources of patient data.

Focused Interview

The focused interview for the musculoskeletal system concerns data related to the structures and functions of that system. Subjective data are gathered during the focused interview. The nurse must be prepared to observe the patient and to listen for cues related to the function of the musculoskeletal system. The nurse may use open-ended and closed questions to obtain information. A number of follow-up questions or requests for descriptions may be required to clarify data or gather missing information. Follow-up questions are intended to identify the sources of problems, duration of difficulties, and measures used to alleviate or manage problems. They also provide clues about the patient's knowledge of his or her own health.

The focused interview guides the physical assessment of the musculoskeletal system. The information is always considered in relation to norms and expectations about musculoskeletal function. Therefore, the nurse must consider age, gender, race, culture, environment, health practices, past and concurrent problems, and therapies when

TABLE 25.4	**Potential Secondary Sources for Patient Data Related to the Musculoskeletal System**
LABORATORY TESTS	**NORMAL VALUES**
Calcium	8.9–10.3 mg/dL
Phosphorus	2.5–4.5 mg/dL
AST/SGOT	Males 8–48 Units/L Females 8–43 Units/L
Alkaline Phosphatase (ALP)	44–147 Units/L
Aldolase	<7.7 Units/L
Creatinine phosphokinase (CPK)	Males 52–336 Units/L Females 38–176 Units/L
Erythrocyte Sedimentation Rate (ESR)	Males <23 mm/hr Females <29 mm/hr
Rheumatoid Factor	<15 IU/mL
Antinuclear antibodies (ANA)	negative
Diagnostic Tests Arthroscopy Bone Density Scan Bone Scan Computed Tomography (CT) Joint Aspiration Magnetic Resonance Imaging (MRI) Myelography X-ray	

framing questions and using techniques to elicit information. In order to address all of the factors when conducting a focused interview, categories of questions related to the status and function of the musculoskeletal system have been developed. These categories include general questions that are asked of all patients; those addressing illness and infection; questions related to symptoms, pain, and behaviors; those related to habits or practices; questions that are specific to patients according to age; those for the pregnant female; and questions that address environmental concerns. One approach to elicit information about symptoms is the OLDCART & ICE method, described in chapter 7; see Figure 7.3 on page 120. ∞

The nurse must consider the patient's ability to participate in the focused interview and physical assessment of the musculoskeletal system. Illness, discomfort, and disease may affect the ability to participate in the interview. Participation in the focused interview may be influenced by the ability to communicate in the same language. Language barriers interfere with the accuracy of data collection and cause anxiety in the patient and examiner. A nurse may have to use a translator in conducting interviews and during the physical assessment. If the patient is experiencing acute pain, recent injury, or anxiety, attention must be focused on relief of discomfort and relief of symptoms before proceeding with the in-depth interview.

Focused Interview Questions	Rationales and Evidence

The following section provides sample questions and bulleted follow-up questions in each of the categories previously mentioned. A rationale for each of the questions is provided. The list of questions is not all-inclusive but represents the types of questions required in a comprehensive focused

interview related to the musculoskeletal system. As these questions are asked, the subjective data obtained help to identify strengths or risks associated with the musculoskeletal system as described in Healthy People 2020.

General Questions

1. **Describe your mobility today, 2 months ago, and 2 years ago.**

   ► This gives patients the opportunity to provide their own perceptions about mobility.

2. **Are you able to carry out all of your regular activities?**
   - Describe the change in your activity.
   - Do you know what is causing the problem?
   - What do you do about the problem?
   - How long has this been happening?
   - Have you discussed this with a healthcare professional?

   ► Musculoskeletal problems affect activities of daily living (ADLs) because of pain or decreased mobility.

3. **Do you have any chronic diseases such as diabetes mellitus, hypothyroidism, sickle cell anemia, lupus, or rheumatoid arthritis?**
   - If so, describe the disease and its progression, treatment, and effects on daily activities.

   ► These conditions can predispose the patient to musculoskeletal problems such as osteomyelitis (Wilmes et al., 2012).

4. **Please describe any musculoskeletal problems of any family member.**
   - What is the disease or problem?
   - Who in the family has had the problem?
   - When was it diagnosed?
   - Describe the treatment.
   - How effective has the treatment been?

   ► Some conditions such as rheumatoid arthritis are genetic or familial and recur in a family (Bax, van Heemst, Huizinga, & Toes, 2011).

Questions Related to Illness, Infection, or Injury

1. **Have you ever been diagnosed with a musculoskeletal illness?**
   - When were you diagnosed with the problem?
   - What treatment was prescribed for the problem?
   - Was the treatment helpful?
   - What kinds of things do you do to help with the problem?
   - Has the problem ever recurred (acute)?
   - How are you managing the disease now (chronic)?

   ► The patient has an opportunity to provide information about a specific illness. If a diagnosed illness is identified, follow-up about the date of diagnosis, treatment, and outcomes is required. Data about each illness identified by the patient are essential to an accurate health assessment. Illnesses can be classified as acute or chronic, and follow-up regarding each classification will differ.

2. **An alternative to question 1 is to list possible musculoskeletal illnesses, such as arthritis, myalgia, and lupus, and ask the patient to respond "yes" or "no" as each is stated.**

   ► This is a comprehensive and easy way to elicit information about all musculoskeletal diagnoses. Follow-up would be carried out for each identified diagnosis as in question 1.

Focused Interview Questions	Rationales and Evidence
3. Have you ever had an infection in your bones, muscles, or joints? • When were you diagnosed with the infection? • When did the problem begin? • What treatment was prescribed? • Was the treatment helpful? • What do you do to help the problem? • Has the problem ever recurred (acute)? • How are you managing the problem now (chronic)?	▶ Osteomyelitis, an infection of the bone, frequently recurs in patients with a history of previous infections (MedlinePlus, 2013).
4. Have you had any fractures (broken bones)? If so, tell me about the frequency, cause, injuries, treatment, and present problems with daily activities.	▶ Older adults who have osteoporosis and osteomalacia (adult vitamin D deficiency) are prone to develop multiple fractures of the bone (Weycker et al., 2013). Physical abuse should be considered when an individual has a history of frequent fractures; however, disease or hereditary illness can predispose fractures.
5. Have you ever experienced any penetrating wounds (punctures from a nail or sharp object, stabbing, or gunshot)? If so, please describe them.	▶ Penetrating wounds may be a causative factor for osteomyelitis (Izadi et al., 2013). Follow-up for questions 4 and 5 would follow the format for questions 1 and 3.

Questions Related to Symptoms, Pain, and Behaviors

When gathering information about symptoms, many questions are required to elicit details and descriptions that assist in the analysis of the data. Discrimination is made in relation to the significance of a symptom, in relation to specific diseases or problems, and in relation to potential follow-up examination or referral. One rationale may be provided for a group of questions in this category.

The following questions refer to specific symptoms and behaviors associated with the musculoskeletal system. For each symptom, questions and follow-up are required. The details to be elicited are the characteristics of the symptom; the onset, duration, and frequency of the symptom; the treatment or remedy for the symptom, including over-the-counter and home remedies; the determination if diagnosis has been sought; the effect of treatments; and family history associated with a symptom or illness.

1. Tell me about any swelling, heat, redness, or stiffness you have had in your muscles or joints.	▶ Swelling, heat, redness, and stiffness are associated with disorders of the musculoskeletal system such as arthritis or sprains (Osborn, Wraa, Watson, & Holleran, 2013).
2. How long have you had the symptom?	▶ Determining the duration of symptoms is helpful in identifying the significance of the symptoms in relation to specific diseases and problems.
3. Do you know what causes the symptom? **4. Does the symptom differ at different times of day?** **5. Have you sought treatment?** **6. When was the treatment sought?** **7. What happened when you sought treatment?**	▶ Questions 3 through 9 elicit information about the need for diagnosis, referral, or continued evaluation of the symptom; information about the patient's knowledge about a current diagnosis or underlying problems; and the patient's response to intervention.

Focused Interview Questions	Rationales and Evidence

8. Was something prescribed or recommended?

9. What was the effect of the remedy?

10. Do you now use, or have you ever used, over-the-counter (OTC) or home remedies for the symptom?

▶ Questions 10 through 13 elicit information about drugs and substances that may relieve symptoms or provide comfort. Some substances may mask symptoms, interfere with the effect of prescribed medication, or harm the patient.

11. What are the OTC or home remedies that you use?

12. How often do you use them?

13. How much of them do you use?

14. Do you experience constipation or abdominal distention?

▶ These diagnostic cues commonly occur in patients who have decreased mobility, atrophy of the abdominal muscles, or spinal deformity.

15. Do you have difficulty breathing? If so, describe.

▶ Spinal deformities, osteoporosis, and any other condition that restricts trunk movement may interfere with normal breathing movements.

Questions Related to Pain

1. Please describe any pain you experience in your bones, muscles, or joints
   - How would you rate the pain on a scale of 0 to 10, with 10 being the worst?
   - When did the pain begin?
   - What were you doing when the pain began?
   - What activities increase the pain?
   - What activities seem to decrease or eliminate the pain?
   - Does this pain radiate from one place to another?
   - Do you experience any unusual sensations along with the pain?

▶ These questions help determine if the pain has a sudden or gradual onset. Also, certain activities such as lifting heavy objects can strain ligaments and vertebrae in the back, causing acute pain. Weight-bearing activities may increase the pain if the patient has degenerative disease of the hip, knee, and vertebrae. The pain from hiatal hernia and from cardiac, gallbladder, and pleural conditions may be referred to the shoulder. Lumbosacral nerve root irritation may cause pain to be felt in the leg. (See Figure 11.5 on page 177 for an illustration of common sites of referred pain.) Sensations of burning, tingling, or prickling (paresthesia) may accompany compression of nerves or blood vessels in that body region.

2. What do you do to relieve the pain?

3. Is that treatment effective?

▶ Questions 2 and 3 are intended to determine if the patient has selected a treatment based on past experience, knowledge of musculoskeletal illness, or use of complementary and alternative medicine and its effectiveness.

Questions Related to Behaviors

1. Do you smoke?
   - If so, how much?
   - How much caffeine do you consume each day?
   - How many cups of coffee, tea, or cola?
   - How much alcohol do you drink?

▶ Smoking, caffeine consumption, and alcohol consumption increase the patient's risk for osteoporosis (University of Maryland Medical Center [UMMC], 2013).

2. Tell me about your exercise program.

▶ A sedentary lifestyle leads to muscle weakness, contributes to poor coordination skills, and predisposes postmenopausal females to osteoporosis (Pervaiz, Cabezas, Downes, Santoni, & Frankle, 2013).

Focused Interview Questions	Rationales and Evidence

Questions Related to Age

The focused interview must reflect the anatomic and physiologic differences that exist along the life span. The following questions are examples of those that would be specific for infants and children, the pregnant female, and the older adult.

Questions Regarding Infants and Children

1. **Were you told about any trauma to the infant during labor and delivery?**
   - If so, describe the trauma.

   ▶ Traumatic births increase the risk for fractures, especially of the clavicle (Dashe, Roocroft, Bastrom, & Edmonds, 2013).

2. **Did the baby require resuscitation after delivery?**

   ▶ Periods of hypoxia or anoxia can result in decreased muscle tone (Orcesi, 2013).

3. **Have you noticed any deformity of the child's spine or limbs or any unusual shape of the child's feet and toes?**
   - If yes, please describe these deformities and any treatment the child has had.

   ▶ Some deformities correct themselves as the child grows. Others may require physical therapy or surgery.

4. **Please describe any dislocations or broken bones the child has had, including any treatment.**

   ▶ Dislocations or broken bones are more common in children with certain developmental disabilities or sensory or motor disorders such as cerebral palsy or Down syndrome. They may also signal physical abuse. The latter will require further investigation.

5. *For the school-age child:* **Do you play any sports at school or after school?**
   - If so, describe the sports activities.

   ▶ Sports activities can cause musculoskeletal injuries, especially if played without adequate adult supervision or the use of protective equipment.

Questions for the Pregnant Female

1. **Please describe any back pain you are experiencing.**
   - Tell me about the effects of the pain on your daily activities.

   ▶ Lordosis may occur in the last months of pregnancy along with complaints of back pain (Chang et al., 2014).

Questions for the Older Adult

1. **Have you noticed any muscle weakness over the past few months?**
   - If so, explain what effect this muscle weakness has on your daily activities.

   ▶ Muscle weakness is common as a person ages, especially in people with sedentary lifestyles.

2. **Have you fallen in the past 6 months?**
   - If so, how many times?
   - What prompted the fall(s)?
   - Describe your injuries.
   - What treatment did you receive?
   - What effect did your injuries have on your daily activities?

   ▶ Older adults have an increased rate of falls because of a change in posture that can affect their balance (Schmid, Van Puymbroeck, & Koceja, 2010). Loss of balance may also be caused by sensory or motor disorders, inner ear infections, the side effects of certain medications, and other factors (Osborn et al., 2013).

3. **Do you use any walking aids such as a cane or walker to help you get around?**
   - If so, please describe the aid or show it to me.

   ▶ These aids help the older adult ambulate, but they can also cause falls, especially if the patient does not use the device properly.

4. *For postmenopausal females:* **Do you take calcium supplements?**

   ▶ Calcium supplementation may slow the development of some of the musculoskeletal changes associated with age, such as osteoporosis.

Focused Interview Questions	Rationales and Evidence

Questions Related to the Environment

Environment refers to both the internal and external environments. Questions related to the internal environment include all of the previous questions and those associated with internal or physiologic responses. Questions regarding the external environment include those related to home, work, or social environments.

Internal Environment

1. **Describe your typical daily diet.**
   - Do you have problems eating or drinking dairy products?
   - If so, describe the problems you experience.

▶ Protein deficiency interferes with bone growth and muscle tone; calcium deficiency predisposes an individual to low bone density, resulting in osteoporosis; and vitamin C deficiency inhibits bone and tissue healing (Osborn et al., 2013). Patients with intolerance to milk products frequently ingest low amounts of calcium, leading to musculoskeletal problems such as osteoporosis.

2. **Have you had any recent gain or loss in weight?**
   - If so, how much weight?

▶ Increased weight puts added stress on the musculoskeletal system. New weight loss (for example, in those having had gastric bypass surgery) increases the risk for osteoporosis (Shapses & Sukumar, 2012).

3. **Are you currently taking any medications such as steroids, estrogen, muscle relaxants, or any other drugs?**

▶ These drugs may cause a variety of symptoms such as weakness, swelling, and increased muscle size that could affect the musculoskeletal system (Wilson, Shannon, & Shields, 2013).

External Environment

1. **How much sunlight do you get each day?**

▶ Twenty minutes of sunshine each day helps the body manufacture vitamin D. Vitamin D deficiency can lead to osteomalacia (Osborn et al., 2013).

2. **What kind of work do you do?**
   - Do you work on a computer?
   - What are your typical workplace lifting requirements?

▶ Frequent repetitive movements may lead to misuse syndromes such as carpal tunnel syndrome, an inflammation of the tissues of the wrist that causes pressure on the median nerve. Work that requires heavy lifting or twisting may lead to lower back problems.

3. **Describe your hobbies or athletic activities.**

▶ Participation in athletic or sports activities can predispose the individual to trauma or "wear and tear" injuries. Sitting for long periods and repetitive motion such as in sewing, crocheting, and woodworking can cause musculoskeletal damage.

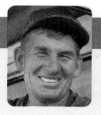

Patient-Centered Interaction

Mr. Alexander French, a 49-year-old truck driver, returns to the pain clinic at 10:30 A.M. accompanied by his wife. His health history includes having been diagnosed with a herniated intervertebral disk at L4–5 about 10 months ago. At that time, he declined surgery and selected the alternative method of treatment, which included wearing a back brace and home exercises to help strengthen his back muscles. Now his chief complaint is back pain radiating to his left leg. The following is an excerpt from the focused interview.

Interview

Nurse: Good morning, Mr. French. I see by your report you are having back pain again. Your last visit was about 3 months ago for a routine follow-up with no pain.

Mr. French: Yes, that is correct. Yes, to both of your thoughts.

Nurse: First, we need to determine your pain level right now and find a comfortable position for you.

Mr. French: Right now my pain is about 4 on a scale of 0 to 10 and it sometimes shoots down my left leg. It was higher at home but I took my pills before coming here. That's why my wife drove and is here with me. I will be able to sit for awhile. When I can't sit any longer, I will tell you.

Nurse: I need more information about the cause, actions you have taken to decrease the pain, and activities since your last visit. Where shall we begin?

Mr. French: I'll start with the cause. I was outside Saturday after it stopped snowing, and I shoveled our front walk. Then I helped the children build a big snowman. I was tired and had a backache that evening but I tried to ignore it.

Nurse: You ignored it?

Mr. French: I should have taken the medicine right away. I should have had my brace on when I was shoveling and building the snowman with the children.

Nurse: You weren't wearing your back brace?

Mr. French: That's right. I wear it every day to work. I never forget since I move heavy boxes from the truck. I had been feeling so good, no problems, and the snow was not heavy. I guess when I lifted the second snowball for the snowman, that did me in though.

Analysis

Several techniques were used to obtain subjective data from the patient. The nurse first clarified the reason for the visit and then determined the patient's pain level and position for comfort. Using open-ended statements and listening to the patient, the nurse encouraged the patient to focus on details of the topics being discussed. However, the nurse introduced several thoughts and questions at one time. This could have hindered the communication process during the interview.

Patient Education

The following are physiologic, behavioral, and cultural risk factors that affect the health of the musculoskeletal system across the life span. Several factors are cited as trends in *Healthy People 2020* documents. The nurse provides advice and education to reduce risks associated with the aforementioned factors and to promote and maintain musculoskeletal health.

LIFESPAN CONSIDERATIONS

Risk Factors	Patient Education
• Diet impacts musculoskeletal health across the age span.	▶ Instruct about healthy diet. Include recommendations for daily calcium intake and to eat a balance of protein, fats, and carbohydrates. Calcium-rich foods include dairy products, green leafy vegetables, and sardines. Vitamins C and D are important for tissue strength, healing, and promoting absorption of calcium. Laying down of bone occurs predominantly in adolescence. Nutrition discussion is critical. Image-conscious females may abstain from dairy and other calcium-rich foods to avoid the fat content in these foods.
• Decreased bone density, muscle strength, and flexibility occur with aging.	▶ Recommend regular exercise according to age and ability to maintain or improve musculoskeletal function.

CULTURAL CONSIDERATIONS

Risk Factors

- Osteoporosis occurs with the greatest frequency in Caucasian and Asian females.

- Systemic lupus erythematosus occurs more frequently in females and those of African descent than in males and Caucasians or Hispanics.

- Sickle cell anemia, an inherited blood disorder, can result in delayed growth and bone damage. Sickle cell anemia occurs in descendants of individuals from Africa, South and Central America, Saudi Arabia, the Mediterranean, and India.

Patient Education

▶ Caucasian and Asian females need to have information about the increased risk of osteoporosis and preventive measures including changes in diet and exercise programs.

▶ Advise at-risk patients to seek information and screening for connective and hematologic diseases that affect joint and musculoskeletal health and function.

▶ Advise at-risk patients to seek information and screening for connective and hematologic diseases that affect joint and musculoskeletal health and function.

ENVIRONMENTAL CONSIDERATIONS

Risk Factors

- Obesity increases the risks of disorders of the bones, muscles, and joints.

- Medication can impact the function and integrity of the musculoskeletal system.

Patient Education

▶ Advise that maintenance of healthy or ideal weight or weight reduction is important in reducing risks of joint disease and injury.
▶ Obesity can create problems with self-esteem and contribute to immobility and isolation. Weight reduction increases body image and mobility.

▶ Advise patients to provide information about their use of alternative, complementary, or prescribed medicine in order to avoid potential harmful interactions or reactions with prescribed therapies.

BEHAVIORAL CONSIDERATIONS

Risk Factors

- Smoking and alcohol use contribute to the development of osteoporosis.

- Sedentary lifestyles increase the risk for musculoskeletal problems.

- Accidents and trauma affect musculoskeletal health and function.

Patient Education

▶ Educate and advise about smoking cessation programs to reduce the incidence of osteoporosis.

▶ Recommend regular exercise according to age and ability to maintain or improve musculoskeletal function.

▶ Educate about how safety practices—in the home, at work, and when participating in sports or athletic activities—are important in reducing traumatic and other musculoskeletal injuries. Safety measures include seat belt use when driving or riding as a passenger in a vehicle. Helmets and protective gear should be used when playing recreational or team sports.

Physical Assessment

Assessment Techniques and Findings

Physical assessment of the musculoskeletal system requires the use of inspection and palpation. During each of the procedures the nurse is gathering data related to the patient's skeleton, joints, musculature, strength, and mobility. Knowledge of normal or expected findings is essential in determining the meaning of the data as the nurse conducts the physical assessment.

Both adults and children who are pre-school age and older have erect posture, an even gait, and symmetry in size and shape of muscles. A healthy individual is capable of active and complete range of motion in all joints. Joints are nonswollen and nontender. Muscle strength is equal bilaterally, and the movements against resistance are smooth and symmetric. The spine is midline and cervical; thoracic and lumbar curves are present. The extremities are of equal length. The arm span is equal to height, and the distance from head to pubis is equal to the distance from pubis to toes.

Physical assessment of the musculoskeletal system follows an organized pattern. It begins with a patient survey and proceeds in a cephalocaudal direction to include inspection; palpation; assessment of range of motion of each joint; and assessment of muscle size, symmetry, and strength.

EQUIPMENT

- examination gown
- clean, nonsterile examination gloves
- examination light
- skin marking pen
- goniometer
- tape measure

HELPFUL HINTS

- Age and agility influence the patient's ability to participate in the assessment.
- It is often more helpful to demonstrate the movements you expect of the patient during this assessment than to use easily misunderstood verbal instructions. A "Simon Says" approach works well, especially with children.
- When assessing range of motion, do not push the joint beyond its normal range.
- Stop when the patient expresses discomfort.
- Measure the joint angle with a goniometer when range of motion appears limited.
- Use an orderly approach: head to toe, proximal to distal, compare the sides of the body for symmetry.
- The musculoskeletal assessment may be exhausting for some patients. Provide rest periods or schedule two sessions.
- Use Standard Precautions.

Techniques and Normal Findings	Abnormal Findings Special Considerations

Survey

A quick survey of the patient enables the nurse to identify any immediate problems and to determine the patient's ability to participate in the assessment.

Inspect the overall appearance, posture, and position of the patient. Observe for deformities, inflammation, and immobility (see Figure 25.17 ■).

► If a patient is experiencing pain or inflammation, these issues must be addressed first. The complete assessment of the musculoskeletal system may have to be delayed until acute problems are attended to. Limited strength and mobility must be considered throughout the assessment.

The posture and position of body parts in obese patients is often the first indication of underlying problems with bones or ligaments. Genu valgus and varus abnormalities suggest cartilage loss in obese patients.

Techniques and Normal Findings	Abnormal Findings Special Considerations

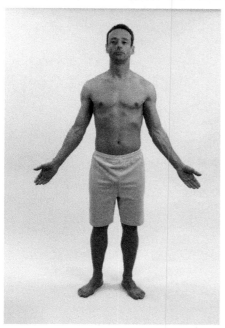 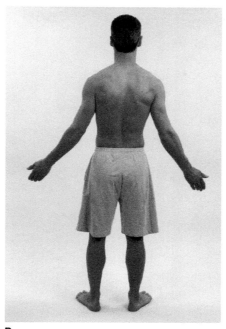 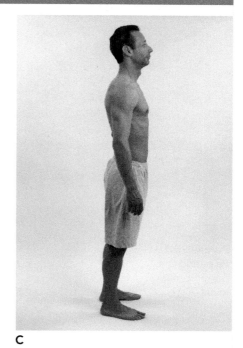

A   B   C

Figure 25.17 Survey and posture of patient. A. Anterior view. B. Posterior view. C. Lateral view.

Assessment of the Joints

1. **Position the patient.**
   - The patient should be in a sitting position and wearing an examination gown.

2. **Instruct the patient.**
   - Explain that you will be touching the patient for the purpose of assessing bones, muscles, and joints and that you will ask the patient to move different parts of the body to determine the mobility of the joints.
   - Explain that part of the assessment will require the patient to move against the resistance you provide. It is helpful to demonstrate or describe the movements expected of the patient for one joint and to apply resistance as the patient repeats the expected movement. Then explain that each joint will be assessed in a similar manner with the same amount of resistance and that you will provide direction with each examination.
   - Explain that the assessment should not cause discomfort and tell the patient to inform you of pain, discomfort, or difficulty with any assessment. Explain that you will provide assistance or support when necessary and can provide rest periods throughout the assessment.
   - Muscle strength should be equal bilaterally and the patient should be able to fully resist the opposing force you apply during testing. Table 25.5 on page 715 provides a scale for rating muscle strength.

3. **Inspect the temporomandibular joint (TMJ) on both sides.**
   - The joints should be symmetric and not swollen or painful.

4. **Palpate the temporomandibular joints.**
   - Place the finger pads of your index and middle fingers in front of the tragus of each ear. Ask the patient to open and close the mouth while you palpate the temporomandibular joints (see Figure 25.18 ■).

► Palpation of the ankle, knee, hip, shoulder, and back is difficult in the obese patient due to increased subcutaneous fat.

► An enlarged or swollen joint shows as a rounded protuberance.

► Discomfort, swelling, crackling sounds, and limited movement of the jaw are unexpected findings that require further evaluation for dental or neurologic problems or TMJ syndrome.

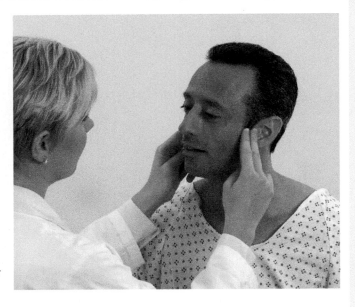

Figure 25.18
Palpating the temporomandibular joints.

- As the patient's mouth opens, your fingers should glide into a shallow depression of the joints. Confirm the smooth motion of the mandible.
- The joint may audibly and palpably click as the mouth opens. This is normal.

5. **Palpate the muscles of the jaw.**
   - Instruct the patient to clench the teeth as you palpate the masseter and temporalis muscles. Confirm that the muscles are symmetric, firm, and nontender.

   ▶ Swelling and tenderness suggest arthritis and myofascial pain syndrome.

6. **Test for range of motion of the temporomandibular joints.**
   - Ask the patient to open the mouth as wide as possible. Confirm that the mouth opens with ease to as much as 3 to 6 cm (1.17 to 2.34 in.) between the upper and lower incisors.
   - With the mouth slightly open, ask the patient to push out the lower jaw, and return the lower jaw to a neutral position. The jaw should protrude and retract with ease.
   - Ask the patient to move the lower jaw from side to side. Confirm that the jaw moves laterally from 1 to 2 cm (0.39 to 0.78 in.) without deviation or dislocation.
   - Ask the patient to close the mouth. The mouth should close completely without pain or discomfort.

   ▶ TMJ dysfunction should be suspected if facial pain and limited jaw movement accompany clicking sounds as the jaw opens and closes.

7. **Test for muscle strength and for motor function of cranial nerve V.**
   - Instruct the patient to repeat the movements in step 6 as you provide opposing force. The patient should be able to perform the movements against your resistance. The strength of the muscles on both sides of the jaw should be equal.
   - For more detailed testing of cranial nerve V, including sensory function, see chapter 26. ∞

Shoulders

1. **With the patient facing you, inspect both shoulders.**
   - Compare the shape and size of the shoulders, clavicles, and scapula. Confirm that they are symmetric and similar in size both anteriorly and posteriorly.

   ▶ Swelling, deformity, atrophy, and misalignment, combined with limited motion, pain, and crepitus (a grating sound caused by bone fragments in joints), suggest degenerative joint disease; traumatized joints (strains, sprains); or inflammatory conditions (rheumatoid arthritis, bursitis, or tendinitis).

Techniques and Normal Findings	Abnormal Findings Special Considerations

2. **Palpate the shoulders and surrounding structures.**

- Begin palpating at the sternoclavicular joint; then move laterally along the clavicle to the acromioclavicular joint.
- Palpate downward into the subacromial area and the greater tubercle of the humerus.
- Confirm that these areas are firm and nontender, the shoulders are symmetric, and the scapulae are level and symmetric.

▶ Shoulder pain without palpation or movement may result from insufficient circulation to the myocardium. This cue, known as *referred pain*, can be a precursor to a myocardial infarction (heart attack). If the patient exhibits other symptoms such as chest pain, indigestion, and cardiovascular changes, medical assistance must be obtained immediately.

3. **Test the range of motion of the shoulders.**

- Instruct the patient to use both arms for the following maneuvers:
- Shrug the shoulders by flexing them forward and upward.
- With the elbows extended, raise the arms forward and upward in an arc. The patient should demonstrate a forward flexion of 180 degrees.
- Return the arms to the sides. Keeping the elbows extended, move the arms backward as far as possible (see Figure 25.19 ■). The patient should demonstrate an extension of as much as 50 degrees.

▶ If the patient expresses discomfort, it is important to determine if the pain is referred. Conditions that increase intra-abdominal pressure, such as hiatal hernia and gastrointestinal disease, may cause pain in the shoulder area. Whenever limitation or increase in range of motion (ROM) is assessed, the goniometer should be used to precisely measure the angle.

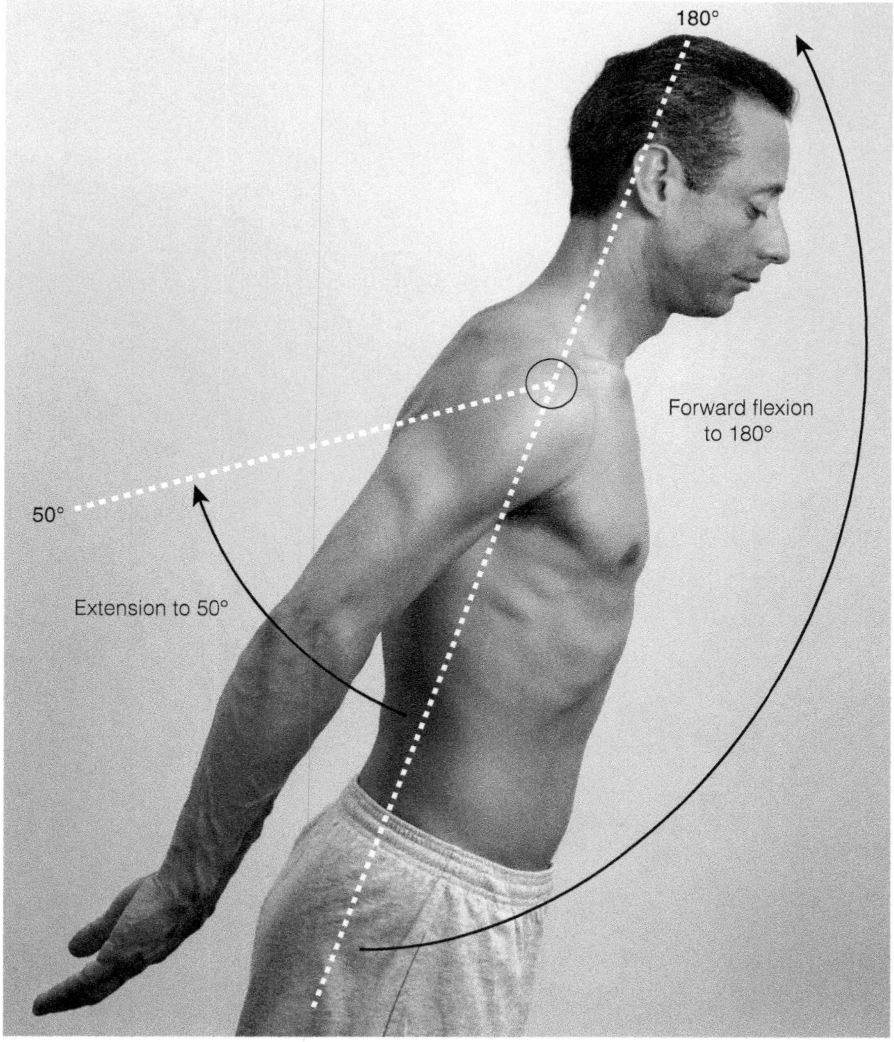

Figure 25.19 Flexion and extension of the shoulders.

- Ask the patient to clasp his or her hands on the back as high above the waist as possible (internal rotation; see Figure 25.20 ■).

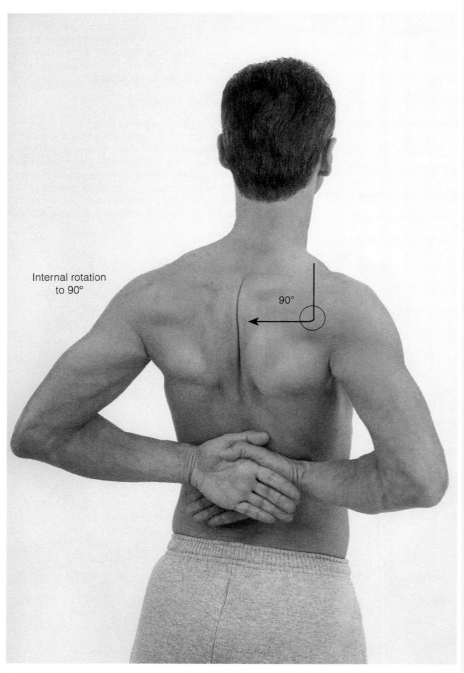

Internal rotation
to 90°

90°

Figure 25.20 Internal rotation of the shoulders.

- Ask the patient to clasp his or her hands behind the head (external rotation; see Figure 25.21 ■).

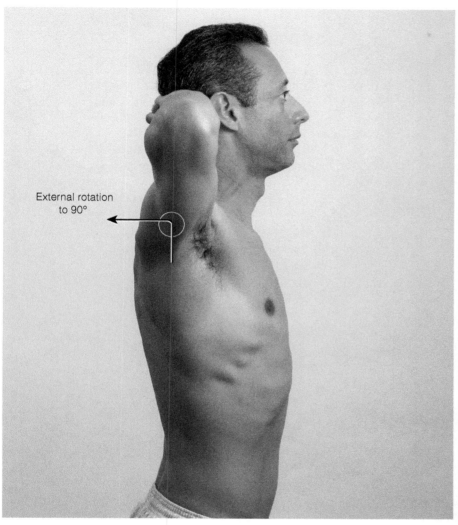

External rotation to 90°

Figure 25.21 External rotation of the shoulders.

- With elbows extended, ask the patient to swing the arms out to the sides in arcs, touching the palms together above the head. The patient should demonstrate abduction of 180 degrees.

▶ In rotator cuff tears, the patient is unable to perform abduction without lifting or shrugging the shoulder. This sign is accompanied by pain, tenderness, and muscle atrophy.

Techniques and Normal Findings	Abnormal Findings Special Considerations

- With the elbows extended, ask the patient to swing each arm toward the midline of the body (see Figure 25.22 ■).
- The patient should demonstrate adduction of as much as 50 degrees.

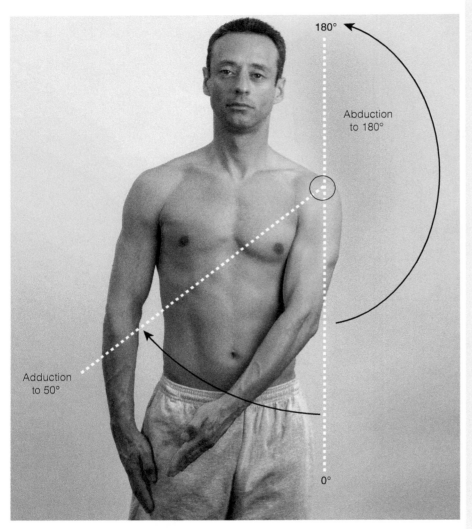

Figure 25.22 Abduction and adduction of the shoulder.

Techniques and Normal Findings	Abnormal Findings Special Considerations

4. Test for strength of the shoulder muscles.

- Instruct the patient to repeat the movements in step 3 as you provide opposing force. The patient should be able to perform the movements against your resistance. The strength of the shoulder muscles on both sides should be equal.

- Muscle strength is rated on a scale of 0 to 5, with 0 representing absence of strength and 5 indicating maximum or normal strength. Table 25.5 includes information about rating muscle strength.

▶ Full resistance during the shoulder shrug indicates adequate cranial nerve XI (spinal accessory) function. See chapter 26 for more details. ∞

TABLE 25.5 **Rating Muscle Strength**

RATING	DESCRIPTION OF FUNCTION	CLASSIFICATION
5	Full range of motion against gravity with full resistance	Normal
4	Full range of motion against gravity with moderate resistance	Good
3	Full range of motion with gravity	Fair
2	Full range of motion without gravity (passive motion)	Poor
1	Palpable muscle contraction but no movement	Trace
0	No muscle contraction	Zero

Elbows

1. Support the patient's arm and inspect the lateral and medial aspects of the elbow.

- The elbows should be symmetric.

▶ Swelling, deformity, or malalignment requires further evaluation. If there is a subluxation (partial dislocation), the elbow looks deformed, and the forearm is misaligned.

2. Palpate the lateral and medial aspects of the olecranon process.

- Use your thumb and middle fingers to palpate the grooves on either side of the olecranon process.

- The joint should be free of pain, thickening, swelling, or tenderness.

▶ In the presence of inflammation, the grooves feel soft and spongy, and the surrounding tissue may be red, hot, and painful.

▶ Inflammatory conditions of the elbow include arthritis, bursitis, and epicondylitis. *Rheumatoid arthritis* may result in nodules in the olecranon bursa or along the extensor surface of the ulna. Nodules are firm, nontender, and not attached to the overlying skin. *Lateral epicondylitis* (tennis elbow) results from constant, repetitive movements of the wrist or forearm. Pain occurs when the patient attempts to extend the wrist against resistance. *Medial epicondylitis* (pitcher's or golfer's elbow) results from constant, repetitive flexion of the wrist. Pain occurs when the patient attempts to flex the wrist against resistance.

Techniques and Normal Findings	Abnormal Findings Special Considerations

3. Test the ROM of each elbow.

- Instruct the patient to perform the following movements:
  - Bend the elbow by bringing the forearm forward and touching the fingers to the shoulder (see Figure 25.23 ■). The elbow should flex to 160 degrees.
  - Straighten the elbow. The lower arm should form a straight line with the upper arm. The elbow in a neutral position is at 0 degree extension. The elbow should extend to 0 degree.
  - Holding the arm straight out, turn the palm upward facing the ceiling, then downward facing the floor (see Figure 25.25 ■). The elbow should supinate and pronate to 90 degrees.

▶ To use the goniometer, begin with the joint in a neutral position and then flex the joint as far as possible. Measure the angle with the goniometer. Fully extend the joint and measure the angle with the goniometer. Compare the goniometer measurements to the expected degree of flexion and extension. See Figure 25.24 ■ for an example.

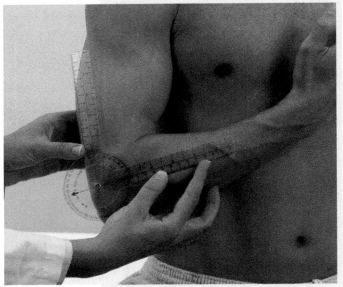

Figure 25.24 Goniometer measure of joint range of motion.

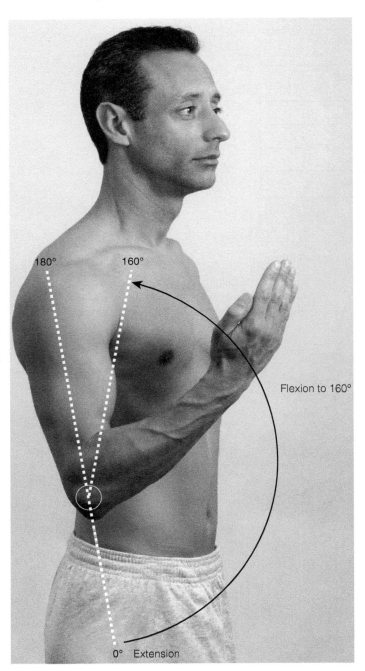

Figure 25.23 Flexion and extension of the elbow.

Techniques and Normal Findings	Abnormal Findings Special Considerations

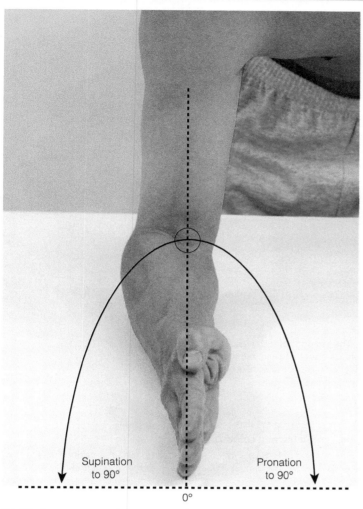

Figure 25.25 Supination and pronation of the elbow.

- The patient should be able to put each elbow through the normal ROM without difficulty or discomfort.

4. **Test for muscle strength.**
   - Stabilize the patient's elbow with your nondominant hand while holding the wrist with your dominant hand.
   - Instruct the patient to flex the elbow while you apply opposing resistance (see Figure 25.26 ■).

Techniques and Normal Findings	Abnormal Findings Special Considerations

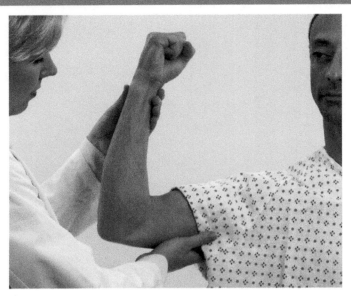

Figure 25.26 Testing muscle strength using opposing force.

- Instruct the patient to extend the elbow against resistance.
- The patient should be able to perform these movements. The strength of the muscles associated with flexion and extension of each elbow should be equal. Muscle strength is measured by testing against the strength of the examiner as resistance is applied.

Wrists and Hands

1. **Inspect the wrists and dorsum of the hands for size, shape, symmetry, and color.**
   - The wrists and hands should be symmetric and free from swelling and deformity. The color should be similar to that of the rest of the body. The ends of either the ulna or radius may protrude further in some individuals.

   ▶ Redness, swelling, or deformity in the joints requires further evaluation. It is important to note any nodules on the hands or wrists or atrophy of the surrounding muscles. In acute rheumatoid arthritis, the wrist, proximal inter-phalangeal, and metacarpophalangeal joints are likely to be swollen, tender, and stiff. As the disease progresses, the proximal interphalangeal joints deviate toward the ulnar side of the hand; the interosseous muscles atrophy; and rheumatoid nodules form, giving the rheumatic hand its characteristic appearance.

2. **Inspect the palms of the hands.**
   - There is a rounded protuberance over the thenar eminence (the area proximal to the thumb).

   ▶ Carpal tunnel syndrome is a nerve disorder in which an inflammation of tissues in the wrist causes pressure on the median nerve (which innervates the hand). Thenar atrophy is a common finding associated with carpal tunnel syndrome; however, some atrophy of the thenar eminence occurs with aging.

3. **Palpate the wrists and hands for temperature and texture.**
   - The temperature of the wrists and hands should be warm and similar to the rest of the body. The skin should be smooth and free of cuts. The skin around the interphalangeal joints may have a rougher texture.

Techniques and Normal Findings

Abnormal Findings
Special Considerations

4. Palpate each joint of the wrists and hands.

- Move your thumbs from side to side gently but firmly over the dorsum, with your fingers resting beneath the area you are palpating (see Figures 25.27A and B ■). As you palpate, make sure you keep the patient's wrist straight.

- To palpate the interphalangeal joints, pinch them gently between your thumb and index finger (see Figure 25.27C ■). All joints should be firm and nontender with no swelling.

- As you palpate, note the temperature of the patient's hand.

▶ A ganglion is a typically painless, round, fluid-filled mass that arises from the tendon sheaths on the dorsum of the wrist and hand. It may require surgery. Ganglia that are more prevalent when the wrist is flexed do not interfere with ROM or function.

▶ A cool temperature in the extremities may indicate compromised vascular function, which may in turn influence muscle strength.

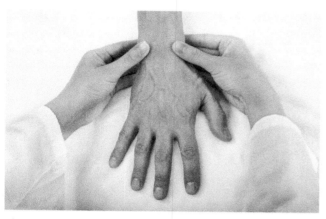

Figure 25.27A Palpating the wrist.

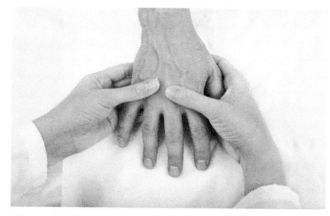

Figure 25.27B Palpating the hand.

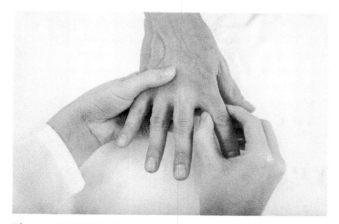

Figure 25.27C Palpating the fingers.

5. Test the ROM of the wrist.

- Instruct the patient to perform the following movements:
  - Straighten the hand (extension).

Techniques and Normal Findings	Abnormal Findings Special Considerations

- Using the wrist as a pivot point, bring the fingers backward as far as possible, and then bend the wrist downward (see Figure 25.28 ■). The wrist should hyperextend to 70 degrees and flex to 90 degrees.

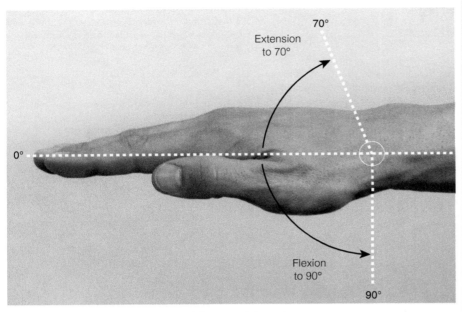

Figure 25.28 Hyperextension and flexion of the wrist.

- Turn the palms down; move the hand laterally toward the fifth finger, then medially toward the thumb (see Figure 25.29 ■). Be sure the movement is from the wrist and not the elbow. Ulnar deviation should reach as much as 55 degrees, and radial deviation should reach as much as 20 degrees.

▶ Abnormalities of wrist flexion or extension may be related to arthritis or other musculoskeletal conditions. Unusual sensations when performing these motions, such as numbness or tingling in the fingers, may be suggestive of carpal tunnel syndrome or other disorders. Abnormalities should be reported to the primary care provider for further evaluation.

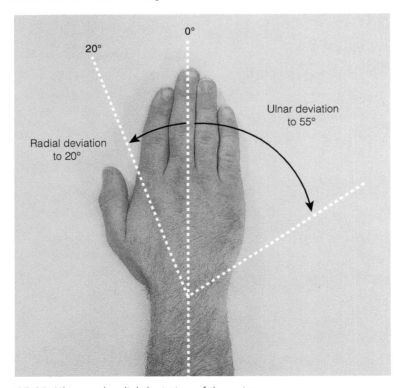

Figure 25.29 Ulnar and radial deviation of the wrist.

Techniques and Normal Findings	Abnormal Findings Special Considerations

- Bend the wrists downward and press the backs of both hands together (*Phalen's test*; see Figure 25.30 ■). This causes flexion of the wrists to 90 degrees. Normally patients experience no symptoms with this maneuver.

▶ When a Phalen's test is performed on individuals with carpal tunnel syndrome, 80% experience pain, tingling, and numbness that radiates to the arm, shoulder, neck, or chest within 60 seconds.

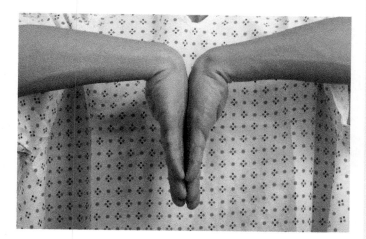

Figure 25.30
Phalen's test.

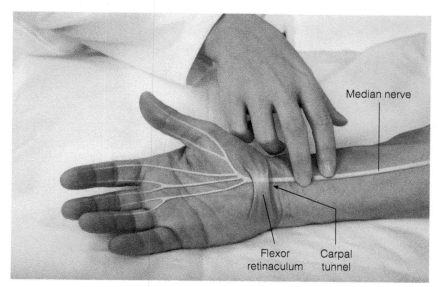

Median nerve

Flexor retinaculum   Carpal tunnel

Figure 25.31 Tinel's sign.

▶ If carpal tunnel syndrome is suspected, it is important to check for Tinel's sign by percussing lightly over the median nerve in each wrist. If carpal tunnel syndrome is present, the patient feels numbness, tingling, and pain along the median nerve (Figure 25.31 ■).

6. **Test the ROM of the hands and fingers.**
   - Instruct the patient to perform the following movements:
     - Make a tight fist with each hand with the fingers folded into the palm and the thumb across the knuckles (thumb flexion).
     - Open the fist and stretch the fingers (extension).

Techniques and Normal Findings	Abnormal Findings Special Considerations

- Point the fingers downward toward the forearm, and then back as far as possible (see Figure 25.32 ■). Fingers should flex to 90 degrees and hyperextend to as much as 30 degrees.

▶ In *Dupuytren's contracture*, the patient is unable to extend the fourth and fifth fingers. This is a progressive, painless, inherited disorder that causes severe flexion in the affected fingers, is usually bilateral, and is more common in middle-aged and older males.

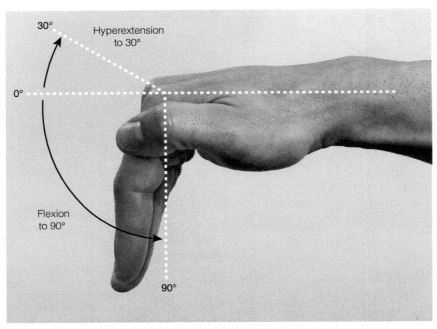

Figure 25.32 Flexion and extension of the fingers.

- Spread the fingers far apart, then back together. Fingers should abduct to 20 degrees and should adduct fully (to touch).
- Move the thumb toward the ulnar side of the hand and then away from the hand as far as possible.
- Touch the thumb to the tip of each of the fingers and to the base of the little finger.

7. **Test for muscle strength of the wrist.**
   - Place the patient's arm on a table with his or her palm facing up.
   - Stabilize the patient's forearm with one hand while holding the patient's hand with your other hand.
   - Instruct the patient to flex the wrist while you apply opposing resistance (see Figure 25.33 ■). The patient should be able to provide full resistance.

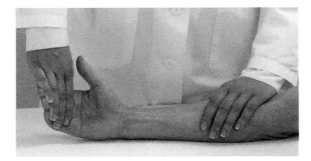

Figure 25.33 Testing the muscle strength of the wrist.

8. **Test for muscle strength of the fingers.**
   - Ask the patient to spread his or her fingers, and then try to force the fingers together.
   - Ask the patient to touch his or her little finger with the thumb while you place resistance on the thumb in order to prevent the movement.

▶ Patients with carpal tunnel syndrome manifest weakness when attempting opposition of the thumb.

Techniques and Normal Findings	Abnormal Findings Special Considerations

Hips

1. **With the patient in a supine position, inspect the position of each hip and leg.**
   - The legs should be slightly apart and the toes should point toward the ceiling. The legs should be of equal length.

2. **Palpate each hip joint and the upper thighs.**
   - The hip joints are firm, stable, and nontender.

3. **Test the ROM of the hips.**

> **ALERT!**
>
> *Do not ask patients who have undergone hip replacement to perform these movements without the permission of the physician, because these motions can dislocate the prosthesis.*

   - Instruct the patient to perform the straight leg raise (SLR) test.
     - Raise one leg straight off the bed or table (see Figure 25.34 ■). The other leg should remain flat on the bed. Hip flexion with straight knee should reach 90 degrees. Return the leg to its original position and repeat this maneuver with the other leg.

▶ External rotation of the lower leg and foot is a classic sign of a fractured femur. Shortening of a limb is associated with hip fracture.

▶ Pain, tenderness, swelling, deformity, limited motion (especially limited internal rotation), and crepitus are diagnostic cues that signal inflammatory or degenerative joint diseases in the hip. A fractured femur should be suspected if the joint is unstable and deformed.

▶ In the patient with a herniated disk, the straight leg raise test may produce the *Lasègue sign*, which includes back and leg pain along the course of the sciatic nerve. Presence of the Lasègue sign is nonspecific and may be indicative of a variety of conditions; as such, follow-up evaluation is required to confirm sciatic nerve involvement (Kraemer, 2009).

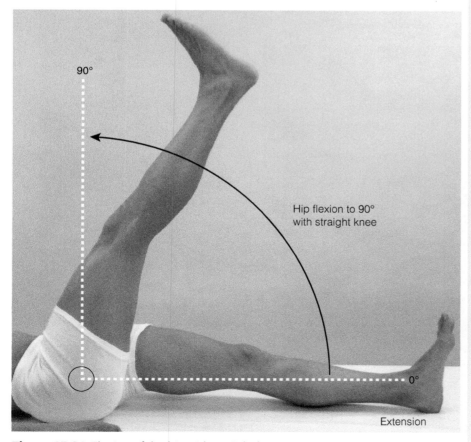

90°

Hip flexion to 90° with straight knee

0°

Extension

Figure 25.34 Flexion of the hip with straight knee.

Techniques and Normal Findings	Abnormal Findings Special Considerations

- Raise the leg with the knee flexed toward the chest as far as it will go (see Figure 25.35 ■). Hip flexion with flexed knee should reach 120 degrees. Return the leg to its original position.

▶ Abnormalities of hip flexion and rotation may be reflective of numerous musculoskeletal conditions, including arthritis, inguinal hernia, and spinal and joint disorders (Micheo, 2010). Abnormalities should be reported to the primary care provider for further evaluation.

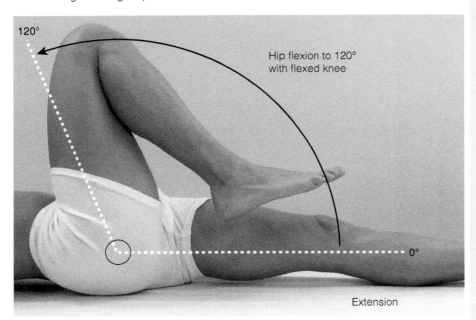

Figure 25.35 Flexion of the hip with flexed knee.

- Move the foot away from the midline as the knee moves toward the midline (see Figure 25.36 ■). Internal hip rotation should reach 40 degrees.

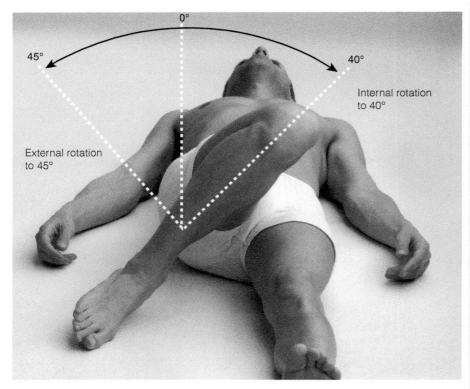

Figure 25.36 Internal and external hip rotation.

Techniques and Normal Findings	Abnormal Findings Special Considerations

- Move the foot toward the midline as the knee moves away from the midline. External hip rotation should reach 45 degrees.
- Move the leg away from the midline (see Figure 25.37 ■), then as far as possible toward the midline. Abduction should reach 45 degrees. Adduction should reach 30 degrees.

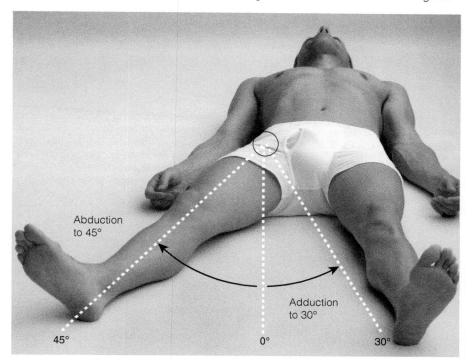

Figure 25.37 Abduction and adduction of the hip.

- Assist the patient to turn onto his or her abdomen. An alternative position could be side lying. With the patient's knee extended, ask the patient to raise each leg backward and up as far as possible (see Figure 25.38 ■). Hips should hyperextend to 15 degrees. (You may also perform this test later, during assessment of the spine, with the patient standing.)

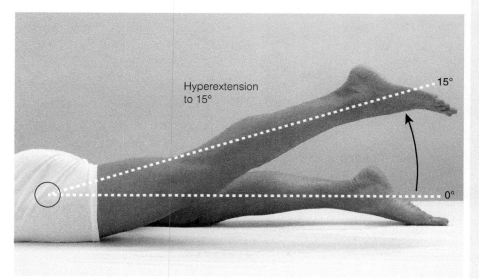

Figure 25.38 Hyperextension of the hip.

► Abnormalities of hip abduction or adduction may be indicative of various injuries, including tearing of the acetabular labrum, which is a ring of cartilage that covers the outer rim of the socket of the hip joint. Injury to this structure may be caused by repetitive motions of hip abduction or adduction, which occur when playing certain sports, such as golf and soccer. Musculoskeletal disorders such as **developmental dysplasia of the hip** (DDH) also are associated with acetabular labrum tears (Micheo, 2010). Abnormalities should be reported to the primary care provider for further evaluation.

Techniques and Normal Findings	Abnormal Findings Special Considerations

4. Test for muscle strength of the hips.
- Assist the patient in returning to the supine position.
- Press your hands on the patient's thighs and ask the patient to raise his or her hip.
- Place your hands outside the patient's knees and ask the patient to spread both legs against your resistance.
- Place your hands between the patient's knees, and ask the patient to bring the legs together against your resistance.

Knees

1. Inspect the knees.
- With the patient in the sitting position, inspect the knees.
- The patella should be centrally located in each knee. The normal depressions along each side of the patella should be sharp and distinct. The skin color should be similar to that of the surrounding areas.

▶ Swelling and signs of fluid in the knee and its surrounding structures require further evaluation. Fluid accumulates in the suprapatellar bursa, the prepatellar bursa, and other areas adjacent to the patella when there is inflammation, trauma, or degenerative joint disease.

2. Inspect the quadriceps muscle in the anterior thigh.
- The muscles should be symmetric.

▶ Atrophy in the quadriceps muscles occurs with disuse or chronic disorders.

3. Palpate the knee.
- Using your thumb, index finger, and middle finger, begin palpating approximately 10 cm (3.9 in.) above the patella with your thumb, index, and middle fingers (see Figure 25.39 ■). Palpate downward, evaluating each area.

▶ Any pain, swelling, thickening, or heat should be noted while palpating the knee. These diagnostic cues occur when the synovium is inflamed. Painless swelling frequently occurs in degenerative joint disease. A painful, localized area of swelling, heat, and redness in the knee is caused by the inflammation of the bursa (bursitis); for example, *prepatellar bursitis* (housemaid's knee).

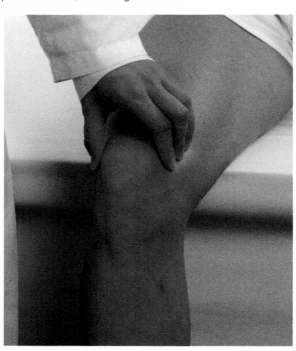

Figure 25.39 Palpating the knee.

- The quadriceps muscle and surrounding soft tissue should be firm and nontender. The suprapatellar bursa is usually not palpable.

Techniques and Normal Findings	Abnormal Findings Special Considerations

4. Palpate the tibiofemoral joint.

- With the patient's knee still in the flexed position, use your thumbs to palpate deeply along each side of the tibia toward the outer aspects of the knee.

▶ Signs of inflammation, including pain and tenderness, occur when the joint is inflamed or damaged and may indicate degenerative joint disease, synovitis, or a torn meniscus. Bony ridges or prominences in the outer aspects of the joint occur with osteoarthritis.

- Then palpate along the lateral collateral ligament.
- The joint should be firm and nontender.

5. Test for the bulge sign.

- This procedure detects the presence of small amounts of fluid (4 to 8 mL or 0.8 to 1.5 tsp) in the suprapatellar bursa.
- With the patient in the supine position, use firm pressure to stroke the medial aspect of the knee upward several times, displacing any fluid (see Figure 25.40 ■).

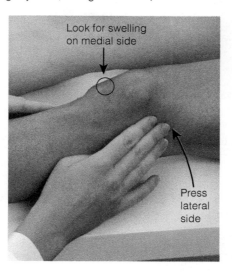

Look for swelling on medial side

Press lateral side

Figure 25.40 Testing for the bulge sign.

- Apply pressure to the lateral side of the knee while observing the medial side.
- Normally no fluid is present.

▶ The medial side of the knee bulges if fluid is in the joint.

6. Perform ballottement.

- **Ballottement** is a technique used to detect fluid or to examine or detect floating body structures. The nurse displaces body fluid and then palpates the return impact of the body structure.

▶ When there are abnormal fluid levels, fluid forced between the patella and femur causes the patella to "float" over the femur. A palpable click is felt when the patella is snapped back against the femur when fluid is present.

- To detect large amounts of fluid in the suprapatellar bursa, firmly grasp the thigh just above the knee with your thumb and fingers. This action causes any fluid in the suprapatellar bursa to move between the patella and the femur.

- With the fingers of your left hand, quickly push the patella downward upon the femur (see Figure 25.41 ■).

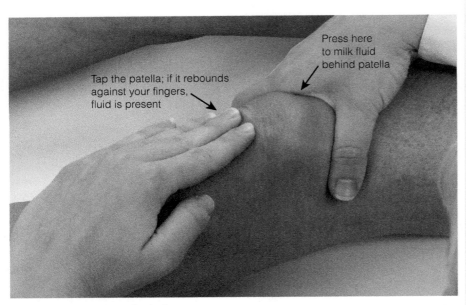

Tap the patella; if it rebounds against your fingers, fluid is present

Press here to milk fluid behind patella

Figure 25.41 Testing for ballottement.

- Normally the patella sits firmly over the femur, allowing little or no movement when pressure is exerted over the patella.

7. **Test the ROM of each knee.**
   - Instruct the patient to bend each knee against the chest as far as possible (flexion) (see Figure 25.42 ■), and then return the knee to its extended position.

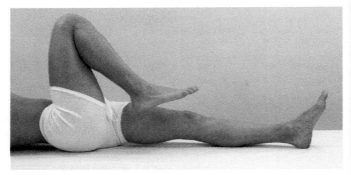

Figure 25.42
Flexion of the knee.

8. **Test for muscle strength.**
   - Instruct the patient to flex each knee while you apply opposing force.
   - Now instruct the patient to extend the knee again.
   - The patient should be able to perform the movement against resistance.
   - The strength of the muscles in both knees should be equal.

9. **Inspect the knee while the patient is standing.**
   - Ask the patient to stand erect. If the patient is unsteady, allow the patient to hold onto the back of a chair.
   - The knees should be in alignment with the thighs and ankles.
   - Ask the patient to walk at a comfortable pace with a relaxed gait.

▶ Look for *genu varum* (bowlegs), *genu valgum* (knock knees), or *genu recurvatum* (excessive hyperextension of the knee with weight bearing due to weakness of quadriceps muscles).

Techniques and Normal Findings	Abnormal Findings Special Considerations

Ankles and Feet

1. Inspect the ankles and feet with the patient sitting, standing, and walking.

- The color of the ankles and feet should be similar to that of the rest of the body. They should be symmetric, and the skin should be unbroken. The feet and toes should be in alignment with the long axis of the lower leg. No swelling should be present, and the patient's weight should fall on the middle of the foot.

▶ The following abnormalities require further evaluation:
- *Gouty arthritis:* The metatarsophalangeal joint of the great toe is swollen, hot, red, and extremely painful.
- ***Hallux valgus*** *(bunion):* The great toe deviates laterally from the midline, crowding the other toes. The metatarsophalangeal joint and bursa become enlarged and inflamed, causing a bunion.
- *Hammertoe:* There is flexion of the proximal interphalangeal joint of a toe, while the distal metatarsophalangeal joint hyperextends. A callus or corn frequently occurs on the surface of the flexed joint from external pressure.
- *Pes planus (flatfoot):* The arch of the foot is flattened, sometimes coming in contact with the floor. The deformity may be noticeable only when an individual is standing and bearing weight on the foot.

2. Palpate the ankles.

- Grasp the heel of the foot with the fingers of both hands while palpating the anterior and lateral aspects of the ankle with your thumbs (see Figure 25.43 ■).
- The ankle joints should be firm, stable, and nontender.

▶ Pain or discomfort on palpation and movement frequently indicate degenerative joint disease.

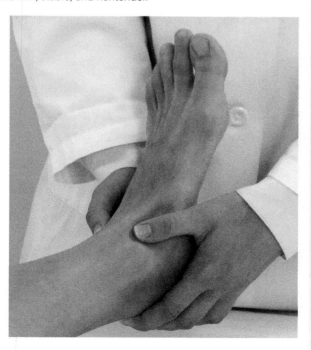

Figure 25.43 Palpating the ankle.

3. Palpate the length of the calcaneal (Achilles) tendon at the posterior ankle.

- The calcaneal tendon should be free of pain, tenderness, and nodules.

▶ Pain and tenderness along the tendon may indicate tendinitis or bursitis. Small nodules sometimes occur in patients with rheumatoid arthritis.

Techniques and Normal Findings	Abnormal Findings Special Considerations

4. Palpate the metatarsophalangeal joints just below the ball of the foot.

- The metatarsophalangeal joints should be nontender.

▶ Pain and discomfort with this maneuver suggest early involvement of rheumatoid arthritis. Acute inflammation of the first metatarsophalangeal joint suggests gout.

5. Deeply palpate each metatarsophalangeal joint.

- The joints should be firm and nontender.

▶ Pain, swelling, or tenderness may be associated with inflammation or degenerative joint disease.

6. Test the ROM of the ankles and feet.

- Instruct the patient to perform the following movements:
  - Point the foot toward the nose. Dorsiflexion should reach 20 degrees.
  - Point the foot toward the floor. Plantar flexion should reach 45 degrees.
  - Point the sole of the foot outward and then inward. The ankle should evert to 20 degrees and invert to 30 degrees (see Figure 25.44 ■).
  - Curl the toes downward (flexion).
  - Spread the toes as far as possible (abduction), and then bring the toes together (adduction).

▶ Limited ROM and painful movement of the foot and ankle without signs of inflammation suggest degenerative joint disease.

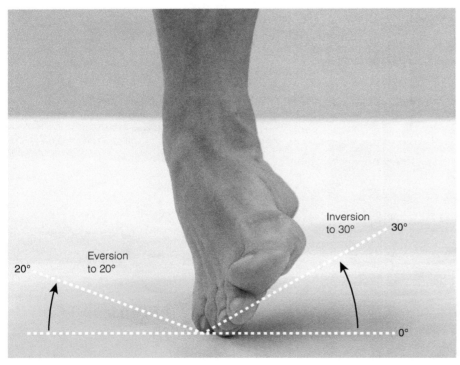

Figure 25.44 Eversion and inversion of the ankles.

7. Test muscle strength of the ankle.

- Ask the patient to perform dorsiflexion and plantar flexion against your resistance.

8. Test muscle strength of the foot.

- Ask the patient to flex and extend the toes against your resistance.

Techniques and Normal Findings	**Abnormal Findings** **Special Considerations**

9. Palpate each interphalangeal joint.

- As you did for the hand, note the temperature of the extremity. Confirm that it is similar to the temperature of the rest of the patient's body.

▶ Pain, swelling, or tenderness may be associated with inflammation or degenerative joint disease.

▶ A temperature in the lower extremities that is significantly cooler than the rest of the body may indicate vascular insufficiency, which in turn may lead to musculoskeletal abnormalities.

Spine

1. Inspect the spine.

- With the patient in a standing position, move around the patient's body to check the position and alignment of the spine from all sides. Confirm that the cervical and lumbar curves are concave, and that the thoracic curve is convex (see Figure 25.45A ■).
- Imagine a vertical line falling from the level of T1 to the gluteal cleft. Confirm that the spine is straight (see Figure 25.45B ■).

▶ Lack of symmetry of the scapulae may indicate thoracic surgery. A scapula may appear higher if a lung has been removed on that side. In addition, the following abnormalities require further evaluation:

- **Kyphosis:** An exaggerated thoracic dorsal curve that causes asymmetry between the sides of the posterior thorax.
- **Lordosis:** An exaggerated lumbar curve that compensates for pregnancy, obesity, or other skeletal changes.
- *Flattened lumbar curve:* A reduced lumbar concavity frequently occurs when spasms affect the lumbar muscles.
- *List:* The spine leans to the left or right. A plumb line drawn from T1 does not fall between the gluteal cleft. This condition may occur with spasms in the paravertebral muscles or a herniated disk.

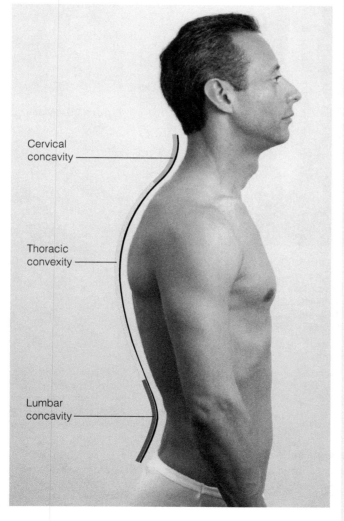

Cervical concavity

Thoracic convexity

Lumbar concavity

Figure 25.45A
Lateral view of spine.

Techniques and Normal Findings	Abnormal Findings Special Considerations

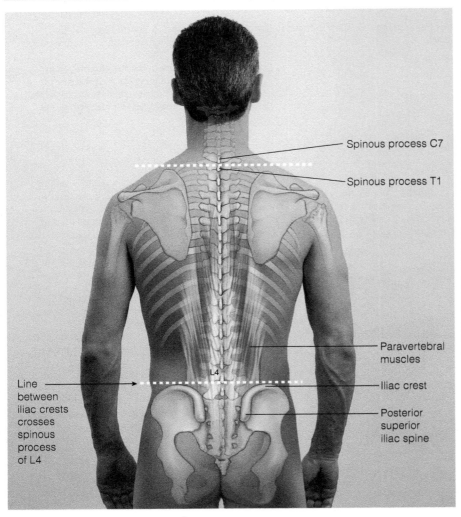

Figure 25.45B Posterior view of spine.

- Spinous process C7
- Spinous process T1
- Paravertebral muscles
- Line between iliac crests crosses spinous process of L4
- Iliac crest
- Posterior superior iliac spine

- Imagine a horizontal line across the top of the scapulae. Confirm that the scapulae are level and symmetric (see Figure 25.45B). Similarly, check that the heights of the iliac crests and the gluteal folds are level (see Figure 25.45B). Ask the patient to bend forward, and assess the alignment of the vertebrae.

2. **Palpate each vertebral process with your thumb.**
    - The vertebral processes should be aligned, uniform in size, firm, stable, and nontender.

3. **Palpate the muscles on both sides of the neck and back.**
    - The neck muscles should be fully developed and symmetric, firm, smooth, and nontender.

- *Scoliosis:* The spine curves to the right or left, causing an exaggerated thoracic convexity on that side. The body compensates, and a plumb line dropped from T1 falls between the gluteal cleft. Unequal leg length may contribute to scoliosis; therefore, if scoliosis is suspected, it is necessary to measure the patient's leg length. With the patient supine, measure the distance from the anterior superior iliac spine to the medial malleolus, crossing the tape measure at the medial side of the knee (Figure 25.46 ■) Spinal abnormalities are depicted in Table 25–7 on page 737.

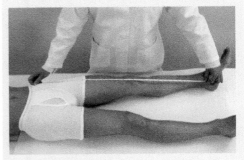

Figure 25.46 Measuring leg length.

▶ A *compression fracture* should be considered if the patient is elderly, complains of pain and tenderness in the back, and has restricted back movement. T8 and L3 are the most common sites for compression fractures.

▶ *Muscle spasms* feel like hardened or knotlike formations. When they occur, the patient may complain of pain and restricted movement. Muscle spasms may be associated with TMJ dysfunction or with *spasmodic torticollis,* a disorder in which the spasms cause the head to be pulled to one side.

4. **Test the ROM of the cervical spine.**
   - Instruct the patient to perform the following movements:
     - Touch the chest with the chin (flexion).
     - Look up toward the ceiling (hyperextension).
     - Attempt to touch each shoulder with the ear on that side, keeping the shoulder level (lateral bending or flexion).
     - Turn the head to face each shoulder as far as possible (rotation).

5. **Test the ROM of the thoracic and lumbar spine.**
   - Sit or stand behind the standing patient. Stabilize the pelvis with your hands and ask the patient to bend sideways to the right and to the left. Right and left lateral flexion should reach 35 degrees (see Figure 25.47 ■).

▶ Limited ROM, crepitation, or pain with movement in the joint requires further evaluation. If the patient complains of sharp pain that begins in the lower back and radiates down the leg, perform the straight leg raise (SLR) test as described on p. 723. If the patient reports pain when performing the SLR test, additional clues as to the origin of the pain may be identified by adding foot dorsiflexion, which may increase the sensation of pain (Magee, 2014). Record the distribution and severity of the pain and the degree of leg elevation at the time the pain occurs. Also record whether dorsiflexion increases the pain. Pain with straight-leg raising may indicate a herniated disk.

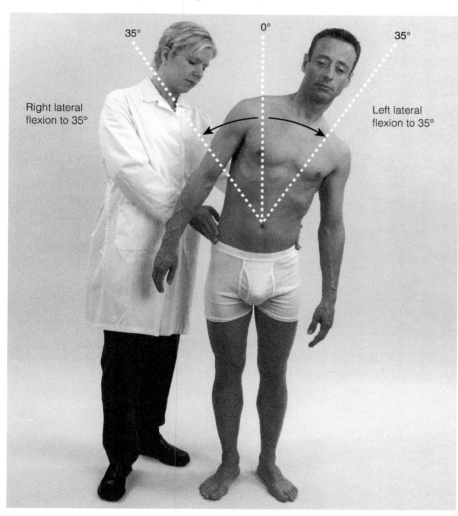

35°   0°   35°

Right lateral flexion to 35°

Left lateral flexion to 35°

Figure 25.47 Lateral flexion of the spine.

Techniques and Normal Findings	Abnormal Findings Special Considerations

● Ask the patient to bend forward and touch the toes (flexion). Confirm that the lumbar concavity disappears with this movement and that the back assumes a single C-shaped convexity (see Figure 25.48 ■).

▶ If the forward bend test reveals unevenness in the height of the posterior rib cage or the scapulae, scoliosis may be present. Abnormalities should be reported to the primary care provider for further evaluation.

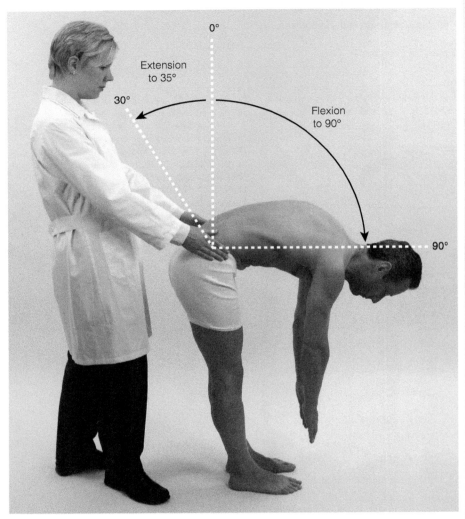

Figure 25.48 Forward flexion of the spine.

Techniques and Normal Findings

- Ask the patient to bend backward as far as is comfortable. Hyperextension should reach 30 degrees.
- Ask the patient to twist the shoulders to the left and to the right. Rotation should reach 30 degrees (see Figure 25.49 ■).

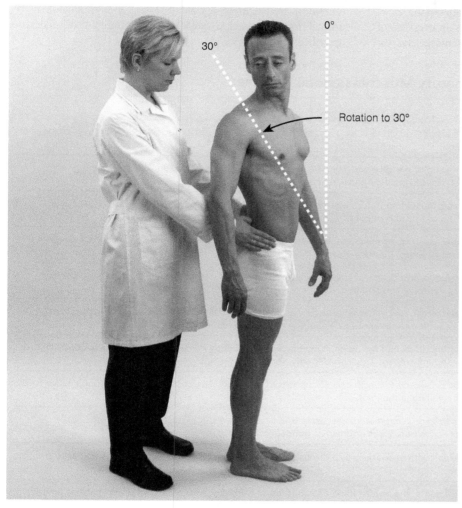

0°

30°

Rotation to 30°

Figure 25.49 Rotation of the spine.

Abnormal Findings Special Considerations

▶ Pain during spinal rotation or decreased mobility during this maneuver may be indicative of various disorders, including degenerative joint disease of the spine or damage to one or more of the intervertebral disks. Abnormalities should be reported to the primary care provider for further evaluation.

Abnormal Findings

bnormal findings of the musculoskeletal system include joint disorders, inflammatory disorders, abnormalities of the spine, and trauma-induced disorders. Table 25.6 provides an overview of common inflammatory diseases that affect the musculoskeletal sys- tem. Table 25.7 summarizes several of the most common traumatic musculoskeletal injuries. A general review of common spinal ab- normalities is provided in Table 25.8. Common joint disorders are described in Table 25.9.

TABLE 25.6 **Overview of Inflammatory Musculoskeletal Diseases**

DISEASE	DESCRIPTION
Osteoarthritis (OA)	In OA the joint cartilage erodes, resulting in pain and stiffness. Disability is associated with osteoarthritic changes in the spine, knees, and hips.
Rheumatoid Arthritis (RA)	Inflammation of the synovium of the joint occurs in RA. The inflammation leads to pain, swelling, damage to the joint, and loss of function. RA affects the hands and feet symmetrically.
Juvenile Rheumatoid Arthritis (JRA)	This form of arthritis occurs in children before age 16 and can affect any body part. Inflammation causes pain, swelling, stiffness, and loss of function of joints. Symptoms may include fever and skin rash.
Systemic Lupus Erythematosus (SLE)	SLE is an autoimmune disease. The autoimmune response results in inflammation and damage to joints and other organs including the kidneys, lungs, blood vessels, and heart.
Scleroderma	In scleroderma there is an overproduction of collagen in the skin or organs, which results in damage to the skin, blood vessels, and joints. Typically, the skin becomes hard and tight.
Fibromyalgia	Fibromyalgia is a chronic disease that is characterized by pain in the muscles and soft tissues that support and surround joints. Pain is experienced in tender points of the head, neck, shoulders, and hips.
Ankylosing Spondylitis (AS)	AS is a chronic inflammatory disease of the spine. It occurs more frequently in males than in females. Fusion of the spine results in stiffness and inflexibility. This disorder may also affect the hips.
Gout	Gout is a type of arthritis caused by uric acid crystal deposits in the joints. The uric acid deposits (tophi) cause inflammation, pain, and swelling in the joint.
Infectious Arthritis	Infectious arthritis refers to joint inflammatory processes that occur as a result of bacterial or viral infection. Infectious arthritis can occur as parvovirus arthritis, as gonococcal arthritis, or in Lyme disease.
Psoriatic Arthritis (PsA)	PsA may occur in individuals with psoriasis, a skin disease. Joint inflammation occurs in the fingers and toes and, occasionally, in the spine.
Bursitis	Bursitis refers to inflammation of the bursae (fluid-filled sacs) that surround joints. The pain of bursitis may limit ROM of the affected area.
Tendinitis	Overuse or inflammatory processes can result in tendinitis. The inflammation of the tendon results in pain and limitation in movement.
Polymyositis	Polymyositis refers to inflammation and weakness in skeletal muscles. This disease can affect the entire body and result in disability.

TABLE 25.7 **Traumatic Musculoskeletal Injuries**

DISORDER	DESCRIPTION
Dislocation	A displacement of the bone from its usual anatomic location in the joint.
Joint Sprain	A stretching or tearing of the capsule or ligament of a joint due to forced movement beyond the joint's normal range.
Fracture	A partial or complete break in the continuity of the bone from trauma.
Muscle Strain	A partial muscle tear resulting from overstretching or overuse of the muscle.

TABLE 25.8	**Common Spinal Abnormalities**

Kyphosis

An exaggeration of the normal convex curve of the thoracic spine that may result from congenital abnormality, rheumatic conditions, compression fractures, or other disease processes including syphilis, tuberculosis, and rickets. Severe kyphosis may occur with aging due to other contributing factors, such as degenerative joint disease, poor posture, or hormonal changes.

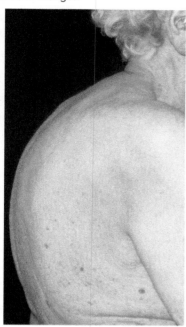

Figure 25.50 Kyphosis.
Source: Dr. P. Marazzi/Science Source.

Scoliosis

A lateral curvature of the spine that may occur congenitally, or as a result of disease, injury, habitual improper posture, unequal leg length, weakening of musculature, or chronic head tilting in visual disorders.

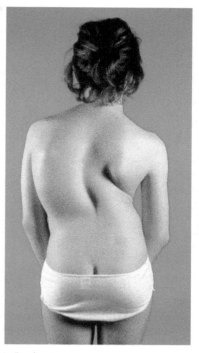

Figure 25.51 Scoliosis.
Source: Princess Margaret Rose Orthopaedic Hospital/Science Source.

Lordosis

An exaggeration of the normal lumbar curve. Lordosis occurs in pregnancy and in obesity to compensate for the protuberance of the abdomen. Benign juvenile lordosis occurs congenitally. Other conditions such as spondylolisthesis may also aid in the formation of lordosis later in life (Kalichman, Li, Hunter, & Been, 2011).

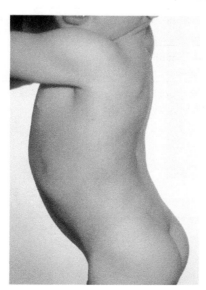

Figure 25.52 Benign juvenile lordosis.
Source: Wellcome Image Library/Custom Medical Stock Photo.

| TABLE 25.9 | **Common Joint Disorders** |

Temporomandibular Joint Syndrome

Inflammation or trauma can result in temporomandibular joint (TMJ) syndrome.

Findings include swelling and crepitus or pain in the TM joint, especially on movement such as opening and closing the mouth.

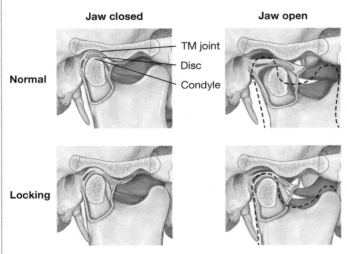

Figure 25.53 Temporomandibular joint (TMJ) syndrome.

Rotator Cuff Tear

Arises from repeated impingement, injury, or falls. Impaired abduction of the glenohumeral joint occurs with a complete tear of the supraspinatus tendon.

Findings include muscle atrophy of the infraspinatus and supraspinatus, tenderness, and pain.

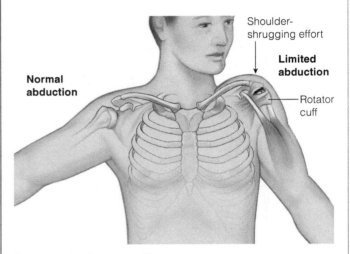

Figure 25.54 Rotator cuff tear.

Olecranon Bursitis

Inflammation of the olecranon bursa at the bony prominence of the elbow that may be caused by trauma or inflammation from rheumatoid or gouty arthritis. Bursitis can develop in a variety of body regions.

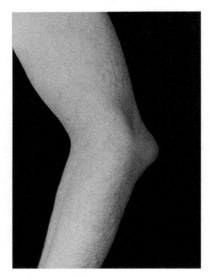

Figure 25.55 Olecranon bursitis.
Source: StockPhotosArt/Fotolia.

Joint Effusion

Inflammatory joint disease results in fluid in the joint capsule, causing joint effusion. Joint effusion produces distention of the tissue around the inflamed joint.

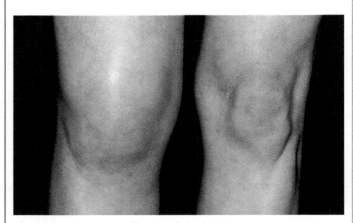

Figure 25.56 Joint effusion of the knee.
Source: Dr. P. Marazzi/Science Source.

TABLE 25.9   **Common Joint Disorders** (continued)

Rheumatoid Nodules

Firm, nontender subcutaneous nodules that often are seen distal to the olecranon bursa in the hands and fingers.

Rheumatoid nodules may occur along the extensor surface of the ulna.

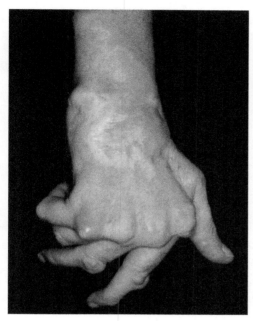

Figure 25.57 Rheumatoid nodules.

Carpal Tunnel Syndrome

Chronic repetitive motion results in compression of the median nerve, which lies inside the carpal tunnel. Decreased motor function leads to atrophy of the thenar eminence. Findings in carpal tunnel syndrome include pain, numbness, and positive Phalen's test.

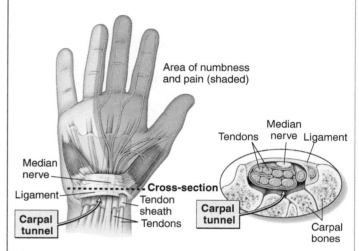

Figure 25.58 Carpal tunnel syndrome.

Dupuytren's Contracture

Flexion contracture of the fingers is a result of hyperplasia of the fascia of the palmar surface of the hand. Impaired ROM is a hallmark of contractures. Dupuytren's contracture may be inherited or occur with diabetes or alcoholic cirrhosis.

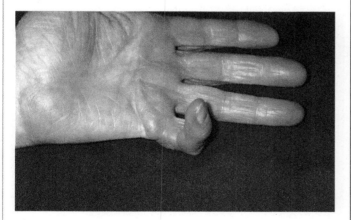

Figure 25.59 Dupuytren's contracture.
Source: Dr. P. Marazzi/Science Source.

Ulnar Deviation

In RA the chronic inflammation of the metacarpophalangeal and interphalangeal joints leads to ulnar deviation. RA can lead to a number of musculoskeletal deformities, the most common of which affect the hands and feet.

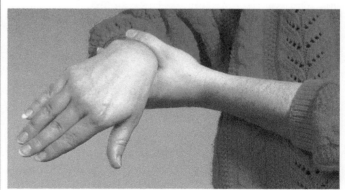

Figure 25.60 Ulnar deviation.

(continued)

TABLE 25.9 **Common Joint Disorders** (continued)

Swan-Neck and Boutonnière Deformities

Flexion contractures associated with rheumatoid arthritis. *Swan-neck contractures* refer to hyperextension of the proximal interphalangeal joints with fixed flexion of the distal interphalangeal joints. *Boutonnière deformities* involve proximal interphalangeal joint flexion in conjunction with distal interphalangeal joint hyperextension.

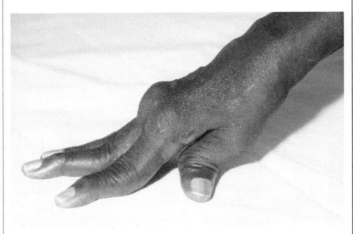

Figure 25.61 Swan-neck and boutonnière deformities.
Source: Sue Ford/Science Source.

Osteoarthritis

OA is associated with the development of Bouchard's and Heberden's nodes, which are hard nodules over the proximal and distal interphalangeal joints.

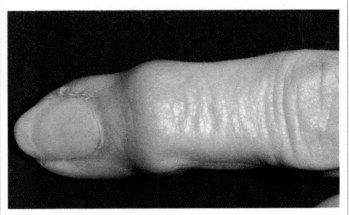

Figure 25.62 Heberden's nodes are found in the distal interphalangeal joints.
Source: Dr. P. Marazzi/Science Source.

Rheumatoid Arthritis

RA results in symmetric fusiform swelling in the soft tissue around the proximal interphalangeal joints. Other symptoms may include pain, fatigue, and morning joint stiffness.

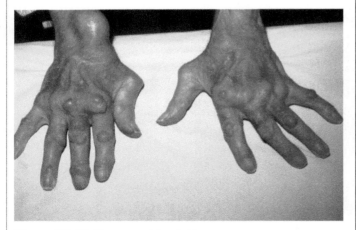

Figure 25.63 Rheumatoid arthritis.
Source: Dr. P. Marazzi/Science Source.

Synovitis

Refers to inflammation of the synovium, which is the tissue that lines the joints. In the knee, effusion within the synovinum results in distention of the suprapatellar area and the lateral aspects of the knee.

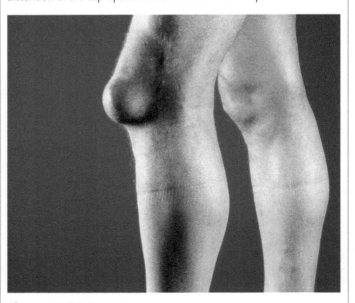

Figure 25.64 Synovitis.
Source: Princess Margaret Rose Orthopaedic Hospital/Science Source.

TABLE 25.9	**Common Joint Disorders** (continued)

Gout

Altered purine metabolism results in inflammation of the joints. Usually seen in the metatarsophalangeal joint of the first toe, gout is manifested in erythema, pain, and edema. Hard nodules (**tophi**) may appear over the joint.

Hallux Valgus (Bunion)

A bunion is a thickening and inflammation of the bone or the bursa of the joint of the great toe that produces lateral displacement of the toe with marked joint enlargement. The big toe may turn toward the second toe. The tissues around the joint may be swollen and tender.

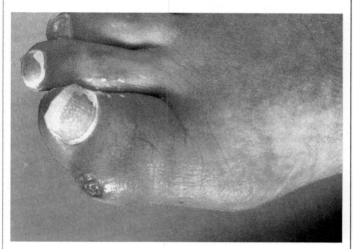

Figure 25.65 Gout.
Source: Wellcome Image Library/Custom Medical Stock Photo.

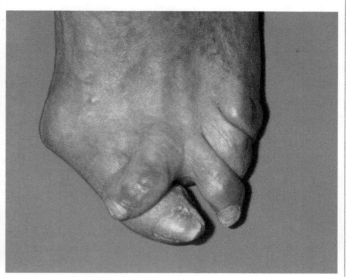

Figure 25.66 Hallux valgus (bunion); also note the hammertoe of the second digit.
Source: Dr. P. Marazzi/Science Source.

Hammertoe

Hammertoe is caused by an imbalance of the muscle and ligament around the toe joint. It may be the result of trauma or genetic factors. This condition also may be caused by wearing certain types of footwear, including narrow-toed shoes, high heels, or shoes that are too small. The middle toe joint becomes fixed in a flexed position. Without treatment, this condition will progressively worsen.

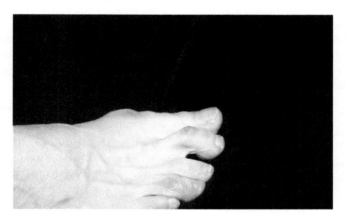

Figure 25.67 Hammertoe.
Source: Roseman/Custom Medical Stock Photo.

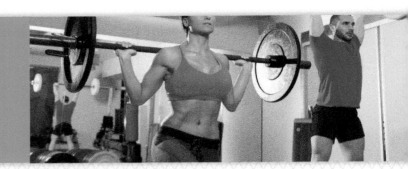

Application Through Critical Thinking

▌ Case Study

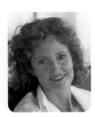

Mrs. Rhonda Barber is a 43-year-old teacher. She visits the clinic for assessment of swelling and stiffness all over, but especially in her hands.

The health history reveals that for several months Mrs. Barber has had some stiffness in her joints when awakening from sleep and after long periods of physical activity "like housework." She became "alarmed" when her hands were "hot, red, and swollen" and that she "could hardly move them." She has had no recent illness but has "felt weak and tired" and has not had much of an appetite lately. She reports no family history of musculoskeletal disease. She reports that she has had regular physical examinations including blood work, and that nothing has been abnormal. Her last exam was 6 months ago. She takes no prescribed medications but has been using Advil and Aleve for the stiffness with moderate relief. She states that she is concerned about her hands because she must write on the board and correct papers. She also fears that "if something is really wrong and I don't get relief, I won't be able to care for my family or myself for that matter."

Physical assessment reveals a well-developed female 5′3″ tall, weighing 120 lb. Her skin is pale and warm. Her gait is steady. She has normal ROM in the upper and lower extremities. ROM of her wrists, hands, and fingers is limited. The joints of her fingers are erythematous, hot, and edematous bilaterally. Her joints are tender to touch and painful upon movement. Pain is 6 to 7 on a scale of 0 to 10.

The nurse suspects that Mrs. Barber may have rheumatoid arthritis. The nurse will obtain laboratory tests and X-rays.

▌ Complete Documentation

The following is a sample documentation from assessment of Rhonda Barber.

SUBJECTIVE DATA: Stiffness in joints when waking and after long periods of physical activity for several months. "Alarmed" when hands were hot, red, swollen, and could hardly move them. No recent illness. Weak, tired, and loss of appetite lately. No family history of musculoskeletal disease. Regular physical examinations with normal results and normal "blood work." Last examination 6 months ago. No prescribed medications. Advil and Aleve for stiffness—moderate relief. Concerned about ability to work as teacher and "if something is really wrong," about ability to care for family.

OBJECTIVE DATA: Well-developed 43-year-old female. 5′3″, 120 lb. Skin pale, warm. Gait steady. Full ROM all extremities except hands and fingers. Joints of fingers erythematous, hot, edematous bilaterally, tender to touch, and painful on movement. Pain 6 to 7 on scale of 0 to 10.

▌ Critical Thinking Questions

1. Describe the thoughts and actions of the nurse that led to the suspicion of rheumatoid arthritis.

2. What information would help in developing a plan of care for Mrs. Barber?

3. How would the nurse discriminate between findings for rheumatoid arthritis and osteoarthritis?

4. As Mrs. Barber ages, what additional age-related changes will she need to be concerned about?

5. What are some strategies that would help Mrs. Barber get through the physical exam portion?

▌ Prepare Teaching Plan

LEARNING NEED: The data in the case study reveal that Mrs. Barber may have rheumatoid arthritis. Her symptoms are typical for rheumatoid arthritis. She will undergo laboratory tests and X-rays to confirm the diagnosis.

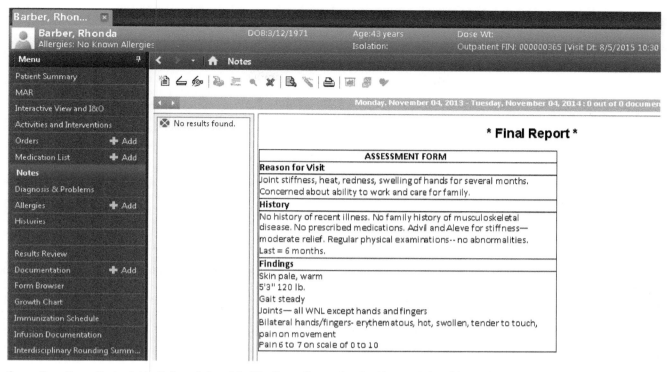

Barber, Rhon... ✕

Barber, Rhonda
Allergies: No Known Allergies

DOB:3/12/1971   Age:43 years   Dose Wt:
                      Isolation: Outpatient FIN: 000000365 [Visit Dt: 8/5/2015 10:30

Menu
Patient Summary
MAR
Interactive View and I&O
Activities and Interventions
Orders   ➕ Add
Medication List   ➕ Add
Notes
Diagnosis & Problems
Allergies   ➕ Add
Histories

Results Review
Documentation   ➕ Add
Form Browser
Growth Chart
Immunization Schedule
Infusion Documentation
Interdisciplinary Rounding Summ...

‹ › · 🏠 Notes

Monday, November 04, 2013 - Tuesday, November 04, 2014 : 0 out of 0 documen

No results found.

* Final Report *

ASSESSMENT FORM
Reason for Visit
Joint stiffness, heat, redness, swelling of hands for several months. Concerned about ability to work and care for family.
History
No history of recent illness. No family history of musculoskeletal disease. No prescribed medications. Advil and Aleve for stiffness—moderate relief. Regular physical examinations-- no abnormalities. Last = 6 months.
Findings
Skin pale, warm 5'3" 120 lb. Gait steady Joints— all WNL except hands and fingers Bilateral hands/fingers- erythematous, hot, swollen, tender to touch, pain on movement Pain 6 to 7 on scale of 0 to 10

Source: From Cerner Electronic Health Record. Copyright © by Cerner Corporation. Used by permission of Cerner Corporation.

The case study provides data that are representative of risks, symptoms, and behaviors of many individuals. Therefore, the following teaching plan is based on the need to provide information to members of any community about arthritis.

GOAL: The participants in this learning program will have increased awareness of risk factors and symptoms associated with arthritis.

OBJECTIVES: At the completion of this learning session, the participants will be able to:

1. Describe arthritis.
2. Identify risk factors associated with arthritis.
3. List the symptoms of arthritis.
4. Discuss strategies in diagnosis and treatment of arthritis.

APPLICATION OF OBJECTIVE 2: Identify risk factors associated with arthritis

Content	Teaching Strategy	Evaluation
• Age. Osteoarthritis risk increases after age 45. • Gender. Females have a higher incidence of arthritis. • Hereditary factors. Family history and genetic factors increase risk for arthritis. • Obesity. Obesity increases risk for arthritis in weight-bearing joints. • Joint injury through sports or repeated stress in some occupations can increase the risk of osteoarthritis. • Joint misalignment or deformity can increase the risk for arthritis.	• Lecture • Discussion • Audiovisual materials • Printed materials Lecture is appropriate when disseminating information to large groups. Discussion allows participants to bring up concerns and to raise questions. Audiovisual materials such as illustrations reinforce verbal presentation. Printed material, especially to be taken away with learners, allows review, reinforcement, and reading at the learner's pace.	• Written examination. May use short answer, fill-in, or multiple-choice items or a combination of items. If these are short and easy to evaluate, the learner received immediate feedback.

▶ References

Bax, M., van Heemst, J., Huizinga, T. W., & Toes, R. E. (2011). Genetics of rheumatoid arthritis: What have we learned? *Immunogenetics, 63*(8), 459–466.

Bikley, L. S. (2008). *Bates' guide to physical examination and history taking* (10th ed.). Philadelphia, PA: Lippincott.

Chang, H. Y., Lai, Y. H., Jensen, M. P., Shun, S. C., Hsiao, F. H., Lee, C. N., & Yang, Y. L. (2014). Factors associated with low back pain changes during the third trimester of pregnancy. *Journal of Advanced Nursing, 70*(5), 1054–1064.

Dashe, J., Roocroft, J. H., Bastrom, T. P., & Edmonds, E. W. (2013). Spectrum of shoulder injuries in skeletally immature patients. *Orthopedic Clinics of North America, 44*(4), 541–551.

Izadi, M., Sadat, S. E., Zamani, M. M., Mousavi, S. A., Jafari, N. J., Fard, M. M., . . . Talakoob, H. (2013). Trauma induced chronic osteomyelitis: Specimens from sinus tract or bone? *Galen Medical Journal, 2*(4), 146–151.

Kalichman, L., Li, L., Hunter, D. J., & Been, E. (2011). Association between computed tomography-evaluated lumbar lordosis and features of spinal degeneration, evaluated in supine position. *Spine Journal, 11*(4), 308–315.

Kraemer, J. (2009). *Intervertebral disk diseases: Causes, diagnosis, treatment and prophylaxis* (3rd ed.). Stuttgart, Germany: Thieme.

Kruger, M. C., Todd, J. M., Schollum, L. M., Kuhn-Sherlock, B., McLean, D. W., & Wylie, K. (2013). Bone health comparison in seven Asian countries using calcaneal ultrasound. *BMC Musculoskeletal Disorders, 14*(1), 81.

Lidar, Z., Behrbalk, E., Regev, G. J., Salame, K., Keynan, O., Schweiger, C., . . . Keidar, A. (2012). Intervertebral disc height changes after weight reduction in morbidly obese patients and its effect on quality of life and radicular and low back pain. *Spine, 37*(23), 1947–1952.

Magee, D. J. (2014). *Orthopedic physical assessment* (6th. ed.). St. Louis, MO: Elsevier.

Marieb, E. (2009). *Essentials of human anatomy and physiology* (9th ed.). Redwood City, CA: Benjamin/Cummings/Pearson Education.

May, A., Pettifor, J. M., Norris, S. A., Ramsay, M., & Lombard, Z. (2013). Genetic factors influencing bone mineral content in a black South African population. *Journal of Bone and Mineral Metabolism, 31*(6), 708–716.

Mayo Clinic. (2013). *Osteoporosis: Definition.* Retrieved from http://www .mayoclinic.org/diseases-conditions/osteoporosis/basics/definition/ con-20019924

Mayo Clinic. (2013). *Tests and procedures: Sed rate (erythrocyte sedimentation rate).* Retrieved from http://www.mayoclinic.org/tests-procedures/sed-rate/basics/ results/prc-20013502

Mayo Foundation for Medical Education and Research. (2014). *Rochester test catalog: 2014 online test catalog.* Available at http://www .mayomedicallaboratories.com/test-catalog/

MedlinePlus. (2013). *Osteomyelitis.* Retrieved from http://www.nlm.nih.gov/ medlineplus/ency/article/000437.htm

Micheo, W. (Ed.) (2010). *Rehabilitation medicine quick reference: Musculoskeletal, sports, and occupational medicine.* New York, NY: Demos Medical Publishing.

Orcesi, S. (2013). The floppy newborn. *Early Human Development, 89,* Supplement 4, S79–S81.

Osborn, K. S., Wraa, C. E., Watson, A., & Holleran, R. S. (2013). *Medical-surgical nursing: Preparation for practice* (2nd ed.). Upper Saddle River, NJ: Pearson.

Pervaiz, K., Cabezas, A., Downes, K., Santoni, B. G., & Frankle, M. A. (2013). Osteoporosis and shoulder osteoarthritis: Incidence, risk factors, and surgical implications. *Journal of Shoulder and Elbow Surgery, 22*(3), e1–e8.

Schmid, A. A., Van Puymbroeck, M., & Koceja, D. M. (2010). Effect of a 12-week yoga intervention on fear of falling and balance in older adults: A pilot study. *Archives of Physical Medicine and Rehabilitation, 91*(4), 576–583.

Shapses, S. A., & Sukumar, D. (2012). Bone metabolism in obesity and weight loss. *Annual Review of Nutrition, 32,* 287–309.

University of Maryland Medical Center (UMMC). (2013). *Osteoporosis.* Retrieved from http://umm.edu/health/medical/reports/articles/osteoporosis

U.S. Department of Health and Human Services (USDHHS). (2014). *Healthy people 2020.* Retrieved from http://www.healthypeople.gov/2020/default.aspx

Weycker, D., Lamerato, L., Schooley, S., Macarios, D., Woodworth, T. S., Yurgin, N., & Oster, G. (2013). Adherence with bisphosphonate therapy and change in bone mineral density among women with osteoporosis or osteopenia in clinical practice. *Osteoporosis International, 24*(4), 1483–1489.

Wilmes, D., Omoumi, P., Squifflet, J., Cornu, O., Rodriguez-Villalobos, H., & Yombi, J. C. (2012). Osteomyelitis pubis caused by Kingella kingae in an adult patient: Report of the first case. *BMC Infectious Diseases, 12*(1), 236.

Wilson, B. A., Shannon, M. T., & Shields, K. M. (2013). *Pearson nurse's drug guide.* Upper Saddle River, NJ: Pearson.

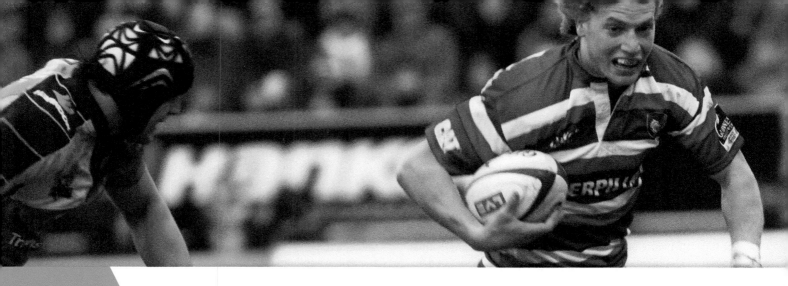

Neurologic System

▶ Learning Outcomes

Upon completion of this chapter, you will be able to:

1. Describe the anatomy and physiology of the neurologic system.

2. Develop questions to be used when completing the focused interview.

3. Describe the techniques required for assessment of the neurologic system.

4. Differentiate normal from abnormal findings in the physical assessment of the neurologic system.

5. Describe developmental, cultural, psychosocial, and environmental variations in assessment techniques and findings of the neurologic system.

6. Discuss the objectives regarding neurologic health as stated in *Healthy People 2020*.

7. Apply critical thinking to the physical assessment of the neurologic system.

Key Terms

analgesia, 778
anesthesia, 778
anosmia, 766
Babinski response, 786
brain stem, 747
central nervous system, 746
cerebellum, 747
cerebrum, 746
clonus, 783
coma, 787
dermatome, 748
diplopia, 767
dysphagia, 771
hypalgesia, 778
hyperesthesia, 778
hypoesthesia, 778
meninges, 746
nuchal rigidity, 787
nystagmus, 767
optic atrophy, 767
papilledema, 767
peripheral nervous system, 746
reflexes, 747

The complex integration, coordination, and regulation of body systems, and, ultimately, all body functions, are achieved through the mechanics of the nervous system. The intricate nature of the nervous system permits the individual to perform all physiologic functions, perform all activities of daily living, function in society, and maintain a degree of independence. A threat to any aspect of neurologic function is a threat to the whole person. A neurologic deficit could alter self-concept, produce anxiety related to decreased function and loss of self-control, and restrict the patient's mobility. Thus, it is essential to assess the psychosocial health status of a patient experiencing a neurologic deficit. Because factors such as diet, alcohol intake, smoking, and other health practices can influence neurologic health, the nurse must consider the patient's self-care practices when assessing the patient's neurologic system. Factors relating to the patient's occupation, environment, and genetic background also contribute to neurologic health. These are among the considerations regarding neurologic health as described in *Healthy People 2020*. Objectives related to the promotion of neurologic health are included in Table 26.2 on page 751.

The nervous system is immature at birth. Many reflexes that are present in the newborn begin to disappear as the system matures. The older adult experiences a decrease in neurologic function; the senses diminish, as do reactions to stimuli. Degeneration of the nervous system may lead to a variety of psychosocial problems such as social isolation, lowered self-esteem, stress, anxiety, and ineffective coping.

A healthy diet, exercise, and rest help ensure optimum neurologic functions. Alcohol causes neurologic impairments ranging from mild sedation to severe motor deficits. Caffeine is a mild stimulant that may cause restlessness, tremors, and insomnia.

A variety of home, work, and environmental factors may cause neurologic impairments. For example, lead-based paint in older homes may cause lead poisoning and encephalopathy in children.

A thorough neurologic assessment gives the nurse detailed data regarding the patient's health status and self-care practices. It is imperative to develop and refine assessment skills regarding the wellness and normal parameters of the neurologic functions in the body. The nurse needs to foster a keen discriminatory skill concerning the subtle changes that could be occurring in the patient. Neurologic assessment is an integral aspect of the patient's health and must be carefully considered when conducting a thorough health assessment.

Anatomy and Physiology Review

The neurologic system, a highly integrated and complex system, is divided into two principal parts: the central nervous system (CNS) and the peripheral nervous system (PNS). The **central nervous system** consists of the brain and the spinal cord, whereas the cranial nerves and the spinal nerves make up the **peripheral nervous system**. The two systems work together to receive an impulse, interpret it, and initiate a response, enabling the individual to maintain a high level of adaptation and homeostasis. The nervous system is responsible for control of cognitive function and both voluntary and involuntary actions.

The basic cell of the nervous system is the *neuron*. This highly specialized cell sends impulses throughout the body. Many of the nerve fibers that have a large diameter or are long in length are covered with a *myelin sheath*. This white, fatty cover helps to protect the neuron while increasing the delivery of a nerve impulse, hence the term *white matter of the nervous system*.

Central Nervous System

The central nervous system (CNS) includes the brain and spinal cord. These structures are described in the following sections.

Brain

The brain is the largest portion of the central nervous system. It is covered and protected by the meninges, the cerebrospinal fluid, and the bony structure of the skull. The **meninges** are three connective tissue membranes that cover, protect, and nourish the central nervous system. The cerebrospinal fluid also helps to nourish the central nervous system; however, its primary function is to cushion the brain and prevent injury to the brain tissue. The brain is made up of the cerebrum, diencephalon, cerebellum, and brain stem (see Figure 26.1 ■).

CEREBRUM The **cerebrum** is the largest portion of the brain. The outermost layer of the cerebrum, the *cerebral cortex*, is composed of gray matter. Responsible for all conscious behavior, the cerebral cortex enables the individual to perceive, remember, communicate, and initiate voluntary movements. The cerebrum consists of the frontal, parietal, occipital, and temporal lobes. The lobes of the cerebrum are illustrated in Figure 26.2 ■.

The frontal lobe of the cerebrum helps control voluntary skeletal movement, speech, emotions, and intellectual activities. The prefrontal cortex of the frontal lobe controls intellect, complex learning abilities, judgment, reasoning, concern for others, and creation of abstract ideas.

The parietal lobe of the cerebrum is responsible for conscious awareness of sensation and somatosensory stimuli, including temperature, pain, shapes, and two-point discrimination—for example, the ability to sense a round versus square object placed in the hand or hot versus cold materials against the skin.

The visual cortex, located in the occipital lobe, receives stimuli from the retina and interprets the visual stimuli in relation to past experiences.

The temporal lobe of the cerebrum is responsible for interpreting auditory stimuli. Impulses from the cochlea are transmitted to the temporal lobe and are interpreted regarding pitch, rhythm, loudness, and perception of what the individual hears. The olfactory cortex is also in the temporal lobe and transmits impulses related to smell.

DIENCEPHALON The diencephalon is composed of the thalamus, hypothalamus, and epithalamus. The **thalamus** is the gateway to the cerebral cortex. All input channeled to the cerebral cortex is processed by the thalamus.

The hypothalamus, an autonomic control center, influences activities such as blood pressure; heart rate; force of heart contraction; digestive motility; respiratory rate and depth; and perception of pain, pleasure, and fear. Regulation of body temperature, food intake, water balance, and sleep cycles are also regulated by the hypothalamus.

The epithalamus helps control moods and sleep cycles. It contains the choroid plexus, where the cerebrospinal fluid is formed.

CEREBELLUM The **cerebellum** is located below the cerebrum and behind the brain stem. It coordinates stimuli from the cerebral cortex to provide precise timing for skeletal muscle coordination and smooth movements. The cerebellum also assists with maintaining equilibrium and muscle tone. The cerebellum receives information about the body position from the inner ear and then sends impulses to the muscles, whose contraction maintains or restores balance.

BRAIN STEM The **brain stem** contains the midbrain, pons, and medulla oblongata. Located between the cerebrum and spinal cord, the brain stem connects pathways between the higher and lower structures. Of the 12 pairs of cranial nerves, 10 originate in the brain stem. As an autonomic control center, the brain stem influences

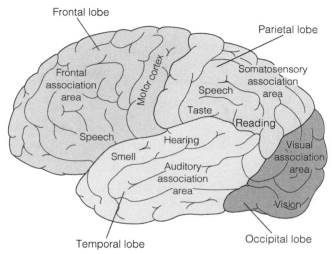

Figure 26.2 Lobes of the cerebrum.

blood pressure by controlling vasoconstriction. It also regulates respiratory rate, depth, and rhythm as well as vomiting, hiccupping, swallowing, coughing, and sneezing.

Spinal Cord

The **spinal cord** is a continuation of the medulla oblongata. About 42 cm (17 in.) in length, it passes through the skull at the foramen magnum and continues through the vertebral column to the first and second lumbar vertebrae. The meninges, cerebrospinal fluid, and bony vertebrae protect the spinal cord. The spinal cord has the ability to transmit sensory impulses to and motor impulses from the brain via the ascending and descending pathways. It also mediates stretch reflexes and reflexes for defecation and urination. Some reflex activity takes place within the spinal cord; however, for this activity to be useful, the brain must interpret it.

Reflexes

Reflexes are stimulus–response activities of the body. They are fast, predictable, unlearned, innate, and involuntary reactions to stimuli. The individual is aware of the results of the reflex activity and not the activity itself. The reflex activity may be simple and take place at the level of the spinal cord, with interpretation at the cerebral level. For example, if the tendon of the knee is sharply stimulated with a reflex hammer, the impulse follows the afferent nerve fibers. A synapse occurs in the spinal cord, and the impulse is transmitted to the efferent nerve fibers, leading to an additional synapse and stimulation of muscle fibers. As the muscle fibers contract, the lower leg moves, causing the knee-jerk reaction. The individual is aware of the reflex after the lower leg moves and the brain has interpreted the activity. Figure 26.3 ■ illustrates two simple reflex arcs.

Peripheral Nervous System

The peripheral nervous system (PNS) includes the 12 pairs of cranial nerves, which take impulses to and from the brain, and the paired spinal nerves, which transmit impulses to and from the spinal cord. They are described in the following paragraphs.

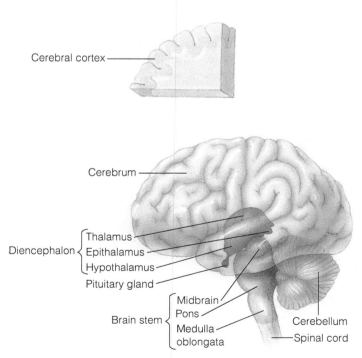

Figure 26.1 Regions of the brain.

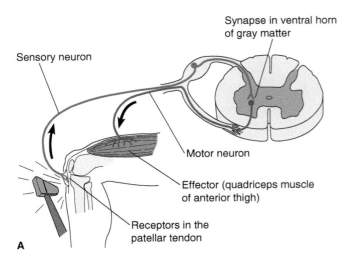

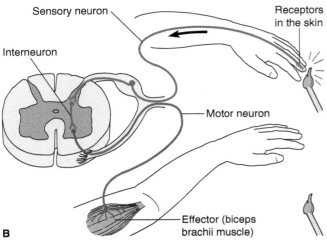

Figure 26.3 Two simple reflex arcs. A. In the two-neuron reflex arc, the stimulus is transferred from the sensory neuron directly to the motor neuron at the point of synapse in the spinal cord. B. In the three-neuron reflex arc, the stimulus travels from the sensory neuron to an interneuron in the spinal cord, and then to the motor neuron. (Sensory nerves are shown in blue; motor nerves, in red.)

Cranial Nerves

The 12 pairs of cranial nerves originate in the brain and serve various parts of the head and neck (see Figure 26.4 ■). The first 2 pairs originate in the anterior brain, and the remaining 10 pairs originate in the brain stem. The vagus nerve is the only cranial nerve to serve a muscle and body region below the neck. The cranial nerves are numbered using roman numerals and many times are discussed by number rather than by name. Composition of the cranial nerve fibers varies, producing sensory nerves, motor nerves, and mixed nerves. A summary of the names, numbers, functions, and activities of the cranial nerves is presented in Table 26.1.

Spinal Nerves

The spinal cord supplies the body with 31 pairs of spinal nerves that are named according to the vertebral level of origin as shown in Figure 26.5 ■ on page 750.

There are 8 pairs of cervical nerves, 12 pairs of thoracic nerves, 5 pairs of lumbar nerves, 5 pairs of sacral nerves, and 1 pair of coccygeal nerves. At the cervical level, the nerves exit superior to the vertebra except for the eighth cervical nerve. This nerve exits inferior to the seventh cervical vertebra. All remaining descending nerves exit the spinal cord and vertebral column inferior to the same-numbered vertebrae. Spinal nerves are all classified as mixed nerves because they contain motor and sensory pathways that produce motor and sensory activities. Each pair of nerves is responsible for a particular area of the body. The nerves provide some overlap of body segments they serve. This overlap is more complete on the trunk than on the extremities.

A **dermatome** is an area of skin innervated by the cutaneous branch of one spinal nerve. All spinal nerves except the first cervical (C1) serve a cutaneous region. The anterior and posterior views of the dermatomes of the body are shown in Figure 26.6 ■ on page 751.

Special Considerations

Throughout the assessment process, the nurse gathers subjective and objective data reflecting the patient's state of health. Using critical thinking and the nursing process, the nurse identifies many factors to be considered when collecting the data. Some of these factors include but are not limited to age, developmental level, race, ethnicity, work history, living conditions, and socioeconomics. Physical wellness and emotional wellness are also among the many factors or special considerations that impact a patient's health status. The following sections describe the ways in which neurologic health is affected by these special considerations.

Health Promotion Considerations

Just as concepts in nursing—such as oxygenation and perfusion—are interrelated, so are body systems. As such, neurologic function overlaps with the function of many other body systems, such as vision, hearing, and smell. Various *Healthy People 2020* objectives related to each of these physiologic functions are discussed in chapters that explore assessment of their respective primary body systems. Alterations in neurologic health also include disorders of central and peripheral nervous system function, such as various forms of dementia and motor nerve disorders. See Table 26.2 on page 751 for examples of *Healthy People 2020* objectives that are designed to promote neurologic health and wellness among individuals across the life span.

Lifespan Considerations

Growth and development are dynamic processes that describe change over time. The following discussion presents specific variations for different age groups across the life span. The structures and functions of the neurologic system undergo change as a result of normal growth and development. Accurate interpretation of subjective and objective data from assessment of the neurologic system is dependent on knowledge of expected variations. The discussion of age-related variations is presented in the following sections.

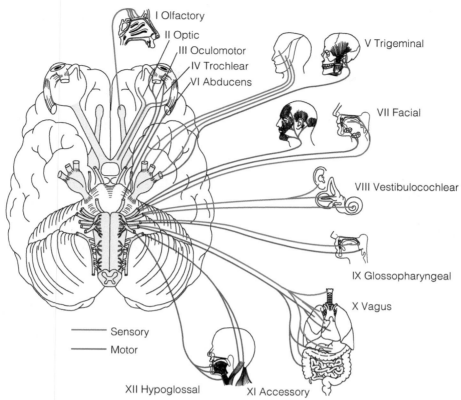

Figure 26.4 Cranial nerves and their target regions. (Sensory nerves are shown in blue; motor nerves, in red.)

TABLE 26.1		**Cranial Nerves**	
NAME	**NUMBER**	**FUNCTION**	**ACTIVITY**
Olfactory	I	Sensory	Sense of smell.
Optic	II	Sensory	Vision.
Oculomotor	III	Motor	Pupillary reflex, extrinsic muscle movement of eye.
Trochlear	IV	Motor	Eye-muscle movement.
Trigeminal	V	Mixed	*Ophthalmic branch:* Sensory impulses from scalp, upper eyelid, nose, cornea, and lacrimal gland. *Maxillary branch:* Sensory impulses from lower eyelid, nasal cavity, upper teeth, upper lip, palate. *Mandibular branch:* Sensory impulses from tongue, lower teeth, skin of chin, and lower lip. Motor action includes teeth clenching, movement of mandible.
Abducens	VI	Mixed	Extrinsic muscle movement of eye.
Facial	VII	Mixed	Taste (anterior two thirds of tongue). Facial movements such as smiling, closing of eyes, frowning. Production of tears and salivary stimulation.
Vestibulocochlear	VIII	Sensory	*Vestibular branch:* Sense of balance or equilibrium. *Cochlear branch:* Sense of hearing.
Glossopharyngeal	IX	Mixed	Produces the gag and swallowing reflexes. Taste (posterior third of the tongue).
Vagus	X	Mixed	Innervates muscles of throat and mouth for swallowing and talking. Other branches responsible for pressoreceptors and chemoreceptor activity.
Accessory	XI	Motor	Movement of the trapezius and sternocleidomastoid muscles. Some movement of larynx, pharynx, and soft palate.
Hypoglossal	XII	Motor	Movement of tongue for swallowing, movement of food during chewing, and speech.

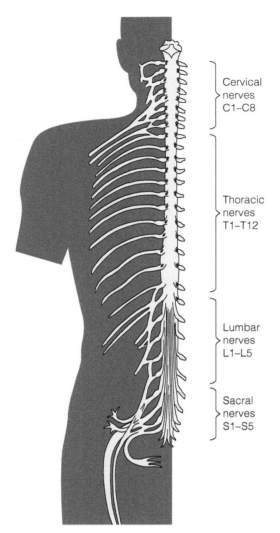

Figure 26.5 Spinal nerves.

Cervical nerves C1–C8

Thoracic nerves T1–T12

Lumbar nerves L1–L5

Sacral nerves S1–S5

Infants and Children

The growth of the nervous system is very rapid during the fetal period. This rate of growth does not continue during infancy. Some research indicates that no neurons are formed after the third trimester of fetal life. It is believed that during infancy the neurons mature, allowing for more complete actions to take place. The cerebral cortex thickens, brain size increases, and myelinization occurs. The maturational advances in the nervous system are responsible for the cephalocaudal and proximal-to-distal refinement of development, control, and movement.

The neonate has several primitive reflexes at birth. These include but are not limited to sucking; stepping; startle (Moro); and the Babinski reflex, in which stimulation of the sole of the foot from the heel toward the toes results in dorsiflexion of the great toe and fanning of other toes. The Babinski reflex and the tonic neck reflex are normal until around 2 years of age. (See Table 26.3, Primitive Reflexes of Early Childhood, on pages 752–753.) By about 1 month of age, the reflexes begin to disappear, and the child takes on more controlled and complex activity.

The cry of the newborn helps place the infant on the health–illness continuum. *Strong* and *lusty* are terms used to describe the cry of a healthy newborn. An absent, weak, or "catlike" or shrill cry usually indicates cerebral disease.

Throughout infancy and the early childhood years, it is important to assess the fine and gross motor skills, language, and personal–social skills of the child. The nurse identifies benchmarks or mileposts related to age and level of functioning and compares the child's actual functioning to an anticipated level of functioning. Developmental delays or learning disabilities may be related to, but are not limited to, neurologic conditions such as fetal alcohol syndrome, autism, and attention deficit disorder.

The Pregnant Female

As the uterus grows to accommodate the fetus, pressure may be placed on nerves in the pelvic cavity, thus producing neurologic changes in the legs. As the pressure is relieved in the pelvis, the changes in the lower extremities are resolved. As the fetus grows, the center of gravity of the female shifts, and the lumbar curvature of the spine is accentuated. This change in posture can place pressure on roots of nerves, causing sensory changes in the lower extremities. These sensory changes are reversible following relief of pressure and postural changes. Hyperactive reflexes may indicate pregnancy-induced hypertension (PIH).

The Older Adult

As the individual ages, many neurologic changes occur. Some of these changes are readily visible, whereas others are internal and are not easily detected. The internal changes could be primary in nature, or secondary to other changes, and contribute to the aging process. In general, the aging process causes a subtle, slow, but steady decrease in neurologic function. These changes can be more pronounced and more troublesome for the individual when they are accompanied by a chronic illness such as heart disease, diabetes, or arthritis. Impulse transmission decreases, as does reaction to stimuli. Reflexes are diminished or disappear, and coordination is not as strong as it once was. Deep tendon reflexes are not as brisk. Coordination and movement may be slower and not as smooth as they were at one time.

The senses—hearing, vision, smell, taste, and touch—are not as acute as they once were. Taste is not as strong; therefore, the older adult tends to use more seasonings on food. Visual acuity and hearing also begin to diminish as the individual ages.

As muscle mass decreases, the older individual moves and reacts more slowly than during youth. The patient's gait may now include short, shuffling, uncertain, and perhaps unsteady steps. The posture of the older adult demonstrates more flexion than in earlier years.

Assessment techniques used with the older adult are the same as those used for the younger or middle-aged adult. However, because the older adult tires more easily, the nurse may need to do the total assessment in more than one visit. The nurse should allow more time than usual when performing the neurologic assessment of the older adult. It is also imperative to obtain a detailed history, because chronic health problems can influence the findings.

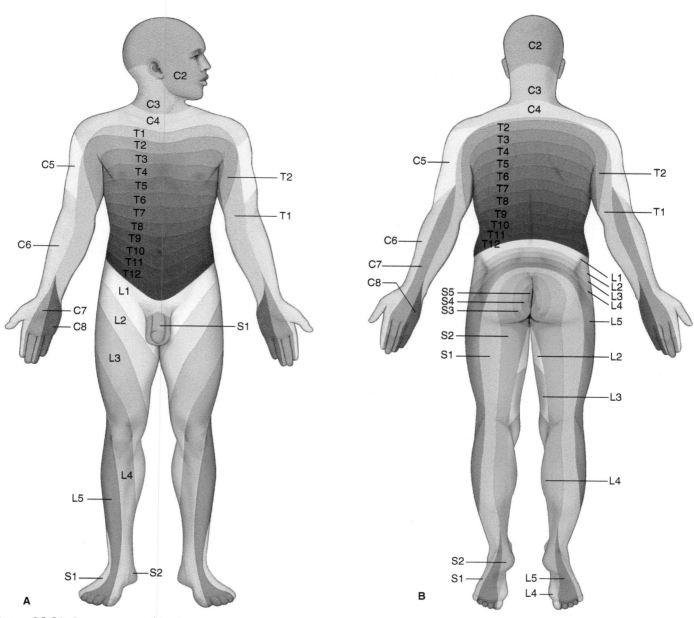

A

Figure 26.6A Dermatomes of body, anterior view.

B

Figure 26.6B Dermatomes of body, posterior view.

TABLE 26.2	Examples of *Healthy People 2020* Objectives Related to Neurologic Health
OBJECTIVE NUMBER	**DESCRIPTION**
DIA-1	(Developmental) Increase the proportion of persons with diagnosed Alzheimer's disease and other dementias, or their caregiver, who are aware of the diagnosis
DIA-2	(Developmental) Reduce the proportion of preventable hospitalizations in persons with diagnosed Alzheimer's disease and other dementias

Source: U.S. Department of Health and Human Services (USDHHS). (2014). *Healthy people 2020*. Retrieved from http://www.healthypeople.gov/2020/default.aspx.

TABLE 26.3	Primitive Reflexes of Early Childhood		
REFLEX	**HOW TO ELICIT**	**AGE WHEN DISAPPEARS**	**EXAMPLE**
Tonic Neck	Turn the infant's head to one side while the infant is supine. The infant will extend the arm and leg on the side the head is turned to while flexing the opposite arm and leg.	2 to 6 months	
Palmar Grasp	Infant will grasp fingers or objects placed in the palm of the hand.	3 to 4 months	
Plantar Grasp	Infant will curl toes when the base of the toes is touched.	6 to 8 months	
Moro (startle)	Infant will extend the arms with the fingers spread and flex the legs with loud sounds or if the infant's body drops suddenly.	4 to 6 months	
Rooting	Lightly stroke the infant's cheek. Infant will turn the head with the mouth open toward the stroked side.	3 to 4 months	

TABLE 26.3	Primitive Reflexes of Early Childhood (continued)		
REFLEX	HOW TO ELICIT	AGE WHEN DISAPPEARS	EXAMPLE
Stepping	Infant will flex the leg and take steps if the infant is upright with the feet touching a surface.	4 to 5 months	
Babinski	Gently stroke the plantar surface of the foot from heel to toe. Infant will extend and fan the toes and flex the foot.	18 to 24 months	

Psychosocial Considerations

Changes in nervous system functioning may alter an individual's ability to control body movements, speech, and elimination patterns and to engage in activities of daily living. Inevitably, these changes will affect the individual's psychosocial health. Patients' self-esteem may suffer as they suddenly or progressively become unable to carry out the roles they previously assumed in their family and society. Another common psychosocial problem associated with neurologic disorders is social isolation. For example, an individual in the first stage of Alzheimer's disease will decline invitations to social functions because the individual feels anxious and confused in unfamiliar surroundings. Such problems indicate a need for improved coping strategies and increased support systems.

As stresses accumulate, an individual becomes increasingly susceptible to neurologic problems, such as forgetfulness, confusion, inability to concentrate, sleeplessness, and tremors. For example, a college senior who is studying for examinations, who is writing applications for graduate school, and who has just broken up with his or her significant other might experience one or all of these symptoms. Chronic stress may also contribute to clinical depression in some patients.

Cultural and Environmental Considerations

Huntington's disease is a genetically transferred neurologic disorder. However, the genetic link to most other degenerative neurologic disorders, such as Alzheimer's disease, multiple sclerosis, myasthenia gravis, and others, is unclear. The incidence of Alzheimer's disease is higher among individuals of African American and Hispanic descent (Alzheimer's Association, 2010).

Research is also inconclusive on the effects of environmental toxins on the development of degenerative neurologic disorders. However, some research indicates that toxins such as carbon monoxide, manganese, and mercury may cause some cases of Parkinson's disease (Caudle, Guillot, Lazo, & Miller, 2012). Peripheral neuropathy (damage to the peripheral nerves) occurs more often among farm workers exposed to the organophosphates in many insecticides (Ross, McManus, Harrison, & Mason, 2013).

Lead poisoning also causes peripheral neuropathy and encephalopathy (Rao, Vengamma, Naveen, & Naveen, 2014). Although not as common as in the past, the risk for lead poisoning still remains high among preschool children who live in old apartments or houses in which walls are painted with lead-based paints. Lead poisoning not only affects those who live in low-cost, inner-city dwellings, but also may occur in wealthy families living in restored older homes.

Gathering the Data

Health assessment of the neurologic system includes gathering subjective and objective data. Subjective data are collected during the patient interview, prior to the physical assessment. During the interview, various communication techniques are used to elicit general and specific information about the status of the patient's neurologic system and ability to function. Health records, results of laboratory tests, X-rays, and imaging reports are important secondary sources to be included in the data-gathering process (Table 26.4). During the physical assessment, the techniques of inspection and palpation, as well as techniques and methods specific to neurologic function, will be used. See Table 26.4 for further information on potential secondary sources of patient data.

Focused Interview

The focused interview for the neurologic system concerns data related to the functions of this body system. Subjective data are collected during the focused interview. The nurse must be prepared to observe the patient and to listen for cues related to the function of the neurologic system. The nurse may use open-ended and closed questions to obtain information. A number of follow-up questions or requests for descriptions may be required to clarify data or gather missing information. Follow-up questions are intended to identify the sources of problems, duration of difficulties, measures to alleviate or manage problems, and clues about the patient's knowledge of his or her own health.

The focused interview guides the physical assessment of the neurologic system. The information is always considered in relation to norms and expectations of neurologic function. Therefore, the nurse must consider age, gender, race, culture, environment, health practices, past and concurrent problems, and therapies when framing questions and using techniques to elicit information. In order to address all of the factors when conducting a focused interview, categories of questions related to the status and function of the neurologic system have been developed. These categories include general questions that are asked of all patients; those addressing illness and infection; questions related to symptoms, pain, and behaviors; those related to habits or practices; questions that are specific for patients according to age; those for the pregnant female; and questions that address environmental concerns. One approach to elicit information about symptoms is the OLDCART & ICE method, described in chapter 7 (see Figure 7.3 on page 120). ∞

The nurse must consider the patient's ability to participate in the focused interview and physical assessment of the neurologic system. Participation in the focused interview is influenced by the ability to communicate in the same language. Language barriers interfere with the accuracy of the data and cause anxiety in the patient. The nurse may have to use a translator in conducting an interview and in the physical assessment. If the patient is experiencing pain, recent injury, or anxiety, attention must focus on relief of symptoms or discomfort before proceeding with an in-depth interview.

TABLE 26.4	Potential Secondary Sources for Patient Data Related to the Neurologic System

Laboratory Tests

Blood tests are used to detect hemorrhage, blood vessel disease, and autoimmune diseases; to monitor therapeutic drug levels; and to detect toxins. These blood tests may include:

Vitamin B_{12} and folate levels

Thyroid, liver, and kidney functions

Vasculitis evaluation

Oral glucose tolerance test

Antibodies to nerve components (e.g., anti-MAG [myelin-associated glycoprotein] antibody)

Antibodies related to celiac disease

Lyme disease

HIV/AIDS

Hepatitis C and B

Analysis of cerebrospinal fluid

Genetic testing for neurologic disease

Diagnostic Tests

Angiography

Carotid Ultrasonography

Computed Tomography (CT)

Discography Elecromyography (EMG)

Electroencepholography (EEG)

Evoked Potentials

Fluoroscopy

Lumbar Puncture

Magnetic Resonance Imaging (MRI)

Neurosonography

Positron Emission Tomography (PET)

X-ray of the skull

| **Focused Interview Questions** | **Rationales and Evidence** |

The following section provides sample questions and bulleted follow-up questions in each of the previously mentioned categories. A rationale for each question is provided. The list of questions is not all-inclusive, but rather represents the types of questions required in a comprehensive focused interview related to the neurologic system. As these questions are asked, the subjective data obtained help to identify patient strengths or risks associated with the neurologic system described in Healthy People 2020.

General Questions

1. **Please complete this sentence: "After I get out of bed in the morning, a typical day in my life includes _____."**

   ▶ The nurse is asking the patient to describe activities of daily living (ADLs). If these data have been obtained in another area of the assessment, the nurse should alter the lead statement accordingly. The patient usually perceives this opening as nonthreatening. It places a focus on activities, self-care practices, and the patient's level of wellness. The nurse can then employ therapeutic communication skills to seek clarification and encourage the patient to relate all of the activities of the day.

2. **Explain what brings you here today.**

   ▶ This open-ended statement allows the patient to state what is important. It increases the patient's control in what may be a stressful situation, thereby producing a less threatening environment. Based on the patient's response, the nurse should adjust the sequence of questions to explore the patient's concern.

3. **Have you had a change in your ability to carry out your daily activities?**
   • Describe the change.
   • Do you know what is causing the change?
   • What do you do about the problem?
   • How long has this been happening?
   • Have you discussed this with your healthcare provider?

   ▶ Neurologic problems can interfere with the ability to carry out ADLs.

4. **Do you have any chronic disease such as diabetes or hypertension?**

   ▶ Chronic diseases such as diabetes and hypertension can predispose patients to neurologic problems (VanGilder, Rosen, Barr, & Huber, 2011).

5. **Do any members of your family now have, or have they ever had, a neurologic problem or disease?**
   • What is the disease or problem?
   • Who in the family has the problem?
   • When was it diagnosed?
   • How has it been treated?
   • How effective has the treatment been?

   ▶ Some conditions are familial and recur in families. For example, certain forms of Alzheimer's disease and amyotrophic lateral sclerosis (ALS, or Lou Gehrig's disease), both of which are discussed later in this chapter, are familial conditions (University of Michigan Health Systems, n.d.).

Questions Related to Illness, Infection, or Injury

1. **Have you ever been diagnosed with a neurologic illness, meningitis, for example?**
   • When were you diagnosed with the problem?
   • What treatment was prescribed for the problem?
   • What kinds of things do you do to help with the problem?
   • Has the problem ever recurred (acute)?
   • How are you managing the disease now (chronic)?

   ▶ The patient has the opportunity to provide information about a specific illness. If a diagnosed illness is identified, follow-up about the date of diagnosis, treatment, and outcomes is required. Data about each illness identified by the patient are essential to an accurate health assessment. Illnesses can be classified as acute or chronic, and follow-up regarding each classification will differ.

2. **An alternative to question 1 is to list possible neurologic illnesses such as stroke, paresis, epilepsy, multiple sclerosis, and myasthenia gravis and ask the patient to respond "yes" or "no" as each is stated.**

   ▶ This is a comprehensive and easy way to elicit information about all neurologic diagnoses. Follow-up would be carried out for each identified diagnosis as in question 1.

Focused Interview Questions	Rationales and Evidence

3. Have you ever had an infection of the neurologic system? Follow-up would be the same as in question number 1.

4. An alternative to question 3 is to list neurologic infections such as poliomyelitis, meningitis, and encephalitis and ask the patient to state "yes" or "no" as each is stated. The rationale is the same as in question 2.

5. Have you ever had an injury to your head or back?
   - If so, please explain what happened.
   - When did this happen?
   - What treatments did you receive?
   - As a result of this injury, what problems do you have today? Follow-up would be the same as in question 1.

▶ The medical history being developed should include past incidents and residual deficits.

Questions Related to Symptoms, Pain, and Behaviors

When gathering information about symptoms, many questions are required to elicit details and descriptions that assist in analysis of the data. Discrimination is made in relation to the significance of a symptom, in relation to specific diseases or problems, and in relation to the potential need for follow-up examination or referral.

The following questions refer to specific symptoms associated with the neurologic system. For each symptom, questions and follow-up are required. The details to be elicited are the characteristics of the symptom; the treatment or remedy for the symptom, including over-the-counter (OTC) and home remedies; the determination if diagnosis has been sought; the effects of treatments; and family history associated with a symptom.

Questions Related to Symptoms

1. Do you have fainting spells?
   - Describe your fainting.

▶ Fainting or loss of consciousness can be associated with neurologic problems (van Dijk & Wieling, 2013).

2. Do you have a history of seizures or convulsions?
   - If so, when did you have your first episode?
   - What happens to you immediately before the seizure?
   - What have you been told about what your body does during the seizure?
   - How do you feel after the seizure?
   - What medications do you take?
   - Do you take your medications regularly?
   - When was the last time you had a seizure?

▶ The patient should be encouraged to identify the type of seizures: partial, complex, or mixed. The questions focus on an aura, muscular activity, postictal period, and use of medications. Lifestyle changes are important, because these individuals need to be cautioned regarding driving and the use of dangerous equipment (Berman & Snyder, 2012).

3. Has your vision changed in any way?
   - Do you ever see two objects when you know there is just one?
   - Are you able to see off to the sides without turning your head?
   - When you go from a bright room to a darker room, do your eyes adjust to the change rapidly?

▶ Changes in vision may indicate problems with the cranial nerves, a brain tumor, increased intracranial pressure, or ocular disease (Osborn, Wraa, Watson, & Holleran, 2013).

4. What changes, if any, have you noticed in your hearing?
   - Have you noticed any ringing in the ears?

▶ Changes in hearing and ringing in the ears (tinnitus) may indicate a problem with the eighth cranial nerve, auditory functions, or aspirin toxicity (Stolzberg, Salvi, & Allman, 2012).

5. Have you noticed any change with your ability to smell or taste?

▶ A change in the ability to smell or taste may also indicate a problem with cranial nerve function (Berman & Snyder, 2012).

Focused Interview Questions	Rationales and Evidence

6. Describe your balance.
- Are you steady on your feet?
- Are you able to perform daily activities without difficulty?
- Is one leg stronger than the other?
- Do you notice any tremors?
- Could you bend down to pick up a straight pin and stand up again?
- Do you drop things easily?
- Do you find yourself being very clumsy—tripping, spilling things, and knocking things over?
- If so, how long have the symptoms been present?
- Are the symptoms continuous?
- Are they getting worse? What do you do to control or limit the symptoms?

▶ All of these questions relate to activities of the cerebellum.

7. Do you have numbness or tingling in any part of your body?
- How long have you had this?
- Do you know what causes it?
- Have you sought treatment?
- What do you do to relieve the problem?

▶ Numbness or tingling may result from neurologic changes alone or as a result of systemic or circulatory disease (Berman & Snyder, 2012).

Questions Related to Pain

1. Are you having any pain?
- If so, where is it?
- When did the pain begin?
- Is the pain constant or intermittent?
- What relieves or decreases the pain?
- What increases the pain?
- Does the pain interfere with your daily activities?
- How would you describe the pain—sharp, dull, acute, burning, stabbing, or stinging?
- On a scale of 0 to 10, with 10 being highest, how would you rate the pain?

▶ Pain, a completely subjective experience, can be acute or chronic. Understanding the patient's view of the pain will help the nurse understand the physiological cause of the pain and will help guide treatment.

2. Do you get headaches?
- If so, describe them.
- Where are they located?
- Are they always in the same area?
- How often do they occur?
- Are you able to function with these headaches?
- What do you think causes your headaches?
- What do you do to help relieve the pain?
- Does this remedy work?
- On a scale of 0 to 10, rate the severity of your headaches.

▶ The nurse is obtaining a medical history to determine if headaches are migraines, tension, cluster, unilateral, bilateral, or associated with other disease. (Refer to chapter 14 for more information on headaches. ∞)

Questions Related to Behaviors

1. Do you now use or have you ever used recreational drugs or alcohol?
- What was the drug or substance?
- When did you use it?
- How long have you used it?
- Have you experienced problems as a result of this drug?
- How much alcohol do you consume?
- For how long?

▶ *Recreational drugs* is a common term used to imply illegal substances. This category could include heroin, cocaine, marijuana, ketamine, oxycodone, and other substances. Use of social drugs and alcohol can create risk for neurologic symptoms or disorders that may be temporary or have long-term consequences.

2. Describe your memory.
- Do you need to make a list or write things down so you won't forget?
- Do you lose things easily?
- What did you do today before you came here?

▶ Memory loss is indicative of some neurologic or psychiatric disease such as Alzheimer's, depression, or stroke. The nurse is developing a baseline regarding the patient's memory and the ability to recall recent and distant events.

Questions Related to Age

The focused interview must reflect the anatomic and physiologic differences that exist along the life span. The following questions are examples of those that would be specific for infants and children, the pregnant female, and the older adult.

Focused Interview Questions	Rationales and Evidence

Questions Regarding Infants and Children

1. **Describe if you can the pregnancy with this child, including any health problems, medications taken, or alcohol or drugs used.**
   - Was the child premature, at term, or late?
   - Describe the birth of the child, including any complications during or shortly after the birth.

   ▶ Problems during the antepartal period, including the use of medications, alcohol, or drugs, may affect the neurologic health of the child. Similarly, complications during or shortly after birth may have residual effects (Berman & Snyder, 2012). For example, research indicates that some cases of epilepsy, a seizure disorder, may be due to prenatal or birth trauma (World Health Organization [WHO], 2012).

2. **Has the child ever had a seizure?**
   - If so, how often has this happened?
   - Describe what happens when the child has a seizure.
   - Has the child had a high fever when the seizures occurred?

   ▶ Seizures in feverish infants and toddlers are not uncommon. Seizures without accompanying fever may indicate a seizure disorder such as epilepsy (National Institute of Neurological Disorders and Stroke, 2014).

3. **Have you noticed any clumsiness in the child's activities? For example, does the child frequently drop things, have difficulty manipulating toys, bump into things, have problems walking or climbing stairs, or fall frequently?**

   ▶ These signs may indicate neurologic disease.

4. **Are you aware of any surfaces in the home that are painted with lead-based paint?**
   - Have you ever seen the child eating paint chips?
   - Have you seen the child chewing on wood surfaces in the home, such as window sills or molding?

   ▶ Lead poisoning may lead to developmental delays, peripheral nerve damage, or brain damage (Grandjean & Landrigan, 2014).

5. **How is the child doing in school?**
   - Does the child seem to be able to concentrate on homework assignments and complete them on time?
   - Have you ever been told that the child has a learning disability?
   - Have you ever been told that the child is hyperactive?
   - Do you agree with this assessment?
   - Why or why not?
   - Have any medications or therapies been prescribed for the hyperactivity?
   - If so, please provide details.

   ▶ Learning and behavioral problems may have a neurologic basis and warrant follow-up.

Questions for the Pregnant Female

1. **Do you have a history of seizures?**
   - Have you had any seizures during this pregnancy or previous pregnancies?
   - If so, how often?

   ▶ Seizures could indicate neurologic pathology or eclampsia (Berman & Snyder, 2012).

2. **Are you taking any vitamins or other nutritional supplements?**
   - Please describe these.

   ▶ Prenatal supplements are important to provide for the neurologic health of the growing fetus. For example, vitamin B6 (pyridoxine) is required for nerve myelination (Mayo Clinic, 2013), and folic acid has been shown to reduce the incidence of neural tube defects (Osterhues, Ali, & Michels, 2013).

Questions for the Older Adult

1. **Do you require more time to perform tasks today than perhaps 2 years ago? Five years ago? Explain.**

   ▶ Endurance decreases with aging; therefore, more time is required for all activities.

2. **When you stand up, do you have trouble starting to walk?**

   ▶ Trouble initiating movement may indicate Parkinson's disease (Wu et al., 2011), which is more common in older adults.

Focused Interview Questions	Rationales and Evidence
3. Do you notice any tremors?	▶ Tremors may indicate motor nerve disease, or they may be attributable to certain medications (Wilson, Shannon, & Shields, 2013) or excessive consumption of caffeine (Seifert, Schaechter, Hershorin, & Lipshultz, 2011).
4. What safety features have you added to your home?	▶ Safety precautions, such as hand rails, grab bars, night lights, and nonslip treads, are essential to prevent neurologic trauma from falls and other accidents.

Questions Related to the Environment

Environment refers to both the internal and external environments. Questions related to the internal environment include all of the previous questions and those associated with internal or physiologic responses. Questions related to the external environment include those related to home, work, or social environments.

Internal Environment

1. Describe your daily diet. • Do you have problems eating or drinking certain products?	▶ The diet provides nutrients and electrolytes responsible for neuromuscular activity and electrical activity in the nervous system.

2. Are you currently taking any medications?
   • What are the medications?
   • Do you use prescribed, OTC, herbal, or culturally derived medications?
   • Do you use home remedies?
	▶ Medications alone can cause neurologic problems. The interaction of medications, herbs, or other products may alter or affect the absorption or effects of prescribed medications (Wilson, Shannon, & Shields, 2013).

External Environment

1. Are you now or have you ever been exposed to environmental hazards such as insecticides, organic solvents, lead, toxic wastes, or other pollutants?
   • If so, which one, when, and for what period of time were you exposed?
   • What treatment did you seek?
   • Are you left with any problems because of the exposure?
	▶ Such exposure could contribute to neurologic deficits and neoplastic activity in the body (Ross, McManus, Harrison, & Mason, 2013).

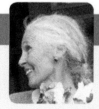

Patient-Centered Interaction

Mrs. Roberta Andoli, age 59, reports to her primary care provider with the chief complaint of weakness of the right side of her face. Her right eye is tearing and she has noticed some drooling. All of the symptoms have developed within the last 3 days. A tentative diagnosis of Bell's palsy is made. The following is an excerpt taken from the focused interview.

Interview

Nurse: Good afternoon, Mrs. Andoli. I would like to talk with you about your reason for coming today.

Mrs. Andoli: My face didn't feel right when I got up today. I can't explain it.

Nurse: Did you notice anything else about your face?

Mrs. Andoli: When I washed my face this morning, I noticed the crease by my nose was gone. When I brushed my teeth the water and toothpaste were dripping out the right side of my mouth. I could not keep the water in on that side.

Nurse: Did you have breakfast this morning?

Mrs. Andoli: Oh yes, I had one cup of tea and cereal with milk, my usual breakfast.

Nurse: Did the tea or cereal milk drip out of your mouth?

Mrs. Andoli: Oh yes, I could have used a bib. I had trouble swallowing and my cereal didn't taste right. I don't know why. My milk was not sour or anything.

Nurse: What other changes have you noticed?	**Analysis**
Mrs. Andoli: When I went to put on eye makeup today, I noticed my right eye was funny.	During the interview, the nurse used several strategies to obtain specific subjective data from the patient. The nurse built on the first statement made by the patient describing feelings of the face. Clarification was sought. Open-ended statements were used to elicit greater information.
Nurse: I'm not sure I know what funny means.	
Mrs. Andoli: My right eye seemed to be opened wider than my left eye this morning. I usually line my eyelids but I didn't this morning. My bottom lid is turned. I don't know what I did. Gee, I'm really a mess.	

Patient Education

The following are physiologic, behavioral, and cultural factors that influence neurologic health across the life span. Several factors are cited as trends in *Healthy People 2020* documents. The nurse provides advice and education to reduce risks associated with the factors mentioned to promote and maintain neurologic health.

LIFESPAN CONSIDERATIONS

Risk Factors	Patient Education
• Low-birth-weight infants are at risk for neurologic problems including intraventricular hemorrhage. African Americans have a higher incidence of low-birth-weight infants.	▶ Advise pregnant females, especially African Americans, to seek and participate in prenatal care to prevent low birth weight.
• Head injuries are common causes of neurologic problems in children.	▶ Educate and inform parents of safety measures for children to prevent head injuries.
• The incidence of epilepsy is highest in children under 10 years of age but occurs and can be chronic across the age span.	▶ Explain to individuals, parents, and children the types of seizures they experience and the medications required for controls and safety measures to prevent accident or injury.
• Reye's syndrome is an illness associated with recovery from viral illness such as influenza, cold, or chickenpox. The development of Reye's syndrome has been linked with the use of aspirin to treat the symptoms of viral illnesses in children. Reye's syndrome results in damage to the brain and generally occurs in children between the ages of 4 and 12.	▶ Educate parents to read medication labels and avoid giving aspirin and products with aspirin to their children to decrease the risk of developing Reye's syndrome.
• Meningitis and encephalitis result from viral or bacterial infections and occur mainly in children and those in crowded living conditions.	▶ Advise patients to follow recommendations for *H. influenzae* and pneumococcal vaccinations to reduce risks for meningitis and encephalitis.
• Older adults have decreased reaction time, resulting in accident and injury.	▶ Instruct all patients regarding safety. Include use of seat belts while traveling in a car or driving and the use of safety devices in the home and at work.

CULTURAL CONSIDERATIONS

Risk Factors

- Hypertension increases the risk for cerebrovascular problems, including stroke. African Americans have a greater incidence of hypertension.

Patient Education

► Educate patients about screening for hypertension and about the importance of diet and exercise to prevent hypertension.

ENVIRONMENTAL CONSIDERATIONS

Risk Factors

- Stress can increase blood pressure, resulting in risk for stroke (brain attack, cerebral vascular accident).

- Medications and remedies, alone or in combinations, may cause neurologic problems or symptoms.

- Stroke (brain attack) occurs with greater frequency in individuals with heart disease, hypertension, and diabetes. Stroke can result in death or functional limitations.

Patient Education

► Educate patients about the benefits of stress reduction techniques, such as meditation, guided imagery, yoga, and massage.

► Educate patients about prescription and over-the-counter medication use, herbs, home remedies, and cultural therapies and the interactions that may lead to neurologic problems.

► Teach patients to recognize and seek help for symptoms of stroke. The American Stroke Association (ASA) recommends using the acronym FAST to help teach patients the signs and symptoms of stroke. As indicated in FAST, if the first three signs and symptoms are present, the individual is advised to seek emergency treatment:
F: Facial drooping
A: Arm weakness
S: Speech difficulty
T: Time to call 9-1-1 (American Heart Association, n.d.).

BEHAVIORAL CONSIDERATIONS

Risk Factors

- Accidents at home, at work, or in social situations can result in neurologic problems.

- Alcohol or drug use increases risks for accidents and injury and neurologic disorders.

Patient Education

► Instruct all patients regarding safety. Include use of seat belts while traveling in a car or driving and safety devices in the home and at work. Also include teaching about use of helmets during sports and recreational activities, including bicycling, to prevent traumatic head injuries.

► Discuss limiting or avoiding the use of alcohol and drugs to reduce the risk of accidents and neurologic problems.

Physical Assessment

Assessment Techniques and Findings

Physical assessment of the neurologic system requires the use of inspection, palpation, auscultation, and special equipment and procedures to test the functions of the system. During each part of the assessment, the nurse is gathering objective data related to the functioning of the patient's central and peripheral nervous systems. The assessment begins with evaluation of the patient's mental status and includes cranial nerves, motor and sensory function, balance, and reflexes. Knowledge of normal or expected findings is essential in interpretation of the data.

Adults and children who are pre-school age or older have erect posture and a smooth gait. Facial expressions correspond to the content and topic of discussion. The speech is clear and vocabulary and word choice are appropriate to age and experience. Adults are well groomed, clean, and attired appropriately for the season and setting. The adult is oriented to person, place, and time and can respond to questions and directions. The adult demonstrates intact short- and long-term memory, is capable of abstract thinking, and can perform calculations. Children should also be able to respond to increasingly difficult questions based on their age. For adults and children, the cranial nerves are intact. Motor function is intact, and movements are coordinated and smooth. Sensory function is demonstrated in the ability to identify touch, pain, heat, and cold; to sense vibrations; to identify objects; and to discriminate between place and points of touch on the body. The response to testing of reflexes is $2+$ on a scale of 0 to $4+$. Carotid arteries are without bruits.

Physical assessment of the neurologic system follows an organized pattern. It begins with assessment of the patient's mental status and proceeds to assessment of cranial nerves, motor and sensory function, reflexes, and auscultation of carotid arteries. Assessment proceeds in a cephalocaudal manner. The nurse tests distal to proximal and moves from gross function to fine function, always comparing corresponding body parts. More than one technique can be used to assess one function.

EQUIPMENT

- examination gown
- clean, nonsterile examination gloves
- cotton wisp
- percussion hammer
- tuning fork
- sterile cotton balls
- penlight
- ophthalmoscope
- stethoscope
- tongue blade
- applicator
- hot and cold water in test tubes
- objects to touch such as coins, paper clips, or safety pins
- substances to smell, for example, vanilla, mint, and coffee
- substances to taste such as sugar, salt, lemon, and grape

HELPFUL HINTS

- Data gathering begins with the initial nurse–patient interaction. As nurses meet patients, they make assessments regarding their general appearance, personal hygiene, and ability to walk and sit down. These activities are related to cerebral function.
- Physical assessment of the neurologic system proceeds in a cephalocaudal and distal-to-proximal pattern and includes comparison of corresponding body parts.
- Several assessments may occur at one time. For example, asking the patient to smile tests cranial nerve VII. The ability to follow directions and initiate voluntary movements tests hearing (cranial nerve VIII) and the functions of the cerebral cortex.
- Provide specific information about what is expected of the patient. Demonstrate movements.
- Explain and demonstrate the purposes and uses of the equipment.
- Use Standard Precautions.

Mental Status

The nurse assesses the mental status of the patient when meeting the patient for the first time. This process begins with taking the health history and continues with each patient contact.

▶ A variety of tools are available to conduct mental status assessment. These tools are described in Table 26.5.

TABLE 26.5	**Tools for Assessment of Mental Status**
TOOL	**ASSESSMENT**
Mini-Mental State Examination (MMSE)	Cognitive status—conducted via interview
Addenbrooke's Cognitive Examination	Detects early dementia
Confusion Assessment Method (CAM)	Tests for delirium
Telephone Interview for Cognitive Status (TICS)	Similar to MMSE, cognitive function assessed via telephone interview
Cornell Scale for Depression in Dementia	Assessment of behavioral problems
Dementia Symptoms Scale	Assessment of behavioral problems
Psychogeriatric Dependency Rating Scale	Assessment of behavioral problems
Hopkins Competency Assessment Test	Assessment of ability to make decisions about health care
General Health Questionnaire	Assessment of emotional disturbance in those with normal cognitive ability
Hamilton Depression Rating Scale	Assessment of depression in patients with impaired cognition
Short Portable Mental Status Questionnaire (SPMSQ)	Assessment of organic brain deficit

1. **Instruct the patient.**
   - Explain to the patient that you will be conducting a variety of tests. Tell the patient that you will provide instructions before beginning each examination. Explain that moving about and changing position during the examination will be required.
   - Provide reassurance that the tests will not cause discomfort; however, the patient must inform you of problems if they arise during any part of the assessment.
   - Identify the types of equipment you will use and describe the purpose in relation to neurologic function.
   - Tell the patient that you will begin the assessment with some general questions about the present and past. Then you will ask the patient to respond to number and word questions.

Techniques and Normal Findings	Abnormal Findings Special Considerations

2. Position the patient.

- The patient should be sitting on the examination table wearing an examination gown (see Figure 26.7 ■).

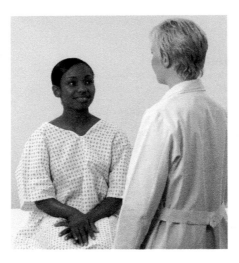

Figure 26.7 Positioning the patient.

3. Observe the patient.

- Look at the patient and note hygiene, grooming, posture, body language, facial expressions, speech, and ability to follow directions.

▶ Inadequate self-care, flatness of affect, and inability to follow directions may be associated with mental illnesses such as depression or schizophrenia, or with neurological abnormalities such as organic brain syndrome. Abnormal facial expressions or body language also may be reflective of neurological or psychiatric disorders.

4. Note the patient's speech and language abilities.

- Throughout the assessment, note the patient's rate of speech, ability to pronounce words, tone of voice, loudness or softness (volume) of voice, and ability to speak smoothly and clearly.
- Assess the patient's choice of words, ability to respond to questions, and ease with which a response is made.

▶ Changes in speech could reflect anxiety, Parkinson's disease, depression, or dysphasia (difficulty speaking).

5. Assess the patient's sensorium.

- Determine the patient's orientation to date, time, place, as well as the need for the physical assessment. Grade the level of alertness on a scale from full alertness to coma.

▶ Neurologic disease can produce a sliding or changing degree of alertness. Change in the level of consciousness may be related to cortical or brain stem disease. A stroke, seizure, or hypoglycemia could also contribute to a change in the level of consciousness (LOC).

6. Assess the patient's memory.

- Ask for the patient's date of birth, names and ages of any children or grandchildren, educational history with dates and events, work history with dates, and job descriptions. Ask questions for which the responses can be verified.

▶ Loss of long-term memory may indicate cerebral cortex damage, which occurs in Alzheimer's disease.

7. Assess the patient's ability to calculate problems.

- Start with a simple problem, such as 4 + 3, 8 ÷ 2, and 15 − 4.

▶ Inability to calculate simple problems may indicate the presence of organic brain disease, or it may simply indicate lack of exposure to mathematical concepts, nervousness, or an incomplete understanding of the examiner's language. In an otherwise unremarkable assessment, a poor response to calculations should not be considered an abnormal finding.

Techniques and Normal Findings	Abnormal Findings Special Considerations

- Progress to more difficult problems, such as $(10 + 4) - 8$, or ask the patient to start with 100 and subtract 7 ($100 - 7 = 93$, $93 - 7 = 86$, $86 - 7 = 79$, and so on).
- Remember to use problems that are appropriate for the patient's developmental, educational, and intellectual levels.
- Asking the patient to calculate change from one dollar for the purchase of items costing 25, 39, and 89 cents is a quick test of calculation.

8. **Assess the patient's ability to think abstractly.**
   - Ask the patient to identify similarities and differences between two objects or topics, such as wood and coal, king and president, orange and apple, and pear and celery. Quote a proverb and ask the patient to explain its meaning. For example:
     - "A stitch in time saves nine."
     - "The empty barrel makes the most noise."
     - "Don't put all your eggs in one basket."
   - Be aware that age and culture influence the ability to explain American proverbs and slang terms.

▶ Responses made by the patient may reflect lack of education, mental retardation, or dementia. Patients with personality disorders and patients with disorders such as schizophrenia or depression may make bizarre responses.

9. **Assess the patient's mood and emotional state.**
   - Observe the patient's body language, facial expressions, and communication technique. The facial expression and tone of voice should be congruent with the content and context of the communication.

▶ Lack of congruence of facial expression and tone of voice with the content and context of communication may occur with neurologic problems, emotional disturbance, or a psychogenic disorder such as schizophrenia or depression.

   - Ask if the patient generally feels this way or if he or she has experienced a change and if so over what period of time.
   - Ask the patient if it is possible to identify an event or incident that fostered the change in mood or emotional state.
   - The patient's mood and emotions should reflect the current situation or response to events that trigger mood change or call for an emotional response (e.g., a change in health status, a loss, or a stressful event).

▶ Lack of emotional response, lack of change in facial expression, and flat tone of voice can indicate problems with mood or emotional responses. Other abnormal findings in relation to mood and emotional state include anxiety, depression, fear, anger, overconfidence, ambivalence, euphoria, impatience, and irritability. Mood disorders include bipolar disorder, anxiety disorders, and major depression.

10. **Assess perceptions and thought processes.**
    - Listen to the patient's statements. Statements should be logical and relevant. The patient should complete his or her thoughts.

▶ Disturbed thought processes can indicate neurologic dysfunction or mental disorder.

    - Assessment of perception includes determining the patient's awareness of reality.

▶ Disturbances in sense of reality can include hallucination and illusion. These are associated with mental disturbances as seen in schizophrenia.

11. **Assess the patient's ability to make judgments.**
    - Determine if the patient is able to evaluate situations and to decide on a realistic course of action. For example, ask the patient about future plans related to employment.

    - The plans should reflect the reality of the patient's health, psychological stability, and family situation and obligations. The patient's responses should reflect an ability to think abstractly.

▶ Impaired judgment can occur in emotional disturbances, schizophrenia, and neurologic dysfunction.

Cranial Nerves

1. **Instruct the patient.**
   - Tell the patient that you will be testing special nerves and the senses of smell, vision, taste, and hearing. Explain that several of the tests will require the patient to close both eyes. You will be asking the patient to make changes in facial expression. Occasionally, you will touch the patient with your hands while using different types of equipment during each test.

2. **Test the olfactory nerve (cranial nerve I).**
   - If you suspect the patient's nares are obstructed with mucus, ask the patient to blow his or her nose.
   - Ask the patient to close both eyes and then apply gentle pressure to the external surface of one naris with his or her index finger. If necessary, the nurse could occlude the patient's naris. Place a familiar odor under the open naris (see Figure 26.8 ■).

▶ **Anosmia**, the absence of the sense of smell, may be due to cranial nerve dysfunction, colds, rhinitis, or zinc deficiency, or it may be genetic. A unilateral change in this sense may be indicative of a brain tumor.

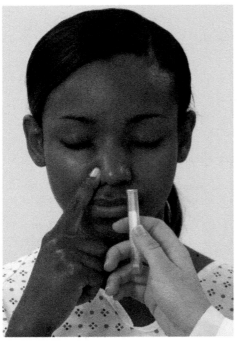

Figure 26.8 Olfactory nerve assessment.

   - Ask the patient to sniff and identify the odor. Use coffee, peppermint, or other scents that are familiar to the patient. Repeat with the other naris.

3. **Test the optic nerve (cranial nerve II).**
   - Test near vision by asking the patient to read from a magazine, newspaper, or prepared card. Observe closeness or distance of page to face. Also note the position of the head.
   - Use the Snellen chart to test distant vision (see Figure 15.7 on page 305 ∞). Color vision may be tested using Ishihara cards, which feature colored dot patterns that contain embedded symbols or numbers.

▶ Pathologic conditions of the optic nerve include retrobulbar neuritis, papilledema, and optic atrophy. **Retrobulbar neuritis** is an inflammatory process of the optic nerve behind the eyeball. Multiple sclerosis is the most common cause.
▶ Inability to distinguish symbols or numbers on one or more of the Ishihara cards is reflective of impaired color vision (University of Maryland Medical Center, 2014).

Techniques and Normal Findings

Abnormal Findings
Special Considerations

- Use the ophthalmoscope to inspect the fundus of the eye. Locate the optic disc and describe the color and shape.
- See chapter 15 for a detailed description of the techniques for all of these activities. ∞

► **Papilledema** (or *choked disc*) is a swelling of the optic nerve as it enters the retina. A symptom of increased intracranial pressure, papilledema can be indicative of brain tumors or intracranial hemorrhage.

► Immediate medical attention is required if intracranial hemorrhage is suspected.

► **Optic atrophy** produces a change in the color of the optic disc and decreased visual acuity. It can be a symptom of multiple sclerosis or brain tumor.

4. **Test the oculomotor, trochlear, and abducens nerves (cranial nerves III, IV, and VI).**
   - Test the six cardinal points of gaze.

► Pathologic conditions include nystagmus, strabismus, diplopia, or ptosis of the upper lid. **Nystagmus** is the constant involuntary movement of the eyeball. A lack of muscular coordination, *strabismus*, causes deviation of one or both eyes. **Diplopia** is double vision. A dropped lid, or *ptosis* of the lid, is usually related to weakness of the muscles.

   - Test direct and consensual pupillary reaction to light (cranial nerve III).
   - Test convergence and accommodation of the eyes.
   - These three tests are described in detail in chapter 15. ∞

5. **Explain the procedure for testing the trigeminal nerve.**
   - Show the patient the cotton wisp. Touch the patient's arm with the wisp and explain that the wisp will feel like that when a body part is touched. Ask the patient to close both eyes.
   - Touch the arm with the wisp. Ask the patient to say "now" when the wisp is felt. Explain that further tests with the wisp will be carried out with the eyes closed, and "now" is to be stated when the wisp is felt.
   - Show the patient the broken tongue blade. Explain that while you touch the arm with the rounded end the sensation is dull, and with the broken end the sensation is sharp.
   - Tell the patient that both eyes must be closed during several tests with the tongue blade.
   - The patient is expected to identify each touch or sensation as sharp or dull.
   - Discard the tongue blade at the completion of the examination.

6. **Test the trigeminal nerve (cranial nerve V).**
   - Test the sensory function.
   - Ask the patient to close both eyes.
   - Touch the patient's face, forehead, and chin with a wisp of cotton (see Figure 26.9 ■).

Techniques and Normal Findings	Abnormal Findings Special Considerations

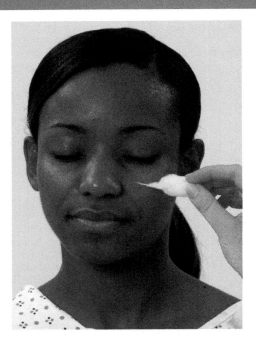

Figure 26.9 Testing sensory function of the trigeminal nerve.

- Direct the patient to say "now" every time the cotton is felt. Repeat the test using sharp and dull stimuli.

- Be random with the stimulation. Do *not* establish a pattern when testing.

- Test the motor function of the nerve. Ask the patient to clench the teeth tightly. Bilaterally palpate the masseter and temporalis muscles, noting muscle strength (see Figure 26.10 ■).
- Ask the patient to open and close the mouth several times. Observe for symmetry of movement of the mandible without deviation from midline.

▶ Document any loss of sensation, pain, or noted fasciculations (fine rapid muscle movements).

▶ Muscle pain, spasms, and deviation of the mandible with movement can indicate myofascial pain dysfunction.

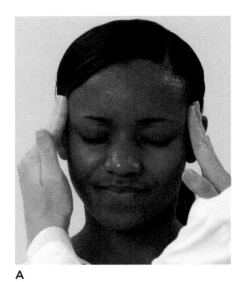

A

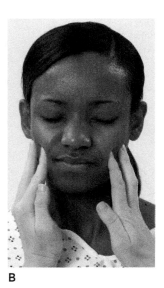

B

Figure 26.10 Testing muscle strength. A. Temporalis muscles. B. Masseter muscles.

Techniques and Normal Findings	Abnormal Findings Special Considerations

7. **Test the facial nerve (cranial nerve VII).**
   - Test the motor activity of the nerve.
   - Ask the patient to perform several functions such as the following: smile, show your teeth, close both eyes, puff your cheeks, frown, and raise your eyebrows (see Figure 26.11 ■).

▶ Asymmetry or muscle weakness may indicate nerve damage. Muscle weakness includes drooping of the eyelid and changes in the nasolabial folds.

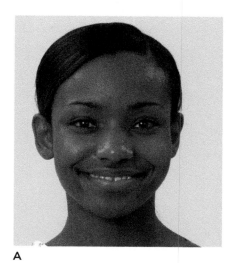
A

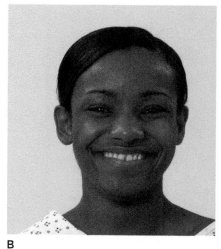
B

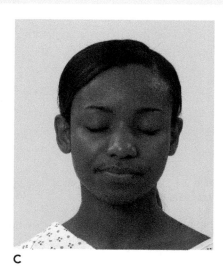
C

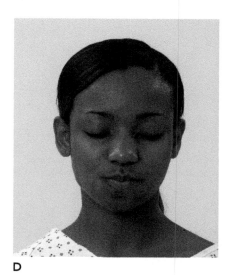
D

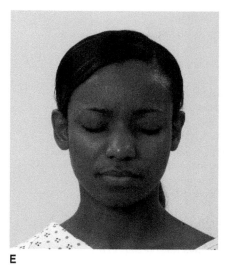
E

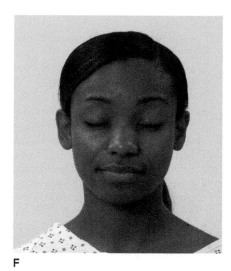
F

Figure 26.11 Testing motor function of cranial nerve VII. A. Smile. B. Show teeth. C. Close both eyes. D. Puff cheeks. E. Frown. F. Raise eyebrows.

- Look for symmetry of facial movements.
- Test the muscle strength of the upper face.
- Ask the patient to close both eyes tightly and keep them closed.

▶ Inability to perform motor tasks could be the result of a lower or upper motor neuron disease.

| Techniques and Normal Findings | Abnormal Findings / Special Considerations |

- Try to open the eyes by retracting the upper and lower lids simultaneously and bilaterally (see Figure 26.12 ■).

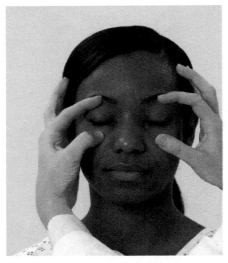

Figure 26.12 Testing the strength of the facial muscles.

- Test the muscle strength of the lower face.
  - Ask the patient to puff the cheeks.
  - Apply pressure to the cheeks, attempting to force the air out of the lips.
- Test the sense of taste.
  - Moisten three applicators and dab one in each of the samples of sugar, salt, and lemon.
  - Touch the patient's tongue with one applicator at a time and ask the patient to identify the taste.
  - Water may be needed to rinse the mouth between tests.
- Test the corneal reflex.
  - This may have been tested with the trigeminal nerve assessment (see Figure 26.9). Cranial nerve VII regulates the motor response of this reflex.

8. **Test the vestibulocochlear nerve (cranial nerve VIII).**
- Test the auditory branch of the nerve by performing the Weber test. This test uses the tuning fork and provides lateralization of the sound.
- Perform the Rinne test. This compares bone conduction of sound with air conduction. Both the Rinne and Weber tests are described in detail in chapter 16 (see pages 352–353). ∞
- The caloric test (or ice water test, as it is sometimes called) tests the vestibular portion of the nerve.
  - This test is usually conducted only when the patient is experiencing dizziness or vertigo. (Consult a neurology text for a description of this technique.)
- Romberg's test assesses coordination and equilibrium. It is discussed later in this chapter on page 775 and in chapter 16, page 353. ∞

9. **Test the glossopharyngeal and vagus nerves (cranial nerves IX and X).**
- Test motor activity.
  - Ask the patient to open the mouth.
  - Depress the patient's tongue with the tongue blade.
  - Ask the patient to say "ah."
- Observe the movement of the soft palate and uvula (see Figure 26.13 ■).
- Normally, the soft palate rises and the uvula remains in the midline.
- Test the gag reflex. This tests the sensory aspect of cranial nerve IX and the motor activity of cranial nerve X.

▶ Tinnitus and deafness are deficits associated with the cochlear or auditory branch of the nerve.

▶ Vertigo is associated with the vestibular portion.

▶ Unilateral palate and uvula movement indicate disease of the nerve on the opposite side.

Techniques and Normal Findings	Abnormal Findings Special Considerations

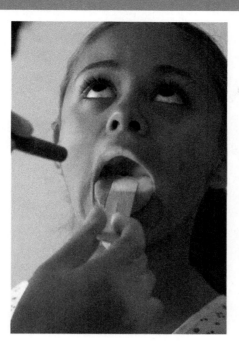

Figure 26.13 Testing cranial nerves IX and X.

▶ Bifid uvula, a condition in which the uvula is split into two segments, occurs in approximately 1 percent of the general population. Although this condition usually is benign, in rare cases, it may be linked to serious genetic disorders, including cleft palate (Liberty et al., 2014).

- Inform the patient that you are going to place an applicator in the mouth and lightly touch the throat.

▶ Patients with a diminished or absent gag reflex have an increased potential for aspiration and need medical evaluation.

- Touch the posterior wall of the pharynx with the applicator.
- Observe pharyngeal movement.
- Test the motor activity of the pharynx.
- Ask the patient to drink a small amount of water and note the ease or difficulty of swallowing.
- Note the quality of the voice or hoarseness when speaking.

▶ **Dysphagia**, difficulty with swallowing, could be related to cranial nerve disease.
▶ Vocal changes could be indicative of lesions, paralysis, or other conditions.

10. **Test the accessory nerve (cranial nerve XI).**
   - Test the trapezius muscle.
   - Ask the patient to shrug the shoulders.
   - Observe the equality of the shoulders, symmetry of action, and lack of fasciculations (see Figure 26.14 ▪).

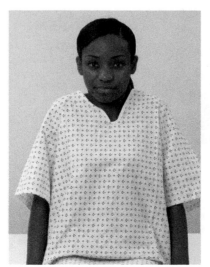

Figure 26.14 Trapezius muscle movement.

Techniques and Normal Findings	Abnormal Findings Special Considerations

- Test the sternocleidomastoid muscle.
  - Ask the patient to turn the head to the right and then to the left (see Figure 26.15 ■).
  - Ask the patient to try to touch the right ear to the right shoulder without raising the shoulder.
  - Repeat with the left shoulder.
  - Observe ease of movement and degree of range of motion.

▶ Abnormal findings include muscle weakness, muscle atrophy, fasciculations, uneven shoulders, and the inability to raise the chin following flexion.

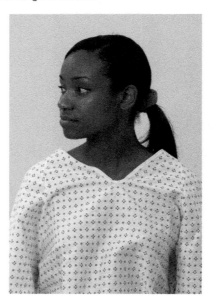

Figure 26.15 Sternocleidomastoid muscle movement.

- Test trapezius muscle strength.
  - Have the patient shrug the shoulders while you resist with your hands (see Figure 26.16 ■).

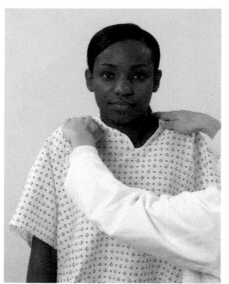

Figure 26.16 Testing the strength of the trapezius muscle against resistance.

- Test sternocleidomastoid muscle strength.
  - Ask the patient to turn the head to the left to meet your hand.
  - Attempt to return the patient's head to midline position (see Figure 26.17 ■).
  - Repeat the preceding steps with the patient turning to the right side.

Techniques and Normal Findings	Abnormal Findings Special Considerations

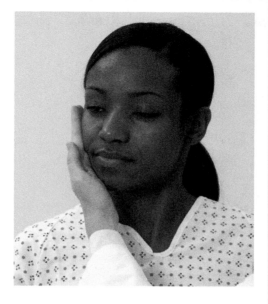

Figure 26.17 Testing the strength of the sternocleidomastoid muscle against resistance.

11. **Test the hypoglossal nerve (cranial nerve XII).**
    - Test the movement of the tongue.
      - Ask the patient to protrude the tongue.
      - Ask the patient to retract the tongue.
      - Ask the patient to protrude the tongue and move it to the right and then to the left.
      - Note ease of movement and equality of movement (see Figure 26.18 ■).

▶ Note atrophy, tremors, and paralysis. An ipsilateral paralysis will demonstrate deviation and atrophy of the involved side.

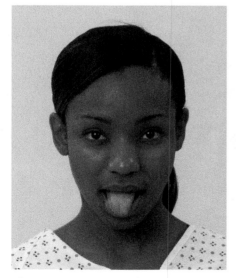 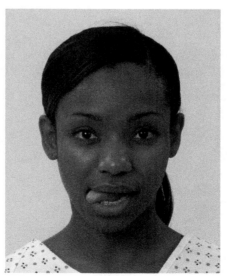

Figure 26.18A Protruding movement of tongue.

Figure 26.18B Lateralization of tongue.

- Test the strength of the tongue.
  - Ask the patient to push against the inside of the cheek with the tip of the tongue.
  - Provide resistance by pressing one or two fingers against the patient's outer cheek (see Figure 26.19 ■).
- Repeat on the other side.

Techniques and Normal Findings	Abnormal Findings Special Considerations

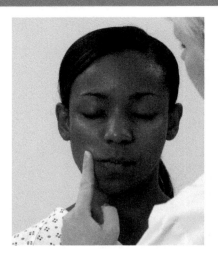

Figure 26.19 Testing the strength of the tongue.

Motor Function

Motor function requires the integrated efforts of the musculoskeletal and the neurologic systems. Assessment of the musculoskeletal system is discussed in detail in chapter 25. ∞ The neurologic aspect of motor function is directly related to activities of the cerebellum, which is responsible for coordination and smoothness of movement, and equilibrium. All of the following tests focus on activities of the cerebellum.

ALERT!

Be ready to support and protect the patient to prevent an accident, injury, or fall.

1. **Assess the patient's gait and balance.**
   - Ask the patient to walk across the room and return (see Figure 26.20 ■).
   - Ask the patient to walk heel to toe (or tandem), by placing the heel of the left foot in front of the toes of the right foot, then the heel of the right foot in front of the toes of the left foot. Be sure the patient is looking straight ahead and not at the floor. Continue this pattern for several yards (see Figure 26.21 ■).

▶ A change in gait could be indicative of drug or alcohol intoxication, motor neuron weakness, or muscle weakness.

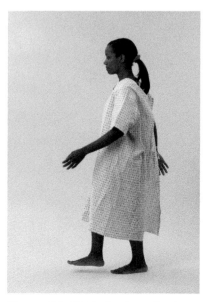

Figure 26.20 Evaluation of gait.

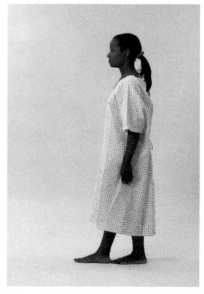

Figure 26.21 Heel-to-toe walk.

- Ask the patient to walk on his or her toes.
- Ask the patient to walk on the heels. Observe the patient's posture. Does the posture demonstrate stiffness or relaxation? Note the equality of steps taken, the pace of walking, the position and coordination of arms when walking, and the ability to maintain balance during all of these activities.

2. **Perform Romberg's test.**
   - **Romberg's test** assesses coordination and equilibrium (cranial nerve VIII).
   - Ask the patient to stand with feet together and arms at the sides. The patient's eyes are open.
   - Stand next to the patient to prevent falls. Observe for swaying.
   - Ask the patient to close both eyes without changing position.
   - Observe for swaying while the patient's eyes are closed. Swaying normally increases slightly when the eyes are closed (see Figure 26.22 ■).

▶ A positive Romberg sign occurs when swaying greatly increases or the patient experiences difficulty maintaining his or her balance. This may indicate disease of the posterior column of the spinal cord.

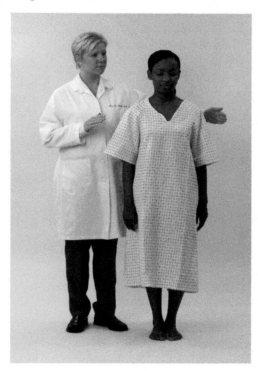

Figure 26.22 Romberg's test for balance.

3. **Perform the finger-to-nose test.**
   - The finger-to-nose test also assesses coordination and equilibrium. It is sometimes called the pass-point test.
   - Ask the patient to resume a sitting position.
   - Ask the patient to extend both arms from the sides of the body.
   - Ask the patient to keep both eyes open.
   - Ask the patient to touch the tip of the nose with the right index finger, and then return the right arm to an extended position.
   - Ask the patient to touch the tip of the nose with the left index finger, and then return the left arm to an extended position.
   - Repeat the procedure several times.
   - Ask the patient to close both eyes and repeat the alternating movements (see Figure 26.23 ■).

Techniques and Normal Findings	Abnormal Findings Special Considerations

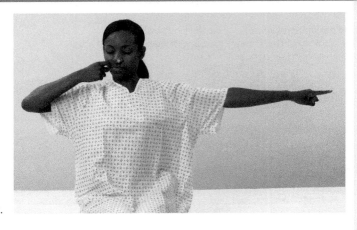

Figure 26.23
Finger-to-nose test.

- Observe the movement of the arms, the smoothness of the movement, and the point of contact of the finger. Does the finger touch the nose, or is another part of the face touched?
- An alternative technique is to have the patient touch the nose with the index finger and then touch the finger of the nurse (see Figure 26.24 ■).

▶ With the eyes closed, the patient with cerebellar disease will reach beyond the tip of the nose because the sense of position is affected.

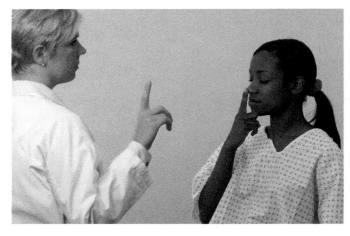

Figure 26.24
Alternative for
finger-to-nose test.

4. **Assess the patient's ability to perform a rapid alternating action.**
   - Ask the patient to sit with the hands placed palms down on the thighs (see Figure 26.25A ■).
   - Ask the patient to turn the hands palms up (see Figure 26.25B ■).

▶ Inability to perform this task could indicate upper motor neuron weakness.

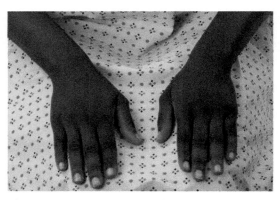

Figure 26.25A Testing rapid alternating movement, palms down.

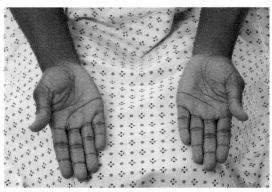

Figure 26.25B Testing rapid alternating movement, palms up.

Techniques and Normal Findings	Abnormal Findings Special Considerations

- Ask the patient to return the hands to a palms-down position.
- Ask the patient to alternate the movements at a faster pace. If you suspect any deficit, test one side at a time.
- Observe the rhythm, rate, and smoothness of the movements.
- Figure 26.26 ■ demonstrates the finger-to-finger test, which is an alternative method to assess coordination.
- Ask the patient to touch the thumb to each finger in sequence with increasing pace.

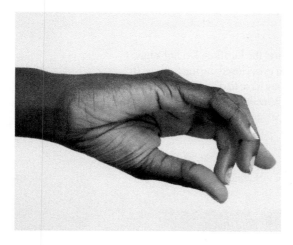

Figure 26.26 Testing coordination using the finger-to-finger test.

5. **Ask the patient to perform the heel-to-shin test.**
   - Assist the patient to a supine position.
   - Ask the patient to place the heel of the right foot below the left knee.
   - Ask the patient to slide the right heel along the shin bone to the ankle.
   - Ask the patient to repeat the procedure, reversing the legs (see Figure 26.27 ■).
   - Observe the smoothness of the action. The patient should be able to move the heel in a straight line so that it does not fall off the lower leg.

▶ Inability to perform this test could indicate disease of the posterior spinal tract.

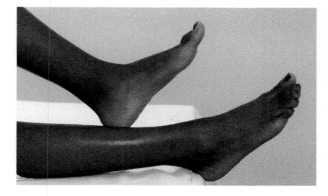

Figure 26.27 Heel-to-shin test.

Sensory Function

This part of the physical assessment evaluates the patient's response to a variety of stimuli. This assessment tests the peripheral nerves, the sensory tracts, and the cortical level of discrimination. A variety of stimuli are used, including light touch, hot/cold, sharp/dull, and vibration. Stereognosis, graphesthesia, and two-point discrimination are also assessed. Each of these assessments is described in the following sections.

Techniques and Normal Findings	Abnormal Findings Special Considerations

ALERT!

The patient may tire during these procedures. If this happens, stop the assessment and continue at a later time. Be sure to test corresponding body parts. Take a distal-to-proximal approach along the extremities. When the patient describes sensations accurately at a distal point, it is usually not necessary to proceed to a more proximal point. If a deficit is detected at a distal point, then it becomes imperative to proceed to proximal points while attempting to map the specific area of the deficit. Repeat testing to determine accuracy in areas of deficits.

Remember, always ask the patient to describe the stimulus and the location. Do not suggest the type of stimulus or location. Tell the patient to keep both eyes closed during testing. To promote full patient understanding and cooperation, you may have to demonstrate what you will be doing and what you expect the patient to do while using a wisp of cotton, the uncovered end of an applicator, or a tongue blade. Specific dermatomes are tested as you assess corresponding locations.

1. **Assess the patient's ability to identify light touch.**
   - Using a wisp of cotton, touch various parts of the body, including feet, hands, arms, legs, abdomen, and face (see Figure 26.28 ■).

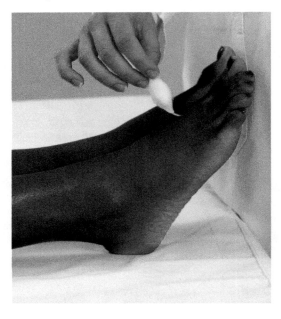

Figure 26.28 Evaluation of light touch.

   - Touch at random locations and use random time intervals.
   - Ask the patient to say "yes" or "now" when the stimulus is perceived. Be sure to test corresponding dermatomes.

▶ **Anesthesia** is the inability to perceive the sense of touch. **Hyperesthesia** is an increased sensation, whereas **hypoesthesia** is a decreased but not absent sensation.

2. **Assess the patient's ability to distinguish the difference between sharp and dull.**
   - Ask the patient to say "sharp" or "dull" when something sharp or dull is felt on the skin.
   - Touch the patient with the uncovered end of an applicator or the irregular edge of a broken tongue blade. The sharp edge is used to identify pain, while the dull edge is a repeat of step 1 (see Figure 26.29A ■).
   - Now touch the patient with the cotton end of the applicator or the smooth edge of a tongue blade (see Figure 26.29B ■).

▶ The absence of pain sensation is called **analgesia**. Decreased pain sensation is called **hypalgesia**. These conditions may result from neurologic disease or circulatory problems such as peripheral vascular disease.

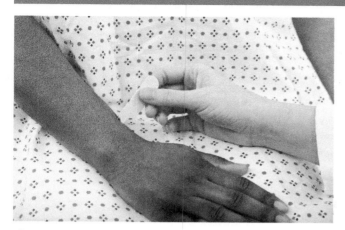

Figure 26.29A Testing the patient's ability to identify sharp sensations.

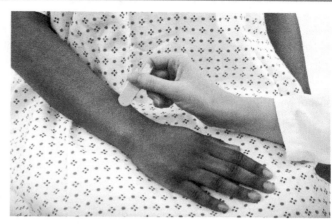

Figure 26.29B Testing the patient's ability to identify dull sensations.

- Alternate between sharp and dull stimulation.
- Touch the patient using random locations, random time intervals, and alternating patterns.
- Be sure to test corresponding body parts. This tests specific dermatomes.
- Discard the applicator or tongue blade.

3. **Assess the patient's ability to distinguish temperature.**
   - Perform this test only if the patient demonstrates an absence or decrease in pain sensation.
   - Randomly touch the patient with test tubes containing warm and cold water.
   - Ask the patient to describe the temperature.
   - Be sure to test corresponding body parts.

4. **Assess the patient's ability to feel vibrations.**
   - Set a tuning fork in motion and place it on bony parts of the body, such as the toes, ankle, knee, iliac crest, spinal process, fingers, sternum, wrists, or elbows (see Figure 26.30 ■).

▶ If an area of decreased or absent sensation is assessed, attempt to map the region to determine if it is associated with a dermatome or peripheral sensory nerve pattern. Diminished sensation may indicate peripheral nerve, polyneuropathy, or CNS involvement.

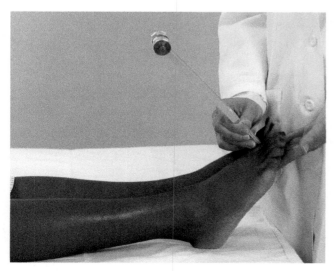

Figure 26.30A Testing the patient's ability to feel vibrations, the toe.

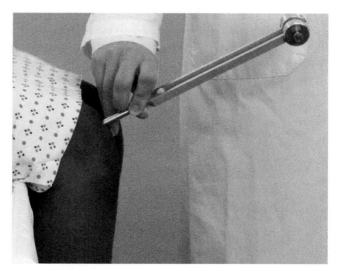

Figure 26.30B Testing the patient's ability to feel vibrations, the knee.

Techniques and Normal Findings	Abnormal Findings Special Considerations

- Ask the patient to say "now" when the vibration is perceived and "stop" when it is no longer felt.
- If the patient's perception is accurate when you test the most distal aspects (toes, ankles, fingers, and wrist), end the test at this time.
- Proceed to proximal points if distal perception is diminished.

► The inability to perceive vibration may indicate neuropathy. This may be associated with aging, diabetes, intoxication, or posterior column disease.

5. **Test stereognosis, the ability to identify an object without seeing it.**
   - Direct the patient to close both eyes. Place a closed safety pin in the patient's right hand and ask the patient to identify it.
   - Place a different object, a key, in the left hand and ask the patient to identify it.
   - Place a coin in the right hand and ask the patient to identify it (see Figure 26.31 ■).

► Inability to identify a familiar object could indicate cortical disease.

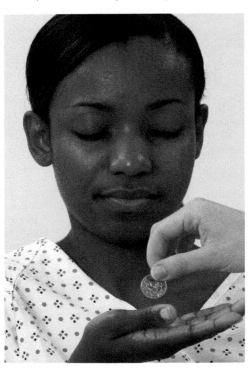

Figure 26.31 Testing stereognosis using a coin.

- Place a different coin in the left hand and ask the patient to identify it.
- The objects you use must be familiar and safe to hold (no sharp objects).
- Test each object independently.

6. **Test graphesthesia, the ability to perceive writing on the skin.**
   - Direct the patient to keep both eyes closed.
   - Using the noncotton end of an applicator or the base of a pen, scribe a number such as 3 into the palm of the patient's right hand (see Figure 26.32 ■).

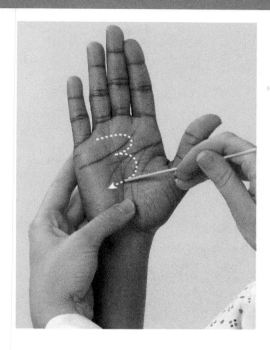

Figure 26.32 Testing graphesthesia.

- Be sure the number faces the patient.
- Ask the patient to identify the number.
- Repeat in the left hand using a different number such as 5 or 2.
- Ask the patient to identify the number.

7. **Assess the patient's ability to discriminate between two points.**
   - Simultaneously touch the patient with two stimuli over a given area (see Figure 26.33 ■).

▶ Inability to perceive a number on the skin may indicate cortical disease.

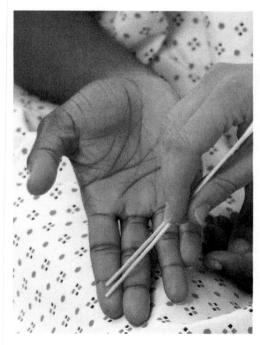

Figure 26.33 Two-point discrimination.

Techniques and Normal Findings	Abnormal Findings / Special Considerations

- Use the unpadded end of two applicators.
- Vary the distance between the two points according to the body region being stimulated. The more distal the location, the more sensitive the discrimination.
- Normally, the patient is able to perceive two discrete points at the following distances and locations:

Fingertips	0.3 to 0.6 cm (0.12 to 0.24 in.)
Hands and feet	1.5 to 2 cm (0.59 to 0.78 in.)
Lower leg	4 cm (1.56 in.)

- Ask the patient to say "now" when the two discrete points of stimulus are first perceived.
- Note the smallest distance between the points at which the patient can perceive two distinct stimuli.
- Discard the applicators.

▶ An inability to perceive two separate points within normal distances may indicate cortical disease.

8. **Assess topognosis, the ability of the patient to identify an area of the body that has been touched.**
   - This need not be a separate test. Include it in any of the previous steps by asking the patient to identify what part of the body was involved. Also ask the patient to point to the area you touched.

▶ Inability of the patient to identify a touched area demonstrates sensory or cortical disease.

9. **Assess kinesthesia, the position sense of joint movement.**
   - Ask the patient to close both eyes. Grasp the great toe. Move the joint into dorsiflexion, plantar flexion, and abduction.
   - Ask the patient to identify the movement (see Figure 26.34 ■).

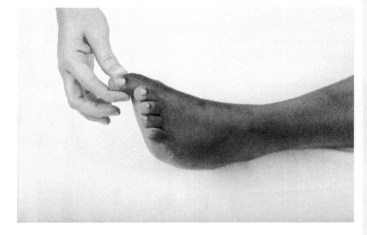

Figure 26.34
Position sense of joint movement.

Reflexes

Reflex testing is usually the last part of the neurologic assessment. The patient is usually in a sitting position; however, you can use a supine position if the patient's physical condition so requires. Position the patient's limbs properly to stretch the muscle partially.

Proper use of the reflex hammer requires practice. Hold the handle of the reflex hammer in your dominant hand between your thumb and index finger. Use your wrist, not your hand or arm, to generate the striking motion. Proper wrist action will provide a brisk, direct, smooth arc for stimulation with the flat or pointed end of the hammer. Stimulate the reflex arc with a brisk tap to the tendon, not the muscle. Through continued practice and experience, you will learn the amount of force to use. Strong force will cause pain, and too little force will not stimulate the arc. After striking the tendon, remove the reflex hammer immediately.

Techniques and Normal Findings	Abnormal Findings / Special Considerations

Evaluate the response on a scale from 0 to 4+:

0	no response
1+	diminished
2+	normal
3+	brisk, above normal
4+	hyperactive

Before concluding that a reflex is absent or diminished, repeat the test. Encourage the patient to relax. You might need to help the patient adjust his position or you might need to strike the tendon with slightly more force. It may be necessary to distract the attention of the patient to achieve muscle relaxation. Distraction, which involves simultaneously performing an isometric activity of a distant muscle group, helps relax the muscle that is being tested and enhances the reflex. For example, ask the patient to pull on his hands (isometric activity) while testing the reflexes of the leg.

1. **Assess the biceps reflex (C5, C6).**
   - Support the patient's lower arm with your nondominant hand and arm. The arm needs to be slightly flexed at the elbow with palm up.
   - Compress the biceps tendon with the thumb of your nondominant hand.
   - Using the pointed side of a reflex hammer, briskly tap your thumb (see Figure 26.35 ■).
   - Look for contraction of the biceps muscle and slight flexion of the forearm.

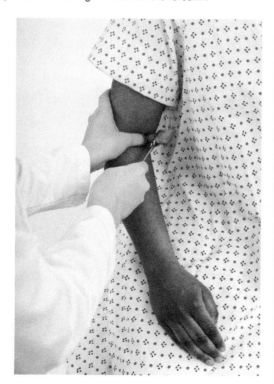

Figure 26.35 Testing the biceps reflex.

2. **Assess the triceps reflex (C6, C7).**
   - Support the patient's elbow with your nondominant hand.
   - Sharply percuss the tendon just above the olecranon process with the pointed end of the reflex hammer (see Figure 26.36 ■).
   - Observe contraction of the triceps muscle with extension of the lower arm.

► Neuromuscular disease, spinal cord injury, or lower motor neuron disease may cause absent or diminished (hypoactive) reflexes.
► Hyperactive reflexes may indicate upper motor neuron disease.
► **Clonus,** rhythmically alternating flexion and extension, confirms upper motor neuron disease.

Techniques and Normal Findings	Abnormal Findings Special Considerations

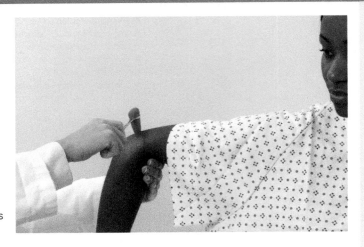

Figure 26.36 Testing the triceps reflex.

3. **Assess the brachioradialis reflex (C5, C6).**
   - Position the patient's arm so the elbow is flexed and the hand is resting on the patient's lap with the palm in a semi-pronating position.
   - Using the flat end of the reflex hammer, briskly strike the tendon toward the radius about 2 or 3 inches above the wrist (see Figure 26.37 ■).
   - Observe flexion of the lower arm and supination of the hand.

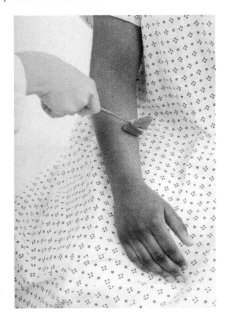

Figure 26.37 Testing the brachioradialis reflex.

4. **Assess the patellar (knee) reflex (L2, L3, L4).**
   - Palpate the patella to locate the patellar tendon inferior to the patella.
   - Briskly strike the tendon with the flat end of the reflex hammer (see Figure 26.38 ■).
   - Note extension of lower leg and contraction of the quadriceps muscle.

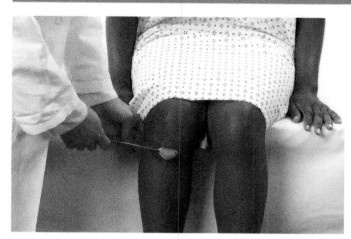

Figure 26.38A Testing patellar reflex, patient in a sitting position.

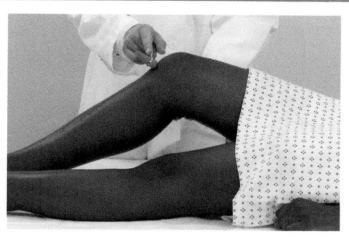

Figure 26.38B Testing patellar reflex, patient in a supine position.

▶ Flex the leg at the knee. Occasionally, the response is not obtained. Distraction such as that depicted in Figure 26.39 ■ may be required.

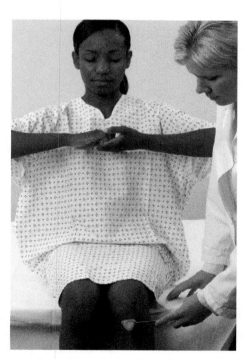

Figure 26.39 Testing patellar reflex using a distraction technique.

5. **Assess the Achilles tendon (ankle) reflex (S1).**
   - Flex the leg at the knee.
   - Dorsiflex the foot of the leg being examined.
   - Hold the foot lightly in the nondominant hand.
   - Strike the Achilles tendon with the flat end of the reflex hammer (see Figure 26.40 ■).

Techniques and Normal Findings	Abnormal Findings Special Considerations

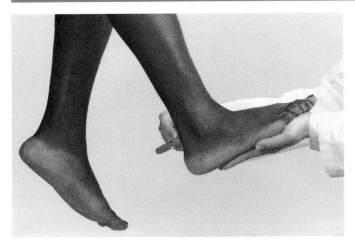

Figure 26.40A Testing the Achilles tendon reflex with patient in a sitting position.

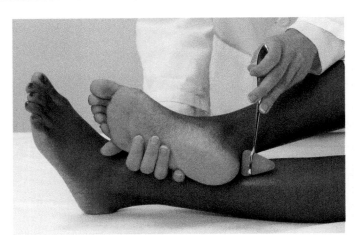

Figure 26.40B Testing the Achilles tendon reflex with patient in a supine position.

- Observe plantar flexion of the foot; the heel will "jump" from your hand.

6. **Assess the plantar reflex (L5, S1).**
   - Position the leg with a slight degree of external rotation at the hip.
   - Stimulate the sole of the foot from the heel to the ball of the foot on the lateral aspect. Continue the stimulation across the ball of the foot to the big toe.
   - Observe for plantar flexion, in which the toes curl toward the sole of the foot (see Figure 26.41 ■). It may be necessary to hold the patient's ankle to prevent movement.

Figure 26.41 Testing the plantar reflex.

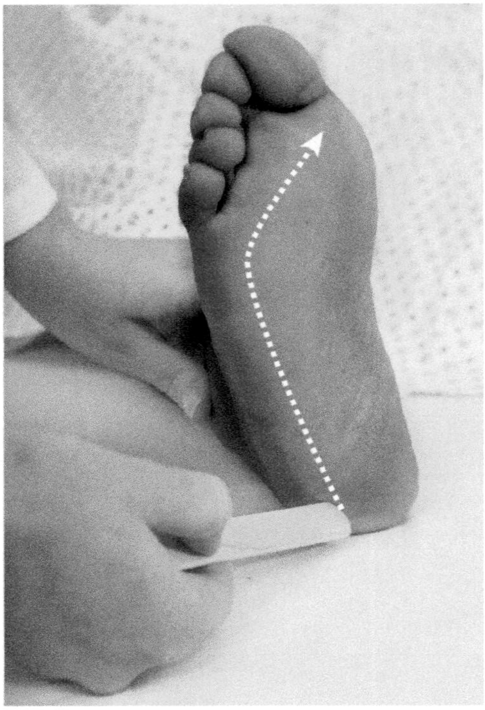

► A **Babinski response** is the fanning of the toes with the great toe pointing toward the dorsum of the foot (see Figure 26.42 ■). This is called dorsiflexion of the toe and is considered an abnormal response in the adult. It may indicate upper motor neuron disease.

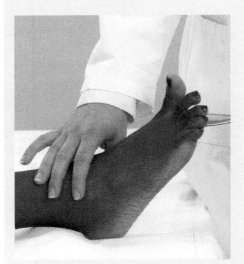

Figure 26.42 A Babinski response in an adult is an abnormal finding.

► A positive Babinski response is considered a normal response in the child until about 2 years of age (see Table 26.3 on page 753).

Techniques and Normal Findings	Abnormal Findings Special Considerations

7. **Assess the abdominal reflexes (T8, T9, T10 for upper and T10, T11, T12 for lower).**

- Using an applicator or tongue blade, briskly stroke the abdomen from the lateral aspect toward the umbilicus (see Figure 26.43 ■).

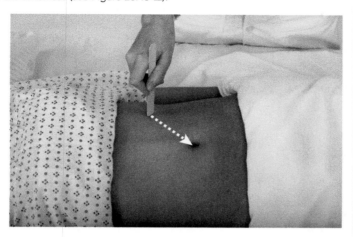

Figure 26.43
Abdominal reflex testing pattern.

- Observe muscular contraction and movement of the umbilicus toward the stimulus.
- Repeat this procedure in the other three quadrants of the abdomen.

▶ Obesity and upper and lower motor neuron pathology can decrease or diminish the response.

Additional Assessment Techniques

Meningeal Assessment

Ask the patient to flex the neck by bringing the chin down to touch the chest. Observe the degree of range of motion and the absence or presence of pain. The patient should be able to flex the neck about 45 degrees without pain.

When the patient complains of pain and has decreased neck flexion, you will observe for *Brudzinski's sign*. With the patient in a supine position, assist the patient with neck flexion. Observe the legs. Brudzinski's sign is positive when neck flexion causes flexion of the legs and thighs.

▶ A positive Brudzinski's sign may be indicative of irritation or inflammation of the meningeal membranes, as in meningitis. **Nuchal rigidity** (severe neck stiffness) is a hallmark of meningitis.

Use of the Glasgow Coma Scale

The *Glasgow Coma Scale* assesses the level of consciousness of the individual on a continuum from alertness to coma (see Figure 26.44 ■). The scale tests three body functions: verbal response, motor response, and eye response. A maximum total score of 15 indicates the person is alert, responsive, and oriented. A total score of 3, the lowest achievable score, indicates a nonresponsive comatose individual.

▶ **Syncope** is a brief loss of consciousness and is usually sudden. **Coma** is a more prolonged state with pronounced and persistent changes.
▶ A patient experiencing any loss of consciousness needs immediate medical interventions.

Techniques and Normal Findings	Abnormal Findings Special Considerations

GLASGOW COMA SCALE

BEST EYE-OPENING RESPONSE
4 = Spontaneously
3 = To speech
2 = To pain
1 = No response
(Record "C" if eyes closed by swelling)

BEST MOTOR RESPONSE to painful stimuli
6 = Obeys verbal command
5 = Localizes pain
4 = Flexion—withdrawal
3 = Flexion—abnormal
2 = Extension—abnormal
1 = No response
(Record best upper limb response)

BEST VERBAL RESPONSE
5 = Oriented × 3
4 = Conversation—confused
3 = Speech—inappropriate
2 = Sounds—incomprehensible
1 = No response
(Record "E" if endotracheal tube in place, "T" if tracheostomy tube in place)

Figure 26.44
Glasgow Coma Scale.

▶ The Glasgow Coma Scale has limitations. For example, a patient with an endotracheal tube or tracheostomy cannot verbally communicate. As a result, the score is carried out according to each individual component of the scale. The verbal response score would then indicate intubation or tracheostomy. In addition, the motor response scale is invalid in a patient with a spinal cord injury, and eye opening may be impossible to assess in those individuals with severe orbital injury.

Abnormal Findings

Problems commonly associated with the neurologic system include changes in motor function, including gait and movement; seizures; spinal cord injury; traumatic brain injury; infections; degenerative disorders; and cranial nerve dysfunction. These conditions are described next and in Tables 26.6 and 26.7.

Seizures

Seizures are sudden, rapid, and excessive discharges of electrical energy in the brain. They are usually centered in the cerebral cortex. Some seizure disorders stem from neurologic problems that occur before or during birth, or they can develop secondary to childhood fevers. In children and adults, seizures can result from a variety of factors including trauma; infections; cerebrovascular disease; environmental toxins; drug overdose; and withdrawal from alcohol, sedatives, or antidepressants. *Epilepsy* is a chronic seizure disorder.

Spinal Cord Injuries

The spinal cord extends from the medulla oblongata of the brain stem. As it continues down the back, the cervical, thoracic, and lumbar vertebrae protect it. Spinal cord injuries result from trauma to the vertebrae, which causes dislocation fractures that in turn compress or transect the spinal cord. The most common causes of this type of trauma are automobile and motorcycle accidents, sports accidents such as football and diving accidents, and penetrating injuries such as stab wounds and gunshots. Generally speaking, the higher the level of the injury, the greater the loss of neurologic function. Injuries to the cervical region are the most common and the most devastating.

TABLE 26.6   Problems with Motor Function

GAIT	MOVEMENT
Ataxic Gait A walk characterized by a wide base, uneven steps, feet slapping, and a tendency to sway. This type of walk is associated with posterior column disease or decreased proprioception regarding extremities. Seen in multiple sclerosis and drug or alcohol intoxication.	**Fasciculation** Commonly called a twitch, this is an involuntary, local, visible muscular contraction. It is not significant when it occurs in tired muscles. It can be associated with motor neuron disease.
Scissors Gait A walk characterized by spastic lower limbs and movement in a stiff, jerky manner. The knees come together; the legs cross in front of one another; and the legs are abducted as the individual takes short, progressive, slow steps. This is seen in individuals with multiple sclerosis.	**Tic** Commonly called a *habit*, a tic is usually psychogenic in nature. The involuntary spasmodic movement of the muscle is seen in a muscle under voluntary control, usually in the face, neck, or shoulders, and increases during stress. Tourette's syndrome is a neurologic disorder characterized by involuntary movements and vocalizations called tics.
Steppage Gait Sometimes called the "foot drop" walk. The individual flexes and raises the knee to a higher-than-usual level, yielding a flopping of the foot when walking. This usually is indicative of lower motor neuron disease. Seen in individuals with alcoholic neuritis and progressive muscular atrophy.	**Tremor** A rhythmic or alternating involuntary movement from the contraction of opposing muscle groups. Tremors vary in degree and are seen in Parkinson's disease, multiple sclerosis, uremia (a form of kidney failure), and alcohol intoxication.
Festination Gait Referred to as the "Parkinson's walk." The individual has stooped posture, takes short steps, and turns stiffly. There is a slow start to the walk and frequent, accelerated steps. This gait is associated with basal ganglia disease.	**Athetoid Movement** A continuous, involuntary, repetitive, slow, "wormlike," arrhythmic muscular movement. The muscles are in a state of hypotoxicity, producing a distortion to the limb. This movement is seen in cerebral palsy.
Dystonia Similar to athetoid movements, dystonia involves larger muscle groups. The twisting movements yield a grotesque change to the individual's posture. Torticollis, or wryneck, is an example of dystonia. Primary dystonia is unrelated to any illness and accounts for almost 50% of all cases. Secondary dystonia can result from trauma, tumor, strokes, or toxins.	**Myoclonus** A continual, rapid, short spasm involving a muscle, part of a muscle, or even a group of muscles. Frequently occurs in an extremity as the individual is falling asleep. Myoclonus is also seen in seizure disorders.

TABLE 26.7   Problems Associated with Dysfunction of Cranial Nerves

CRANIAL NERVE		DYSFUNCTION
I	Olfactory	Unilateral or bilateral anosmia.
II	Optic	Optic atrophy, papilledema, amblyopia, field defects.
III	Oculomotor	Diplopia, ptosis of lid, dilated pupil, inability to focus on close objects.
IV	Trochlear	Convergent strabismus, diplopia.
V	Trigeminal	Tic douloureux, loss of facial sensation, decreased ability to chew, loss of corneal reflex, decreased blinking.
VI	Abducens	Diplopia, strabismus.
VII	Facial	Bell's palsy, decreased ability to distinguish tastes.
VIII	Vestibulocochlear	Tinnitus, vertigo, deafness.
IX	Glossopharyngeal	Loss of "gag" reflex, loss of taste, difficulty swallowing.
X	Vagus	Loss of voice, impaired voice, difficulty swallowing.
XI	Accessory	Difficulty with shrugging of shoulders, inability to turn head to left and right.
XII	Hypoglossal	Difficulty with speech and swallowing, inability to protrude tongue.

TRAUMATIC BRAIN INJURY

Traumatic brain injury (TBI) is an acquired brain injury in which damage to the brain results from a sudden, forceful impact to the brain. TBI commonly results from motor vehicle accidents, sports injuries, blasts, and other accidents. It may also occur during violence such as a gunshot wound or blow to the head or during abuse. Depending on the extent and location of the damage, symptoms can be mild, moderate, or severe.

Subjective findings:

- Headache.
- Confusion.
- Dizziness.
- Fatigue.
- Sensory problems (e.g., blurred vision, tinnitus, bad taste in mouth, light or sound sensitivity).
- Cognitive problems (e.g., inability to concentrate, mood swings, depression, aggression, etc.).

Objective findings:

- Vomiting.
- Seizures.
- Unconsciousness.
- Slurred speech.
- Dilation of pupils (NINDS, 2014b).

Infections of the Neurologic System

Infections of the neurologic system include meningitis, myelitis, brain abscess, and Lyme disease. Each of these is described in the following paragraphs.

MENINGITIS

Meningitis is caused by a virus or bacteria that infect the coverings, or meninges, of the brain or spinal cord. Meningitis may result from a penetrating wound, fractured skull, or upper respiratory infection, or it may occur secondary to facial or cranial surgery.

In some cases, meningitis may spread to the underlying brain tissues, causing encephalitis. *Encephalitis* is defined as an inflammation of the tissue of the brain. It usually results from a virus, which may be transmitted by ticks or mosquitoes, or it may result from a childhood illness such as chickenpox or the measles.

Subjective findings:

- Headache or stiff neck.
- Nausea.
- Photophobia.
- Confusion.

Objective findings:

- Fever.
- Irritability.
- Vomiting.
- Seizures.
- Coma (CDC, 2014).

MYELITIS

Myelitis is an inflammation of the spinal cord. Poliomyelitis and herpes zoster infection are two common causes. It may develop after an infection such as measles or gonorrhea, or it may follow vaccination for rabies.

Subjective findings:

- Lower neck or back pain.
- Muscle weakness.
- Abnormal sensations such as numbness, tingling, or burning.

Objective findings:

- Paralysis.
- Urinary retention.
- Loss of bowel control (Mayo Clinic, 2014).

BRAIN ABSCESS

A brain abscess is usually the result of a systemic infection. It is marked by an accumulation of pus in the brain cells. Most brain abscesses develop secondary to a primary infection. Others result from skull fractures or penetrating injuries, such as a gunshot wound.

Subjective findings:

- Headache.
- Stiff neck.
- Nausea or vomiting.

Objective findings:

- Fever.
- Seizures.
- Papilledema.
- Focal neurologic deficits or hemiparesis.
- Altered level of consciousness (Miranda, Castellar-Leones, Elzain, & Moscote-Salazar, 2013).

LYME DISEASE

Lyme disease is an infection caused by a spirochete transmitted by a bite from an infected tick that lives on deer. If untreated, Lyme disease may cause neurologic disorders including but not limited to Bell's palsy, visual disturbances, and nerve damage in the extremities.

Subjective findings:

- Arthritis.
- Headache or neck stiffness.
- Flu-like symptoms (fatigue, chills, fever, joint aches).
- Dizziness.
- Heart palpitations (CDC, 2013).

Objective findings:

- Bull's eye rash (erythema migrans).
- Swollen lymph nodes.
- Fever (CDC, 2013).

Degenerative Neurologic Disorders

Degenerative neurologic disorders include Alzheimer's disease, amyotrophic lateral sclerosis, Huntington's disease, multiple sclerosis, myasthenia gravis, and Parkinson's disease. These are discussed in the following paragraphs.

ALZHEIMER'S DISEASE

Alzheimer's disease is a progressive degenerative disease of the brain that leads to dementia. Although it is more common in people over age 65, its onset may occur as early as middle adulthood.

Subjective findings:

- Memory loss, particularly of recent events.
- Hallucinations.
- Paranoid fantasies (in later stage of disease).

Objective findings:

- Shortened attention span.
- Confusion.
- Disorientation.
- Wandering.

AMYOTROPHIC LATERAL SCLEROSIS

Amyotrophic lateral sclerosis (ALS), commonly known as Lou Gehrig's disease, is a chronic degenerative disease involving the cerebral cortex and the motor neurons in the spinal cord. The result is a progressive wasting of skeletal muscles that eventually leads to death. Although the cause is unknown, research has implicated viral infection. Certain forms of ALS are familial (University of Michigan Health Systems, n.d.).

Subjective findings:

- Muscle weakness.
- Muscle cramping.
- Shortness of breath.

Objective findings:

- Muscle fasciculations (twitching).
- Difficulty speaking (dysphonia).
- Impaired movement of limbs.

HUNTINGTON'S DISEASE

Huntington's disease is an inherited disorder characterized by uncontrollable jerking movements, called *chorea*, which literally means dance. It typically progresses to mental deterioration and, ultimately, death. Symptoms usually first appear in early middle age; thus, those with Huntington's disease often have had children before they know they have the disorder.

Subjective findings:

- Difficulty with reasoning.
- Difficulty swallowing (dysphagia).
- Disinhibition.

Objective findings:

- Muscle rigidity.
- Choreiform movements (involuntary, irregular, jerking movements).
- Slow movements (bradykinesia).

MULTIPLE SCLEROSIS

Multiple sclerosis is the deterioration of the protective sheaths, composed of myelin, of the nerve tracts in the brain and spinal cord. The first attack usually occurs between the ages of 20 and 40. Some individuals experience repeated attacks that progress in severity. In these individuals, permanent disability with progressive neuromuscular deficits develops.

Subjective findings:

- Blurred vision.
- Transient tingling sensations.
- Numbness.
- Weakness (sometimes limited to one limb or one side of the body).

Objective findings:

- Slurred speech.
- Wide, uneven gait (ataxia).
- Tremors.

MYASTHENIA GRAVIS

Myasthenia gravis is a chronic neuromuscular disorder involving increasing weakness of voluntary muscles with activity and some abatement of symptoms with rest. Onset is gradual and usually occurs in adolescence or young adulthood. The precise etiology is unknown, but it is believed that myasthenia gravis is an *autoimmune* disorder; that is, the individual's immune system attacks the individual's own normal cells rather than foreign pathogens.

Subjective findings:

- Diplopia (double vision).
- Dysphagia (difficulty swallowing).
- Difficulty speaking (dyphasia).

Objective findings:

- Ptosis (drooping eyelids).
- Flat affect.
- Weak, monotone voice.

PARKINSON'S DISEASE

Parkinson's disease is a degeneration of the basal nuclei of the brain, which are collections of nerve cell bodies deep within the white matter of the cerebrum. These nuclei are responsible for initiating and stopping voluntary movement. Although the precise etiology is unknown, research indicates that environmental toxins, such as carbon monoxide or certain metals, may cause some cases of Parkinson's disease. It may also result from previous encephalitis.

Subjective findings:

- Difficulty speaking (dysphasia).
- Decrease in unconscious movements, such as blinking.
- Impaired sense of balance.
- Muscle pain.

Objective findings:

- Slowed movements (bradykinesia).
- Muscle rigidity.
- Rhythmic shaking of the hands.
- Pill-rolling tremor of the forefinger and thumb.
- Mask-like facial expression.

Application Through Critical Thinking

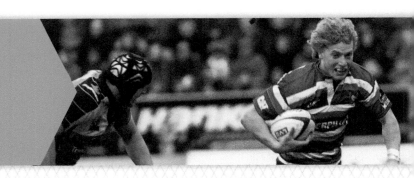

▌ Case Study

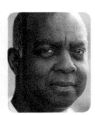

Mr. John Phelps, age 65, is an African American male who comes to the community health clinic. He and his wife Helen recently celebrated their 40th wedding anniversary. He has a 35-year-old daughter, a 32-year-old son, and three grandchildren. Mr. Phelps retired 4 months ago from a busy accounting firm where he worked as a certified public accountant (CPA) for 25 years. He and his wife have been planning their retirement and are looking forward to traveling across the country to visit family.

Mr. Phelps's chief complaint is tremors that seem to be getting worse over the past few months. He noticed the tremors about 6 months ago and thought they were related to fatigue, since the office was very busy and he was working late hours. He anticipated that the tremors would stop after he retired and became rested. Mrs. Phelps indicates that her husband's handwriting has become small and almost illegible and that she had to write several checks

for him last week. She also comments that her husband seems depressed about his recent retirement, since he has a "blank look" on his face and his speech is slow. Mari Chung, RN, conducts a focused interview and then proceeds with the physical assessment. She gathers the following objective and subjective data:

- Mood swings
- Tremors, movement of thumb and index finger in a circular fashion
- Shuffling gait, falls easily
- Constipation
- Fatigue
- Loss of 10 lb
- Drooling
- Speaks in a monotone; voice slow, weak, and soft
- Rigidity during passive range of motion (ROM)

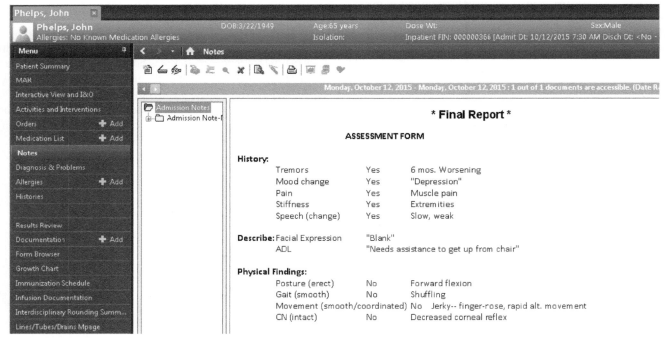

- Jerky movements
- Muscle pain and soreness
- Decrease in corneal response
- Posture not erect, forward flexion
- Unable to perform finger-to-nose test and rapid alternating movement
- Difficulty standing from sitting position without assistance

Ms. Chung consults with the clinic physician. After further evaluation, Mr. Phelps is admitted to the neurologic unit of the community hospital with a diagnosis of Parkinson's disease.

▌Complete Documentation

The following is sample documentation from the health assessment of John Phelps.

SUBJECTIVE DATA: Complains of tremors, getting worse over 6 months. He has had some change in his moods, has lost some weight, and is constipated frequently. He has occasional drooling. Experiences muscle pain and soreness. Requires assistance to get up

from a chair and falls easily. Wife states writing increasingly illegible. She reports he has become depressed, has a "blank look," and has slow speech.

OBJECTIVE DATA: Posture not erect—favored flexion, shuffling gait, jerky movements. Voice monotone, slow, weak, soft. Decreased corneal response. Rigidity during passive ROM. Unable to perform finger-to-nose and rapid alternating movement tests. Drooling. Weight loss 10 lbs. in past three months.

▌Critical Thinking Questions

1. What data were considered in the medical diagnosis of Parkinson's disease?
2. What additional data would be required to confirm a diagnosis of Parkinson's disease?
3. What are the nursing considerations for Mr. Phelps?
4. What psychosocial considerations should the nurse be aware of when assessing Mr. Phelps?
5. What environmental considerations should the nurse screen for in this case?

APPLICATION OF OBJECTIVE 4: Discuss strategies in management of Parkinson's disease

Content	Teaching Strategy	Evaluation
• Medication is used to manage problems with tremor and movement. • Surgery may improve movement. • Deep brain stimulation refers to implantation of a device to reduce trembling. • Self-care includes a healthy diet. Fiber reduces problems with constipation. Including folate in the diet or as a supplement may protect against Parkinson's disease. Eating and swallowing carefully reduces risk of choking. • Regular exercise improves mobility, balance, range of motion, and emotional well-being. • Reduce the risk of injury from falls by making the home environment safe (no throw rugs, install handrails and grab bars). • Seek assistance from physical and occupational therapists for guidelines to improve ease of ambulation and carrying out daily tasks. • Communication requires speaking louder than believed necessary. Practice reading aloud. Seek assistance from a speech pathologist.	• Lecture • Discussion • Audiovisual materials • Printed materials Lecture is appropriate when disseminating information to large groups. Discussion allows participants to bring up concerns and to raise questions. Audiovisual materials such as illustrations reinforce verbal presentation. Printed materials, especially to be taken away with learners, allow review, reinforcement, and reading at the learner's pace.	• Written examination. May use short answer, fill-in, or multiple-choice items or a combination of items. If these are short and easy to evaluate, the learner receives immediate feedback.

▌ Prepare Teaching Plan

LEARNING NEED: The data in the case study revealed that Mr. Phelps has signs and symptoms of Parkinson's disease. His symptoms include tremors, weight loss, fatigue, constipation, falling, and others. He was admitted to the hospital and will begin treatment for his problem. He and his wife will require education about the disease and his care upon discharge.

The case study provides data that are representative of risks, symptoms, and behaviors of many individuals. Therefore, the following teaching plan is based on the need to provide information to members of any community about Parkinson's disease.

GOAL: The participants in this learning program will have increased knowledge about Parkinson's disease and its management.

OBJECTIVES: At the completion of this learning session, the participants will be able to:

1. Describe Parkinson's disease.
2. Identify risk factors associated with Parkinson's disease.
3. List the symptoms of Parkinson's disease.
4. Discuss strategies in management of Parkinson's disease.

▌ References

Alzheimer's Association. (2010). 2010 Alzheimer's disease facts and figures. *Alzheimer's & Dementia: The Journal of the Alzheimer's Association, 6*(2), 158–194.

American Heart Association (AHA). (n.d.). *Think you are having a stroke? Call 9-1-1 immediately!* Retrieved from http://strokeassociation.org/STROKEORG/WarningSigns/Stroke-Warning-Signs-and-Symptoms_UCM_308528_SubHomePage.jsp

Berman, A., & Snyder, S. (2012). *Kozier and Erb's Fundamentals of nursing: Concepts, process, and practice* (9th ed.). Upper Saddle River, NJ: Prentice Hall.

Bikley, L. S. (2012). *Bates' guide to physical examination and history taking* (11th ed.). Philadelphia, PA: Lippincott.

Caudle, W. M., Guillot, T. S., Lazo, C. R., & Miller, G.W. (2012). Industrial toxicants and Parkinson's disease. *Neurotoxicology, 33*(2), 178–188.

Centers for Disease Control and Prevention (CDC). (2013). Signs and symptoms of lyme disease. Retrieved from http://www.cdc.gov/lyme/signs_symptoms/index.html

Centers for Disease Control and Prevention (CDC). (2014). Meningitis. Retrieved from http://www.cdc.gov/meningitis/index.html

Grandjean, P., & Landrigan, P. J. (2014). Neurobehavioural effects of developmental toxicity. *The Lancet Neurology, 13*(3), 330–338.

Gray, H. (2004). *Gray's anatomy.* New York: Barnes & Noble Books.

Hockenberry, M., & Wilson, D. (2007). *Wong's nursing care of infants and children* (8th ed.). St. Louis, MO: C. V. Mosby.

Liberty, G., Shaul, C., Anteby, E. Y., Zohav, E., Cohen, S. M., Boldes, R., & Yagel, S. (2014). OP28. 05: 2D and 3D ultrasound imaging of the fetal normal and bifid uvula. *Ultrasound in Obstetrics & Gynecology, 44*(S1), 152.

Lucile Packard Children's Hospital. (2008). *Neurological disorders, seizures, and epilepsy.* Retrieved from http://www.lpch.org/diseasehealthinf/healthlibrary/neuro/seizep.htm

Marieb, E. (2008). *Essentials of human anatomy and physiology* (9th ed.). Redwood City, CA: Benjamin/Cummings/Pearson Education.

Mayo Clinic. (2013). *Drugs and supplements: Vitamin B6 (pyridoxine).* Retrieved from http://www.mayoclinic.org/drugs-supplements/vitamin-b6/background/hrb-20058788

Mayo Foundation for Medical Education and Research. (2014). *Rochester test catalog: 2014 online test catalog.* Available at http://www.mayomedicallaboratories.com/test-catalog/

Miranda, H. A., Castellar-Leones, S. M., Elzain, M. A., & Moscote-Salazar, L. R. (2013). Brain abscess: Current management. *Journal of Neurosciences in Rural Practice, 4*(Suppl 1), S67–S81.

National Institute of Neurological Disorders and Stroke. (2014). *Febrile seizures fact sheet.* Retrieved from http://www.ninds.nih.gov/disorders/febrile_seizures/detail_febrile_seizures.htm

Neurologic disorders. (2008). Retrieved from http://www.pch.org/diseases healthinfo/healthlibrary/neuro.html

Osborn, K. S., Wraa, C. E., Watson, A., & Holleran, R. S. (2013). *Medical-surgical nursing: Preparation for practice* (2nd ed.). Upper Saddle River, NJ: Pearson.

Osterhues, A., Ali, N. S., & Michels, K. B. (2013). The role of folic acid fortification in neural tube defects: A review. *Critical Reviews in Food Science and Nutrition, 53*(11), 1180–1190.

Rao, J. B., Vengamma, B., Naveen, T., & Naveen, V. (2014). Lead encephalopathy in adults. *Journal of Neurosciences in Rural Practice, 5*(2), 161–163.

Ross, S. M., McManus, I. C., Harrison, V., & Mason, O. (2013). Neurobehavioral problems following low-level exposure to organophosphate pesticides: A systematic and meta-analytic review. *Critical Reviews in Toxicology, 43*(1), 21–44.

Seifert, S. M., Schaechter, J. L., Hershorin, E. R., & Lipshultz, S. E. (2011). Health effects of energy drinks on children, adolescents, and young adults. *Pediatrics, 127*(3), 511–529.

Stolzberg, D., Salvi, R. J., & Allman, B. L. (2012). Salicylate toxicity model of tinnitus. *Frontiers in Systems Neuroscience, 6*(28), 1–12.

Tortora, G. J., & Derrickson, B. H. (2009). *Principles of anatomy and physiology* (12th ed.). New York: John Wiley & Sons.

U.S. Department of Health and Human Services (USDHHS). (2014). *Healthy people 2020.* Retrieved from http://www.healthypeople.gov/2020/default.aspx

University of Maryland Medical Center (2014). *Color vision test.* Retrieved from http://umm.edu/health/medical/ency/articles/color-vision-test

University of Michigan Health Systems. (n.d.). *Genetic disorders: Neurogenetics.* Retrieved from http://www.uofmhealth.org/medical-services/neurogenetics

U.S. Department of Health and Human Services (USDHHS). (2010). *Healthy people 2020.* Retrieved from http://www.healthypeople.gov/2020/default.aspx

van Dijk, J. G., & Wieling, W. (2013). Pathophysiological basis of syncope and neurological conditions that mimic syncope. *Progress in Cardiovascular Diseases, 55*(4), 345–356.

VanGilder, R. L., Rosen, C. L., Barr, T. L., & Huber, J. D. (2011). Targeting the neurovascular unit for treatment of neurological disorders. *Pharmacology & Therapeutics, 130*(3), 239–247.

Wilson, B. A., Shannon, M. T., & Shields, K. M. (2013). *Pearson nurse's drug guide.* Upper Saddle River, NJ: Pearson.

World Health Organization (WHO). (2012). *Epilepsy: Fact sheet N₀ 999.* Retrieved from http://www.who.int/mediacentre/factsheets/fs999/en/

Wu, T., Wang, L., Hallett, M., Chen, Y., Li, K., & Chan, P. (2011). Effective connectivity of brain networks during self-initiated movement in Parkinson's disease. *Neuroimage, 55*(1), 204–215.

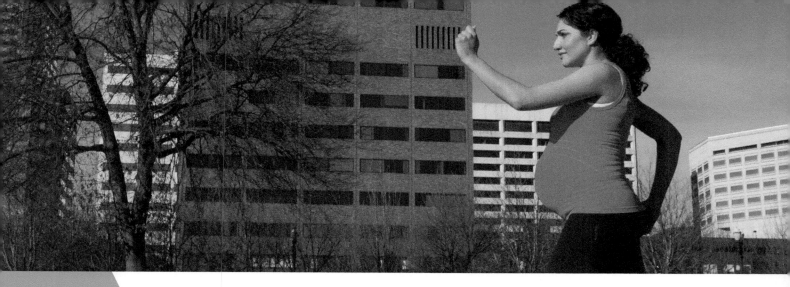

Learning Outcomes

Upon completion of the chapter, you will be able to:

1. Describe the anatomy and physiology specific to assessment of the pregnant and postpartum female.

2. Illustrate the anatomic and physiologic variations in body systems that guide assessment in pregnancy and postpartum.

3. Practice questions used when completing the focused interview.

4. Demonstrate the techniques used in the assessment of the pregnant and postpartum female.

5. Differentiate normal from abnormal findings in the focused interview and physical assessment of the pregnant female.

6. Teach patients about health promotion and education topics related to care of the pregnant female.

7. Apply the objectives in *Healthy People 2020* to the pregnant female.

8. Apply critical thinking to the physical assessment of the pregnant and postpartum female patient.

Key Terms

Through the actions of the nurse, pregnancy and the postpartum period offer a unique opportunity for health promotion, disease prevention, and changes in lifestyle behaviors. For the vast majority of childbearing females, pregnancy and postpartum are normal processes that can be enhanced through education, health care, and supportive intervention. Changes in personal lifestyle behaviors and health care can influence not only the course of the pregnancy and the health of mother and child but also the health behaviors of the entire family in the future. Knowledge of variations in body systems during the three trimesters of pregnancy and postpartum periods will enable the nurse to differentiate normal from abnormal changes. The risk for and development of many pathologic conditions in pregnancy and postpartum can be ascertained and prevented by a careful, thorough interview. Past medical, obstetric, gynecologic, family, genetic, and social history will influence the focus of the physical assessment and teaching. Knowledge of lifestyle and health practices, nutrition and exercise history, environmental exposures, and current symptoms will also guide assessment and teaching.

The physical assessment also provides an opportunity for patient education and clarification of misperceptions. Cultural, familial, and personal beliefs can be discussed as appropriate during the history taking and physical assessment. Whether the nurse is perceived as kind and personal, or cold and bureaucratic, as knowledgeable and helpful, or ill informed and ineffective, will influence the patient's willingness and ability to implement health recommendations. This life transition is also an opportunity for sharing much joy and excitement with childbearing families. The nurse can influence a whole generation through caring, accurate, and appropriate assessment and intervention (see Figure 27.1 ■).

Healthy People 2020 objectives focus on the areas of family planning, fetal and infant deaths, maternal deaths and illnesses, prenatal care, and breast-feeding. Objectives related to contraception, reproductive health, prenatal care, and fetal health are included in Table 27.1 on page 806.

Anatomy and Physiology Review

In order to implement programs of maternal–infant care to promote health, the nurse must understand the adaptations that occur in the female body during pregnancy and postpartum. The anatomic and

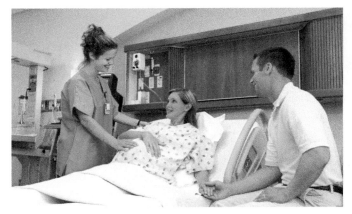

Figure 27.1 Nurse with pregnant patient and partner.
Source: Jupiterimages/Stockbyte/Getty Images.

physiologic changes during the 40 weeks of pregnancy serve three important functions:

- Maintain normal maternal physiologic function.
- Meet maternal metabolic needs as she adapts to the pregnancy.
- Meet the growth and development needs of the fetus.

An assessment of the changes in each body system during pregnancy and postpartum will enable the nurse to interpret findings in the interview and assessment.

The Placenta

The physiologic and anatomic changes in pregnancy are due to the hormones secreted by the fetus and placenta and the mechanical effects of the growing fetus. The human placenta is a unique organ that promotes and provides for fetal growth and development. Its functions include metabolism, transport of gases and nutrients, and secretion of hormones. It develops from the fertilized ovum but generally also includes the maternal uterine lining at the site of implantation. The **placenta** is an ovoid organ that weighs approximately one sixth the weight of the fetus and covers one third of the inner surface area of the uterus at term. Implantation of the fertilized egg, called a *blastocyst*, in the endometrium or lining of the uterus begins 6 days after fertilization. The umbilical blood vessels and placenta

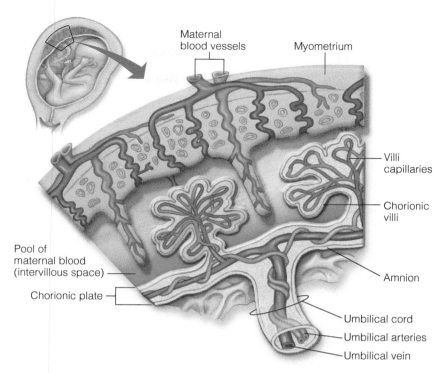

Figure 27.2 Cross section of the placenta.

develop. Two arteries and a vein exit the fetus at the umbilicus, forming the umbilical cord, and insert in the center of the placenta (see Figure 27.2 ■). The fetal vessels branch out into treelike chorionic villi where the fetal capillaries are the sites of exchange between the maternal and fetal circulations. The fetal and maternal circulations are kept essentially separate by the placental membrane covering the villi. The exchange of nutrients from the maternal to the fetal circulation takes place here, as well as passage of waste products such as carbon dioxide and uric acid from the fetal to maternal circulation. The placenta, in conjunction with the fetus and maternal uterine lining, also produces hormones such as human chorionic gonadotropin (hCG), estrogen, progesterone, relaxin, prolactin, and other hormones.

Fetal Development

Pregnancy is divided into three trimesters, each lasting approximately 13 weeks (3 months in lay terms). The age of the developing human can be referred to in weeks beyond fertilization (as used in discussion of fetal development) or in weeks from the last normal menstrual period, more commonly known as **gestational age**.

The first 2 weeks after fertilization are the early embryo stage, and disruptions in development at this stage, such as from environmental agents, usually cause death or miscarriage. From 2 to 8 weeks after fertilization, the **embryo** is in the stage of *organogenesis*. During this period a **teratogen**, an agent such as a virus, a drug, a chemical, or radiation that causes malformation of an embryo or **fetus**, may induce major congenital anomalies. After the completion of 8 weeks until birth, the developing human is referred to as the fetus (see Figure 27.3 ■).

By the end of the first trimester, all major systems have formed. **Viability**, the point at which the fetus can survive outside the uterus, may occur as early as 22 weeks or at the weight of 500 g. During the fetal period the body grows, and differentiation of tissues, organs, and systems occurs.

Although fetal movement can be detected as early as 7 weeks through diagnostic techniques, **quickening**, the fluttery initial sensations of fetal movement perceived by the mother, usually occurs at approximately 18 weeks, possibly earlier in females who have given birth before.

The fetal heart begins beating at 22 days. During assessment, the fetal heartbeat can be heard via Doppler starting between 7 and 12 weeks of pregnancy, and with a **fetoscope**, a specialized stethoscope for listening to fetal heart sounds, beginning at approximately 18 weeks of gestation. The *uterine souffle*, the sound of the uterine arteries, which is synchronous with the maternal pulse, may be heard, as well as the *funic souffle*, the sound of the umbilical vessels that is synchronous with the fetal heartbeat.

Fetal circulation prior to birth has three shunts that enable the fetus to maximize oxygenation from the maternal circulation since lungs are not yet functional for oxygen exchange. Oxygenated blood from the placenta is carried via the umbilical vein to the fetus, entering at the umbilicus. The fetal liver is partially bypassed by the **ductus venosus**, so that highly oxygenated blood continues on to the heart. More highly oxygenated blood flows into the second shunt, the **foramen ovale**, which connects the fetal right atrium to the fetal left atrium. The other half of the blood continues to the right ventricle. The more highly oxygenated blood from the umbilical vein continues to the left ventricle and is shunted across the **ductus arteriosus** into the descending aorta. In this way, only a small part

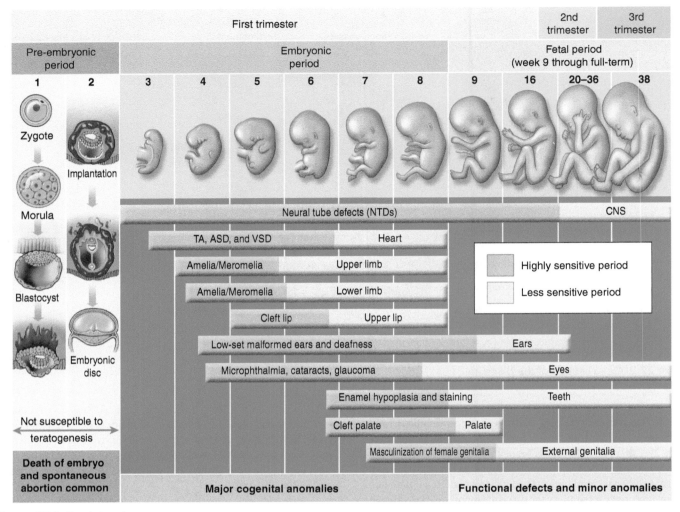

Figure 27.3 Fetal development.

of the blood flow enters the pulmonary bed. The oxygenated blood then perfuses the rest of the fetal body and returns to the placenta via the umbilical arteries (see Figure 27.4 ■).

Reproductive System Changes

In addition to the fetus and placenta, extensive changes occur in the reproductive organs. The uterus, cervix, fallopian tubes, and vagina undergo massive changes in size and function.

Uterus

The uterus is profoundly transformed in pregnancy. The crisscross muscle fibers of the body of the uterus increase in size and number due to the effects of progesterone and estrogen. The uterus increases in size from 70 grams (2.5 oz) to 1,000 grams (2.2 lb), and from 7.5 cm (3 in.) long, 5 cm (2 in.) wide, and 2.5 cm (1 in.) deep to 25 cm (10 in.) long, 20 cm (8 in.) wide, and 22.5 cm (9 in.) deep; its capacity increases from 10 mL to 5,000 mL. During the second and third trimesters, the growing fetus also mechanically expands the uterus.

Early in pregnancy the uterus retains its nonpregnant pear shape but becomes more globular by 12 weeks. Bimanual palpation is used to assess the size of the uterus during the early weeks. The

early sizes can be compared to fruits: 6 weeks, a lemon; 8 weeks, a small orange; 10 weeks, a large orange; and 12 weeks, a grapefruit. The growing uterus can be palpated abdominally by about 10 to 12 weeks, at which time the top of the uterus, or **fundus**, is slightly above the symphysis pubis. The female begins to "show" externally at approximately 14 to 16 weeks, later for a **primigravida**, a female pregnant for the first time, and earlier for a **multigravida**, a female who has been pregnant two or more times. At 16 weeks, the fundus is halfway between the symphysis and umbilicus. Between 20 and 22 weeks, the fundus reaches the umbilicus. Fundal height increases until 38 weeks. The distance from the symphysis pubis to the fundus is measured with a measuring tape to assess fetal growth and dating in pregnancy. **McDonald's rule** for estimating fetal growth states that after 20 weeks in pregnancy, the weeks of gestation approximately equal the **fundal height** in centimeters (see Figure 27.5 ■). Between 38 and 40 weeks **lightening**, or the descent of the fetal head into the pelvis, occurs, and the fundal height drops slightly.

The decidua or lining of the uterus becomes four times thicker during pregnancy. Amenorrhea, or the absence of menstruation, is one of the first signs that pregnancy has occurred. Throughout pregnancy the uterus softens, as does the region that connects the body of the uterus and cervix, referred to as **Hegar's sign**.

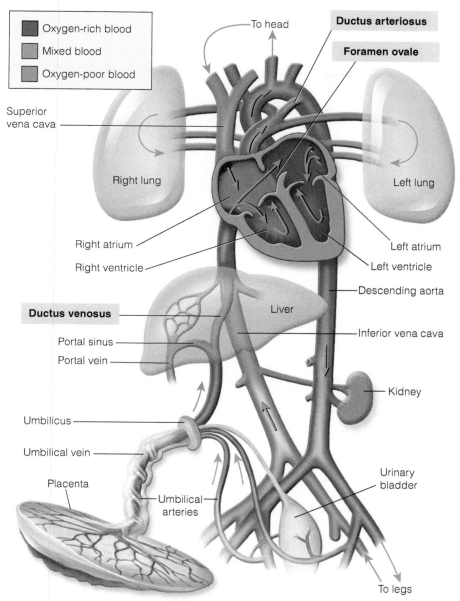

Figure 27.4 Fetal circulation.

Piskacek's sign is the irregular shape of the uterus due to the implantation of the ovum. The contractility of the uterus increases due to the action of estrogen. **Braxton-Hicks contractions**, painless and unpredictable contractions of the uterus that do not dilate the cervix, start in the first trimester, are palpable to the nurse by the second trimester, and are felt by the mother usually starting in the third trimester. **Ballottement**, a technique of palpation, where the examiner's hand is used to push against the uterus and detect the presence or position of a fetus by its return impact, can be elicited after about 20 weeks because the **amniotic fluid**, a clear, slightly yellowish liquid that surrounds the fetus, is greater in comparison to the still small fetus.

Cervix and Vagina

The cervix, or opening of the uterus, develops a protective **mucous plug** during pregnancy, due to the action of progesterone, which also causes **leukorrhea**, a profuse, nonodorous, nonpainful vaginal discharge that protects against infection. Increased glycogen in vaginal cells predisposes the mother to yeast infections in pregnancy. **Goodell's sign** is the softening of the cervix starting at about 6 weeks. At the same time, increased vascularity causes the cervix and vagina to appear bluish (**Chadwick's sign**). Due to these changes, the cervix is more friable and may bleed slightly with sexual intercourse or vaginal examination. Near the end of pregnancy, cervical **ripening**, or softening, and **effacement**, or thinning, occur in preparation for labor. Progressive **dilation**, or opening of the cervix, does not usually occur until the onset of active labor. Externally, the labia majora, labia minora, clitoris, and vaginal introitus enlarge because of hypertrophy and increased vascularity.

Changes in Breasts

One of the first symptoms in pregnancy is breast tenderness, enlargement, and tingling, which is noticeable at 4 to 6 weeks' gestation. These changes are caused by the growth of the alveoli and

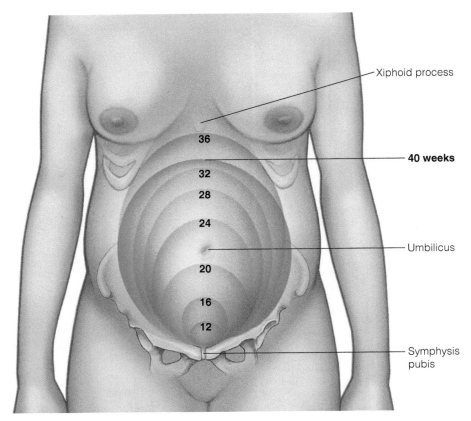

Figure 27.5 Fundal height in pregnancy.

ductal system and the deposition of fat in the breasts under the influence of estrogen and progesterone. The nipple and the **areola**, the pink circle around the nipple, darken in color in pregnancy, and the sebaceous glands on the areola, **Montgomery's tubercles**, enlarge and produce a secretion that protects and lubricates the nipples. With the doubling of the blood flow to the breasts, the vascular network above the breasts enlarges and becomes more visible. **Colostrum**, a yellowish specialized form of early breast milk, is produced starting in the second trimester and is replaced by mature milk during the early days of lactation after the delivery of the baby (see Figure 27.6 ■).

Respiratory System Changes

Mechanical and biochemical changes during pregnancy allow the respiratory needs of both mother and fetus to be met. The enlarging uterus lifts the diaphragm up 4 cm (1.034 in.), the transverse diameter of the chest increases, the ribs flare, and the subcostal angle increases. The increasing hormonal levels of progesterone and relaxin allow these changes in the thorax.

The respiratory-stimulating properties of progesterone contribute to the following:

- A slight increase in respiratory rate of about two breaths per minute
- A lowered threshold for carbon dioxide, contributing to a sense of dyspnea by the pregnant female
- Decreased airway resistance

- Increased tidal volume and inspiratory capacity
- Decreased expiratory volume

The vital capacity is unchanged, but oxygen consumption is increased 20% to 60%. The pregnant female may report great fatigue, particularly in the first trimester, due to these changes. Hyperventilation may occur, and rales in the base of the lung may be heard as a result of compression by the growing uterus.

Cardiovascular and Hematologic System Changes

The most significant hematologic change is an increase in blood and plasma volume of 30% to 50% beginning at 6 to 8 weeks, which is greater in multiple pregnancies. This change is facilitated by three factors:

- The increased progesterone leads to decreased venous tone.
- The increased progesterone combined with increased estrogen results in increased sodium retention and an increase in total body water.
- The shunt of blood to uteroplacental circulation provides physical space for increased plasma volume.

Other hematologic changes include the following:

- A 25% to 33% increase in red blood cells (RBCs)
- Decrease in hemoglobin and hematocrit, or **physiologic anemia**, caused by the plasma volume increase outpacing the increase in RBCs

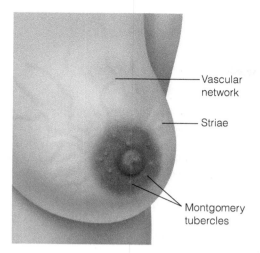

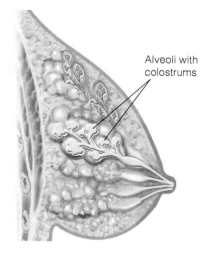

Vascular
network

Striae

Montgomery
tubercles

Alveoli with
colostrums

Figure 27.6 Breast changes in pregnancy.

- Gradual increase in reticulocytes
- Increased white blood cells (WBCs)
- Hypercoagulable state caused by increased activity of most coagulation factors and decreased activities of factors that inhibit coagulation

Physical changes in the cardiac system include cardiac enlargement caused by the increased blood volume and accompanying increase in cardiac output. The upward displacement of the diaphragm by the growing uterus shifts the heart upward and to the left. Most pregnant females will have an S1 sound that is louder. Systolic murmurs are usually heard. Due to increased blood flow, a murmur over the mammary vessels, the **mammary souffle**, is occasionally heard. The heart rate gradually increases by 10 to 20 beats per minute (beats/min) over the course of the pregnancy.

Blood pressure remains the same at the beginning of pregnancy. The decrease in vascular resistance leads to a decrease in diastolic blood pressure that reaches its nadir, or lowest point, during the second trimester and gradually returns to baseline by the time of delivery.

The changes in hemodynamics can cause orthostatic stress when the female changes position from sitting to standing or lying to sitting. **Supine hypotension syndrome**, also known as the vena cava syndrome, occurs when pressure from the pregnant uterus compresses the aorta and the inferior vena cava when the female is in the supine position (see Figure 27.7 ■). She may experience dizziness, syncope, and a significant drop in heart rate and blood pressure.

Decreased peripheral resistance leads to increased filling in the legs, but the pressure of the growing uterus on the femoral veins restricts venous return, leading to increased dependent edema and varicosities in the legs, vulva, and rectum (hemorrhoids).

Integumentary System Changes

Hormonal and mechanical factors cause the integumentary changes seen with pregnancy. Categories of change include alterations in pigmentation, connective tissue, vascular system, secretory glands, skin, hair, and pruritus. The changes are not usually pathologic but are a source of concern to expectant mothers.

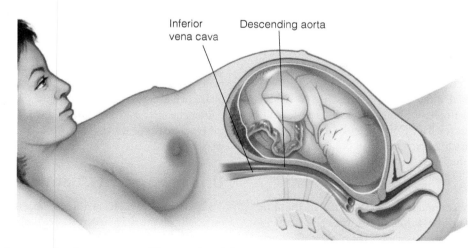

Inferior
vena cava

Descending aorta

Figure 27.7 Supine hypotension in pregnancy. The weight of the uterus compresses the vena cava, trapping blood in the lower extremities.

Alterations in pigmentation, the most common integumentary changes in pregnancy, are caused by the increase in estrogen and progesterone early in pregnancy and by the increase in placental hormones and melanocyte-stimulating hormone, as well as others, later in pregnancy. Any areas of pigmentation in the body will usually become darker for females of all skin colors, including the areolae, axillae, perineum, and inner thighs. The *linea alba*, a tendinous line that extends midline from the symphysis pubis to the xiphoid, darkens with the progression of the fundus up through the abdomen and becomes the **linea nigra**. *Melasma*, also called chloasma or the "mask of pregnancy," occurs in a butterfly pattern over the forehead, nose, and cheeks. There is a strong genetic predisposition for this condition, and it is also seen with the use of combined oral contraceptive pills. Freckles, nevi, and scars may also darken in pregnancy.

A change in connective tissue is **striae gravidarium**, also known as stretch marks, pinkish-purplish streaks that are depressions in the skin. Caused by the stretching of the collagen in skin, they develop in the second half of pregnancy and fade to silver in the postpartum; unlike most integumentary changes, they do not resolve completely after pregnancy. They may develop in the lower abdomen, breasts, thighs, and buttocks.

Vascular alterations that affect the integumentary system are spider angiomas or nevi and palmar erythema. Spider angiomas or nevi are arterioles dilated at the center, with branches radiating outward, appearing on the face, neck, and arms. They fade after pregnancy but do not usually disappear. They often occur with palmar erythema, a reddening or mottling of the palms or fleshy side of the fingers, which occurs after the first trimester, has a genetic predisposition, and regresses by the first week after birth.

Alterations in secretory glands in pregnancy include a decrease in apocrine sweat gland activity in the axillae, abdomen, and genitalia. The eccrine sweat glands in the palms, soles, and forehead increase in activity due to increases in thyroid and metabolic activity, allowing for dissipation of increased heat. Some females experience a "glow" in their skin during pregnancy, while some experience an increase in acne due to increased sebaceous gland activity.

A skin change that sometimes occurs in the second half of pregnancy is the development of soft, pedunculated, flesh-colored or pigmented skin tags. Although a common occurrence in the general population, elevated hormones may cause an increase in the formation. They occur on the sides of the face and neck, on the upper axillae, between and under the breasts, and in the groin, often where skin rubs against clothing or skin rubs against skin. These may or may not have to be removed after delivery.

Due to the hormonal influence of estrogen in pregnancy, more hairs enter the growth phase. Some females experience mild hirsutism and report thicker hair. Consequently, more than the usual number of hairs reach maturity and fall out in the postpartum period during months 1 to 5. Usually all hair regrows by 6 to 15 months postpartum. Occasionally nails become soft or more brittle.

Pruritus (itching) is common in the abdomen in the third trimester, and if severe must be distinguished from rare dermatologic disorders in pregnancy such as cholestasis of pregnancy, pruritic urticarial papules and plaques of pregnancy (PUPPP), herpes gestationis, and prurigo of pregnancy. Figure 27.8 ■ depicts several of the integumentary changes in pregnancy.

Changes in the Ear, Nose, Throat, and Mouth

An increase in estrogen increases vascularity throughout the body in pregnancy. Increased vascularity of the middle ear may cause a feeling of fullness or earaches. Increased blood flow (hyperemia) to the sinuses can cause rhinitis and epistaxis. The sense of smell is heightened in pregnancy. Edema of the vocal cords may cause hoarseness or deepening of the voice. Hyperemia of the throat can lead to an increase in snoring. In the mouth, small blood vessels and connective tissue increase. Gingivitis or inflammation of the gums occurs in many females. This leads to bleeding and discomfort with brushing and eating. Occasionally a hyperplastic overgrowth forms a mass on the gums called epulis, which bleeds easily and recedes after birth.

Gastrointestinal System Changes

Nausea and vomiting are common beginning at 4 to 6 weeks and usually resolve by 12 weeks' gestation. The exact cause is unknown, although hormonal and psychologic factors have been implicated. Other gastrointestinal changes occur during the second and third trimesters. *Ptyalism*, an increase in saliva production, may occasionally occur with nausea and vomiting. The pregnant female may also report pica, an abnormal craving for and ingestion of nonnutritive substances such as starch, dirt, or ice. Mechanical pressure from the growing uterus contributes to displacement of the small intestine and reduces motility. The increased secretion of progesterone further reduces motility because of decreased gastric tone and increased smooth muscle relaxation; thus, the emptying time of the stomach and bowel is prolonged, and constipation is common. Progesterone's relaxing effect on smooth muscle also accounts for the prolonged emptying time of the gallbladder, and gallstone formation may result. *Pyrosis*, or heartburn, the regurgitation of the acidic contents of the stomach into the esophagus, is related to the enlarging uterus displacing the stomach upward and to the relaxation of the esophageal sphincter. Hemorrhoids are another common finding in the third trimester, resulting from the increasing size of the uterus creating pressure on the pelvic veins. If the mother is constipated, the pressure on the venous structures from straining to move the bowels can also lead to hemorrhoids.

Nutritional demands of the pregnancy and fetus increase the maternal requirements. Each day, the mother requires an increased intake of 300 calories and 15 g or more of protein. Most nutrient requirements increase from 20% to 100%. The recommended weight gain for females of average weight is 25 to 35 lb, 28 to 40 lb if underweight, 15 to 25 lb if overweight, and 11 to 20 lb if obese.

Urinary System Changes

The growing uterus causes displacement of the ureters and kidneys, especially on the right side. A slower flow of urine through the ureters causes physiologic **hydronephrosis** and **hydroureter**. Estrogen causes increased bladder vascularity, predisposing the mucosa

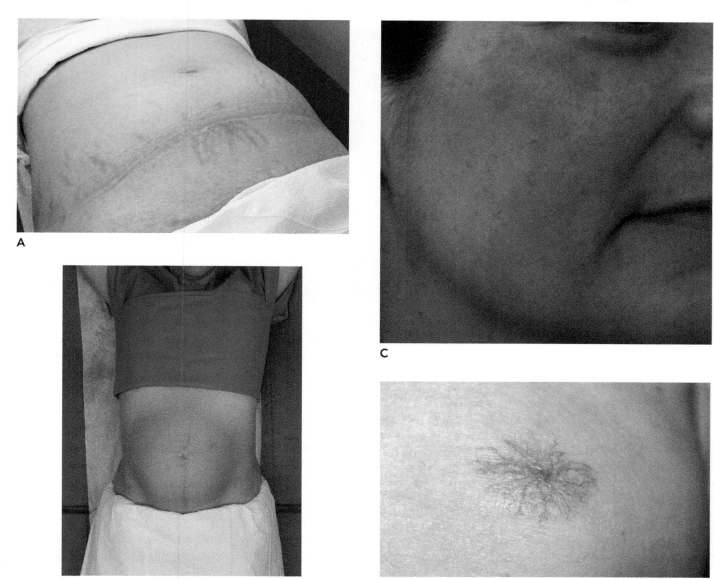

Figure 27.8 Integumentary changes in pregnancy. A. Striae. B. Linea nigra. C. Melasma. D. Spider angioma.
Source: D: SPL/Custom Medical Stock Photo.

to bleed more easily. Urinary frequency occurs in the first trimester as the uterus grows and puts pressure on the bladder. Relief from frequency occurs after the uterus moves out of the pelvis, only to return in the third trimester when the enlarged uterus again presses on the bladder.

The functional changes in the urinary system include the following:

- Increased renal blood flow by 35% to 60%
- Increased glomerular filtration rate by as much as 50% above prepregnancy levels
- Decreased reabsorption of filtered glucose in the renal tubules, contributing to glycosuria
- Increased tubular reabsorption of sodium, promoting necessary retention of fluid

- Decreased bladder tone due to the effects of progesterone on smooth muscle, and increased capacity
- Dilation of ureters, leading to increased risk of urinary tract infection
- Nocturia, increased urination at night, due to dependent edema resolving while recumbent

Musculoskeletal Changes

Anatomic changes in the musculoskeletal system result from the influence of hormones, growth of the fetus, and maternal weight gain. Round ligaments, which attach to the uterus just under the fallopian tubes and insert in the groin, may cause sharp, shooting lower abdominal and groin pain in early pregnancy as the uterus enlarges. As pregnancy advances, the growing uterus tilts the pelvis forward,

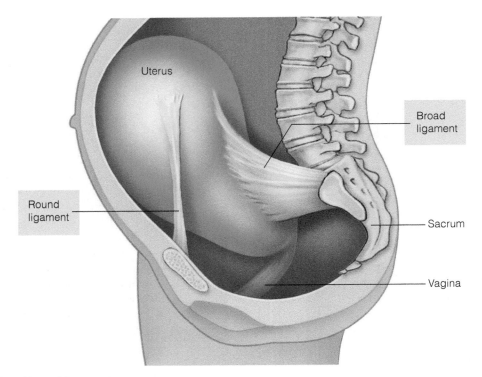

Figure 27.9 Round and broad ligaments.

increasing the lumbosacral curve and creating a gradual lordosis, and the stretching of the broad ligament attaching the uterus to the sacrum may cause back pain (see Figure 27.9 ■). The enlarging breasts pull the shoulders forward, and the patient may assume a stoop-shouldered stance. The pelvic joints and ligaments are relaxed by progesterone and relaxin. The rectus abdominis muscles that run vertically down the midline of the abdomen may separate during the third trimester. This is called **diastasis recti abdominis** and may allow the abdominal contents to protrude (see Figure 27.10 ■). The weight of the uterus and breasts, along with the relaxation of the pelvic joints, changes the patient's center of gravity, stance, and gait. Muscle cramps and ligament injury are more frequent in pregnancy. Shoe size, especially width, may increase permanently.

Neurologic System Changes

Neurologic changes frequently associated with pregnancy include the following:

- Increase in frequency of vascular headaches
- Entrapment neuropathies due to mechanical pressures in the peripheral nervous system
  - Sciatica, pain, numbness, or tingling feeling in the thigh, caused by pressure of the growing uterus on the sciatic nerve
  - Carpal tunnel syndrome, pressure on the median nerve beneath the carpal ligament of the wrist, causing burning, tingling, and pain in the hand

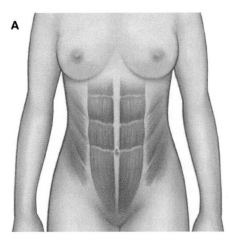

Normal rectus abdominis

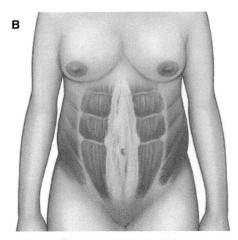

Diastasis recti abdominis

Figure 27.10 Diastasis recti in pregnancy. A. Normal position in nonpregnant female. B. Diastasis recti abdominis in pregnant female.

- Change in the corneal curvature, increased corneal thickness/edema, or change in tear production, causing changes in optical prescription
- Increased total sleep time and insomnia in first and third trimesters
- Leg cramps, which may be caused by inadequate intake of calcium
- Dizziness and light-headedness, which may be associated with supine hypotension syndrome and vasomotor instability

Endocrine System Changes

Changes in the endocrine system facilitate the metabolic functions that maintain maternal and fetal health throughout the pregnancy. Human chorionic gonadotropin (hCG), the hormone that is detected by pregnancy tests, is secreted by tissue surrounding the embryo soon after implantation. It serves as a messenger to the corpus luteum to maintain progesterone and estrogen production until the placenta starts to produce these hormones at approximately 5 weeks. It also may be involved in the suppression of maternal immunologic rejection of the fetal tissue.

The fetus and placenta become additional sites for synthesis and metabolism of hormones. The pituitary, thyroid, parathyroid, and adrenal glands enlarge because of estrogen stimulation and increased vascularity. Increases in the production of thyroid hormones, particularly T_3 and T_4, increase the basal metabolic rate (BMR), cardiac output, vasodilation, heart rate, and heat intolerance. The BMR may increase by eightfold.

Changes also occur in the metabolism of protein, glucose, and fats due to the increasing production of human placental lactogen (hPL) by the placenta. Throughout pregnancy, protein is metabolized more efficiently to meet fetal needs. In the second trimester, insulin production increases in response to the rising glucose levels and falls to nonpregnant levels at the end of pregnancy. In addition, the mother's body tissues develop a decreased sensitivity to insulin, sometimes referred to as the diabetogenic state of pregnancy. This ensures an adequate supply of glucose, which the fetus requires in large amounts. A disruption in this delicate homeostatic balance results in gestational diabetes mellitus (GDM). A form of glucose-sparing called accelerated starvation causes the metabolism of fats stored in pregnancy, which makes more glucose available to the fetus but puts the pregnant female at greater risk of ketosis; ketones are harmful to the fetal brain. Pregnant females are at increased risk of lipolysis during pregnancy secondary to hypoglycemia or prolonged fasting.

After birth, *oxytocin*, secreted by the posterior pituitary, stimulates uterine contractions and causes milk ejection in the mammary glands. Prolactin, secreted by the anterior pituitary, increases production of breast milk after delivery.

Special Considerations

Although pregnancy is considered a healthy state, the mother requires extra care to ensure a healthy pregnancy for both the mother and the infant. Factors such as previous pregnancies and miscarriages, presence of sexually transmitted infections, chronic maternal conditions, and maternal nutrition all contribute to potential complications in pregnancy. In addition, sexually active females who do not want to be pregnant are a growing concern and may require additional education and counseling to help prevent unwanted pregnancies and help the mother adapt emotionally to the realities of pregnancy and childbirth.

Health Promotion Considerations

Several *Healthy People 2020* goals and objectives focus on conception, pregnancy, and maternal and infant health. For example, *Healthy People 2020* desires to increase family planning services for women, including providing contraceptive and reproductive services, education, and counseling. This goal also focuses on providing education about sexually transmitted infections (STIs) and human immunodeficiency virus (HIV), including how to prevent transmission to the newborn. Goals related to the health of the mother, infant, and child include decreasing fetal, infant, and maternal death through decreased use of alcohol, cigarettes, and illicit drugs; decreased transmission of HIV and other infections; and increased prenatal care. See Table 27.1 for examples of *Healthy People 2020* objectives that target pregnancy and maternal and infant health.

Developmental Considerations

Although traditionally most women who are pregnant are between the ages of 20 and 35, an increasing number of younger adolescents (age 19 and under) and older women (age 36 and above) are becoming pregnant.

Adolescent Females

Adolescent pregnancies have declined over the past several decades, but in 2013, over 275,000 babies were born to young women age 19 and under (Hamilton, Martin, Osterman, & Curtin, 2014). Of these adolescent pregnancies, 17 percent were multigravida, and 82 percent were unplanned. For adolescents, teaching about abstinence, safe sex, and contraception are important topics. Once the adolescent has become pregnant, nursing care must include substantial emotional counseling and support in addition to the typical nursing responsibilities. Options for care and support of the infant must be discussed, including who will care for the infant while the mother is in school, who will provide financial support for the infant's needs, the potential role of the baby's father in providing support, and the possibility of giving the baby up for adoption.

Older Women

Because many women are getting married later or choosing to wait to have children, pregnancies in older women have become more common. Although many women over the age of 35 deliver healthy babies, complications are more common in pregnant women of this age group. Women over the age of 35 may take longer to become pregnant, and the use of in vitro fertilization increases the chance of having a multiple pregnancy. Women over the age of 35 are more likely to develop complications such as gestational diabetes and high blood pressure. These conditions can lead to fetal complications such as large-for-gestational-age, placental problems, and infant death due to preeclampsia. Women over the age of 35 may also be at risk for delivering a low-birth-weight baby

TABLE 27.1	Examples of *Healthy People 2020* Objectives Related to the Pregnant Female
OBJECTIVE NUMBER	**DESCRIPTION**
FP-1	Increase the proportion of pregnancies that are intended
FP-2	Reduce the proportion of females experiencing pregnancy despite use of a reversible contraceptive method
FP-8	Reduce pregnancies among adolescent females
FP-9	Increase the proportion of adolescents aged 17 years and under who have never had sexual intercourse
FP-13	Increase the proportion of adolescents who talked to a parent or guardian about reproductive health topics before they were 18 years old
HIV-8	Reduce perinatally acquired HIV and AIDS cases
MICH-1	Reduce the rate of fetal and infant deaths
MICH-5	Reduce the rate of maternal mortality
MICH-6	Reduce maternal illness and complications due to pregnancy (complications during hospitalized labor and delivery)
MICH-7	Reduce cesarean births among low-risk (full-term, singleton, and vertex presentation) women
MICH-8	Reduce low birth weight (LBW) and very low birth weight (VLBW).
MICH-9	Reduce preterm births
MICH-10	Increase the proportion of pregnant women who receive early and adequate prenatal care
MICH-11	Increase abstinence from alcohol, cigarettes, and illicit drugs among pregnant women
MICH-14	Increase the proportion of women of childbearing potential with intake of at least 400 mcg of folic acid from fortified foods or dietary supplements
MICH-21	Increase the proportion of infants who are breastfed
MICH-25	Reduce the occurrence of fetal alcohol syndrome (FAS)
NWS-22	Reduce iron deficiency among pregnant females

Source: U.S. Department of Health and Human Services (USDHHS). (2014). *Healthy people 2020.* Retrieved from http://www.healthypeople.gov/2020/default.aspx.

or delivering prematurely. They are also more likely than younger women to need a C-section, and the risk of pregnancy loss is higher. In addition, older women are at higher risk of giving birth to an infant with chromosomal abnormalities such as Trisomy-21, which causes Down Syndrome (Mayo Clinic, 2014). Therefore, nursing care of older women should include discussions about potential complications associated with age, options for genetic testing, and the importance of testing for gestational diabetes and high blood pressure.

The Postpartum Female

The critical role of the nurse in assisting patients through the maternity cycle continues after the birth with postpartum assessment.

Anatomy and Physiology Review

During the postpartum period, the reproductive organs return to the nonpregnant state through the process of involution.

Immediately after the birth of the placenta, the uterine fundus is located midway between the symphysis pubis and the umbilicus. The fundus rises to the umbilicus by 12 hours later, and decreases approximately 1 cm or fingerbreadth per day until it is nonpalpable externally by 10 days. The contracted uterus is firm, preventing postpartum hemorrhage through ligation of the uterine arteries by the contraction. The uterus is longer and wider in mothers who have a cesarean section and shorter in mothers who breast-feed.

The uterine lining or endometrium returns to the nonpregnant state through the process of a postpartum vaginal discharge called lochia. The initial *lochia rubra* contains blood from the placental site, amniotic membrane, cells from the decidua basalis, vernix and lanugo from the infant's skin, and meconium. It is dark red and has a fleshy odor and lasts anywhere from 2 days to 18 days. Next, the discharge becomes pinkish and is called *lochia serosa*. It is composed of blood, placental site exudates, erythrocytes, leukocytes, cervical mucus, microorganisms, and decidua and lasts approximately a week. Finally, the discharge becomes whitish-yellow, *lochia alba,* and is composed of leukocytes, mucus, bacteria, epithelial cells, and decidua. Most females will have vaginal discharge from 10 days to 5 or 6 weeks.

The cervix closes over the next 2 weeks, and the vagina regains its folds or rugae. Decreased lubrication and lacerations or surgical incisions to the perineum cause discomfort. Hemorrhoids may occur during pregnancy due to increased pelvic pressure or pushing during childbirth. Gastric motility slows during labor and resumes afterward. Bowel movements usually restart after 2 to 3 days postpartum. The urethra may be bruised, swollen, or damaged by childbirth or episiotomy.

The hormones estrogen and progesterone, secreted by the placenta, decrease rapidly after birth. Prolactin, which controls milk production, increases after birth, causing milk production to occur within 2 to 3 days after birth. Oxytocin acts on the smooth muscle of the uterus, causing contractions needed for uterine involution. Oxytocin also stimulates the muscle cells surrounding the breast alveoli, causing them to eject milk into the ducts during breast-feeding. In non–breast-feeding mothers, menses return at 6 to 10 weeks postpartum. In lactating mothers, menses usually do not return for 12 or more weeks; with exclusive breast-feeding and introduction of solid foods after 6 months, amenorrhea may last a year or more. Eighty percent of first menses in lactating mothers are preceded by anovulatory cycles due to the action of prolactin. These hormonal swings, combined with role changes and exhaustion, contribute to emotional fragility, expressed as "baby blues."

After birth, the non–breast-feeding mother will experience breast engorgement when the transitional milk starts to be produced by days 2 to 3 and is not emptied by a suckling baby. The breast-feeding mother who puts the baby to breast soon after birth will first secrete colostrum, which is higher in protein and immunoglobulin and lower in fat and carbohydrate than the transitional milk that will start to be secreted by days 2 to 3. Mature milk will be produced by about 2 weeks postpartum. Breast-feeding mothers who exclusively breast-feed frequently as demanded by their infants should not experience breast engorgement.

In the circulatory system, it may take up to 6 weeks for slowed blood velocity and relaxed veins to return to the nonpregnant state, so a risk of thromboembolism remains during the postpartum period. In the renal system, diuresis occurs on days 2 to 5, and decreased bladder tone and urinary retention can be worsened by birth trauma.

The BUBBLESHE Head-to-Toe Postpartum Assessment

With all the physiologic changes occurring in the postpartum period, a thorough postpartum assessment plays an important role in health care. The mnemonic BUBBLESHE can be used to remember the steps in assessing a postpartum patient.

B   Breast
U   Uterus
B   Bowel
B   Bladder
L   Lochia
E   Episiotomy/perineum
S   Support system
H   Homans' sign and extremities
E   Emotional state

In preparation for the postpartum assessment, the nurse gathers the following supplies: lab coat, stethoscope, black ink pen, and penlight. Prior to entering the room, it is important to review the data needed to fill out the assessment flow sheet (data on pain, urinary tract infection [UTI] symptoms, voiding, stooling, flatus, bleeding, support system, bonding, etc.) as well as the physical assessment. Establishing a good rapport with the patient is important, along with the physical assessment. The nurse should project caring and confidence and use eye contact.

Throughout all aspects of the assessment, the nurse must be sure to maintain the patient's privacy and dignity.

Assess the vital signs, and auscultate the lungs, the heart, and the abdomen. Inspect the IV/saline lock site. Examine the patient's breasts, palpate for costovertebral angle tenderness, and palpate the fundus to determine the height and firmness. Assess the surgical incision for the woman who delivered by cesarean section.

Inspect the lower extremities for vascular changes, perform the Homans' test, and assess for edema. Place the patient in a lateral position to inspect the perineum for an episiotomy and the rectum for any tears. The acronym REEDA (redness, ecchymosis, edema, discharge, and approximation) is useful for assessing wound healing or the presence of inflammation or infection.

Psychosocial Considerations

A female's adaptation to pregnancy will depend heavily on their development within a social environment. For many females, the support of a boyfriend, husband, or other family member is essential to their ability to cope with the physical and emotional changes they are experiencing. This support system is especially important for females who undergo postpartum depression. The pregnant female's socioeconomic status also contributes to their health during pregnancy, because mothers without access to regular health care during pregnancy will not have adequate care if complications occur before, during, or after birth.

Cultural and Environmental Considerations

At the time of pregnancy and birth, females in all stages of acculturation to the mainstream culture will hear the call of their roots. Culturally competent nurses will know specifics about individual cultural groups, not to stereotype patients but to gain a perspective on what issues might pertain to the individual. Table 27.2 summarizes beliefs about pregnancy, childbirth, the postpartum period, and the newborn for cultural, racial, and ethnic groups. Sources of diversity within groups include timing of immigration, urban or rural origin, socioeconomic status, educational level, religion, strength of ethnic identity, family style, and personal characteristics.

TABLE 27.2	Cultural Beliefs and Childbearing		
CULTURE (U.S. POPULATION, 2010)	**PREGNANCY**	**BIRTH**	**POSTPARTUM/ NEWBORN**
African Americans (42.0 million)	Pregnancy is respected and highly valued; pica occasionally occurs; late entry to care seen in teen and low socioeconomic groups.	Usually in the hospital; typically presents late in labor with father of baby (FOB) and female relatives; FOB usually unlikely to provide labor support spontaneously.	Rest encouraged; female relative, especially maternal grandmother, will stay with new mother; herbal teas used; avoidance of drafts practiced; breast-feeding uncommon; mothers are typically caregivers. May refuse a bath or shower until bleeding stops.
Native Americans (5.2 million)	High birth rate; pregnancy is sacred period with traditional rituals and taboos such as avoiding negative thoughts, dead animals, inactivity; pregnancy seen as normal process that does not require medical intervention; also entry to care problems related to transportation and health problems; smoking, fetal alcohol syndrome, and diabetes significant problems.	Usually in hospital, occasionally birth center; medicine person may be called upon to assist; certified nurse-midwives attend many deliveries with emphasis on active participation; placenta and umbilical cord may be saved for burial. Stoicism is encouraged for labor pains. Father may perform certain rituals and be absent following birth.	Lying-in period observed in some tribes; acculturation decreasing use of such traditional practices as mothering helper after birth; infants wrapped tightly in blankets or cradleboards; amulets or juniper bracelets to provide protection to infant may be used. Umbilical cord often saved for spiritual ritual.
Arab Americans (1.5 million)	Chastity until marriage highly valued and enforced; pregnancy brings increased social status; strenuous activity is avoided; strong emotions believed to hurt pregnancy; cravings are satisfied; care sought for confirmation of pregnancy and problems but not preventive care.	Husband does not participate in labor support but is close by; female relatives provide labor support; a rug to bite on may be used for pain, and herbal drinks offered; vocalization and prayers allowed; placenta considered part of human remains and burial preferred.	A 40-day lying-in period observed; postpartal females considered impure and no sexual intercourse while bleeding; may fear bathing or showering; strenuous activity and drafts avoided; breast-feeding for 2 years common, but some may believe colostrum is harmful; special foods encouraged including fresh goat's milk, candied sesame seed butter, and chicken soup; infant wrapped with cotton umbilical band and massaged with olive oil; amulet pouches pinned to clothing.
Central Americans (4.0 million)	Pregnant females given attention; avoidance of cool air, "hot" foods, strong emotions, and moonlight recommended in some Latin cultures.	Loud vocalization of pain common; pregnant woman's mother and female relatives often present for birth; fathers usually passive.	*La cuarenta*, a 40-day lying-in period, may be observed; "cold" foods, drafts, strong emotional states avoided; foods offered may include chicken soup, bananas, and meat; herbal teas and baths may be used for mother and child; public breast-feeding accepted.
Chinese (4.0 million)	Good nutrition, activity restriction, and positive thought during pregnancy recommended; iron supplements believed to harden bones and complicate delivery; may use ginseng in third trimester; prenatal care expected and practiced.	Father and family members may wait outside delivery room; mothers may be reluctant to vocalize pain or ask for pain medication because silence is believed to protect the baby from evil spirits.	One-month postpartum period observed; goal of decreasing yin or cold air through consumption of "hot" foods such as ginger, chicken soup, eggs, fish, pork recommended; rice wine avoided for 2 weeks; no going outdoors and windows are kept closed; bathing or showering is often forbidden in the first 30 days; grandmothers provide support and advice. Breast-feeding is encouraged, but colostrum is considered "dirty."
Colombians (908,734)	Usual activities and diet maintained until term; some believe fright should be avoided and cravings satisfied.	Females may eat and drink little during labor due to fear of vomiting; family members not expected to be present at delivery; analgesia welcome but not expected by low-income women.	*Quarentena* for 40 days observed; if women go outside, may cover ears with cotton; breast-feeding common, but not usually over a year; amulets against evil eye such as bead bracelet may be used.

TABLE 27.2   Cultural Beliefs and Childbearing (continued)

CULTURE (U.S. POPULATION, 2010)	PREGNANCY	BIRTH	POSTPARTUM/ NEWBORN
Cubans (1.8 million)	Avoidance of loud noises, strenuous activities, and people with deformities recommended; fresh fruit and low-salt foods recommended. May be fearful of evil eye or strangers touching their belly.	Pregnant woman's mother present; acculturated fathers may participate; prefer physician provider; pain expressed loudly.	Mother and infant housebound for 41 days; pregnant woman's mother and sisters provide care; new mother protected from stress. Baby may be dressed in red to prevent effects from evil eye. Breast-feeding is common.
Filipinos (3.4 million)	Pampering pregnant females is a social value; prolonged sitting or sleeping discouraged; sexual intercourse taboo during last 2 months of pregnancy; in late pregnancy, "slippery" foods such as fresh eggs encouraged for easier birth. Jewelry, especially necklaces, are prohibited during pregnancy.	Traditionally, fathers not present; pregnant women encouraged to be assertive and vocal during labor; traditional placental burial not usually practiced in U.S. hospitals. Foot massages are encouraged to relieve pain.	Bathing and activity are restricted in the postpartum period of 10 days; breast-feeding, sometimes to toddlerhood, is common; pelvic binder may be used for 6 weeks; cold drinks and cold drafts avoided; *hilot* may provide massage and perineal hygiene; religious medals or tiger tooth pendant may be pinned to infant's clothing.
Koreans (1.7 million)	Seaweed soup is popular pregnancy food, but many foods are forbidden, including duck, eggs, crab, and rabbit; rest promoted. May prefer same-sex medical providers.	Traditionally stoic, Koreans in North America are more vocal in modern times; fathers traditionally not present; only warm food and water consumed; no ice chips should be given.	Exposure to cold and water avoided in postpartum period of 3 to 8 weeks; perineal ice packs may be refused; strong preference for sons; infant's whole body covered to prevent exposure to cold air. Mother may consume a seaweed soup daily.
Mexicans (31.8 million)	Moderate activity is encouraged; medications including iron and vitamins may be avoided. Excellent self-care promoted, including exercise; rest; good nutrition; and avoidance of smoking, drugs, and alcohol. Grandmothers and female relatives provide domestic support in late pregnancy.	Loud verbal repetition of "aye, yie, yie" used for pain relief; ambulation recommended; fathers present at birth but do not provide labor support.	*La cuarentena*, a 40-day lying-in period, observed; new mothers discouraged from getting out of bed for several hours after birth; showers discouraged for several days; breast-feeding common; chiles and beans avoided; herbal teas offered to infant; admiring infant without touching puts infant at risk of evil eye.
Puerto Ricans (4.6 million)	Pregnant females indulged; cravings and morning sickness common; some females refrain from sexual activity in the second and third trimesters; extended family may be involved in prenatal care.	Hygiene and modesty valued in labor; extended family present in labor.	During the *cuarentena*, family assists mother; hair not washed during this period; chicken broths and other soups offered to mother; bottle-feeding more common; beans, eggs, and starches avoided during breast-feeding; amulet neck chain may be worn by infant.
South Asian Indians (3.2 million)	Pregnancy is healthy state; heavy lifting and shock proscribed; grandmothers important source of advice; Ayurvedic practitioners consume "cold" foods such as milk products, fruits, and vegetables; pregnant woman may return to her mother's home at end of pregnancy; medicinal oils and massage may be given to pregnant women; Hindus have a special ritual for pregnant women in third trimester.	Light eating advised during labor; traditionally fathers not involved in birthing process; sex of child not told to mother until after placenta delivers; ambulation encouraged in early labor; afterbirth burial traditions not usually observed in North America; Muslim male relatives recite words in right and left ear of newborn to confirm child is Muslim.	A lying-in period of 40 to 56 days is observed; special cooling dishes provided to new mother using ingredients such as herbs and clarified butter; birth celebration party may be held; infant charms may be worn to ward off evil eye; massage for mother and child may be provided; breast-feeding for 6 months to 2 years encouraged.

(continued)

TABLE 27.2　Cultural Beliefs and Childbearing (continued)

CULTURE (U.S. POPULATION, 2010)	PREGNANCY	BIRTH	POSTPARTUM/ NEWBORN
Vietnamese (1.7 million)	A regimen of "cold" and "hot," and "tonic" and "wind" foods is recommended during pregnancy; sexual intercourse taboo; male personnel may intimidate females in prenatal care.	Father not traditionally present at birth; female relatives provide support; laboring females stoic; natural childbirth preferred, but anesthesia accepted.	Recuperation period is 3 months; mothers do not take full shower for 1 to 3 months; hot, salty towels may be applied to vaginal area; breast-feeding common for up to 1 year, with "cold" or "windy" foods avoided; the newborn should not be given compliments due to fear of evil spirits; the head of the newborn should not be touched.
Japanese (1.3 million)	A nutritious diet is followed; the mother is encouraged to seek early prenatal care. Prenatal care is given by both midwives and OB doctors. Positive thinking and music are encouraged.	Mothers are encouraged to consume foods rich in protein and carbohydrates during labor. Only quiet expressions of pain are acceptable; loud expressions of pain are considered shameful. Father's role during birth may vary; instead, female family members and health professionals provide care and support.	Breast-feeding is encouraged but starts the day after birth. Special foods recommended include carp fish soup, mochi, miso, spinach, and other green vegetables. Mothers and babies are not to leave home for 2–4 weeks. A special naming ceremony is performed when the baby is 7 days old (called "oshichia"); only close family and friends attend. A ritual called "Hesono O" is performed in which the baby's umbilical cord is placed in a wooden box and kept to signify hopes for a good mother–child relationship.
Native Hawaiian and other Pacific Islanders (1.2 million)	Prenatal care is accepted; may prefer to use traditional or natural medicines.	The father is involved in the childbirth process; female family members are also present for support. Mothers may want to walk or swim to speed up the labor process. C-sections are not preferred.	Family may request umbilical cord and/or placenta because of spiritual value. Rest is encouraged. Breast-feeding is encouraged, but bottle-feeding is acceptable. Mothers may avoid green vegetables and other foods that are believed to contribute to colic.
Dominicans (1.4 million)	Pregnancy is considered a normal life process, and the entire family is involved. Mothers are often afraid to share traditional practices that are being used and are afraid to disagree with advice from the healthcare professional. Due to fear of deportation, health care is often sought late in pregnancy. Baby could be lost if mother's cravings are not satisfied.	C-sections may be popular, as vaginal birth carries a high sense of fear.	The mother should have a 40-day postpartum rest period (cuarentena); the mother and baby should not be outside, as this protects the baby from viruses and the evil eye; mothers should not use chemicals. Breastfeeding is encouraged, mother may eat salt fish to increase milk production. Baby is dressed in a cross-shaped band (faja) and a talisman (azabache) to ward off evil spirits. Babies may be given special spices to help them sleep; a moist piece of cloth or mother's hair can be stuck to the baby's forehead to help stop hiccups.

Sources: Adapted from St. Hill, P., Lipson, J. G., & Meleis, A. I. (2003). Caring for women cross-culturally. Philadelphia: F.A. Davis; Lipson, J. G., Dibble, S. L., & Minarik, P. A. (1996). Culture & nursing care. San Francisco: UCSF Nursing Press; U.S. Census Bureau. (2010). 2010 Census Briefs. Retrieved from http://www.census.gov/2010census/data/; Hawaii Community College. (n.d.). Japanese culture: Beliefs and practices during pregnancy, birth, and postpregnancy. Retrieved from http://www.hawcc.hawaii.edu/nursing/RNJapanese03.html; Health Care Chaplaincy. (2013). Handbook of patients' spiritual and cultural values for health care professionals. Retrieved from http://www.healthcarechaplaincy.org/userimages/Cultural%20Sensitivity%20handbook%20from%20HealthCare%20Chaplaincy%20%20(3-12%202013).pdf; The Bronx Health Link. (2011). Pregnancy, childbirth, and baby care across cultures: Understanding, respecting, and serving immigrants in the Bronx. 2011 Annual Forum. Retrieved from http://www.bronxhealthlink.org/tbhl/education/pregnancy_childbirth_and_baby_care:en-us.pdf; and McHale, C. (n.d.). Pregnancy, birth, and neonatal care practices in the Dominican Republic and Haiti. Retrieved from http://delivery-child-birth.knoji.com/pregnancy-birth-and-neonatal-care-practices-in-the-dominican-republic-haiti/.

Gathering the Data

The role of the nurse in assessment of the pregnant female includes collecting subjective data from the focused interview. Objective data are obtained from the physical assessment. Objective data are also obtained from secondary sources such as health records, the results of laboratory tests, and radiologic and ultrasound studies. Preparation includes gathering equipment, positioning, and informing the patient about the physical assessment.

Focused Interview

At the first prenatal visit, a very thorough interview is conducted. Important information that may dramatically affect the health of the fetus and mother can be obtained; the quality of the relationship with the patient for the entire pregnancy is begun. The environment for the interview should be comfortable, quiet, private, and relaxing.

For the purposes of identification, statistics, billing, and record keeping, collect the demographic information listed in Box 27.1 for each pregnant patient. For discussion of cultural considerations related to the patient interview, see chapter 4. ∞

Box 27.1 Demographic Information

- Complete name and nickname (knowing a nickname helps during stressful situations such as labor).
- Address
- Date of birth (screens for age-related complications)
- Race or ethnicity (screens for race/ethnicity-related genetic disorders)
- Occupation, hours worked per week, activities at work (screens for occupational hazards to the mother and fetus)
- Marital or relationship status (patient's support system)

- Baby's father's name (patient's support system)
- Partner's name, if that is a different person (patient's support system)
- Emergency contact and their phone number
- People residing in same residence as patient (patient's support system)
- Religion (relates to maternity care, such as attitudes toward blood products)
- Number of years of school completed (assists in the development of the teaching plan)

Focused Interview Questions

Rationales and Evidence

The following sections provide sample questions for each of the categories identified above. A rationale and evidence for each of the questions is provided. The list of questions is not comprehensive but represents the type of questions required in a comprehensive prenatal focused interview.

Questions Related to Confirmation of Pregnancy

Prior to the provision of a prenatal interview and physical assessment, it must be ensured that the patient is indeed pregnant. Pregnancy can be determined through urine and serum pregnancy tests as well as signs and symptoms of pregnancy.

Urine pregnancy tests test for the beta subunit of hCG and can be accurate 7 days after implantation, or can indicate pregnancy before the missed menstrual period. These tests produce results in 1 to 5 minutes and are 99% accurate. Serum pregnancy tests may indicate pregnancy as soon as 7 to 9 days after ovulation, or just after implantation. This test can be qualitative, with a value of positive or negative, or quantitative, with a level of hCG reported. Serum progesterone can also be obtained if necessary; nonviable pregnancies have lower levels than normal pregnancies.

Presumptive signs of pregnancy are symptoms the patient reports that may have multiple causes other than pregnancy. These presumptive signs include amenorrhea; breast tenderness; nausea and vomiting; frequent urination; quickening; or the patient's perception of fetal movement, skin changes, and fatigue. Probable signs are elicited by the nurse and have few causes other than pregnancy. Probable signs include positive pregnancy test, abdominal enlargement, Piskacek's sign, Hegar's sign, Goodell's sign, Chadwick's sign, and Braxton-Hicks contractions. Positive signs of pregnancy have no possible explanation other than pregnancy. These include hearing the fetal heart with Doppler, fetoscope, or ultrasound; fetal movements verified by the examiner; and visualization of the fetus via ultrasound or radiology.

Focused Interview Questions	Rationales and Evidence

Questions Related to Menstrual History

1. **When was the date of your last menstrual period?**

▶ The estimated date of birth (EDB), also known as the estimated date of delivery (EDD), estimated date of confinement (EDC), or due date, is usually calculated by using the first day of the last menstrual period (LMP), which may also be useful in estimating gestational age (American Pregnancy Association [APA], 2007).

2. **Do you know the date you ovulated?**

▶ This can help determine due date.

3. **Do you know the date you conceived?**

▶ This also can assist in dating the pregnancy.

4. **Were you using any methods of contraception at the time you conceived?**

▶ Although oral contraceptive pills have not shown any adverse effects on pregnancy, their use does affect the timing of ovulation. An intrauterine device (IUD) in place at the time of conception can cause complications in the pregnancy (Kim et al., 2010).

5. **Describe your usual menstrual cycle.**

▶ The typical menstrual cycle is 28 days in length. Prolonged, shortened, or irregular menstrual cycles affect the EDB. If the LMP was not normal for the patient, it may have been implantation bleeding or a menstrual dysfunction. Some prenatal charts ask for last NORMAL menstrual period (LNMP) to assist in dating the pregnancy.

6. **Have you had any cramping, bleeding, or spotting since your LMP?**

▶ Cramping, bleeding, or spotting may indicate a problem with hormonal support of the endometrium and may lead to a spontaneous abortion (Ladewig, London, & Davidson, 2014).

7. **How old were you when you got your first menstrual period?**

▶ The number of years since **menarche**, or age of the first menstrual period, helps determine physical maturity of the patient.

Calculating Estimated Date of Birth and Gestational Weeks

A pregnancy lasts approximately 266 days from conception, or 280 days from the LMP, based on a 28-day cycle. **Nägele's rule** can be used to compute the EDB based on the LMP (Box 27.2). To use this approximate guide to determine the due date, 7 days are added to the day of the month of the first day of the LMP, 3 is subtracted from the number of the month (12 is added to the month number if the LMP occurs in January, February, or March), and the year of the due date is the year of the LMP, plus 1 year if January 1 is passed during the pregnancy.

A gestational wheel is a two-layer round computational device, usually made of laminated paper, that can also be used to compute the EDB and weeks of gestation. Each day of the month in the year has a line on the outer wheel, and each day of the week of the pregnancy has a line on the inner wheel. Zero weeks and days indicate the LMP, and exactly 40 weeks indicates the EDB on the inner wheel. If the zero or LMP line on the inner wheel is aligned with the date of the LMP on the outer wheel, the EDB can be found by determining which date lines up with exactly 40 weeks. If the LMP or EDB is correctly lined up with its date on the outer wheel, the current date on the outer wheel will line up with the gestational age (e.g., 36 weeks and 4 days, often recorded as 36.4 or 36 4/7, based on a 7-day week).

| **Focused Interview Questions** | **Rationales and Evidence** |

Box 27.2 Using Nägele's Rule to Compute an Estimated Date of Birth (EDB)

EXAMPLE: LMP = January 29, 2015
Rule = first day of LMP + 7, number of month − 3 (year of LMP + 1 if January 1 is passed during pregnancy)

Jan 29
   30   Day 1   Month Dec = 12th month
   31   2   Jan = 13 (if LMP is in January, February, or March, add 12 to month to
                            prevent negative number)
Feb 1   3   Feb = 14
    2   4   14 − 3 = 11 = November
    3   5
    4   6
    5   7
Due date = November 5, 2015

The third way that the EDB can be determined is through the use of ultrasound ("sonograms") in the first half of pregnancy. The EDB should be shared as soon as it is determined with the patient, along with its degree of certainty. The fact that a due date actually is the middle day of a month straddling the due date by 2 weeks on each side should be emphasized (+/− 2 weeks of the date determined).

Obstetric and Gynecologic History

1. **Have you experienced any discomfort or unusual occurrences since your LMP?**

▶ The patient's response allows the nurse to evaluate whether the symptoms reported are expected or if they suggest development of a complication. The patient will most likely report subjective signs of pregnancy, such as absence of menstrual periods, nausea, vomiting, breast tenderness, fatigue, abdominal enlargement, or urinary frequency. Patient teaching and other nursing interventions can also be identified.

Questions Related to Reaction to Pregnancy

1. **Was this pregnancy planned?**

▶ Confirmation of pregnancy usually causes ambivalent feelings whether or not the pregnancy was planned. If the pregnancy was unplanned, the nurse needs to assess the mother's desire to maintain the pregnancy and explain available options (Ladewig et al., 2014).

2. **How do you feel about this pregnancy? How does your family and partner [if applicable] feel about the pregnancy?**

▶ This discussion can strengthen the relationship between the nurse and the patient and provide important cues to the home environment of the patient.

Questions Related to Past Obstetric History

1. **Have you been pregnant before? If so, how many times?**

▶ Multiparity, especially if there have been more than three previous pregnancies, increases the maternal risks of antepartal and postpartal hemorrhage and fetal/neonatal anemia (London et al., 2014). Teaching needs are also affected by the patient's previous experiences.

Focused Interview Questions	Rationales and Evidence
2. Have you had any spontaneous or induced abortions? • If so, how far along in weeks were you? • Did you have any follow-up such as a D&C (dilation and curettage procedure)?	► Previous history of persistent spontaneous abortion (miscarriage or stillbirth) places the patient at higher risk for subsequent spontaneous abortions (London et al., 2014). Induced abortions may cause trauma to the cervix and may interfere with cervical dilation and effacement during labor (Ladewig et al., 2014).
3. Describe any previous pregnancies, including the length of the pregnancy, the length of labor, problems during pregnancy, medications taken during pregnancy, prenatal care received, type of birth, and your perception of the experience.	► Discussion of the patient's previous pregnancies helps the nurse anticipate needs and complications of the current pregnancy.
4. Describe your birth experience, including labor or delivery complications, the infant's condition at birth, the infant's weight, and whether the infant required additional treatment or special care after birth.	► Reviewing the patient's previous birth experience(s) helps to anticipate needs and complications of the current pregnancy and to assess the patient's current knowledge base and the success with which the patient integrated the previous birth experience into her life experiences. An example of a previous complication that would impact the current pregnancy is group B streptococcus (GBS) colonization. If a patient has a history of GBS colonization of the vagina in a previous pregnancy, her baby has a risk for early-onset infection that has serious morbidity and mortality, so she will need to be treated in labor with antibiotics (Davidson, London, & Ladewig, 2012).
5. Do you attend or plan to attend prenatal education classes?	► Assessment of prenatal education provides information on the patient's current knowledge base and attitude toward education for self-care.
6. What are your expectations for this pregnancy?	► Identification of the patient's desires helps the nurse provide guidance in formulating the birth plan in the present pregnancy.

Questions Related to Past Gynecologic History

1. When was your most recent Pap smear and what was the result?	► Abnormal Pap smears must be followed up during pregnancy as at any time.
2. At what age did you become sexually active?	► This influences risk for certain conditions.
3. What is your current number of sexual partners?	► This addresses risk for sexually transmitted infections.
4. How would you describe your sexual orientation: heterosexual, bisexual, or lesbian?	► This addresses risk for sexually transmitted infections.
5. What types of safer sex methods do you use and how often do you use them?	► This determines how much teaching in this area is required.
6. What methods of birth control have you used in the past? How satisfied were you with each method?	► This will influence teaching on this topic later in the pregnancy.
7. Have you ever had a sexually transmitted disease (STD)? • What was the treatment? • Were your partners treated and notified?	► Untreated STDs can cause complications in pregnancy (Davidson et al., 2012).

Focused Interview Questions	Rationales and Evidence
8. Were you exposed to diethylstibestrol (DES) while your mother was pregnant with you?	▶ Females with exposure to DES, given from the 1940s to 1970s to prevent miscarriage, may have uterine anomalies (CDC, n.d.).
9. Have you had any problems with or surgeries on your breasts, vagina, fallopian tubes, ovaries, or urinary tract?	▶ Problems in the genitourinary system may impact pregnancy. Fibroids will affect the measurement of fundal height during pregnancy (Davidson et al., 2012). Some types of vaginitis, particularly bacterial vaginosis, can cause preterm labor (Ladewig et al., 2014). Surgery on the breasts may impact the ability to breast-feed.
10. Have you ever been raped? Did you receive any care afterward?	▶ A history of sexual abuse is linked to complications in pregnancy and may influence a patient's psychologic adaptation to pregnancy (Ladewig et al., 2014).
11. Do you have a history of infertility?	▶ Many causes of previous infertility can impact the current pregnancy. For example, pelvic inflammatory disease increases a patient's risk of an ectopic pregnancy (Davidson et al., 2012).

Questions Related to Past Medical/Surgical History and Family History

1. Have you or any members of your family or your partner's family had any of the following conditions:	▶ The nurse needs to assess the family medical history to identify and investigate risk factors thoroughly. ▶ Preexisting maternal conditions may increase maternal and fetal risk. ▶ Previous corrective surgery may impact the course and/or outcome of the pregnancy.
• Hypertension	▶ Mild-to-moderate hypertension poses the risk of intrauterine growth restriction (IUGR) and fetal death (Davidson et al., 2012). When combined with smoking, there is an increased risk of placental abruption, when the placenta shears off the uterus, which is highly dangerous to mother and child (London et al., 2014).
• Heart disease/congenital heart disease	▶ More women with congenital heart disease are surviving into childbearing age, thus adding cardiac risk to their pregnancy (Davidson et al., 2012).
• Asthma	▶ The nurse should ask if asthma is well controlled and how stable medication levels have been, and note which medications are currently being used. Asthma can cause fetal growth restriction and may necessitate serial ultrasounds to follow growth in the intrapartum period (London et al., 2014). Meperidine and morphine for pain relief, and prostaglandin $F_{2\alpha}$ to control postpartum hemorrhage, are not recommended for use by patients with asthma (Davidson et al., 2012).

Focused Interview Questions	Rationales and Evidence
• Kidney or gallbladder problems	▶ Previous occurrences of urinary tract infection may increase risk for asymptomatic bacteriuria, the presence of bacteria in the urine without the usual cystitis symptoms of urinary frequency, burning upon urination, and flank pain. Asymptomatic bacteriuria may lead to pyelonephritis (kidney infection) (Davidson et al., 2012). UTIs in pregnancy are associated with preterm labor and low birth weight (Ladewig et al., 2014). Gallbladder problems may be exacerbated in pregnancy.
• Diabetes mellitus	▶ Pregestational diabetes (diabetes that was present before the pregnancy) is associated with fetal anomalies and pregnancy loss (London et al., 2014).
• Blood or bleeding disorders	▶ Blood disorders such as anemia are associated with UTIs, preterm delivery, low birth weight, preeclampsia, and perinatal mortality (London et al., 2014). Females with sickle cell anemia and thalassemia have an increase in maternal and perinatal mortality and morbidity. If the patient has sickle cell trait, she may have an increase in UTIs and iron and folate deficiency anemia. Monitor female patients with thalassemia minor for anemia; females with thalassemia major are often infertile (Davidson et al., 2012).
• Hepatitis	▶ If a pregnant patient has a past history of hepatitis B and is part of the 6% to 10% who go on to become carriers, there is a risk of transmission to the newborn as well as to her sexual partners. The infant should receive hepatitis B immunoglobulin as well as the hepatitis B virus (HBV) vaccine (Davidson et al., 2012).
• Cancer	▶ If cancer of the cervix was treated with cone biopsy, the patient is at risk for preterm labor (Davidson et al., 2012).
• Infectious diseases such as HIV	▶ HIV transmission to the newborn can be dramatically reduced by treatment in pregnancy (Ladewig et al., 2014).
• Tuberculosis (TB)	▶ TB treatment in pregnancy decreases neonatal mortality and morbidity (CDC, 2012).
• Chickenpox	▶ If the patient does not report a history of varicella (chickenpox) and is not immune by blood test, she is susceptible to infection during pregnancy. Chickenpox, or varicella, can cause abnormalities in the fetus if contracted between 8 and 20 weeks in pregnancy (Mayo Clinic, 2012a). Varicella-zoster immune globulin can be given to exposed mothers and infants but not to pregnant women (CDC, 2011).
• Allergies	▶ Allergies are identified in the prenatal period in the case that medications are recommended during the perinatal period. The nurse should note the type of reaction.
2. **What medications have you taken since your LMP?**	▶ This will help identify any teratogenic exposures as well as medications for illnesses and symptoms. Drugs in pregnancy are rated in risk categories A, B, C, D, and X (Box 27.3).

| Focused Interview Questions | Rationales and Evidence |

Box 27.3 Drugs in Pregnancy: Risk Categories

A: Adequate and well-controlled studies in pregnant women have not shown an increased risk of fetal abnormalities. Example drugs: folic acid, levothyroxine.

B: Animal studies have revealed no evidence of harm to the fetus; however, there are no adequate and well-controlled studies in pregnant women, or animal studies have shown an adverse effect, but adequate and well-controlled studies in pregnant women have failed to demonstrate a risk to the fetus. Example drugs: acetaminophen, chlorpheniramine, pseudoephedrine, loperamide, aluminum hydroxide/magnesium hydroxide, amoxicillin, ondansetron, metformin, insulin.

C: Animal studies have shown an adverse effect and there are no adequate and well-controlled studies in pregnant women, or no animal studies have been conducted and there are no adequate and well-controlled studies in pregnant women. Example drugs: guaifenesin, dextromethorphan, calcium carbonate, fluconazole, albuterol, sertraline, fluoxetine.

D: Adequate well-controlled or observational studies in pregnant women have demonstrated a risk to the fetus. However, the benefits of therapy may outweigh the potential risk. Example drugs: aspirin, paroxetine, lithium, phenytoin.

X: Adequate well-controlled or observational studies in animals or pregnant women have demonstrated positive evidence of fetal abnormalities. The use of the product is contraindicated in women who are or who may become pregnant. Example drugs: isotretinoin, thalidomide.

3. **Have you ever had a blood transfusion?**

▶ This will help identify increased risk for abnormal antibody reactions or bloodborne pathogens.

4. **What infections and immunizations have you had?**

▶ Some infections, including chicken pox and rubella, can cause birth defects (Ladewig et al., 2014). If the patient has hepatitis B, her newborn may need hepatitis B immunoglobulin and vaccine after birth (Davidson et al., 2012). Prior immunizations and exposures affect the patient's risk for contracting certain infections during pregnancy.

5. **Have you had any surgeries such as:**
   • Breast reduction/enhancement

▶ Breast-feeding is usually possible following pedicle reduction surgery (Cruz & Korchin, 2007); however, the amount of milk produced may be lower. Women who have undergone this surgery will need encouragement and be observed for physiologic engorgement and milk production (Lawrence & Lawrence, 2011). Women who have had reduction surgery through the free nipple technique may not be able to breast-feed because the ducts have been disrupted. Breast augmentation carries a risk of lactation failure (Cruz & Korchin, 2010).

   • Back

▶ Thoracic or lumbar spinal surgery that has scarred, distorted, or obliterated the epidural space will not allow the use of an epidural for either analgesia or anesthesia.

   • Hip

▶ Hip surgery may impact the ability of the patient to use stirrups in the lithotomy position.

Focused Interview Questions	Rationales and Evidence
• Bariatric	▶ Bariatric surgery is either restrictive or restrictive/malabsorptive. This can cause nutritional deficiencies (ACOG, 2013). These women will still need to consume about 1,500 calories each day, necessitating dietary counseling. These women also need to be checked regularly for nutrient deficiencies, particularly folic acid, calcium, iron, and vitamin B_{12}. There is a trend for increased risk of small-for-gestational-age infants. Previous bariatric surgery is not an indication for delivery via cesarean section (Kominiarek, 2011).
• Uterine	▶ Previous uterine surgery may dictate delivery via cesarean section without labor (Landon & Lynch, 2011).
• Other prior surgeries?	▶ Any previous surgeries should be discussed in regard to the impact they may have on pregnancy and subsequent delivery.
6. **Review of systems questions: For each body system, the nurse should discuss benign as well as worrisome changes in pregnancy. For example: Describe any changes you have experienced regarding your skin, digestion, bowel function, muscles and joints, or vision.**	▶ This discussion will ensure that the pregnant patient recalls each system and provides an important teaching opportunity.

Questions Related to Genetic Information

In order to obtain information to determine genetic risk factors, the nurse will ask the patient about three generations of her family. This is called a *medical family tree* or *genetic pedigree*. These questions refer to her brothers and sisters, her mother and father, her aunts and uncles on both sides, her grandparents and their siblings, all of her children, and all of her cousins on both sides. This information is also needed for the baby's father's family.

1. **Please tell me the date of birth and, if applicable, death as well as any health problems or diseases for each of these individuals. For those who have died, tell me what the cause was and date of death.**	▶ Three generations of medical history are needed to determine recessive as well as dominant genetic diseases (London et al., 2014).
2. **Do you or the baby's father, or anybody in your families, have any of the following conditions:** • Sickle cell anemia or trait • Thalassemia • Down syndrome • Cystic fibrosis • Huntington's disease • Muscular dystrophy • Tay-Sachs • Hemophilia • Any other blood or genetic disorders	▶ Sometimes charting the medical family tree will not jog the memory of the patient, but a specific mention of the condition will. ▶ Tay-Sachs occurs more frequently in Ashkenazi Jews, cystic fibrosis trait occurs in 1 in 29 northern European Caucasians, and the sickle cell trait occurs in 1 in 8 African Americans (see Table 27.3).
3. **What is your ethnic background?**	

Questions Related to Lifestyle and Social Health Practices

1. **How much do you smoke per day? Does anyone in your household smoke?**	▶ Smoking doubles the risk of a low-birth-weight baby and increases the risk of ectopic pregnancy or placental complications. It also increases the infant's risk of sudden infant death syndrome (SIDS), asthma, and autism after birth. Secondhand smoke exposure also may contribute to low birth weight (Ladewig et al., 2014).

TABLE 27.3 Genetic Disorders and Traits with Increased Frequency by Ethnicity

ETHNIC DESCENT/ GEOGRAPHIC LOCATION	GENETIC DISORDERS AND TRAITS WITH INCREASED FREQUENCY
Africans	Sickle cell anemia Alpha- and beta-thalassemia G6PD Fy (Duffy) antigen Rh positive Arcus corneae Café au lait spots Clubbing of digits Polydactyly Vitiligo Abnormal separation of sutures Earlobe absent Keloid Hereditary hypertrophic osteoarthropathy Scaphocephaly Alpha-antitrypsin deficiency
Europeans	Cystic fibrosis Neural tube defects Congenital spherocytic anemia PTC taster Red-green color vision defect Alpha$_1$-antitrypsin deficiency Baldness Cleft lip and palate Hemophilia A Congenital dislocation of the hip Hereditary spherocytosis Phenylketonuria XYY syndrome
Ashkenazi Jews	Tay-Sachs disease Niemann-Pick disease Gaucher's disease Canavan's disease Torsion dystonia Familial dysautonomia Nonclassical 21-hydroxylase deficiency Bloom syndrome Hereditary breast cancer
Sephardic and Oriental Jews	G6PD Familial Mediterranean fever Gaucher's disease Beta-thalassemia Laron-type dwarfism
Puerto Rican	Sickle cell anemia
Mediterranean	Sickle cell anemia Alpha-thalassemia
Southeast Asian	Alpha-thalassemia Beta-thalassemia
Italian	Beta-thalassemia
Greek	Beta-thalassemia
Middle Eastern	Sickle cell anemia
French Canadian	Tay-Sachs disease Familial hypercholesterolemia
Lebanese	Familial hypercholesterolemia
Denmark	Alpha$_1$- antitrypsin deficiency
Hispanic	Sickle cell anemia
Scotland	Phenylketonuria
Finland	Phenylketonuria Gyrate atrophy
Japan	Phenylketonuria

Sources: Mahowald, M. B., McKusick, V. A., Scheuerle, A. S., & Aspinwall, T. J. (2001). *Genetics in the clinic: Clinical, ethical, and social implications for primary care.* St. Louis, MO: Mosby; Lea, D. H., Jenkins, J. F., & Francomano, C. A. (1998). *Genetics in clinical practice: New directions for nursing and health care.* Boston: Jones & Bartlett; and Nussbaum, R. L., McInnes, R. R., & Willard, H. F. (2007). *Thompson & Thompson genetics in medicine* (7th ed.). Philadelphia: Saunders.

Focused Interview Questions	Rationales and Evidence
2. Since the start of pregnancy, how many alcoholic drinks have you consumed each day?	▶ Any amount of alcohol consumption during pregnancy can cause fetal alcohol syndrome and related disorders composed of physical, neurologic, and behavioral defects in the infant (Davidson et al., 2012).
3. What recreational drugs have you used since your LMP? This includes marijuana, cocaine, heroin, prescription painkillers, methadone, and so on.	▶ Cocaine and other drugs have been shown to cause miscarriage and multiple fetal defects (Davidson et al., 2012).
4. Have you ever been emotionally or physically abused by your partner or someone important to you? ● Within the last year, have you been pushed, shoved, slapped, hit, kicked, or otherwise physically hurt by someone? ● If yes, by whom? ● Within the last year, have you been forced to have sex? ● If yes, by whom? ● Are you afraid of your partner or anyone else?	▶ All female patients should be screened during each trimester for abuse. At least 4% to 8% of females report abuse during pregnancy, which makes abuse more common than most complications screened for in pregnancy such as diabetes and hypertension. Abuse can cause miscarriage, fetal trauma, maternal stress, smoking, and drug abuse. Risk factors for abuse in pregnancy include unintended pregnancy, unhappiness with pregnancy, young maternal age, single maternal status, higher parity, late or absent entry to care, and substance abuse. The nurse should notify the physician or midwife of any positive findings and work together to develop a plan of care (CDC, 2013).

Questions Related to Nutrition and Exercise History

1. What kind of exercise do you currently engage in? How many days per week for how many minutes do you do it?	▶ Current recommendations state all pregnant patients should be screened for risk factors such as heart disease, lung disease, cervix that dilates prematurely, preterm labor, multiple births, frequent vaginal bleeding, placenta previa, and hypertension. If no high-risk conditions exist, all normal pregnant patients should be counseled to engage in an accumulated 30 minutes of moderate exercise on most, if not all, days each week. Exercise in pregnancy can prevent complications, such as GDM, and build stamina for labor. Sports that are not safe in pregnancy include soccer, vigorous racquet sports, gymnastics, basketball, ice hockey, horseback riding, kickboxing, downhill skiing, and scuba diving. Females should not perform any exercises that require lying on the back after the first trimester (Davidson et al., 2012).

ALERT!

If a pregnant female experiences any of the following conditions during exercise, she should stop exercising and call her healthcare provider:

● *bleeding from the vagina*
● *difficulty or labored breathing BEFORE exercising*
● *dizziness, headache, or chest pain*
● *muscle weakness, calf pain, or swelling*
● *preterm labor symptoms*
● *decreased movement of the fetus*
● *leakage of fluid from the vagina*

Focused Interview Questions

2. Describe everything you have consumed for the past 24 hours. Include water, vitamins, and supplements.

TABLE 27.4 **Dietary Reference Intakes (DRIs): Estimated Average Requirements of Major Nutrients by Women's Age Groups and in Pregnancy**

FEMALE RDA (BY AGE)	14–18	19–30	31–50	51+	PREGNANT
Calcium (mg/d)	1,100	800	800	1,000	800
Protein (g/kg/d)	0.71	0.66	0.66	0.66	0.88
Vitamin E (mg/d)	12	12	12	12	12
Vitamin A (mcg/d)	485	500	500	500	550
Vitamin C (mg/d)	60	60	60	60	70
Thiamin (mg/d)	0.9	0.9	0.9	0.9	1.2
Riboflavin (mg/d)	0.9	0.9	0.9	0.9	1.2
Niacin (mg/d)	11	11	11	11	14
Vitamin B_6 (mg/d)	1.0	1.1	1.1	1.3	1.6
Folate (mcg/d)	330	320	320	320	520
Vitamin B_{12} (mcg/d)	2.0	2.0	2.0	2.0	2.2
Iron (mg/d)	7.9	8.1	8.1	5	22
Zinc (mg/d)	7.3	6.8	6.8	6.8	9.5
Selenium (mcg/d)	45	45	45	45	49

Source: Food and Nutrition Board, Institute of Medicine, National Academies. (2011). *Dietary Reference Intakes (DRIs): Estimated Average Requirements.* Retrieved from http://iom.edu/Activities/Nutrition/SummaryDRIs/~/media/Files/Activity%20Files/Nutrition/DRIs/1_%20EARs.pdf.

Rationales and Evidence

▶ During pregnancy, females should include the following in their diet: four or more servings (1/2 cup each) of fruits and vegetables for vitamins and minerals; six or more servings of whole-grain or enriched bread and cereal for energy; four or more servings of milk and milk products for calcium; and three or more servings of meat, poultry, fish, eggs, nuts, dried beans, and peas for protein (see Table 27.4 for daily reference intakes [DRIs] in pregnancy). Patients often need education on portion size: for example, one serving equals one slice of bread, a potato the size of a computer mouse, 3/4 cup of juice, 1 cup milk, 2 to 3 oz of meat or poultry, 11/2 cup beans, or 1/2 cup vegetables (Davidson et al., 2012).

Caffeine is a stimulant found in coffee, tea, chocolate, and many medications. In large quantities it may cause miscarriage or low-birth-weight babies and dehydration for the mother and should be avoided. Calcium needs increase 40% in pregnancy. Dairy foods are an excellent source of calcium; other excellent sources include collard greens, sesame seed meal, blackstrap molasses, bok choy and other greens, soybeans, and tortillas. It is important that females consume 8 glasses of water each day. Sodium, 2,000 to 8,000 mg, is a required nutrient in pregnancy; pregnant females should salt foods to taste and not consume overly processed highly salted foods.

Females should avoid consuming nonfood items such as clay, cornstarch, laundry starch, dry milk of magnesia, paraffin, coffee grounds, or ice. Pregnant females should also avoid these foods: swordfish, shark, king mackerel, and tilefish due to potentially risky levels of mercury; more than 6 oz of albacore ("white") tuna per week; game fish unless first checking its safety with the local health department; raw fish, especially shellfish (oysters, clams); undercooked meat, poultry, or seafood; hot dogs and deli meats (such as ham, salami, and bologna); soft-scrambled eggs and all foods made with raw or lightly cooked eggs; soft cheeses such as Brie, feta, Camembert, Roquefort, and Mexican style, unless they are labeled as made with pasteurized milk; unpasteurized milk and any foods made from it; unpasteurized juices; and raw sprouts, especially alfalfa sprouts, because there is a danger of salmonellosis and *E. coli* infections (Davidson et al., 2012). Everyone, but especially pregnant females, should practice safe food handling, including hand washing, keeping refrigerator temperature below 40°F, cleaning the refrigerator regularly, refrigerating and freezing food promptly, and avoiding cross-contamination between cooked and uncooked foods to avoid listeriosis and other foodborne infections (FSIS, 2013).

Focused Interview Questions

| Rationales and Evidence |

Focused Interview Questions

ALERT!

Great nutrition is vital to the health of every mother and fetus during pregnancy. The nurse should give the patient a "gold spoon" (plastic, of course) to remind her how valuable every bite is during pregnancy.

Questions Related to Environmental Exposure

1. **What kind of chemicals are you exposed to in your home and workplace?**

Rationales and Evidence

Some herbal supplements and vitamin supplements can be a problem during pregnancy. As research in herbs in pregnancy is continuing, it is recommended that females check with their healthcare provider prior to consuming herbal teas and supplements. A partial list of common herbs known to be harmful in pregnancy includes aloe vera, black cohosh, blue cohosh, dong quai, goldenseal, pennyroyal, saw palmetto, yohimbe, passion flower, and Roman chamomile (APA, 2013). Although most healthcare providers recommend that pregnant patients consume a prenatal vitamin during pregnancy, some vitamin supplements (such as vitamin A) can cause harm if consumed beyond the RDA (Ladewig et al., 2014).

▶ To prevent birth defects and miscarriage, pregnant females should avoid cigarette smoke, lead (in water and paint), carbon monoxide, mercury, pesticides, insect repellents, some oven cleaners, solvents such as alcohol and degreasers, paint, paint thinners, benzene, and formaldehyde. If the pregnant female must be around these substances, she should minimize her exposure by ensuring good ventilation, wearing protective gear such as a face mask and gloves, and checking with the water or health department about the quality of the drinking water. For X-rays, 5 rads is the level of exposure believed to be necessary to cause birth defects; dental, chest, or mammogram X-rays are less than 0.02 rads of exposure (Williams & Fletcher, 2010). Federal guidelines prohibit exposure in the workplace to more than 0.5 rad accumulated during pregnancy, if the pregnant female has notified her employer of her pregnancy (U.S. Nuclear Regulatory Commission [NRC], 1999).

Patient-Centered Interaction

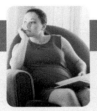

Olu Adams, age 16, presents for a return prenatal visit at 20 weeks' gestation. The prenatal record indicates that this is her first pregnancy, she lives with her parents in a nearby apartment building, and she is in 10th grade. Besides her unplanned adolescent pregnancy, the problems identified so far in this pregnancy include a UTI that was treated with antibiotics and a total weight gain of 10 lb; she is 5′7″ tall and weighed 120 lb at the beginning of the pregnancy.

Interview

Nurse: Hi, Ms. Adams. Have a seat and tell me how you have been doing since your last visit.

The nurse leads the patient to a chair in the examination room and pulls up a stool to sit beside the patient. The teenager stares down at her lap.

Ms. Adams: Fine.

Nurse: Have you had any vaginal bleeding, contractions, or pelvic pressure?

The patient shrugs.

> **Nurse:** Any more problems with peeing, like burning, or peeing more frequently than usual?

The patient shakes her head.

> **Nurse:** Is your mom or the baby's father in the waiting room?

Ms. Adams: Nah.

> **Nurse:** Ms. Adams?

Nurse waits for Olu to look up.

> Have you felt the baby move yet? It would feel like a little tickle on the middle of your belly.

Ms. Adams: (Face lights up, her voice is louder.) **Yes, I am feeling that! Is it the baby?**

> **Nurse:** Yes, it probably is. Tell me about it.

Ms. Adams: In the mornings for about the last week I feel something brushing my insides. And I don't feel so sick anymore.

> **Nurse:** Well, that is certainly good news. Why don't you sit on the exam table and we will listen to the baby's heartbeat and see how much your baby has grown since the last visit.

Ms. Adams: I hope you can tell me how big the baby is now.

ALERT!

Research indicates that patients are often not clear on the signs of preterm labor.

The nurse should discuss the signs of preterm labor with all patients at every prenatal visit after 20 weeks.

- *More than six contractions per hour. This may feel like "the baby balling up," menstrual cramps, backache, or diarrhea.*
- *Leaking fluid, vaginal bleeding, or increased vaginal discharge.*
- *Pelvic pressure, heaviness, or suprapubic pain.*

Analysis

The nurse was appropriate in sitting beside the patient and providing a time away from the examination table for questions. Her initial question about preterm contractions was probably not well understood by a patient of this age and education level. The nurse's question about urinary symptoms was at a more appropriate level, but yes/no questions to teenagers or any uncommunicative patient are not the best choice. The nurse tried to elicit information about the patient's family, but again with a closed question. When the patient became more animated about quickening, the nurse wisely provided an open-ended question that led to a more productive interchange with the patient. The nurse can now go on to find out what the patient knows about topics that are relevant at this point in pregnancy: symptoms of preterm labor, continuing importance of good nutrition, results of laboratory tests from last visit, and fetal development, among other possible topics. During pregnancy, a great deal of teaching is done with the pregnant patient and her family. In order to ensure that all topics are covered, many obstetric practices use a teaching checklist (Box 27.4).

Box 27.4 Pregnancy Teaching Checklist

GESTATIONAL AGE/ TIMING OF VISIT	TEACHING TOPICS
Initial prenatal visit	Welcome Types of providers and scope of practice Hours of office/clinic Phone number, after-hours contact number Warning signs in first trimester Schedule of prenatal care and laboratory studies Safe medications in pregnancy Resources: Pregnancy and childbirth classes Nutritional requirements in pregnancy; request 3-day food diary Exercise in pregnancy Discomforts in pregnancy and relief measures Dental care Abuse screen Benefits of breast-feeding Bathing and clothing
Second prenatal visit	Explanation of test results Discuss 3-day food diary Psychologic adaptation to pregnancy Body mechanics
Throughout pregnancy	Fetal growth and development Sexuality/partner relationship Traveling while pregnant
15 to 20 weeks	Second trimester laboratory testing Genetic testing Ultrasound Warning signs in second trimester Abuse screen
21 to 34 weeks	Preterm labor signs Preparation for birth Car seats Breast-feeding instructions if appropriate Home preparation for newborn 28 week testing
35 to 42 weeks	Signs of labor Sibling preparation for birth Abuse screen Breast preparation 36 week testing

Patient Education

During pregnancy, the advice and education provided by the nurse regarding physiologic, cultural, behavioral, and environmental risk factors is especially vital. Risk factors and *Healthy People 2020* objectives can be used to formulate nursing actions for health promotion and patient education.

LIFESPAN CONSIDERATIONS: PREGNANCY

Risk Factors	Patient Education
• Pregnancy discomforts include vomiting, breast tenderness, leukorrhea, changes in nasal mucosa, excessive salivation, edema, varicosities, hemorrhoids, constipation, backache, leg cramps, dizziness, and dyspnea.	▶ Provide information about specific remedies for each experience. ▶ Counsel patients to seek healthcare intervention for prolonged or unusual symptoms. ▶ Instruct patients regarding hygiene, body mechanics, and other measures to reduce the risk of injury and discomfort during pregnancy. ▶ Counsel patients to include fiber and fluids in daily intake to reduce risks for gastrointestinal (GI) and genitourinary (GU) problems. ▶ Recommend supportive undergarments and devices to reduce breast-related problems.

CULTURAL CONSIDERATIONS

Risk Factors	Patient Education
• African American mothers experience much higher rates of infant mortality, compared to non-Hispanic white mothers. • Asian American and Pacific Islander women experience language barriers in some prenatal care settings. • Hispanic women have an increased risk of developing gestational diabetes.	▶ Encourage early and regular prenatal care. ▶ Implement culturally competent care models. ▶ Provide translation services. ▶ Encourage early screening. ▶ Provide education about diet and exercise.

BEHAVIORAL CONSIDERATIONS

Risk Factors	Patient Education
• Decreased rest contributes to anxiety and health problems.	▶ Advise patients of the need for 8 to 10 hours of sleep. ▶ Recommend a side-lying position during pregnancy.
• Restrictive clothing may lead to problems with circulation or falls.	▶ Advise the patient to select and wear loose-fitting, cotton clothing. ▶ Explain the importance of low-heeled, supportive footwear in preventing slips, falls, and injury.
• Food selection and the amount of intake have consequences for the health of the fetus and mother.	▶ Provide recommended dietary guidelines for pregnant and postpartal patients. ▶ Advise pregnant patients to take folic acid to promote fetal growth and prevent maternal anemia.
• Lack of exercise increases the risk of obesity, gestational diabetes, and pregnancy discomfort.	▶ Provide guidelines for safe and effective exercise in pregnancy. ▶ Provide a list of prohibited athletic activities in pregnancy.

BEHAVIORAL CONSIDERATIONS

Risk Factors	Patient Education
• Lack of information for travel can lead to fetal or maternal injury.	▶ Advise patients to avoid air travel in the final weeks of pregnancy. ▶ Counsel patients to use safety equipment as recommended for pregnancy.
• Substance abuse is harmful to the fetus and mother.	▶ Provide information about the hazards of substance abuse. ▶ Counsel or provide recommendations for smoking cessation and addiction services. ▶ Advise patients to consult with healthcare providers before using OTC medications and products.
• Questions about sexual activity during pregnancy can increase anxiety.	▶ Provide information about sexual activity during pregnancy.
• Pregnant couples may have little experience with safe and effective parenting skills.	▶ Recommend attendance at childbirth education and parenting classes throughout the pregnancy.

ENVIRONMENTAL CONSIDERATIONS

Risk Factors	Patient Education
• Substances such as cancer treatment drugs, lead, ethylene glycol ethers, and ionizing radiation can affect the health of the mother and fetus.	▶ Teach patients how to recognize and avoid hazardous substances.
• Some foods, such as seafood, raw fish, and cheese, may affect the health of the mother and fetus during pregnancy.	▶ Provide details about foods to avoid during pregnancy. ▶ Educate patients regarding hand hygiene, food preparation, and other hygiene measures.
• Infectious diseases during pregnancy can harm the fetus.	▶ Counsel patients to avoid exposure to infectious diseases, such as measles, chickenpox, and hepatitis.

Nutritional Assessment

A comprehensive nutritional history is important when assessing the nutritional health of a pregnant female. Diet recall and food frequency questionnaires remain important tools to use to assess intake. Assessment of the pre-conception diet should also be obtained in general detail because it provides the foundation for nutritional health in early pregnancy and beyond. Table 27.5 outlines specific data to be assessed when conducting a nutritional history of a pregnant female. Lactation needs are also addressed.

Physical Assessment

The assessment of a pregnant female should include parameters to assess the nutritional health of the patient and weight gain patterns necessary to support a healthy pregnancy.

Anthropometric Measurements

Weight, weight history, and gestational weight gain pattern and amount are important considerations during pregnancy. Preconception weight, height, and body mass index (BMI) are necessary to determine gestational weight gain goals. The importance of achieving gestational weight gain goals needs to be stressed. Excessive gestational weight gain in some women may result in retained weight after childbirth. If the retained weight is not lost prior to the next pregnancy, the woman then starts subsequent pregnancies at higher weights, thus contributing to the higher weight status among American women (Walker, 2007). In pregnant adolescents, **gynecologic age** should be determined to assess whether linear growth may still be occurring. Gynecologic age is the difference between current age and age at menarche. Young women with a gynecologic age of 3 years or less are considered to still be completing linear growth and will have competing nutritional needs between

TABLE 27.5 Nutritional History Data for Gestation and Lactation

Assess for Specific Foods and Nutrients

- Folic acid—fortified flour and cereals, orange juice, green leafy vegetables, legumes
- Calcium and vitamin D—dairy, fortified juices, fortified soy products
- Iron—meats, poultry, shellfish, fortified cereals and grains, legumes, dried fruit
- Vitamin B_{12} if vegan—must be synthetic, plant sources not bioavailable
- Vitamin A—dairy, fish, meats
- Fluids, include alcohol and water intake
- Caffeine—coffee, tea, cola and other soda, cocoa, chocolate, over-the-counter (OTC) medications
- Mercury—recommendation is to eat 8 to 12 oz/week of a variety of fish that are lower in mercury, such as salmon, shrimp, pollock, light canned tuna, tilapia, catfish, and cod

Assess for Eating Patterns and Behaviors

- Weight gain with any prior pregnancies
- Restrictive eating, missed meals, dieting attempts
- Cultural beliefs related to food and pregnancy
- Food aversions
- Pica
- Gastrointestinal complaints and any resultant alterations in diet

Assess for Supplement Use

- Prenatal vitamin compliance
- Iron supplement compliance
- Other vitamins—high intake of vitamin A is teratogenic
- Herbs—most untested in pregnant or lactating females
- Remedies for any pregnancy symptoms

their own growth and that of the fetus. Recent trends in obesity among childbearing women dictated the need to revise weight gain guidelines for pregnant women. On June 1, 2009, the Institute of Medicine, a division of the National Academy of Sciences, issued new guidelines for weight gain during pregnancy. These current guidelines are listed in Table 27.6. Weight gain guidelines for other racial and ethnic groups have had insufficient research focus to establish a consensus. For each patient, the nurse should develop individual weight gain guidelines, with the prevention of excess weight gain an important focus.

During the physical assessment, the nurse can screen for factors for low weight gain patterns. Smoking, alcohol consumption, drug use, lack of social support, and depression have all been associated with low weight gain. An adolescent trying to hide a pregnancy may be at risk for low weight gain.

The nurse can also ask questions about the presence of physical symptoms that may be affecting nutritional status. Gastrointestinal discomfort, nausea and vomiting, constipation, and heartburn occur during pregnancy and can alter dietary intake and food tolerance. Follow-up questions should seek information on remedies used to relieve symptoms. A pregnant female with a history of an eating disorder and hyperemesis gravidarum should be screened for current signs of an eating disorder. Box 27.5 outlines physical findings with an eating disorder.

Laboratory Measurements

Laboratory assessment of the pregnant female should routinely include screening for iron deficiency anemia. The increased iron needs during pregnancy put many females at risk for iron deficiency. Hemoglobin and hematocrit decrease until the end of the second trimester due to expansion of blood volume and red cell mass during pregnancy. Pregnancy-specific standards for normal hemoglobin and hematocrit values should be used (Table 27.7).

Assessment for gestational diabetes is performed between weeks 24 and 28. More recently, the American College of Obstetricians and Gynecologists (ACOG) and the American Diabetes Association (ADA) recommend that women who are considered obese by their prepregnant BMI and/or have risk factors associated

TABLE 27.6 Gestational Weight Gain Recommendations

BMI (PREPREGNANCY)	TOTAL GAIN (LB)	FIRST TRIMESTER GAIN (TOTAL LB)	WEEKLY GAIN FOR SECOND AND THIRD TRIMESTER (LB/WK)
Underweight <18.5	28–40	1.1–4.4	1 (1–1.3)
Normal Weight 18.5–24.9	25–35	1.1–4.4	1 (0.8–1)
Overweight 25–29.9	15–25	1.1–4.4	0.6 (0.5–0.7)
Obese (includes all classes ≥30)	11–20	1.1–4.4	0.5 (0.4–0.6)
Twins	35–45	1 lb/week first 20 weeks	1 lb/week after 20 weeks
Triplets	50–60	1 lb/week first 20 weeks	1.5 lb/week after 20 weeks

Source: Adapted from the IOM and National Research Council of the National Academies, 2009.

Box 27.5 Clinical Findings Consistent with Eating Disorders

General Eating Disorder Findings
- Body dissatisfaction. Ask: "How do you feel about your weight?" followed by "Have you ever tried to gain or lose weight? Tell me what you did."
- Constipation
- Bloating
- Fatigue

Bulimia/Binge-Purge Behavior	**Anorexia/Restrictive Eating Behavior**
• Bloodshot eyes • Broken blood vessels on the face • Swollen parotid glands or "chipmunk cheeks" • Dental erosion • Hoarse voice • Scarring on the dorsal surface of the hand from teeth during purge attempts • Poor or lacking gag reflex • Weight fluctuations	• Cold intolerance • Lanugo, soft white hair growth on body • Pedal edema • Dry skin • Alopecia • Bradycardia • Hypotension • Amenorrhea in nonpregnant postmenarcheal females • Loss of strength and muscle tone

TABLE 27.7 Gestational Hemoglobin and Hematocrit References for Anemia

	FIRST AND THIRD TRIMESTERS	SECOND TRIMESTER
Hemoglobin (g/dL)	<11	<10.5
Hematocrit (%)	<33	<32

Source: Centers for Disease Control and Prevention. (2011). *What is PedNSS/PNSS?: PNSS health indicators.* Retrieved from http://www.cdc.gov/pednss/what_is/pnss_health_indicators.htm

with gestational diabetes mellitus (GDM) should be screened at the first prenatal visit or early on in the first trimester. If the initial screening is negative, they should be rescreened between 24 and 28 weeks. A fasting plasma glucose level above 105 mg/dL and a 1-hour glucose greater than 180 mg/dL following ingestion of a 100-g glucose load is considered positive for GDM. Both the nutritional health of the mother and the outcome of the pregnancy can be negatively affected if diet changes are not instituted in females found to have gestational diabetes.

Plasma lipid levels increase during pregnancy as normal physiology and may be unrelated to nutrition, requiring no intervention.

Special consideration should be given to screen for plasma lead in females who report **pica**, the eating of nonfood items or ice, because consumption of earth or clay can be a source of environmental contamination. Females following a **vegan** diet with no consumption of animal products are at risk for vitamin B_{12} deficiency unless the diet is fortified or supplemented. Plant sources of vitamin B_{12} are not considered biologically available. Women without added synthetic vitamin B_{12} should be assessed for vitamin B_{12} status. Pregnant females with a history of phenylketonuria should have a plasma assay for phenylalanine to screen for elevated levels. Elevated phenylalanine levels are harmful to fetal brain development.

Physical Assessment

The room should be warm and private. For prenatal blood tests, a variety of collection tubes and collection equipment will be required and differs for each site.

Assessment Techniques and Findings

The nurse should ask the patient to empty her bladder and explain how to collect a clean-catch urine specimen. If this is the patient's first gynecologic assessment, the nurse should explain the components and general purposes of the physical assessment to the patient, using pictures and the equipment as necessary, and ask the patient if she has any special needs or questions about the exam. It is important to provide privacy while the patient puts on the gown with the opening in back and lays a drape across her lap.

For the initial parts of the physical assessment the patient can be sitting (see Figure 27.11 ■) and later will be assisted to a semi-Fowler's position on the examination table. During the

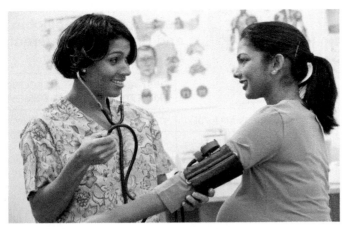

Figure 27.11 Blood pressure measurement in pregnancy.
Source: Jon Feingersh/Vetta/Getty Images.

pelvic part of the assessment, the patient should be assisted to the lithotomy position. Some patients may need to have this assessment in the side-lying position with top knee bent. The nurse assists the patient in placing her feet in the stirrups, which should be padded if possible. The legs should be symmetrically and comfortably positioned. The patient can then be instructed to move her buttocks down to the end of the table until about 0.5 inch is hanging over the edge. For the initial part of the pelvic assessment, it is helpful to tell the patient what she will feel before the nurse touches her ("You will feel me touching your leg, you will feel me touching your labia," etc.). Some patients will be more relaxed if they assist in the insertion of the speculum (see Figure 27.12 ■).

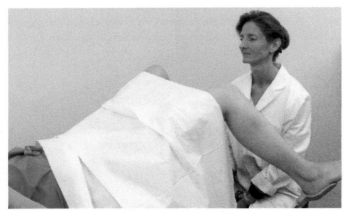

Figure 27.12 Pregnant female in lithotomy position.

EQUIPMENT

- examination gown and drape
- sphygmomanometer
- adjustable light source
- high-performance stethoscope
- centimeter tape measure
- reflex hammer
- fetoscope or fetal Doppler and ultrasonic gel
- urine collection containers
- urine testing strips
- perineal cleansing wipes
- otoscope and specula
- tongue depressor

For the pelvic assessment, the nurse will need the following materials:

- clean, nonsterile examination gloves
- labeled slides and fixative or labeled containers for cytology
- slide for vaginitis check
- potassium hydroxide solution
- saline drops
- plastic or metal speculum
- spatula
- cytology brush or cervical broom
- tissues
- hand mirror (optional per patient preference)
- water-soluble lubricant
- cervical culture swabs

HELPFUL HINTS

- Ask the patient to empty her bladder before the assessment.
- Explain the purposes and processes of each part of the assessment. Use pictures or diagrams as needed.
- Assist the patient to the sitting, lying, and lithotomy positions.
- Explain what the patient will feel before touching her.
- The nurse must be sure to maintain the patient's dignity throughout the assessment.
- The side-lying position may be used to inspect the perineum and rectum of the postpartum patient.
- Use Standard Precautions throughout the assessment.

| Techniques and Normal Findings | Abnormal Findings Special Considerations |

General Survey

1. **Measure the patient's height and weight.**
   - At the initial exam, take these measurements to establish a baseline. In the first trimester, the patient should gain 4 to 6 lb. The patient should gain 1 lb per week in both the second and the third trimesters, for a total weight gain of about 25 to 35 lb, if she is normal weight at conception.

   ▶ A gain of 6.6 lb or more per month may be associated with a large for gestational age baby or developing preeclampsia. A gain of less than 2.2 lb per month may cause preterm birth, a small for gestational age infant, or IUGR.

2. **Assess the patient's general appearance and mental status.**
   - Tiredness and ambivalence are normal in early pregnancy. Most females express well-being and energy during the second trimester. During the third trimester, most report increased fatigue and concern regarding the upcoming birth.

   ▶ It is important to watch for signs of depression such as decreased appetite; persistent feelings of sadness, guilt, or worry; and suicidal thoughts.

3. **Take the patient's vital signs.**
   - The respiratory rate may increase slightly during pregnancy, the heart rate increases, and the blood pressure may drop to below prepregnancy baseline during the second trimester.

   ▶ For women who typically have blood pressure in the normal range, blood pressure should not be greater than 140/90. Elevated blood pressure could be a sign of gestational hypertension or, if accompanied by significant proteinuria, preeclampsia. Note that the pregnant woman's blood pressure should be compared to her blood pressure in a non-pregnant state to determine if she has chronic hypertension or if her elevated blood pressure may be related to gestational hypertension or preeclampsia.

ALERT!

As preeclampsia worsens, multiple systems of the body are affected, producing symptoms such as (from head to toe) the following:

- *headache unrelieved by acetaminophen*
- *blurred vision, dizziness, or vision changes*
- *dyspnea, or difficulty breathing*
- *epigastric (upper abdominal) pain*
- *nausea, vomiting, or malaise ("I don't feel right")*
- *sudden weight gain or sudden, severe edema of face, hands, and legs*
- *Signs noted by healthcare providers include hypertension greater than 140/90, proteinuria ≥ +1, oliguria (decreased urine output), hyperreflexia, and abnormal laboratory values such as elevated liver enzymes and uric acid.*

4. **Test the patient's urine for glucose and protein.**
   - Occasional mild glycosuria or trace protein can be normal findings in pregnancy.

   ▶ Persistent glycosuria may indicate gestational diabetes and necessitates follow-up. Greater than trace protein may indicate preeclampsia. If the patient has lost weight, it is important to check the urine for ketones, indicating ketoacidosis, which is harmful to the fetus.

5. **Observe the patient's posture.**
   - Increasing lordosis is a normal adaptation to pregnancy.

6. **Assist the patient to a sitting position.**

Techniques and Normal Findings	Abnormal Findings Special Considerations

Skin, Hair, and Nails

1. **Observe the skin, hair, and nails for changes associated with pregnancy.**
   - These include linea nigra, striae, melasma, spider nevi, palmar erythema, and darkened areola and perineum. Softening and thinning of nails is common. Hair may become thicker in pregnancy.

▶ Bruises may indicate physical abuse. Lesions may indicate infection. Scars along veins may indicate intravenous drug abuse.

Head and Neck

1. **Inspect and palpate the neck.**
   - Slight thyroid gland enlargement is normal in pregnancy.

▶ Enlarged or tender lymph nodes may indicate infection or cancer. Marked thyroid gland enlargement may indicate hyperthyroidism.

Eyes, Ears, Nose, Mouth, and Throat

1. **Inspect the eyes and ears.**
   - There are no visible changes associated with pregnancy.

▶ Redness or discharge may indicate infection.

2. **Inspect the nose.**
   - Increased swelling of nasal mucosa and redness may accompany the increased estrogen of pregnancy.

▶ Epistaxis may occur if the vascular increase is extreme.

3. **Inspect the mouth.**
   - Hypertrophy of gum tissue is normal.

▶ Epulis nodules, which are formed by hyperplastic tissue overgrowth on the gums, or poor dentition warrant referral to a dentist. Pale gums may indicate anemia. Redness or exudates may indicate infection.

4. **Inspect the throat.**
   - The throat should appear pink and smooth.

Thorax and Lungs

1. **Inspect, palpate, percuss, and auscultate the chest.**
   - Note diaphragmatic expansion and character of respirations. Later in pregnancy, pressure from the growing uterus produces a change from abdominal to thoracic breathing.

   - Observe for symmetric expansion with no retraction or bulging of the intercostal spaces. Confirm that the lungs are clear in all fields.

▶ Unequal expansion or intercostal retractions are signs of respiratory distress. Rales, rhonchi, wheezes, rubs, and absent or unequal sounds may indicate pulmonary disease.

Heart

1. **Auscultate the heart.**
   - Confirm that the rhythm is regular and that the rate is from 70 to 90 beats/min. The heart rate in pregnancy increases 10 to 20 beats/min above the baseline. Short systolic murmurs are due to increased blood volume and displacement of the heart.

▶ Irregular rhythm, dyspnea, or markedly decreased activity tolerance may indicate cardiac disease.

2. **Position the patient.**
   - Assist the patient into a semi-Fowler's position for the next portion of the assessment, and pull out the bottom of the table extension so the patient may lie backwards on the slightly elevated head rest.

Techniques and Normal Findings	Abnormal Findings Special Considerations

Breasts and Axillae

1. **Inspect the breasts.**
   - Normal changes include enlargement, increased venous pattern, enlarged Montgomery tubercles, presence of colostrum after 12 weeks, striae, and darkening of nipple and areola (see Figure 27.6).

   ▶ Flat or inverted nipples can be treated with breast shells in the last month of pregnancy.
   ▶ Bloody discharge or fixed, unchanging masses or skin retraction could indicate breast cancer.

2. **Palpate the breasts and axillae.**
   - Breasts are more tender to touch and more nodular during pregnancy.

Extremities

1. **Inspect and palpate the extremities.**
   - Varicose veins in the lower extremities are normal with pregnancy. Mild dependent edema of the hands and ankles is common in pregnancy. Inspect and palpate the extremities for raised or tender veins. Palpate for ankle or lower leg edema.

   ▶ Raised, hard, tender, warm, painful, or reddened veins may indicate thrombophlebitis. Marked edema may indicate preeclampsia.

Neurologic System

1. **Percuss the deep tendon reflexes.**
   - Reflexes should be +1 or +2 and bilaterally equal.
   - Refer to chapter 26 for more details. ∞

   ▶ Hyperreflexia and clonus are signs of preeclampsia.

Abdomen and Fetal Assessment

1. **Inspect and palpate the abdomen.**
   - The uterus becomes an abdominal organ after 12 weeks in pregnancy. Uterine contractions are palpable after the first trimester. Palpate uterine contractions by laying both hands on the abdomen. The *frequency* of contractions is determined by measuring the interval from the beginning of one contraction to the beginning of the next contraction. Indent the uterus with a finger to measure *intensity* or strength of contractions. The strength can be classified as mild, moderate, or strong. These distinctions can be described by comparing the rigidity of the uterus to the firmness of certain other body features. Mild contractions are comparable to the firmness of the nose, moderate contractions feel like the chin, and strong contractions are as hard and unyielding as the forehead. The *duration* of contractions is measured from the beginning to the end of the contraction.

   ▶ Liver enlargement is abnormal.
   ▶ More than five contractions per hour may indicate preterm labor.

2. **Assess fetal growth through fundal height assessment.**
   - Prior to 20 weeks, fundal height is measured by indicating the number of fingerbreadths or centimeters above the symphysis pubis or below the umbilicus. Once the uterus rises above the umbilicus, a tape measure is used.
   - The 0 line of the measuring tape is placed at the superior edge of the symphysis pubis.
   - The other hand is placed at the xiphoid with the ulnar surface against the abdomen. When the superior edge of the uterus is encountered by the descending hand, the top of the uterus has been located.
   - The measuring tape is stretched from the top of the symphysis pubis to the fundus. The superior aspect of the tape is held between the middle fingers of the hand that is resting perpendicular to the fundus. The fundal height in centimeters is noted and compared to the weeks of pregnancy. Uterine size in centimeters is approximately equal to the weeks of pregnancy. The uterus should measure within 2 units of the weeks of pregnancy (see Figure 27.13 ■).

   ▶ If the uterus is more than 2 cm larger or smaller than the weeks of pregnancy, a growth disorder such as intrauterine growth retardation (IUGR), multiple gestation, amniotic fluid disorders, incorrect dating, fetal malpresentation, or anomalies may be occurring.
   ▶ An unexpectedly large uterus also may be indicative of macrosomia, a condition in which the newborn is substantially larger than average, characterized by a weight of more than 8 pounds at birth. Babies born with macrosomia are at greater risk for health disorders, including hyperglycemia and childhood obesity (Mayo Clinic, 2012b).

Techniques and Normal Findings	Abnormal Findings Special Considerations

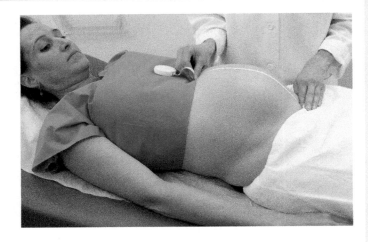

Figure 27.13
Fundal height
measurement.

3. **Assess fetal activity.**
   - After 24 weeks, fetal movement is palpable by the examiner. Maternal perception of movement occurs between 16 and 18 weeks in pregnancy.

4. **Assess fetal lie, presentation, and position.**
   - **Leopold's maneuvers** utilize a specialized palpation of the abdomen sequence to answer a series of questions to determine the position of the fetus in the abdomen and pelvis after 28 weeks' gestation.
   - *First Leopold's maneuver: What is in the fundus?* With the patient in a supine position, stand facing her head. Place the ulnar surface of both hands on the fundus, with the fingertips pointing toward the midline. Palpate the shape and firmness of the contents of the upper uterus. A longitudinal lie will find the head or breech in the fundus. A round, firm mass is the fetal head. A soft, irregular mass is the fetal breech. Nothing in the fundus indicates a transverse lie. The fetus can also be oblique, at an oblique angle to the midline (see Figure 27.14 ■).

▶ The *fetal alarm signal* occurs when there is no fetal movement for 8 hours, fewer than 10 movements in 12 hours, a change in the usual pattern of movements, or a sudden increase in violent fetal movements followed by a complete cessation of movement. Immediate evaluation of the fetus should take place.

▶ Leopold's maneuver may be useful in recognizing fetal macrosomia, which increases both the difficulty of vaginal delivery and the risk of injury to the baby during the delivery and process (Mayo Clinic, 2012b).

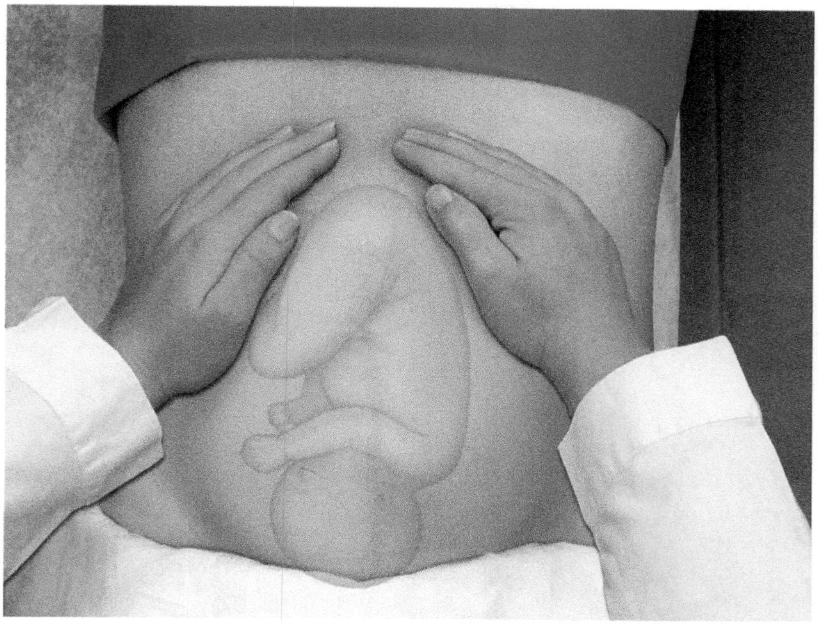

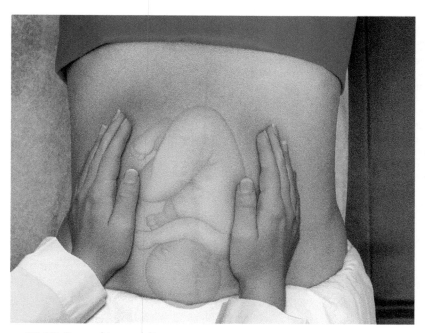

Figure 27.14 First Leopold's maneuver.

- *Second Leopold's maneuver: Where is the fetal back?* Move the hands down the sides of the abdomen along the uterine contour. A smooth, long, firm, continuous outline is found on the side with the fetal back. Irregular, lumpy, moving parts are found on the side with the fetal small parts, or feet and hands. Note whether the back is found on the patient's left or right side; if an indentation about the size of a dinner plate is seen at the midline and movements are at the center of the abdomen, the fetal back may be against the mother's spine (posterior position) (see Figure 27.15 ■).

Figure 27.15 Second Leopold's maneuver.

Techniques and Normal Findings	Abnormal Findings Special Considerations

- *Third Leopold's maneuver: What part of the fetus is presenting at the pelvis?* Next, slide your hands down to the area above the symphysis pubis to determine the "presenting" part of the fetus, the part of the fetus entering the pelvic inlet. Palpate the shape and firmness of the presenting part. Use the thumb and third finger of one hand to grasp the presenting part. This may require pressing into the area above the symphysis pubis with some pressure. Try to move the presenting part with one hand and see if the part of the fetus in the fundus moves with it using the other hand. If the breech is presenting, the whole mass of the fetus will move when the presenting part is moved, and it will feel irregular and soft above the symphysis pubis. If a hard, round, independently movable mass is palpated in the pelvis, it is the head (see Figure 27.16 ■).

▶ A face presentation or forehead presentation may delay the progression of labor and lengthen delivery time (MedlinePlus, 2012). In some cases, cesarean section may be necessary.

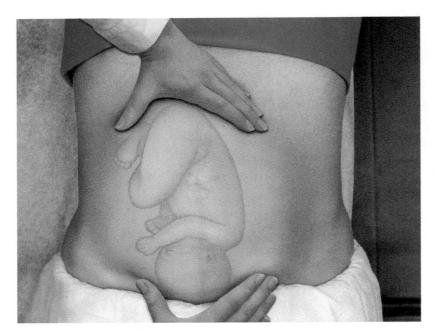

Figure 27.16 Third Leopold's maneuver.

- *Fourth Leopold's maneuver: How deep in the pelvis is the presenting part?* Now, face the patient's feet. Place the ulnar surface of your two hands on each side of the patient's abdomen. Follow the uterine/fetal contour to the pelvic brim. If the fingers come together above the superior edge of the symphysis pubis, the presenting part is floating above the pelvic inlet. If the fingers snap over the brim of the pelvis before coming together, the presenting part has descended into the pelvis. A prominent part on one side is the *cephalic prominence* if the presenting part is the fetal head; this indicates a face presentation if felt on the same side as the back. If a prominence is felt on both sides, the forehead is presenting. If no prominence is felt or the prominence is felt on the same side as the small parts, the fetus is well flexed, with the chin on the chest (flexion) (see Figure 27.17 ■).

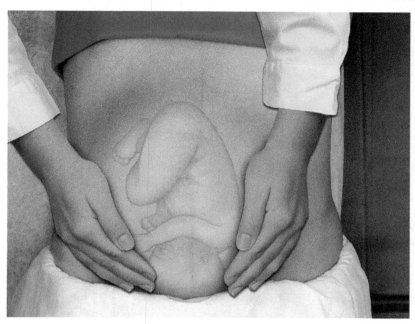

Figure 27.17 Fourth Leopold's maneuver.

- *Fetal position.* The position of the fetus is the relationship of the presenting part to the four quadrants of the maternal pelvis. The fetus can be in the left or right half of the maternal pelvis and in the anterior, posterior, or transverse portion of the pelvis. Three notations are used to designate the fetal position. The first notation is L or R for left or right, indicating in which half of the maternal pelvis the presenting part is found. The second notation is a letter abbreviating the part of the fetus that is presenting at the top of the pelvis. The most common notations for presenting part are O, indicating occiput, or the back of the head in a flexed position; S, indicating sacrum for a breech presentation; Sc, indicating scapula in a transverse lie; and M, indicating mentum or face presentation. The third notation indicates if the presenting part is in the anterior, posterior, or transverse portion of the pelvis. For example, a position of LOA indicates that the presenting part is the occiput, and it is in the left half of the anterior part of the pelvis.

5. **Estimate fetal weight.**
   - Estimating fetal weight by abdominal palpation is only an approximation. It is done in conjunction with fundal height measurement and ultrasound to detect growth abnormalities.
   - Use Leopold's maneuvers to assess fetal size. Experience can be gained by palpating undressed term and preterm infants in the nursery. Compare your estimates with the known weights of the infants.

6. **Auscultate fetal heart rate.**
   - Once the position of the fetus has been determined, the fetal heart tones (FHTs) can be located. They are usually heard loudest over the left scapula of the fetus, so this is the area that should be auscultated (see Figure 27.18 ■).

► Large for gestational age (LGA) or small for gestational age (SGA) infants must be further evaluated.

Techniques and Normal Findings	Abnormal Findings Special Considerations

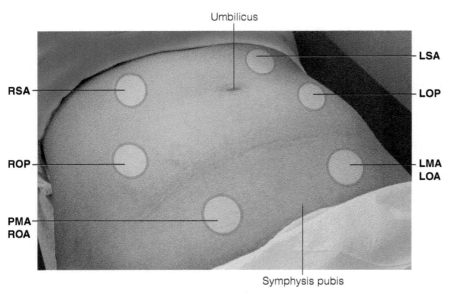

Umbilicus

LSA
LOP
RSA
ROP
LMA
LOA
PMA
ROA

Symphysis pubis

Figure 27.18 Location of fetal heart tones for various fetal positions.

- Place the fetoscope or fetal Doppler in the location where the FHTs are most likely to be heard given the findings of Leopold's maneuvers. Place ultrasonic gel, warmed if possible, on the Doppler prior to placement on the abdomen.

- Auscultate the FHT for 1 minute.

▶ If the fetal heartbeat is not found by 12 weeks with a fetal Doppler, or 20 weeks with a fetoscope, ultrasound evaluation of the fetal viability may be indicated. Other causes could be incorrect dating of pregnancy or retroverted uterus.
▶ Irregular heartbeats, tachycardia (heart rate above 160 beats/min), bradycardia (heart rate below 120 beats/min, or 110 beats/min in postterm fetuses), or decelerations in fetal heart rate below the baseline should be followed up with electronic fetal monitoring.

7. **Assist the patient into the lithotomy position for the next portion of the assessment.**

External Genitalia

1. **Inspect the external genitalia.**
   - Normal findings include enlargement of the clitoris and labia, gaping vaginal introitus for multiparas (patients who have given birth before), scars on perineum from previous births, small hemorrhoids, and darkened pigmentation (see Figure 27.19 ■).
   - Ask the patient to bear down, and note any bulges of the vaginal walls or cervix outside the vagina.

▶ Varicosities can occur in the labia and upper thighs. Lesions may indicate sexually transmitted infection. Redness may indicate vaginitis.
▶ The cervix or vaginal walls may protrude from the vagina in cases of uterine, bladder (cystocele), or rectal (rectocele) prolapse. If the cervix is at the introitus, it is graded as a first-degree uterine prolapse. In a second-degree prolapse, the uterus descends through the introitus. In a third-degree prolapse, the entire uterus is outside the vagina.

Techniques and Normal Findings	Abnormal Findings Special Considerations

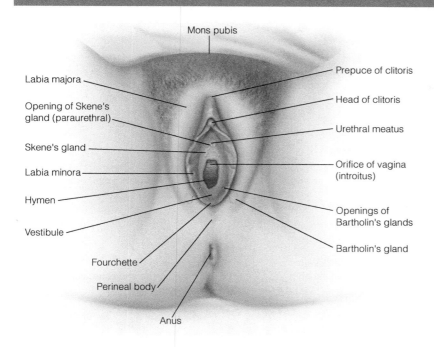

Figure 27.19 External female genitalia.

2. **Palpate Bartholin's gland, urethra, and Skene's glands.**

   - Insert a gloved index finger into the vagina. Press thumb and index finger together at the 5 o'clock and 7 o'clock positions at the vaginal introitus. Note any masses or discharge (see Figure 27.20 ■).

   - Insert the index finger into the vagina and press upward toward the urethra. Milk the urethra and Skene's glands for discharge or swelling.

▶ Note any masses or discharge that may indicate infection.

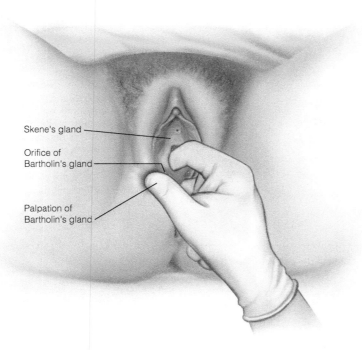

Figure 27.20 Palpation of Bartholin's gland, urethra, and Skene's glands.

Techniques and Normal Findings	Abnormal Findings Special Considerations

Inspection of Vagina and Cervix

1. **Observe the vagina.**
   - The vagina may also be bluish in pregnancy. Note the color, consistency, odor, and amount of discharge. Increased whitish, odorless discharge (leukorrhea) is normal in pregnancy.

   ▶ White, clumping discharge or gray, green, bubbly, fishy smelling discharge is indication of vaginitis or sexually transmitted infections. The patient may complain of itching, burning, dyspareunia or pain on intercourse, or pelvic pain.

2. **Visualize the cervix.**
   - Select the appropriate speculum for the patient. Lubricate the speculum with water or a water-based gel lubricant. (See chapter 24 for more instructions on inserting the speculum. ∞)
   The speculum can be warmed by warm water, the nurse's hands, the light source, or a heating pad kept in the speculum drawer.

   ▶ A speculum that is too cold or too warm is detrimental to the patient's comfort.

3. **Inspect the cervix.**
   - Expected changes in pregnancy include a bluish coloring called Chadwick's sign, or a slitlike cervical opening (os) for multiparas. The shape of the os should match the obstetric history. The os will usually be round and about the size of a pencil tip for a primigravida. The os is usually slitlike in multigravidas. Note any lacerations, ulcerations, erosions, polyps, or other masses on the cervix.

   ▶ Note any dilation of the cervix.
   ▶ Polyps may rupture and cause vaginal bleeding during pregnancy.

   - Note the color and texture of the cervix, and note the character and amount of any discharge from the os.

   ▶ A rough, reddened texture may represent the growth of cells from the internal cervical canal to the outside of the os (ectopy). It is seen in multiparas and females who use oral contraceptives. If the speculum is pushed too deeply into the fornices or corners of the vagina, the internal canal may also appear; this eversion should be eliminated by pulling the speculum back slightly.

   - If the cervix is covered with secretions, and you will be obtaining a Papanicolaou (Pap) smear, use a gauze pad on a sponge stick or a large swab to blot the cervix.
   - Note the size, position, shape, and any friability (bleeding) of the cervix. The cervix should be 2 to 3 cm in diameter.

   ▶ During pregnancy, the cervix is friable, meaning that it is easily eroded and at greater risk for bleeding.

4. **Obtain the Pap smear and cervical cultures.**
   - See chapter 24 for guidelines. ∞

   ▶ Due to the risks of sexually transmitted infections to the fetus during pregnancy, cervical cultures are frequently obtained. The cervical brush is the best method for collection of endocervical cells during pregnancy. Cotton swabs interfere with the growth of chlamydia.

5. **Proceed to pelvic assessment.**
   - Unlock and remove the speculum.

   ▶ If the speculum is not closed prior to removal, there is uncomfortable stretching for the patient.

Palpation of Pelvis

Some nurses with advanced training assess the size and shape of the pelvis to screen for problems during birth.

1. **Assess the angle of the pubic arch.**
   - Place the thumbs at the midline of the lower border of the symphysis pubis (see Figure 27.21 ■). Follow the edge of the pubic bone down to the ischial tuberosity. Estimate the angle of the pubic arch. A pubic arch greater than 90 degrees is best for vaginal birth.

   ▶ An angle less than 90 degrees may be more difficult for a fetus to navigate in labor.

Techniques and Normal Findings	Abnormal Findings Special Considerations

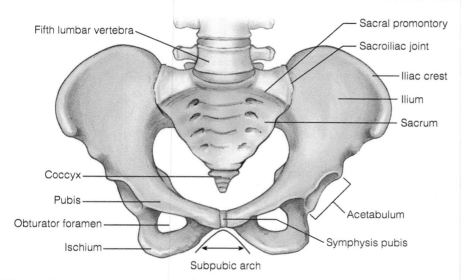

Figure 27.21 Internal structures of the female pelvis for landmarks.

2. **Lubricate the gloved fingers.**
   - Apply a teaspoon or more of lubricating jelly to the index and middle fingers.

3. **Estimate the angle of the subpubic arch.**
   - Insert the index and middle fingers slightly into the vagina, palmar side up. Keep the fingers separated slightly to prevent pressure on the urethra. Palpate the inner surface of the symphysis pubis. Using both thumbs, externally trace the descending sides of the pubis down to the tuberosities. The symphysis pubis should be at least two fingerbreadths wide, and parallel to the sacrum, without any abnormal thickening (see Figure 27.22 ■).

   ▶ An anterior or posterior tilting, or width less than two fingerbreadths, is abnormal.

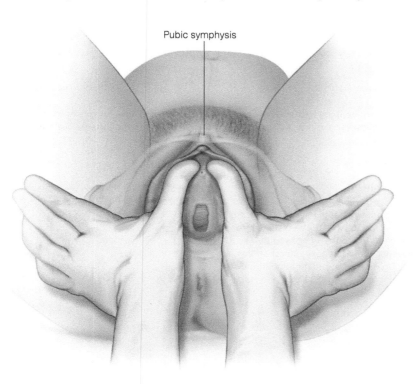

Figure 27.22 Estimation of angle of subpubic arch.

Techniques and Normal Findings	Abnormal Findings Special Considerations

4. Assess the interspinous diameter.

- Turn the fingers to the side and follow the lateral walls of the pelvis to the ischial spine. (As the fingers go deeper into the vagina, ensure that the thumb stays away from the perineum.) Determine if the spine is blunt, flat, or sharp. Sweep your fingers across the pelvis to the opposite ischial spine. Average diameter is approximately 10.5 cm (see Figure 27.23 ■).

▶ A pointy ischial spine can impede labor.
▶ A smaller diameter may mean a contracted pelvis.

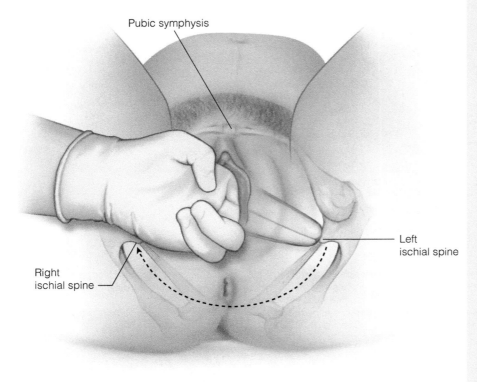

Pubic symphysis

Left ischial spine

Right ischial spine

Figure 27.23 Assessing the interspinous diameter.

5. Assess the curvature of the sacrum.

- Sweep your fingers upward as far as you can reach. Determine if the sacrum is concave, flat, or convex. Note if the coccyx at the posterior end of the sacrum is movable or fixed by pressing down on it.

▶ A hollow sacrum provides more room for the fetus moving through the pelvis.

6. Measure the diagonal conjugate.

- Next, position the fingers in the back of the vagina next to the cervix. Drop your wrist so your fingers are at an upward angle of 45 degrees.
- Reach as far toward the sacrum as you can, and raise your wrist until your hand touches the symphysis pubis. If your fingers reach the sacral promontory, note the distance from the tip of your middle finger touching the sacral promontory to the symphysis pubis. If you cannot reach the sacral promontory, the diagonal conjugate is greater than the length of your examining fingers. The diagonal conjugate is an approximation of the pelvic inlet and should be greater than 11.5 cm (see Figure 27.24 ■).

▶ A diagonal conjugate of less than 11.5 cm may prevent a vaginal birth.

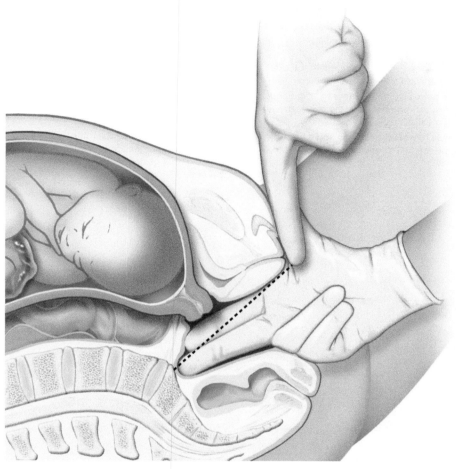

Figure 27.24 Measuring the diagonal conjugate.

Palpation of Cervix, Uterus, Adnexa, and Vagina

1. **Assess the cervix.**
   - Run your fingers around the cervix, and feel the length, width, consistency, and opening. The cervix is usually 1.5 to 2 cm long and 2 to 3 cm wide. In multiparas, the outside of the os may be open up to 2 to 3 cm.

   ▶ The cervix is softer during pregnancy (Goodell's sign). It becomes even softer and jellylike as the patient approaches labor. The outer opening of the cervix may be open but the internal os should be closed prior to term, 37 weeks of pregnancy or more. A shortened cervix is also a symptom or predictor of possible preterm labor.

   - Assess the texture and position of the cervix. It should be smooth.

   ▶ Note the roughness of ectopy or any nodules or masses. Nabothian cysts may become infected or be a sign of cervicitis. Normal variations include a retroverted uterus, which will have an anterior cervix, and an anteverted uterus, which will have a posterior cervix.

   - Move the cervix from side to side with your fingers.

   ▶ Cervical motion tenderness (CMT) is a sign of pelvic inflammatory disease and other abnormalities.

Techniques and Normal Findings	Abnormal Findings Special Considerations

2. Perform bimanual palpation of the uterus.

- Place the nondominate hand on the abdomen halfway between the umbilicus and the symphysis pubis. Press the palmar surface of the fingers toward the fingers in the vagina.
- Insert the fingers of the dominate hand into the vagina. Move the fingers to the sides of the cervix, palmar surfaces upward, and press upward toward the abdomen.
- Estimate the size, consistency, and shape of the uterus captured between your hands. The uterus softens in pregnancy, and the isthmus, the area between the cervix and the upper body of the uterus, is compressible (Hegar's sign).
- The uterus will feel about the size of an orange at 10 weeks' gestation and a grapefruit at 12 weeks' gestation. If the gestation is beyond the first trimester, abdominal fundal height measurement is used (see Figure 27.25 ■).

▶ If the uterine size is not consistent with what is expected for the gestation, then incorrect dating, multiple gestation, or fibroids are suspected.

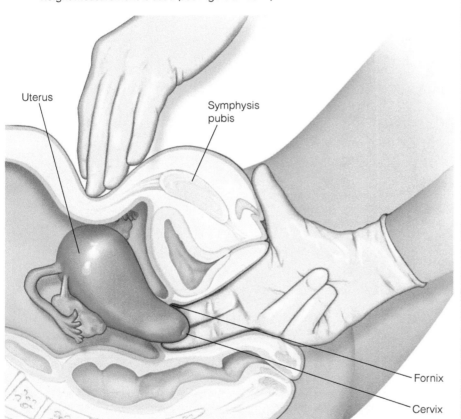

Uterus

Symphysis pubis

Fornix

Cervix

Figure 27.25 Bimanual palpation of the uterus.

3. Palpate the adnexa.

- The fallopian tubes and ovaries, or adnexa, sometimes cannot be palpated, especially after the uterus enters the abdominal cavity as pregnancy progresses.

▶ Any adnexal masses are abnormal and require referral. Bilateral pain is a symptom of pelvic inflammatory disease. During pregnancy an enlarged fallopian tube could indicate ectopic or tubal pregnancy and must be referred to a physician.

4. Assess vaginal tone.

- Withdraw your fingers to just below the cervix, and ask the patient to squeeze her muscles around your fingers as hard and long as she can. Normal strength is demonstrated by a snug squeeze lasting a few seconds and with upward movement. This provides an opportunity to teach the patient about pelvic floor strengthening exercises.

Techniques and Normal Findings	Abnormal Findings Special Considerations

Anus and Rectum

1. Perform the rectovaginal exam.

- The exam is sometimes deferred, but it enables the nurse to evaluate internal structures more deeply and is especially important if any fistulas are noted in the vagina, or if an early pregnancy is in a retroflexed or retroverted uterus.

2. Measure the intertuberous diameter of the pelvic outlet.

- This part of the pelvic assessment is done at the end of the internal exam. As you gently withdraw your hand, make a fist with your thumb on the downward side, and press it in between the ischial tuberosities. A diameter of 11 cm is average, and 8.5 cm or greater usually is adequate. You must know the diameter of your fist to make this determination (see Figure 27.26 ■).

▶ A diameter smaller than 8.5 cm may inhibit fetal descent during expulsion.

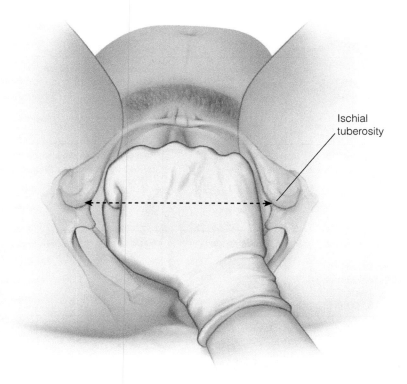

Ischial tuberosity

Figure 27.26 Assessing the pelvic outlet.

3. Inspect the rectum.

- Hemorrhoids are common in pregnancy.

▶ Thrombosed hemorrhoids are tender, swollen, and bluish in color.

▶ *Candida* (yeast), moving trichomonads, or epithelial cells covered with black bacterial spots are abnormal findings.

▶ Potassium hydroxide (KOH) will destroy cell membranes and other structures, but not the hyphae of *Candida* infections.

4. Conclude the exam.

- Dispose of speculum, swabs, and gloves in a biohazard container. Use the tissue to wipe the patient's perineum, or offer tissues to her to do so. Offer your hand to assist her to the sitting position, and leave the room so she can dress in privacy. Share your findings with her.

Laboratory Tests in Pregnancy

Several types of laboratory tests can be performed during pregnancy. Table 27.8 provides information about these various tests, when they should be performed during pregnancy, the normal and abnormal values, and any patient education that is needed as follow-up.

TABLE 27.8   **Tests in Pregnancy**

NAME OF TEST	TIMING OF TEST IN PREGNANCY	NORMAL VALUE	ABNORMAL VALUES	SPECIAL TEACHING
Blood Type, Rh Factor, and Antibody Screen	Initial obstetric (OB) visit and 28 weeks for Rh-negative females	A, B, AB, O, Rh+ or −; no irregular antibodies	Irregular antibodies found	If not her first pregnancy, inquire about previous Rh immune globulin (RhoGAM) administration if Rh−.
Hematocrit	Initial OB visit and 36 weeks	First trimester: 31.0%–41.0% Second trimester: 30.0%–39.0% Third trimester: 28.0%–40.0%	Outside range	Eat iron-rich foods. Report any bleeding.
Hemoglobin	Initial OB visit and 36 weeks	First trimester: 11.6–13.9 g/dL Second trimester: 9.7–14.8 g/dL Third trimester: 9.5–15.0 g/dL	Outside range	Effects of pregnancy on iron needs and possible need for iron supplements.
RBC	Initial OB visit	First trimester: 3.42–4.55 million/mcL Second trimester: 2.81–4.49 million/mcL Third trimester: 2.71–4.43 million/mcL	Outside range	Red cell indices will also be examined to R/O hemoglobinopathies.
WBC	Initial OB visit	First trimester: 5,700–13,600/mcL Second trimester: 5,600–14,800/mcL Third trimester: 5,900–16,900/mcL	Outside range	Report signs of infection.
Platelets	Initial OB visit	First trimester: 174–391 billion/L Second trimester: 155–409 billion/L Third trimester: 146–429 billion/L	Outside range	Report abnormal bleeding from gums, bruising.
HIV	Offered at initial OB visit and prn	Negative	Positive, confirmed by further testing: Western blot	Specific informed consent obtained prior to testing. Advise of dramatic decrease in vertical (mother to child) transmission with medication.
Hepatitis B	Initial OB visit	Negative	Positive	Inform patient of sexual transmissibility. Explain importance of prophylaxis for infant.
Gonorrhea	Initial OB visit; third trimester if high risk	Negative	Positive	Educate patient about infection. Empathetic listening if test is positive. Stress importance of compliance and partner treatment.
Chlamydia	Initial OB visit; third trimester if high risk	Negative	Positive	Address STD prevention.
Rubella Titer	Initial OB visit	Immune	Nonimmune	Recommend maternal immunization after birth. Stress the avoidance of pregnancy for 3 months after immunization. Avoid first-trimester exposure to infection due to risk of congenital rubella syndrome.

TABLE 27.8   Tests in Pregnancy (continued)

NAME OF TEST	TIMING OF TEST IN PREGNANCY	NORMAL VALUE	ABNORMAL VALUES	SPECIAL TEACHING
Tuberculin Skin Testing	Initial OB visit if high risk	Negative	Positive induration > 10 mm in non-immunocompromised patient	Educate mother about infection. Teach respiratory precautions. Encourage smoking cessation.
Urinalysis	Every OB visit	Negative	Presence of protein, glucose, ketones, RBCs, WBCs	Urine collected should be a clean-catch midstream sample.
Urine Culture	Initial OB visit	Negative	Positive bacteria > 100,000 colony-forming units (CFUs)	Wipe from front to back during toileting. Report urgency, flank pain, frequency, burning upon urination.
Papanicolaou Smear	Initial OB visit	Negative	Epithelial cell abnormalities or neoplasms present	Refrain from intercourse or douching 2 to 3 days prior to test (for accuracy). Discuss individualized schedule of testing.
RPR/VDRL FTA-ABS (Syphilis)	Initial OB visit; third trimester	Nonreactive	Reactive FTA-ABS reports a ratio	Educate about infection stages and treatment; advise compliance and abstinence during treatment; reinforce importance of follow-up.
Multiple Marker Genetic Screen	15 to 20 weeks' gestation; first trimester for PAPP-A and Free Beta	No increased risk	Elevated risk	Discuss conditions screened for and limitations of test. Emphasize need for diagnostic testing if screen is positive.
Alpha fetoprotein (AFP) screening test for neural tube defects	16–18 weeks	< 40 micrograms/liter	Low level possible chromosomal abnormalities; Elevated levels positive for neural tube defects	Abnormal results necessitate further diagnostic testing for explanation.
Amniocentesis	11–20 weeks Third trimester for fetal lung maturity	No genetic abnormalities L/S ratio >2:1 Positive Phosphatidylglycerol (PG) Positive Phosphatidylinositol (PI)	Genetic abnormalities Ratio < 2:1 Negative PG & PI	A risk of <1% pregnancy loss exists; abnormal results will necessitate a decision about pregnancy termination Normal value will allow safe early delivery
Chorionic villus sampling	10–12 weeks	No genetic abnormalities	Genetic abnormalities	Same as amniocentesis; questionable results may require more testing.
50-g Glucose Challenge Test (GCT)	24 to 28 weeks; may be done at initial prenatal visit for patients with increased risk of gestational diabetes mellitus (GDM)	≤140 mg/dL	>140	Not fasting; blood drawn exactly 1 hour after glucose is drunk.
3-Hour GTT (100 g glucose given)	Follow-up to elevated 50 g GCT	Fasting <95 mg/dL 1-hr <180 mg/dL 2-hr <155 mg/dL 3-hr <140 mg/dL	Two or more values met or exceeded	Three days of unrestricted carbohydrates and physical activity; fasting prior to test; no smoking or caffeine before and during test; inform re: schedule of blood draws.
Group B Streptococcus	Third trimester/35 to 37 weeks	Positive	Negative	Intravenous (IV) antibiotics will be given in active labor to decrease risk of transmission to infant.
Ultrasound	Optional, frequently at 15 to 20 weeks, dependent on rationale	Normal	Abnormal	Patient can decide whether gender of child should be revealed; some ultrasound studies require vaginal probe; nuchal translucency test at 11 weeks is to screen for chromosomal abnormalities.

Abnormal Findings

Disease processes can result in abnormal assessment findings or abnormal laboratory results. Cultural variations may lead to unexpected psychosocial adaptation and behaviors if the nurse is not familiar with cultural groups and sources of variation.

process to detect complications, identify risk factors, and effectively implement treatment if complications develop. Table 27.9 describes the common complications of pregnancy.

Common Complications in Pregnancy

During pregnancy the role of the nurse is to educate the patient to prevent complications of pregnancy and to assist in the screening

TABLE 27.9 Common Complications in Pregnancy

COMPLICATION	DESCRIPTION	SUBJECTIVE DATA	OBJECTIVE DATA
First Trimester			
Spontaneous Abortion	Loss of pregnancy; lay term is miscarriage.	• Patient complains of low back or abdominal pain.	• Vaginal bleeding accompanied by cramping and loss of fetus, placenta, and membranes through dilated cervix. • No heart tones heard when expected. • Fundal height less than expected.
Ectopic Pregnancy	Implantation of fertilized ovum in fallopian tube or other abnormal location.	• Patient complains of pelvic pain. • Bimanual exam reveals tenderness in adnexa.	• Vaginal bleeding. • Mass palpated near uterus. • Gestational sac smaller than expected size for gestational age.
Anemia	Deficiency in iron, folate, or B12.	• Patient reports fatigue, light-headedness, pica, cold intolerance.	• Abnormal iron values in complete blood count (CBC). • Tachycardia.
Substance Abuse	Use of illicit drugs, alcohol.	• Positive screening questionnaire. • Patient reports irregular prenatal care.	• Inappropriate affect. • Possibly preterm labor.
Molar Pregnancy/ Gestational Trophoblastic Disease	Abnormal growth of placental trophoblast.	• Patient reports nausea or vomiting. • Patient reports pelvic pressure or pain.	• Vaginal bleeding. • Fundal height large for dates. • Fetal heart tones not heard at appropriate time.
Mood Disorders	Depression.	• Patient reports depressed mood, diminished interest in activities, sleep disorders, fatigue, decreased concentration, suicidal ideation.	• Weight changes.
Second and Third Trimester			
Premature Dilation of the Cervix	Passive, painless dilation of cervix during second trimester.	• History of second-trimester loss.	• Short cervix. • Abnormal cervical ultrasound findings.
Preeclampsia	Multisystem reaction to vasospasm.	• Patient reports severe headaches or changes in vision. • Patient reports upper abdominal pain and nausea or vomiting.	• Elevated blood pressure above 140/90 after 20 weeks. • Proteinuria >1 dipstick. • Pathologic edema of face, hands, and abdomen unresponsive to bed rest.

TABLE 27.9 **Common Complications in Pregnancy (continued)**

COMPLICATION	DESCRIPTION	SUBJECTIVE DATA	OBJECTIVE DATA
Gestational Diabetes	Glucose intolerance during pregnancy.	• Patient reports positive history of gestational diabetes.	• Abnormal glucose tolerance test. • Glycosuria.
Preterm Labor	Uterine contractions at 20 to 37 weeks that cause cervical change.	• Patient reports constant low backache and pelvic or abdominal pressure. • Patient reports change in cervical/vaginal discharge.	• Uterine contractions more frequent than every 10 minutes. • Progressive cervical change: effacement > 80%, dilation > 2 cm. • Short cervix. • Positive fetal fibronectin or salivary estriol test.
Intrauterine Growth Restriction	Fetal growth below norms.	• Patient may report feeling that her baby is too small.	• Fundal height less than expected. • Weight gain less than recommended.
Placental Abnormalities	Abnormal placental implantation including placenta previa, when placenta is implanted over cervix, and abruptio placenta, when placenta detaches from uterus.	• Patient reports abdominal pain.	• Vaginal bleeding. • Nonreassuring fetal heart rate pattern. • Abnormal ultrasound.

Common Complications in the Postpartum Period

Several common complications are found during the postpartum period. These complications are discussed in Table 27.10.

TABLE 27.10 **Common Complications in the Postpartum Period**

COMPLICATION	DESCRIPTION	SUBJECTIVE DATA	OBJECTIVE DATA
Postpartum Hemorrhage	Estimated blood loss (EBL) greather than 500 mL at birth for vaginal delivery or greater than 1,000 mL after cesarean birth.	• Patient reports vaginal bleeding that saturates more than one menstrual pad per hour.	• A 10% decrease in hematocrit between admission and postpartum. • Uterine fundus may be relaxed or "boggy," even after circular massage, if caused by uterine atony. • If hemorrhage caused by lacerations of the genital tract, fundus may be firm with continued bleeding.
Preeclampsia	High blood pressure often accompanied by organ damage.	• Patient reports headaches, blurred vision, abdominal pain, dyspnea.	• Elevated blood pressure. • Excessive edema in hands or face. • Proteinuria greater than +1.
Subinvolution of the Uterus	Slower than expected return of the uterus to prepregnant size.	• Patient reports continued uterine bleeding. • Patient reports pelvic or back pain. • Patient reports fatigue or malaise.	• Uterine fundus is above expected level. • At 6 weeks postpartum, uterus has not returned to nonpregnant size.

(continued)

TABLE 27.10	Common Complications in the Postpartum Period (continued)		
COMPLICATION	**DESCRIPTION**	**SUBJECTIVE DATA**	**OBJECTIVE DATA**
Disseminated Intravascular Coagulation (DIC)	Blood disorder in which clotting proteins become overactive and are depleted rapidly.	• Patient reports bruising easily. • Patient reports spontaneous bleeding.	• Bleeding from intravenous (IV) site, gums, or nose. • Petechiae. • Tachycardia. • Diaphoresis. • Decreased platelets and abnormal clotting factor values.
Endometriosis	Lining of the uterus (endometrium) grows ectopically.	• Patient reports chills. • Patient reports extreme pelvic pain upon fundus assessment. • Patient reports increased or foul-smelling lochia.	• Fever. • Tachycardia.
Deep Vein Thrombophlebitis	Blood clot forms in a vein, typically in the legs but also in the arms or neck.	• Patient reports unilateral pain in lower (or upper) extremity.	• Warmth, redness, or swelling over a vein. • Vein feels cordlike. • Homan's sign may be positive.
Hematoma	A localized collection of blood outside the blood vessels.	• Patient reports pain in the perineum.	• Perineum is bulging or bluish.
Mastitis	Infection in the breast tissue.	• Patient reports mastalgia (breast pain).	• Unilateral red streaks on breast. • Presence of flu-like symptoms, including fever.

Application Through Critical Thinking

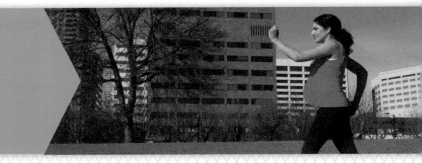

▶ Case Study

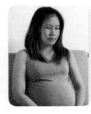

Susan Li, gravida 1, para 1, age 22, is married to a 23-year-old sales clerk who is required to work as much as possible due to family financial problems. She has 2 years of college education and was working as a waitress prior to this pregnancy. She speaks very good English. Her only local family member is her sister, who also works full time. The rest of her family is in China. She gave birth to a 7 lb 4 oz female infant 24 hours ago. Her blood loss at birth was 400 mL, and her placenta delivered intact. A first-degree laceration occurred during birth and was repaired, and a small cluster hemorrhoid developed during the pushing stage of labor. She had an unmedicated birth and breast-fed her baby girl in the delivery room, and two times since for approximately 5 minutes each time. No family members have been to see her since the birth.

▶ Complete Documentation

The case study information is documented in the sample EHR below.

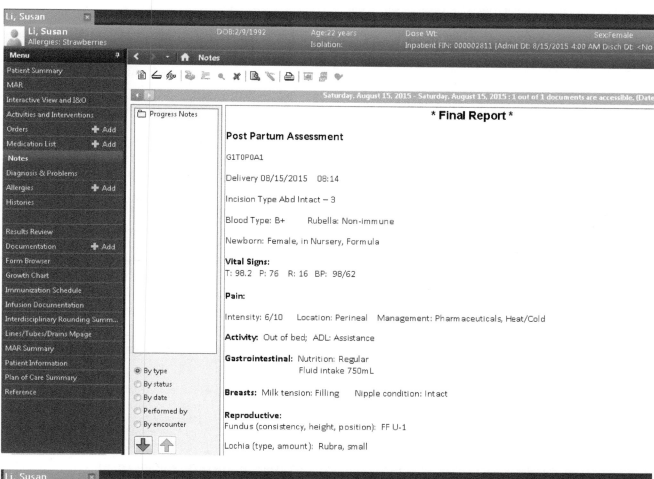

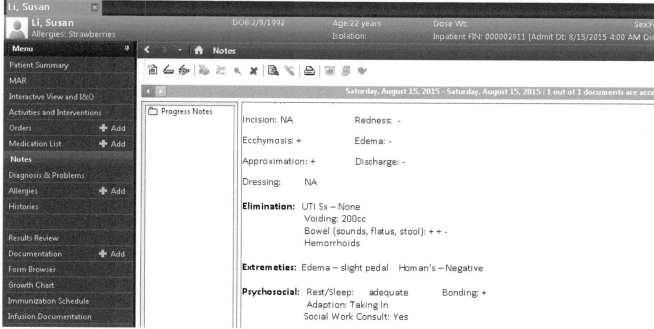

▶ Critical Thinking Questions

1. What should the nurse's priority assessments for Susan be during this postpartum assessment exam at 24 hours after birth?

2. Susan complains that her stitches and hemorrhoids are painful at the level of 7 on a 10-point pain scale. Describe the recommended nursing assessment and relief measures.

3. At 5 weeks postpartum, Susan's sister brings her to the clinic nurse. Susan tells the nurse she feels hopeless and overwhelmed and has been irritable and anxious for the past 3 weeks. What should the nurse's action be?

4. What psychosocial consideration are applicable to this situation?

5. What cultural beliefs should be considered in Susan Li's case?

▶ Prepare Teaching Plan

LEARNING NEED: Ms. Li has just delivered her first child. She is physically stable but is experiencing severe perineal pain. She has a small hemorrhoid that may be contributing to her pain. She has begun breast-feeding but has not established it yet. She is receiving no support from her family at this time. Like most new mothers, she has pain, self-care, knowledge deficit, social support, and breast-feeding needs that must be addressed by the nurse. The following teaching plan is focused on individual care and education for Ms. Li.

GOAL: The new mother will demonstrate safe-care of herself and her newborn, as the family will experience a successful transition to new parenthood.

OBJECTIVES: Upon completion of this educational session, the participant will be able to:

1. Identify two pharmacologic and two nonpharmacologic measures for perineal pain relief.

2. Describe the components of good latch in breast-feeding, the recommended feeding frequency during the first week of life, and indicators of adequate breast-feeding.

3. List three ways in which family members, friends, and community nurses can provide social support to the new mother and family.

4. Demonstrate the use of a sitz bath and other measures for hemorrhoidal pain relief.

5. Explain the difference in baby blues, postpartum depression, and postpartum psychosis, and list two resources for additional help.

APPLICATION OF OBJECTIVE 1: Identify two pharmacologic and two nonpharmacologic measures for perineal pain relief

Content	Teaching Strategy and Rationale	Evaluation
• Sutures are reabsorbed by the body and do not need to be removed.	• Discussion	• Patient verbalizes understanding. For example, patient states, "I should call the midwife if my stitches start hurting more."
• Ibuprofen or acetaminophen may be used safely by breast-feeding mothers for perineal pain relief. Witch hazel pads assist with drying, and anesthetic sprays may provide topical relief.	• Audiovisual materials	• Patient provides counterdemonstration. For example, patient sets up sitz bath unassisted in nurse's presence.
	• Printed materials	
	• Group instruction	
	• Individual discussion allows the patient to verbalize specific concerns as well as fears.	• Nurse observes patient. For example, nurse observes patient put infant to breast and obtain good latch, unassisted.
• Cold packs, a peribottle filled with warm water and squirted on the perineum, and sitz baths are also used to decrease perineal pain.	• Videos on the postpartum unit can allow patients to schedule the timing of the teaching, and provide visual instructions for those with limited English.	
• Do not sit cross-legged (tailor-sit) or place undue stretching on stitches until they have healed.		
• Pain should stay the same or get better each day.	• Printed materials can reinforce teaching performed by the nurse and provide a reference for the patient later.	
• Increased perineal pain should be reported to the healthcare provider.	• Small teaching groups provide support and can be more time efficient to ensure that all the basic components of postpartum care are taught to all patients. Large lecture classes are not appropriate for new mother-infant dyads.	
• Good hand-washing technique and frequency should be maintained.		

▶ References

Alden, K.R., Lowdermilk, D. L., Cashion, M.C., & Perry, S. E. (2012). *Maternity & women's health care* (10th ed.). St. Louis, MO: Mosby.

American College of Obstetricians and Gynecologists (ACOG). (2013). *Obesity in pregnancy.* Retrieved from http://www.acog.org/Resources-And-Publications/Committee-Opinions/Committee-on-Obstetric-Practice/Obesity-in-Pregnancy

American Pregnancy Association. (2007). *Calculating conception.* Retrieved from http://americanpregnancy.org/duringpregnancy/calculatingdates.html

American Pregnancy Association. (2013). *Herbs and pregnancy.* Retrieved from http://americanpregnancy.org/pregnancyhealth/naturalherbsvitamins.html

Barnhard, Y., Bar-Hava, I., & Divon, M. Y. (1996). Accuracy of intrapartum estimates of fetal weight effect of oligohydramnios. *Journal of Reproductive Medicine, 41,* 907–910.

Biancuzzo, M. (2003). *Breastfeeding the newborn: Clinical strategies for nurses* (2nd ed.). St. Louis, MO: Mosby.

Blackburn, S. (2013). *Maternal, fetal, and neonatal physiology* (4th ed.). Maryland Heights, MO: Saunders.

Centers for Disease Control and Prevention. (2011). *Chickenpox and pregnancy.* Retrieved from http://www.cdc.gov/pregnancy/infections-chickenpox.html

Centers for Disease Control and Prevention. (2012). *Fact sheets: Tuberculosis and pregnancy.* Retrieved from http://www.cdc.gov/TB/publications/factsheets/specpop/pregnancy.htm

Centers for Disease Control and Prevention. (2013). *Intimate partner violence during pregnancy: A guide for clinicians.* Retrieved from http://www.cdc.gov/reproductivehealth/violence/IntimatePartnerViolence/

Centers for Disease Control and Prevention. (2014). *Folic acid.* Retrieved from http://www.cdc.gov/ncbddd/folicacid/index.html

Centers for Disease Control and Prevention. (n.d.) *About DES.* Retrieved from http://www.cdc.gov/des/consumers/about/index.html

Chamblin, C. (2006). Breastfeeding after breast reduction: What nurses and moms need to know. *AWHONN Lifelines, 10*(1), 42–48.

Creasy, R. K., Resnik, R., Iams, J. D., Lockwood, C. J., Moore, T. R., & Greene, M. F. (Eds.). (2014). *Maternal-fetal medicine* (7th ed.). Philadelphia: Saunders.

Cruz, N. I., & Korchin, L. (2007). Lactational performance after breast reduction with different pedicles. *Plastic and Reconstructive Surgery, 120*(1), 35–40.

Cruz, N. I., & Korchin, L. (2010). Breastfeeding after augmentation mammaplasty with saline implants. *Annals of Plastic Surgery, 64*(5), 530–533.

Cunningham, F. G. (2010). Appendix B: Laboratory values in normal pregnancy. In J. T. Queenan, J. C. Hobbins, & C. Y. Spong (Eds.), *Protocols for high-risk pregnancies: An evidence-based approach* (5th ed.) (pp. 587–595). Oxford, UK: Wiley-Blackwell.

Cunningham, F., Leveno, K., Bloom, S., Spong, C. Y., & Dashe, J. (2014). *Williams obstetrics* (24th ed.). New York: McGraw-Hill.

Davidson, M. R., London, M. L., & Ladewig, P. A. W. (2012). *Olds' maternal-newborn nursing & women's health across the lifespan* (9th ed.). Upper Saddle River, NJ: Pearson.

Engstrom, J. L. (1993). Fundal height measurement: Part 1—Techniques for measuring fundal height. *Journal of Nurse-Midwifery, 38*(1), 5–16.

Engstrom, J. L., & McFarlin, B. L. (1993). Fundal height measurement: Part 2—Intra- and interexaminer reliability of three measurement techniques. *Journal of Nurse-Midwifery, 38*(1), 17–22.

Engstrom, J. L., Piscioneri, L., Low, L., McShane, H., & McFarlin, B. (1993). Fundal height measurement: Part 3—The effect of maternal position on fundal height measurements. *Journal of Nurse-Midwifery, 38*(1), 25–27.

Freda, M., Andersen, F., Damus, K., & Merkatz, I. R. (1993). Are there differences in information given to private and public prenatal patients? *American Journal of Obstetrics and Gynecology, 169*(1), 155–160.

Godlee, F. (2004). *Clinical evidence concise* (12th ed.). London: BMJ.

Green, C. J. (2012). *Maternal newborn nursing care plans.* Sudbury, MA: Jones & Bartlett.

Hale, T. W. (2004). *Medications and mother's milk: A manual of lactational pharmacology* (11th ed.). Amarillo, TX: Pharmasoft Medical.

Hamilton, B. E., Martin, J. A., Osterman, M. J. K., & Curtin, S. C. (2014). Births: Preliminary data for 2013. *National Vital Statistics Reports 63*(2), 1–20. Retrieved from http://www.cdc.gov/nchs/data/nvsr/nvsr63/nvsr63_02.pdf

Institute of Medicine and National Research Council. (2009). *Weight gain during pregnancy: Reexamining the guidelines.* Washington, DC: The National Academies Press.

James, D. C., & Maher, M. A. (2009). Caring for the extremely obese woman during pregnancy and birth. *MCN: The American Journal of Maternal Child Nursing, 34*(1), 24–30.

Kim, S. K., Romero, R., Kusanovic, J. P., Erez, O., Vasibuch, E., Mazaki-Tovi, S., . . . Hassan, S. S. (2010). The prognosis of pregnancy conceived despite the presence of an intrauterine device (IUD). *Journal of Perinatal Medicine, 38*(1), 45–53.

King, T. L., Brucker, M. C., Kriebs, J. M., & Fahey, J. O. (2015). *Varney's midwifery* (5th ed.). Burlington, MA: Jones & Bartlett.

Kominiarek, M. A. (2011). Preparing for and managing a pregnancy after bariatric surgery. *Seminars in Perinatology, 35*(6), 356–361.

Ladewig, P. A. W., London, M. L., & Davidson, M. R. (2014). *Contemporary maternal-newborn nursing care* (8th ed.). Upper Saddle River, NJ: Pearson.

Landon, M. B., & Lynch, C. D. (2011). Optimal timing and mode of delivery after cesarean with previous classical incision or myomectomy: A review of the data. *Seminars in Perinatology, 35*(5), 257–261.

Lawrence, R. A., & Lawrence, R. M. (2011). *Breastfeeding: A guide for the medical profession.* Maryland Heights, MO: Elsevier.

Lea, D. H., Jenkins, J. F., & Francomano, C. A. (1998). *Genetics in clinical practice: New directions for nursing and health care.* Boston: Jones & Bartlett.

Leitich, H., Brunbauer, M., Bodner-Adler, B., Kaider, A., Egarter, C., & Husslein, P. (2003). Antibiotic treatment of bacterial vaginosis in pregnancy: A meta-analysis. *American Journal of Obstetrics and Gynecology, 188*(3), 752–758.

Lipson, J. G., Dibble, S. L., & Minarik, P. A. (1996). *Culture & nursing care.* San Francisco: UCSF Nursing Press.

Littleton, L. Y., & Engebretson, J. C. (2002). *Maternal, neonatal, and women's health nursing.* Albany, NY: Delmar.

London, M. L., Ladewig, P. A. W., Davidson, M. R., Ball, J. W., Bindler, R. C. M., & Cowen, K. J. (2014). *Maternal & child nursing care* (4th ed.). Upper Saddle River, NJ: Pearson.

Luxner, K. L. (2005). *Delmar's maternal-infant nursing care plans* (2nd ed.). Clifton Park, NY: Thomson Delmar Learning.

Mahowald, M. B., McKusick, V. A., Scheuerle, A. S., & Aspinwall, T. J. (2001). *Genetics in the clinic: Clinical, ethical, and social implications for primary care.* St. Louis, MO: Mosby.

Mamelle, N., Segueilla, M., Munoz, F., & Berland, M. (1997). Prevention of preterm birth in clients with symptoms of preterm labor—The benefits of psychological support. *American Journal of Obstetrics and Gynecology, 177*(4), 947–952.

March of Dimes. (2014). *Smoking during pregnancy.* Retrieved from http://www.marchofdimes.com/pregnancy/smoking-during-pregnancy.aspx

Margulies, R., & Miller, L. (2001). Fruit size as a model for teaching first trimester uterine sizing in bimanual examination. *American College of Obstetricians and Gynecologists, 98*(2), 341–344.

Mattson, S., & Smith, J. E. (2011). *Core curriculum for maternal-newborn nursing* (4th ed.). St. Louis, MO: Saunders.

Mayo Clinic. (2012a). *What are the risks associated with chicken pox and pregnancy?* Retrieved from http://www.mayoclinic.org/healthy-living/pregnancy-week-by-week/expert-answers/chickenpox-and-pregnancy/faq-20057886

Mayo Clinic. (2012b). *Fetal macrosomia: Complications.* Retrieved from http://www.mayoclinic.org/diseases-conditions/fetal-macrosomia/basics/complications/con-20035423

Mayo Clinic. (2014). *Pregnancy nutrition: Healthy-eating basics.* Retrieved from http://www.mayoclinic.org/healthy-living/pregnancy-week-by-week/in-depth/pregnancy-nutrition/art-20046955

McCance, K. L., & Huether, S. E. (2015). *Pathophysiology* (7th ed.). St. Louis, MO: Mosby.

McFarlin, B. (1994). Intrauterine growth retardation: Etiology, diagnosis, and management. *Journal of Nurse-Midwifery, 39*(2), 52S–65S.

MedlinePlus. (2012). *Delivery presentations.* Retrieved from http://www.nlm.nih.gov/medlineplus/ency/patientinstructions/000621.htm

MedlinePlus. (2013). *Alpha fetoprotein.* Retrieved from http://www.nlm.nih.gov/medlineplus/ency/article/003573.htm

MedlinePlus. (2014). *Glucose screening and tolerance tests during pregnancy.* Retrieved from http://www.nlm.nih.gov/medlineplus/ency/article/007562.htm

Miller, D. W., Yeast, J. D., & Evans, R. L. (2003). The unavailability of prenatal records at hospital presentation. *Obstetrics & Gynecology, 101*(4), 87S.

Miller, S. M., & Isabel, J. M. (2002). Prenatal screening tests facilitate risk assessment. *MLO: Medical Laboratory Observer, 34*(2), 8–11, 14–16, 19–21.

Moore, K. L., Persaud, T. V. N., & Torchia, M. G. (2013). *Before we are born: Essentials of embryology and birth defects* (8th ed.). Philadelphia: Saunders.

Nussbaum, R. L., McInnes, R. R., & Willard, H. F. (2007). *Thompson & Thompson genetics in medicine* (7th ed.). Philadelphia: Saunders.

Ogden, C. L., Carroll, M. D., Curtin, L. R., McDowell, M. A., Tabak, C. J., & Flegal, K. M. (2006*). JAMA: Journal of the American Medical Association, 295*(13), 1549–1555.

Robertson, L., Flinders, C., & Godfrey, B. (1986). *The new Laurel's kitchen: A handbook of vegetarian cookery and nutrition.* Petaluma, CA: Nilgiri Press.

Rorie, J. L., Paine, L. L., & Barger, M. K. (1993). Primary care for women: Cultural competence in primary care services. *Journal of Nurse-Midwifery, 41*(2), 92–100.

Sarwer, D. B., Allison, K. C., Gibbons, L. M., Markowitz, J. T., & Nelson, D. B. (2006). Pregnancy and obesity: A review and agenda for future research. *Journal of Women's Health, 15*(6), 720–733.

Siega-Riz, A., Siega-Riz, A., & Laraia, B. (2006). The implications of maternal overweight and obesity on the course of pregnancy and birth outcomes. *Maternal & Child Health Journal, 10*(5), S153–156.

Sinclair, C. (2004). *A midwife's handbook.* St. Louis, MO: Saunders.

Smith, S. A., Hulsey, T., & Goodnight, W. (2008). Effects of obesity on pregnancy. *JOGNN: Journal of Obstetric, Gynecologic, & Neonatal Nursing, 37*(2), 176–184.

Smith, S. M. & McKinney, E. S. (2014). *Foundations of maternal-newborn and women's health nursing.* (6th ed.). St. Louis, MO: Elsevier.

Star, W. L., Shannon, M. T., Lommel, L. L., & Gutierrez, Y. M. (1999). *Ambulatory obstetrics* (3rd ed.). San Francisco: UCSF Nursing Press.

St. Hill, P., Lipson, A., & Meleis, A. I. (2003). *Caring for women cross-culturally.* Philadelphia: F. A. Davis.

Toppenberg, K. S., Hill, D. A., & Miller, D. P. (1999). Safety of radiographic imaging during pregnancy. *Am Fam Physician, 59*(7), 1813–1818.

University of Rochester Medical Center. (n.d.) *Lecithin-sphingomyelin ratio (amniotic fluid).* Retrieved from http://www.urmc.rochester.edu/encyclopedia/content.aspx?ContentTypeID=167&ContentID=ls_ratio

U.S. Census Bureau. (2010). *2010 Census Briefs.* Retrieved from http://www.census.gov/2010census/data/

U.S. Department of Agriculture, Food Safety and Inspection Service (FSIS). (2013). *Protect your baby and yourself from listeriosis.* Retrieved from http://www.fsis.usda.gov/wps/portal/fsis/topics/food-safety-education/get-answers/food-safety-fact-sheets/foodborne-illness-and-disease/protect-your-baby-and-yourself-from-listeriosis/ct_index

U.S. Department of Health and Human Services (USDHHS). (2014). *Healthy people 2020.* Retrieved from http://www.healthypeople.gov/2020/default.aspx

U.S. Nuclear Regulatory Commission (NRC). (1999). *Instruction concerning prenatal radiation exposure.* Retrieved from http://pbadupws.nrc.gov/docs/ML0037/ML003739505.pdf

U.S. Preventive Services Task Force. (2008). *Screening for bacterial vaginosis in pregnancy to prevent preterm delivery.* Retrieved from http://www.uspreventiveservicestaskforce.org/uspstf/uspsbvag.htm

Walker, L. O. (2007). Managing excessive weight gain during pregnancy and the postpartum period. *JOGNN: Journal of Obstetric, Gynecologic, & Neonatal Nursing, 36*(5), 490–500.

Walsh, L. V. (2001). *Midwifery: Community-based care during the childbearing year.* Philadelphia: Saunders.

Whitley, N. (1985). *A manual of clinical obstetrics.* Philadelphia: Lippincott.

Williams, P. M. & Fletcher, S. (2010). Health effects of prenatal radiation exposure. *American Family Physician, 82*(5), 488–493.

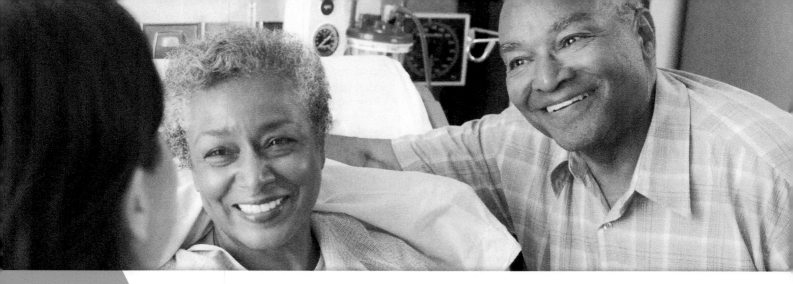

The Hospitalized Patient

▌ Learning Outcomes

Upon completion of the chapter, you will be able to:

1. Differentiate the types of assessment carried out with the hospitalized patient.

2. Conduct a rapid and routine assessment of a hospitalized patient.

3. Apply knowledge and skills in the assessment of a hospitalized patient.

4. Apply critical thinking to assessment of the hospitalized patient.

Introduction

The nursing process has been recognized as the systematic and cyclic process used by the nurse to plan and provide care for patients. Assessment, the first step of the nursing process, is a dynamic and fluid activity. Analysis of the data gathered in the assessment phase of the nursing process requires critical thinking and application of knowledge about health, illness, and factors that influence a person's response to changes in his or her health status. Only with detailed assessment and accurate analysis of data can nursing care plans be developed to meet the specific needs of the patient.

The depth and breadth of assessment of the hospitalized patient varies with both the purpose of the assessment and the health status of the patient. In nonemergent situations, nurses conduct complete (comprehensive) health assessments of patients on admission.

When the patient is in distress, or in special circumstances, such as following surgery, a more focused and limited assessment is carried out. Routine, or ongoing assessments, occur throughout the patient's hospital stay. These ongoing assessments include shift-by-shift assessments as well as assessments to ascertain patient response to a treatment or intervention. In practice, each patient encounter includes assessment in relation to current and expected status, change, and progress.

Hospitalized patients undergo frequent assessments; therefore, it is important that the nurse communicates effectively regarding the type and purpose of the assessment. In addition, the nurse must be sure to have all the required equipment and must be able to use physical assessment techniques with efficiency and competence. Hospitals often have policies to guide the types and frequencies of assessments required in accordance with medical diagnoses or parameters for laboratory findings, monitor readings, patient condition, or administration of medication.

Application of the nursing process is specific for each patient. Integration of assessment data with other knowledge about a patient is essential to planning care. The knowledge base about the patient will include health problems (i.e., current and coexisting medical diagnoses); age; gender; nutritional status; results of laboratory and diagnostic testing; documentation and communication with other members of the healthcare team; medication regimens; and functional capabilities. Additionally, the knowledge base includes psychosocial factors and concerns including, for example, the presence of a support system, knowledge about the health problems, coping abilities, cultural preferences, and spirituality. This knowledge base assists the nurse in making judgments about assessment findings in relation to expected norms in each patient encounter.

The following pages present two types of assessment of the hospitalized patient: a rapid assessment and a routine or initial assessment. Remember to apply all concepts of patient safety, Standard Precautions, and professional standards in each patient encounter, in professional communication, and in documentation of assessment data. Assessment procedures that apply to National Patient Safety Goals are noted throughout and explained in Table 28.1.

The Rapid Assessment

The rapid assessment requires 1 minute or less to complete. This type of assessment is often used as an initial assessment of a group of patients in a nursing assignment. The nurse uses the collected data to prioritize his or her actions and interventions. As a beginning student, the rapid assessment of a single patient is helpful in reducing anxiety because priorities can be established alone or in collaborative discussion with the faculty, preceptor, or staff. In addition, documentation of data from the rapid assessment establishes a baseline for ongoing patient interaction and care.

Sequence

Perform hand hygiene (NPSG.07.01.01).

Note isolation precautions, latex allergies, or fall precautions.

Enter the room.

TABLE 28.1	**Selected Hospital National Patient Safety Goals**
NPSG.01.01.01	Use at least two methods of patient identification. For example, use the patient's name *and* date of birth. The patient's room number is not an acceptable means of identification. Verification of the patient's identity ensures that each patient gets the correct medicine and treatment.
NPSG.03.06.01	Confirm the patient's medication regimen with the patient or the patient's primary caregiver. Record and report correct information about the patient's current medication regimen. Review any newly-prescribed medications and check for duplications, omissions, and contraindications. Prior to discharging the patient, provide written instructions for administration of each medication. Make sure the patient or the primary caregiver understands the directions for medication administration. Teach the patient or primary caregiver to bring an up-to-date medication list to every healthcare appointment.
NPSG.06.01.01	Make improvements to ensure that alarms on medical equipment are heard and responded to on time.
NPSG.07.01.01	Use the hand cleaning guidelines from the Centers for Disease Control and Prevention or the World Health Organization. Set goals for improving hand cleaning. Use the goals to improve hand cleaning.
NPSG.07.04.01	Use proven guidelines to prevent infection of the blood from central lines.
NPSG.07.05.01	Use proven guidelines to prevent infection after surgery.
NPSG.07.06.01	Use proven guidelines to prevent infections of the urinary tract that are caused by catheters.

Source: The Joint Commission. (2014). *Hospital National Patient Safety Goals.* Retrieved from http://www.jointcommission.org/assets/1/6/2014_HAP_NPSG_E.pdf.

Identify yourself and explain that you will be providing care for a given time period.

Ask the patient's name and identify the patient using at least two patient identifiers, such as wrist band and identification number (NPSG.01.01.01).

Note the location of the patient (bed, chair, bathroom).

If in bed, is it in the lowest position and is the call bell in reach?

Observe for level of consciousness.

Observe for signs of distress.

Observe skin color and respiratory effort.

Observe posture, facial expression, and symmetry.

Observe the patient's response to your introduction.

Observe speech for clarity.

Place a hand on the patient and assess skin temperature.

Note any equipment that is immediately visible.

Explain that you will return shortly.

Discuss with the faculty, preceptor, or staff, as needed.

Document findings.

The Routine or Initial Assessment

The routine or initial assessment is used to gather more in-depth data about a patient for whom care will be provided. Data gathered in the initial assessment will guide the direction of care and inform the nurse about the need for, as well as the type and frequency of, continuing assessment.

1. **Introduction**

    Perform hand hygiene (NPSG.07.01.01).

    Enter the room.

    Identify yourself and explain that you will be providing care for a given length of time.

    Ask the patient's name and identify the patient using at least two patient identifiers, such as wristband and identification number (NPSG.01.01.01, see Figure 28.1 ■).

    Note the patient's location (bed, chair, or bathroom).

    Note that call bell is in reach.

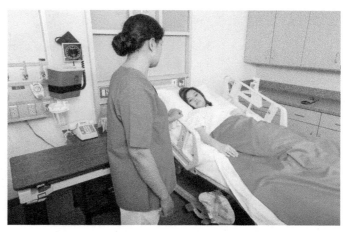

Figure 28.2 The nurse observing the patient in bed.

2. **General Appearance**

    Observe the following:

    Level of consciousness

    Respiratory status

    Skin color

    Nutritional status

    Facial expression—symmetry and appropriateness

    Body posture and position; relaxation, comfort, or pain

    Clarity, fluency, quality, and appropriateness of speech

    Hygiene and grooming

    Response to your introduction in relation to hearing and congruence with situation (see Figure 28.2 ■)

3. **Measurement**

    Temperature

    Pulses—radial, dorsalis pedis bilaterally

    Respiration

    Blood pressure (bilaterally if not contraindicated) (see Figure 28.3 ■)

    Pain—use of rating scale. Correlate with administration of pain medication if so indicated (NPSG.03.06.01).

    Pulse oximetry

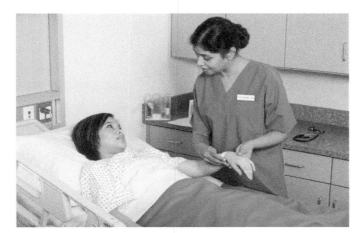

Figure 28.1 The nurse confirms the patient's identification.

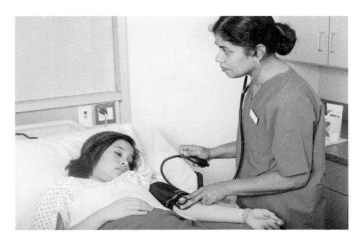

Figure 28.3 The nurse checking vital signs.

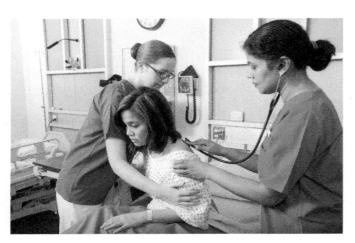

Figure 28.4 Auscultation of the posterior thorax.

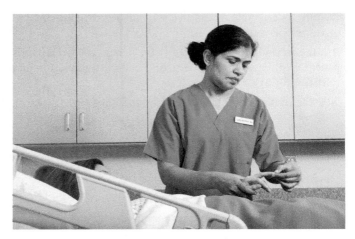

Figure 28.6 Assessment of capillary refill.

4. **Respiratory System**

   Respiratory effort

   Oxygen therapy—mask, nasal cannula; check placement and flowmeter (NPSG.06.01.01).

   Auscultate breath sounds—posterior and anterior. Seek assistance for positioning if required (see Figure 28.4 ■).

   Assess for coughing; if productive, assess sputum.

5. **Cardiovascular System**

   Auscultate apical pulse for rate and rhythm (see Figure 28.5 ■).

   Assess heart sounds in five auscultatory areas.

   Assess for capillary refill (see Figure 28.6 ■).

   Assess for peripheral edema.

   Assess intravenous (IV) site (NPSG.07.04.01), and if IV fluid is running, verify that it is the correct solution and rate (NPSG.03.06.01).

6. **Abdomen**

   Inspect for contour, skin color, and pulsations.

   Auscultate bowel sounds.

Palpate and percuss.

Assess the time of the most recent bowel elimination and/or flatus.

Assess drains, tubes, dressings, when indicated (NPSG.07.05.01, see Figure 28.7 ■).

7. **Genitourinary**

   Assess urine output—voiding—frequency and amount, or catheter drainage amount (NPSG.07.06.01).

   Assess the color and clarity of urine (see Figure 28.8 ■).

8. **Skin**

   Palpate skin temperature, moisture.

   Assess skin turgor (see Figure 28.9 ■).

   Assess for lesions.

   Assess wounds and incision lines if present (NPSG.07.05.01).

   Utilize standardized tools to determine risk for skin problems (scales/questionnaires).

   Assess functioning of any devices applied on the skin or used to prevent pressure (NPSG.06.01.01).

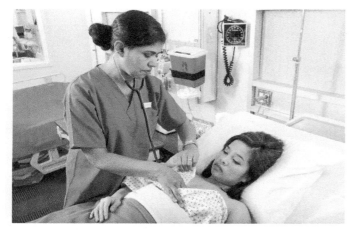

Figure 28.5 Auscultation of the apical pulse.

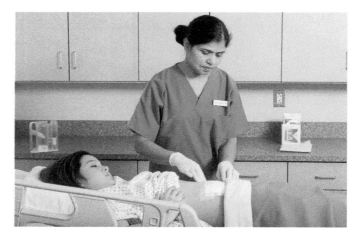

Figure 28.7 Assessment of an abdominal dressing.

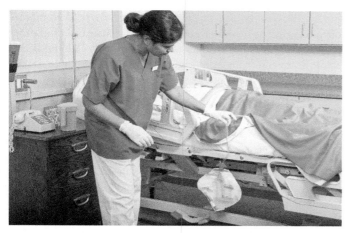

Figure 28.8 Assessment of urinary catheter drainage.

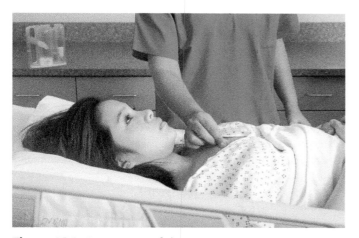

Figure 28.9 Assessment of skin turgor.

9. **Activity**

Assess symmetry and coordination of movements throughout the assessment.

Assess the ability to move self to sitting and standing positions.

Assess for presence of and use of assistive devices.

Use standardized measures to evaluate risk for falls.

Assess the environment for hazards related to mobility.

10. **Documentation**

Discuss with the faculty, preceptor, or staff, as needed (see Figure 28.10 ■).

Document findings according to agency policy.

Special Considerations

Some populations of patients require special care when hospitalized, including children, patients with communication barriers, and dying patients. In children, vital sign measurements may require smaller equipment than used for an adult, and normal ranges for vital signs vary with age and developmental level (see chapter 10 ∞). Children may need the nurse to use simpler

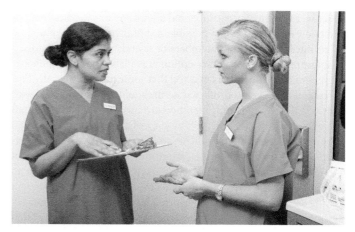

Figure 28.10 Discussion of patient assessment.

language to describe assessments and elicit responses, such as saying "tummy" or "belly" rather than "abdomen." Children may also need additional comfort measures during assessment such as holding hands with a parent or sitting on a parent's lap; conversation, toys, or television as a distraction; and manipulating or touching the equipment in order to calm fears about unknown objects (see Figure 28.11 ■). When possible, children should be given an opportunity to make choices about their care, and older children should be given the opportunity to be assessed without parents present (see chapter 7 ∞). Nurses must also consider the cultural or spiritual beliefs of the parents that may affect the assessment and care of children. Some populations may require care by a same-sex provider. Always consult with parents or guardians about assessment procedures before conducting an assessment on children. Determining which adult is the correct person with whom to discuss the child's care may require additional assessment and interviewing. Discussing a parent's observations of their child may also add subjective data to the assessment that will be valuable in providing appropriate care.

Patients with communication barriers include patients who do not speak English as their first language (ESL patients) and deaf or hard-of-hearing patients who require commuication through American Sign Language. Before assessing these patients, an interpreter should be found who can communicate with the patient to

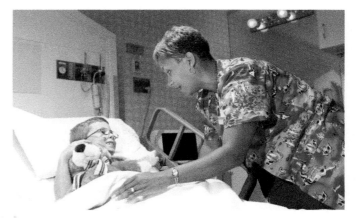

Figure 28.11 Children may need additional comfort measures while hospitalized.
Source: Jupiterimages/Stockbyte/Thinkstock/Getty Images

describe assessment procedures and obtain answers to assessment or interview questions. When possible, a staff member should be used as an interpreter. Family members or friends should only be used as interpreters when no other option is available, because some patients and family members may feel that some topics, especially topics related to the genitourinary system, should not be discussed with others in the family. Family members are also more likely than a staff member to change the interpretation of what the patient is saying if they do not agree with the patient's answer, or change the interpretation of what the provider is saying if they do not want the patient to know specific information about his or her condition. Using an appropriate interpreter can provide emotional care to the patient during assessments and help the provider obtain more accurate assessment information. When assessing these patients, confirm that the patient understands the assessment procedures and questions before beginning the assessment.

Dying patients and their family members also require special care in the hospital. Patients who are dying will require not only physical care but also emotional care. These patients should be treated with respect and be allowed to participate in choices about their care as much as possible. Assessments should include interview questions related to the patient's emotional state to determine if counseling or spiritual care is needed. Spending extra time with dying patients to help them feel like they are not alone may provide added comfort during this transition. Nurses should also assess the emotional state of family members and friends who are present to determine if emotional care or information about death, dying, and funeral preparations are needed. This is especially important if the patient is a child or if the death is sudden or unexpected. The nurse

should also ask the patient or family about advanced healthcare directives such as living wills or do-not-recuscitate orders in order to determine appropriate goals and interventions. Cultural beliefs about death and dying also need to be assessed and incorporated into any nursing interventions.

Summary

This chapter presents an overview of two types of assessments required when applying the nursing process in the care of the hospitalized patient. Hospitalized patients undergo frequent assessments; therefore, it is important that the nurse communicates effectively and uses physical assessment techniques with efficiency and competence. Two types of assessments of the hospitalized patient are presented in the chapter. The first is a rapid assessment, requiring 1 minute or less to complete. This type of assessment is often used as an initial assessment to prioritize actions and interventions. The second type of assessment is a routine or initial assessment and is used to gather more in-depth data about a patient for whom care will be provided.

The chapter reminds you that analysis of the data requires critical thinking and application of knowledge about health, illness, and the factors that influence a person's response to changes in his or her health status. Only with detailed assessment and accurate analysis of data can nursing care plans be developed to meet the specific needs of the patient. In addition, special considerations are needed when assessing some patients, including children, patients with communication barriers, and dying patients.

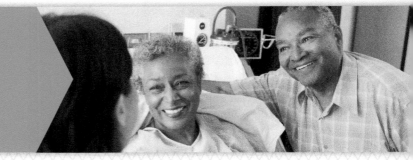

Application Through Critical Thinking

▌ Case Study

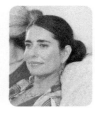

Mrs. Janelle Hoskins is a 34-year-old admitted to the emergency department via ambulance following a bicycle accident. The assessment in the emergency department revealed that Mrs. Hoskins was alert and oriented, stating she had pain "all over" at a level of 8 on a scale of 0 to 10. Further assessment and diagnostic testing revealed a fractured left tibia and fibula, abrasions on both hands, contusions in the chest and abdomen, and a deep laceration on the right lower extremity lateral to the upper

border of the patella. Mrs. Hoskins denies any history of acute or chronic illness, takes medication for seasonal allergies, uses oral birth control medication, and takes one ibuprofen for occasional pain or headache. She denies drug or alcohol use and has never been hospitalized.

Mrs. Hoskins was admitted to the hospital and underwent an open reduction–internal fixation (ORIF) of the fracture of the tibia and fibula and closure of the right lower-leg laceration. Her postsurgical treatment plan includes bed rest, use of an incentive spirometer, medication for pain, increasing from a liquid to regular diet as tolerated, intravenous therapy with dextrose in saline at a slow rate, and Foley catheter drainage.

You, a student nurse, have been assigned to care for Mrs. Hoskins 26 hours postsurgery. You received information about Mrs. Hoskins and her diagnoses and treatments and had an opportunity to prepare for her care. A brief discussion about her injuries, surgery, and treatments occurred in a preclinical conference.

Your first encounter with Mrs. Hoskins included a rapid assessment. Upon entering the room, you introduced yourself and told Mrs. Hoskins that you would be providing her care. You made some observations. Your findings were as follows:

Mrs. Hoskins was supine in bed; her eyes opened when you entered the room. She nodded to acknowledge your introduction. While checking the identification band, you noted hot skin. The patient's face appeared flushed. Her breathing was shallow. Mrs. Hoskins was supine and held herself in a rigid posture. She had covers over her; the left leg appeared to be elevated on a pillow. An IV was running via a pump and urine was in the collection bag. Mrs. Hoskins said, "Okay, I'll be here" very quietly when you explained that you would return shortly to begin assessment and care.

You will now meet with your faculty to discuss your findings and proceed with clinical interventions for Mrs. Hoskins.

Complete Documentation

SUBJECTIVE DATA: Acknowledged your presence by opening eyes, spoke in quiet voice.

OBJECTIVE DATA: Supine, face flushed, hot skin to touch, shallow breathing, supine, rigid posture, left leg elevated, IV running, Foley catheter draining.

Critical Thinking Questions

1. What assessments would you expect to complete in a rapid assessment for Mrs. Hoskins?

2. What is the difference between a rapid assessment and a routine or initial assessment?

3. What information will your faculty expect you to provide about the findings?

4. How will those findings influence your continued assessment of the patient?

5. What further information do you need about findings from your rapid assessment?

Upon your return to Mrs. Hoskins bedside, you carried out further assessment and documented the findings as follows:

SUBJECTIVE DATA: "I feel awful, I am afraid to move, I hurt all over; it hurts to move, to breathe, and even when someone touches me." Asking for pain medication. States "then I can sleep, I am so exhausted. Please don't tell me you have to do anything much, I can't take it." States "I don't want to eat or drink, I'll take one sip of water if you insist." When asked if she had used the incentive spirometer, she replied "that thing, I don't even know what it is or why it is here."

Pain assessment:

Onset: "It has been hurting all along."

Location: "Left leg and chest."

Duration: "My leg keeps getting worse and my chest hurts a lot more than it did during the night."

Characteristics: "Left leg 8, chest 6 on scale of 0 to 10. It is throbbing and pressure."

Aggravating factors: "Oh, if I try to move everything hurts and my chest hurts when I breathe."

Relieving factors: "It seems to help if I stay still; the medication helped a lot."

Treatment: "I had the medication—I don't know when I had it, I need more now."

Impact on ADLs: "I just don't want to do anything; don't ask me to."

Coping strategies: "I just keep still, try to sleep, and ask for medication."

Emotional impact: "This pain is wearing me out, I want it to go away, I can't think about anything and I should be finding out about when I will be able to get out of here, right now, I don't care."

OBJECTIVE DATA: Temperature 100.2 oral. B/P 128/82, pulse 88, RR 24, shallow. Pulse Oximetry 95. Nail bed refill immediate. Auscultation of the lungs is limited to the anterior chest, sounds are distant and difficult to assess. Abdomen is soft with rare bowel sounds. Skin dry with erythema, lips dry. Ecchymosis on chest and abdomen, dressing right lower leg dry and intact, left leg in a cast to thigh. Toes warm bilaterally, no edema.

Foley draining dark yellow urine, 60 mL in collection bag. IV site intact and dextrose in saline running as ordered. Patient lies still throughout the assessment. Answers questions slowly, grimaces when moving.

Prepare Teaching Plan

LEARNING NEED: Mrs. Hoskins was admitted to the hospital following a bicycle accident. She sustained several injuries. She has contusions to the chest and abdomen and had surgery to close a laceration on her right leg and to repair a fracture of the left tibia and fibula. The data indicate a need to learn about use of the incentive spirometer.

GOAL: Mrs. Hoskins will effectively use the incentive spirometer to reduce risks of respiratory problems.

OBJECTIVES: At the completion of the learning session Mrs. Hoskins will be able to:

1. Describe the purpose of incentive spirometry.

2. Correctly demonstrate use of the incentive spirometer.

3. Follow the recommendations for frequency of use of the incentive spirometer.

APPLICATION OF OBJECTIVE 2: Correctly demonstrate use of the incentive spirometer

Content	Teaching Strategy and Rationale	Evaluation
<ul><li>Use a sitting position.</li><li>Hold the spirometer in an upright position.</li><li>Exhale normally.</li><li>Seal the lips tightly around the mouthpiece.</li><li>Breathe in slowly to elevate the balls or cylinder; hold breath for 2 seconds in first attempts, increasing to 6 seconds, and hold the ball or cylinder elevated if possible.</li><li>Avoid brisk, shallow breaths. Long, slow breaths, keeping the ball of cylinder elevated, achieve the greatest lung expansion.</li><li>A nose clip can be used if you have difficulty breathing only through your mouth.</li><li>Remove the mouthpiece and exhale normally.</li><li>Cough after use of the incentive spirometer.</li><li>Relax and take several normal breaths before using the spirometer again.</li><li>Clean the mouthpiece with water and dry after use.</li></ul>	<ul><li>Demonstration and practice allow hands-on experience, repetition, and immediate feedback.</li></ul>	<ul><li>Mrs. Hoskins follows each step of the procedure correctly.</li></ul>

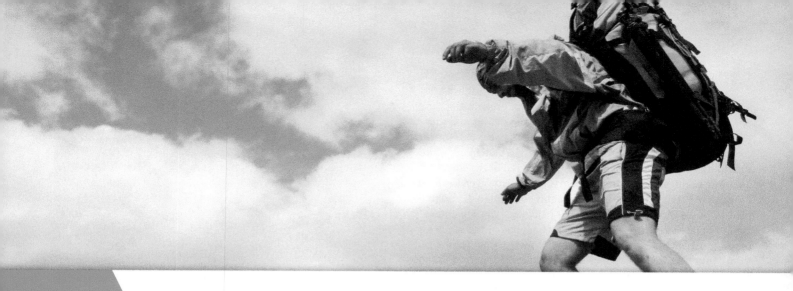

The Complete Health Assessment

▶ Learning Outcomes

Upon completion of the chapter, you will be able to:

1. Use professional communication skills to gather subjective data in a health history.

2. Apply knowledge and skill in gathering objective data in a general survey and physical assessment of a patient.

3. Apply critical thinking to the complete health assessment.

This chapter is designed to help you perform a complete health assessment. Conducting a complete health assessment requires effective communication, organization, use of knowledge from the natural and behavioral sciences and nursing, efficient and accurate performance of physical assessment techniques, recognition of verbal and nonverbal patient cues, and the abilities to interpret and document findings. For the student, a complete health assessment may seem difficult. However, learning to conduct a complete health assessment is essential in developing plans to meet the healthcare needs of patients. Planning and organization are steps to a successful assessment. Plan the sequence of steps; gather the necessary equipment; review documentation forms; and have pen and paper or a computer or tablet ready to record data or to write reminders or notes for yourself to clarify points, to prompt follow-up in specific areas, and to help in orderly and concise documentation.

The complete health assessment includes the interview, general survey, assessment of vital signs, and physical assessment of all body systems. Complete health assessments may be needed for several reasons, including annual physicals, well-child checkups, and sports exams. Complete health assessments may also be necessary when patients have symptoms with an unknown or uncommon cause; the complete health assessment can then be used to help diagnose an acute or chronic condition that requires treatment. Recall that findings are influenced by a number of factors including age, gender, developmental level, genetic makeup, culture, religion, psychologic and emotional status, and the patient's internal and external environments.

The following pages describe one sequence for the complete health assessment. There are a variety of sequences that may be employed. This sequence minimizes the number of position changes for the patient. The complete health assessment should be approached with confidence and a professional demeanor. This important part of professional nursing practice will become easier with practice.

The complete health assessment begins with the first patient encounter. Observations made during your introduction and while settling down for the interview provide data as part of the general survey and may provide cues about the patient. Always begin by introducing yourself, stating the purpose of the complete health assessment, and including assurances regarding the confidentiality of the information. Follow guidelines for patient safety and use Standard Precautions throughout the assessment. In the initial encounter and during the interview, the patient is clothed and sits facing the nurse.

Sequence

1. The Health History

Complete the interview (see Figure 29.1 ■).

Include all areas and address cultural and spiritual assessments.

For children, ask about the child's grade level and school.

The data are subjective; document in the patient's own words.

2. Appearance and Mental Status

Compare stated age with appearance.

Assess level of consciousness.

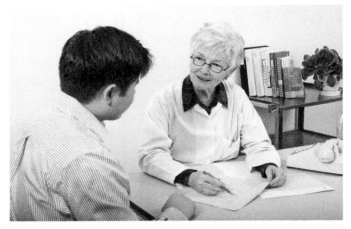

Figure 29.1 The patient participating in the health history.

Observe body build, height and weight in relation to age, lifestyle, and health.

Observe facial expression, posture, and position and observe mobility.

Observe overall hygiene and grooming.

Note body odor and breath odor.

Note signs of health or illness (skin color, signs of pain).

Assess attitude, attentiveness, affect, mood, and appropriateness of responses.

Listen for quantity, quality, relevance, and organization of speech.

At the completion of the interview, have the patient change into an examination gown. Provide privacy to the patient. Have the patient empty the bladder; if required, provide a container and instructions for collecting a urine specimen.

3. Measurements

Measure height.

Measure weight (see Figure 29.2 ■).

Measure skinfold thickness.

Calculate the body mass index (BMI).

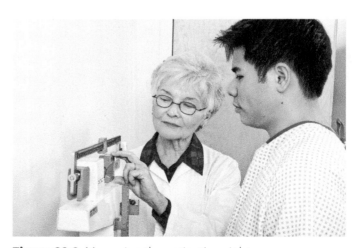

Figure 29.2 Measuring the patient's weight.

Assess vision with the Snellen Chart and Jaeger Card (cranial nerve II). For children who cannot read, assess vision using age-appropriate symbols or other available tools.

4. **Vital Signs**

Assess the radial pulses.

Count respirations.

Take the temperature.

Measure the blood pressure bilaterally.

Assess for pain. For young children, use a faces pain rating scale rather than a numerical scale.

5. **Skin, Hair, and Nails**

Inspect the skin on the face, neck, and upper and lower extremities (other skin areas will be assessed as part of the systems assessment).

Inspect for color and uniformity of color.

Inspect and palpate skin.

Palpate for skin temperature, moisture, turgor, and edema (see Figure 29.3 ■).

Inspect, palpate, measure, and describe lesions.

Inspect the hair on the scalp and body.

Palpate scalp hair for texture and moisture.

Inspect the fingernails for curvature, angle, and color.

Palpate the nails for texture and capillary refill.

6. **Head, Neck, and Related Lymphatics**

Inspect the skull for size, shape, and symmetry.

Observe facial expressions and symmetry of facial features and movements (cranial nerves V and VII).

Palpate the skull and lymph nodes of the head and neck (see Figure 29.4 ■).

Palpate the muscles of the face (cranial nerve V).

Assess facial response to sensory stimulation (cranial nerve V).

Inspect the neck for symmetry, pulsations, swelling, or masses.

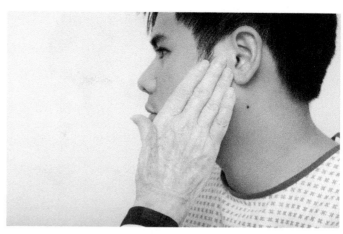

Figure 29.4 Palpating the preauricular lymph nodes.

Assess range of motion and strength of muscles against resistance. Observe as the patient moves the head forward and back and side to side and shrugs the shoulders (cranial nerve XI).

Palpate the trachea.

Palpate the thyroid for symmetry and masses.

Palpate and auscultate the carotid arteries, one at a time (see Figure 29.5 ■).

7. **Eyes**

Inspect the external eye.

Inspect the pupils for color, size, shape, and equality.

Test the visual fields (cranial nerve II).

Test extraocular movements (cranial nerves III, IV, VI).

Test pupillary reaction to light and accommodation (cranial nerve III) (see Figure 29.6 ■).

Darken the room and use the ophthalmoscope to assess the red reflex, optic disc, retinal vessels, retinal background, macula, and fovea centralis.

8. **Ears, Nose, Mouth, and Throat**

Inspect the external ears.

Palpate the auricle and tragus of each ear.

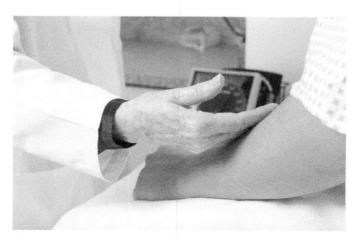

Figure 29.3 Palpating skin moisture.

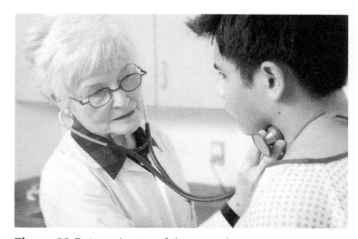

Figure 29.5 Auscultation of the carotid artery.

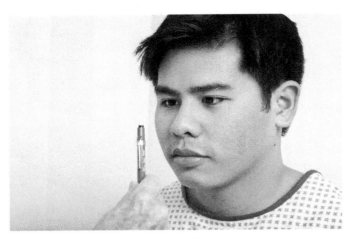

Figure 29.6 Testing for accommodation.

Use an otoscope to inspect each external ear canal and the tympanic membrane (see Figure 29.7 ■).

Test hearing using the whisper, Weber, and Rinne tests (cranial nerve VIII).

Assess patency of the nares.

Test sense of smell (cranial nerve I).

Use a nasal speculum or otoscope with speculum attachment to inspect the internal nose.

Palpate the nose and sinuses.

Palpate the temporal artery.

Palpate the temporomandibular joint (TMJ) as the patient opens and closes the mouth.

Inspect the lips.

Use a penlight to inspect the tongue, palates, buccal mucosa, gums, teeth, the opening to the salivary glands, tonsils, and oropharynx.

Test the sense of taste (cranial nerve VII).

Wearing gloves, palpate the tongue, gums, and floor of the mouth.

Observe the uvula for position and mobility as the patient says "ah," and test the gag reflex (cranial nerves IX, X).

Observe as the patient protrudes the tongue (cranial nerve XII).

9. **The Respiratory System, Breasts, and Axillae**

Inspect the skin of the posterior chest.

Inspect the posterior chest for symmetry, musculoskeletal development, and thoracic configuration.

Observe respiratory excursion.

Auscultate posterior lung sounds.

Palpate and percuss the costovertebral angle for tenderness.

Palpate for thoracic expansion and tactile fremitus.

Inspect and palpate the scapula and spine.

Percuss the posterior thorax (see Figure 29.8 ■).

Percuss for diaphragmatic excursion.

Inspect the skin of the anterior chest.

Inspect the anterior chest for symmetry and musculoskeletal development.

Assess range of motion and movement against resistance of the upper extremities (see Figure 29.9 ■).

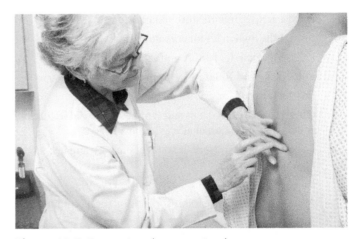

Figure 29.8 Percussing the posterior thorax.

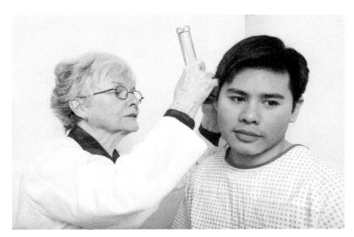

Figure 29.7 Using the otoscope.

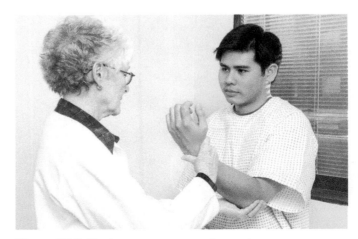

Figure 29.9 Testing movement against resistance.

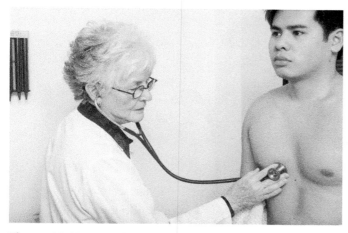

Figure 29.10 Auscultating the anterior thorax.

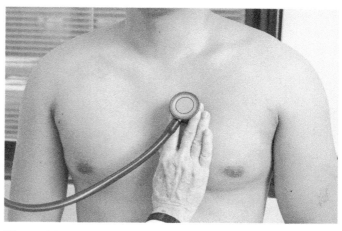

Figure 29.12 Using the bell to auscultate the pulmonic area.

Inspect the breasts for symmetry, mobility, masses, dimpling, and nipple retraction. Ask the post-pubescent female to lift arms over her head, press her hands on her hips, and lean forward as you inspect.

Auscultate anterior lung sounds (see Figure 29.10 ■).

Palpate the axillary, supraclavicular, and infraclavicular lymph nodes.

Palpate the breasts and nipples (see Figure 29.11 ■).

Palpate the anterior chest.

Percuss the anterior thorax.

10. The Cardiovascular System

Inspect the neck for jugular pulsations or distention.

Inspect and palpate the chest for pulsations, lifts, or heaves.

Use the bell and diaphragm of the stethoscope to auscultate for heart sounds (Figure 29.12 ■).

At each area of auscultation distinguish the rate, rhythm, and location of S1 and S2 sounds.

Palpate the apical pulse and note the intensity and location.

11. The Abdomen

Inspect the skin of the abdomen.

Inspect the abdomen for symmetry, contour, and movement or pulsation.

Auscultate the abdomen for bowel sounds.

Auscultate the abdomen for vascular sounds.

Palpate the liver, spleen, and kidneys.

Palpate to determine if tenderness, masses, or distention are present.

Palpate the inguinal region for pulses, lymph nodes, and presence of hernias.

Percuss the abdomen in all quadrants (see Figure 29.13 ■).

Percuss the abdomen to determine liver and spleen size.

12. The Musculoskeletal System

Test range of motion and strength in the hips, knees, ankles, and feet (see Figure 29.14 ■).

Assist the patient to a standing position.

Inspect the skin of the posterior legs.

Perform the Romberg test.

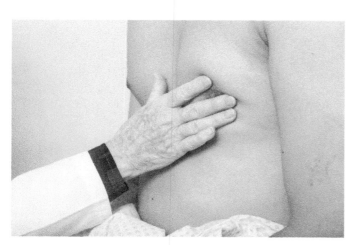

Figure 29.11 Palpating the nipple.

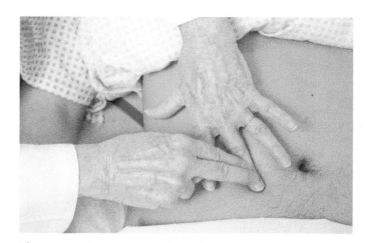

Figure 29.13 Percussion of the abdomen.

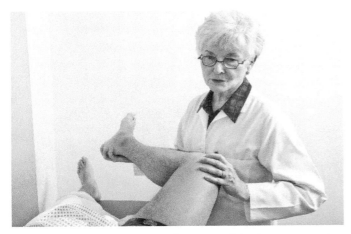

Figure 29.14 Testing range of motion of the lower extremity.

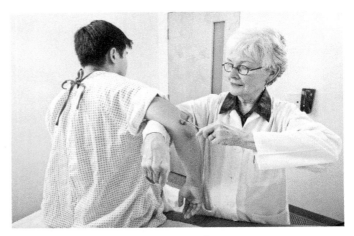

Figure 29.16 Testing the triceps reflex.

Observe as the patient walks in a natural gait.

Observe the patient walking heel to toe.

Observe the patient stand on the right foot, then the left foot with eyes closed.

Observe as the patient performs a shallow knee bend.

Stand behind the patient and observe the spine as the patient touches the toes.

Test range of motion of the spine.

13. The Neurologic System

Assess sensory function. Include light touch, tactile location, pain, temperature, vibratory sense, kinesthetic sensation, and tactile discrimination (see Figure 29.15 ■).

Test position sense.

Test cerebellar function with finger-to-nose test.

Test cerebellar function with heel-shin test.

Test stereognosis and graphesthesia.

Test tendon reflexes bilaterally and compare (see Figure 29.16 ■). Recall that reflexes in newborns will differ from reflexes in children and adults.

14A. The Female Reproductive System

Inspect the amount, distribution, and characteristics of pubic hair.

Inspect the clitoris, urethral orifice, and vaginal orifice (see Figure 29.17 ■).

Palpate Bartholin's glands.

Assess the integrity of the pelvic musculature.

Insert a speculum and examine the internal genitalia.

Inspect the cervix for shape of the os, color, size, and position.

For post-pubescent females, obtain a specimen for a Papinicolaou smear.

Inspect the vaginal walls.

Perform a bimanual examination.

Palpate the rectum and rectovaginal walls.

Observe and test stool for occult blood.

14B. The Male Reproductive System

Observe the amount, distribution, and characteristics of pubic hair.

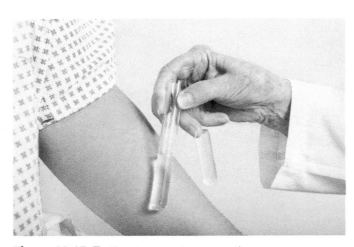

Figure 29.15 Testing temperature sensation.

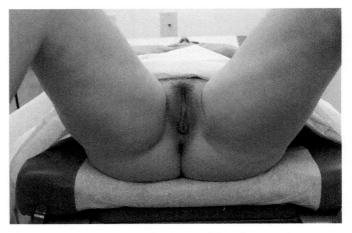

Figure 29.17 Inspecting the external female genitalia.

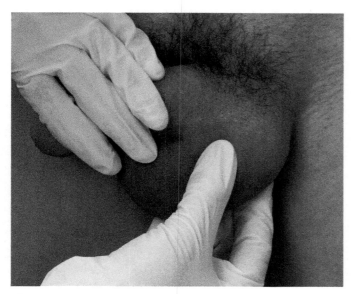

Figure 29.18 Palpating the testes.

Inspect the penile shaft, glans, and urethral meatus.

Observe the color and position of the urethral meatus.

Inspect the scrotum for appearance, size, and symmetry.

Palpate the scrotum, testicles, epididymis, and spermatic cord. If a mass is present, then transilluminate (see Figure 29.18 ■).

Inspect the sacrococcygeal and perianal areas.

Palpate the rectal walls and prostate gland.

Observe any stool and test for occult blood.

Document findings from the comprehensive health assessment according to agency policy. Include all concepts of patient safety, Standard Precautions, and professional standards in the documentation of assessment data. Documentation is important; the data documented from the complete assessment establish a baseline for ongoing patient interaction and care.

Summary

This chapter presents information related to the complete health assessment. This assessment requires application of knowledge and skills acquired in the study and practice of the individual elements of the interview, general survey, assessment of vital signs, and physical assessment of all body systems. You are reminded to consider the characteristics of the individual patient, including, but not limited to, age, gender, and developmental level in planning and organizing your approach to the assessment. One sequence, minimizing the number of position changes for the patient, is presented. The sequence begins with the first patient encounter and then follows an organized approach to collection of subjective and objective data. Conducting a complete health assessment becomes easier with practice, and learning to conduct a complete health assessment is essential to meeting the specific healthcare needs of patients of all ages and in varied settings.

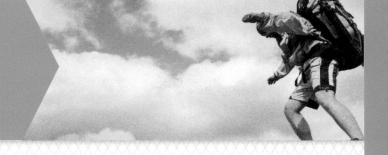

Application Through Critical Thinking

▶ Case Study

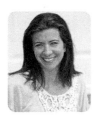

Mrs. Amparo Bellisimo arrives at the health center. In her phone call to arrange for a visit, she stated she had abdominal pain and some coughing. Mrs. Bellisimo was last seen at the center 9 months ago for a complete health assessment. In preparation for her assessment, her health history was reviewed (see, for example, "Documentation of a Health History" in chapter 8 ∞). Mrs. Bellisimo is not in acute distress and states she is comfortable enough to answer questions about all parts of her health since her previous assessment. The nurse completes the health history and performs a general survey and measurement of vital signs.

▶ Complete Documentation

SUBJECTIVE DATA: Health History

Date: March 24th

Biographic Data: Unchanged

Present Health/Illness: Reason for seeking care: "I have some stomach pain, I have a little cough, I've had diarrhea," and very quietly she tells you, "I have some itching in my private area, by my vagina. This all started last week. We were on vacation and I got sick. I went to an urgi-center and they said I had sinusitis and gave me an antibiotic. I had been having pressure in my head, my nose was congested, I had a bad headache and earache. At first I thought I was allergic to something, but it was really uncomfortable and I didn't want to ruin our vacation, so I went to see if I could get medicine. I have been taking the antibiotic for 5 days and some saline nose drops, but I really feel awful, and now I have to go back to work."

Health Beliefs and Practices: Denies change

Health Patterns: Denies change

Medications: No change except antibiotic 5 days, saline nose drops 5 days

Past History: No change

Family History: Mother recently diagnosed with hypertension

Psychosocial History: No change

Review of Systems: Denies changes except as noted in reason for visit

> **Head and Neck:** Sinusitis—headache, pressure, runny nose, earache—improved since antibiotic
>
> **Respiratory:** Cough
>
> > **Onset:** It started with the sinus thing but is worse.
> >
> > **Location:** A throaty and chest cough.
> >
> > **Duration:** I just seem to cough a lot, but nothing comes up.
> >
> > **Characteristics:** I have a little clear mucus in my throat in the morning; it's a dry cough.
> >
> > **Aggravating factors:** I don't know—it just comes on sometimes.
> >
> > **Relieving factors:** Being still.
> >
> > **Treatment:** I haven't really done anything; I figured I better see what's what.
> >
> > **Impact on ADLs:** I am okay but really too tired to do much.
> >
> > **Coping strategies:** I'm trying to be calm; my husband has been really good about all of it and he brought me here.
> >
> > **Emotional impact:** I'm worried that I have something serious, I'm a little nervous.

> **Abdomen**
>
> 1. Stomach pain
>
> > **Onset:** 3 days ago.
> >
> > **Location:** Lower stomach, sometimes one side or the other but right now mostly the left.
> >
> > **Duration:** It hurts most of the time.
> >
> > **Characteristics:** Sore, achy 3 to 5 on a scale of 0 to 10.
> >
> > **Aggravating factors:** I'm not sure; it may be with the diarrhea.
> >
> > **Relieving factors:** When I'm still and not coughing or going to the bathroom it is okay.
> >
> > **Treatment:** I really did not know what to do.
> >
> > **ICE**—As above.
>
> 2. Diarrhea
>
> > **Onset:** 4 days ago—after I was at the urgi-center.
> >
> > **Duration:** It was once a day; now I have had diarrhea about 2 or 3 times a day.
> >
> > **Characteristics:** Light brown watery stuff; depends on what I eat.
> >
> > **Aggravating factors:** I really don't know—it seems eating may cause me to go, but not always.
> >
> > **Relieving factors:** I haven't done anything—it's just happening.
> >
> > **Treatment:** I haven't taken anything—I was always told to let it out.
> >
> > **ICE**—As above.

> **Reproductive**—Vaginal itch, LMP 2 weeks ago
>
> > **Onset:** 2 days ago.
> >
> > **Location:** Vagina and all around.
> >
> > **Duration:** It's itchy almost all the time—it seems to be getting worse.
> >
> > **Characteristics:** Itching and burning.
> >
> > **Aggravating factors:** Nothing really.
> >
> > **Relieving factors:** It seems a little better after I shower.
> >
> > **Treatment:** I didn't know what to do.
> >
> > **ICE**—As above.

OBJECTIVE DATA: Mrs. Bellisimo is alert and oriented with clear speech; uses concise and clear responses to questions. She is fully mobile and has a steady gait. Her skin color is suntanned with pink undertones; she has bluish skin color below the eyes. She is well-groomed and admits to being nervous. She coughed occasionally during the interview and held her abdomen during the cough. The cough was dry and the episodes were 10 to 20 seconds long.

Vital Signs: Temperature 98.8 oral, B/P 118/74, Pulse 88, RR 20. Pain—abdomen 3 to 5 (scale 0 to 10). Height 5′2″ Weight 122 lb. Skin warm and dry

Mrs. Bellisimo voided and provided a urine specimen as she changed into a gown for the physical assessment.

▶ Critical Thinking Questions

1. Identify the pattern/approach you would use to conduct the physical assessment of Mrs. Bellisimo.

2. Describe any changes required for any particular body system and the reason for the change.

3. Identify additional information that may be helpful in planning care for Mrs. Bellisimo.

4. What situations require complete health assessments?

5. What factors influence findings in the physical assessment?

▶ Prepare Teaching Plan

LEARNING NEED: The data in this case study include symptoms of diarrhea and vaginal itching in a patient receiving antibiotic therapy. This indicates that Mrs. Bellisimo may not have knowledge about the impact of antibiotics on the physiology of the body systems. Mrs. Bellisimo needs to learn more about antibiotic therapy and how to decrease risks associated with antibiotics.

GOAL: Mrs. Bellisimo will incorporate measures to reduce risks of complications associated with antibiotic therapy.

OBJECTIVES: At the completion of this learning session, Mrs. Bellisimo will be able to:

1. Describe the impact of antibiotics on body systems.

2. Identify measures to reduce the risk of complications associated with antibiotic therapy.

APPLICATION OF OBJECTIVE 1: Describe the impact of antibiotics on body systems		
Content	**Teaching Strategy**	**Evaluation**
• Antibiotics alter the normal flora (microorganisms/bacteria) in the bowel and vagina and can affect the pH of vaginal secretions, leaving the female more susceptible to yeast infections.	One-to-one discussion encourages learner participation, permits reinforcement of content, and is appropriate for sensitive subject matter.	Mrs. Bellisimo can describe the impact of antibiotics in her own words.

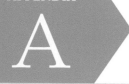

Standard Precautions for Blood and Bodily Fluid Exposure

Background

Standard Precautions are designed to reduce the risk of transmission of microorganisms from both recognized and unrecognized sources of infection in hospitals. Standard Precautions apply to (1) blood; (2) all body fluids, secretions, and excretions except sweat, regardless of whether or not they contain visible blood; (3) nonintact skin; and (4) mucous membranes.

Standard Precautions

Use Standard Precautions, or the equivalent, for the care of all patients.

A. Hand Hygiene

1. Wash hands after touching blood, body fluids, secretions, excretions, and contaminated items, whether or not gloves are worn. Wash hands immediately after gloves are removed, between patient contacts, and when otherwise indicated to avoid transfer of microorganisms to other patients or environments. It may be necessary to wash hands between tasks and procedures on the same patient to prevent cross-contamination of different body sites.

2. If hands are not visibly contaminated, or following removal of visible contaminants with plain (nonantimicrobial) soap and water, the preferred method of hand hygiene is with an alcohol-based hand rub. Healthcare providers should be aware that frequent use of an alcohol-based hand rub following handwashing with a nonantimicrobial soap may increase the incidence of dermatitis. As an alternative, healthcare providers may use plain (nonantimicrobial) soap and water for routine hand hygiene.

3. Use an antimicrobial agent or a waterless antiseptic agent for specific circumstances (e.g., control of outbreaks or hyperendemic infections), as defined by the infection control program.

B. Gloves

Wear gloves (clean, nonsterile gloves are adequate) when there is potential for touching blood, body fluids, secretions, excretions, and contaminated items. Put on clean gloves just before touching mucous membranes and nonintact skin. Change gloves between tasks and procedures on the same patient after contact with material that may contain a high concentration of microorganisms. Remove gloves promptly after use, before touching noncontaminated items and environmental surfaces, and before going to another patient, and perform hand hygiene immediately to avoid transfer of microorganisms to other patients or environments.

C. Mask, Eye Protection, Face Shield

Wear a mask and eye protection or a face shield to protect mucous membranes of the eyes, nose, and mouth during procedures and patient-care activities that are likely to generate splashes or sprays of blood, body fluids, secretions, and excretions, including during endotracheal intubation and when suctioning respiratory secretions.

D. Gown

Wear a gown (a clean, nonsterile gown is adequate) to protect skin and to prevent soiling of clothing during procedures and patient-care activities that are likely to generate splashes or sprays of blood, body fluids, secretions, or excretions. Select a gown that is appropriate for the activity and amount of fluid likely to be encountered. Remove a soiled gown as promptly as possible, and wash hands to avoid transfer of microorganisms to other patients or environments.

E. Patient Care Equipment

Handle used patient care equipment soiled with blood, body fluids, secretions, and excretions in a manner that prevents skin and mucous membrane exposures, contamination of clothing, and transfer of microorganisms to other patients and environments. Ensure that reusable equipment is not used for the care of another patient until it has been cleaned and reprocessed appropriately. Ensure that single-use items are discarded properly. Follow manufacturers' instructions for cleaning of all reusable equipment, including computers and personal digital assistants (PDAs).

F. Environmental Controls

Ensure that the hospital has adequate procedures for the routine care, cleaning, and disinfection of environmental surfaces, beds, bedrails, bedside equipment, and other frequently touched surfaces, and ensure that these procedures are being followed.

G. Linen

Handle, transport, and process used linen soiled with blood, body fluids, secretions, and excretions in a manner that prevents skin and mucous membrane exposures and contamination of clothing, and that avoids transfer of microorganisms to other patients and environments.

H. Occupational Health and Bloodborne Pathogens

1. Take care to prevent injuries when using needles, scalpels, and other sharp instruments or devices; when handling sharp instruments after procedures; when cleaning used instruments; and

when disposing of used needles. Never recap used needles, or otherwise manipulate them using both hands, or use any other technique that involves directing the point of a needle toward any part of the body; rather, use either a one-handed "scoop" technique or a mechanical device designed for holding the needle sheath. Do not remove used needles from disposable syringes by hand, and do not bend, break, or otherwise manipulate used needles by hand. Place used disposable syringes and needles, scalpel blades, and other sharp items in appropriate puncture-resistant containers, which are located as close as practical to the area in which the items were used, and place reusable syringes and needles in a puncture-resistant container for transport to the reprocessing area.

2. Use mouthpieces, resuscitation bags, or other ventilation devices as an alternative to mouth-to-mouth resuscitation methods in areas where the need for resuscitation is predictable.

I. Patient Placement

Place a patient who contaminates the environment or who does not (or cannot be expected to) assist in maintaining appropriate hygiene or environmental control in a private room. If a private room is not available, consult with infection control professionals regarding patient placement or other alternatives.

Source: Excerpted from Guidelines for Isolation Precautions in Hospitals, January 1996. Centers for Disease and Precaution http://www.cdc.gov/ncidod/hip/ISOLAT/std_prec_excerpt.htm. *These precautions last reviewed by CDC in 2007.*
Source: Excerpted from Guideline for Isolation Precautions: Preventing Transmission of Infectious Agents in Healthcare Settings 2007. Centers for Disease Control and Prevention. http://www.cdc.gov/hicpac/pdf/isolation/Isolation2007.pdf

Standard Precautions[†]

Use Standard Precautions for the care of all patients.

Airborne Precautions

In addition to Standard Precautions, use Airborne Precautions for patients known or suspected to have serious illnesses transmitted by airborne droplet nuclei. Examples of such illnesses include:

- Measles
- Varicella (including disseminated zoster)[†]
- Tuberculosis‡

Droplet Precautions

In addition to Standard Precautions, use Droplet Precautions for patients known or suspected to have serious illnesses transmitted by large particle droplets. Examples of such illnesses include:

- Invasive *Haemophilus influenzae* type B disease, including meningitis, pneumonia, epiglottitis, and sepsis
- Invasive *Neisseria meningitidis* disease, including meningitis, pneumonia, and sepsis

Other serious bacterial respiratory infections spread by droplet transmission, including:

- Diphtheria (pharyngeal)
- Mycoplasma pneumonia
- Pertussis (whooping cough)
- Pneumonic plague (until patients have received 48 hours of therapy)
- Streptococcal (group A) pharyngitis, pneumonia, or scarlet fever in infants and young children

Serious viral infections spread by droplet transmission, including:

- Adenovirus[†]
- Influenza

- Mumps
- Parvovirus B19
- Rubella

Contact Precautions

In addition to Standard Precautions, use Contact Precautions for patients known or suspected to have serious illnesses easily transmitted by direct patient contact or by contact with items in the patient's environment. Examples of such illnesses include:

Gastrointestinal, respiratory, skin, or wound infections or colonization with multidrug-resistant bacteria judged by the infection control program, based on current state, regional, or national recommendations, to be of special clinical and epidemiologic significance.

Enteric infections with a low infectious dose or prolonged environmental survival, including:

- *Clostridium difficile*
- For diapered or incontinent patients: enterohemorrhagic *Escherichia coli* O157:H7, *Shigella*, hepatitis A, or rotavirus

Respiratory syncytial virus, parainfluenza virus, or enteroviral infections in infants and young children

Skin infections that are highly contagious or that may occur on dry skin, including:

- Diphtheria (cutaneous)
- Herpes simplex virus (neonatal or mucocutaneous)
- Impetigo
- Major (noncontained) abscesses, cellulitis, or decubiti
- Pediculosis
- Scabies
- Staphylococcal furunculosis in infants and young children
- Zoster (disseminated or in the immunocompromised host)[†]

Viral/hemorrhagic conjunctivitis

- Viral hemorrhagic infections (Ebola, Lassa, or Marburg)

Source: Excerpted from Guideline for Isolation Precautions: Preventing Transmission of Infectious Agents in Healthcare Settings 2007. Centers for Disease Control and Prevention. http://www.cdc.gov/hicpac/pdf/isolation/Isolation2007.pdf
† Certain infections require more than one type of precaution.

Blood Pressure Standards for Girls Ages 1 to 17 Years

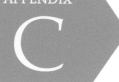

TABLE C.1 **Blood Pressure Levels for Girls by Age and Height Percentile. Use the child's height percentile for the age and sex from a standard growth chart. A blood pressure value at 50th percentile for the child's age, sex, and height percentile is considered the midpoint of the normal range. A reading above the 95th percentile indicates hypertension.**

AGE (YEAR)	BP PERCENTILE	Systolic BP (mmHg) Percentile of Height							Diastolic BP (mmHg) Percentile of Height						
		5TH	10TH	25TH	50TH	75TH	90TH	95TH	5TH	10TH	25TH	50TH	75TH	90TH	95TH
1	90th	97	97	98	100	101	102	103	52	53	53	54	55	55	56
	95th	100	101	102	104	105	106	107	56	57	57	58	59	59	60
2	90th	98	99	100	101	103	104	105	57	58	58	59	60	61	61
	95th	102	103	104	105	107	108	109	61	62	62	63	64	65	65
3	90th	100	100	102	103	104	106	106	61	62	62	63	64	64	65
	95th	104	104	105	107	108	109	110	65	66	66	67	68	68	69
4	90th	101	102	103	104	106	107	108	64	64	65	66	67	67	68
	95th	105	106	107	108	110	111	112	68	68	69	70	71	71	72
5	90th	103	103	105	106	107	109	109	66	67	67	68	69	69	70
	95th	107	107	108	110	111	112	113	70	71	71	72	73	73	74
6	90th	104	105	106	108	109	110	111	68	68	69	70	70	71	72
	95th	108	109	110	111	113	114	115	72	72	73	74	74	75	76
7	90th	106	107	108	109	111	112	113	69	70	70	71	72	72	73
	95th	110	111	112	113	115	116	116	73	74	74	75	76	76	77
8	90th	108	109	110	111	113	114	114	71	71	71	72	73	74	74
	95th	112	112	114	115	116	118	118	75	75	75	76	77	78	78
9	90th	110	110	112	113	114	116	116	72	72	72	73	74	75	75
	95th	114	114	115	117	118	119	120	76	76	76	77	78	79	79
10	90th	112	112	114	115	116	118	118	73	73	73	74	75	76	76
	95th	116	116	117	119	120	121	122	77	77	77	78	79	80	80
11	90th	114	114	116	117	118	119	120	74	74	74	75	76	77	77
	95th	118	118	119	121	122	123	124	78	78	78	79	80	81	81
12	90th	116	116	117	119	120	121	122	75	75	75	76	77	78	78
	95th	119	120	121	123	124	125	126	79	79	79	80	81	82	82
13	90th	117	118	119	121	122	123	124	76	76	76	77	78	79	79
	95th	121	122	123	124	126	127	128	80	80	80	81	82	83	83
14	90th	119	120	121	122	124	125	125	77	77	77	78	79	80	80
	95th	123	123	125	126	127	129	129	81	81	81	82	83	84	84
15	90th	120	121	122	123	125	126	127	78	78	78	79	80	81	81
	95th	124	125	126	127	129	130	131	82	82	82	83	84	85	85
16	90th	121	122	123	124	126	127	128	78	78	79	80	81	81	82
	95th	125	126	127	128	130	131	132	82	82	83	84	85	85	86
17	90th	122	122	123	125	126	127	128	78	79	79	80	81	81	82
	95th	125	126	127	129	130	131	132	82	83	83	84	85	85	86

BP, blood pressure

The 90th percentile is 1.28 SD, 95th percentile is 1.645 SD, and the 99th percentile is 2.326 SD over the mean.

National Heart, Lung, and Blood Institute. (2004). Blood pressure tables for children and adolescents from the fourth report on the diagnosis, evaluation, and treatment of high blood pressure in children and adolescents. www.nhlbi.nih.gov/guidelines/hypertension/child_tbl.htm, accessed 9/25/2014.

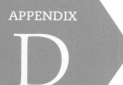

TABLE D.1 **Blood Pressure Levels for Boys by Age and Height Percentile. Use the child's height percentile for the age and sex from a standard growth chart. A blood pressure value at 50th percentile for the child's age, sex, and height percentile is considered the midpoint of the normal range. A reading above the 95th percentile indicates hypertension.**

AGE (YEAR)	BP PERCENTILE	Systolic BP (mmHg) Percentile of Height							Diastolic BP (mmHg) Percentile of Height						
		5TH	10TH	25TH	50TH	75TH	90TH	95TH	5TH	10TH	25TH	50TH	75TH	90TH	95TH
1	90th	94	95	97	99	100	102	103	49	50	51	52	53	53	54
	95th	98	99	101	103	104	106	106	54	54	55	56	57	58	58
2	90th	97	99	100	102	104	105	106	54	55	56	57	58	58	59
	95th	101	102	104	106	108	109	110	59	59	60	61	62	63	63
3	90th	100	101	103	105	107	108	109	59	59	60	61	62	63	63
	95th	104	105	107	109	110	112	113	63	63	64	65	66	67	67
4	90th	102	103	105	107	109	110	111	62	63	64	65	66	66	67
	95th	106	107	109	111	112	114	115	66	67	68	69	70	71	71
5	90th	104	105	106	108	110	111	112	65	66	67	68	69	69	70
	95th	108	109	110	112	114	115	116	69	70	71	72	73	74	74
6	90th	105	106	108	110	111	113	113	68	68	69	70	71	72	72
	95th	109	110	112	114	115	117	117	72	72	73	74	75	76	76
7	90th	106	107	109	111	113	114	115	70	70	71	72	73	74	74
	95th	110	111	113	115	117	118	119	74	74	75	76	77	78	78
8	90th	107	109	110	112	114	115	116	71	72	72	73	74	75	76
	95th	111	112	114	116	118	119	120	75	76	77	78	79	79	80
9	90th	109	110	112	114	115	117	118	72	73	74	75	76	76	77
	95th	113	114	116	118	119	121	121	76	77	78	79	80	81	81
10	90th	111	112	114	115	117	119	119	73	73	74	75	76	77	78
	95th	115	116	117	119	121	122	123	77	78	79	80	81	81	82
11	90th	113	114	115	117	119	120	121	74	74	75	76	77	78	78
	95th	117	118	119	121	123	124	125	78	78	79	80	81	82	82
12	90th	115	116	118	120	121	123	123	74	75	75	76	77	78	79
	95th	119	120	122	123	125	127	127	78	79	80	81	82	82	83
13	90th	117	118	120	122	124	125	126	75	75	76	77	78	79	79
	95th	121	122	124	126	128	129	130	79	79	80	81	82	83	83
14	90th	120	121	123	125	126	128	128	75	76	77	78	79	79	80
	95th	124	125	127	128	130	132	132	80	80	81	82	83	84	84
15	90th	122	124	125	127	129	130	131	76	77	78	79	80	80	81
	95th	126	127	129	131	133	134	135	81	81	82	83	84	85	85
16	90th	125	126	128	130	131	133	134	78	78	79	80	81	82	82
	95th	129	130	132	134	135	137	137	82	83	83	84	85	86	87
17	90th	127	128	130	132	134	135	136	80	80	81	82	83	84	84
	95th	131	132	134	136	138	139	140	84	85	86	87	87	88	89

BP, blood pressure

The 90th percentile is 1.28 SD, 95th percentile is 1.645 SD, and the 99th percentile is 2.326 SD over the mean.

National Heart, Lung, and Blood Institute. (2004). Blood pressure tables for children and adolescents from the fourth report on the diagnosis, evaluation, and treatment of high blood pressure in children and adolescents. www.nhlbi.nih.gov/guidelines/hypertension/child_tbl.htm, accessed 9/25/2014.

Mini Nutritional Assessment
MNA®

Nestlé
Nutrition Institute

Last name: _____ First name: _____

Sex: _____ Age: _____ Weight, kg: _____ Height, cm: _____ Date: _____

Complete the screen by filling in the boxes with the appropriate numbers.
Add the numbers for the screen. If score is 11 or less, continue with the assessment to gain a Malnutrition Indicator Score.

Screening

A Has food intake declined over the past 3 months due to loss of appetite, digestive problems, chewing or swallowing difficulties?
0 = severe decrease in food intake
1 = moderate decrease in food intake
2 = no decrease in food intake   ☐

B Weight loss during the last 3 months
0 = weight loss greater than 3kg (6.6lbs)
1 = does not know
2 = weight loss between 1 and 3kg (2.2 and 6.6 lbs)
3 = no weight loss   ☐

C Mobility
0 = bed or chair bound
1 = able to get out of bed / chair but does not go out
2 = goes out   ☐

D Has suffered psychological stress or acute disease in the past 3 months?
0 = yes   2 = no   ☐

E Neuropsychological problems
0 = severe dementia or depression
1 = mild dementia
2 = no psychological problems   ☐

F Body Mass Index (BMI) (weight in kg) / (height in m²)
0 = BMI less than 19
1 = BMI 19 to less than 21
2 = BMI 21 to less than 23
3 = BMI 23 or greater   ☐

Screening score (subtotal max. 14 points)   ☐☐
12-14 points: Normal nutritional status
8-11 points: At risk of malnutrition
0-7 points: Malnourished

For a more in-depth assessment, continue with questions G-R

Assessment

G Lives independently (not in nursing home or hospital)
1 = yes   0 = no   ☐

H Takes more than 3 prescription drugs per day
0 = yes   1 = no   ☐

I Pressure sores or skin ulcers
0 = yes   1 = no   ☐

J How many full meals does the patient eat daily?
0 = 1 meal
1 = 2 meals
2 = 3 meals   ☐

K Selected consumption markers for protein intake
• At least one serving of dairy products
  (milk, cheese, yoghurt) per day   yes ☐ no ☐
• Two or more servings of legumes
  or eggs per week   yes ☐ no ☐
• Meat, fish or poultry every day   yes ☐ no ☐
0.0 = if 0 or 1 yes
0.5 = if 2 yes
1.0 = if 3 yes   ☐.☐

L Consumes two or more servings of fruit or vegetables per day?
0 = no   1 = yes   ☐

M How much fluid (water, juice, coffee, tea, milk...) is consumed per day?
0.0 = less than 3 cups
0.5 = 3 to 5 cups
1.0 = more than 5 cups   ☐.☐

N Mode of feeding
0 = unable to eat without assistance
1 = self-fed with some difficulty
2 = self-fed without any problem   ☐

O Self view of nutritional status
0 = views self as being malnourished
1 = is uncertain of nutritional state
2 = views self as having no nutritional problem   ☐

P In comparison with other people of the same age, how does the patient consider his / her health status?
0.0 = not as good
0.5 = does not know
1.0 = as good
2.0 = better   ☐.☐

Q Mid-arm circumference (MAC) in cm
0.0 = MAC less than 21
0.5 = MAC 21 to 22
1.0 = MAC 22 or greater   ☐.☐

R Calf circumference (CC) in cm
0 = CC less than 31
1 = CC 31 or greater   ☐

Assessment (max. 16 points)   ☐☐.☐

Screening score   ☐☐.☐

Total Assessment (max. 30 points)   ☐☐.☐

Malnutrition Indicator Score
24 to 30 points   ☐   Normal nutritional status
17 to 23.5 points   ☐   At risk of malnutrition
Less than 17 points   ☐   Malnourished

References
1. Vellas B, Villars H, Abellan G, et al. Overview of the MNA® - Its History and Challenges. J Nutr Health Aging. 2006; 10:456-465.
2. Rubenstein LZ, Harker JO, Salva A, Guigoz Y, Vellas B. Screening for Undernutrition in Geriatric Practice: Developing the Short-Form Mini Nutritional Assessment (MNA-SF). J. Geront. 2001; 56A: M366-377
3. Guigoz Y. The Mini-Nutritional Assessment (MNA®) Review of the Literature - What does it tell us? J Nutr Health Aging. 2006; 10:466-487.

For more information: www.mna-elderly.com

Glossary

abdomen The largest cavity of the body that contains organs and structures belonging to various systems of the body

abduction Movement of a limb away from the midline or median plane of the body, along the frontal plane

accessory digestive organs The structures connected to the alimentary canal by ducts—the liver, gallbladder, and pancreas—that contribute to the digestive process of foods

accommodation The ability of the eye to automatically adjust clear vision from far to near or a variety of distances

acetabulum A rounded cavity on the right and left lateral sides of the pelvic bone

acini cells Glandular tissue in each breast that produce milk

acrocyanosis A normal finding in newborns and infants in which during times of stress, especially exposure to cold environments, the hands and feet appear cyanotic and are often accompanied by increased mottling of the distal arms and legs

acromegaly A disorder caused by overproduction of growth hormone by the pituitary gland. The result may be enlargement of the skull and cranial bones; enlargement of the lower jaw; and enlargement of the lips, tongue, hands, and feet.

actinic keratoses Normal aging growths, especially in fair skins, that are considered precancerous; they appear as calluslike red, yellow, or flesh-colored plaques on exposed areas such as ears, cheeks, lips, nose, upper extremities, or balding scalp

acute pain Pain that lasts only through the expected recovery period from illness, injury, or surgery, whether it has a sudden or slow onset and regardless of the intensity

adduction The movement of a limb toward the body midline

adolescence The period between 11 and 21 years of age

adolescent The transition period from childhood to adulthood, 12 to 19 or 20 years of age

adventitious sounds Added sounds heard during auscultation of the chest. These sounds are superimposed on normal breath sounds and may indicate underlying airway problems or diseases.

aerobic exercise Activity in which oxygen is metabolized to produce energy

air conduction The transmission of sound through the tympanic membrane to the cochlea and auditory nerve

alimentary canal A continuous, hollow, muscular tube, that begins at the mouth and terminates at the anus

Allen's test Test used to determine patency of the radial and ulnar arteries

alopecia Hair loss caused by an immune-mediated attack on the hair follicles

alopecia areata Sudden patchy or complete loss of body hair for unknown cause. Occurs most often on scalp although it may occur over the entire body.

amniotic fluid A clear, slightly yellowish liquid that surrounds the fetus during pregnancy

anabolism A condition that occurs when the intake of protein and calories exceeds the nitrogen loss

anaerobic exercise Activity in which the energy required is provided without using inspired oxygen

analgesia The absence of pain sensation

anesthesia The inability to perceive the sense of touch

angle of Louis Also called the sternal angle. A horizontal ridge formed at the point where the manubrium joins the body of the sternum.

angular stomatitis A clinical finding of poor nutrition; cracks at the corner of the mouth

anorexia nervosa A complex psychosocial and physiologic problem characterized by a severely restricted intake of nutrients and a low body weight

anosmia The absence of the sense of smell, which may be due to cranial nerve dysfunction, colds, rhinitis, or zinc deficiency, or it may be genetic

anteflexion Abnormal variations of uterine position in which the uterus folded forward at about a 90-degree angle, and the cervix is tilted downward

anterior fontanelle A small diamond-shaped area, also known as a "soft spot," located at the top of the skull where the bones of the skull have not as yet closed. This area protects the brain during birth and allows for skull and brain growth during infancy.

anterior triangle A landmark area of the anterior neck bordered by the mandible, the midline of the neck, and the anterior aspect of the sternocleidomastoid muscles

anteversion Normal uterine position where the uterus is tilted forward, cervix tilted downward

anthropometrics Any scientific measurement of the body

anus The terminal end of the large intestine exiting the body

apical impulse The anatomic point at which the heartbeat is most easily palpated; located at the apex of the heart. Also referred to as point of maximal impulse (PMI).

apocrine glands Glands in the axillary and anogenital regions that are dormant until the onset of puberty and produce a secretion made up of water, salts, fatty acids, and proteins, which is released into hair follicles

aqueous humor A clear, fluidlike substance found in the anterior segment of the eye that helps maintain ocular pressure

arcus senilis A light gray ring around the outer pupil due to the deposition of lipids

areola A circular pigmented field of wrinkled skin containing the nipple

arterial aneurysm A bulging or dilation caused by a weakness in the wall of an artery

arterial insufficiency Inadequate arterial circulation, usually due to the buildup of fatty plaque or calcification of the arterial wall

arteries Tubular elastic-walled vessels that carry oxygenated blood throughout the body

ascites An abnormal collection of fluid in the peritoneal cavity

assessment The first step of the nursing process. This includes the collection, organization, and validation of subjective and objective data.

assimilation The adoption and incorporation of characteristics, customs, and values of the dominant culture by those new to that culture

astigmatism A condition in which the refraction of light is spread over a wide area rather than on a distinct point on the retina

atlas The first cervical vertebra, which carries the skull

atopic dermatitis (Eczema) A chronic skin disorder characterized by intense itching, patches, erythema, and papules that typically begins in the first year of life

atrioventricular (AV) node Cluster of specialized cells located between the atria and ventricles that receives electrical impulses from the sinoatrial (SA) node and transmits the electrical impulses to the bundle of His; capable of initiating electrical impulses in the event of SA node failure

atrioventricular (AV) valves Valves that separate the atria from the ventricles within the heart

atrophic papillae A clinical finding of poor nutritional health

attending Giving full-time attention to verbal and nonverbal messages

auricle The external portion of the ear

auscultation Using a stethoscope to listen to the sounds produced by the body

axillary tail (Tail of Spence) Breast tissue that extends superiolaterally into the axilla

axis The second cervical vertebra (C2), which supports the movement of the head

azotemia A buildup of wastes in the bloodstream due to renal dysfunction

Babinski response The fanning of the toes with the great toe pointing toward the dorsum of the foot; considered an abnormal response in the adult that may indicate upper motor neuron disease

ballottement A palpation technique used to detect fluid or examine floating body structures by using the hand to push against the body

Bartholin's glands (Greater vestibular glands) Glands located posteriorly at the base of the vaginal vestibule that produce mucus, which is released into the vestibule and actively promotes sperm motility and viability following intercourse

Bell's palsy A temporary disorder affecting cranial nerve VII and producing a unilateral facial paralysis

blepharitis Inflammation of the eyelids

blood pressure Pressure caused by waves of blood as it ebbs and flows within the systemic arteries

Blumberg's sign The experience of sharp, stabbing pain as the compressed area returns to a noncompressed state

bone conduction The transmission of sound through the bones of the skull to the cochlea and auditory nerve

borborygmi Stomach growling; caused by contraction muscles in the stomach and intestines

brain stem Located between the cerebrum and spinal cord, contains the midbrain, pons, and medulla oblongata and connects pathways between the higher and lower structures

Braxton-Hicks contractions Painless and unpredictable contractions of the uterus that do not dilate the cervix

bronchial sounds Loud, high-pitched sounds heard in the upper airways and region of the trachea. Expiration is longer in duration than inspiration

bronchophony Auscultation of voice sounds, patient says "ninety-nine" and normal lung sound will be muffled

bronchovesicular sounds Sounds that are medium in loudness and pitch, heard as ausculation moves from the large central airways toward the periphery of the lungs. Inspiration and expiration are equal in duration.

bruit A group of heart sounds that elicit a loud blowing sound. This is an abnormal finding, most often associated with a narrowing or stricture of the carotid artery usually associated with atherosclerotic plaque.

bulbourethral glands (Cowper's glands) Small, round glands located below the prostate within the urethral sphincter; just before ejaculation, they secrete a clear mucus into the urethra that lubricates the urethra and increases its alkaline environment

bulimia nervosa An eating disorder characterized by binge eating and purging or another compensatory mechanism to prevent weight gain

bundle branches Expressways of conducting fibers that spread the electrical current through the ventricular myocardial tissue

bundle of His Pathway of cardiac tissue that receives electrical impulses from the atrioventricular (AV) node and transmits the electrical impulses to the ventricles

bursae Small, synovial fluid–filled sacs that protect ligaments from friction

calcaneus A tarsal bone of the foot, also known as the heel bone

calculi Stones that block the urinary tract, usually composed of calcium, struvite, or a combination of magnesium, ammonium, phosphate, and uric acid content in water

capillaries The smallest vessels of the circulatory system that exchange gases and nutrients between the arterial and venous systems

caput succedaneum A condition that is characterized by edema that results from a collection of fluid in the tissue at the top of the skull

cardiac conduction system The heart's conduction system, which can initiate an electrical charge and transmit that charge via cardiac muscle fibers throughout the myocardial tissue

cardiac cycle The events of one complete heartbeat, the contraction and relaxation of the atria and ventricles

cardiac output The amount of blood ejected from the left ventricle over 1 minute

cartilaginous joint Bones joined by cartilage

catabolism A condition that occurs when there is a negative nitrogen balance

cataract A condition in which the lens continues to thicken and yellow, forming a dense area that reduces lens clarity resulting in a loss of central vision

central nervous system (CNS) Nervous system of the body that consists of the brain and the spinal cord

cephalocaudal Head to toe, direction

cephalohematomas Blood collections inside of the skull's periosteum that do not cross suture lines

cerebellum Located below the cerebrum and behind the brain stem, it coordinates stimuli from the cerebral cortex to provide precise timing for skeletal muscle coordination and smooth movements; also assists with maintaining equilibrium and muscle tone

cerebrovascular accident (CVA, stroke, brain attack) Interruption or occlusion of cerebral blood flow resulting in impaired delivery of oxygen and nutrients to the brain cells. This condition may be fatal. Neurologic deficits following CVA may be temporary or permanent, and may range from mild to severe.

cerebrum The largest portion of the brain, responsible for all conscious behavior

cerumen Yellow-brown wax secreted by glands in the external auditory canal

cervical os The inferior opening; the vaginal end of the canal

cervix Round part of the uterus that projects 2.5 cm into the vagina

Chadwick's sign Vascular congestion that creates a blue-purple blemish or change in cervical coloration

cheilitis Angular stomatitis; inflammation of the lip

cheilosis An abnormal condition of the lips characterized by scaling of the surface and by the formation of fissures in the corners of the mouth

cherry angiomas Vascular lesions, nonsignificant tiny red spots, either macules or papules, rarely larger than 3 to 4 mm, seen usually on the trunk

chloasma A skin condition that develops during pregnancy resulting in hyperpigmented patches on the face. Also referred to as melasma, gravidum, or "the mask of pregnancy"

choanal atresia A congenital defect that results in a thin membrane that obstructs the nasal passages

choroid The middle layer, the vascular-pigmented layer of the eye

chronic pain Pain that is prolonged, usually recurring or persisting over 6 months or longer, and interferes with functioning

circumduction Movement in which the limb describes a cone in space: while the distal end of the limb moves in a circle, the joint itself moves only slightly in the joint cavity

claudication Pain in the thigh, calf, or buttocks that is caused by arterial insufficiency; may be a sign of peripheral vascular disease

clitoris The primary organ of sexual stimulation in females, it is a small, elongated mound of erectile tissue located at the anterior of the vaginal vestibule

clonus Rhythmically alternating flexion and extension; confirms upper motor neuron disease

clubbing Flattening of the angle of the nail and enlargement of the tips of the fingers is a sign of oxygen deprivation in the extremities

coarctation of the aorta A congenital cardiac defect in the newborn that results in the narrowing of the aorta with decreased femoral pulses and bounding upper extremity pulses, and causes discrepancies in blood pressure and oxygen saturation between the upper and lower extremities

cochlea A spiraling chamber in the inner ear that contains the receptors for hearing

cognitive theory How people learn to think, reason, and use language

cold sores Vesicle that occurs on the lip or corner of the mouth. Caused by a herpes simplex virus.

colostrum A thick, yellowish specialized form of early breast milk that is produced starting in the second trimester and replaced by mature milk during the early days of lactation after the delivery of the baby

coma A prolonged state of unconciousness with pronounced and persistent changes

complete health assessment Includes the interview, general survey, assessment of vital signs, and physical assessment of all body systems

communication Exchange of information, feelings, thoughts, and ideas

concreteness Speaking to the patient in specific terms rather than in vague generalities

confidentiality Protecting information, sharing only to those directly involved in patient care

consanguinity Union between closely related individuals; intimate relationship between two people who share a common ancestor.

consensual constriction The simultaneous response of one pupil to the stimuli applied to the other

convergence Movement of the two eyes so that the coordination of an image falls at corresponding points of the two retinas

cornea The clear, transparent part of the sclera that forms the anterior part of the eye, considered to be the window of the eye

cortex The outer portion of each kidney composed of over 1 million nephrons, which form urine

costovertebral angle (CVA) The area on the lower back formed by the vertebral column and the downward curve of the last posterior rib

cranial sutures Palpable gaps between the bones of the skull

craniosynostosis A condition that results in cranial deformity due to premature fusion of the cranial bones

cremasteric reflex A reflexive action that may cause the testicles to migrate upward temporarily; cold hands, a cold room, or the stimulus of touch could cause this response

crepitation A crackling, rattling, or grating sound

critical thinking A process of purposeful and creative thinking about resolutions of problems or the development of ways to manage situations

cryptorchidism The failure of one or both testicles to descend through the inguinal canal during the final stages of fetal development

cues Bits of information that hint at the possibility of a health problem

cultural competence The capacity of nurses or health service delivery systems to effectively understand and plan for the needs of a culturally diverse patient or group

culture The nonphysical traits, such as values, beliefs, attitudes, and customs, that are shared by a group of people and passed from one generation to the next

Cushing's syndrome Abnormality where increased adrenal hormone production leads to a rounded "moon" face, ruddy cheeks, prominent jowls, and excess facial hair

cutaneous pain Pain that originates in the skin or subcutaneous tissue

cuticle A fold of epidermal skin along the base of the nail that protects the root and sides of each nail

cystocele A hernia that is formed when the urinary bladder is pushed into the anterior vaginal wall

dandruff White or gray dead, scaly skin flakes of epidermal cells

database The collected objective and subjective gathered about a patient's medical history and physical assessment findings, recorded electronically or in writing as part of the patient's record.

deep somatic pain Pain that is diffuse and arises from ligaments, tendons, bones, blood vessels, and nerves, which tends to last longer than cutaneous pain

depression For the musculoskeletal system, this is the movement in which the elevated part is moved downward to its original position

dermatome An area of skin innervated by the cutaneous branch of one spinal nerve

dermis A layer of connective tissue that lies just below the epidermis

development An orderly, progressive increase in the complexity of the total person. It involves the continuous, irreversible, complex evolution of intelligence, personality, creativity, sociability, and morality

developmental dysplasia of the hip A congenital disorder that results from inadequate development of the hip socket

diaphoresis Profuse perspiration or sweating that may occur during exertion, fever, pain, and emotional stress and in the presence of some metabolic disorders such as hyperthyroidism

diastasis recti abdominis The rectus abdominis muscles that run vertically down the midline of the abdomen may separate during the third trimester and may allow the abdominal contents to protrude

diastole The phase of ventricular relaxation in which the ventricles relax and are filled as the atria contract. This is also associated with the bottom number of a blood pressure reading.

diastolic pressure The lowest arterial blood pressure of the cardiac cycle occurring when the heart is at rest

diet recall A remembrance of all food, beverages, and nutritional supplements or products consumed in a set period such as a 24-hour period

dilation Progressive opening of the cervix

diplopia Double vision

disability A physical or mental impairment that limits one or more of a person's life activities. People with disabilities may be in need of healthcare services by reason of mental health, physical, sensory, developmental, age, or illness concerns.

dislocation A displacement of the bone from its usual anatomical location in the joint

diversity The state of being different

documentation The recording of information about a patient. This is a legal document used to plan care, to communicate information between and among healthcare providers, and to monitor quality of care

dorsiflexion Flexion of the ankle so that the superior aspect of the foot moves in an upward direction

Down syndrome A chromosomal defect that causes varying degrees of mental retardation; its prominent facial features include slanted eyes, a flat nasal bridge, a flat nose, a protruding tongue, and a short neck

ductus arteriosus The third shunt in fetal circulation that shunts blood into the descending aorta

ductus venosus A shunt in fetal circulation that enables the fetus to maximize oxygenation from the maternal circulation

dullness A flat percussion tone that is soft and of short duration

dysphagia Difficulty swallowing

dyspnea Shortness of breath or difficulty getting one's breath

dysreflexia An alteration in urinary elimination that affects patients with spinal cord injuries at level T7 or higher

ecchymosis Bruising resulting from the escape of blood from a ruptured blood vessel into the tissues

eccrine glands Glands that produce a clear perspiration mostly made up of water and salts, which they release into funnel-shaped pores at the skin surface

ectropion Eversion of the lower eyelid and eyelashes; causes include muscle weakness, scarring, facial paralysis, eyelid growths, congenital disorders, surgery, radiation, and certain medications

eczema (Atopic dermatitis) A chronic skin disorder characterized by intense itching, patches, erythema, and papules, typically beginning in the first year of life

edema Accumulation of fluid in the tissues or in a body cavity

effacement Thinning of the cervix occurring near the end of pregnancy in preparation for labor

egophony Ausculation of voice sounds; when patient says "E," normal lungs sound like "eeeeee"

elder abuse A term referring to a knowing, intentional, or negligent act that causes harm or risk of harm to an older adult

electrocardiogram (ECG) Electrical representations of the cardiac cycle are documented by deflections on recording paper

elevation Lifting or moving superiorly along a frontal plane

embryo Child during any development stage of pregnancy prior to birth

emmetropia The normal refractive condition of the eye

empathy Understanding, being aware, being sensitive to the feelings, thoughts, and/or experiences of another

encoding The process of formulating a message for transmission to another person

endocardium The innermost layer of the heart, a smooth layer that provides an inner lining for the chambers of the heart

entropion Inversion of the eyelid and eyelashes; causes include muscle weakness, inflammation, infection, muscle spasm, or congenital or developmental complications

enuresis Involuntary urination, such as bed-wetting, that occurs after 4 years of age

epicardium The outer layer of the heart wall that is also called the visceral pericardium

epidermis The outer layer of skin on the body

epididymis A comma- or crescent-shaped system of ductules emerging posteriorly from the testis that holds the sperm during maturation

epididymitis A common infection in males characterized by a dull, aching pain

epiphyseal plates Plates located in the ends of the bones

epispadias A condition in which the urethral meatus is located on the superior aspect of the glans

epitrochlear nodes Lymph nodes located on the medial surface of the arm above the elbow that drain the ulnar surface of the forearm and the third, fourth, and fifth digits

esophagitis Inflammatory process of the esophagus, caused by a variety of irritants

esophoria Inward turning of the eye toward the nose

ethnicity The awareness of belonging to a group in which certain characteristics or aspects such as culture and biology differentiate the members of one group from another

ethnocentrism The tendency to believe one's way of life, values, beliefs, and customs are superior to those of others

eupnea The regular, even-depth, rhythmic pattern of inspiration and expiration; normal breathing

eustachian tube The bony and cartilaginous auditory tube that connects the middle ear with the nasopharynx. This helps to equalize the air pressure on both sides of the tympanic membrane

eversion A movement in which the sole of the foot is turned laterally

evidenced-based nursing practice An approach to decision making, intervention, and nursing care that requires integration of clinical expertise with the best evidence from systematic research and regard for the concerns and choices of the patient

exophoria Outward turning of the eye

extension A bending movement around a joint that increases the angle between the bone of the limb at the joint

false reassurance The patient is assured of a positive outcome with no basis for believing in it

fetal alcohol syndrome (FAS) Congenital condition caused by exposure to high levels of alcohol during fetal development. Fetal defects may include mental retardation, developmental delays, and physical deformities.

fetoscope A specialized stethoscope for listening to fetal heart sounds, beginning at approximately 18 weeks of gestation

fetus The developing product of conception, usually from the eighth week until birth

fever blisters Lesions or blisters on the lips may be caused by the herpes simplex virus

fibrous joint Bones joined by fibrous tissue

fifth vital sign The assessment of pain with other vital sign evaluations

flag sign Dyspigmentation of the mouth or a part of the mouth

flatness A dull percussion tone that is soft and has a short duration

flexion A bending movement that decreases the angle of the joint and brings the articulating bones closer together

focused interview An interview that enables the nurse to clarify points, to obtain missing information, and to follow up on verbal and nonverbal cues identified in the health history

follicular hyperkeratosis Goose bump–like flesh, can be related to vitamin A deficiency

food deserts Low-income, urban or rural areas that lack access to healthy, affordable food. When food is available, it is generally high calorie food of poor nutritional quality, such as found in fast food restaurants and convenience stores.

food frequency questionnaire A questionnaire that assesses intake of a variety of food groups on a daily, weekly, or longer basis

food security A parameter used in nutritional assessment, free access to adequate and safe food

foramen ovale The second shunt in fetal circulation prior to birth that connects the fetal right atrium to the fetal left atrium

formal teaching Organized information sharing that occurs in response to an identified learning need of an individual, group, or community

fracture A partial or complete break in the continuity of the bone from trauma

fremitus The palpable vibration on the chest wall when the patient speaks

friction rub A rough, grating sound caused by the rubbing together of organs or an organ rubbing on the peritoneum

functional assessment An observation to gather data while the patient is performing common or routine activities

fundal height Size of the fundus; after 20 weeks of pregnancy, the weeks of gestation equal the fundal height in centimeters

fundus The inner back surface of the internal eye

galactorrhea Lactation not associated with childbearing or breast-feeding

general survey Impressions based on what is seen, heard, or smelled during the initial phase of assessment

genital warts Raised, moist, cauliflower-shaped papules

genu valgum Knock knees, a condition of the musculoskeletal system where the knees touch each other but the ankles do not

genu varum Bowlegs, a condition of the musculoskeletal system where the ankles touch each other but the knees do not

genuineness The ability to present oneself honestly and spontaneously

geography The country, region, section, community, or neighborhood in which one was born and raised or in which one currently resides or works

gestational age The age of the fetus, which can be referred to in weeks from the last normal menstrual period

gliding The simplest type of joint movements. One flat bone surface glides or slips over another similar surface. The bones are merely displaced in relation to one another

glomerulus Tufts of capillaries of the kidneys that filter more than 1 liter (1 L) of fluid each minute. Plural glomeruli.

glossitis Inflammation or redness of the tongue. Often seen in malnutrition.

goiter Enlargement of the thyroid gland that is commonly visible as swelling of the anterior neck. The cause is often lack of iodine intake.

Goodell's sign An increase in cervical vascularity that contributes to the softening of the cervix during pregnancy

growth Measurable physical change and increase in size; indicators of growth include height, weight, bone size, and dentition

gynecologic age The difference between one's current age and age at menarche

gynecomastia Benign temporary breast enlargement in one or both breasts in males

hair A thin, flexible, elongated fiber composed of dead, keratinized cells that grow out in a columnar fashion

hallux valgus The great toe is abnormally adducted at the metatarsophalangeal joint

health A state of complete physical, mental, and social well-being

health assessment A systematic method of collecting data about a patient for the purpose of determining the patient's current and ongoing health status, predicting risks to health, and identifying health-promoting activities

healthcare-associated infections (HAIs) An infection that results directly from the delivery of healthcare services in a facility such as a clinic, hospital, or long-term care facility

health disparities Gaps in the quality of health and health care that mirror differences in socioeconomic status, racial and ethnic background, and levels of education

health history Information about the patient's health in his or her own words and based on the patient's own perceptions. Includes biographic data, perceptions about health, past and present history of illness and injury, family history, a review of systems, and health.

health pattern A set of related traits, habits, or acts that affect a patient's health

health promotion Behavior motivated by the desire to increase well-being and actualize human potential

Healthy People 2020 A report and program sponsored by the United States Department of Health and Human Services focusing on health promotion of individuals, families, and communities

heart An intricately designed pump composed of a meticulous network of synchronized structures. The heart is responsible for receiving unoxygenated blood from the body and returning oxygenated blood to the body.

heart murmurs Atypical sounds of the heart often indicating a functional or structural abnormality

Hegar's sign The softening of the uterus and the region that connects the body of the uterus and cervix that occurs throughout pregnancy

helix The external large rim of the auricle of the ear

hematuria Blood in the urine

hemorrhoids A mass of dilated veins in swollen tissue caused by continuous overdistention of the bowel and straining to pass stools

hepatitis An inflammatory process of the liver caused by viruses, bacteria, chemicals, or drugs

heritage A range of meanings, behaviors, and contemporary activities that are drawn from a combination of an individual's culture, inherited traditions, objects, and monuments

heritage consistency The extent to which one's lifestyle reflects one's traditional heritage, as well as the degree to which the individual identifies with his traditional heritage

heritage inconsistency The degree to which an individual adopts and implements beliefs and practices obtained by way of acculturation into a dominant or host culture

hernia A protrusion of an organ or structure through an abnormal opening or weakened area in a body wall

hirsutism Male-pattern hair growth in women; often associated with polycystic ovarian syndrome, Cushing's syndrome, congenital adrenal hyperplasia, androgen-secreting tumors, or certain medications

holism Considering more than the physiologic health status of a patient, including all factors that impact the patient's physical and emotional well-being

Homans' sign Diagnostic maneuver in which pain may increase with sharp dorsiflexion of the foot

hydrocephalus The enlargement of the head caused by inadequate drainage of cerebrospinal fluid, resulting in abnormal growth of the skull

hydronephrosis An enlargement of the kidney caused by an obstruction, as in kidney stone or pregnancy

hydroureter An enlargement of the ureter caused by an obstruction, as in kidney stone or pregnancy

hymen A thin layer of skin within the vagina

hyoid A bone that is suspended in the neck approximately 2 cm (1 in.) above the larynx

hypalgesia Decreased pain sensation

hyperalgesia Excessive sensitivity to pain

hyperesthesia An increased sensation

hyperextension A bending of a joint beyond 180 degrees

hyperopia A condition in which the light rays focus behind the retina. Also called farsightedness.

hyperresonance Abnormally loud auscultatory tone that is low and of long duration

hyperthermia Body temperature that is greater than expected. Also called a fever, it may be caused by an infection, trauma, surgery, or a malignancy.

hyperthyroidism The excessive production of thyroid hormones, resulting in enlargement of the gland, exophthalmos (bulging eyes), fine hair, weight loss, diarrhea, and other alterations

hypodermis A cellular layer of subcutaneous tissue consisting of loose connective tissue. Stores approximately half of the body's fat cells, cushions the body against trauma, insulates the body from heat loss, and stores fat for energy.

hypoesthesia A decreased but not absent sensation

hypospadias A condition in which the urethral meatus is located on the underside of the glans

hypothermia Body temperature that is less than expected. This is usually a response to prolonged exposure to cold

hypothyroidism Metabolic disorder causing enlarged thyroid due to iodine deficiency

immunocompetence A biochemical assessment laboratory measurement used in nutritional assessment. A depressed immune status can result from malnutrition, disease, medication, or other disease treatments.

incontinence The inability to retain urine; may be classified as functional, reflex, stress, urge, or total

infant A child from 1 month of age through 11 months of age

infective endocarditis A condition caused by bacterial infiltration of the lining of the heart's chambers

informal teaching Occurs as a natural part of a patient encounter, may provide instructions, explain a question or procedure, or reduce anxiety

inguinal hernia When a separation of the abdominal muscle exists, the weak points of these canals afford an area for the protrusion of the intestine into the groin region

innocent murmurs Heart sounds that arise from increased blood flow across normal heart structures in children; they are grades I–II/VI in intensity, are systolic (with the exception of the venous hum), and are usually not associated with thrills or other cardiac symptoms

inspection The skill of observing the patient in a deliberate, systematic manner

interactional skills Actions that are used during the encoding/decoding process to obtain and disseminate information, develop relationships, and promote understanding of self and others

interdependent relationship Relationships in which the individual establishes bonds with others based on some single factor such as trust or a common goal

interpretation of findings Making determinations about all of the data collected in the health assessment process

interview Subjective data gathering, including the health history and focused interview, that include primary and secondary sources

intimate partner violence Physical, sexual, or psychological harm by a current or former partner or spouse that can occur among heterosexual or same-sex couples and does not require sexual intimacy

intractable pain Pain that is highly resistant to relief

introitus Vaginal opening

inversion A movement in which the sole of the foot is turned medially or inward

iris The circular, colored muscular aspect of the eye's middle layer located in the anterior portion of the eye

iritis Inflammation of the iris that is characterized by redness around the iris and cornea, decreased vision, and deep, aching pain; pupil is often irregular

joint (Articulation) The point where two or more bones in the body meet

keratin A fibrous protein that gives the epidermis its tough, protective qualities

kidneys Bean-shaped organs located in the retroperitoneal space on either side of the vertebral column

koilonychia A clinical finding of poor nutrition; spoon-shaped ridges in the cardia

kyphosis An exaggerated thoracic dorsal curve that causes asymmetry between the sides of the posterior thorax

labia A dual set of liplike structures lying on either side of the vagina

labial adhesion A condition common in preadolescent females that occurs when the labia minora fuse together

lambdoidal sutures Palpable gaps between the bones of the skull that separate the temporal and occipital bones

landmarks Thoracic reference points and specific anatomic structures used to help provide an exact location for the assessment findings and an accurate orientation for documentation of findings

lanugo A fine, downy fine hair in newborns that is most prominent on the upper chest, shoulders, and back

laryngomalacia Congenital defect of the cartilage in the larynx

left atrium The left atrium of the heart is the chamber that receives oxygenated blood from the pulmonary system

left ventricle The left ventricle, the most powerful of all heart chambers, pumps the oxygenated blood outward through the aorta to the periphery of the body

lens A flexible, transparent, biconvex (convex on both surfaces) structure situated directly behind the pupil that separates the anterior and posterior segments of the eye; responsible for fine focusing of images

Leopold's maneuvers A special palpation sequence of the pregnant female's abdomen used to determine the position of the fetus after 28 weeks' gestation

leukorrhea A profuse, nonodorous, nonpainful vaginal discharge that protects against infection

lightening The descent of the fetal head into the pelvis

linea nigra A dark line running from the umbilicus to the pubic area that may occur during pregnancy; often accompanied by increased pigmentation of the areolae and nipples

linguistic competence The ability of an organization and its members to effectively communicate and convey information in such a way that diverse audiences may easily comprehend the intended meaning

listening Paying undivided attention to what the patient says and does

lobule A small flap of flesh at the inferior end of the auricle of the ear

lordosis An exaggerated lumbar curve of the spine that compensates for pregnancy, obesity, or other skeletal changes

lunula A moon-shaped crescent that appears on the nail body over the thickened nail matrix

lymph Clear fluid that passes from the intercellular spaces of the body tissue into the lymphatic system

lymphedema Swelling that is caused by some degree of lymphatic system obstruction

lymphadenopathy The enlargement of lymph nodes that is often caused by infection, allergies, or a tumor

lymphatic vessels Vessels that extend from the capillaries. Their purpose is to collect lymph in organs and tissues.

lymph nodes Rounded lymphoid tissues that are surrounded by connective tissue. Lymph nodes are located along the lymphatic vessels in the body.

macrocephaly Any child whose head circumference is above the 95th percentile; the condition is associated with hydrocephalus, brain tumor, and increased intracranial pressure

macula Appears as a hyperpigmented spot on the temporal aspect of the retina and is responsible for central vision

malnutrition An imbalance, whether a deficit or excess, of the required nutrients of a balanced diet

mammary ridge "Milk line," which extends from each axilla to the groin

mammary souffle A murmur over the mammary vessel due to increased blood flow, occasionally heard during pregnancy

manual compression test A maneuver to determine the length of varicose veins

manubrium The superior or upper portion of the sternum

mapping The process of dividing the abdomen into quadrants or regions for the purpose of examination

Marfan's syndrome A degenerative disease of the connective tissue, which over time may cause the ascending aorta to either dilate or dissect, leading to abrupt death

mastalgia Breast pain

mastoiditis Inflammation of the mastoid that may occur secondary to a middle ear or a throat infection

McDonald's rule A method for estimating fetal growth that states that after 20 weeks in pregnancy, the weeks of gestation approximately equal the fundal height in centimeters

mediastinal space The area where the heart sits obliquely within the thoracic cavity between the lungs and above the diaphragm

mediastinum Part of the thorax, or thoracic cavity, that contains the heart, trachea, esophagus, and major blood vessels of the body

medulla The inner portion of the kidney, composed of structures called pyramids and calyces

melanin Skin pigment produced in the melanocytes in the stratum basale

menarche Age of first menstrual period

meninges Three connective tissue membranes that cover, protect, and nourish the central nervous system

metabolic syndrome A combination of disorders that increase the risk of developing cardiovascular disease and diabetes. It is characterized by excess abdominal fat, hypertension, dyslipidemia, and insulin-resistant glucose metabolism.

microcephaly Any child whose head circumference is below the 5th percentile, may be caused by genetic disorders or intrauterine exposure to cocaine or alcohol

middle adulthood The period of a person's life when 40 to 65 years of age

midposition Uterine position, which lies parallel to the tailbone, with the cervix pointed straight

milia Harmless skin markings on newborns; areas of tiny white facial papules due to sebum that collects in the openings of hair follicles

Mini-Mental State Examination (MMSE) A screening instrument of cognitive reasoning for detecting dementia and delirium relating to organic disease

miosis Excessive or prolonged constriction of the pupil of the eye

mixed-status family A family in which one or more family members are undocumented immigrants and other family members are citizens, lawful permanent residents, or immigrants with another form of temporary legal immigration status

Mongolian spots Gray, blue, or purple spots in the sacral and buttocks areas of newborns that fade during the first year of life

Montgomery's glands (tubercles) The sebaceous glands on the areola, which enlarge and produce a secretion that protects and lubricates the nipples

mucous plug A protective covering of the cervix that develops during pregnancy due to progesterone

multigravida A female who has been pregnant two or more times

muscular dystrophy An X-linked genetic disorder that results in progressive loss of muscle function

mydriasis Excessive or prolonged dilation of the pupil of the eye

myocardium The second, thick, muscular layer of the heart, made up of bundles of cardiac muscle fibers reinforced by a branching network of connective tissue fibers called the fibrous skeleton of the heart

myopia (Nearsightedness) A condition in which the light rays focus in front of the retina

Nägele's rule A formula that can be used to compute the fetus' expected date of birth (EDB) based on the mother's last menstrual period (LMP)

nails Thin plates of keratinized epidermal cells that shield the distal ends of the fingers and toes

nasal polyps Smooth, pale, benign growths found along the turbinates of the nose

neuropathic pain Pain resulting from current or past damage to the peripheral or central nervous system rather than a particular stimulus

neuropathy Nerve damage or dysfunction that may lead to weakness or numbness

newborns Children between birth and 1 month of age

nociception The physiologic processes related to pain perception

nociceptors The receptors that transmit pain sensation

nocturia Nighttime urination

nonverbal communication Nonspoken language used to share information and ideas. This may include gestures, facial expressions, and mannerisms that inform others of emotions, feelings, and responses.

nuchal rigidity Stiffness of the neck as experienced when the meningeal membranes are irritated or inflamed

nursing diagnosis The second step of the nursing process, whereby the nurse uses critical thinking and applies knowledge from the sciences and other disciplines to analyze and synthesize the data

nursing process A systematic, rational, dynamic, and cyclic process used by the nurse for planning and providing care for the patient

nutritional health Using vitamins, foods, nutrients, or herbs to achieve or maintain good health

nystagmus Rapid fluttering or constant involuntary movement of the eyeball

obesity Weight of 20% or more above recommended body weight

obesity paradox The condition where both obesity and nutrient deficiencies occur simultaneously in a person

objective data Data observed or measured by the professional nurse, also known as overt data or signs since they are detected by the nurse. These data can be seen, felt, heard, or measured.

older adulthood The period of a person's life when over 65 years of age

oliguria Diminished volume of urine

onycholysis Separation of the nail plate from the nail bed

opposition The movement of touching the thumb to the tips of the other fingers of the same hand

optic atrophy Degeneration of the optic nerve resulting in a change in the color of the optic disc and decreased visual acuity

optic disc The creamy yellow area on the retina of the eye where the optic nerve leaves the eye

orchitis Inflammation of the testicles

orthopnea Difficulty breathing (dyspnea) when supine that is relieved by sitting upright

ossicles Bones of the middle ear: the malleus, the incus, and the stapes

otitis externa Swimmer's ear, infection of the outer ear or ear canal

otitis media Middle ear infections

ovaries Almond-shaped glandular structures that produce ova as well as estrogen and progesterone

overnutrition Excessive intake or storage of essential nutrients

overweight A weight of 10% to 20% in excess of recommended body weight

oxygen saturation The percentage of oxygen in the blood

pain A highly unpleasant sensation that affects a person's physical health, emotional health, and well-being

pain rating scale Assessment of the intensity of pain using a standardized measurement tool. The tools, which may be numbers, words, or pictures, provide the patient the opportunity to describe the degree of discomfort.

pain reaction Responses to pain, including the autonomic nervous system and behavioral responses to pain

pain sensation The acknowledgment of pain, often known as pain threshold

pain threshold The point at which the sensation of pain is perceived

pain tolerance The maximum amount and duration of pain that an individual is able to endure without relief

palate The anterior portion of the roof of the mouth formed by bones

palpation The skill of assessing the patient through the sense of touch to determine specific characteristics of the body

palpebrae The eyelid

palpebral fissure The opening between the upper and lower eyelids

papilledema Swelling and protrusion of the blind spot of the eye caused by edema

paranasal sinuses Mucus-lined, air-filled cavities that surround the nasal cavity and perform the same air-processing functions of filtration, moistening, and warming

paraphrasing Restating the patient's basic message to test whether it was understood

paraurethral glands (Skene's glands) Glands located just posterior to the urethra that open into the urethra and secrete a fluid that lubricates the vaginal vestibule during sexual intercourse

Parkinson's disease A chronic, progressive movement disorder characterized by the malfunction and death of brain neurons and subsequent decrease in dopamine production. Primarily affects neurons located in the substantia nigra, which is involved in motor control.

paronychia An inflammation of the cuticle, sometimes caused by infection

patient record A legal document used to plan care, to communicate information between and among healthcare providers, and to monitor quality of care

peau d'orange "Orange peel" appearance caused by edema from blocked lymphatic drainage in advanced cancer

pediculosis capitis Small parasitic insects that live on the scalp and neck, often called head lice

pedigree A graphic representation or diagram that depicts both medical history and genetic relationships. In a pedigree, each family member is represented by a symbol, using a circle for females and a square for males

pellagra A photosensitive symmetric rash caused by a diet that is deficient in niacin

penis The male organ used for both elimination of urine and ejaculation of sperm during reproduction

percentiles Comparisons of various measurement values used to assess growth rate and healthy weights versus height

percussion "Striking through" a body part with an object, fingers, or reflex hammer, ultimately producing a measurable sound

pericardium A thin sac composed of a fibroserous material that surrounds the heart

perineum The space between the vaginal opening and anal area or between the scrotum and anus

periorbital edema Swelling of the soft tissue in the periorbital area. Often, the swelling is found in the dependent tissue space.

peripheral nervous system (PNS) System of the body that consists of the cranial nerves and spinal nerves

peripheral vascular system Blood vessels of the body that together with the heart and the lymphatic vessels make up the body's circulatory system

peritoneum A thin, double layer of serous membrane in the abdominal cavity

peritonitis A local or generalized inflammatory process of the peritoneal membrane of the abdomen

petechiae Pinpoint hemorrhages on the skin, can be related to vitamin C deficiency

Peyronie's disease Disease that causes the shaft of the penis to be crooked during an erection

phantom pain Painful sensation experienced in a missing body part (amputation) or paralyzed area

phimosis Condition in which the foreskin of a penis cannot be fully retracted

physical assessment Hands-on examination of the patient; components are the survey and examination of systems

physical environment Consists of all the things that are experienced through the individual's senses and some harmful elements such as radiation, ozone, and radon

physiologic anemia Decrease in hemoglobin and hematocrit caused by plasma volume increase outpacing the increase in red blood cells (RBCs)

pica Abnormal craving for or eating of nonfood items such as chalk or dirt

pinguecula Yellowish nodules that are thickened areas of the bulbar conjunctiva caused by prolonged exposure to sun, wind, and dust. They may be on either side of the pupil and cause no problems.

pinna The external portion of the ear

Piskacek's sign The irregular shape of the uterus due to the implantation of the ovum

placenta A vascular organ that connects the developing fetus to the uterine lining; facilitates the delivery of oxygen and nutrients from mother to fetus, and allows for the release of fetal carbon dioxide and other metabolic waste products.

plantar flexion Extension of the ankle (pointing the toes) away from the body

pleximeter The device (or finger) that accepts the tap or blow from a hammer (or tapping finger)

plexor A hammer or tapping finger used to strike an object

positive regard The ability to appreciate and respect another person's worth and dignity with a nonjudgmental attitude

posterior fontanelle A small diamond-shaped "soft spot" on the infant's skull located in the superior occiput that protects the brain during birth and allows for skull and brain growth during infancy

posterior triangle A landmark area of the posterior neck bordered by the trapezius muscle, the sternocleidomastoid muscle, and the clavicle

preinteraction The period before first meeting with the patient in which the nurse reviews information and prepares for the initial interview

presbycusis High-frequency hearing loss that occurs over time. Often associated with aging.

presbyopia Decreased ability of the eye lens to change shape to accommodate for near vision

preschooler A child between 3 and 5 years of age

pressure ulcer Localized region of damaged or necrotic tissue caused by the exertion of pressure over a bony prominence

primary lesions The initial lesion of a disease

primary prevention Interventions that occur to promote health and well-being before a problem occurs

primary source The patient is the best source because he or she can describe personal symptoms, experiences, and factors leading to the current concerns

primigravida A female pregnant for the first time

proband The individual around whom a pedigree is created

prolapsed uterus Condition in which the uterus may protrude right at the vaginal wall with straining, or it may hang outside of the vaginal wall without any straining

pronation Movement of the forearm so that the palm faces down, posteriorly or inferiorly

prostate gland Organ that borders the urethra near the lower part of the bladder; it lies just anterior to the rectum and is composed of glandular structures that continuously secrete a milky, alkaline solution

protein-calorie malnutrition A nutrient deficiency resulting from undernutrition

protraction A nonangular anterior movement in a transverse plane

pruritus Itching, usually due to dry skin, that may increase with age

psychoanalytic theory Defines the structure of personality as consisting of three parts: the id, the ego, and the superego

psychologic distress A mental condition that can be brought about by many factors including loss of spouse and friends through death or illness, loss of occupation or living arrangement due to functional disability, loss of body image, loss of favored recreation, or loss of any other item of significance

psychosocial functioning The way a person thinks, feels, acts, and relates to self and others. It is the ability to cope and tolerate stress, and the capacity for developing a value and belief system.

psychosocial health Being mentally, emotionally, socially, and spiritually well

psychosocial theory States that culture and society influence development across the entire life span

pterygium An opacity of the bulbar conjunctiva that can grow over the cornea and block vision

ptosis One eyelid drooping

pulse Wave of pressure felt at various points in the body due to the force of the blood against the walls of the arteries

pupil Opening in the center of the iris that allows light to enter the eye

Purkinje fibers Fibers that fan out and penetrate into the myocardial tissue to spread the current into the tissues themselves

purpura Flat, reddish-blue, irregularly shaped extensive patches of varying size

quickening The fluttery initial sensations of fetal movement perceived by the mother

race The identification of an individual or group by shared genetic heritage and biologic or physical characteristics

radiating pain Pain perceived at one location that then extends to nearby tissues

rales/crackles Discontinuous sounds that are intermittent, nonmusical, and brief

rapid assessment A type of assessment, requiring 1 minute or less to complete, often used as an initial assessment of a group of patients in a nursing assignment. The nurse uses the collected data to prioritize her actions and interventions

Raynaud's disease A condition in which the arterioles in the fingers develop spasms, causing intermittent skin pallor or cyanosis and then rubor (red color)

rectal prolapse A condition caused by continuous overdistention of the bowel and straining to pass stools, whereby the lower rectal tissue may be forced out of the body through the anus

rectocele A hernia that is formed when the rectum pushes into the posterior vaginal wall

referred pain Pain felt in a part of the body that is considerably removed or distant from the area actually causing the pain

reflecting A communication technique used in letting the patient know that the nurse empathizes with the thoughts, feelings, or experiences expressed

reflexes An automatic stimulus–response that involves a nerve impulse passing from a peripheral nerve receptor to the spinal cord and then outward to an effector muscle without passing through the brain. The muscle typically contracts following stimulation of the nerve receptor.

resonance A long, low-pitched hollow sound elicited with percussion over the lungs

respiratory cycle Consists of an inspiratory and expiratory phase of breathing

respiratory rate The number of times the individual inhales and exhales during a 1-minute period

retina The third and innermost membrane, the sensory portion of the eye, a direct extension of the optic nerve

retraction A nonangular posterior movement in a transverse plane

retrobulbar neuritis An inflammatory process of the optic nerve behind the eyeball

retroflexion Abnormal variation of uterine position in which the uterus is folded backward at about a 90-degree angle, cervix tilted upward

retroversion Normal variation of uterine position in which the uterus is tilted backward, cervix tilted upward

rhonchi A range of whistling or snoring sounds heard during auscultation when there is some type of airway obstruction. Types of rhonchi include sibilant wheezes, sonorous rhonchi, and stridor.

rickets A clinical finding associated with poor nutritional health resulting in bowed legs

right atrium A thin-walled chamber located above and slightly to the right of the right ventricle that forms the right border of the heart. The right atrium receives unoxygenated blood from the periphery of the body.

right ventricle Part of the heart formed triangularly that comprises much of the anterior or sternocostal surface of the heart. The right ventricle pushes unoxygenated blood out to the pulmonary vessels. This is where oxygenation occurs.

ripening Softening of the cervix near the end of pregnancy in anticipation of birth

role development The individual's capacity to identify and fulfill the social expectations related to the variety of roles assumed in a lifetime

Romberg's test A test that assesses coordination and equilibrium

rotation The turning movement of a bone around its own long axis

routine or initial assessment Used to gather more in-depth data about a patient for whom care will be provided. Data gathered in the initial assessment guides the direction of care and informs the nurse about the need for, as well as the type and frequency of, continuing assessment.

S1 The first heart sound (lub) is heard when the AV valves close. Closure of these valves occurs when the ventricles have been filled.

S2 The second heart sound (dub) occurs when the aortic and pulmonic valves close; they close when the ventricles have emptied their blood into the aorta and pulmonary arteries

sagittal suture Palpable gap between the bones of the skull that lies in the middle of the skull and crosses the anterior and posterior fontanelles

school age A child between 6 and 10 years old

sclera The outermost layer of the eye, an extremely dense, hard, fibrous membrane that helps to maintain the shape of the eye

scoliosis A lateral curvature of the lumbar or thoracic spine that is more common in children with neuromuscular deficits

scorbutic gums Swollen, red gums related to vitamin C deficiency

scrotum A loosely hanging, pliable, pear-shaped pouch of darkly pigmented skin located behind the penis that houses the testes, which produce sperm

sebaceous glands Oil glands that secrete sebum, an oily secretion, which generally is released into hair follicles

seborrheic keratoses Benign, greasy, wartlike lesions that are yellow-brown in color; they can appear anywhere on the body but are seen more frequently on the neck, chest, and back

secondary lesions Skin condition or changes to the skin that occurs following a primary lesion

secondary prevention Focus on early diagnosis of health problems and prompt treatment with the restoration of health

secondary source A person or record beyond the patient that provides additional information about the patient

seizures Sudden and rapid physical manifestations (as convulsions or loss of consciousness), resulting from excessive discharges of electrical energy in the brain

self-concept The beliefs and feelings one holds about oneself

self-directed violence (SDV) Behavior committed by and aimed at oneself that results in deliberate actual or potential self-harm.

semilunar valves Valves that separate the ventricles from the vascular system

seminal vesicles A pair of saclike glands, located between the bladder and rectum, that are the source of 60% of the semen produced

senescence Defined as the deterioration of organ and bodily functions over time

senile lentigines (Liver spots) Patchy pale spots of pigment loss or denser spots of color. These skin discolorations due to melanocyte clumping are relatively small in size.

sexual identity A self-assigned description that comprises the most significant aspects of an individual's sexual life, including sexual attractions, behaviors, desires, and fantasies

sexual orientation An individual's predisposition toward affiliation, affection, bonding, thoughts, or sexual fantasies in relationship to members of the same sex, the other sex, both sexes, or neither sex

sexual orientation label Designation that may be used to describe an individual's sexual orientation; for example, straight (or heterosexual), gay, lesbian, and bisexual

sinoatrial (SA) node The node located at the junction of the superior vena cava and right atrium that initiates the electrical impulse; natural "pacemaker" of the heart

sinus arrhythmia (Heart period variability) Presents with heart rate increases during inspiration and decreases during expiration

smegma A white, cheesy sebaceous matter that collects between the glans of the penis and the foreskin

social determinants of health The situations in which a person is born, lives, works, and ages as well as the systems in place to deal with illness

social environment Interactions between individuals and others as well as the institutions in an individual's community, including churches, schools, transportation systems, and protective services

somatic protein Another term for muscle mass or skeletal muscle

spermatic cord A cord composed of fibrous connective tissue; its purpose is to form a protective sheath around the nerves, blood vessels, lymphatic structures, and muscle fibers associated with the scrotum

spermatocele A cyst located in the epididymis

sphygmomanometer An instrument used to measure arterial blood pressure

spinal cord A continuation of the medulla oblongata that has the ability to transmit impulses to and from the brain via the ascending and descending pathways

sprain A stretching or tearing of the capsule or ligament of a joint due to forced movement beyond the joint's normal range

sternum The flat, narrow center bone of the upper anterior chest

strabismus A condition in which the axes of the eyes cannot be directed at the same object

strain A partial muscle tear resulting from overstretching or overuse of the muscle

stress Perceived or physical response to environmental factors. It is the body's response to thoughts and feelings that may result in a behavioral or physiologic response

striae (Stretch marks) A change in connective tissue resulting in silvery, shiny, irregular markings on the skin. Often seen in obesity, pregnancy, and ascites

striae gravidarium Also known as stretch marks, these pinkish-purplish skin depressions in connective tissue develop in the second half of pregnancy

stroke volume The amount of blood that is ejected with every heartbeat

subculture Groups that exist within a larger culture. Subcultures are composed of individuals who have a distinct identity based on some characteristic such as occupation, a medical problem, or a specific ethnic heritage.

subjective data Information that the patient experiences and communicates to the nurse, known as covert data or symptoms

subluxation A partial dislocation of the bones in a joint such as the head of the radius that may occur when a child is dangled by his or her hands

suicidal ideation Considering, planning, or thinking about committing suicide

summarizing Tying together the various messages that the patient has communicated throughout the interview

supination Movement of the forearm so that the palm faces up, anteriorly or superiorly

supine hypotension syndrome (Vena cava syndrome) Occurs when pressure from the pregnant uterus compresses the aorta and the inferior vena cava when the female is in the supine position

suspensory ligament (Cooper's ligaments) Ligaments that extend from the connective tissue layer, through the breast, and attach to the fascia underlying the breast

sutures Nonmovable joints that connect two bones

syncope Brief loss of consciousness, usually sudden

synovial joint Bones separated by a fluid-filled joint cavity

systole The phase of ventricular contraction in which the ventricles have been filled, then contract to expel blood into the aorta and pulmonary arteries. This is also associated with the top number of a blood pressure reading.

systolic pressure The highest arterial blood pressure during the height of a ventricular contraction; the first number in a blood pressure reading

temperature The degree of hotness or coldness within the body as measured by a thermometer.

tendons Tough fibrous bands that attach muscle to bone, or muscle to muscle

teratogen An agent that causes birth defects, such as a virus, a drug, a chemical, or radiation

terminal hair Dark, coarse, long hair that appears on eyebrows, the scalp, and the pubic region

tertiary prevention Activity aimed at restoring the individual to the highest possible level of health and functioning

testes Two firm, rubbery, olive-shaped structures that manufacture sperm and are thus the primary male sex organs

thalamus The largest subdivision of the diencephalon, which is the gateway to the cerebral cortex. The location where all input channeled to the cerebral cortex is processed.

thelarche Breast budding, often the first pubertal sign in females

thrill A soft vibratory sensation assessed by palpation with either the fingertips or palm flattened to the chest

thyroid gland The largest gland of the endocrine system which is butterfly shaped and is located in the anterior portion of the neck

toddler Child who is at least 1 year old but who has not yet reached 3 years of age

tophi Gout-related hard nodules that may appear over the joint

torticollis A spasm of the sternocleidomastoid muscle on one side of the body, which often results from birth trauma

tracheal sounds Harsh, high-pitched sounds heard over the trachea when the patient inhales and exhales

tracheomalacia Congenital defect of the cartilage in the trachea

tragus A small projection on the external ear that is positioned in front of the external auditory canal

transgender Also referred to as *gender nonconforming*, individuals who identify themselves and live as the gender that is not associated with their birth gender

trichotillomania Compulsive hair twisting or plucking

tympanic membrane Also called the eardrum, this membrane separates the external ear and middle ear

tympany A loud, high-pitched, drumlike tone of medium duration characteristic of an organ that is filled with air

ulcerative colitis A recurrent inflammatory process causing ulcer formation in the lower portions of the large intestine and rectum

umbilical hernia A protrusion at the umbilicus, visible at birth

undernutrition Insufficient intake or storage of essential nutrients. Also referred to as malnutrition.

uniform language The consistent use of accepted terminology by all individuals involved in documenting any aspect of the patient's care, including patient data that pertains to assessment and treatment

ureters Mucus-lined narrow tubes approximately 25 to 30 cm (10 to 12 in.) in length and 6 to 12 mm (0.25 to 0.5 in.) in diameter whose major function is transporting urine from the kidney to the urinary bladder

urethra A mucus-lined tube that transports urine from the urinary bladder to the exterior

urethral stricture Condition indicated by pinpoint appearance of the urinary meatus

urinary retention A chronic state in which the patient cannot empty his or her bladder

uterine tubes Ducts on either side of the uterus' fundus; also known as fallopian tubes

uterus A pear-shaped, hollow, muscular organ that is located centrally in the pelvis between the neck of the bladder and the rectal wall

uvula A fleshy pendulum that hangs from the edge of the soft palate in the back of the mouth. The uvula moves with swallowing, breathing, and phonation.

vagina A long, tubular, muscular canal that extends from the vestibule to the cervix at the inferior end of the uterus, its major function is serving as the female organ of copulation, the birth canal, and the channel for the exit of menstrual flow

varicocele A varicose enlargement of the veins of the spermatic cord causing a soft compressible mass in the scrotum. This may lead to male infertility.

varicosities Distended and dilated veins that have a diminished blood flow and an increased intravenous pressure

vegan Dietary choice in which no animal products are consumed

veins Tubular, walled vessels that carry deoxygenated blood from the body periphery back to the heart

vellus hair Pale, fine, short hair that appears over the entire body except for the lips, nipples, palms of hands, soles of feet, and parts of external genitals

venous insufficiency Inadequate circulation in the venous system usually due to incompetent valves in deep veins or a blood clot in the veins

verbal communication Spoken language to share information and ideas

vernix caseosa A cheesy white substance that coats the skin surfaces at birth

vesicular sounds Soft and low-pitched breath sounds heard over the periphery; inspiration is longer than expiration

viability The point at which the fetus can survive outside the uterus

visceral layer of pericardium The inner layer, which lines the surface of the heart

visceral pain Pain that results from stimulation of pain receptors deep within the body such as the abdominal cavity, cranium, or the thorax

visual field Refers to the total area of vision in which objects can be seen while the eye remains focused on a central point

vital signs The systematic measurement of temperature, pulse, respirations, blood pressure, and pain status

vitiligo A skin condition identified by patchy, depigmented skin over various areas of the body

vitreous humor A refractory medium, a clear gel within the eye that helps maintain the intraocular pressure and the shape of the eye, and transmits light rays through the eye

vulnerable populations Groups that are not well integrated into the U.S. healthcare system because of racial, ethnic, cultural, economic, geographic, or health characteristics

wellness A state of life that is balanced, personally satisfying, and characterized by the ability to adapt and to participate in activities that enhance quality of life

wheezes High-pitched squeaky or sibilant breath sounds heard on expiration

whispered pectoriloquy Auscultation of voice sounds, patient whispers "one, two, three," normal lung sounds will be faint, almost indistinguishable

xanthelasma Soft, yellow plaques on the lids at the inner canthus, which are sometimes associated with high cholesterolemia

xerophthalmia A clinical finding of poor nutrition, dry mucosa

young adult The period of a person's life between 20 and 40 years of age

Photo Credits

Chapter Opener Sources

1 Schmid Christophe/Shutterstock
2 Monkey Business Images/Shutterstock
3 Dmitriy Shironosov/Shutterstock
4 Supri Suharjoto/Shutterstock
5 moodboard/Alamy
6 Monkey Business Images/Shutterstock
7 KidStock/Blend Images/Corbis
8 Andresr/Shutterstock
9 Sergey Rusakov/Shutterstock
10 fotosearch/SuperStock
11 Sandro Donda/Shutterstock

12 Aurora Open/SuperStock
13 Gallo Images/SuperStock
14 OJO Images/SuperStock
15 Fotosearch/Getty Images
16 moodboard/SuperStock
17 heshphoto/Getty Images
18 Exactostock/SuperStock
19 Suzanne Tucker/Shutterstock
20 Datacraft Co. Ltd/Getty Images
21 eurobanks/Shutterstock
22 DreamPictures/Shannon Faulk/SuperStock
23 KidStock/Blend Images/Getty Images

24 heKtor/Shutterstock
25 holbox/Shutterstock
26 Daniel Goodings/Shutterstock
27 Blend Images/SuperStock
28 Monkey Business Images/Shutterstock
29 Kapu/Shutterstock
COV Pete Saloutos/Corbis

Patient-Centered Interaction Sources

13 SW Productions/Getty Images
15 Stockbyte/Getty Images
16 Getty Images
17 Ryan McVay/Getty Images
18 Stockdisc/Getty Images

19 Doug Menuez/Getty Images
20 George Doyle/Getty Images
21 Dennis Wise/Getty Images
22 Ryan McVay/Getty Images
23 manley099/Getty Images

24 Zero Creatives/Getty Images
25 Mark Andersen/Getty Images
26 Mark Romanelli/Getty Images
27 Geoff Manasse/Getty Images

Case Study Sources

1 Lisa Peardon/Getty Images
2 Irena Misevic/Shutterstock
3 stockdisc/Getty Images
4 Eric Raptosh Photograph/Corbis
5 holbox/Shutterstock
6 Andy Dean Photography/Shutterstock
7 Kevin Peterson/Getty Images
8 Datacraft Co., Ltd/Getty Images
9 Gelpi JM/Shutterstock
10 Digital Vision/Getty Images

11 oliveromg/Shutterstock
12 imtmphoto/Shutterstock
13 Jess Alford/Getty Images
14 Jack Q./Shutterstock
15 Konstantin Sutyagin/Shutterstock
16 Ryan McVay/Getty Images
17 Samuel Borges Photography/Shutterstock
18 Digital Vision/Getty Images
19 Jeff Cleveland/Shutterstock

20 Caroline Woodham/Getty Images
21 Phase4Studios/Shutterstock
22 Cheryl Savan/Shutterstock
23 Goodluz/Shutterstock
24 George Doyle/Getty Images
25 Ryan McVay/Getty Images
26 Ryan McVay/Getty Images
27 graphixmania/Shutterstock
28 OJO Images/SuperStock
29 Stuart Monk/Shutterstock

Index